# NURSING DIAGNOSIS HANDBOOK

***A Guide to Planning Care***

# NURSING DIAGNOSIS HANDBOOK

## *A Guide to Planning Care*

*Betty J. Ackley, MSN, EdS, RN*
*Gail B. Ladwig, MSN, RN, CHTP*

*Seventh Edition*

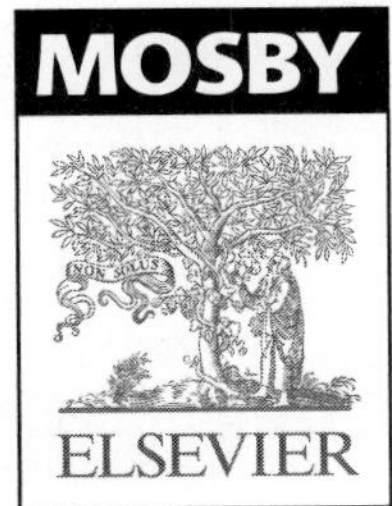

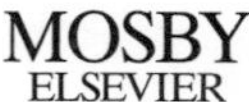

11830 Westline Industrial Drive
St. Louis, Missouri 63146

NURSING DIAGNOSIS HANDBOOK: A GUIDE TO PLANNING CARE, SEVENTH EDITION

0-323-03664-3



**NOTICE**

Neither the Publisher nor the Authors assume any responsibility for any loss or injury and/or damage to persons or property arising out of or related to any use of the material contained in this book. It is the responsibility of the treating practitioner, relying on independent expertise and knowledge of the patient, to determine the best treatment and method of application for the patient.

Previous editions copyrighted 1993, 1995, 1997, 1999, 2002, 2004

**International Standard Book Number 0-323-03664-3**

*Acquisitions Editor:* Sandra Clark Brown
*Senior Developmental Editor:* Cindi Anderson
*Publishing Services Manager:* Deborah L. Vogel
*Project Manager:* Katherine Hinkebein
*Designer:* Paula Ruckenbrod

Printed in the United States of America

Last digit is the print number: 9 8 7 6 5 4 3 2 1

*To:*

Dale Ackley, the greatest guy in the world, without whose support this book would have never happened, and my daughter, Dr. Dawn Goulding, and her husband, Cameron. Dale and Dawn have been the joy of my life.

Jerry Ladwig, my wonderful husband, who after 40 years is still supportive and helpful—I couldn't have done this book without him; our children and their spouses and all our wonderful grandchildren—Jerry, Kathy, Alexandra, Elizabeth, and Benjamin; Chrissy, John, Sean, and Ciara; Jenny, Jim, Abby, Katelyn, and Blake; and Amy, Scott, and Ford Michael—the greatest family anyone could ever hope for.

A special thank-you to our nursing students, who teach us every day, and our nursing faculty colleagues—"friends are one of life's most precious gifts." Also, a special thank-you to all the contributors who have devoted their time and talent to help "students think like nurses."

**Health**

Fleeting Fragile, like the
Wind
When it blows you feel it
When it's still you don't know
It's there
Fleeting, Fragile, grasp it
Hold it

G. Ladwig 1/31/05, HH

## ABOUT THE AUTHORS

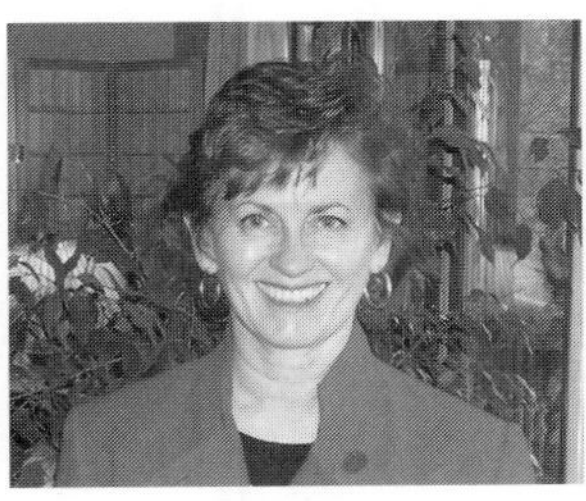

**Betty Ackley** has worked in nursing for more than 35 years in many capacities. She has been a staff nurse on a CCU unit, medical ICU unit, respiratory ICU unit, intensive care unit, and stepdown unit. She has worked on a gynecological surgery floor and an orthopedic floor, and she spent many years working in oncology. She also has been in management, has been in nursing education in a hospital, and for the last 31 years has been a professor of nursing at Jackson Community College. She has taught medical-surgical nursing, medical terminology, fundamentals of nursing, nursing management, and nutrition. Currently she is teaching an online nutrition course that is taken by students from throughout the United States as well as international students at intervals.

Betty has presented nationally and internationally in the areas of nursing diagnosis, nursing process, and online learning. In 2000 she was named Faculty of the Year at her college. She has written NCLEX-RN questions for the national licensure examination four times and is an expert in the area of testing and NCLEX preparation.

Betty obtained her BSN from Michigan State University, MS in nursing from University of Michigan, and education specialist degree from Michigan State University. She will be starting a PhD program in nursing soon.

Her free time is spent exercising, especially spinning and Pilates. She is certified in teaching spinning and plans to teach Pilates in the near future. In addition, she loves to travel, read, garden, and learn anything new!

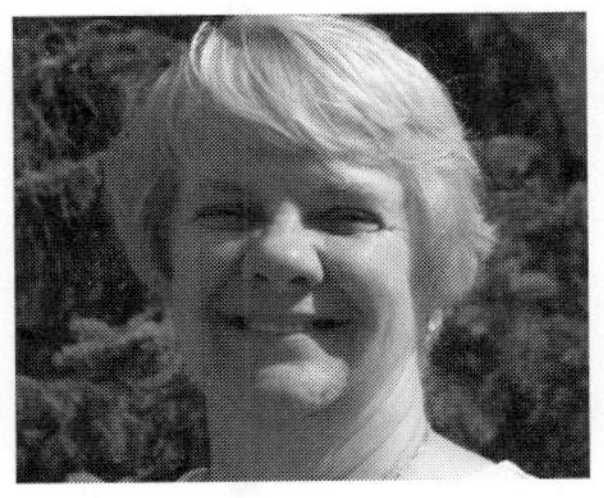

**Gail Ladwig** is a Professor Emeritus of Jackson Community College. During her tenure there she served four years as the Department Chair of Nursing and as a nurse consultant for Continuing Education.

She has taught classroom and clinical at JCC in fundamentals, medical-surgical nursing, mental health, and a transfer course for BSN students. In addition, she has taught online courses in pharmacology and a hybrid course (partially online) for BSN transfer students. More recently she taught pathophysiology online for the Medical University of South Carolina.

Gail worked as a staff nurse in medical-surgical nursing and intensive care before beginning her teaching career. She has a master's degree in psychiatric mental health nursing from Wayne State University. Her master's research was published in the *International Journal of Addictions.*

She has presented nationally and internationally on many topics including nursing diagnosis, computerized care planning, and holistic nursing topics. She is certified as a Healing Touch practitioner and is co-owner and founder of Holistic Choices, specializing in alternative presentations and Healing Touch and Guided Imagery treatments.

Gail is the mother of four children and grandmother of nine. She has been married to Jerry for almost 41 years. She is passionate about her family and the profession of nursing.

# CONTRIBUTORS

**Donna Algase, PhD, RN, FAAN**
Professor of Nursing
University of Michigan School of Nursing
Ann Arbor, Michigan

**Sharon Baranoski, MSN, RN, CWOCN**
Director of Clinical Programs and Development
Silver Cross Hospital and Medical Centers
Joliet, IL

**Lisa Burkhart, MPH, PhD, RN**
Assistant Professor
Marcella Niehoff School of Nursing
Center for Spiritual Leadership in Health Care
Loyola University Chicago
Chicago, Illinois

**Mary DeWys, RN, BS**
Infant Development Specialist
Devos Children's Hospital
Grand Rapids, Michigan

**Terri Ellis, RN, MSN**
Clinical Quality Specialist
W.A. Foote Memorial Hospital
Addison, Michigan

**Brenda Emick-Herring, RN, MSN, CRRN**
Admission Liaison for the Iowa Rehabilitation Network
Staff Development Specialist for Central Iowa Health System
Des Moines, Iowa

**Arlene T. Farren, RN, MA, AOCN**
Assistant Professor
Department of Nursing
College of Staten Island/City University of New York
Staten Island, New York

**Judith A. Floyd, PhD, RN, FAAN**
Associate Dean for Research
Wayne State University
Detroit, Michigan

**Terri Foster, RN, BSN, CNOR**
Unit Educator HA/OR/PACU/CSP/Anesthesia/Ortho Services/Scheduled Care
Foote Hospital
Jackson, Michigan

**Judith Gentz, RN, CS, NP**
President, Nurse Practitioner Care, Inc.
Grass Lake, Michigan

**Barbara A. Given, RN, PhD, FAAN**
University Distinguished Professor
College of Nursing
Michigan State University
East Lansing, Michigan

**Mikel Gray Jr., PhD, CUNP, CCCN, FAAN**
Professor of Nursing
Department of Urology
University of Virginia
Charlottesville, Virginia

**Elizabeth Henneman, RN, PhD**
Assistant Professor
University of Massachusetts School of Nursing
Amherst, Maryland

**T. Heather Herdman, RN, PhD**
President-Elect, NANDA-International
Assitant Professor of Nursing
Bellin College of Nursing
Green Bay, Wisconsin

**Kimberly Hickey, MSN, RN**
Clinical Nurse Specialist, Gerontology
University of Michigan Health System
Ann Arbor, Michigan

**Teresa Howell, MSN, ARHP**
Assistant Professor of Nursing
Morehead State University
Morehead, Kentucky

**Linda Hutson, RN, SANE-A**
Nurse Manager, Emergency Department
Sexual Assault Nurse Examiner
Mercy Hospital Anderson
Cincinnati, Ohio

**Ann C. Keeley, RN, MN, CNS/PMH**
Assistant Professor
Georgia Baptist College of Nursing
Mercer University
Atlanta, Georgia

**Marcia LaHaie, MSN, RN, OCN**
Hematology/Oncology Nurse Coordinator
Veterans Administration
Ann Arbor Health Care Center
Ann Arbor, Michigan

**Scott Chisholm Lamont, BSN, RN, CCRN, CFRN, ENC(C)**
Adjunct Lecturer and Clinical Instructor
Department of Nursing
Dominican University of California
San Rafael, California

**Margaret Lunney, RN, PhD**
Professor and Graduate Programs Coordinator
Department of Nursing
College of Staten Island
Staten Island, New York

**Margo McCaffrey, RN, MS, FAAN**
Consultant in the Nursing Care of Patients with Pain
Los Angeles, California

**Graham J. McDougall Jr., PhD, RN, APRN, BC, FAAN**
Associate Professor
Gerontological Nurse Practitioner
School of Nursing
The University of Texas at Austin
Principal Investigator
SeniorWISE
Austin, Texas

**Pamela H. Mitchell, PhD, RN, CNRN, FAAN**
Elizabeth S. Soule Distinguished Professor of Nursing and Health Promotion
Professor of Biobehavioral Nursing and Health Systems
Associate Dean for Research
University of Washington School of Nursing
Seattle, Washington

**Leslie H. Nicoll, PhD, MBA, RN, BC**
Maine Desk LLC—Professional Editorial Services
Editorial Office for CIN and JHPN
Portland, Maine

**Chris Pasero, MS, RN, FAAN**
Consultant in the Nursing Care of Patients with Pain
El Dorado Hills, California

**Paula R. Sherwood, RN, PhD, CNRN**
Research Assistant Professor
School of Nursing
University of Pittsburgh
Pittsburgh, Pennsylvania

**P. Ann Solari-Twadell, RN, PhD, MPA, FAAN**
Assistant Professor
Director, Center for Spiritual Leadership in Health Care
Marcella Neihoff School of Nursing
Loyola University Chicago
Chicago, Illinois

**Michele Walters, RN, MSN, ARNP**
Assistant Professor of Nursing
Morehead State University
Morehead, Kentucky

**Linda S. Williams, MSN, RNBC**
Professor of Nursing
Jackson Community College
Jackson, Michigan

## Consultant in home care—contributor of home care interventions

**Kathleen L. Patusky, PhD, APRN-BC**
Assistant Professor
College of Health and Human Sciences, School of Nursing
Georgia State University
Atlanta, Georgia

## Consultant in culturally competent nursing care

**Marina Martinez-Kratz, RN, MS**
Professor of Nursing
Jackson Community College

## Consultant in nursing research utilization

**Beth Ann Swann, PhD, CRNP**
Special Projects Coordinator and Adjunct Assistant Professor
University of Pennsylvania School of Nursing
Rydal, Pennsylvania

## Consultants to previous editions

**Elizabeth L. Foster, MS, RN,** Consultant in home care—contributor of home care interventions—Third through fifth editions

**Ann F. Jacobson, PhD, RN,** Consultant in nursing research utilization—Third edition

**Debra Martinez, BSW,** Consultant in culturally competent nursing care—Fifth edition

**Brenda J. Wagner, PhD, RN,** Consultant in nursing research utilization—Third edition

**Elizabeth H. Winslow, PhD, RN, FAAN,** Consultant in nursing research utilization—Third edition

## The authors would also like to thank the following individuals for their contributions to earlier editions:

Jill Barnes, MS, RNCS
Victoria L. Cole-Schonlau, DNSc, MPA, RN
Sandra Cunningham, MS, RN, CCRN, CS
Jane Maria Curtis, MSN, CAN, RN
Gwethalyn B. Edwards, MSN, RN
Pamela M. Emery, BS, RNFA, CNOR, RN
Nancy English, PhD, RN
Roslyn Fine, MS, CCC, SLP
Mary A. Fuerst-DeWys, BS, RN
J. Keith Hampton, MSN, RN, CS
Mary Henrikson, MN, RNC, ARNP
Kathie D. Hesnan, BSN, RN, CETN
Constance Hollman, MA, EdS
Leslie Kalbach, MN, RN, CETN
Helen Kelley, MSN, RN, CHTP, HNC, NP
Diane Krasner, PhD, RN, CWOCN, CWS, FAAN
Carroll A. Lutz, MA, BSN, RN
Leslie Lysaght RN, MS, CS
Mary Markle, MSN, RNC
Marty J. Martin, MSN, RN
Michelle Masta, RN, BSN
Cathy McClean, RN, BSN
Vicki McClurg, MN, RN
Beverly Pickett, MA, BS, RN, CHTP, HNC
Nancee B. Radtke, MSN, RN
Judith S. Rizzo, MS, RN, CS
Pam B. Schweitzer, MS, RN, CS
Suzanne Skowronski, MSN, RN
Teepa Snow, MS, OTR-L, FAOTA
Martha A. Spies, MSN, RN
Kathy A. Stimac O'Brien, MSN, RN
Linda Straight, MA, RN
Terry VandenBosch, PhD, RN, CS
Catherine Vincent, MSN, RN
Virginia Wall, RN, MN, IBCLC
Peggy A. Wetsch, RN, MSN, CNA
Fran Wistom, MSN, RN, CSW, CPN
Janet Woodruff, BSN, RN
Kathy Wyngarden, MSN, FNP Certificate, RN

# PREFACE

*Nursing Diagnosis Handbook: A Guide to Planning Care* is a convenient reference to help the practicing nurse or nursing student make a nursing diagnosis and write a care plan with ease and confidence. This handbook helps nurses correlate nursing diagnoses with known information about clients on the basis of assessment findings, established medical, surgical, or psychiatric diagnoses, and the current treatment plan.

Making a nursing diagnosis and planning care are complex processes that involve diagnostic reasoning and critical thinking skills. Nursing students and practicing nurses cannot possibly memorize the extensive list of defining characteristics, related factors, and risk factors for the 172 diagnoses approved by NANDA-International. This book correlates suggested nursing diagnoses with what nurses know about clients and offers a care plan for each nursing diagnosis.

Section I, Nursing Diagnosis, the Nursing Process, and Evidence-Based Nursing, explains how the nurse formulates a nursing diagnosis using assessment findings. In Section II, Guide to Nursing Diagnoses, the nurse can look up symptoms and problems and their suggested nursing diagnoses for more than 1300 client symptoms, medical, surgical and psychiatric diagnoses, diagnostic procedures, surgical interventions, and clinical states. In Section III, Guide to Planning Care, the nurse can find care plans for all nursing diagnoses suggested in Section II. In this edition, we have included the suggested nursing outcomes from the Nursing Outcomes Classification (NOC) and interventions from the Nursing Interventions Classification (NIC) by the Iowa Intervention Project. We are excited about this work and believe it is a significant addition to the nursing process to further define nursing practice.

New special features of the seventh edition of *Nursing Diagnosis Handbook: A Guide to Planning Care* include the following:

- Five new nursing diagnoses recently approved by NANDA-I
- Revisions made by NANDA-I in existing nursing diagnoses
- Revised NOC outcomes for each nursing diagnosis, including the rating scale
- Revised NIC interventions for each nursing diagnosis
- Labeling of nursing research as EBN (Evidence-Based Nursing) and clinical research as EB (Evidence-Based) to identify the source of evidence-based rationales
- Addition of pediatric interventions to appropriate care plans
- Even more culturally appropriate interventions added to care plans as relevant
- An associated EVOLVE Course Management System that includes critical thinking case studies; worksheets; and the ability to post a class syllabus, outline, and lecture notes, share e-mail, and encourage student participation through chat rooms and discussion boards
- An instructor's CD and PowerPoint lecture slides

The following features of *Nursing Diagnosis Handbook: A Guide to Planning Care* are also included:

- Suggested nursing diagnoses for more than 1300 clinical entities including signs and symptoms, medical diagnoses, surgeries, maternal-child disorders, mental health disorders, and geriatric disorders
- An EVOLVE Courseware System with the Ackley Care Plan Constructor that helps the student or nurse write a nursing care plan, including links to websites for client education
- Rationales for nursing interventions that are based on nursing research and literature

- Nursing references identified for each care plan
- A complete list of NOC outcomes on the EVOLVE website
- A complete list of NIC interventions on the EVOLVE website
- Nursing care plans that contain many holistic interventions
- Care plans for **Caregiver Role Strain** and **Fatigue** written by two national experts, Dr. Barbara Given and Dr. Paula Sherwood
- Care plans for **Pain** written by two national experts on pain, Margo McCaffery and Christine Pasero
- Care plans for **Rape-trauma syndrome** written by national expert Linda Hutson
- Care plans for **Spirituality** written by national experts Ann Solari-Twadell and Lisa Burkhart
- Care Plans for **Religiosity** written by national expert Dr. Lisa Burkhart
- Care plans for **Skin integrity** written by national expert Dr. Sharon Baranoski
- Care plans for **Community** written by national expert Dr. Margaret Lunney
- Care plan for **Impaired Memory** written by national expert Dr. Graham McDougall
- Care plans for **Incontinence** written by national expert Dr. Mikel Gray
- Care plan for **Decreased Intracranial adaptive capacity** written by national expert Dr. Pamela Mitchell
- Care plan for **Latex Allergy response** written by national expert Dr. Leslie Nicoll
- Care plan for **Wandering** written by national expert Dr. Donna Algase
- A format that facilitates analyzing signs and symptoms by the process already known by nurses, which involves using defining characteristics of nursing diagnoses to make a diagnosis
- Use of NANDA-I terminology and approved diagnoses
- Inclusion of three additional nursing diagnoses, **Grieving, Impaired Comfort,** and **Supportive Family Role Performance,** not currently on the NANDA-I list but very helpful to nursing practice
- An alphabetical format for Sections II and III, which allows rapid access to information
- Nursing care plans for all nursing diagnoses listed in Section II
- Specific geriatric interventions in appropriate plans of care
- Specific client/family teaching interventions in each plan of care
- Information on culturally competent nursing care included where appropriate
- Inclusion of commonly used abbreviations (e.g., AIDS, MI, CHF) and cross-references to the complete term in Section II
- Contributions by leading nurse experts from throughout the United States, who together represent all of the major nursing specialties and have extensive experience with nursing diagnoses and the nursing process

We acknowledge the work of NANDA-I, which is used extensively throughout this text. In some cases the authors and contributors have modified the NANDA-I work to increase ease of use. The original NANDA-I work can be found in *NANDA-I Nursing Diagnoses: Definitions & Classification 2005-2006.* Several contributors are the original authors of the nursing diagnoses established by NANDA-I. These contributors include the following:

Dr. Margaret Lunney
**Ineffective community Coping**
**Readiness for enhanced community Coping, Effective Therapeutic regimen management, Ineffective Therapeutic regimen management, Ineffective community Therapeutic regimen management, Ineffective family Therapeutic regimen management**

Lisa Burkhart, PhD, RN
**Spiritual distress**
**Readiness for enhanced Spiritual well-being**
**Impaired Religiosity**, **Risk for Impaired Religiosity,** and **Readiness for enhanced Religiosity**

Dr. Pamela H. Mitchell
**Decreased Intracranial adaptive capacity**

Brenda Emick-Herring
**Impaired bed Mobility**
**Impaired Transfer ability**
**Impaired Walking**

Vicki E. McClurg, Mary Henrikson, and Virginia R. Wall—First through fifth editions
**Effective Breastfeeding**
**Ineffective Breastfeeding**
**Interrupted Breastfeeding**

Kathy Wyngarden—First through third editions
**Risk for impaired parent/infant/child Attachment**
**Impaired wheelchair Mobility**

We and the consultants and contributors trust that nurses will find this seventh edition of *Nursing Diagnosis Handbook: A Guide to Planning Care* a valuable tool that simplifies the process of diagnosing clients and planning for their care, thus allowing nurses more time to provide evidence-based care that speeds each client's recovery.

# ACKNOWLEDGMENTS

We would like to thank the following people at Mosby: Sandra Brown, Acquisitions Editor, who supported us with this seventh edition of the text with intelligence and kindness; Cindi Anderson, Senior Developmental Editor, who was a continual support and constant source of wise advice and who is frankly wonderful; and a special thank-you to Katherine Hinkebein for project management of this edition.

We acknowledge with gratitude the nursing students and graduates of Jackson Community College who made us think and shared a very special time with us; the nurses at W.A. Foote Memorial Hospital, Doctors Hospital, Chelsea Hospital, The Jackson County Medical Care Facility, Arbor Manor Care Center, Countryside Care Center, and Lifeways, as well as the professionals in community nursing agencies who have helped us educate students and who have served as role models for excellence in nursing care; and finally, each other, for perseverance, patience, and friendship.

Care has been taken to confirm the accuracy of information presented in this book. However, the authors, editors, and publisher cannot accept any responsibility for consequences resulting from errors or omissions of the information in this book and make no warranty, express or implied, with respect to its contents. The reader should use practices suggested in this book in accordance with agency policies and professional standards. Every effort has been made to ensure the accuracy of the information presented in this text.

We hope you find this text useful in your nursing practice.

Betty J. Ackley
Gail B. Ladwig

# HOW TO USE NURSING DIAGNOSIS HANDBOOK: A GUIDE TO PLANNING CARE

## ASSESS
Assess the client using the format provided by the clinical setting. Collect data including client's symptoms, clinical state, and known medical or psychiatric diagnoses.

## DIAGNOSIS
Turn to Section II, Guide to Nursing Diagnoses, and locate the client's symptoms, clinical state, medical or psychiatric diagnoses, and anticipated or prescribed diagnostic studies or surgical interventions (listed in alphabetical order). Note suggestions for appropriate nursing diagnoses.

Use Section III, Guide to Planning Care, to evaluate each suggested nursing diagnosis and "related to" etiology statement. Section III is a listing of care plans according to NANDA-I, arranged alphabetically by diagnostic concept, for each nursing diagnosis referred to in Section II. Determine the appropriateness of each nursing diagnosis by comparing the Defining Characteristics and Risk Factors to the client data collected.

## DETERMINE OUTCOMES
Use Section III, Guide to Planning Care, to find appropriate outcomes for the client. Use either the NOC outcomes with the associated rating scales, or Client Outcomes as desired.

## PLAN INTERVENTIONS
Use Section III, Guide to Planning Care, to find appropriate interventions for the client. Use either the NIC interventions or Nursing Interventions as found in that section.

## GIVE NURSING CARE
Administer nursing care following the plan of care based on the interventions.

## EVALUATE NURSING CARE
Evaluate nursing care administered using either the NOC outcomes or Client Outcomes. If the outcomes were not met, and the nursing interventions were not effective, it may be appropriate to reassess the client and determine if the appropriate nursing diagnoses were made.

## DOCUMENT
Document all of the previous steps using the format provided in the clinical setting.

# CONTENTS

SECTION

# I

# Nursing Process, Nursing Diagnosis, and Evidence-Based Nursing

Section I is an overview of the nursing process and evidence-based nursing. It includes how to make a nursing diagnosis and how to plan nursing care.

The nursing process is an organizing framework for professional nursing practice. It is very similar to the steps used in scientific reasoning and problem solving. Critical thinking is used as part of the process.

Components of the five key steps in the Nursing Process include:

1. Performing a nursing **A**ssessment
2. Making nursing **D**iagnoses
3. **P**lanning; formulating and writing outcome/goal statements and determining appropriate nursing interventions
4. **I**mplementing care
5. **E**valuating the nursing care that has been given (making necessary revisions)

An easy way to remember the steps of the Nursing Process is to use an acronym: **ADPIE.** ADPIE stands for **A**ssessment, **D**iagnosis, **P**lanning, **I**mplementation, and **E**valuation. The process can be visualized as a circular, continuous process (Figure I-1).

A concept that has been added to the nursing process is basing nursing practice on evidence or research. This concept is called *evidence-based nursing* (EBN). EBN uses a critical appraisal of the most relevant research, the nurse's own clinical expertise, and client preferences to provide care of the highest quality possible (Melnyk and Fineout-Overholt, 2004).

In this text the abbreviation **EBN** is used when interventions have rationale supported by nursing research. The abbreviation **EB** is used when interventions have rationale for research that has been gleaned from other disciplines.

This book focuses on an essential part of the nursing process: how to make and use a nursing diagnosis. A nursing diagnosis is a clinical judgment about individual, family, or community responses to actual or potential health problems or life processes. Nursing diagnoses provide the basis for selection of nursing interventions to achieve outcomes for which the nurse is accountable (NANDA-I, 2005).

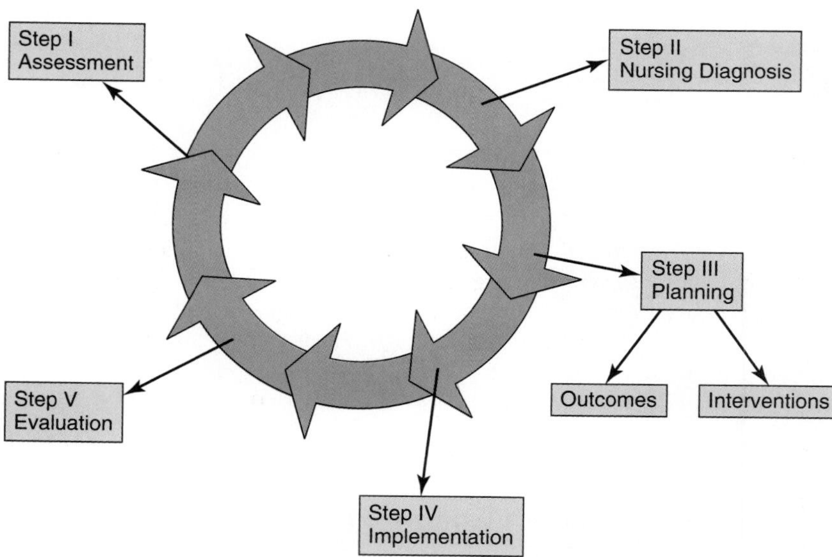


**Figure I-1**
The nursing process.

The nursing diagnoses that are used throughout this book are taken from NANDA-International (NANDA-I, 2005). The complete nursing diagnosis list by the NNN Taxonomy of Nursing practice by domains, classes, diagnosis, outcomes, interventions, and NANDA can be found on the Evolve site.

The following is an overview and practical application of the steps of the nursing process. The steps are listed in the usual order in which they are performed.

## STEP 1: ASSESSMENT (ADPIE)

Assessment involves performing a thorough holistic nursing assessment of the client. This is the first step needed to make an appropriate nursing diagnosis. This is done using the assessment format adopted by the facility or educational institution in which the practice is situated. Several organizational approaches to assessment are available, including Gordon's Functional Health Patterns (see Appendix B) and head-to-toe and body systems approaches. Regardless of the approach used, the nurse assesses the client, being alert for symptoms that will help formulate a nursing diagnosis.

Assessment information is obtained first by taking a thorough health and medical history. To elicit as many symptoms as possible, the nurse should use open-ended rather than yes or no questions during this part of the assessment. The client should be asked questions such as the following:

"Describe what you are feeling."
"How long have you been feeling this way?"
"When did the symptoms start?"
"Describe the symptoms."

These types of questions will encourage the client to give more information about his or her situation. Listen carefully for cues and record relevant information that the client shares.

Information is also obtained by performing a physical assessment and noting diagnostic test results. If the client is critically ill or unable to respond verbally, much of the information will be gathered from the physical assessment and diagnostic test results, and possibly from the client's significant others. The information from each of these sources is used to formulate a nursing diagnosis. All of this information needs to be carefully documented on the forms provided by the agency or school of nursing. HIPPA regulations need to be followed to protect client confidentiality. When the assessment is complete, proceed to the next step.

## STEP 2: NURSING DIAGNOSIS (ADPIE)

### Formulating a Nursing Diagnosis with Related Factors and Defining Characteristics

A working nursing diagnosis may have two or three parts. The two-part system consists of the nursing diagnosis and the "related to" statement. "Related factors are factors that appear to show some type of patterned relationship with the nursing diagnosis: such factors may be described as antecedent to, associated with, relating to, contributing to, or abetting." (NANDA-I, 2005)

The three-part system consists of the nursing diagnosis, the "related to" statement, and the defining characteristics, which are "Observable cues/inferences that cluster as manifestations of an actual or wellness nursing diagnosis." (NANDA-I, 2005)

Some nurses refer to the three-part diagnostic statement as the PES system:

**P** (problem)—The nursing diagnosis, or label; a concise term or phrase that represents a pattern of related cues
**E** (etiology)—"Related to" (r/t) phrase or etiology; related cause or contributor to the problem
**S** (symptoms)—Defining characteristics phrase; symptoms that the nurse identified in the assessment

## Application and Examples of Making a Nursing Diagnosis

When the assessment is complete, identify common patterns/symptoms of response to actual or potential health problems and select an appropriate Nursing Diagnosis label using critical thinking skills.

A. Highlight or underline the relevant symptoms.
B. Make a short list of the symptoms.
C. Cluster similar symptoms.
D. Analyze/interpret the symptoms.
E. Select a Nursing Diagnosis label that fits with the appropriate related factors and defining characteristics.

Consider the following case study.

### A. Underline the Symptoms

A 73-year-old man has been admitted to the unit with a diagnosis of chronic obstructive pulmonary disease (COPD). He states that he has "difficulty breathing when walking short distances." He also states that his "heart feels like it is racing" at the same time. He states that he is "tired all the time," and while talking to you, he is continually wringing his hands and looking out the window.

### B. List the Symptoms

chronic obstructive pulmonary disease (COPD); "difficulty breathing when walking short distances"; "heart feels like it is racing"; "tired all the time"; continually wringing his hands and looking out the window.

### C. Cluster Symptoms

chronic obstructive pulmonary disease (COPD)
"difficulty breathing when walking short distances"
"heart feels like it is racing"
"tired all the time"

continually wringing his hands
looking out the window

### D. Analyze

#### Interpret the "Subjective Symptoms" (What the Client Has Stated)

- "difficulty breathing when walking short distances" = dyspnea
- "heart feels like it is racing" = dysrhythmia
- "tired all the time" = fatigue

#### Interpret the "Objective Symptoms" (Observable Information)

- continually wringing his hands = (extraneous movement, hand/arm movements; defining characteristics of **Anxiety**)
- looking out the window = (poor eye contact, glancing about; defining characteristics of **Anxiety**)

### E. Select the Nursing Diagnosis Label

In Section II, look up *dyspnea* or *dysrhythmia*, (these are chosen because they are high priority) and you will find the nursing diagnosis **Activity intolerance** listed with these symptoms. Is this diagnosis appropriate for this client?

To validate that the diagnosis **Activity intolerance** is appropriate for the client, turn to Section III, and read the NANDA-I definition of the nursing diagnosis **Activity intolerance,** which is "Insufficient physiological or psychological energy to endure or complete required or desired daily activities." When reading the definition, ask, "Does this definition describe the symptoms demonstrated by the client?" If the appropriate nursing diagnosis has been selected, the definition should describe the condition that has been observed.

The client should also have defining characteristics for this particular diagnosis. Are the client symptoms that you identified in the list of defining characteristics?

Another way to use this text and to help validate the diagnosis is to look up the client's medical diagnosis in Section II. This client had a medical diagnosis of COPD. Is **Activity intolerance** listed with this medical diagnosis?

The process of identifying significant symptoms, clustering or grouping them into logical patterns, and then choosing an appropriate nursing diagnosis involves diagnostic reasoning (critical thinking) skills that must be learned in the process of becoming a nurse. This text serves as a tool to help the learner in this process.

## "Related to" Phrase or Etiology

The second part of the nursing diagnosis is the "related to" (r/t) phrase. This phrase states what may be causing or contributing to the nursing diagnosis, commonly referred to as the *etiology.* Pathophysiological and psychosocial changes, such as developmental age and cultural and environmental situations, may be causative or contributing factors. Ideally the etiology, or cause, of the nursing diagnosis is something that can be treated by a nurse. When this is the case, the diagnosis is identified as an independent nursing diagnosis. If medical intervention is also necessary, it might be identified as a collaborative diagnosis. A carefully written, individualized r/t statement enables the nurse to plan nursing interventions that will assist the client in accomplishing goals and return to a state of optimum health.

For each suggested nursing diagnosis, the nurse should refer to the statements listed under the heading "Related Factors (r/t)" in Section III. These r/t factors may or may not be appropriate for the individual client. If they are not appropriate, the nurse should develop and write an r/t statement that is appropriate for the client. A two-part statement could be made here:

P = Activity intolerance
E = r/t Imbalance between oxygen supply and demand

## Defining Characteristics Phrase

The defining characteristics phrase is the third part of the three-part diagnostic system, and it consists of the signs and symptoms that have been gathered during the assessment phase. The phrase "as evidenced by" (aeb) may be used to connect the etiology (r/t) with the defining characteristics. The use of identifying defining characteristics is similar to the process the physician uses when making a medical diagnosis. For example, the physician who observes the following signs and symptoms—diminished inspiratory and expiratory capacity of the lungs, complaints of dyspnea on exertion, difficulty in inhaling and exhaling deeply, and sometimes chronic cough—may make the medical diagnosis of COPD. This same process is used to identify the nursing diagnosis of **Activity intolerance.**

## Put It All Together: Writing the Three-Part Nursing Diagnosis Statement

**P**—Choose the label (nursing diagnosis) using the guidelines explained previously. A list of nursing diagnosis labels can be found in Section II and on the inside back cover.
**E**—Write an r/t phrase (etiology). These can be found in Section II.
**S**—Write the defining characteristics (signs and symptoms). A list of the signs and symptoms associated with each nursing diagnosis can be found in Section III.

Using the information from the above case study/example, the nursing diagnostic statement would be as follows:

P—**Activity intolerance**
E—Related to imbalance between oxygen supply and demand
S—Verbal reports of fatigue, exertional dyspnea ("difficulty breathing when walking"), and dysrhythmia ("racing heart")

Consider a second case study:

### A. Underline the Symptoms

A 45-year-old woman comes to the clinic and asks for medication to help her sleep. She states she is worrying about too much and states, "It takes me about an hour to get to sleep, and it is very hard to fall asleep. I feel like I can't do anything because I am so tired. My husband passed away recently."

### B. Make a Short List of the Symptoms

asks for medication to help her sleep; states she is worrying about too much; "It takes me about an hour to get to sleep; it is very hard to fall asleep; I feel like I can't do anything because I am so tired; My husband passed away recently."

### C. Cluster Similar Symptoms

asks for medication to help her sleep
"It takes me about an hour to get to sleep."
"It is very hard to fall asleep."
"I feel like I can't do anything because I am so tired."

states she is worrying about too much
"My husband passed away recently."

### D. Analyze/Interpret the Symptoms

#### Subjective Symptoms

- Asks for medication to help her sleep, "It takes me about an hour to get to sleep; it is very hard to fall asleep. I feel like I can't do anything because I am so tired." (all defining characteristics = verbal complaints of difficulty with sleeping)
- States she is worrying about too much (anxiety)
- "My husband passed away recently." **(Risk for dysfunctional Grieving)**

### E. Select a Nursing Diagnosis with Related Factors and Defining Characteristics

Look up **Sleep** in Section II. Listed under the heading "Sleep Pattern Disorders" in Section II is the following information:

**Disturbed Sleep pattern** (nursing diagnosis) r/t sensory alterations internal factors (illness, psychological stress), external factors (environmental changes, social cues)

This client states she is worrying too much, which could be considered psychological stress.
Look up **Disturbed Sleep pattern** in Section III.
Check the definition: Time-limited disruption of sleep (natural periodic suspension of consciousness)
Does this describe the client in the case study? What are the related factors? What are the symptoms?
Make the diagnostic statement:

**P—Disturbed Sleep pattern**
**E**—r/t "worrying too much," "My husband passed away recently"
**S**—difficulty falling asleep, "I am so tired, I can't do anything"

After the diagnostic statement is written, proceed to the next step: planning.

## STEP 3: PLANNING (ADPIE)

This phase consists of **writing measurable client outcomes and nursing interventions** to accomplish the outcomes. Before this can be done, if the client has more than one diagnosis, the priority of the nursing diagnoses must be determined. The highest priority nursing diagnoses can be determined by using Maslow's hierarchy of needs. In this hierarchy, priority is generally given to immediate problems that may be life threatening. For example, **Activity intolerance**, a physiological need, may be a higher priority than **Grieving**, a love and belonging need. Refer to Appendix A, Nursing Diagnoses Arranged by Maslow's Hierarchy of Needs, for assistance in prioritizing nursing diagnoses.

It is here that you might pose a "clinical question" to incorporate the concept of EBN. *What are some of the most effective ways to help a patient who has intolerance to activity? What does the research say? What has helped this person in the past? How can the outcomes be measured using standards of practice for a patient with intolerance to activity?*

### Outcomes

After the appropriate priority of the nursing diagnoses is determined, outcomes are developed: "Nursing-sensitive outcome is an individual, family or community state, behavior or perception that is measured along a continuum in response to nursing interventions. The outcomes are variable concepts that can be measured along a continuum, which means the outcomes are stated as concepts that reflect a patient, family caregiver, family, or community actual state rather than expected goals. It also means that the outcomes are neutral; that is, they don't specify the desired state, although they can be used to set goals. This retains the variability of the outcome and allows measurement of the patient condition at any point in time." (Moorhead, Johnson, & Maas, 2004).

If at all possible, the nurse involves the client in determining appropriate outcomes.

Development of appropriate outcomes can be done one of two ways: using the Nursing Outcomes Classification (NOC) or writing an outcome statement, both of which are included in this book in Section III. There are suggested outcome statements for each nursing diagnosis in this text that can be used as written or modified as necessary to meet the needs of the client.

The Evolve site includes a listing of additional NOC outcomes. "Each outcome has a group of indicators that are used to determine patient status in relation to the outcome. A *nursing-sensitive patient outcome indicator* is defined as a more concrete individual, family or community state, behavior or perception that serves as a cue for measuring an outcome" (Moorhead, Johnson, & Maas, 2004). The use of NOC outcomes can be very helpful to the nurse because they contain a five-point Likert-type rating scale that can be used to evaluate progress toward achieving the outcome. In this text the rating scale is listed, along with some of the more common indicators. As an example, the rating scale for the outcome **Sleep** is shown in Table I-1.

Because the NOC outcomes are very specific, they enhance the nursing process by helping the nurse record change after interventions have been performed. The nurse can choose to have clients rate their own progress using the Likert-type rating scale. This involvement can help increase client motivation to progress toward outcomes.

After client outcomes are selected and discussed with a client, the nurse plans nursing care and estab-

TABLE I-1

## NOC Outcome—Sleep

*Definition:* Natural periodic suspension of consciousness during which the body is restored.

| Sleep | Severely Compromised 1 | Substantially Compromised 2 | Moderately Compromised 3 | Mildly Compromised 4 | Not Compromised 5 |
|---|---|---|---|---|---|
| Hours of sleep (at least 5 hr/24 hr)* | 1 | 2 | 3 | 4 | 5 |
| Observed hours of sleep | 1 | 2 | 3 | 4 | 5 |
| Sleep pattern | 1 | 2 | 3 | 4 | 5 |
| Sleep quality | 1 | 2 | 3 | 4 | 5 |
| Sleep quantity | 1 | 2 | 3 | 4 | 5 |
| Sleep efficiency (ratio of sleep time/total time trying) | 1 | 2 | 3 | 4 | 5 |
| Sleep routine | 1 | 2 | 3 | 4 | 5 |
| Sleeps through the night consistently | 1 | 2 | 3 | 4 | 5 |
| Feels rejuvenated after sleep | 1 | 2 | 3 | 4 | 5 |
| Wakeful at appropriate times | 1 | 2 | 3 | 4 | 5 |
| EEG | 1 | 2 | 3 | 4 | 5 |
| EMG | 1 | 2 | 3 | 4 | 5 |
| EOG | 1 | 2 | 3 | 4 | 5 |

| | Severe | Substantial | Moderate | Mild | None | NA |
|---|---|---|---|---|---|---|
| Interrupted sleep | 1 | 2 | 3 | 4 | 5 | |
| Inappropriate napping | 1 | 2 | 3 | 4 | 5 | |
| Sleep apnea | 1 | 2 | 3 | 4 | 5 | |
| Dependence on sleep aids | 1 | 2 | 3 | 4 | 5 | |

*Appropriate for adults

*EEG,* Electroencephalogram; *EMG,* electromyogram; *EOG,* electro-oculogram.

From Moorhead S, Johnson M, Maas M: *Nursing outcomes classification (NOC),* ed 3, St Louis, 2004, Mosby.

lishes a means that will help the client achieve the selected outcomes. The usual means are nursing interventions.

## Interventions

Interventions are like road maps directing the best ways to provide nursing care. The more clearly a nurse writes an intervention, the easier it will be to complete the journey and arrive at the destination of successful client outcomes.

To increase the chance that the chosen interventions will be effective, nurses are now using EBN, which is using interventions that are supported as effective in helping clients through nursing research. Development of EBN is an ongoing process that should involve all nurses to determine the best nursing interventions to provide nursing care. To implement EBN, nurses must work together and follow the strategies outlined in Box I-1.

This text includes EBN interventions whenever possible, along with references to research to validate their usefulness. This is an important part of EBN. It looks at standard protocol and determines if the protocol is effective based on gathered evidence. This evidence ranges along a continuum from anecdotal experience of provider and consumer, institutional protocols, organizational guidelines, consensus

### BOX I-1 STRATEGIES FOR IMPLEMENTING EVIDENCE-BASED NURSING PRACTICE

1. Pose clinical questions (e.g., What is the best way to provide oral care for clients receiving chemotherapy?).
2. Collect and review literature that is relevant from appropriate studies or systematic reviews in the area of the clinical question.
3. Critically appraise the evidence for relevance and applicability. Systematic reviews or meta-analyses can be most helpful because they summarize many research studies. For individual studies, randomized clinical trials are generally the gold standard for producing the best evidence. Ask a number of questions as part of the review of the research, including the following: How large was the treatment effect? How precise is the estimate of the treatment effect? Will the results help me care for my client(s)? Is the treatment feasible in our setting? Were all clinically important outcomes considered, including possible harm as well as benefit?
4. Develop practice guidelines using the best evidence currently available.
5. Establish measurable outcomes that can be used to determine the effectiveness of the guidelines.
6. Measure the current outcomes based on existing practice so that there is a "before" measurement to show that evidenced practice made a difference.
7. Implement the practice guidelines.
8. Measure the proposed outcomes after the practice guidelines have been implemented.
9. Evaluate the effectiveness of the practice guidelines and determine where use should be continued or revisions should be made in the guidelines.
10. Pose the next clinical question.

Adapted from Cullum N: Evaluation of studies of treatment or prevention interventions, *Evid Based Nurs* 4:7, 2001; Melnyk BM and Fineout-Overholt E: *Evidence-based practice in nursing and healthcare: a guide to best practice,* Philadelphia, 2004, Lippincott-Lippincott-Williams & Wilkens; and Melnyk BM et al: Evidenced-based practice: the past, the present, and recommendations for the millennium, *Pediatr Nurs* 26(1):79, 2000.

groups, and single-study results to highly structured systematic reviews (Swan, McGinley, & Lang, 2002).

Every attempt has been made to supply the most current research for the nursing interventions. Some references may have earlier dates because they are classic studies that have not been replicated. For example, in the Spiritual care plans, the work by Koenig, Pargament, Fry, Reed, Engebretson, and Dossey is considered seminal work. The clinical practice guidelines from AANA (1998), ASA (1999), the joint task force statement for all the allergy associations (1998), and NIOSH (1998) have not been updated since their original publication dates. However, in reviewing them, the content is still current and appropriate, and no new evidence supercedes any of their guidelines.

"Theoretical perspectives may be used as a source of evidence. Many theories and models are based on past research and have strong consensus among people in the field (also evidence). Sometimes this type of evidence is better than one small research study with the inherent biases that are present in small research studies." (Lunney, 2005)

If you are aware of or have information on more current research, we encourage you to submit the information to customer.support@elsevier.com. We appreciate your interest in keeping this text up-to-date and current and your support of providing the best "evidence" for state of the art nursing practice.

Many of the cultural interventions presented are general and are repeated throughout the text. Cultural groups are not homogeneous, and individual variation must always be considered when working with culturally diverse individuals. As such, the cultural interventions were developed to reflect the following assumptions:

- All work with culturally diverse individuals requires individualized assessment to avoid relying on stereotypes and other misrepresentations of culture.
- An awareness of how one's own cultural background and experiences, attitudes, values, and biases influence the application of the nursing process and the care provided is crucial to providing culturally competent care.
- Confronting one's own comfort with differences that exist between oneself and one's patients in race, ethnicity, culture, and beliefs is mandatory.
- Awareness of the stereotypes and preconceived notions that one may hold toward other culturally diverse groups will enhance care.
- Specific knowledge and information about the life experiences, cultural heritage, and historical background of diverse groups will guide a nursing approach.
- An understanding of how race, culture, ethnicity, and so forth may affect the manifestation of illness, help-seeking behavior, and the appropriateness or inappropriateness of nursing approaches.
- Respect for clients' religious and spiritual beliefs and values, indigenous helping practices, and the community help-giving networks will enhance the nurse-patient relationship.
- Awareness of institutional barriers that prevent or restrict culturally different clients from using health services is necessary.
- Knowledge of the models of minority and majority identity, and understanding how these models relate to the nurse-patient relationship and the nursing process is pertinent.
- An understanding of how racism and discrimination influence the use of and perceptions of the health care system is required (Galanti, 1997).

Nurses in all clinical settings make hundreds of clinical decisions every day. Patients are sometimes assessed from minute to minute and sometimes over a period of months depending on the nature of the practice. In so doing, nurses identify patient problems/diagnoses based on assessment and collection of patient data. Next, nurses decide on and provide complex nursing interventions. Accurate diagnosis and selection of interventions based on searching and evaluating evidence at the point of care is essential (Swan & Boruch, 2004; Swan, Lang, & McGinley, 2004). Nurses can find evidence to guide their practice in many places. The Agency for Healthcare Research and Quality (AHRQ), formerly the Agency for Health Care Policy and Research (AHCPR), began producing clinical practice guidelines in 1989. Clinical practice guidelines are defined as "systematically developed statements to assist practitioners and patient decisions about appropriate health care for specific clinical circumstances" (IOM, p.38). Although AHRQ no longer develops guidelines, it supports the National Guidelines Clearinghouse (NGC). The NGC is a comprehensive database of evidence-based clinical practice guidelines and related documents produced by the AHRQ in partnership with the American Medical Association (AMA) and the American Association of Health Plans (AAHP). The NGC mission is to provide physicians, nurses, and other health professionals, health care providers, health plans, integrated delivery systems, purchasers, and others an accessible mechanism for obtaining objective, detailed information on clinical practice guidelines and to further their dissemination, implementation, and use. There are currently 13,765 guidelines in the clearinghouse with new and frequent additions. The guidelines are easily accessed at www.guideline.gov. Both professionals and consumers use this resource to access the guidelines and information for specific health problems. In addition, AHRQ sponsors the National Quality Measures Clearinghouse (NQMC). The NQMC is an on-line evidence-based quality measures warehouse with 541 measures and measure sets (www.qualitymeasures.ahrq.gov).

The journal *Evidence-Based Nursing* is another rich and useful resource. This journal is devoted to helping nurses identify and appraise high quality, clinically relevant research. The journal selects from the health-related literature articles reporting studies and reviews that warrant immediate attention by nurses attempting to keep pace with their practice and delivering quality care (www.evidencebased-nursing.com). *The Annual Review of Nursing Research* is very useful. Many nursing journals now publish practice guidelines based on reviews of nursing research that are helpful to the nurse heading in the direction of EBN.

In an effort to support nursing knowledge worldwide, Sigma Theta Tau International (STTI) (www.stti.iupui.edu/library), through the Virginia Henderson International Library, provides the *Registry of Nursing Research* (RNR) as a resource to its members. The RNR is an electronic research resource that contains information and abstracts from more than 13,000 studies. As part of an evidence-based practice initiative, the *Online Journal of Knowledge Synthesis for Nursing* (OJKSN) has added a new clinical column. This column includes exemplars of EBN practice (Capasso, Burke, Stanley, & Abbott, 2002). In March 2004, STTI introduced its new journal, *WORLDviews on Evidence-Based Nursing*, an international source of information for using EBN practice to improve patient care.

A new Web-based evidence resource is www.globalevidence.com. This website provides a searchable database of online resources, organizations, and institutions related to evidence for practice, research, education, and evaluation, both nationally and internationally. It promotes the advancement of the use of evidence in clinical practice by providing a central information source and communication channel.

Some of the multiple helpful websites on evidence-based care include:

- *The Joanna Briggs Institute for Evidence-Based Nursing and Midwifery.* This site identifies areas in which nurses need summarized evidence on which to base their practice, facilitates systematic reviews of international research, undertakes multisite randomized controlled clinical trials in areas in which research is needed, and prepares easy-to-read summaries of best practice in the form of Practice Information Sheets based on the results of systematic reviews. Website: www.joannabriggs.edu.au
- *The University of York Centre for Evidence-Based Nursing.* This center works with nurse clinicians,

researchers, educators, and managers to identify EBN through research and systematic reviews. Website: www.york.ac.uk/depts/hstd/centres/evidence/ev-intro.htm

- *The Sarah Cole Hirsh Institute for Best Nursing Practices Based on Evidence.* This institute works to educate and assist nurses, health care providers, and health care organizations in the implementation of evidence-based practices and it continues to build a repository of best nursing practices. Website: fpb.cwru.edu/HirshInstitute/
- *The Cochrane Collaboration.* This international collaboration facilitates the creation, maintenance, and dissemination of more than 1000 systematic reviews of the effects of health care interventions in multiple conditions. More than 60 interdisciplinary working groups and collaborative review groups are composed of people from around the world who share an interest in developing and maintaining systematic reviews relevant to a particular health area. Website: www.cochrane.org
- *The Campbell Collaboration.* Similar to the Cochrane Collaboration, this international organization aims to produce, disseminate, and continuously update systematic reviews of studies of the effectiveness of social and behavioral interventions. Website: www.campbellcollaboration.org
- *Netting the Evidence.* A ScHARR Introduction to Evidence-Based Practice on the Internet, this is an alphabetical list of more than 150 websites related to evidence-based practice. Website: www.shef.ac.uk/~scharr/ir/netting/%

When using EBN, it is vitally important that the clients' concerns and individual situations be taken under consideration (website: www.ahcpr.gov). The nurse must always use critical thinking when applying EBN guidelines to any particular nursing situation. Each client is unique in his or her needs and capabilities. Prescriptive guidelines can be applied inappropriately, resulting in increased problems for the client (Mitchell, 1999). The goal is to provide the best care based on input from researchers, practitioners, and the recipients of care.

Section III supplies choices of interventions for each nursing diagnosis. The interventions are identified as independent (autonomous actions that are initiated by the nurse in response to a nursing diagnosis) or collaborative (actions that the nurse performs in collaboration with other health care professionals and that may require a physician's order and may be in response to both medical and nursing diagnoses). The nurse may choose the interventions appropriate for the client and individualize them accordingly or determine additional interventions. This text also contains several suggested Nursing Interventions Classification (NIC) interventions for each nursing diagnosis to help the reader see how NIC is used along with NOC and nursing diagnoses. The NIC interventions are a comprehensive, standardized classification of treatments that nurses perform. The classification includes both physiological and psychosocial interventions and covers all nursing specialties. A listing of NIC interventions is included on the Evolve site. For more information about NIC interventions, the reader is referred to the NIC text, which is identified in the reference list (McCloskey & Bulechek, 2004).

## Putting It All Together—Writing the Care Plan

The final planning phase is writing the actual care plan, including prioritized nursing diagnostic statements, outcomes, and interventions. To ensure continuity of care, the plan must be written and shared with all health care personnel caring for the client. This text provides rationales, most of which are research based, to validate that the interventions are appropriate and workable. Because it usually takes at least 1 year from the time a manuscript is accepted for publication for it to appear in print, we have provided many websites as references for rationales and client/family teaching. In this time of rapid change in health care, we cannot wait a year for access to vital information. Today some material appears only in electronic form (Sparks & Rizzolo, 1998). Websites for client/family teaching are available at the EVOLVE website. A sample care plan is illustrated in Figure I-2.

- NOC Outcomes
- Client Outcomes
- NIC Interventions
- Nursing Interventions and Rationales
- Home Care Interventions
- Client/Family Teaching
- Websites for Education
- References

Create the Care Plan

< Main page

## Nursing Diagnosis: Activity intolerance

Linda L. Straight

NANDA Definition: Insufficient physiological or psychological energy to endure or complete required or desired daily activities

Defining Characteristics: Verbal report of fatigue or weakness, abnormal heart rate or blood pressure response to activity, exertional discomfort or dyspnea, electrocardiographic changes reflecting dysrhythmias or ischemia

Related Factors: Bed rest or immobility; generalized weakness; sedentary lifestyle; imbalance between oxygen supply and demand

### NOC Outcomes (Nursing Outcomes Classification)

Suggested NOC Labels

- ☐ Endurance
- ☐ Energy Conservation
- ☐ Activity Tolerance
- ☐ Self-Care: Activities of Daily Living (ADLs)

### Client Outcomes

- ☐ Participates in prescribed physical activity with appropriate increases in heart rate, blood pressure, and breathing rate; maintains monitor patterns (rhythm and ST segment) within normal limits
- ☐ States symptoms of adverse effects of exercise and reports onset of symptoms immediately
- ☐ Maintains normal skin color and skin is warm and dry with activity
- ☐ Verbalizes an understanding of the need to gradually increase activity based on testing, tolerance, and symptoms
- ☐ Expresses an understanding of the need to balance rest and activity
- ☐ Demonstrates increased activity tolerance

### NIC Interventions (Nursing Interventions Classification)

Suggested NIC Labels

- ☐ Energy Management
- ☐ Activity Therapy

### Nursing Interventions and Rationales

- ☐ Determine cause of activity intolerance (see Related Factors) and determine whether cause is physical, psychological, or motivational. *Determining the cause of a disease can help direct appropriate interventions.*
- ▲ ☐ Assess client daily for appropriateness of activity and bed rest orders. *Inappropriate prolonged bed rest orders may contribute to activity intolerance. A review of 39 studies on bed rest resulting from 15 disorders demonstrated that bed rest for treatment of medical conditions is associated with worse outcomes than early mobilization (Allen, Glasziou, Del Mar, 1999).*

### Client/Family Teaching

- ☐ Instruct client on rationale and techniques for avoiding activity intolerance.
- ☐ Teach client to use controlled breathing techniques with activity.
- ☐ Teach client the importance and method of coughing, clearing secretions.
- ☐ Instruct client in the use of relaxation techniques during activity.
- ☐ Help client with energy conservation and work simplification techniques in ADLs.
- ☐ Teach client the importance of proper nutrition.
- ☐ Describe to client the symptoms of activity intolerance, including which symptoms to report to the physician.
- ☐ Explain to client how to use assistive devices or medications before or during activity.
- ☐ Help client set up an activity log to record exercise and exercise tolerance.

Websites for Education: See the **EVOLVE** website for World Wide Web resources for client education.

References

Create the Care Plan

**Figure I-2**
**Activity intolerance** care plan from the EVOLVE site.

## STEP 4: IMPLEMENTATION (ADPIE)

The implementation phase of the nursing process is the actual initiation of the nursing care plan. Client outcomes are achieved by the performance of the nursing interventions. During this phase the nurse continues to assess the client to determine whether the interventions are effective. An important part of this phase is documentation. The nurse should use the facility's tool for documentation and record the results of implementing nursing interventions. Documentation is also necessary for legal reasons because in a legal dispute, *if it wasn't charted, it wasn't done.*

## STEP 5: EVALUATION (ADPIE)

Although evaluation is listed as the last phase of the nursing process, it is actually an integral part of each phase and something the nurse does continually. When evaluation is performed as the last phase, the nurse refers to the client's outcomes and determines whether they were met. If the outcomes were not met, the nurse begins again with assessment and determines the reason they were not met. Were the outcomes attainable? Was the wrong nursing diagnosis made? Should the interventions be changed? At this point the nurse can look up any new symptoms or conditions that have been identified and adjust the care plan as needed. When using EBN, it is at this point the nurse determines whether the practice that was followed was effective. Necessary revisions may be made at this time.

Many health care providers are using critical pathways to plan nursing care. The use of nursing diagnoses should be an integral part of any critical pathway to ensure that nursing care needs are being assessed and appropriate nursing interventions are planned and implemented.

The use of nursing diagnoses, NOC outcomes, and NIC interventions ensures that nurses are speaking a common language when providing nursing care. This system also is easily computerized for simplified documentation and analysis of patterns of care. Nursing diagnosis is the essence of nursing, used to ensure that clients receive excellent, holistic nursing care.

Just as nurses continually evaluate the interventions and outcomes of care delivered, so too must they continually evaluate the evidence and the quality of the evidence, including both the quality of individual studies and the strength of the body of evidence. There are several systems to rank the hierarchical levels of evidence by grading/interpreting the strength of individual studies using a numeric or alpha rating. Melnyk and Fineout-Overholt (2004) recommend a Level I through Level VII rating system for the hierarchy of evidence, Level I represents evidence from a systematic review or meta-analysis through Level VII representing evidence from opinion of authorities and/or reports from expert committees. The strength of the body of evidence is rated based on quality, quantity, and consistency. Quality refers to the aggregate of quality ratings for each research study based on the extent to which bias was minimized. Quantity refers to the magnitude of effect and the numbers of studies. Consistency refers to the extent to which similar findings for any given topic are reported using similar and different study designs (AHRQ, 2002). After rating the quality of the evidence, nurses must ask: (1) Is the evidence valid?; (2) If valid, is this evidence important?; and (3) If valid and important, can the evidence be applied through nursing interventions to a given client?

The nursing process is continually evolving. In this text, our goal is to present state-of-the-art information to assist the nurse and nursing student to provide the best nursing care possible.

## REFERENCES

Agency for Healthcare Research and Quality (AHRQ): *Evidence-based practice outcomes and effectiveness,* retrieved from the World Wide Web March 16, 2003, available online at: www.ahcpr.gov/clinic/outcomix.htm.

Agency for Healthcare Research and Quality (AHRQ): Systems to rate the strength of scientific evidence, *Evid Rep/Technol Assess* 47, 2002.

Capasso V et al: Clinical column: unit-based specialty vascular transitional home care program: an example of evidence-based nursing practice, *Online J Knowl Synth Nurs* (Feb 11):3, 2002.
Cullum N: Evaluation of studies of treatment or prevention interventions, *Evid Based Nurs* 4:7, 2001.
Galanti G: *Caring for patients from different cultures,* Philadelphia, 1997, University of Pennsylvania.
Lunney M: Personal communication, March 15, 2005.
McCloskey JC, Bulechek GM: *Nursing interventions classification (NIC),* ed 4, St Louis, 2004, Mosby.
Melnyk BM: Evidence-based practice: the past, the present, and recommendations for the millennium, *Pediatr Nurs* 26(1):79, 2000.
Melnyk BM, Fineout-Overholt E: *Evidence-based practice in nursing and healthcare: a guide to best practice,* Philadelphia, 2004, Lippincott-Williams & Wilkins.
Moorhead S, Johnson M, Maas M: *Nursing outcomes classification (NOC),* ed 3, St Louis, 2004, Mosby.
Mitchell GJ: Evidenced-based practice: critique and alternative view, *Nurs Sci Q* 12(1):, 1999.
North American Nursing Diagnosis Association-International (NANDA-I): *Nursing diagnoses: definitions and classification, 2005-2006,* Philadelphia, 2005, Author.
Sparks SM, Rizzolo MA: World Wide Web search tools, *Image J Nurs Sch* 30(2):167-171, 1998.
Swan BA, McGinley AM, Lang NM: Ambulatory care nursing practice: developing and contributing to the evidence base, *Nurs Econ$* 20(2):83-87, 2002.
Swan BA, Boruch RF: Quality of evidence: usefulness in measuring the quality of health care, *Medical Care* 42(suppl 2):II-12-II-20, 2004.
Swan BA, Lang NM, McGinley AM: Access to quality health care: links between evidence, nursing language, and informatics, *Nurs Econ* 22(6):325-332, 2004.
Weinick RM, Jacobs EA, Stone LC, Ortega AN, Burstin H: Hispanic healthcare disparities: challenging the myth of a monolithic Hispanic population, *Medical Care* 42(4):313-320, 2004.

SECTION

# II

# Guide to Nursing Diagnoses

Section II is an alphabetical listing of client symptoms, client problems, medical diagnoses, psychiatric diagnoses, and clinical states. Use this section to find suggestions for nursing diagnoses for your client.

First assess the client using the format provided by the clinical setting. Then use this section to locate the client's symptoms, problems, clinical state, diagnoses, surgeries, and diagnostic testing. Note suggestions given for appropriate nursing diagnoses.

Using information found in Section III, evaluate each suggested nursing diagnosis to see if it is appropriate for the client.

# A

## Abdominal Distention

Acute **Pain** r/t retention of air, gastrointestinal secretions

**Constipation** r/t decreased activity, decreased fluid intake, decreased fiber intake, pathological process

Delayed **Surgical** recovery r/t pain, nausea

Imbalanced **Nutrition**: less than body requirements r/t nausea, vomiting

**Nausea** r/t irritation of gastrointestinal tract

## Abdominal Hysterectomy

*See Hysterectomy*

## Abdominal Pain

Acute **Pain** r/t injury, pathological process

Imbalanced **Nutrition**: less than body requirements r/t unresolved pain

*See cause of Abdominal Pain*

## Abdominal Perineal Resection

Risk for perioperative positioning **Injury** r/t prolonged surgery, lithotomy position

*See Abdominal Surgery; Colostomy*

## Abdominal Surgery

Acute **Pain** r/t surgical procedure

**Constipation** r/t decreased activity, decreased fluid intake, anesthesia, narcotics

Imbalanced **Nutrition**: less than body requirements r/t high metabolic needs, decreased ability to ingest or digest food

Ineffective **Health** maintenance r/t knowledge deficit regarding self-care after surgery

Ineffective **Tissue** perfusion: peripheral r/t immobility, abdominal surgery resulting in stasis of blood flow

Risk for **Infection** r/t invasive procedure

*See Surgery, Perioperative Care; Surgery, Postoperative Care; Surgery, Preoperative Care*

## Abdominal Trauma

Acute **Pain** r/t abdominal trauma

Deficient **Fluid** volume r/t hemorrhage

Disturbed **Body** image r/t scarring, change in body function, need for temporary colostomy

Ineffective **Breathing** pattern r/t abdominal distention, pain

Risk for **Infection** r/t possible perforation of abdominal structures

## Abortion, Induced

Acute **Pain** r/t surgical intervention

Chronic low **Self-esteem** disturbance r/t feelings of guilt

Chronic **Sorrow** r/t loss of potential child

Compromised family **Coping** r/t unresolved feelings about decision

Ineffective **Health** maintenance r/t deficient knowledge regarding self-care following abortion

Risk for delayed **Development** r/t unplanned or unwanted pregnancy

Risk for imbalanced **Fluid** volume r/t possible hemorrhage

Risk for **Infection** r/t open uterine blood vessels, dilated cervix

Risk for **Post-trauma** syndrome r/t psychological trauma of abortion

Risk for **Spiritual** distress r/t perceived moral implications of decision

**Spiritual** distress r/t perceived moral implications of decision

## Abortion, Spontaneous

Acute **Pain** r/t uterine contractions, surgical intervention

Chronic **Sorrow** r/t loss of potential child

Disabled family **Coping** r/t unresolved feelings about loss

Disturbed **Body** image r/t perceived inability to carry pregnancy, produce child

**Fear** r/t implications for future pregnancies

**Grieving** r/t loss of fetus

Ineffective **Coping** r/t personal vulnerability

Ineffective **Health** maintenance r/t deficient knowledge regarding self-care following abortion

Interrupted **Family** processes r/t unmet expectations for pregnancy and childbirth

Risk for deficient **Fluid** volume r/t hemorrhage

Risk for **Infection** r/t septic or incomplete abortion of products of conception, open uterine blood vessels, dilated cervix

Risk for **Post-trauma** syndrome r/t psychological trauma of abortion

Risk for **Spiritual** distress r/t loss of fetus

**Self-esteem** disturbance r/t feelings of failure, guilt

## Abruptio Placentae <36 Weeks

Acute **Pain** r/t irritable uterus, hypertonic uterus

**Anxiety** r/t unknown outcome, change in birth plans

Death **Anxiety** r/t unknown outcome, hemorrhage/pain

**Fear** r/t threat to well-being of self and fetus

Impaired **Gas** exchange: placental r/t decreased uteroplacental area

Impaired **Tissue** integrity: maternal r/t possible uterine rupture

Interrupted **Family** process r/t unmet expectations for pregnancy/childbirth

Ineffective **Health** maintenance r/t deficient knowledge regarding self-care with disorder

Risk for deficient **Fluid** volume r/t hemorrhage

Risk for disproportionate **Growth** r/t uteroplacental insufficiency

Risk for ineffective **Tissue** perfusion: fetal r/t uteroplacental insufficiency

Risk for **Infection** r/t partial separation of placenta

## Abscess Formation

Impaired **Tissue** integrity r/t altered circulation, nutritional deficit/excess

Ineffective **Health** maintenance r/t deficient knowledge regarding self-care with abscess

Ineffective **Protection** r/t inadequate nutrition, abnormal blood profile, drug therapy, depressed immune function

## Abuse, Child

*See Child Abuse*

## Abuse, Spouse, Parent, or Significant Other

**Anxiety** r/t threat to self-concept, situational crisis of abuse

**Caregiver** role strain r/t chronic illness, self-care deficits, lack of respite care, extent of caregiving required

Compromised family **Coping** r/t abusive patterns

Defensive **Coping** r/t low self-esteem

Disturbed **Sleep** pattern r/t psychological stress

Impaired verbal **Communication** r/t psychological barriers of fear

Interrupted **Family** process: alcoholism r/t inadequate coping skills

**Post-trauma** syndrome r/t history of abuse

**Powerlessness** r/t lifestyle of helplessness

Risk for **Post-trauma** syndrome r/t inadequate social support

Risk for self-directed **Violence** r/t history of abuse

**Self-esteem** disturbance r/t negative family interactions

## Accessory Muscle Use (to Breathe)

Ineffective **Breathing** pattern r/t compromised lung function, neuromuscular impairment, pain, musculoskeletal impairment, perception/cognitive impairment, anxiety, decreased energy, fatigue

*See Asthma; Bronchitis; COPD; Respiratory Infections, Acute Childhood*

## Accident Prone

Acute **Confusion** r/t altered level of consciousness

Adult **Failure** to thrive r/t fatigue

Ineffective **Coping** r/t personal vulnerability, situational crises

Risk for **Injury** r/t history of accidents

## Achalasia

Acute **Pain** r/t stasis of food in esophagus

Impaired **Swallowing** r/t neuromuscular impairment

Ineffective **Coping** r/t chronic disease

Risk for **Aspiration** r/t nocturnal regurgitation

## Acidosis, Metabolic

Acute **Pain**: headache r/t neuromuscular irritability

Decreased **Cardiac** output r/t dysrhythmias from hyperkalemia

Disturbed **Thought** processes r/t central nervous system depression

Imbalanced **Nutrition**: less than body requirements r/t inability to ingest, absorb nutrients

Impaired **Memory** r/t electrolyte imbalance

Ineffective **Tissue** perfusion: cardiopulmonary r/t progressive shock

Risk for **Injury** r/t disorientation, weakness, stupor

## Acidosis, Respiratory

**Activity** intolerance r/t imbalance between oxygen supply and demand

Disturbed **Thought** processes r/t central nervous system depression

Impaired **Gas** exchange r/t ventilation perfusion imbalance

Impaired **Memory** r/t hypoxia

A

Risk for decreased **Cardiac** output r/t dysrhythmias associated with respiratory acidosis

## Acne

Disturbed **Body** image r/t biophysical changes associated with skin disorder

Impaired **Skin** integrity r/t hormonal changes (adolescence, menstrual cycle)

Ineffective management of **Therapeutic** regimen r/t deficient knowledge (medications, personal care, cause)

## Acquired Immunodeficiency Syndrome

*See AIDS (Acquired Immunodeficiency Syndrome)*

## Acromegaly

Disturbed **Body** image r/t changes in body function and appearance

Impaired physical **Mobility** r/t joint pain

Ineffective **Airway** clearance r/t airway obstruction by enlarged tongue

**Sexual** dysfunction r/t changes in hormonal secretions

## Activity Intolerance

**Activity** intolerance r/t bedrest/immobility, generalized weakness, sedentary lifestyle, imbalance between oxygen supply/demand, pain

## Activity Intolerance, Potential to Develop

Risk for **Activity** intolerance r/t deconditioned status, presence of circulatory/respiratory problems, inexperience with activity

## Acute Abdomen

Acute **Pain** r/t pathological process

Deficient **Fluid** volume r/t air and fluids trapped in bowel, inability to drink

*See cause of Acute Abdomen*

## Acute Alcohol Intoxication

Disturbed **Thought** processes r/t central nervous system depression

Dysfunctional **Family** processes: alcoholism r/t abuse of alcohol

Ineffective **Breathing** pattern r/t depression of the respiratory center

Risk for **Aspiration** r/t depressed reflexes with acute vomiting

Risk for **Infection** r/t impaired immune system from altered nutrition

## Acute Back

Acute **Pain** r/t back injury

**Anxiety** r/t situational crisis, back injury

**Constipation** r/t decreased activity

Impaired physical **Mobility** r/t pain

Ineffective **Coping** r/t situational crisis, back injury

Ineffective **Health** maintenance r/t deficient knowledge regarding self-care with painful back

## Acute Confusion

*See Confusion, Acute*

## Acute Respiratory Distress Syndrome

*See ARDS (Acute Respiratory Distress Syndrome)*

## Adams-Stokes Syndrome

*See Dysrhythmia*

## Addiction

*See Alcoholism; Drug Abuse*

## Addison's Disease

**Activity** intolerance r/t weakness, fatigue

Deficient **Fluid** volume r/t failure of regulatory mechanisms

Disturbed **Body** image r/t increased skin pigmentation

Imbalanced **Nutrition**: less than body requirements r/t chronic illness

Ineffective **Health** maintenance r/t deficient knowledge

Risk for **Injury** r/t weakness

## Adenoidectomy

Acute **Pain** r/t surgical incision

Impaired **Comfort** r/t effects of anesthesia, nausea, vomiting

Ineffective **Airway** clearance r/t hesitation/reluctance to cough secondary to pain

Ineffective **Health** maintenance r/t deficient knowledge of postoperative care

**Nausea** r/t anesthesia effects, drainage from surgery

Risk for **Aspiration** r/t postoperative drainage, impaired swallowing

Risk for deficient **Fluid** volume r/t decreased intake secondary to painful swallowing, effects of anesthesia

Risk for imbalanced **Nutrition**: less than body requirements r/t hesitation/reluctance to swallow

## Adhesions, Lysis of

*See Abdominal Surgery*

## Adjustment Disorder

**Anxiety** r/t inability to cope with psychosocial stressor

Disturbed personal **Identity** r/t psychosocial stressor (specific to individual)

Impaired **Adjustment** r/t assault to self-esteem

Impaired **Social** interaction r/t absence of significant others or peers

Situational low **Self-esteem** r/t change in role function

## Adjustment Impairment

Impaired **Adjustment** r/t disability requiring change in lifestyle, inadequate support systems, impaired cognition, sensory overload assault to self-esteem, altered locus of control, incomplete grieving

## Adolescent, Pregnant

**Anxiety** r/t situational and maturational crisis, pregnancy

Decisional **Conflict**: keeping child versus giving up child versus abortion r/t lack of experience with decision-making, interference with decision-making, multiple or divergent sources of information, lack of support system

Deficient **Knowledge** r/t pregnancy, infant growth and development, parenting

Delayed **Growth** and development r/t pregnancy

Disabled family **Coping** r/t highly ambivalent family relationships, chronically unresolved feelings of guilt, anger, despair

Disturbed **Body** image r/t pregnancy superimposed on developing body

**Fear** r/t labor and delivery

**Health**-seeking behaviors r/t desire for optimal maternal and fetal outcome

Imbalanced **Nutrition**: less than body requirements r/t lack of knowledge of nutritional needs during pregnancy and as growing adolescent

Impaired **Social** interaction r/t self-concept disturbance

Ineffective **Coping** r/t situational and maturational crisis, personal vulnerability

Ineffective **Denial** r/t fear of consequences of pregnancy becoming known

Ineffective **Health** maintenance r/t deficient knowledge with denial of pregnancy, desire to keep pregnancy secret, fear

Ineffective **Role** performance r/t pregnancy

Interrupted **Family** processes r/t unmet expectations for adolescent, situational crisis

**Noncompliance** r/t denial of pregnancy

Risk for **Constipation** r/t hormone effect, inadequate fiber in diet, inadequate fluid in diet

Risk for delayed **Development** r/t unplanned or unwanted pregnancy

Risk for impaired parent-infant **Attachment** r/t anxiety associated with the parent role

Risk for impaired **Parenting** r/t adolescent parent, unplanned or unwanted pregnancy, single parent

Risk for urge urinary **Incontinence** r/t pressure on bladder by growing uterus

Situational low **Self-esteem** r/t feelings of shame and guilt about becoming/being pregnant

**Social** isolation r/t absence of supportive significant other(s)

## Adoption, Giving Child Up for

Chronic **Sorrow** r/t loss of relationship with child

Decisional **Conflict** r/t unclear personal values or beliefs, perceived threat to value system, support system deficit

Disturbed **Sleep** pattern r/t depression or trauma of relinquishment of child

Ineffective **Coping** r/t final decision

Interrupted **Family** processes r/t conflict within family regarding relinquishment of child

**Grieving** r/t loss of child, loss of role of parent

Readiness for enhanced **Spiritual** well-being r/t harmony with self, regarding final decision

Risk for **Post-trauma** syndrome r/t psychological trauma of relinquishment of child

Risk for **Spiritual** distress r/t perceived moral implications of decision

**Social** isolation r/t making choice that goes against values of significant other(s)

## Adrenal Crisis

Deficient **Fluid** volume r/t insufficient ability to reabsorb water

Delayed **Surgical** recovery r/t inability to respond to stress

Ineffective **Protection** r/t inability to tolerate stress

*See Addison's Disease; Shock*

## Advance Directives

Anticipatory **Grieving** r/t possible loss of self, significant other

A

Death **Anxiety** r/t planning for end-of-life health decisions

Decisional **Conflict** r/t unclear personal values or beliefs, perceived threat to value system, support system deficit

Readiness for enhanced **Spiritual** well-being r/t harmonious interconnectedness with self, others, higher power/God

## Affective Disorders

Adult **Failure** to thrive r/t altered mood state

Chronic low **Self-esteem** r/t repeated unmet expectations

Chronic **Sorrow** r/t chronic mental illness

**Constipation** r/t inactivity, decreased fluid intake

Disturbed **Sleep** pattern r/t inactivity

Dysfunctional **Grieving** r/t lack of previous resolution of former grieving response

**Fatigue** r/t psychological demands

**Hopelessness** r/t feeling of abandonment, long-term stress

Ineffective **Coping** r/t dysfunctional grieving

Ineffective **Health** maintenance r/t lack of ability to make good judgments regarding ways to obtain help

Risk for **Loneliness** r/t pattern of social isolation, feelings of low self-esteem

Risk for **Suicide** r/t panic state

**Self-care** deficit: specify r/t depression, cognitive impairment

**Sexual** dysfunction r/t loss of sexual desire

**Social** isolation r/t ineffective coping

*See specific disorder: Depression; Dysthymic Disorder; Manic Disorder, Bipolar I*

## Age-Related Macular Degeneration

*See Macular Degeneration*

## Aggressive Behavior

**Fear** r/t real or imagined threat to own well-being

Risk for other-directed **Violence** r/t antisocial character, battered woman, catatonic excitement, child abuse, manic excitement, organic brain syndrome, panic states, rage reactions, suicidal behavior, temporal lobe epilepsy, toxic reactions to medication

Risk for self-directed **Violence** r/t antisocial character, battered woman, catatonic excitement, child abuse, manic excitement, organic brain syndrome, panic states, rage reactions, suicidal behavior, temporal lobe epilepsy, toxic reactions to medication

## Aging

Adult **Failure** to thrive r/t depression, apathy, fatigue

Anticipatory **Grieving** r/t multiple losses, impending death

Chronic **Sorrow** r/t multiple losses

Death **Anxiety** r/t fear of unknown, loss of self, impact on significant others

Disturbed **Sensory** perception: visual or auditory r/t aging process

Functional urinary **Incontinence** r/t impaired vision, impaired cognition, neuromuscular limitations, altered environmental factors

**Health**-seeking behaviors r/t knowledge about medication, nutrition, exercise, coping strategies

Impaired **Dentition** r/t ineffective oral hygiene; barriers to self-care, professional care; nutritional deficits; dietary habits; selected prescription medications; chronic use of tobacco, coffee, tea, red wine; lack of knowledge regarding dental health

Impaired **Memory** r/t fluid and electrolyte imbalance, neurological disturbances, excessive environmental disturbances, anemia, acute or chronic hypoxia, decreased cardiac output

Ineffective management of **Therapeutic** regimen r/t deficient knowledge: medication, nutrition, exercise, coping strategies

Ineffective **Thermoregulation** r/t aging

Readiness for enhanced community **Coping** r/t providing social support and other resources identified as needed for elderly client

Readiness for enhanced family **Coping** r/t ability to gratify needs, address adaptive tasks

Readiness for enhanced **Knowledge** of: specify r/t need to improve health

Readiness for enhanced **Nutrition** r/t need to improve health

Readiness for enhanced **Sleep** r/t need to improve sleep

Readiness for enhanced **Spiritual** well-being r/t one's experience of life's meaning, harmony with self, others, higher power/God, environment

Readiness for enhanced **Urinary** elimination r/t need to improve health

Risk for **Caregiver** role strain r/t inability to handle increasing needs of significant other

Risk for **Injury** r/t disturbed sensory perception

Risk for **Loneliness** r/t inadequate support system, role transition, health alterations, depression, fatigue

**Sleep** deprivation r/t aging-related sleep stage shifts

## Agitation

Acute **Confusion** r/t side effects of medication, hypoxia, decreased cerebral perfusion, alcohol abuse or withdrawal, substance abuse or withdrawal, sensory deprivation, sensory overload

**Sleep** deprivation r/t sundown syndrome

## Agoraphobia

**Anxiety** r/t real or perceived threat to physical integrity

**Fear** r/t leaving home, going out in public places

Impaired **Social** interaction r/t disturbance in self-concept

Ineffective **Coping** r/t inadequate support systems

**Social** isolation r/t altered thought process

## Agranulocytosis

Delayed **Surgical** recovery r/t abnormal blood profile

Ineffective **Health** maintenance r/t deficient knowledge of protective measures to prevent infection

Ineffective **Protection** r/t abnormal blood profile

## AIDS (Acquired Immunodeficiency Syndrome)

Anticipatory **Grieving**: family/parental r/t potential/impending death of loved one

Anticipatory **Grieving**: individual r/t loss of physiopsychosocial well-being

Disturbed **Body** image r/t chronic contagious illness, cachexia

**Caregiver** role strain r/t unpredictable illness course, presence of situation stressors

Chronic **Pain** r/t tissue inflammation and destruction

Chronic **Sorrow** r/t living with long-term chronic illness

Death **Anxiety** r/t fear of premature death

**Diarrhea** r/t inflammatory bowel changes

Disturbed **Energy** field r/t chronic illness

**Fatigue** r/t disease process, stress, poor nutritional intake

**Fear** r/t powerlessness, threat to well-being

**Hopelessness** r/t deteriorating physical condition

Imbalanced **Nutrition**: less than body requirements r/t decreased ability to eat and absorb nutrients secondary to anorexia, nausea, diarrhea; pathology in gastrointestinal tract

Ineffective **Health** maintenance r/t deficient knowledge regarding transmission of infection, lack of exposure to information, misinterpretation of information

Ineffective **Protection** r/t risk for infection secondary to inadequate immune system

Ineffective **Sexuality** pattern r/t possible transmission of disease

Interrupted **Family** processes r/t distress about diagnosis of human immunodeficiency virus (HIV) infection

Risk for deficient **Fluid** volume r/t diarrhea, vomiting, fever, bleeding

Risk for impaired **Oral** mucous membranes r/t immunological deficit

Risk for impaired **Skin** integrity r/t immunological deficit, diarrhea

Risk for **Infection** r/t inadequate immune system

Risk for **Loneliness** r/t social isolation

Risk for **Spiritual** distress r/t physical illness

Situational low **Self-esteem** r/t crisis of chronic contagious illness

**Social** isolation r/t self-concept disturbance, therapeutic isolation

**Spiritual** distress r/t challenged beliefs or moral system

*See AIDS, Child; Cancer; Pneumonia*

## AIDS Dementia

Chronic **Confusion** r/t viral invasion of nervous system

Disturbed **Thought** processes r/t viral infection in the brain

*See Dementia*

## AIDS, Child

Impaired **Parenting** r/t congenital acquisition of infection secondary to intravenous (IV) drug use, multiple sexual partners, history of contaminated blood transfusion

**Parental** role conflict r/t interruption of family life due to home care regimen, intimidation with invasive or restrictive modalities

Risk for delayed **Development** r/t chronic illness

Risk for disproportionate **Growth** r/t chronic illness

*See AIDS (Acquired Immunodeficiency Syndrome); Child with Chronic Condition; Hospitalized Child; Terminally Ill Child, Adolescent; Terminally Ill Child, Infant/Toddler; Terminally Ill Child, Preschool Child; Terminally Ill Child, School-Age Child/Preadolescent; Terminally Ill Child/Death of Child, Parent*

## Airway Obstruction/Secretions

Ineffective **Airway** clearance r/t decreased energy; fatigue; tracheobronchial infection, obstruction, secretions; perceptual/cognitive impairment; trauma; decreased force of cough because of aging

## Alcohol Withdrawal

Acute **Confusion** r/t effects of alcohol withdrawal

**Anxiety** r/t situational crisis, withdrawal

Chronic low **Self-esteem** r/t repeated unmet expectations

Disturbed **Sensory** perception: visual, auditory, kinesthetic, tactile, olfactory r/t neurochemical imbalance in brain

Disturbed **Sleep** pattern r/t effect of depressants, alcohol withdrawal, anxiety

Disturbed **Thought** processes r/t potential delirium tremors

Dysfunctional **Family** processes: alcoholism r/t abuse of alcohol

Imbalanced **Nutrition**: less than body requirements r/t poor dietary habits

Ineffective **Coping** r/t personal vulnerability

Ineffective **Health** maintenance r/t deficient knowledge regarding chronic illness or effects of alcohol consumption

Risk for deficient **Fluid** volume r/t excessive diaphoresis, agitation, decreased fluid intake

Risk for other-directed **Violence** r/t substance withdrawal

Risk for self-directed **Violence** r/t substance withdrawal

## Alcoholism

Acute **Confusion** r/t alcohol abuse

**Anxiety** r/t loss of control

Chronic **Confusion** r/t neurological effects of chronic alcohol intake

Defensive **Coping** r/t alcoholism

Ineffective **Denial** r/t refusal to acknowledge alcoholism

Disturbed **Sleep** pattern r/t irritability, nightmares, tremors

Dysfunctional family **Coping:** alcoholism r/t codependency issues

Imbalanced **Nutrition**: less than body requirements r/t anorexia

Impaired **Adjustment** r/t lack of motivation to change behaviors

Impaired **Home** maintenance r/t memory deficits, fatigue

Impaired **Memory** r/t alcohol abuse

Ineffective **Coping** r/t use of alcohol to cope with life events

Ineffective **Protection** r/t malnutrition, sleep deprivation

Interrupted **Family** process: alcoholism r/t alcohol abuse

**Powerlessness** r/t alcohol addiction

Risk for **Injury** r/t alteration in sensory/perceptual function

Risk for **Loneliness** r/t unacceptable social behavior

Risk for other-directed **Violence** r/t reactions to substances used, impulsive behavior, disorientation, impaired judgment

Risk for self-directed **Violence** r/t reactions to substances used, impulsive behavior, disorientation, impaired judgment

**Self-esteem** disturbance r/t failure at life events

**Social** isolation r/t unacceptable social behavior, values

## Alcoholism, Dysfunctional Family Processes

Dysfunctional **Family** processes: alcoholism r/t abuse of alcohol, genetic predisposition, lack of problem-solving skills, inadequate coping skills, family history of alcoholism, resistance to treatment, biochemical influences, addictive personality

## Alkalosis

*See Metabolic Alkalosis*

## Allergies

Ineffective **Health** maintenance r/t deficient knowledge regarding allergies

Latex **Allergy** r/t hypersensitivity to natural rubber latex

Risk for latex **Allergy** r/t repeated exposure to products containing latex

## Alopecia

Deficient **Knowledge** r/t self-care needed to promote hair growth

Disturbed **Body** image r/t loss of hair, change in appearance

## Altered Mental Status

*See Confusion, Acute; Confusion, Chronic; Impaired Memory*

## ALS (Amyotrophic Lateral Sclerosis)

*See Amyotrophic Lateral Sclerosis*

## Alzheimer's Type Dementia

Adult **Failure** to thrive r/t difficulty in reasoning, judgment, memory, concentration

Disturbed **Thought** processes r/t chronic organic disorder

**Caregiver** role strain r/t duration and extent of caregiving required

Chronic **Confusion** r/t Alzheimer's disease

Compromised family **Coping** r/t interrupted family processes

Disturbed **Sleep** pattern r/t neurological impairment, daytime naps

**Fear** r/t loss of self

**Hopelessness** r/t deteriorating condition

Impaired **Environmental** interpretation syndrome r/t Alzheimer's disease

Impaired **Home** maintenance r/t impaired cognitive function, inadequate support systems

Impaired **Memory** r/t neurological disturbance

Impaired physical **Mobility** r/t severe neurological dysfunction

Ineffective **Health** maintenance r/t deficient knowledge of caregiver regarding appropriate care

**Powerlessness** r/t deteriorating condition

Risk for **Injury** r/t confusion

Risk for **Loneliness** r/t potential social isolation

Risk for other-directed **Violence** r/t frustration, fear, anger

Risk for **Relocation** stress syndrome r/t impaired psychosocial health, decreased health status

**Self-care** deficit: specify r/t psychological-physiological impairment

**Social** isolation r/t fear of disclosure of memory loss

**Wandering** r/t cognitive impairment, frustration, physiological state

*See Dementia*

## AMD (Age-Related Macular Degeneration)

*See Macular Degeneration*

## Amenorrhea

Imbalanced **Nutrition**: less than body requirements r/t inadequate food intake

Risk for **Sexual** dysfunction r/t altered body function

*See Sexuality, Adolescent*

## AMI (Acute Myocardial Infarction)

*See MI (Myocardial Infarction)*

## Amnesia

Acute **Confusion** r/t alcohol abuse, delirium, dementia, drug abuse

Dysfunctional **Family** processes: alcoholism r/t alcohol abuse, inadequate coping skills

Impaired **Memory** r/t excessive environmental disturbance, neurological disturbance

**Post-trauma** syndrome r/t history of abuse, catastrophic illness, disaster, accident

## Amniocentesis

**Anxiety** r/t threat to self and fetus, unknown future

Decisional **Conflict** r/t choice of treatment pending results of test

Risk for **Infection** r/t invasive procedure

## Amnionitis

*See Chorioamnionitis*

## Amniotic Membrane Rupture

*See Premature Rupture of Membranes*

## Amputation

Acute **Pain** r/t surgery, phantom limb sensation

Chronic **Pain** r/t surgery, phantom limb sensation

Chronic **Sorrow** r/t grief associated with loss of body part

Disturbed **Body** image r/t negative effects of amputation, response from others

**Grieving** r/t loss of body part, future lifestyle changes

Impaired physical **Mobility** r/t musculoskeletal impairment, limited movement

Impaired **Skin** integrity r/t poor healing, prosthesis rubbing

Ineffective **Health** maintenance r/t deficient knowledge of care of stump, rehabilitation

Ineffective **Tissue** perfusion: peripheral r/t impaired arterial circulation

Risk for deficient **Fluid** volume: hemorrhage r/t vulnerable surgical site

A

## Amyotrophic Lateral Sclerosis (ALS)

Chronic **Sorrow** r/t chronic illness

Death **Anxiety** r/t impending progressive loss of function leading to death

Decisional **Conflict**: ventilator therapy r/t unclear personal values or beliefs, lack of relevant information

Impaired spontaneous **Ventilation** r/t weakness of muscles of respiration

Impaired **Swallowing** r/t weakness of muscles involved in swallowing

Impaired verbal **Communication** r/t weakness of muscles of speech, deficient knowledge of ways to compensate and alternative communication devices

Ineffective **Breathing** pattern r/t compromised muscles of respiration

Risk for **Aspiration** r/t impaired swallowing

Risk for **Spiritual** distress r/t chronic debilitating condition

*See Neurological Disorders*

## Anal Fistula

*See Hemorrhoidectomy*

## Anaphylactic Shock

Impaired spontaneous **Ventilation** r/t acute airway obstruction

Ineffective **Airway** clearance r/t laryngeal edema, bronchospasm

Latex **Allergy** response r/t abnormal immune mechanism response

*See Shock*

## Anasarca

Excess **Fluid** volume r/t excessive fluid intake, cardiac/renal dysfunction, loss of plasma proteins

Risk for impaired **Skin** integrity r/t impaired circulation to skin

*See cause of Anasarca*

## Anemia

**Anxiety** r/t cause of disease

Delayed **Surgical** recovery r/t decreased oxygen supply to body, increased cardiac workload

**Fatigue** r/t decreased oxygen supply to the body, increased cardiac workload

Impaired **Memory** r/t anemia

Ineffective **Health** maintenance r/t deficient knowledge regarding nutritional and medical treatment of anemia

Ineffective **Protection** r/t bleeding disorder

Risk for **Injury** r/t alteration in peripheral sensory perception

## Anemia, in Pregnancy

**Anxiety** r/t concerns about health of self and fetus

**Fatigue** r/t decreased oxygen supply to the body, increased cardiac workload

Ineffective **Health** maintenance r/t deficient knowledge regarding nutrition in pregnancy

Risk for delayed **Development** r/t reduction in the oxygen-carrying capacity of blood

Risk for **Infection** r/t reduction in oxygen-carrying capacity of blood

## Anemia, Sickle Cell

*See Anemia; Sickle Cell Anemia/Crisis*

## Anencephaly

*See Neurotube Defects*

## Aneurysm, Abdominal Surgery

Risk for deficient **Fluid** volume: hemorrhage r/t potential abnormal blood loss

Risk for ineffective **Tissue** perfusion: peripheral or renal r/t impaired arterial circulation

Risk for **Infection** r/t invasive procedure

*See Abdominal Surgery*

## Aneurysm, Cerebral

*See Craniectomy/Craniotomy; Subarachnoid Hemorrhage (if aneurysm has ruptured)*

## Anger

**Anxiety** r/t situational crisis

Defensive **Coping** r/t inability to acknowledge responsibility for actions and results of actions

**Fear** r/t environmental stressor, hospitalization

**Grieving** r/t significant loss

Impaired **Adjustment** r/t assault to self-esteem, disability requiring change in lifestyle, inadequate support system

**Powerlessness** r/t health care environment

Risk for other-directed **Violence** r/t history of violence, rage reaction

Risk for **Post-trauma** syndrome r/t inadequate social support

Risk for self-directed **Violence** r/t history of violence, history of abuse, rage reaction

## Angina Pectoris

**Activity** intolerance r/t acute pain, dysrhythmias

Acute **Pain** r/t myocardial ischemia

**Anxiety** r/t situational crisis

Decreased **Cardiac** output r/t myocardial ischemia, medication effect, dysrhythmia

**Grieving** r/t pain, lifestyle changes

Ineffective **Coping** r/t personal vulnerability to situational crisis of new diagnosis, deteriorating health

Ineffective **Denial** r/t deficient knowledge of need to seek help with symptoms

Ineffective **Health** maintenance r/t deficient knowledge of care of angina condition

Ineffective **Sexuality** pattern r/t disease process, medications, loss of libido

## Angiocardiography (Cardiac Catheterization)

*See Cardiac Catheterization*

## Angioplasty, Coronary

Decreased **Cardiac** output r/t ventricular ischemia, dysrhythmias

**Fear** r/t possible outcome of interventional procedure

Ineffective **Health** maintenance r/t deficient knowledge regarding care following procedures, measures to limit coronary artery disease

Risk for deficient **Fluid** volume r/t possible damage to coronary artery, hematoma formation, hemorrhage

Risk for ineffective **Tissue** perfusion: peripheral/cardiopulmonary r/t vasospasm, hematoma formation

## Anomaly, Fetal/Newborn (Parent Dealing with)

**Anxiety** r/t threat to role functioning, situational crisis

Chronic **Sorrow** r/t loss of ideal child

Decisional **Conflict**: interventions for fetus/newborn r/t lack of relevant information, spiritual distress, threat to value system

Deficient **Knowledge** r/t limited exposure to situation

Effective **Therapeutic** regimen management r/t verbalized intent to reduce risk factors for progression of illness and sequelae associated with anomaly

**Fear** r/t real or imagined threat to baby, implications for future pregnancies, powerlessness

**Hopelessness** r/t long-term stress, deteriorating physical condition of child, lost spiritual belief

Disabled family **Coping** r/t chronically unresolved feelings about loss of perfect baby

Impaired **Parenting** r/t interruption of bonding process

Ineffective **Coping** r/t personal vulnerability in situational crisis

Interrupted **Family** processes r/t unmet expectations for perfect baby, lack of adequate support systems

Parental role **Conflict** r/t separation from newborn, intimidation with invasive or restrictive modalities, specialized care center policies

**Powerlessness** r/t complication threatening fetus/newborn

Risk for disorganized **Infant** behavior r/t congenital disorder

Risk for dysfunctional **Grieving** r/t loss of perfect child

Risk for impaired parent/infant/child **Attachment** r/t ill infant who is unable to effectively initiate parental contact as result of altered behavioral organization

Risk for impaired **Parenting** r/t interruption of bonding process; unrealistic expectations for self, infant, or partner; perceived threat to own emotional survival; severe stress; lack of knowledge

Risk for **Spiritual** distress r/t lack of normal child to raise and carry on family name

**Self-esteem** disturbance r/t perceived inability to produce a perfect child

**Social** isolation r/t alterations in child's physical appearance, altered state of wellness

**Spiritual** distress r/t test of spiritual beliefs

## Anorectal Abscess

Acute **Pain** r/t inflammation of perirectal area

Disturbed **Body** image r/t odor and drainage from rectal area

Risk for **Constipation** r/t fear of painful elimination

## Anorexia

Deficient **Fluid** volume r/t inability to drink

Delayed **Surgical** recovery r/t inadequate nutritional intake

Imbalanced **Nutrition**: less than body requirements r/t loss of appetite, nausea, vomiting

## Anorexia Nervosa

**Activity** intolerance r/t fatigue, weakness

Chronic low **Self-esteem** r/t repeated unmet expectations

A

**Constipation** r/t lack of adequate food, fiber, and fluid intake

Defensive **Coping** r/t psychological impairment, eating disorder

**Diarrhea** r/t laxative abuse

Disabled family **Coping** r/t highly ambivalent family relationships

Disturbed **Body** image r/t misconception of actual body appearance

Disturbed **Thought** processes r/t anorexia, impaired nutrition

Imbalanced **Nutrition**: less than body requirements r/t inadequate food intake

Ineffective **Denial** r/t fear of consequences of therapy, possible weight gain

Ineffective family **Therapeutic** regimen management r/t family conflict, excessive demands on family associated with complexity of condition and treatment

Ineffective **Sexuality** pattern r/t loss of libido from malnutrition

Interrupted **Family** processes r/t situational crisis

Risk for **Infection** r/t malnutrition resulting in depressed immune system

Risk for **Spiritual** distress r/t low self-esteem

*See Maturational Issues, Adolescent*

## Anosmia (Smell, Loss of Ability to)

Disturbed **Sensory** perception: olfactory r/t altered sensory reception, transmission, integration

Imbalanced **Nutrition**: less than body requirements r/t loss of appetite associated with loss of smell

## Antepartum Period

*See Pregnancy, Normal; Prenatal Care, Normal*

## Anterior Repair, Anterior Colporrhaphy

Risk for urge urinary **Incontinence** r/t trauma to bladder

**Urinary** retention r/t edema of urinary structures

*See Vaginal Hysterectomy*

## Anticoagulant Therapy

**Anxiety** r/t situational crisis

Ineffective **Health** maintenance r/t deficient knowledge regarding precautions to take with anticoagulant therapy

Ineffective **Protection** r/t altered clotting function from anticoagulant

Risk for deficient **Fluid** volume: hemorrhage r/t altered clotting mechanism

## Antisocial Personality Disorder

Defensive **Coping** r/t excessive use of projection

Disturbed **Thought** processes r/t internal turmoil and conflict (intrusive thinking)

**Hopelessness** r/t abandonment

Impaired **Social** interaction r/t sociocultural conflict, chemical dependence, inability to form relationships

Ineffective **Coping** r/t frequently violating the norms and rules of society

Ineffective family **Therapeutic** regimen management r/t excessive demands on family

Risk for impaired **Parenting** r/t inability to function as parent or guardian, emotional instability

Risk for **Loneliness** r/t inability to interact appropriately with others

Risk for other-directed **Violence** r/t history of violence

Risk for **Self-mutilation** r/t self-hatred, depersonalization

**Spiritual** distress r/t separation from religious/cultural ties

## Anuria

*See Renal Failure*

## Anxiety

**Anxiety** r/t threat to or change in role status, unmet needs, interpersonal transmission/contagion, situational/maturational crisis, threat of death, threat to or change in health status, threat to or change in interaction patterns, threat to or change in role function, threat to self-concept, unconscious conflict regarding essential values/goals of life, threat to or change in environment, stress, threat to or change in economic status, substance abuse

Risk for **Powerlessness** r/t anxiety

Risk for situational low **Self-esteem** r/t anxiety

## Anxiety Disorder

**Anxiety** r/t unmet security and safety needs

Death **Anxiety** r/t fears of unknown, powerlessness

Decisional **Conflict** r/t low self-esteem, fear of making a mistake

Defensive **Coping** r/t overwhelming feelings of dread

Disabled family **Coping** r/t ritualistic behavior, actions

Disturbed **Energy** field r/t hopelessness, helplessness, fear

Disturbed **Sleep** pattern r/t psychological impairment, emotional instability

Disturbed **Thought** processes r/t anxiety

Ineffective **Coping** r/t inability to express feelings appropriately

Ineffective **Denial** r/t overwhelming feelings of hopelessness, fear, threat to self

**Powerlessness** r/t lifestyle of helplessness

Risk for **Spiritual** distress r/t psychological distress

**Self-care** deficit r/t ritualistic behavior, activities

**Sleep** deprivation r/t prolonged psychological discomfort

## Aortic Aneurysm Repair (Abdominal Surgery)

*See Abdominal Surgery; Aneurysm, Abdominal Surgery*

## Aortic Valvular Stenosis

*See Congenital Heart Disease/Cardiac Anomalies*

## Aphasia

**Anxiety** r/t situational crisis of aphasia

Impaired verbal **Communication** r/t decrease in circulation to brain

Ineffective **Coping** r/t loss of speech

Ineffective **Health** maintenance r/t deficient knowledge regarding information on aphasia and alternative communication techniques

## Aplastic Anemia

**Activity** intolerance r/t imbalance between oxygen supply and demand

**Anxiety** r/t deficient knowledge of disease process and treatment

Delayed **Surgical** recovery r/t risk for infection

Impaired **Protection** r/t inadequate immune function

Risk for **Infection** r/t inadequate immune function

## Apnea in Infancy

*See Premature Infant (Child); Premature Infant (Parent); SIDS*

## Apneustic Respirations

Impaired **Breathing** pattern r/t perception/cognitive impairment, neurological impairment

*See cause of Apneustic Respirations*

## Appendectomy

Acute **Pain** r/t surgical incision

Deficient **Fluid** volume r/t fluid restriction, hypermetabolic state, nausea, vomiting

Ineffective **Health** maintenance r/t deficient knowledge regarding self-care following appendectomy

Risk for **Infection** r/t perforation/rupture of appendix, surgical incision, peritonitis

*See Hospitalized Child; Surgery, Postoperative*

## Appendicitis

Acute **Pain** r/t inflammation

Deficient **Fluid** volume r/t anorexia, nausea, vomiting

Delayed **Surgical** recovery r/t risk for infection

Risk for **Infection** r/t possible perforation of appendix

## Apprehension

**Anxiety** r/t threat to self-concept, threat to health status, situational crisis

Death **Anxiety** r/t apprehension over loss of self, consequences to significant others

## AMD (Age-Related Macular Degeneration)

*See Macular Degeneration*

## ARDS (Acute Respiratory Distress Syndrome)

Death **Anxiety** r/t seriousness of physical disease

Delayed **Surgical** recovery r/t complications associated with respiratory pathology

Impaired **Gas** exchange r/t damage to alveolar-capillary membrane, change in lung compliance

Impaired spontaneous **Ventilation** r/t damage to alveolar capillary membrane

Ineffective **Airway** clearance r/t excessive tracheobronchial secretions

*See Child with Chronic Condition; Ventilator Client*

## Arrhythmia

*See Dysrhythmia*

## Arterial Insufficiency

Delayed **Surgical** recovery r/t ineffective tissue perfusion

Ineffective **Tissue** perfusion: peripheral r/t interruption of arterial flow

## Arthritis

**Activity** intolerance r/t chronic pain, fatigue, weakness

Chronic **Pain** r/t progression of joint deterioration

Chronic **Sorrow** r/t presence of chronic condition

Disturbed **Body** image r/t ineffective coping with joint abnormalities

A

Impaired physical **Mobility** r/t musculoskeletal impairment

Ineffective **Health** maintenance r/t deficient knowledge regarding care of arthritis

Risk for **Spiritual** distress r/t presence of chronic condition

**Self-care** deficit: specify r/t pain, musculoskeletal impairment

*See JRA (Juvenile Rheumatoid Arthritis)*

## Arthrocentesis

Acute **Pain** r/t invasive procedure

## Arthroplasty (Total Hip Replacement)

Acute **Pain** r/t tissue trauma associated with surgery

**Constipation** r/t immobility

Impaired physical **Mobility** r/t decreased muscle strength, surgery

Impaired **Walking** r/t decreased muscle strength, surgery

Risk for **Infection** r/t invasive surgery, foreign object in body, anesthesia, immobility with stasis of respiratory secretions

Risk for **Injury** r/t interruption of arterial blood flow, dislocation of prosthesis

Risk for perioperative positioning **Injury** r/t immobilization, muscle weakness

Risk for **Peripheral** neurovascular dysfunction r/t orthopedic surgery

*See Surgery, Perioperative; Surgery, Postoperative; Surgery, Preoperative*

## Arthroscopy

Ineffective **Health** maintenance r/t deficient knowledge regarding procedure, postoperative restrictions

## Ascites

Chronic **Pain** r/t altered body function

Imbalanced **Nutrition**: less than body requirements r/t loss of appetite

Ineffective **Breathing** pattern r/t increased abdominal girth

Ineffective **Health** maintenance r/t deficient knowledge of care with condition of ascites

*See cause of Ascites; Cancer; Cirrhosis*

## Asphyxia, Birth

Anticipatory **Grieving** r/t loss of "perfect" child, concern of loss of future abilities

**Fear** (parental) r/t concern over safety of infant

Impaired **Gas** exchange r/t poor placental perfusion, lack of initiation of breathing by newborn

Impaired spontaneous **Ventilation** r/t brain injury

Ineffective **Breathing** pattern r/t depression of breathing reflex secondary to anoxia

Ineffective **Coping** r/t uncertainty of child outcome

Ineffective **Tissue** perfusion: cerebral r/t poor placental perfusion or cord compression resulting in lack of oxygen to brain

Risk for delayed **Development** r/t lack of oxygen to brain

Risk for disorganized **Infant** behavior r/t lack of oxygen to brain

Risk for disproportionate **Growth** r/t lack of oxygen to brain

Risk for impaired parent/infant **Attachment** r/t ill infant who is unable to initiate parental contact, hospitalization in critical care environment

Risk for **Injury** r/t lack of oxygen to brain

Risk for **Post-trauma** syndrome: parental r/t psychological trauma of sudden potential for loss of newborn

## Aspiration, Danger of

Risk for **Aspiration** r/t reduced level of consciousness; depressed cough or gag reflexes; presence of tracheostomy or endotracheal tube; incomplete lower esophageal sphincter; presence of gastrointestinal tubes or tube feedings; medication administration; situations hindering elevation of upper body; increased intragastric pressure; increased gastric residual; decreased gastrointestinal motility; delayed gastric emptying; impaired swallowing; facial, oral, or neck surgery or trauma; wired jaws

## Assault Victim

**Post-trauma** syndrome r/t assault

**Rape-trauma** syndrome r/t rape

Risk for **Post-trauma** syndrome r/t perception of event, inadequate social support, nonsupportive environment, diminished ego strength, duration of event

Risk for **Spiritual** distress r/t physical, psychological stress

## Assaultive Client

Disturbed **Thought** process r/t use of hallucinogenic substance, psychological disorder

Ineffective **Coping** r/t lack of control of impulsive actions

Risk for **Injury** r/t confused thought process, impaired judgment

Risk for other-directed **Violence** r/t paranoid ideation, anger

## Asthma

**Activity** intolerance r/t fatigue, energy shift to meet muscle needs for breathing to overcome airway obstruction

**Anxiety** r/t inability to breathe effectively, fear of suffocation

Disturbed **Body** image r/t decreased participation in physical activities

Impaired **Home** maintenance r/t deficient knowledge regarding control of environmental triggers

Ineffective **Airway** clearance r/t tracheobronchial narrowing, excessive secretions

Ineffective **Breathing** pattern r/t anxiety

Ineffective **Coping** r/t personal vulnerability to situational crisis

Ineffective **Health** maintenance r/t deficient knowledge regarding physical triggers, medications, treatment of early warning signs

**Sleep** deprivation r/t ineffective breathing pattern

*See Child with Chronic Condition; Hospitalized Child*

## Ataxia

**Anxiety** r/t change in health status

Disturbed **Body** image r/t staggering gait

Impaired physical **Mobility** r/t neuromuscular impairment

Risk for **Injury** r/t gait alteration

## Atelectasis

Impaired **Gas** exchange r/t decreased alveolar-capillary surface

Ineffective **Breathing** pattern r/t loss of functional lung tissue, depression of respiratory function or hypoventilation because of pain

## Athlete's Foot

Impaired **Skin** integrity r/t effects of fungal agent

Ineffective **Health** maintenance r/t deficient knowledge regarding treatment and prevention of athlete's foot

*See Itching*

## ATN (Acute Tubular Necrosis)

*See Renal Failure*

## Atrial Fibrillation

*See Dysrhythmia*

## Atrial Septal Defect

*See Congenital Heart Disease/Cardiac Anomalies*

## Attention Deficit Disorder

Disabled family **Coping** r/t significant person with chronically unexpressed feelings of guilt, anxiety, hostility, and despair

Impaired **Adjustment** r/t intense emotional state

Risk for delayed **Development** r/t behavior disorders

Risk for impaired **Parenting** r/t lack of knowledge of factors contributing to child's behavior

Risk for **Loneliness** r/t social isolation

Risk for **Spiritual** distress r/t poor relationships

**Self-esteem** disturbance r/t difficulty in participating in expected activities

**Social** isolation r/t unacceptable social behavior

## Autism

Compromised family **Coping** r/t parental guilt over etiology of disease, inability to accept or adapt to child's condition, inability to help child and other family members seek treatment

Delayed **Growth** and development r/t inability to develop relations with other human beings, inability to identify own body as separate from those of other people, inability to integrate concept of self

Disturbed personal **Identity** r/t inability to distinguish between self and environment, inability to identify own body as separate from those of other people, inability to integrate concept of self

Disturbed **Thought** processes r/t inability to perceive self or others, cognitive dissonance, perceptual dysfunction

Impaired **Social** interaction r/t communication barriers, inability to relate to others

Impaired verbal **Communication** r/t speech and language delays

Risk for delayed **Development** r/t autism

Risk for **Loneliness** r/t health alterations, change in cognition

Risk for other-directed **Violence** r/t frequent destructive rages toward others secondary to extreme response to changes in routine, fear of harmless things

Risk for self-directed **Violence** r/t frequent destructive rages toward self, secondary to extreme response to changes in routine, fear of harmless things

Risk for **Self-mutilation** r/t autistic state

*See Child with Chronic Condition; Mental Retardation*

## Autonomic Dysreflexia

**Autonomic** dysreflexia r/t bladder distention, bowel distention, noxious stimuli

Risk for **Autonomic** dysreflexia r/t bladder distention, bowel distention, noxious stimuli

## Autonomic Hyperreflexia

*See Autonomic Dysreflexia*

# B

## Back Pain

Acute **Pain** r/t back injury

**Anxiety** r/t situational crisis, back injury

Chronic **Pain** r/t back injury

Disturbed **Energy** field r/t chronic pain

Impaired physical **Mobility** r/t pain

Ineffective **Coping** r/t situational crisis, back injury

Ineffective **Health** maintenance r/t deficient knowledge regarding prevention of further injury, proper body mechanics

Risk for **Constipation** r/t decreased activity, side effect of pain medication

Risk for **Disuse** syndrome r/t severe pain

## Bacteremia

Ineffective **Protection** r/t compromised immune system

*See Infection; Infection, Potential for*

## Barrel Chest

*See Aging (if appropriate); COPD (Chronic Obstructive Pulmonary Disease)*

## Bathing/Hygiene Problems

Bathing/hygiene **Self-care** deficit r/t intolerance to activity, decreased strength and endurance, pain, discomfort, perceptual or cognitive impairment, neuromuscular impairment, musculoskeletal impairment, depression, severe anxiety

Impaired bed **Mobility** r/t chronic physically limiting condition

## Battered Child Syndrome

Acute **Pain** r/t physical injuries

Chronic low **Self-esteem** r/t lack of positive feedback, excessive negative feedback

Chronic **Sorrow** r/t situational crises

Deficient **Diversional** activity r/t diminished/absent environmental or personal stimuli

Delayed **Growth** and development: regression versus delayed r/t diminished/absent environmental stimuli, inadequate caretaking, inconsistent responsiveness by caretaker

Disturbed **Sleep** pattern r/t hypervigilance, anxiety

Dysfunctional **Family** processes: alcoholism r/t inadequate coping skills

**Fear** r/t threat of punishment for perceived wrongdoing

Imbalanced **Nutrition**: less than body requirements r/t inadequate caretaking

Impaired **Skin** integrity r/t altered nutritional state, physical abuse

**Post-trauma** syndrome r/t physical abuse, incest, rape, molestation

Risk for **Aspiration** r/t propped bottle

Risk for delayed **Development** r/t shaken baby, abuse

Risk for disproportionate **Growth** r/t abuse

Risk for **Poisoning** r/t inadequate safeguards, lack of proper safety precautions, accessibility of illicit substances secondary to impaired home maintenance

Risk for **Post-trauma** syndrome r/t physical abuse, incest, rape, molestation

Risk for **Self-mutilation** r/t feelings of rejection, dysfunctional family

Risk for **Suffocation** r/t unattended child, unsafe environment

Risk for **Trauma** r/t inadequate precautions, cognitive or emotional difficulties

**Sleep** deprivation r/t prolonged psychological discomfort

**Social** isolation: family imposed r/t fear of disclosure of family dysfunction and abuse

## Battered Person

*See Abuse, Spouse, Parent, or Significant Other*

## Bed Mobility, Impaired

Impaired bed **Mobility** r/t intolerance to activity, decreased strength and endurance, pain or discomfort, perceptual or cognitive impairment, neuromuscular impairment, musculoskeletal impairment, depression, severe anxiety

## Bedbugs, Infestation

Impaired **Home** maintenance r/t deficient knowledge regarding prevention of bedbug infestation

Impaired **Skin** integrity r/t bites of bedbugs

*See Itching*

## Bedrest, Prolonged

Deficient **Diversional** activity r/t prolonged bedrest

Impaired bed **Mobility** r/t neuromuscular impairment

Risk for **Disuse** syndrome r/t prolonged immobility

Risk for **Loneliness** r/t prolonged bedrest

**Social** isolation r/t prolonged bedrest

## Bedsores

*See Pressure Ulcer*

## Bedwetting

*See Enuresis; Toilet Training*

## Bell's Palsy

Acute **Pain** r/t inflammation of facial nerve

Disturbed **Body** image r/t loss of motor control on one side of face

Imbalanced **Nutrition**: less than body requirements r/t difficulty with chewing

Risk for **Injury** (eye) r/t dysfunction of facial nerve

## Benign Prostatic Hypertrophy

*See BPH (Benign Prostatic Hypertrophy); Prostatic Hypertrophy*

## Bereavement

Chronic **Sorrow** r/t death of loved one, chronic illness, disability

Disturbed **Sleep** pattern r/t grief

Dysfunctional **Grieving** r/t death of a loved one

**Grieving** r/t loss of significant person

Risk for **Spiritual** distress r/t death of a loved one

## Biliary Atresia

**Anxiety** r/t surgical intervention, possible liver transplantation

Imbalanced **Nutrition**: less than body requirements r/t decreased absorption of fat and fat-soluble vitamins, poor feeding

Impaired **Comfort** r/t pruritus, nausea

Risk for impaired **Skin** integrity r/t pruritus

Risk for ineffective **Breathing** pattern r/t enlarged liver, development of ascites

Risk for **Injury**: bleeding r/t vitamin K deficiency, altered clotting mechanisms

*See Child with Chronic Condition; Cirrhosis (as complication); Hospitalized Child; Terminally Ill Child, Adolescent; Terminally Ill Child, Infant/Toddler; Terminally Ill Child, Preschool Child; Terminally Ill Child, School-Age Child/Preadolescent; Terminally Ill Child/Death of Child, Parent*

## Biliary Calculus

*See Cholelithiasis*

## Biliary Obstruction

*See Jaundice*

## Biopsy

**Fear** r/t outcome of biopsy

Ineffective **Health** maintenance r/t deficient knowledge regarding biopsy site, further needed health care

## Bioterrorism

Risk for **Infection** r/t exposure to harmful biological agent

Risk for **Injury** r/t harmful chemical agent exposure

Risk for **Post-trauma** syndrome r/t perception of event of bioterrorism

## Bipolar Disorder I (Most Recent Episode, Depressed or Manic)

Chronic low **Self-esteem** r/t repeated unmet expectations

Disturbed **Energy** field r/t disharmony of mind, body, spirit

Dysfunctional **Grieving** r/t lack of previous resolution of former grieving response

**Fatigue** r/t psychological demands

Impaired **Adjustment** r/t low state of optimism

Ineffective **Coping** r/t dysfunctional grieving

Ineffective **Health** maintenance r/t lack of ability to make good judgments regarding ways to obtain help

Risk for **Loneliness** r/t stress, conflict

Risk for **Spiritual** distress r/t mental illness

**Self-care** deficit: specify r/t depression, cognitive impairment

**Social** isolation r/t ineffective coping

*See Depression; Manic Disorder, Bipolar I*

## Birth Asphyxia

*See Asphyxia, Birth*

## Birth Control

*See Contraceptive Method*

## Bladder Cancer

**Urinary** retention r/t clots obstructing urethra

*See Cancer; TURP*

B

## Bladder Distention

**Urinary** retention r/t high urethral pressure caused by weak detrusor, inhibition of reflex arc, blockage, strong sphincter

## Bladder Training

Disturbed **Body** image r/t difficulty in maintaining control of urinary elimination

Functional urinary **Incontinence** r/t altered environment; sensory, cognitive, mobility deficit

Ineffective **Health** maintenance r/t deficient knowledge regarding incontinence self-care

Stress urinary **Incontinence** r/t degenerative change in pelvic muscles and structural supports

Urge urinary **Incontinence** r/t decreased bladder capacity, increased urine concentration, overdistention of bladder

## Bleeding Tendency

Ineffective **Protection** r/t abnormal blood profile, drug therapies

Risk for delayed **Surgical** recovery r/t bleeding tendency

## Blepharoplasty

Disturbed **Body** image r/t effects of surgery

Ineffective **Health** maintenance r/t deficient knowledge regarding postoperative care of surgical area

## Blindness

Disturbed **Sensory** perception: visual r/t altered sensory reception, transmission, integration

Impaired **Home** maintenance r/t decreased vision

Ineffective **Role** performance r/t alteration in health status (change in visual acuity)

Interrupted **Family** processes r/t shift in health status of family member (change in visual acuity)

Risk for delayed **Development** r/t vision impairment

Risk for **Injury** r/t sensory dysfunction

**Self-care** deficit r/t inability to see to be able to perform activities of daily living

*See Vision Impairment*

## Blood Disorder

Ineffective **Protection** r/t abnormal blood profile

*See cause of Blood Disorder*

## Blood Pressure Alteration

*See Hypertension; Hypotension; HTN*

## Blood Transfusion

**Anxiety** r/t possibility of harm from transfusion

*See Anemia*

## Body Dysmorphic Disorder

Disturbed **Body** Image r/t over involvement in physical appearance

## Body Image Change

Disturbed **Body** image r/t psychosocial, biophysical, cognitive/perceptual, cultural, spiritual, developmental changes; illness; trauma or injury; surgery; illness treatment

## Body Temperature, Altered

Risk for imbalanced **Body** temperature r/t extremes of age or weight, exposure to cold or hot environment, dehydration, change in activity, effects of medication, dysfunction of body temperature regulation center

## Bone Marrow Biopsy

Acute **Pain** r/t bone marrow aspiration

**Fear** r/t unknown outcome of results of biopsy

Ineffective **Health** maintenance r/t deficient knowledge of expectations following procedure, disease treatment following biopsy

*See disease necessitating bone marrow biopsy (e.g., Leukemia)*

## Borderline Personality Disorder

**Anxiety** r/t perceived threat to self-concept

Defensive **Coping** r/t difficulty with relationships, inability to accept blame for own behavior

Disturbed **Thought** processes r/t poor reality testing

Ineffective **Coping** r/t use of maladjusted defense mechanisms (e.g., projection, denial)

Ineffective family **Therapeutic** regimen management r/t manipulative behavior of client

**Powerlessness** r/t lifestyle of helplessness

Risk for **Caregiver** role strain r/t inability of care receiver to accept criticism, care receiver taking advantage of others to meet own needs or having unreasonable expectations

Risk for self-directed **Violence** r/t feelings of need to punish self, manipulative behavior

Risk for **Self-mutilation** r/t ineffective coping, feelings of self-hatred

Risk for **Spiritual** distress r/t poor relationships associated with behaviors attributed to borderline personality disorder

**Social** isolation r/t immature interests

## Boredom

Deficient **Diversional** activity r/t environmental lack of diversional activity

**Social** isolation r/t altered state of wellness

## Botulism

Deficient **Fluid** volume r/t profuse diarrhea

Ineffective **Health** maintenance r/t deficient knowledge regarding prevention of botulism, care following episode

## Bowel Incontinence

**Bowel** incontinence r/t decreased awareness of need to defecate, loss of sphincter control, fecal impaction

## Bowel Obstruction

Acute **Pain** r/t pressure from distended abdomen

**Constipation** r/t decreased motility, intestinal obstruction

Deficient **Fluid** volume r/t inadequate fluid volume intake, fluid loss in bowel

Imbalanced **Nutrition**: less than body requirements r/t nausea, vomiting

## Bowel Resection

*See Abdominal Surgery*

## Bowel Sounds, Absent or Diminished

**Constipation** r/t decreased or absent peristalsis

Deficient **Fluid** volume r/t inability to ingest fluids, loss of fluids in bowel

Delayed **Surgical** recovery r/t inability to obtain adequate nutritional status

## Bowel Sounds, Hyperactive

**Diarrhea** r/t increased gastrointestinal motility

## Bowel Training

**Bowel** incontinence r/t loss of control of rectal sphincter

Ineffective **Health** maintenance r/t deficient knowledge regarding treatment of bowel incontinence

## BPH (Benign Prostatic Hypertrophy)

Disturbed **Sleep** pattern r/t nocturia

Ineffective **Health** maintenance r/t deficient knowledge regarding self-care with prostatic hypertrophy

Risk for **Infection** r/t urinary residual postvoiding, bacterial invasion of bladder

Risk for urge urinary **Incontinence** r/t detrusor muscle instability with impaired contractility, involuntary sphincter relaxation

**Urinary** retention r/t obstruction

*See Prostatic Hypertrophy*

## Bradycardia

Decreased **Cardiac** output r/t slow heart rate supplying inadequate amount of blood for body function

Ineffective **Health** maintenance r/t deficient knowledge of condition, effects of cardiac medications

Ineffective **Tissue** perfusion: cerebral r/t decreased cardiac output secondary to bradycardia, vagal response

Risk for **Injury** r/t decreased cerebral tissue perfusion

## Bradypnea

Ineffective **Breathing** pattern r/t neuromuscular impairment, pain, musculoskeletal impairment, perception/cognitive impairment, anxiety, fatigue/decreased energy, effects of drugs

*See cause of Bradypnea*

## Brain Injury

*See Intracranial Pressure, Increased*

## Brain Surgery

*See Craniectomy/Craniotomy*

## Brain Tumor

Acute **Pain** r/t pressure from tumor

Anticipatory **Grieving** r/t potential loss of physiosocial-psychosocial well-being

Decreased **Intracranial** adaptive capacity r/t presence of brain tumor

Disturbed **Sensory** perception: specify r/t tumor growth compressing brain tissue

Disturbed **Thought** processes r/t altered circulation, destruction of brain tissue

**Fear** r/t threat to well-being

Risk for **Injury** r/t sensory-perceptual alterations, weakness

*See Cancer; Chemotherapy; Child with Chronic Condition; Craniectomy/Craniotomy; Hospitalized Child; Radiation Therapy; Terminally Ill Child, Adolescent; Terminally Ill Child, Infant/Toddler; Terminally Ill Child, Preschool Child; Terminally Ill Child, School-Age Child/Preadolescent; Terminally Ill Child/Death of Child, Parent*

## Braxton Hicks Contractions

**Activity** intolerance r/t increased perception of contractions with increased gestation

**Anxiety** r/t uncertainty about beginning labor

Disturbed **Sleep** pattern r/t contractions when lying down

**Fatigue** r/t lack of sleep

B

Ineffective **Sexuality** patterns r/t fear of contractions

Stress urinary **Incontinence** r/t increased pressure on bladder with contractions

## Breast Biopsy

**Fear** r/t potential for diagnosis of cancer

Ineffective **Health** maintenance r/t deficient knowledge regarding appropriate postoperative care of breasts

Risk for **Spiritual** distress r/t fear of diagnosis of cancer

## Breast Cancer

Chronic **Sorrow** r/t diagnosis of cancer, loss of body integrity

Death **Anxiety** r/t diagnosis of cancer

**Fear** r/t diagnosis of cancer

Ineffective **Coping** r/t treatment, prognosis

Risk for **Spiritual** distress r/t fear of diagnosis of cancer

**Sexual** dysfunction r/t loss of body part, partner's reaction to loss

*See Cancer; Chemotherapy; Mastectomy; Radiation Therapy*

## Breast Lumps

**Fear** r/t potential for diagnosis of cancer

Ineffective **Health** maintenance r/t deficient knowledge regarding appropriate care of breasts

## Breast Pumping

**Anxiety** r/t interrupted breastfeeding

Decisional **Conflict** r/t infant feeding method

Disturbed **Body** image r/t individual response to breastfeeding process

Ineffective **Health** maintenance r/t deficient knowledge regarding breast milk expression and storage

Risk for impaired **Skin** integrity r/t high suction

Risk for **Infection** r/t contaminated breast pump parts, incomplete emptying of breast

## Breastfeeding, Effective

Effective **Breastfeeding** r/t basic breastfeeding knowledge, normal breast structure, normal infant oral structure, infant gestational age >34 weeks, support sources, maternal confidence

## Breastfeeding, Ineffective

Impaired **Swallowing** r/t prematurity of infant

Ineffective **Breastfeeding** r/t prematurity, infant anomaly, maternal breast anomaly, previous breast surgery, previous history of breastfeeding failure, infant receiving supplemental feedings with artificial nipple, poor infant sucking reflex, nonsupportive partner/family, deficient knowledge, interruption in breastfeeding, maternal anxiety or ambivalence

Ineffective **Infant** feeding pattern r/t prematurity of infant

*See Painful Breasts, Sore Nipples; Painful Breasts, Engorgement*

## Breastfeeding, Interrupted

Interrupted **Breastfeeding** r/t maternal or infant illness, prematurity, maternal employment, contraindications to breastfeeding (e.g., drugs, true breast milk jaundice), need to abruptly wean infant

## Breath Sounds, Decreased or Absent

*See Atelectasis; Pneumothorax*

## Breathing Pattern Alteration

Ineffective **Breathing** pattern r/t neuromuscular impairment, pain, musculoskeletal impairment, perception/cognitive impairment, anxiety, decreased energy/fatigue

## Breech Birth

**Anxiety**: maternal r/t threat to self, infant

**Fear**: maternal r/t danger to infant, self

Impaired **Gas** exchange: fetal r/t compressed umbilical cord

Ineffective **Tissue** perfusion: cerebral r/t compressed umbilical cord

Risk for **Aspiration**: fetal r/t birth of body before head

Risk for delayed **Development** r/t compressed umbilical cord

Risk for impaired **Tissue** integrity: fetal r/t difficult birth

Risk for impaired **Tissue** integrity: maternal r/t difficult birth

## Bronchitis

**Anxiety** r/t potential chronic condition

**Health**-seeking behavior r/t wish to stop smoking

Ineffective **Airway** clearance r/t excessive thickened mucus secretion

Ineffective **Health** maintenance r/t deficient knowledge regarding care of condition

## Bronchopulmonary Dysplasia

**Activity** intolerance r/t imbalance between oxygen supply and demand

Excess **Fluid** volume r/t sodium and water retention

Imbalanced **Nutrition**: less than body requirements r/t poor feeding, increased caloric needs secondary to increased work of breathing

*See Child with Chronic Condition; Hospitalized Child; Respiratory Conditions of the Neonate*

## Bronchoscopy

Risk for **Aspiration** r/t temporary loss of gag reflex

Risk for **Injury** r/t complication of pneumothorax, laryngeal edema, hemorrhage (if biopsy done)

## Bruits, Carotid

Ineffective **Tissue** perfusion: cerebral r/t interruption of carotid blood flow

Risk for **Injury** r/t loss of motor, sensory, visual function

## Bryant's Traction

*See Traction and Casts*

## Buck's Traction

*See Traction and Casts*

## Buerger's Disease

*See Peripheral Vascular Disease*

## Bulimia

Chronic low **Self-esteem** r/t lack of positive feedback

Defensive **Coping** r/t eating disorder

Disturbed **Body** image r/t misperception about actual appearance, body weight

**Fear** r/t food ingestion, weight gain

Imbalanced **Nutrition**: less than body requirements r/t induced vomiting

Compromised family **Coping** r/t chronically unresolved feelings of guilt, anger, hostility

**Noncompliance** r/t negative feelings toward treatment regimen

**Powerlessness** r/t urge to purge self after eating

*See Maturational Issues, Adolescent*

## Bunion

Ineffective **Health** maintenance r/t deficient knowledge regarding appropriate care of feet

## Bunionectomy

Impaired physical **Mobility** r/t sore foot

Impaired **Walking** r/t pain associated with surgery

Ineffective **Health** maintenance r/t deficient knowledge regarding postoperative care of feet

Risk for **Infection** r/t surgical incision, advanced age

## Burns

Acute **Pain** r/t burn injury, treatments

Anticipatory **Grieving** r/t loss of bodily function, loss of future hopes and plans

Deficient **Diversional** activity r/t long-term hospitalization

Delayed **Surgical** recovery r/t ineffective tissue perfusion

Disturbed **Body** image r/t altered physical appearance

**Fear** r/t pain from treatments, possible permanent disfigurement

**Hypothermia** r/t impaired skin integrity

Imbalanced **Nutrition**: less than body requirements r/t increased metabolic needs, anorexia, protein and fluid loss

Impaired physical **Mobility** r/t pain, musculoskeletal impairment, contracture formation

Impaired **Skin** integrity r/t injury of skin

Ineffective **Tissue** perfusion: peripheral r/t circumferential burns, impaired arterial/venous circulation

**Post-trauma** syndrome r/t life-threatening event

Risk for deficient **Fluid** volume r/t loss from skin surface, fluid shift

Risk for ineffective **Airway** clearance r/t potential tracheobronchial obstruction, edema

Risk for **Infection** r/t loss of intact skin, trauma, invasive sites

Risk for **Peripheral** neurovascular dysfunction r/t eschar formation with circumferential burn

Risk for **Post-trauma** syndrome r/t perception, duration of event that caused burns

*See Hospitalized Child; Safety, Childhood*

## Bursitis

Acute **Pain** r/t inflammation in joint

Impaired physical **Mobility** r/t inflammation in joint

## Bypass Graft

*See Coronary Artery Bypass Grafting*

# C

## Cachexia

Adult **Failure** to thrive r/t imbalanced nutrition: less than body requirements

Imbalanced **Nutrition**: less than body requirements r/t inability to ingest food because of biological factors

Ineffective **Protection** r/t inadequate nutrition

C

## Calcium Alteration

*See Hypercalcemia; Hypocalcemia*

## Cancer

**Activity** intolerance r/t side effects of treatment, weakness from cancer

Anticipatory **Grieving** r/t potential loss of significant others, high risk for infertility

Chronic **Pain** r/t metastatic cancer

Chronic **Sorrow** r/t chronic illness of cancer

Compromised family **Coping** r/t prolonged disease or disability progression that exhausts supportive ability of significant others

**Constipation** r/t side effects of medication, altered nutrition, decreased activity

Death **Anxiety** r/t unresolved issues regarding dying

Decisional **Conflict** r/t selection of treatment choices, continuation/discontinuation of treatment, "do not resuscitate" decision

Disturbed **Body** image r/t side effects of treatment, cachexia

Disturbed **Sleep** pattern r/t anxiety, pain

**Fear** r/t serious threat to well-being

**Hopelessness** r/t loss of control, terminal illness

Imbalanced **Nutrition**: less than body requirements r/t loss of appetite, difficulty swallowing, side effects of chemotherapy, obstruction by tumor

Impaired **Oral** mucous membranes r/t chemotherapy, effects of radiation, oral pH changes, decreased oral secretions

Impaired physical **Mobility** r/t weakness, neuromusculoskeletal impairment, pain

Impaired **Skin** integrity r/t immunological deficit, immobility

Ineffective **Coping** r/t personal vulnerability in situational crisis, terminal illness

Ineffective **Denial** r/t dysfunctional grieving process

Ineffective **Health** maintenance r/t deficient knowledge regarding prescribed treatment

Ineffective **Protection** r/t cancer suppressing immune system

Ineffective **Role** performance r/t change in physical capacity, inability to resume prior role

**Powerlessness** r/t treatment, progression of disease

Readiness for enhanced **Spiritual** well-being r/t desire for harmony with self, others, higher power/God when faced with serious illness

Risk for **Disuse** syndrome r/t severe pain, change in level of consciousness

Risk for impaired **Home** maintenance r/t lack of familiarity with community resources

Risk for **Infection** r/t inadequate immune system

Risk for **Injury** r/t bleeding secondary to bone marrow depression

Risk for **Spiritual** distress r/t physical illness of cancer

**Self-care** deficit: specify r/t pain, intolerance to activity, decreased strength

**Social** isolation r/t hospitalization, lifestyle changes

**Spiritual** distress r/t test of spiritual beliefs

*See Chemotherapy; Child with Chronic Condition; Hospitalized Child; Radiation Therapy; Terminally Ill Child, Adolescent; Terminally Ill Child, Infant/Toddler; Terminally Ill Child, Preschool Child; Terminally Ill Child, School-Age Child/Preadolescent; Terminally Ill Child/Death of Child, Parent*

## Candidiasis, Oral

Impaired **Oral** mucous membranes r/t overgrowth of infectious agent, depressed immune function

Ineffective **Health** maintenance r/t deficient knowledge regarding care of infected mouth

## Capillary Refill Time, Prolonged

Impaired **Gas** exchange r/t ventilation perfusion imbalance

Ineffective **Tissue** perfusion: peripheral r/t interruption of arterial or venous flow

*See Shock*

## Cardiac Arrest

**Post-trauma** syndrome r/t sustaining serious life event

*See cause of Cardiac Arrest*

## Cardiac Catheterization

**Anxiety** r/t invasive procedure, uncertainty of outcome of procedure

Decreased **Cardiac** output r/t ventricular ischemia, dysrhythmia

Impaired **Comfort** r/t postprocedure restrictions, invasive procedure

Ineffective **Health** maintenance r/t deficient knowledge regarding procedure, postprocedure care, treatment and prevention of coronary artery disease

Risk for ineffective **Tissue** perfusion r/t impaired arterial or venous circulation

Risk for **Injury**: hematoma r/t invasive procedure

Risk for **Peripheral** neurovascular dysfunction r/t vascular obstruction

## Cardiac Disorders

Decreased **Cardiac** output r/t cardiac disorder

*See specific cardiac disorder*

## Cardiac Disorders in Pregnancy

**Activity** intolerance r/t cardiac pathophysiology, increased demand secondary to pregnancy, weakness, fatigue

**Anxiety** r/t unknown outcomes of pregnancy, family well-being

Compromised family **Coping** r/t prolonged hospitalization/maternal incapacitation that exhausts supportive capacity of significant others

Death **Anxiety** r/t potential danger of condition

**Fatigue** r/t metabolic demands, psychological and emotional demands

**Fear** r/t potential maternal effects, potential poor fetal/maternal outcome

Ineffective **Coping** r/t personal vulnerability

Ineffective **Health** maintenance r/t deficient knowledge regarding treatment, restrictions with cardiac disorder

Ineffective **Role** performance r/t changes in lifestyle, expectations secondary to disease process with superimposed pregnancy

Interrupted **Family** processes r/t hospitalization, maternal incapacitation, changes in roles

**Powerlessness** r/t illness-related regimen

Risk for delayed **Development** r/t poor maternal oxygenation

Risk for disproportionate **Growth** r/t poor maternal oxygenation

Risk for excess **Fluid** volume r/t compromised regulatory mechanism with increased afterload, preload, circulating blood volume

Risk for imbalanced **Fluid** volume r/t sudden changes in circulation following delivery of placenta

Risk for impaired **Gas** exchange r/t pulmonary edema

Risk for ineffective **Tissue** perfusion: fetal r/t poor maternal oxygenation

Risk for **Spiritual** distress r/t fear of diagnosis for self and infant

Situational low **Self-esteem** r/t situational crisis, pregnancy

**Social** isolation r/t limitations of activity, bed rest/hospitalization, separation from family and friends

## Cardiac Dysrhythmia

*See Dysrhythmia*

## Cardiac Output Decrease

Decreased **Cardiac** output r/t cardiac dysfunction

## Cardiac Tamponade

Decreased **Cardiac** output r/t fluid in pericardial sac

*See Pericarditis*

## Cardiogenic Shock

Decreased **Cardiac** output r/t decreased myocardial contractility, dysrhythmia

*See Shock*

## Caregiver Role Strain

**Caregiver** role strain r/t pathophysiological factors, developmental factors, psychosocial factors, situational factors

Risk for **Caregiver** role strain r/t pathophysiological factors, developmental factors, psychosocial factors, situational factors

## Carious Teeth

*See Cavities in Teeth*

## Carotid Endarterectomy

**Fear** r/t surgery in vital area

Ineffective **Health** maintenance r/t deficient knowledge regarding postoperative care

Risk for ineffective **Airway** clearance r/t hematoma compressing trachea

Risk for ineffective **Tissue** perfusion: cerebral r/t hemorrhage, clot formation

Risk for **Injury** r/t possible hematoma formation

## Carpal Tunnel Syndrome

Chronic **Pain** r/t unrelieved pressure on median nerve

Impaired physical **Mobility** r/t neuromuscular impairment

**Self-care** deficit: bathing/hygiene, dressing/grooming, feeding r/t pain

## Carpopedal Spasm

*See Hypocalcemia*

## Casts

Deficient **Diversional** activity r/t physical limitations from cast

Ineffective **Health** maintenance r/t deficient knowledge regarding cast care, personal care with cast

Impaired physical **Mobility** r/t limb immobilization

Impaired **Walking** r/t cast(s) on lower extremities, fracture of bones

Risk for impaired **Skin** integrity r/t unrelieved pressure on skin

C

Risk for **Peripheral** neurovascular dysfunction r/t mechanical compression from cast

**Self-care** deficit: bathing/hygiene, dressing/grooming, feeding r/t presence of cast(s) on upper extremities

**Self-care** deficit: toileting r/t presence of cast(s) on lower extremities

## Cataract Extraction

**Anxiety** r/t threat of permanent vision loss, surgical procedure

Disturbed **Sensory** perception: vision r/t edema from surgery

Ineffective **Health** maintenance r/t deficient knowledge regarding postoperative restrictions

Risk for **Injury** r/t increased intraocular pressure, accommodation to new visual field

*See Vision Impairment*

## Cataracts

Disturbed **Sensory** perception: vision r/t altered sensory input

*See Vision Impairment*

## Catatonic Schizophrenia

Imbalanced **Nutrition**: less than body requirements r/t decrease in outside stimulation, loss of perception of hunger, resistance to instructions to eat

Impaired **Memory** r/t cognitive impairment

Impaired physical **Mobility** r/t cognitive impairment, maintenance of rigid posture, inappropriate/bizarre postures

Impaired verbal **Communication** r/t muteness

**Social** isolation r/t inability to communicate, immobility

*See Schizophrenia*

## Catheterization, Urinary

Ineffective **Health** maintenance r/t deficient knowledge of normal sensation of catheter in place, care of catheter

Risk for **Infection** r/t invasive procedure

## Cavities in Teeth

Impaired **Dentition** r/t ineffective oral hygiene, barriers to self-care, economic barriers to professional care, nutritional deficits, dietary habits

Ineffective **Health** maintenance r/t lack of knowledge regarding prevention of dental disease secondary to high-sugar diet, giving infants/toddlers with erupted teeth bottles of milk at bedtime, lack of fluoride treatments, inadequate or improper brushing of teeth

## Cellulitis

Acute **Pain** r/t inflammatory changes in tissues from infection

Impaired **Skin** integrity r/t inflammatory process damaging skin

Ineffective **Health** maintenance r/t lack of knowledge regarding prevention of further incidences of infection

Ineffective **Tissue** perfusion: peripheral r/t edema

## Cellulitis, Periorbital

Acute **Pain** r/t edema and inflammation of skin/tissues

Disturbed **Sensory** perception: visual r/t decreased visual fields secondary to edema of eyelids

**Hyperthermia** r/t infectious process

Impaired **Skin** integrity r/t inflammation/infection of skin/tissues

*See Hospitalized Child*

## Central Line Insertion

Ineffective **Health** maintenance r/t deficient knowledge regarding precautions to take when central line in place

Risk for **Infection** r/t invasive procedure

## Cerebral Aneurysm

*See Craniectomy/Craniotomy; Intracranial Pressure, Increased; Subarachnoid Hemorrhage*

## Cerebral Palsy

Chronic **Sorrow** r/t presence of chronic disability

Deficient **Diversional** activity r/t physical impairments, limitations on ability to participate in recreational activities

Imbalanced **Nutrition**: less than body requirements r/t spasticity, feeding or swallowing difficulties

Impaired physical **Mobility** r/t spasticity, neuromuscular impairment/weakness

Impaired **Social** interaction r/t impaired communication skills, limited physical activity, perceived differences from peers

Impaired verbal **Communication** r/t impaired ability to articulate/speak words secondary to facial muscle involvement

Risk for delayed **Development** r/t chronic illness

Risk for disproportionate **Growth** r/t chronic illness

Risk for **Falls** r/t impaired physical mobility

Risk for impaired **Parenting** r/t caring for child with overwhelming needs resulting from chronic change in health status

Risk for **Injury** r/t muscle weakness, inability to control spasticity

Risk for **Spiritual** distress r/t psychic and psychological stress associated with chronic illness

**Self-care** deficit: specify r/t neuromuscular impairments, sensory deficits

*See Child with Chronic Condition*

## Cerebrovascular Accident

*See CVA (Cerebrovascular Accident)*

## Cervicitis

Ineffective **Health** maintenance r/t deficient knowledge regarding care and prevention of condition

Ineffective **Sexuality** patterns r/t abstinence during acute stage

Risk for **Infection** r/t spread of infection, recurrence of infection

## Cesarean Delivery

Acute **Pain** r/t surgical incision, decreased or absent peristalsis secondary to anesthesia, manipulation of abdominal organs during surgery

**Anxiety** r/t unmet expectations for childbirth, unknown outcome of surgery

Disturbed **Body** image r/t surgery, unmet expectations for childbirth

**Fear** r/t perceived threat to own well-being

Impaired **Comfort**: nausea, vomiting, pruritus r/t side effects of systemic or epidural narcotics

Impaired physical **Mobility** r/t pain

Ineffective **Health** maintenance r/t deficient knowledge regarding postoperative care

Ineffective **Role** performance r/t unmet expectations for childbirth

Interrupted **Family** processes r/t unmet expectations for childbirth

Risk for deficient **Fluid** volume r/t increased blood loss secondary to surgery

Risk for imbalanced **Fluid** volume r/t loss of blood

Risk for **Infection** r/t surgical incision, stasis of respiratory secretions secondary to general anesthesia

Risk for **Post-trauma** syndrome r/t emergency condition to save life of mother or baby

Risk for **Urinary** retention r/t regional anesthesia

Situational low **Self-esteem** r/t inability to deliver child vaginally

## Chemical Dependence

*See Alcoholism; Drug Abuse*

## Chemotherapy

Death **Anxiety** r/t chemotherapy not accomplishing desired results

Delayed **Surgical** recovery r/t compromised immune system

Disturbed **Body** image r/t loss of weight, loss of hair

**Fatigue** r/t disease process, anemia, drug effects

Imbalanced **Nutrition**: less than body requirements r/t side effects of chemotherapy

Impaired **Oral** mucous membranes r/t effects of chemotherapy

Ineffective **Health** maintenance r/t deficient knowledge regarding action, side effects, way to integrate chemotherapy into lifestyle

Ineffective **Protection** r/t suppressed immune system, decreased platelets

**Nausea** r/t effects of chemotherapy

Risk for deficient **Fluid** volume r/t vomiting, diarrhea

Risk for ineffective **Tissue** perfusion r/t anemia

Risk for **Infection** r/t immunosuppression

*See Cancer*

## Chest Pain

Acute **Pain** r/t myocardial injury, ischemia

Decreased **Cardiac** output r/t ventricular ischemia

**Fear** r/t potential threat of death

*See Angina Pectoris; MI (Myocardial Infarction)*

## Chest Tubes

Acute **Pain** r/t presence of chest tubes, injury

Impaired **Gas** exchange r/t decreased functional lung tissue

Ineffective **Breathing** pattern r/t asymmetrical lung expansion secondary to pain

Risk for **Injury** r/t presence of invasive chest tube

## Cheyne-Stokes Respiration

Ineffective **Breathing** pattern r/t critical illness

*See cause of Cheyne-Stokes Respiration*

## CHF (Congestive Heart Failure)

**Activity** intolerance r/t weakness, fatigue

**Constipation** r/t activity intolerance

Decreased **Cardiac** output r/t impaired cardiac function

Excess **Fluid** volume r/t impaired excretion of sodium and water

**Fatigue** r/t disease process

**Fear** r/t threat to one's own well-being

Impaired **Gas** exchange r/t excessive fluid in interstitial space of lungs, alveoli

Ineffective **Health** maintenance r/t deficient knowledge regarding care of disease

**Powerlessness** r/t illness-related regimen

*See Child with Chronic Condition; Congenital Heart Disease/Cardiac Anomalies; Hospitalized Child*

## Chickenpox

*See Communicable Diseases, Childhood*

## Child Abuse

Acute **Pain** r/t physical injuries

Chronic low **Self-esteem** r/t lack of positive feedback, excessive negative feedback

Deficient **Diversional** activity r/t diminished or absent environmental/personal stimuli

Delayed **Growth** and development: regression versus delayed r/t diminished/absent environmental stimuli, inadequate caretaking, inconsistent responsiveness by caretaker

Disturbed **Sleep** pattern r/t hypervigilance, anxiety

**Fear** r/t threat of punishment for perceived wrongdoing

Imbalanced **Nutrition**: less than body requirements r/t inadequate caretaking

Impaired **Parenting** r/t psychological impairment, physical or emotional abuse of parent, substance abuse, unrealistic expectations of child

Impaired **Skin** integrity r/t altered nutritional state, physical abuse

Ineffective community **Therapeutic** regimen management r/t deficits in community regarding prevention of child abuse

Interrupted **Family** process: alcoholism r/t inadequate coping skills

**Post-trauma** syndrome r/t physical abuse, incest, rape, molestation

Risk for delayed **Development** r/t shaken baby, abuse

Risk for disproportionate **Growth** r/t abuse

Risk for **Poisoning** r/t inadequate safeguards, lack of proper safety precautions, accessibility of illicit substances secondary to impaired home maintenance

Risk for **Suffocation** r/t unattended child, unsafe environment

Risk for **Trauma** r/t inadequate precautions, cognitive or emotional difficulties

**Social** isolation: family imposed r/t fear of disclosure of family dysfunction and abuse

## Child Neglect

*See Child Abuse; Failure to Thrive, Nonorganic*

## Child with Chronic Condition

**Activity** intolerance r/t fatigue associated with chronic illness

Chronic low **Self-esteem** r/t actual or perceived differences; peer acceptance; decreased ability to participate in physical, school, and social activities

Chronic **Pain** r/t physical, biological, chemical, or psychological factors

Chronic **Sorrow** r/t developmental stages and missed opportunities or milestones that bring comparisons with social or personal norms, unending caregiving as reminder of loss

Compromised family **Coping** r/t prolonged over concern for child; distortion of reality regarding child's health problem, including extreme denial about its existence or severity

Decisional **Conflict** r/t treatment options, conflicting values

Deficient **Diversional** activity r/t immobility, monotonous environment, frequent/lengthy treatments, reluctance to participate, self-imposed social isolation

Deficient **Knowledge** r/t knowledge/skill acquisition regarding health practices, acceptance of limitations, promotion of maximal potential of child, self-actualization of rest of family

Delayed **Growth** and development r/t regression or lack of progression toward developmental milestones secondary to frequent or prolonged hospitalization, inadequate or inappropriate stimulation, cerebral insult, chronic illness, effects of physical disability, prescribed dependence

Disabled family **Coping** r/t prolonged disease or disability progression that exhausts supportive capacity of significant people

Disturbed **Sleep** pattern: child or parent r/t time-intensive treatments, exacerbation of condition, 24-hour care needs

**Hopelessness**: child r/t prolonged activity restriction, long-term stress, lack of involvement in or passively allowing care secondary to parental overprotection

Imbalanced **Nutrition**: less than body requirements r/t anorexia, fatigue secondary to physical exertion

Imbalanced **Nutrition**: more than body requirements r/t effects of steroid medications on appetite

Impaired **Home** maintenance r/t overtaxed family members (e.g., exhausted, anxious)

Impaired **Social** interaction r/t developmental lag/ delay, perceived differences

Ineffective **Coping**: child r/t situational or maturational crises

Ineffective **Health** maintenance r/t exhausting family resources (finances, physical energy, support systems)

Ineffective **Sexuality** patterns: parental r/t disrupted relationship with sexual partner

Interrupted **Family** processes r/t intermittent situational crisis of illness, disease, hospitalization

Parental role **Conflict** r/t separation from child as a result of chronic illness, home care of child with special needs, interruptions of family life resulting from home care regimen

**Powerlessness**: child r/t health care environment, illness-related regimen, lifestyle of learned helplessness

Readiness for enhanced family **Coping** r/t impact of crisis on family values, priorities, goals, or relationships; changes in family choices to optimize wellness

Risk for delayed **Development** r/t chronic illness

Risk for disproportionate **Growth** r/t chronic illness

Risk for impaired **Parenting** r/t impaired/ disrupted bonding, caring for child with perceived overwhelming care needs

Risk for **Infection** r/t debilitating physical condition

**Social** isolation: family r/t actual or perceived social stigmatization, complex care requirements

## Childbirth

*See Labor, Normal; Postpartum, Normal Care*

## Chills

**Hyperthermia** r/t infectious process

## Chlamydia Infection

*See STD (Sexually Transmitted Disease)*

## Choking/Coughing with Feeding

Impaired **Swallowing** r/t neuromuscular impairment

Risk for **Aspiration** r/t depressed cough and gag reflexes

## Cholasma

Disturbed **Body** image r/t change in skin color

## Cholecystectomy

Acute **Pain** r/t trauma from surgery

Imbalanced **Nutrition**: less than body requirements r/t high metabolic needs, decreased ability to digest fatty foods

Ineffective **Health** maintenance r/t deficient knowledge regarding postoperative care

Risk for deficient **Fluid** volume r/t restricted intake, nausea, vomiting

Risk for ineffective **Breathing** pattern r/t proximity of incision to lungs resulting in pain with deep breathing

*See Abdominal Surgery*

## Cholelithiasis

Acute **Pain** r/t obstruction of bile flow, inflammation in gallbladder

Imbalanced **Nutrition**: less than body requirements r/t anorexia, nausea, vomiting

Ineffective **Health** maintenance r/t deficient knowledge regarding care of disease

## Chorioamnionitis

Anticipatory **Grieving** r/t guilt about potential loss of ideal pregnancy and birth

**Anxiety** r/t threat to self and infant

**Hyperthermia** r/t infectious process

Risk for delayed **Growth** and development r/t risk of preterm birth

Risk for **Infection** transmission from mother to fetus r/t infection in fetal environment

Situational low **Self-esteem** r/t guilt about threat to infant's health

## Chronic Confusion

*See Confusion, Chronic*

## Chronic Lymphocytic Leukemia

*See Cancer; Chemotherapy; Leukemia*

## Chronic Obstructive Pulmonary Disease

*See COPD (Chronic Obstructive Pulmonary Disease)*

## Chronic Pain

*See Pain, Chronic*

## Chronic Renal Failure

*See Renal Failure*

## Chvostek's Sign

*See Hypocalcemia*

C

## Circumcision

Acute **Pain** r/t surgical intervention

Ineffective **Health** maintenance r/t deficient knowledge (parental) regarding care of surgical area

Risk for deficient **Fluid** volume r/t hemorrhage

Risk for **Infection** r/t surgical wound

## Cirrhosis

Chronic low **Self-esteem** r/t chronic illness

Chronic **Pain** r/t liver enlargement

Chronic **Sorrow** r/t presence of chronic illness

**Diarrhea** r/t dietary changes, medications

Disturbed **Thought** processes r/t chronic organic disorder with increased ammonia levels, substance abuse

**Fatigue** r/t malnutrition

Imbalanced **Nutrition**: less than body requirements r/t loss of appetite, nausea, vomiting

Ineffective **Health** maintenance r/t deficient knowledge regarding correlation between lifestyle habits and disease process

Ineffective management of **Therapeutic** regimen r/t denial of severity of illness

Ineffective **Protection** r/t risk of impaired blood coagulation, bleeding from portal hypertension

**Nausea** r/t irritation to gastrointestinal system

Risk for deficient **Fluid** volume: hemorrhage r/t abnormal bleeding from esophagus

Risk for impaired **Oral** mucous membranes r/t altered nutrition

Risk for impaired **Skin** integrity r/t altered nutritional state, altered metabolic state

Risk for **Injury** r/t substance intoxication, potential delirium tremors

## CJD (Creutzfeldt-Jakob Disease)

Acute **Pain** r/t neck (nuchal) rigidity, inflammation of meninges, headache, kinesthetic

Decreased **Intracranial** adaptive capacity r/t sustained increase in intracranial pressure

Delayed **Growth** and development r/t brain damage secondary to infectious process, increased intracranial pressure

Disturbed **Sensory** perception: hearing r/t central nervous system infection, ear infection

Disturbed **Sensory** perception: kinesthetic r/t central nervous system infection

Disturbed **Thought** processes r/t inflammation of brain, fever

Excess **Fluid** volume r/t increased intracranial pressure, syndrome of inappropriate antidiuretic hormone (SIADH)

Impaired **Comfort** r/t central nervous system inflammation

Impaired **Comfort**: photophobia r/t increased sensitivity to external stimuli secondary to central nervous system inflammation

Impaired physical **Mobility** r/t neuromuscular or central nervous system insult

Ineffective **Airway** clearance r/t seizure activity

Ineffective **Tissue** perfusion: cerebral r/t inflamed cerebral tissues and meninges, increased intracranial pressure

Risk for **Aspiration** r/t seizure activity

Risk for **Falls** r/t neuromuscular dysfunction

Risk for **Injury** r/t seizure activity

## Cleft Lip/Cleft Palate

Acute **Pain** r/t surgical correction, elbow restraints

Chronic **Sorrow** r/t loss of perfect child, birth of child with congenital defect

**Fear**: parental r/t special care needs, surgery

**Grieving** r/t loss of perfect child, birth of child with congenital defect

Imbalanced **Nutrition**: less than body requirements r/t inability to feed with normal techniques

Impaired **Oral** mucous membranes r/t surgical correction

Impaired physical **Mobility** r/t imposed restricted activity, use of elbow restraints

Impaired **Skin** integrity r/t incomplete joining of lip, palate ridges

Impaired verbal **Communication** r/t inadequate palate function, possible hearing loss from infected eustachian tubes

Ineffective **Airway** clearance r/t common feeding and breathing passage, postoperative laryngeal, incisional edema

Ineffective **Breastfeeding** r/t infant anomaly

Ineffective **Health** maintenance r/t lack of parental knowledge regarding feeding techniques, wound care, use of elbow restraints

Ineffective **Infant** feeding pattern r/t cleft lip, cleft palate

Risk for **Aspiration** r/t common feeding and breathing passage

Risk for deficient **Fluid** volume r/t inability to take liquids in usual manner

Risk for delayed **Development** r/t inadequate nutrition resulting from difficulty feeding

Risk for disproportionate **Growth** r/t inability to feed with normal techniques

Risk for disturbed **Body** image r/t disfigurement, speech impediment

Risk for **Infection** r/t invasive procedure, disruption of eustachian tube development, aspiration

## Clotting Disorder

**Fear** r/t threat to well-being

Ineffective **Health** maintenance r/t deficient knowledge regarding treatment of disorder

Ineffective **Protection** r/t clotting disorder

Risk for deficient **Fluid** volume r/t uncontrolled bleeding

*See Anticoagulant Therapy; DIC (Disseminated Intravascular Coagulation); Hemophilia*

## Cocaine Abuse

Disturbed **Thought** processes r/t excessive stimulation of nervous system by cocaine

Ineffective **Breathing** pattern r/t drug effect on respiratory center

Ineffective **Coping** r/t inability to deal with life stresses

*See Substance Abuse*

## Cocaine Baby

*See Crack Baby*

## Codependency

**Caregiver** role strain r/t codependency

Decisional **Conflict** r/t support system deficit

Ineffective **Coping** r/t inadequate support systems

Ineffective **Denial** r/t unmet self-needs

Impaired verbal **Communication** r/t psychological barriers

**Powerlessness** r/t lifestyle of helplessness

## Cognitive Deficit

Disturbed **Thought** processes r/t neurological impairment

## Cold, Viral

Impaired **Comfort**: sore throat, aching, nasal discomfort r/t viral infection

Ineffective **Health** maintenance r/t deficient knowledge regarding care of viral condition, prevention of further infections

## Colectomy

Acute **Pain** r/t recent surgery

**Constipation** r/t decreased activity, decreased fluid intake

Imbalanced **Nutrition**: less than body requirements r/t high metabolic needs, decreased ability to ingest/digest food

Ineffective **Health** maintenance r/t deficient knowledge regarding procedure, postoperative care

Risk for **Infection** r/t invasive procedure

*See Abdominal Surgery*

## Colitis

Acute **Pain** r/t inflammation in colon

Deficient **Fluid** volume r/t frequent stools

**Diarrhea** r/t inflammation in colon

*See Crohn's Disease; Inflammatory Bowel Disease*

## Collagen Disease

*See specific disease (e.g., Lupus Erythematosus; JRA)*

*See Congenital Heart Disease/Cardiac Anomalies*

## Colostomy

Disturbed **Body** image r/t presence of stoma, daily care of fecal material

Ineffective **Health** maintenance r/t deficient knowledge regarding care of stoma, integrating colostomy care into lifestyle

Ineffective **Sexuality** patterns r/t altered body image, self-concept

Risk for **Constipation** r/t inappropriate diet

Risk for **Diarrhea** r/t inappropriate diet

Risk for impaired **Skin** integrity r/t irritation from bowel contents

Risk for **Social** isolation r/t anxiety about appearance of stoma and possible leakage

## Colporrhaphy, Anterior

*See Vaginal Hysterectomy*

## Coma

Death **Anxiety**: significant others r/t unknown outcome of coma state

Disturbed **Thought** processes r/t neurological changes

Ineffective family **Therapeutic** regimen management r/t complexity of therapeutic regimen

C

Interrupted **Family** processes r/t illness/disability of family member

Risk for **Aspiration** r/t impaired swallowing, loss of cough/gag reflex

Risk for **Disuse** syndrome r/t altered level of consciousness impairing mobility

Risk for impaired **Oral** mucous membranes r/t dry mouth

Risk for impaired **Skin** integrity r/t immobility

Risk for **Injury** r/t potential seizure activity

Risk for **Spiritual** distress: significant others r/t loss of ability to relate to loved one, unknown outcome of coma

**Self-care** deficit: specify r/t neuromuscular impairment

Total urinary **Incontinence** r/t neurological dysfunction

*See cause of Coma*

## Comfort, Loss of

Impaired **Comfort** r/t injury agent

## Communicable Diseases, Childhood (Measles, Mumps, Rubella, Chickenpox, Scabies, Lice, Impetigo)

Acute **Pain** r/t impaired skin integrity, edema

Deficient **Diversional** activity r/t imposed isolation from peers, disruption in usual play activities, fatigue, activity intolerance

Impaired **Comfort** r/t hyperthermia secondary to infectious disease process, pruritus secondary to skin rash or subdermal organisms

Ineffective **Health** maintenance r/t nonadherence to appropriate immunization schedules, lack of prevention of transmission of infection

Risk for **Infection**: transmission to others r/t contagious organisms

*See Meningitis/Encephalitis; Respiratory Infections, Acute Childhood; Reye's Syndrome*

## Communication

Readiness for enhanced **Communication** r/t expressed willingness to enhance communication; ability to speak or write a language; ability to form words, phrases, and language; ability to express thoughts and feelings; ability to use and interpret nonverbal cues appropriately; expression of satisfaction with ability to share information and ideas with others

## Communication Problems

Impaired verbal **Communication** r/t decrease in circulation to brain, brain tumor, physical barrier (e.g., tracheostomy, intubation), anatomical defect, impaired hearing, cleft palate, psychological barriers (e.g., psychosis, lack of stimuli), cultural difference, developmentally related or age-related factors, side effects of medication, environmental barriers, absence of significant others, altered perceptions, lack of information, stress, alteration of self-esteem or self-concept, physiological conditions, alteration of central nervous system, weakening of musculoskeletal system, emotional conditions

## Community Coping

Ineffective community **Coping** r/t natural or manmade disasters; ineffective or nonexistent community systems (e.g., lack of emergency medical, transportation, or disaster planning systems), deficits in community social support services and resources, inadequate resources for problem solving

Readiness for enhanced community **Coping** r/t community sense of power to manage stressors, social supports available, resources available for problem solving

## Community Management of Therapeutic Regimen

Ineffective community **Therapeutic** regimen management r/t inadequate community resources

## Compartment Syndrome

Acute **Pain** r/t pressure in compromised body part

**Fear** r/t possible loss of limb, damage to limb

Ineffective **Tissue** perfusion: peripheral r/t increased pressure within compartment

## Compulsion

*See Obsessive-Compulsive Disorder*

## Conduction Disorders (Cardiac)

*See Dysrhythmia*

## Confusion, Acute

Acute **Confusion** r/t >70 years of age with hospitalization, alcohol abuse, delirium, dementia, drug abuse

Adult **Failure** to thrive r/t confusion

Impaired **Memory** r/t fluid and electrolyte imbalance, neurological disturbances, excessive environmental disturbances, anemia, acute or chronic hypoxia, decreased cardiac output

## Confusion, Chronic

Adult **Failure** to thrive r/t confusion

Chronic **Confusion** r/t Alzheimer's disease, Korsakoff's psychosis, multiinfarct dementia, cerebrovascular accident, head injury

Disturbed **Thought** processes r/t organic mental disorder, disruption of cerebral arterial blood flow, chemical imbalance, intoxication

Impaired **Memory** r/t fluid and electrolyte imbalance, neurological disturbances, excessive environmental disturbances, anemia, acute or chronic hypoxia, decreased cardiac output

## Congenital Heart Disease/Cardiac Anomalies

### ACYANOTIC

Patent ductus arteriosus, atrial/ventricular septal defect, pulmonary stenosis, endocardial cushion defect, aortic valvular stenosis, coarctation of aorta

### CYANOTIC

Tetralogy of Fallot, tricuspid atresia, transposition of great vessels, truncus arteriosus, total anomalous pulmonary venous return, hypoplastic left lung

**Activity** intolerance r/t fatigue, generalized weakness, lack of adequate oxygenation

Decreased **Cardiac** output r/t cardiac dysfunction

Delayed **Growth** and development r/t inadequate oxygen and nutrients to tissues

Excess **Fluid** volume r/t cardiac defect, side effects of medication

Imbalanced **Nutrition**: less than body requirements r/t fatigue, generalized weakness, inability of infant to suck and feed, increased caloric requirements

Impaired **Gas** exchange r/t cardiac defect, pulmonary congestion

Ineffective **Breathing** pattern r/t pulmonary vascular disease

Interrupted **Family** processes r/t ill child

Risk for deficient **Fluid** volume r/t side effects of diuretics

Risk for delayed **Development** r/t inadequate oxygen and nutrients to tissues

Risk for disorganized **Infant** behavior r/t invasive procedures

Risk for disproportionate **Growth** r/t inadequate oxygen and nutrients to tissues

Risk for ineffective **Thermoregulation** r/t neonatal age

Risk for **Poisoning** r/t potential toxicity of cardiac medications

*See Child with Chronic Condition; Hospitalized Child*

## Congestive Heart Failure

*See CHF (Congestive Heart Failure)*

## Conjunctivitis

Acute **Pain** r/t inflammatory process

Disturbed **Sensory** perception r/t change in visual acuity resulting from inflammation

Risk for **Injury** r/t change in visual acuity

## Consciousness, Altered Level of

Acute **Confusion** r/t alcohol abuse, delirium, dementia, drug abuse

Adult **Failure** to thrive r/t altered level of consciousness

Chronic **Confusion** r/t multiinfarct dementia, Korsakoff's psychosis, head injury, Alzheimer's disease, cerebrovascular accident

Decreased **Intracranial** adaptive capacity r/t brain injury

Disturbed **Thought** processes r/t neurological changes

Impaired **Memory** r/t neurological disturbances

Ineffective **Tissue** perfusion: cerebral r/t increased intracranial pressure, decreased cerebral perfusion

Risk for **Aspiration** r/t impaired swallowing, loss of cough/gag reflex

Risk for **Disuse** syndrome r/t impaired mobility resulting from altered level of consciousness

Risk for impaired **Oral** mucous membranes r/t dry mouth

Risk for impaired **Skin** integrity r/t immobility

**Self-care** deficit: specify r/t neuromuscular impairment

Total urinary **Incontinence** r/t neurological dysfunction

*See cause of Altered Level of Consciousness*

## Constipation

**Constipation** r/t decreased fluid intake, decreased intake of foods containing bulk, inactivity, immobility, deficient knowledge of appropriate bowel routine, lack of privacy for defecation

## Constipation, Perceived

Perceived **Constipation** r/t cultural or family health beliefs, faulty appraisal, impaired thought processes

C

## Constipation, Risk for

Risk for **Constipation** r/t functional factors impeding defecation, inappropriate diet, psychological factors, physical factors, medications

## Continent Ileostomy (Kock Pouch)

Imbalanced **Nutrition**: less than body requirements r/t malabsorption

Ineffective **Coping** r/t stress of disease, exacerbations caused by stress

Ineffective **Health** maintenance r/t deficient knowledge regarding postoperative care

Risk for **Injury** r/t failure of valve, stomal cyanosis, intestinal obstruction

*See Abdominal Surgery*

## Contraceptive Method

Decisional **Conflict**: method of contraception r/t unclear personal values or beliefs, lack of experience or interference with decision-making, lack of relevant information, support system deficit

**Health-seeking** behaviors r/t requesting information about available and appropriate birth control methods

Ineffective **Sexuality** patterns r/t fear of pregnancy

## Conversion Disorder

**Anxiety** r/t unresolved conflict

Disturbed personal **Identity** r/t overwhelming stress

**Hopelessness** r/t long-term stress

Impaired **Adjustment** r/t multiple stressors

Impaired physical **Mobility** r/t physical conversion symptom

Impaired **Social** interaction r/t altered thought process

Ineffective **Coping** r/t personal vulnerability

Ineffective **Role** performance r/t physical conversion system

**Powerlessness** r/t lifestyle of helplessness

Risk for **Injury** r/t physical conversion symptom

**Self-esteem** disturbance r/t unsatisfactory or inadequate interpersonal relationships

## Convulsions

**Anxiety** r/t concern over controlling convulsions

Impaired **Memory** r/t neurological disturbance

Ineffective **Health** maintenance r/t deficient knowledge regarding need for medication and care during seizure activity

Risk for **Aspiration** r/t impaired swallowing

Risk for delayed **Development** r/t seizures

Risk for disturbed **Thought** processes r/t seizure activity

Risk for **Injury** r/t seizure activity

*See Seizure Disorders, Adult; Seizure Disorders, Childhood*

## COPD (Chronic Obstructive Pulmonary Disease)

**Activity** intolerance r/t imbalance between oxygen supply and demand

Interrupted **Family** processes r/t role changes

**Anxiety** r/t breathlessness, change in health status

Chronic low **Self-esteem** r/t chronic illness

Chronic **Sorrow** r/t presence of chronic illness

Death **Anxiety** r/t seriousness of medical condition, difficulty being able to "catch breath," feeling of suffocation

**Health-seeking** behaviors r/t wish to stop smoking

Imbalanced **Nutrition**: less than body requirements r/t decreased intake because of dyspnea, unpleasant taste in mouth left by medications

Impaired **Gas** exchange r/t ventilation-perfusion inequality

Impaired **Social** interaction r/t social isolation secondary to oxygen use, activity intolerance

Ineffective **Airway** clearance r/t bronchoconstriction, increased mucus, ineffective cough, infection

Ineffective **Health** maintenance r/t deficient knowledge regarding care of disease

**Noncompliance** r/t reluctance to accept responsibility for changing detrimental health practices

**Powerlessness** r/t progressive nature of disease

Risk for **Infection** r/t stasis of respiratory secretions

**Self-care** deficit: specify r/t fatigue secondary to increased work of breathing

**Sleep** deprivation r/t breathing difficulties when lying down

## Coping

Readiness for enhanced **Coping** r/t defining stressors as manageable; seeking social support; using a broad range of problem-oriented and emotion-oriented strategies; using spiritual resources; acknowledging power; seeking knowledge of new strategies; being aware of possible environmental changes

## Coping Problems

Defensive **Coping** r/t superior attitude toward others, difficulty establishing or maintaining relationships, hostile laughter or ridicule of others, difficulty in reality-testing perceptions, lack of follow-through or participation in treatment or therapy

Ineffective **Coping** r/t gender differences in coping strategies, inadequate level of confidence in ability to cope, uncertainty, inadequate social support created by characteristics of relationships, inadequate level of perception of control, inadequate resources available, high degree of threat, disturbance in pattern of tension release, inadequate opportunity to prepare for stressor, inability to conserve adaptive energies, disturbance in appraisal of threat

*See Community Coping; Family Problems*

## Corneal Reflex, Absent

Risk for **Injury** r/t accidental corneal abrasion, drying of cornea

## Corneal Transplant

Risk for **Infection** r/t invasive procedure; surgery

Readiness for enhanced **Therapeutic** regimen management r/t describes need to rest and avoid strenuous activities during healing phase

## Coronary Artery Bypass Grafting

Acute **Pain** r/t traumatic surgery

Decreased **Cardiac** output r/t dysrhythmia, depressed cardiac function, increased systemic vascular resistance

Deficient **Fluid** volume r/t intraoperative fluid loss, use of diuretics in surgery

**Fear** r/t outcome of surgical procedure

Ineffective **Health** maintenance r/t deficient knowledge regarding postprocedure care, lifestyle adjustment after surgery

Risk for perioperative positioning **Injury** r/t hypothermia, extended supine position

## Costovertebral Angle Tenderness

*See Kidney Stone; Pyelonephritis*

## Cough, Effective/Ineffective

Ineffective **Airway** clearance r/t decreased energy, fatigue, normal aging changes

*See Bronchitis; COPD (Chronic Obstructive Pulmonary Disease); Pulmonary Edema*

## Crack Abuse

*See Cocaine Abuse*

## Crack Baby

Delayed **Growth** and development r/t effects of maternal use of drugs, neurological impairment, decreased attentiveness to environmental stimuli

**Diarrhea** r/t effects of withdrawal, increased peristalsis secondary to hyperirritability

Disorganized **Infant** behavior r/t prematurity, pain, lack of attachment

Disturbed **Sensory** perception: specify r/t hypersensitivity to environmental stimuli

Disturbed **Sleep** pattern r/t hyperirritability, hypersensitivity to environmental stimuli

Imbalanced **Nutrition**: less than body requirements r/t feeding problems; uncoordinated/ineffective suck and swallow; effects of diarrhea, vomiting, colic

Impaired **Parenting** r/t impaired/lack of attachment behaviors, inadequate support systems

Ineffective **Airway** clearance r/t pooling of secretions secondary to lack of adequate cough reflex

Ineffective **Infant** feeding pattern r/t prematurity, neurological impairment

Ineffective **Protection** r/t effects of maternal substance abuse

Risk for delayed **Development** r/t substance abuse

Risk for disproportionate **Growth** r/t substance use/abuse

Risk for impaired parent-infant **Attachment** r/t parent's inability to meet infant's needs, substance abuse

Risk for **Infection** (skin, meningeal, respiratory) r/t effects of withdrawal

## Crackles in Lungs, Coarse

Ineffective **Airway** clearance r/t excessive secretions in airways, ineffective cough

*See cause of Coarse Crackles*

## Crackles in Lungs, Fine

Ineffective **Breathing** pattern r/t fatigue, surgery, decreased energy

*See Bronchitis or Pneumonia (if from pulmonary infection); CHF (Congestive Heart Failure) (if cardiac in origin); Infection*

## Craniectomy/Craniotomy

Acute **Pain** r/t recent surgery, headache

Adult **Failure** to thrive r/t altered cerebral tissue perfusion

Decreased **Intracranial** adaptive capacity r/t brain injury, intracranial hypertension

**Fear** r/t threat to well-being

Impaired **Memory** r/t neurological surgery

Ineffective **Tissue** perfusion: cerebral r/t cerebral edema, decreased cerebral perfusion, increased intracranial pressure

C

Risk for disturbed **Thought** processes r/t neurophysiological changes

Risk for **Injury** r/t potential confusion

*See Coma (if relevant)*

## Crepitation, Subcutaneous

*See Pneumothorax*

## Crisis

Anticipatory **Grieving** r/t potential significant loss

**Anxiety** r/t threat to or change in environment, health status, interaction patterns, situation, self-concept, or role-functioning; threat of death of self or significant other

Compromised family **Coping** r/t situational or developmental crisis

Death **Anxiety** r/t feelings of hopelessness associated with crisis

Disturbed **Energy** field r/t disharmony caused by crisis

**Fear** r/t crisis situation

Ineffective **Coping** r/t situational or maturational crisis

Risk for **Spiritual** distress r/t physical or psychological stress, natural disasters, situational losses, maturational losses

Situational low **Self-esteem** r/t perception of inability to handle crisis

**Spiritual** distress r/t intense suffering

## Crohn's Disease

Acute **Pain** r/t increased peristalsis

**Anxiety** r/t change in health status

**Diarrhea** r/t inflammatory process

Imbalanced **Nutrition**: less than body requirements r/t diarrhea, altered ability to digest and absorb food

Ineffective **Coping** r/t repeated episodes of diarrhea

Ineffective **Health** maintenance r/t deficient knowledge regarding management of disease

**Powerlessness** r/t chronic disease

Risk for deficient **Fluid** volume r/t abnormal fluid loss with diarrhea

## Croup

*See Respiratory Infections, Acute Childhood*

## Cryosurgery for Retinal Detachment

*See Retinal Detachment*

## Cushing's Syndrome

**Activity** intolerance r/t fatigue, weakness

Disturbed **Body** image r/t change in appearance from disease process

Excess **Fluid** volume r/t failure of regulatory mechanisms

Ineffective **Health** maintenance r/t deficient knowledge regarding needed care

Risk for **Infection** r/t suppression of immune system secondary to increased cortisol

Risk for **Injury** r/t decreased muscle strength, osteoporosis

**Sexual** dysfunction r/t loss of libido

## CVA (Cerebrovascular Accident)

Adult **Failure** to thrive r/t neurophysiological changes

**Anxiety** r/t situational crisis, change in physical or emotional condition

**Caregiver** role strain r/t cognitive problems of care receiver, need for significant home care

Chronic **Confusion** r/t neurological changes

**Constipation** r/t decreased activity

Disturbed **Body** image r/t chronic illness, paralysis

Disturbed **Sensory** perception: visual, tactile, kinesthetic r/t neurological deficit

Disturbed **Thought** processes r/t neurophysiological changes

**Grieving** r/t loss of health

Impaired **Home** maintenance r/t neurological disease affecting ability to perform activities of daily living (ADLs)

Impaired **Memory** r/t neurological disturbances

Impaired physical **Mobility** r/t loss of balance and coordination

Impaired **Social** interaction r/t limited physical mobility, limited ability to communicate

Impaired **Swallowing** r/t neuromuscular dysfunction

Impaired **Transfer** ability r/t limited physical mobility

Impaired verbal **Communication** r/t pressure damage, decreased circulation to brain in speech center informational sources

Impaired **Walking** r/t loss of balance and coordination

Ineffective **Coping** r/t disability

Ineffective **Health** maintenance r/t deficient knowledge regarding self-care following CVA

Interrupted **Family** process r/t illness, disability of family member

Reflex **Incontinence** r/t loss of feeling to void

Risk for **Aspiration** r/t impaired swallowing, loss of gag reflex

Risk for **Disuse** syndrome r/t paralysis

Risk for impaired **Skin** integrity r/t immobility

Risk for **Injury** r/t disturbed sensory perception

**Self-care** deficit: specify r/t decreased strength and endurance, paralysis

Total urinary **Incontinence** r/t neurological dysfunction

Unilateral **Neglect** r/t disturbed perception from neurological damage

## Cyanosis, Central with Cyanosis of Oral Mucous Membranes

Impaired **Gas** exchange r/t alveolar-capillary membrane changes

## Cyanosis, Peripheral with Cyanosis of Nail Beds

Ineffective **Tissue** perfusion r/t interruption of arterial flow, severe vasoconstriction, cold temperatures

Risk for **Peripheral** neurovascular dysfunction r/t condition causing disruption in circulation

## Cystic Fibrosis

**Activity** intolerance r/t imbalance between oxygen supply and demand

**Anxiety** r/t dyspnea, oxygen deprivation

Chronic **Sorrow** r/t presence of chronic disease

Disturbed **Body** image r/t changes in physical appearance, treatment of chronic lung disease (clubbing, barrel chest, home oxygen therapy)

Imbalanced **Nutrition**: less than body requirements r/t anorexia; decreased absorption of nutrients, fat; increased work of breathing

Impaired **Gas** exchange r/t ventilation-perfusion imbalance

Impaired **Home** maintenance r/t extensive daily treatment, medications necessary for health, mist/ oxygen tents

Ineffective **Airway** clearance r/t increased production of thick mucus

Risk for **Caregiver** role strain r/t illness severity of care receiver, unpredictable course of illness

Risk for deficient **Fluid** volume r/t decreased fluid intake, increased work of breathing

Risk for delayed **Development** r/t chronic illness

Risk for disproportionate **Growth** r/t chronic illness

Risk for **Infection** r/t thick, tenacious mucus; harboring of bacterial organisms; debilitated state

Risk for **Spiritual** distress r/t presence of chronic disease

*See Child with Chronic Condition; Hospitalized Child; Terminally Ill Child, Adolescent; Terminally Ill Child, Infant/Toddler; Terminally Ill Child, Preschool Child; Terminally Ill Child, School-Age Child/Preadolescent; Terminally Ill Child/Death of Child, Parent*

## Cystitis

Acute **Pain**: dysuria r/t inflammatory process in bladder

Impaired **Urinary** elimination: frequency r/t urinary tract infection

Ineffective **Health** maintenance r/t deficient knowledge regarding methods to treat and prevent urinary tract infections

Risk for urge urinary **Incontinence** r/t infection in bladder

## Cystocele

Ineffective **Health** maintenance r/t deficient knowledge regarding personal care, Kegel exercises to strengthen perineal muscles

Risk for urge urinary **Incontinence** r/t lack of bladder support

Stress urinary **Incontinence** r/t prolapsed bladder

Urge urinary **Incontinence** r/t prolapsed bladder

## Cystoscopy

Ineffective **Health** maintenance r/t deficient knowledge regarding postoperative care

Risk for **Infection** r/t invasive procedure

**Urinary** retention r/t edema in urethra obstructing flow of urine

# D

## Deafness

Disturbed **Sensory** perception: auditory r/t alteration in sensory reception, transmission, integration

Impaired verbal **Communication** r/t impaired hearing

Risk for delayed **Development** r/t impaired hearing

Risk for **Injury** r/t alteration in sensory perception

## Death

Risk for sudden infant **Death** syndrome (SIDS) r/t modifiable risk factors such as infants placed to sleep in the prone or side-lying position, prenatal and/or postnatal infant smoke exposure, infant overheating/ overwrapping, soft underlayment/loose articles in the sleep environment, delayed or nonattendance of prenatal care; potentially modifiable risk factors such as low birth weight, prematurity, young maternal age; nonmodifiable risk factors such as male gender, ethnicity (e.g., African American, Native American race of mother), seasonality of SIDS deaths (higher in winter and fall months); peaking of SIDS mortality between infant ages of 2 and 4 months

D

## Death, Oncoming

Anticipatory **Grieving** r/t loss of significant other

Compromised family **Coping** r/t client's inability to provide support to family

Death **Anxiety** r/t unresolved issues surrounding dying

**Fear** r/t threat of death

Ineffective **Coping** r/t personal vulnerability

**Powerlessness** r/t effects of illness, oncoming death

Readiness for enhanced **Spiritual** well-being r/t desire of client and family to be in harmony with each other and higher power/God

**Social** isolation r/t altered state of wellness

**Spiritual** distress r/t intense suffering

*See Terminally Ill Child, Adolescent; Terminally Ill Child, Infant/Toddler; Terminally Ill Child, Preschool Child; Terminally Ill Child, School-Age Child/Preadolescent; Terminally Ill Child/Death of Child, Parent*

## Decisions, Difficulty Making

Decisional **Conflict** r/t support system deficit, perceived threat to value system, multiple or divergent sources of information, lack of relevant information, unclear personal values/beliefs

## Decubitus Ulcer

*See Pressure Ulcer*

## Deep Vein Thrombosis

*See DVT (Deep Vein Thrombosis)*

## Defensive Behavior

Defensive **Coping** r/t nonacceptance of blame, denial of problems or weakness

Ineffective **Denial** r/t inability to face situation realistically

## Dehiscence, Abdominal

Acute **Pain** r/t stretching of abdominal wall

Delayed **Surgical** recovery r/t altered circulation, malnutrition, opening in incision

**Fear** r/t threat of death, severe dysfunction

Impaired **Skin** integrity r/t altered circulation, malnutrition, opening in incision

Impaired **Tissue** integrity r/t exposure of abdominal contents to external environment

Risk for imbalanced **Fluid** volume r/t altered circulation associated with opening of wound and exposure of abdominal contents

Risk for **Infection** r/t loss of skin integrity

## Dehydration

Deficient **Fluid** volume r/t active fluid volume loss

Impaired **Oral** mucous membranes r/t decreased salivation, fluid deficit

Ineffective **Health** maintenance r/t deficient knowledge regarding treatment and prevention of dehydration

*See cause of Dehydration*

## Delirium

Acute **Confusion** r/t effects of medication, response to hospitalization, alcohol abuse, substance abuse, sensory deprivation or overload

Adult **Failure** to thrive r/t delirium

Disturbed **Thought** processes r/t head trauma, altered metabolic state, substance abuse, sleep deprivation, sensory deprivation or overload

Impaired **Memory** r/t delirium

Risk for **Injury** r/t altered level of consciousness

**Sleep** deprivation r/t nightmares

## Delirium Tremens (DT)

*See Alcohol Withdrawal*

## Delivery

*See Labor, Normal*

## Delusions

Acute **Confusion** r/t alcohol abuse, delirium, dementia, drug abuse

Adult **Failure** to thrive r/t delusional state

**Anxiety** r/t content of intrusive thoughts

Disturbed **Thought** processes r/t mental disorder

Impaired verbal **Communication** r/t psychological impairment, delusional thinking

Ineffective **Coping** r/t distortion and insecurity of life events

Risk for other-directed **Violence** r/t delusional thinking

Risk for self-directed **Violence** r/t delusional thinking

## Dementia

Adult **Failure** to thrive r/t depression, apathy

Chronic **Confusion** r/t neurological dysfunction

Chronic **Sorrow** r/t chronic mental illness

Disturbed **Sleep** pattern r/t neurological impairment, naps during the day

Imbalanced **Nutrition**: less than body requirements r/t psychological impairment

Impaired **Environmental** interpretation syndrome r/t dementia

Impaired **Home** maintenance r/t inadequate support system

Impaired physical **Mobility** r/t neuromuscular impairment

Interrupted **Family** process r/t disability of family member

Risk for **Caregiver** role strain r/t number of caregiving tasks, duration of caregiving required

Risk for **Falls** r/t diminished mental status

Risk for impaired **Skin** integrity r/t altered nutritional status, immobility

Risk for **Injury** r/t confusion, decreased muscle coordination

**Self-care** deficit: specify r/t psychological or neuromuscular impairment

Total urinary **Incontinence** r/t neuromuscular impairment

## Denial of Health Status

Ineffective **Denial** r/t lack of perception about health status effects of illness

Ineffective management of **Therapeutic** regimen r/t denial of seriousness of health situation

## Dental Caries

Impaired **Dentition** r/t ineffective oral hygiene, barriers to self-care, economic barriers to professional care, nutritional deficits, dietary habits

Ineffective **Health** maintenance r/t lack of knowledge regarding prevention of dental disease secondary to high-sugar diet, giving infants or toddlers with erupted teeth bottles of milk at bedtime, lack of fluoride treatments, inadequate or improper brushing of teeth

## Dentition Problems

*See Dental Caries*

## Depression (Major Depressive Disorder)

Adult **Failure** to thrive r/t depression

Chronic low **Self-esteem** r/t repeated unmet expectations

Chronic **Sorrow** r/t unresolved grief

**Constipation** r/t inactivity, decreased fluid intake

Death **Anxiety** r/t feelings of lack of self-worth

Disturbed **Energy** field r/t disharmony

Disturbed **Sleep** pattern r/t inactivity

Dysfunctional **Grieving** r/t lack of previous resolution of former grieving response

**Fatigue** r/t psychological demands

**Hopelessness** r/t feeling of abandonment, long-term stress

Impaired **Environmental** interpretation syndrome r/t severe mental functional impairment

Ineffective **Coping** r/t dysfunctional grieving

Ineffective **Health** maintenance r/t lack of ability to make good judgments regarding ways to obtain help

**Powerlessness** r/t pattern of helplessness

Risk for **Suicide** r/t panic state

**Self-care** deficit: specify r/t depression, cognitive impairment

**Sexual** dysfunction r/t loss of sexual desire

**Social** isolation r/t ineffective coping

## Dermatitis

**Anxiety** r/t situational crisis imposed by illness

Impaired **Comfort**: pruritus r/t inflammation of skin

Impaired **Skin** integrity r/t side effect of medication, allergic reaction

Ineffective **Health** maintenance r/t deficient knowledge regarding methods to decrease inflammation

## Despondency

**Hopelessness** r/t long-term stress

*See Depression*

## Destructive Behavior Toward Others

Impaired **Adjustment** r/t intense emotional state

Ineffective **Coping** r/t situational crises, maturational crises, personal vulnerability

Risk for other-directed **Violence** r/t history of violence, neurological impairment, cognitive impairment, history of childhood abuse, history of witnessing family violence, cruelty to animals, firesetting, history of alcohol/drug abuse, pathological intoxication, psychotic symptomatology, motor vehicle offenses, impulsivity, availability or possession of weapon, body language

## Developmental Concerns

Delayed **Growth** and development r/t prescribed dependence, indifference, separation from significant other(s), environmental and stimulation deficiencies, effects of physical disability, inadequate caretaking, inconsistent responsiveness, multiple caretakers

**INDIVIDUAL**

Risk for delayed **Development** r/t prematurity, seizures, congenital or genetic disorders, positive drug screening test, brain damage (e.g., hemorrhage in postnatal period, shaken baby, abuse, accident), vision impairment, hearing impairment or frequent otitis media, chronic illness, technology dependence, failure to thrive, inadequate nutrition, foster or adopted child, lead poisoning, chemotherapy, radiation therapy, natural disaster, behavior disorders, substance abuse

**ENVIRONMENTAL**

Risk for delayed **Development** r/t poverty, violence

**CAREGIVER**

Risk for delayed **Development** r/t abuse, mental illness, mental retardation or severe learning disability

## Diabetes in Pregnancy

*See Gestational Diabetes*

## Diabetes Insipidus

Deficient **Fluid** volume r/t inability to conserve fluid

Ineffective **Health** maintenance r/t deficient knowledge regarding care of disease, importance of medications

## Diabetes Mellitus

Adult **Failure** to thrive r/t undetected disease process

Disturbed **Sensory** perception r/t ineffective tissue perfusion

Imbalanced **Nutrition**: less than body requirements r/t inability to use glucose (type 1 [insulin-dependent] diabetes)

Imbalanced **Nutrition**: more than body requirements r/t excessive intake of nutrients (type 2 diabetes)

Ineffective **Health** maintenance r/t deficient knowledge regarding care of diabetic condition

Ineffective management of **Therapeutic** regimen r/t complexity of therapeutic regimen

Ineffective **Tissue** perfusion: peripheral r/t impaired arterial circulation

**Noncompliance** r/t restrictive lifestyle; changes in diet, medication, exercise

**Powerlessness** r/t perceived lack of personal control

Risk for disturbed **Thought** processes r/t hypoglycemia, hyperglycemia

Risk for impaired **Skin** integrity r/t loss of pain perception in extremities

Risk for **Infection** r/t hyperglycemia, impaired healing, circulatory changes

Risk for **Injury**: hypoglycemia or hyperglycemia r/t failure to consume adequate calories, failure to take insulin

**Sexual** dysfunction r/t neuropathy associated with disease

## Diabetes Mellitus, Juvenile (IDDM Type I)

Acute **Pain** r/t insulin injections, peripheral blood glucose testing

Disturbed **Body** image r/t imposed deviations from biophysical and psychosocial norm, perceived differences from peers

Imbalanced **Nutrition**: less than body requirements r/t inability of body to adequately metabolize and use glucose and nutrients, increased caloric needs of child to promote growth and physical activity participation with peers

Impaired **Adjustment** r/t inability to participate in normal childhood activities

Ineffective **Health** maintenance r/t parental/child deficient knowledge regarding dietary management, medication administration, physical activity, and interaction between the three; daily changes in diet, medications, activity associated with child's growth spurts and needs; need to instruct other caregivers and teachers regarding signs and symptoms of hypoglycemia or hyperglycemia and treatment

Risk for delayed **Development** r/t chronic illness

Risk for disproportionate **Growth** r/t chronic illness

Risk for **Noncompliance** r/t disturbed body image, impaired adjustment secondary to adolescent maturational crises

*See Diabetes Mellitus; Child with Chronic Condition; Hospitalized Child*

## Diabetic Coma

Deficient **Fluid** volume r/t hyperglycemia resulting in polyuria

Disturbed **Thought** processes r/t hyperglycemia, presence of excessive metabolic acids

Ineffective management of **Therapeutic** regimen r/t lack of understanding of preventive measures, adequate blood sugar control

Risk for **Infection** r/t hyperglycemia, changes in vascular system

*See Diabetes Mellitus*

## Diabetic Ketoacidosis

*See Ketoacidosis, Diabetic*

## Diabetic Retinopathy

Disturbed **Sensory** perception r/t change in sensory reception

**Grieving** r/t loss of vision

Ineffective **Health** maintenance r/t deficient knowledge regarding preserving vision with treatment if possible, use of low-vision aids

*See Vision Impairment*

## Dialysis

*See Hemodialysis; Peritoneal Dialysis*

## Diaphoresis

Impaired **Comfort** r/t excessive sweating

## Diaphragmatic Hernia

*See Hiatus Hernia*

## Diarrhea

**Diarrhea** r/t infection, change in diet, gastrointestinal disorders, stress, medication effect, impaction

## DIC (Disseminated Intravascular Coagulation)

Deficient **Fluid** volume: hemorrhage r/t depletion of clotting factors

**Fear** r/t threat to well-being

Ineffective **Protection** r/t abnormal clotting mechanism

Risk for ineffective **Tissue** perfusion: peripheral r/t hypovolemia from profuse bleeding, formation of microemboli in vascular system

## Digitalis Toxicity

Decreased **Cardiac** output r/t drug toxicity affecting cardiac rhythm, rate

Ineffective management of **Therapeutic** regimen r/t deficient knowledge regarding action, appropriate method of administration of digitalis

## Dilation and Curettage (D & C)

Acute **Pain** r/t uterine contractions

Ineffective **Health** maintenance r/t deficient knowledge regarding postoperative self-care

Risk for deficient **Fluid** volume: hemorrhage r/t excessive blood loss during or after procedure

Risk for ineffective **Sexuality** patterns r/t painful coitus, fear associated with surgery on genital area

Risk for **Infection** r/t surgical procedure

## Discharge Planning

Deficient **Knowledge** r/t lack of exposure to information for home care

Impaired **Home** maintenance r/t family member's disease or injury interfering with home maintenance

Ineffective **Health** maintenance r/t lack of material sources

## Discomforts of Pregnancy

Acute **Pain**: leg cramps r/t nerve compression, calcium/phosphorus/potassium imbalance

**Constipation** r/t decreased gastrointestinal tract motility, pressure from enlarged uterus, supplementary iron

Disturbed **Body** image r/t pregnancy-induced body changes

Disturbed **Sleep** pattern r/t psychological stress, fetal movement, muscular cramping, urinary frequency, shortness of breath

**Fatigue** r/t hormonal, metabolic, body changes

Impaired **Comfort** r/t hormonal changes (nausea, ptyalism, leukorrhea, urinary frequency), enlarged uterus (shortness of breath, abdominal distention, pruritus, reduced bladder capacity), increased vascularization (nasal stuffiness, varicosities)

**Nausea** r/t hormone effect

Risk for **Constipation** r/t decreased intestinal motility, inadequate fiber in diet

Risk for **Injury** r/t faintness and/or syncope secondary to vasomotor lability or postural hypotension, venous stasis in lower extremities

Risk for urge urinary **Incontinence** r/t hormone effect, pressure on bladder from growing uterus

Stress urinary **Incontinence** r/t enlarged uterus, fetal movement

## Dislocation

Acute **Pain** r/t dislocation of a joint

Risk for **Injury** r/t unstable joint

**Self-care** deficit: specify r/t inability to use a joint

## Dissecting Aneurysm

**Fear** r/t threat to well-being

*See Abdominal Surgery; Aneurysm, Abdominal Surgery*

## Disseminated Intravascular Coagulation

*See DIC (Disseminated Intravascular Coagulation)*

D

## Dissociative Identity Disorder (Not Otherwise Specified)

**Anxiety** r/t psychosocial stress

Disturbed personal **Identity** r/t inability to distinguish self caused by multiple personality disorder, depersonalization, disturbance in memory

Disturbed **Sensory** perception: kinesthetic r/t underdeveloped ego

Disturbed **Thought** processes r/t repressed anxiety

Impaired **Memory** r/t altered state of consciousness

Ineffective **Coping** r/t personal vulnerability in crisis of accurate self-perception

*See Multiple Personality Disorder*

## Distress

**Anxiety** r/t situational crises, maturational crises

Death **Anxiety** r/t denial of one's own mortality or impending death

Disturbed **Energy** field r/t disruption in flow of energy as result of pain, depression, fatigue, anxiety, stress

## Disuse Syndrome, Potential to Develop

Risk for **Disuse** syndrome r/t paralysis, mechanical immobilization, prescribed immobilization, severe pain, altered level of consciousness

## Diversional Activity, Lack of

Deficient **Diversional** activity r/t environmental lack of diversional activity as in frequent hospitalizations, lengthy treatments

## Diverticulitis

Acute **Pain** r/t inflammation of bowel

**Constipation** r/t dietary deficiency of fiber and roughage

Deficient **Knowledge** r/t diet needed to control disease, medication regimen

**Diarrhea** r/t increased intestinal motility secondary to inflammation

Imbalanced **Nutrition**: less than body requirements r/t loss of appetite

Risk for deficient **Fluid** volume r/t diarrhea

## Dizziness

Decreased **Cardiac** output r/t dysfunctional electrical conduction

Impaired physical **Mobility** r/t dizziness

Ineffective **Tissue** perfusion: cerebral r/t interruption of cerebral arterial blood flow

Risk for **Injury** r/t difficulty maintaining balance

## Domestic Violence

**Anxiety** r/t threat to self-concept, situational crisis of abuse

**Caregiver** role strain r/t chronic illness, self-care deficits, lack of respite care, extent of caregiving required

Compromised family **Coping** r/t abusive patterns

Defensive **Coping** r/t low self-esteem

Disturbed **Sleep** pattern r/t psychological stress

Impaired verbal **Communication** r/t psychological barriers of fear

Interrupted **Family** processes: alcoholism r/t inadequate coping skills

**Post-trauma** syndrome r/t history of abuse

**Powerlessness** r/t lifestyle of helplessness

Risk for **Post-trauma** syndrome r/t inadequate social support

Risk for self-directed **Violence** r/t history of abuse

**Self-esteem** disturbance r/t negative family interactions

## Down Syndrome

*See Child with Chronic Condition; Mental Retardation*

## Dress Self (Inability to)

Dressing/grooming **Self-care** deficit r/t intolerance to activity, decreased strength and endurance, pain, discomfort, perceptual or cognitive impairment, neuromuscular impairment, musculoskeletal impairment, depression, severe anxiety

## Dribbling of Urine

Stress urinary **Incontinence** r/t degenerative changes in pelvic muscles and structural supports

## Drooling

Impaired **Swallowing** r/t neuromuscular impairment, mechanical obstruction

Risk for **Aspiration** r/t impaired swallowing

## Drug Abuse

**Anxiety** r/t threat to self-concept, lack of control of drug use

Disturbed **Sensory** perception: specify r/t substance intoxication

Disturbed **Sleep** pattern r/t effects of medications

Disturbed **Thought** processes r/t mind-altering effects of drugs

Imbalanced **Nutrition**: less than body requirements r/t poor eating habits

Impaired **Adjustment** r/t failure to intend to change behavior

Impaired **Social** interaction r/t disturbed thought processes from drug abuse

Ineffective **Coping** r/t situational crisis

**Noncompliance** r/t denial of illness

**Powerlessness** r/t feeling unable to change patterns of abuse

Risk for **Injury** r/t hallucinations, drug effects

Risk for **Violence** r/t poor impulse control

**Sexual** dysfunction r/t actions and side effects of drug abuse

**Sleep** deprivation r/t prolonged psychological discomfort

**Spiritual** distress r/t separation from religious, cultural ties

## Drug Withdrawal

Acute **Confusion** r/t effects of substance withdrawal

**Anxiety** r/t physiological withdrawal

Disturbed **Sensory** perception: specify r/t substance intoxication

Disturbed **Sleep** pattern r/t effects of medications

Imbalanced **Nutrition**: less than body requirements r/t poor eating habits

Ineffective **Coping** r/t situational crisis, withdrawal

**Noncompliance** r/t denial of illness

Risk for **Injury** r/t hallucinations

Risk for **Violence** r/t poor impulse control

*See Drug Abuse*

## Dry Eye

*See Conjunctivitis; Keratoconjunctivitis Sicca*

## DT (Delirium Tremens)

*See Alcohol Withdrawal*

## DVT (Deep Vein Thrombosis)

Acute **Pain** r/t vascular inflammation, edema

**Constipation** r/t inactivity, bedrest

Delayed **Surgical** recovery r/t impaired physical mobility

Impaired physical **Mobility** r/t pain in extremity, forced bed rest

Ineffective **Health** maintenance r/t deficient knowledge regarding self-care needs, treatment regimen, outcome

Ineffective **Tissue** perfusion: peripheral r/t interruption of venous blood flow

*See Anticoagulant Therapy*

## Dying Client

*See Terminally Ill Child, Adolescent; Terminally Ill Child, Infant/Toddler; Terminally Ill Child, Preschool Child; Terminally Ill Child, School-Age Child/Preadolescent; Terminally Ill Child/Death of Child, Parent*

## Dysfunctional Eating Pattern

Imbalanced **Nutrition**: less than body requirements r/t psychological factors

Risk for imbalanced **Nutrition**: more than body requirements r/t observed use of food as reward or comfort measure

*See Anorexia Nervosa; Bulimia; Maturational Issues, Adolescent*

## Dysfunctional Family Unit

*See Family Problems*

## Dysfunctional Grieving

Dysfunctional **Grieving** r/t actual or perceived loss

## Dysfunctional Ventilatory Weaning

Dysfunctional **Ventilatory** weaning response r/t physical, psychological, situational factors

## Dysmenorrhea

Ineffective **Health** maintenance r/t deficient knowledge regarding prevention and treatment of painful menstruation

**Nausea** r/t prostaglandin effect

Acute **Pain** r/t cramping from hormonal effects

## Dyspareunia

**Sexual** dysfunction r/t lack of lubrication during intercourse, alteration in reproductive organ function

## Dyspepsia

Acute **Pain** r/t gastrointestinal disease, consumption of irritating foods

**Anxiety** r/t pressures of personal role

Ineffective **Health** maintenance r/t deficient knowledge regarding treatment of disease

## Dysphagia

Impaired **Swallowing** r/t neuromuscular impairment

Risk for **Aspiration** r/t loss of gag or cough reflex

## Dysphasia

Impaired **Social** interaction r/t difficulty in communicating

Impaired verbal **Communication** r/t decrease in circulation to brain

## Dyspnea

**Activity** intolerance r/t imbalance between oxygen supply-demand

**Anxiety** r/t ineffective breathing pattern

Disturbed **Sleep** pattern r/t difficulty breathing, positioning required for effective breathing

**Fear** r/t threat to state of well-being, potential death

Impaired **Gas** exchange r/t alveolar-capillary damage

Ineffective **Breathing** pattern r/t compromised cardiac/pulmonary function, decreased lung expansion, neurological impairment affecting respiratory center, extreme anxiety

**Sleep** deprivation r/t ineffective breathing pattern

## Dysrhythmia

**Activity** intolerance r/t decreased cardiac output

**Anxiety/fear** r/t threat of death, change in health status

Decreased **Cardiac** output r/t altered electrical conduction

Ineffective **Health** maintenance r/t deficient knowledge regarding self-care with disease

Ineffective **Tissue** perfusion: cerebral r/t interruption of cerebral arterial flow secondary to decreased cardiac output

## Dysthymic Disorder

Chronic low **Self-esteem** r/t repeated unmet expectations

Disturbed **Sleep** pattern r/t anxious thoughts

Ineffective **Coping** r/t impaired social interaction

Ineffective **Health** maintenance r/t inability to make good judgments regarding ways to obtain help

Ineffective **Sexuality** pattern r/t loss of sexual desire

**Social** isolation r/t ineffective coping

*See Depression*

## Dystocia

Acute **Pain** r/t difficult labor, medical interventions

**Anxiety** r/t difficult labor, deficient knowledge regarding normal labor pattern

**Fatigue** r/t prolonged labor

**Grieving** r/t loss of ideal labor experience

Ineffective **Coping** r/t situational crisis

**Powerlessness** r/t perceived inability to control outcome of labor

Risk for deficient **Fluid** volume r/t hemorrhage secondary to uterine atony

Risk for delayed **Development** r/t difficult labor and birth

Risk for disproportionate **Growth** r/t difficult labor and birth

Risk for impaired **Tissue** integrity: maternal and fetal r/t difficult labor

Risk for ineffective **Tissue** perfusion: cerebral (fetal) r/t difficult labor and birth

Risk for **Infection** r/t prolonged rupture of membranes

Risk for **Post-trauma** syndrome r/t sudden emergency during delivery of infant

Situational low **Self-esteem** r/t perceived inability to have normal labor and delivery

## Dysuria

Impaired **Urinary** elimination r/t urinary tract infection

Risk for urge urinary **Incontinence** r/t detrusor hyperreflexia from cystitis, urethritis

# E

## E. Coli Infection

Deficient **Knowledge** r/t how to prevent disease; care of self with serious illness

**Fear** r/t serious illness, unknown outcome

*See Gastroenteritis; Gastroenteritis, Child*

## Ear Surgery

Acute **Pain** r/t edema in ears from surgery

Disturbed **Sensory** perception: hearing r/t invasive surgery of ears, dressings

Ineffective **Health** maintenance r/t deficient knowledge regarding postoperative restrictions, expectations, care

Risk for delayed **Development** r/t hearing impairment

Risk for **Injury** r/t dizziness from excessive stimuli to vestibular apparatus

*See Hospitalized Child*

## Earache

Acute **Pain** r/t trauma, edema, infection

Disturbed **Sensory** perception: auditory r/t altered sensory reception, transmission, integration

## Eclampsia

**Fear** r/t threat of well-being to self and fetus

Interrupted **Family** processes r/t unmet expectations for pregnancy and childbirth

Risk for **Aspiration** r/t seizure activity

Risk for delayed **Development** r/t uteroplacental insufficiency

Risk for disproportionate **Growth** r/t uteroplacental insufficiency

Risk for excess **Fluid** volume r/t decreased urine output secondary to renal dysfunction

Risk for imbalanced **Fluid** volume r/t retained fluid, decreased renal activity

Risk for ineffective **Tissue** perfusion: fetal r/t uteroplacental insufficiency

Risk for **Injury**: maternal r/t seizure activity

## ECT (Electroconvulsive Therapy)

Decisional **Conflict** r/t lack of relevant information

**Fear** r/t real or imagined threat to well-being

Impaired **Memory** r/t effects of treatment

*See Depression*

## Ectopic Pregnancy

Acute **Pain** r/t stretching or rupture of implantation site

Chronic **Sorrow** r/t loss of pregnancy, potential loss of fertility

Death **Anxiety** r/t emergency condition, hemorrhage

Deficient **Fluid** volume r/t loss of blood

Disturbed **Body** image r/t negative feelings about body and reproductive functioning

**Fear** r/t threat to self, surgery, implications for future pregnancy

Ineffective **Role** performance r/t loss of pregnancy

Risk for ineffective **Coping** r/t loss of pregnancy

Risk for **Infection** r/t traumatized tissue, blood loss

Risk for interrupted **Family** processes r/t situational crisis

Risk for **Spiritual** distress r/t grief process

Situational low **Self-esteem** r/t loss of pregnancy, inability to carry pregnancy to term

## Eczema

Acute **Pain**: pruritus r/t inflammation of skin

Disturbed **Body** image r/t change in appearance from inflamed skin

Impaired **Skin** integrity r/t side effect of medication, allergic reaction

Ineffective **Health** maintenance r/t deficient knowledge regarding how to decrease inflammation and prevent further outbreaks

## ED (Erectile Dysfunction)

*See Erectile Dysfunction; Impotence*

## Edema

Excess **Fluid** volume r/t excessive fluid intake, cardiac dysfunction, renal dysfunction, loss of plasma proteins

Ineffective **Health** maintenance r/t deficient knowledge regarding treatment of edema

Risk for impaired **Skin** integrity r/t impaired circulation, fragility of skin

*See cause of Edema*

## Elderly

*See Aging*

## Elderly Abuse

*See Abuse, Spouse, Parent, or Significant Other*

## Electroconvulsive Therapy

*See ECT*

## Emaciated Person

Adult **Failure** to thrive r/t imbalanced nutrition: less than body requirements

Imbalanced **Nutrition**: less than body requirements r/t inability to ingest food, digest food, absorb nutrients because of biological, psychological, economic factors

## Embolectomy

**Fear** r/t threat of great bodily harm from embolus

Ineffective **Tissue** perfusion: specify r/t presence of embolus

Risk for deficient **Fluid** volume: hemorrhage r/t postoperative complication, surgical area

*See Surgery, Postoperative Care*

## Emboli

*See Pulmonary Embolism*

## Emesis

**Nausea** r/t chemotherapy, irritation of gastrointestinal system, stimulation of neuropharmacological mechanisms, viral infection

*See Vomiting*

## Emotional Problems

*See Coping Problems*

## Empathy

**Health**-seeking behaviors r/t desire to attain maximum level of health

Readiness for enhanced community **Coping** r/t social supports, being available for problem solving

Readiness for enhanced family **Coping** r/t basic needs met, desire to move to higher level of health

Readiness for enhanced **Spiritual** well-being r/t desire to establish interconnectedness through spirituality

## Emphysema

*See COPD (Chronic Obstructive Pulmonary Disease)*

## Emptiness



Chronic **Sorrow** r/t unresolved grief

**Social** isolation r/t inability to engage in satisfying personal relationships

**Spiritual** distress r/t separation from religious/cultural ties

## Encephalitis

*See Meningitis/Encephalitis*

## Endocardial Cushion Defect

*See Congenital Heart Disease/Cardiac Anomalies*

## Endocarditis

**Activity** intolerance r/t reduced cardiac reserve, prescribed bedrest

Acute **Pain** r/t biological injury, inflammation

Decreased **Cardiac** output r/t inflammation of lining of heart and change in structure of valve leaflets, increased myocardial workload

Ineffective **Health** maintenance r/t deficient knowledge regarding treatment of disease, preventive measures against further incidence of disease

Ineffective **Tissue** perfusion: cardiopulmonary/peripheral r/t high risk for development of emboli

Risk for imbalanced **Nutrition**: less than body requirements r/t fever, hypermetabolic state associated with fever

## Endometriosis

Acute **Pain** r/t onset of menses with distention of endometrial tissue

Anticipatory **Grieving** r/t possible infertility

Ineffective **Health** maintenance r/t deficient knowledge about disease condition, medications, other treatments

**Nausea** r/t prostaglandin effect

**Sexual** dysfunction r/t painful coitus

## Endometritis

Acute **Pain** r/t infectious process in reproductive tract

**Anxiety** r/t prolonged hospitalization, fear of unknown

**Hyperthermia** r/t infectious process

Ineffective **Health** maintenance r/t deficient knowledge regarding condition, treatment, antibiotic regimen

## Enuresis

Ineffective **Health** maintenance r/t unachieved developmental task, neuromuscular immaturity, diseases of urinary system, infections or illnesses such as diabetes mellitus or insipidus, regression in developmental stage secondary to hospitalization or stress, parental deficient knowledge regarding involuntary urination at night after age 6, fluid intake at bedtime, lack of control during sound sleep, male gender

*See Toilet Training*

## Environmental Interpretation Problems

Adult **Failure** to thrive r/t impaired environmental interpretation syndrome

Chronic **Confusion** r/t impaired environmental interpretation syndrome

Disturbed **Thought** processes r/t lack of orientation to person, place, time, circumstances

Impaired **Environmental** interpretation syndrome r/t dementia, Parkinson's disease, Huntington's disease, depression, alcoholism

Impaired **Memory** r/t environmental disturbances

Risk for **Injury** r/t lack of orientation to person, place, time, circumstances

## Epididymitis

Acute **Pain** r/t inflammation in scrotal sac

**Anxiety** r/t situational crisis, pain, threat to future fertility

Ineffective **Health** maintenance r/t deficient knowledge regarding treatment for pain and infection

Ineffective **Sexuality** patterns r/t edema of epididymis and testes

## Epiglottitis

*See Respiratory Infections, Acute Childhood (Croup, Epiglottis, Pertussis, Pneumonia, Respiratory Syncytial Virus)*

## Epilepsy

**Anxiety** r/t threat to role functioning

Impaired **Memory** r/t seizure activity

Ineffective **Health** maintenance r/t deficient knowledge regarding seizures and seizure control

Ineffective **Therapeutic** regimen management r/t deficient knowledge regarding seizure control

Risk for **Aspiration** r/t impaired swallowing, excessive secretions

Risk for delayed **Development** r/t seizure disorder

Risk for disturbed **Thought** processes r/t excessive, uncontrolled neurological stimuli

Risk for **Injury** r/t environmental factors during seizure

*See Seizure Disorders, Adult; Seizure Disorders, Childhood*

## Episiotomy

Acute **Pain** r/t tissue trauma

**Anxiety** r/t fear of pain

Disturbed **Body** image r/t fear of resuming sexual relations

Impaired physical **Mobility** r/t pain, swelling, tissue trauma

Impaired **Skin** integrity r/t perineal incision

Risk for **Infection** r/t tissue trauma

**Sexual** dysfunction r/t altered body structure, tissue trauma

## Epistaxis

**Fear** r/t large amount of blood loss

Risk for deficient **Fluid** volume r/t excessive fluid loss

## Epstein-Barr Virus

*See Mononucleosis*

## Erectile Dysfunction (ED)

Readiness for enhanced **Knowledge** of treatment information for erectile dysfunction

**Self-esteem** disturbance r/t physiological crisis, inability to practice usual sexual activity

**Sexual** dysfunction r/t altered body function

*See Impotence*

## Esophageal Varices

Deficient **Fluid** volume: hemorrhage r/t portal hypertension, distended variceal vessels that can easily rupture

**Fear** r/t threat of death

*See Cirrhosis*

## Esophagitis

Acute **Pain** r/t inflammation of esophagus

Ineffective **Health** maintenance r/t deficient knowledge regarding treatment of disease

## ETOH Withdrawal

*See Alcohol Withdrawal*

## Evisceration

*See Dehiscence, Abdominal*

## Exposure to Hot or Cold Environment

Risk for imbalanced **Body** temperature r/t exposure

## External Fixation

Disturbed **Body** image r/t trauma, change to affected part

Risk for **Infection** r/t pressure of pins on skin surface

*See Fracture*

## Eye Surgery

**Anxiety** r/t possible loss of vision

Disturbed **Sensory** perception: visual r/t surgical procedure

Ineffective **Health** maintenance r/t deficient knowledge regarding postoperative activity, medications, eye care

Risk for **Injury** r/t impaired vision

**Self-care** deficit r/t impaired vision

*See Hospitalized Child; Vision Impairment*

# F

## Failure to Thrive, Adult

Adult **Failure** to thrive r/t depression, apathy, fatigue

## Failure to Thrive, Nonorganic

Chronic low **Self-esteem**: parental r/t feelings of inadequacy, support system deficiencies, inadequate role model

Delayed **Growth** and development r/t parental deficient knowledge, lack of stimulation, nutritional deficit, long-term hospitalization

Disorganized **Infant** behavior r/t lack of boundaries

Disturbed **Sleep** pattern r/t inconsistency of caretaker, lack of quiet environment

Imbalanced **Nutrition**: less than body requirements r/t inadequate type/amounts of food for infant, inappropriate feeding techniques

Impaired **Parenting** r/t lack of parenting skills, inadequate role modeling

Risk for delayed **Development** r/t failure to thrive

Risk for disproportionate **Growth** r/t failure to thrive

Risk for impaired parent/infant **Attachment** r/t inability of parents to meet infant's needs

**Social** isolation r/t limited support systems, self-imposed situation

## Falls, Risk for

Risk for **Falls** r/t history of falls, physiological factors, cognitive impairment, medication effect, unsafe environment, young child or older adult

## Family Presence

Family **Presence** r/t resuscitation or invasive procedures being performed on family member

## Family Problems

Compromised family **Coping** r/t inadequate or incorrect information or understanding by primary person, temporary preoccupation by significant person who is trying to manage emotional conflicts and personal suffering and is unable to perceive or act effectively in regard to client's needs, temporary family disorganization and role changes, other situational or developmental crises the significant person may be facing, little support provided by client for primary person, prolonged disease or disability progression that exhausts supportive capacity of significant people

Disabled family **Coping** r/t significant person with chronically unexpressed feelings such as guilt, anxiety, hostility, despair; dissonant discrepancy of coping styles for dealing with adaptive tasks by significant person and client or among significant people; highly ambivalent family relationships; arbitrary handling of family's resistance to treatment, which tends to solidify defensiveness as it fails to deal adequately with underlying anxiety

Ineffective family **Therapeutic** regimen management r/t complexity of health care system, complexity of therapeutic regimen, decisional conflicts, economic difficulties, excessive demands made on individual or family, family conflict

Interrupted **Family** processes r/t situation transition and/or crises, developmental transition and/or crises

Readiness for enhanced family **Coping** r/t needs sufficiently gratified, adaptive tasks effectively addressed to enable goals of self-actualization to surface

## Family Process

Readiness for enhanced **Family** processes r/t expressed willingness to enhance family dynamics; family functioning that meets physical, social, and psychological needs of family members; activities that support the safety and growth of family members; adequate communication; relationships that are generally positive; interdependence with community; accomplishment of family task; family roles that are flexible and appropriate for developmental stages; evident respect for family members; adaptation of family to change; maintenance of boundaries of family members; energy level of family that supports activities of daily living; evident family resilience; balance between autonomy and cohesiveness

## Fatigue

Disturbed **Energy** field r/t disharmony

**Fatigue** r/t decreased or increased metabolic energy production, overwhelming psychological or emotional demands, increased energy requirements to perform ADLs, excessive social and/or role demands, states of discomfort, altered body chemistry

## Fear

Death **Anxiety** r/t fear of death

**Fear** r/t identifiable physical or psychological threat to person

## Febrile Seizures

*See Seizure Disorders, Childhood*

## Fecal Impaction

*See Impaction of Stool*

## Fecal Incontinence

**Bowel** incontinence r/t neurological impairment, gastrointestinal disorders, anorectal trauma

## Feeding Problems, Newborn

Disorganized **Infant** behavior r/t prematurity, immature neurological system

Impaired **Swallowing** r/t prematurity

Ineffective **Breastfeeding** r/t prematurity, infant anomaly, maternal breast anomaly, previous breast surgery, previous history of breastfeeding failure, infant receiving supplemental feedings with artificial nipple, poor infant sucking reflex, nonsupportive partner and family, deficient knowledge, maternal anxiety or ambivalence

Ineffective **Infant** feeding pattern r/t prematurity, neurological impairment or delay, oral hypersensitivity, prolonged NPO (nothing by mouth) status

Interrupted **Breastfeeding** r/t maternal or infant illness, prematurity, maternal employment, contraindications to breastfeeding, need to abruptly wean infant

Risk for delayed **Development** r/t inadequate nutrition

Risk for disproportionate **Growth** r/t feeding problems

Risk for imbalanced **Fluid** volume r/t inability to take in adequate amount of fluids

## Femoral Popliteal Bypass

Acute **Pain** r/t surgical trauma, edema in surgical area

**Anxiety** r/t threat to or change in health status

Ineffective **Tissue** perfusion: peripheral r/t impaired arterial circulation

Risk for deficient **Fluid** volume: hemorrhage r/t abnormal blood loss

Risk for **Infection** r/t invasive procedure

Risk for **Peripheral** neurovascular dysfunction r/t vascular surgery, emboli

## Fetal Alcohol Syndrome

*See Infant of Substance-Abusing Mother*

## Fetal Distress/Nonreassuring Fetal Heart Rate Pattern

**Fear** r/t threat to fetus

Ineffective **Tissue** perfusion: fetal r/t interruption of umbilical cord blood flow

Ineffective **Tissue** perfusion: placental r/t small or old placenta, interference with gas exchange transplacentally

## Fever

**Hyperthermia** r/t infectious process, damage to hypothalamus, exposure to hot environment, medications, anesthesia, inability or decreased ability to perspire

## Fibrocystic Breast Disease

*See Breast Lumps*

## Filthy Home Environment

Impaired **Home** maintenance r/t individual or family member disease or injury, insufficient family organization or planning, impaired cognitive or emotional functioning, lack of knowledge, economic factors

## Financial Crisis in the Home Environment

Impaired **Home** maintenance r/t insufficient finances

## Fistulectomy

*See Hemorrhoidectomy (same nursing care)*

## Flail Chest

**Anxiety** r/t difficulty breathing

Impaired spontaneous **Ventilation** r/t paradoxical respirations

Ineffective **Breathing** pattern r/t chest trauma

## Flashbacks

**Post-trauma** syndrome r/t catastrophic event

Risk for **Post-trauma** syndrome r/t occupation (e.g., police, fire, rescue, corrections, emergency room staff, mental health), exaggerated sense of responsibility, perception of event, survivor's role in event, displacement from home, inadequate social support, nonsupportive environment, diminished ego strength, duration of event

## Flat Affect

Adult **Failure** to thrive r/t apathy

**Hopelessness** r/t prolonged activity restriction creating isolation, failing or deteriorating physiological condition, long-term stress, abandonment, lost belief in transcendent values or higher power/God

Risk for **Loneliness** r/t social isolation, lack of interest in surroundings

*See Dysthymic Disorder*

## Flesh-Eating Bacteria

*See Necrotizing Fascitis*

## Fluid Balance

Readiness for enhanced **Fluid** balance r/t expressed willingness to enhance fluid balance; stable weight; moist mucous membranes; food and fluid intake adequate for daily needs; straw-colored urine with specific gravity within normal limits; good tissue turgor; no excessive thirst; urine output appropriate for intake; no evidence of edema or dehydration

## Fluid Volume Deficit

Deficient **Fluid** volume r/t active fluid loss, failure of regulatory mechanisms

## Fluid Volume Excess

Excess **Fluid** volume r/t compromised regulatory mechanism, excess sodium intake

## Fluid Volume Imbalance, Risk for

Risk for imbalanced **Fluid** volume r/t major invasive surgeries

## Foodborne Illness

Deficient **Fluid** volume r/t active fluid loss

Deficient **Knowledge** r/t care of self with serious illness, prevention of further incidences of foodborne illness

**Diarrhea** r/t infectious material in gastrointestinal tract

**Nausea** r/t contamination irritating stomach

*See Gastroenteritis; Gastroenteritis, Child; E. Coli Infection*

## Foreign Body Aspiration

Impaired **Home** maintenance r/t insufficient family organization or planning, lack of resources or support systems, inability to maintain orderly and clean surroundings

Ineffective **Airway** clearance r/t obstruction of airway

Ineffective **Health** maintenance r/t parental deficient knowledge regarding small toys, pieces of toys, nuts, balloons

Risk for **Suffocation** r/t inhalation of small object

*See Safety, Childhood*

## Formula Feeding

Decisional **Conflict**: maternal r/t multiple or divergent sources of information, values conflict, support system deficit

**Grieving**: maternal r/t loss of desired breastfeeding experience

Ineffective **Health** maintenance r/t maternal deficient knowledge regarding formula feeding

Risk for **Constipation:** infant r/t iron-fortified formula

Risk for imbalanced **Nutrition**: more than body requirements r/t composition of formula and bottle feeding, overuse of food for reward or comfort measures

Risk for **Infection**: infant r/t lack of passive maternal immunity, supine feeding position

## Fracture

Acute **Pain** r/t muscle spasm, edema, trauma

Deficient **Diversional** activity r/t immobility

Impaired physical **Mobility** r/t limb immobilization

Impaired **Walking** r/t limb immobility

Ineffective **Health** maintenance r/t deficient knowledge regarding care of fracture

Risk for impaired **Skin** integrity r/t immobility, presence of cast

Risk for ineffective **Tissue** perfusion r/t immobility, presence of cast

Risk for **Peripheral** neurovascular dysfunction r/t mechanical compression, treatment of fracture

## Fractured Hip

*See Hip Fracture*

## Frequency of Urination

Impaired **Urinary** elimination r/t anatomical obstruction, sensory-motor impairment, urinary tract infection

Risk for urge urinary **Incontinence** r/t effects of medications, caffeine, alcohol, aging

Stress urinary **Incontinence** r/t degenerative change in pelvic muscles and structural support

Urge urinary **Incontinence** r/t decreased bladder capacity, irritation of bladder stretch receptors causing spasm, alcohol, caffeine, increased fluids, increased urine concentration, overdistended bladder

**Urinary** retention r/t high urethral pressure caused by weak detrusor, inhibition of reflex arc, strong sphincter, blockage

## Frostbite

Acute **Pain** r/t decreased circulation from prolonged exposure to cold

Impaired **Skin** integrity r/t freezing of skin

Impaired **Tissue** integrity r/t freezing of skin

Ineffective **Tissue** perfusion r/t damage to extremities from prolonged exposure to cold

*See Hypothermia*

## Frothy Sputum

*See CHF (Congestive Heart Failure); Pulmonary Edema; Seizure Disorders, Adult; Seizure Disorders, Childhood*

## Fusion, Lumbar

Acute **Pain** r/t discomfort at bone donor site, surgical operation

**Anxiety** r/t fear of surgical procedure, possible recurring problems

Impaired physical **Mobility** r/t limitations from surgical procedure, presence of brace

Ineffective **Health** maintenance r/t deficient knowledge regarding postoperative mobility restrictions, body mechanics

Risk for **Injury** r/t improper body mechanics

Risk for perioperative positioning **Injury** r/t immobilization

# G

## Gag Reflex, Depressed or Absent

Impaired **Swallowing** r/t neuromuscular impairment

Risk for **Aspiration** r/t depressed cough/gag reflex

## Gallop Rhythm

Decreased **Cardiac** output r/t decreased contractility of heart

## Gallstones

*See Cholelithiasis*

## Gangrene

Delayed **Surgical** recovery r/t obstruction of arterial flow

**Fear** r/t possible loss of extremity

Ineffective **Tissue** perfusion: peripheral r/t obstruction of arterial flow

## Gas Exchange, Impaired

Impaired **Gas** exchange r/t ventilation-perfusion imbalance

## Gastric Surgery

Risk for **Injury** r/t inadvertent insertion of nasogastric tube through gastric incision line

*See Abdominal Surgery*

## Gastric Ulcer

*See GI Bleed (Gastrointestinal Bleeding); Ulcer, Peptic*

## Gastritis

Acute **Pain** r/t inflammation of gastric mucosa

Imbalanced **Nutrition**: less than body requirements r/t vomiting, inadequate intestinal absorption of nutrients, restricted dietary regimen

Risk for deficient **Fluid** volume r/t excessive loss from gastrointestinal tract secondary to vomiting, decreased intake

## Gastroenteritis

Acute **Pain** r/t increased peristalsis causing cramping

Deficient **Fluid** volume r/t excessive loss from gastrointestinal tract secondary to diarrhea, vomiting

**Diarrhea** r/t infectious process involving intestinal tract

Imbalanced **Nutrition**: less than body requirements r/t vomiting, inadequate intestinal absorption of nutrients, restricted dietary intake

Ineffective **Health** maintenance r/t deficient knowledge regarding treatment of disease

**Nausea** r/t irritation to gastrointestinal system

*See Gastroenteritis, Child*

## Gastroenteritis, Child

Impaired **Skin** integrity: diaper rash r/t acidic excretions on perineal tissues

Ineffective **Health** maintenance r/t lack of parental knowledge regarding fluid and dietary changes

Risk for delayed **Development** r/t inadequate nutrition

*See Gastroenteritis; Hospitalized Child*

## Gastroesophageal Reflux

Acute **Pain** r/t irritation of esophagus from gastric acids

**Anxiety**: parental r/t possible need for surgical intervention (Nissen fundoplication, gastrostomy tube)

Deficient **Fluid** volume r/t persistent vomiting

Imbalanced **Nutrition**: less than body requirements r/t poor feeding, vomiting

Ineffective **Airway** clearance r/t reflux of gastric contents into esophagus and tracheal or bronchial tree

Ineffective **Health** maintenance r/t deficient knowledge regarding antireflux regimen (e.g., positioning, oral or enteral feeding techniques, medications), possible home apnea monitoring

Risk for **Aspiration** r/t entry of gastric contents in tracheal or bronchial tree

Risk for impaired **Parenting** r/t disruption in bonding secondary to irritable or inconsolable infant

*See Child with Chronic Condition; Hospitalized Child*

## Gastrointestinal Hemorrhage

*See GI Bleed (Gastrointestinal Bleeding)*

## Gastroschisis/Omphalocele

Anticipatory **Grieving** r/t threatened loss of infant, loss of perfect birth or infant secondary to serious medical condition

Impaired **Gas** exchange r/t effects of anesthesia, subsequent atelectasis

Ineffective **Airway** clearance r/t complications of anesthetic effects

Risk for deficient **Fluid** volume r/t inability to feed secondary to condition, subsequent electrolyte imbalance

Risk for **Infection** r/t disrupted skin integrity with exposure of abdominal contents

Risk for **Injury** r/t disrupted skin integrity, ineffective protection

## Gastrostomy

Risk for impaired **Skin** integrity r/t presence of gastric contents on skin

*See Tube Feeding*

## Genital Herpes

*See Herpes Simplex II*

## Genital Warts

*See STD (Sexually Transmitted Disease)*

## Gestational Diabetes (Diabetes in Pregnancy)

**Anxiety** r/t threat to self and/or fetus

Impaired fetal **Nutrition**: more than body requirements r/t excessive glucose uptake

Impaired maternal **Nutrition**: less than body requirements r/t decreased insulin production and glucose uptake in cells

Ineffective **Health** maintenance: maternal r/t deficient knowledge regarding care of diabetic condition in pregnancy

**Powerlessness** r/t lack of control over outcome of pregnancy

Risk for delayed **Development**: fetal r/t endocrine disorder of mother

Risk for disproportionate **Growth**: fetal r/t endocrine disorder of mother

Risk for impaired **Tissue** integrity: fetal r/t macrosomia, congenital defects, birth injury

Risk for impaired **Tissue** integrity: maternal r/t delivery of large infant

*See Diabetes Mellitus*

## GI Bleed (Gastrointestinal Bleeding)

Acute **Pain** r/t irritated mucosa from acid secretion

Deficient **Fluid** volume r/t gastrointestinal bleeding

**Fatigue** r/t loss of circulating blood volume, decreased ability to transport oxygen

**Fear** r/t threat to well-being, potential death

Imbalanced **Nutrition**: less than body requirements r/t nausea, vomiting

Risk for ineffective **Coping** r/t personal vulnerability in crisis, bleeding, hospitalization

## Gingivitis

Impaired **Dentition** r/t ineffective oral hygiene, barriers to self-care

Impaired **Oral** mucous membrane r/t ineffective oral hygiene

## Glaucoma

Deficient **Knowledge** r/t treatment and self-care for disease

Disturbed **Sensory** perception: visual r/t increased intraocular pressure

*See Vision Impairment*

## Glomerulonephritis

Acute **Pain** r/t edema of kidney

Excess **Fluid** volume r/t renal impairment

Imbalanced **Nutrition**: less than body requirements r/t anorexia, restrictive diet

Ineffective **Health** maintenance r/t deficient knowledge regarding care of disease

## Gonorrhea

Acute **Pain** r/t inflammation of reproductive organs

Ineffective **Health** maintenance r/t deficient knowledge regarding treatment and prevention of disease

Risk for **Infection** r/t spread of organism throughout reproductive organs

*See STD (Sexually Transmitted Disease)*

## Gout

Chronic **Pain** r/t inflammation of affected joint

Impaired physical **Mobility** r/t musculoskeletal impairment

Ineffective **Health** maintenance r/t deficient knowledge regarding medications and home care

## Grand Mal Seizure

*See Seizure Disorders, Adult; Seizure Disorders, Childhood*

## Grandiosity

Defensive **Coping** r/t inaccurate perception of self and abilities

## Grandparents Raising Grandchildren

**Anxiety** r/t change in role status

Compromised family **Coping** r/t family role changes

Decisional **Conflict** r/t support system deficit

Ineffective family **Therapeutic** regimen management r/t excessive demands on individual/family

Ineffective **Role** performance r/t role transition

Interrupted **Family** processes r/t family roles shift

Parental role **Conflict** r/t change in parental role

Readiness for enhanced **Parenting** r/t physical and emotional needs of children are met

Risk for impaired **Parenting** r/t role strain

Risk for **Powerlessness** r/t aging

Risk for **Spiritual** distress r/t life change

## Graves' Disease

*See Hyperthyroidism*

## Grieving

Anticipatory **Grieving** r/t anticipated significant loss

Chronic **Sorrow** r/t unresolved grief

Dysfunctional **Grieving** r/t actual or perceived significant loss

**Grieving** r/t actual significant loss; change in life status, style, or function

## Groom Self (Inability to)

Dressing/grooming **Self-care** deficit: r/t intolerance to activity, decreased strength and endurance pain, discomfort, perceptual or cognitive impairment, neuromuscular impairment, musculoskeletal impairment, depression, severe anxiety

## Growth and Development Lag

Delayed **Growth** and development r/t inadequate caretaking, indifference, inconsistent responsiveness, multiple caretakers, separation from significant others, environmental and stimulation deficiencies, effects of physical disability, prescribed dependence

**PRENATAL**

Risk for disproportionate **Growth** r/t congenital/genetic disorders, maternal nutrition, multiple gestation, teratogen exposure, substance use/abuse

**INDIVIDUAL**

Risk for disproportionate **Growth** r/t infection, prematurity, malnutrition, organic and inorganic factors, caregiver and/or individual maladaptive feeding behaviors, anorexia, insatiable appetite, infection, chronic illness, substance abuse

**ENVIRONMENTAL**

Risk for disproportionate **Growth** r/t deprivation, teratogen, lead poisoning, poverty, violence, natural disasters

*See Developmental Concerns*

## Guillain-Barré Syndrome

Impaired spontaneous **Ventilation** r/t weak respiration muscles

*See Neurological Disorders*

## Guilt

Anticipatory **Grieving** r/t potential loss of significant person, animal, prized material possession

Chronic **Sorrow** r/t unresolved grieving

Dysfunctional **Grieving** r/t actual loss of significant person, animal, prized material possession

Readiness for enhanced **Spiritual** well-being r/t desire to be in harmony with self, others, higher power/God

Risk for **Post-trauma** syndrome r/t exaggerated sense of responsibility for traumatic event

**Self-esteem** disturbance r/t unmet expectations of self

# H

## Hair Loss

Disturbed **Body** image r/t psychological reaction to loss of hair

Imbalanced **Nutrition**: less than body requirements r/t inability to ingest food because of biological, psychological, economic factors

## Halitosis

Impaired **Dentition** r/t ineffective oral hygiene

Impaired **Oral** mucous membranes r/t ineffective oral hygiene

## Hallucinations

Acute **Confusion** r/t alcohol abuse, delirium, dementia, mental illness, drug abuse

Adult **Failure** to thrive r/t altered mental status

**Anxiety** r/t threat to self-concept

Disturbed **Thought** processes r/t inability to control bizarre thoughts

Ineffective **Coping** r/t distortion and insecurity of life events

Risk for other-directed **Violence** r/t catatonic excitement, manic excitement, rage/panic reactions, response to violent internal stimuli

Risk for self-directed **Violence** r/t catatonic excitement, manic excitement, rage/panic reactions, response to violent internal stimuli

Risk for **Self-mutilation** r/t command hallucinations

## Head Injury

Acute **Confusion** r/t brain injury

Decreased **Intracranial** adaptive capacity r/t brain injury

Disturbed **Sensory** perception r/t pressure damage to sensory centers in brain

Disturbed **Thought** processes r/t pressure damage to brain

Ineffective **Breathing** pattern r/t pressure damage to breathing center in brain stem

Ineffective **Tissue** perfusion: cerebral r/t effects of increased intracranial pressure

*See Neurological Disorders*

## Headache

Acute **Pain** r/t lack of knowledge of pain control techniques or methods to prevent headaches

Disturbed **Energy** field r/t disharmony

Ineffective management of **Therapeutic** regimen r/t lack of knowledge, identification and elimination of aggravating factors

## Health Maintenance Problems

Ineffective **Health** maintenance r/t significant alteration in communication skills, lack of ability to make deliberate and thoughtful judgments, perceptual or cognitive impairment, ineffective coping, dysfunctional grieving, unachieved developmental tasks, ineffective family coping, disabling spiritual distress, lack of material resources

## Health-Seeking Person

**Health-seeking** behaviors r/t expressed desire for increased control of own personal health

## Hearing Impairment

Disturbed **Sensory** perception: auditory r/t altered state of auditory system

Impaired verbal **Communication** r/t inability to hear own voice

**Social** isolation r/t difficulty with communication

H

## Heart Failure

*See CHF (Congestive Heart Failure)*

## Heart Surgery

*See Coronary Artery Bypass Grafting*

## Heartburn

Acute **Pain**: heartburn r/t gastroesophageal reflux

Ineffective **Health** maintenance r/t deficient knowledge regarding information about factors that cause esophageal reflex

**Nausea** r/t gastrointestinal irritation

Risk for imbalanced **Nutrition**: less than body requirements r/t pain after eating

## Heat Stroke

Chronic **Sorrow** r/t unresolved grief

Deficient **Fluid** volume r/t profuse diaphoresis

Disturbed **Thought** processes r/t hyperthermia, increased oxygen needs

**Hopelessness** r/t prolonged activity restriction creating isolation, failing or deteriorating physiological condition, long-term stress, abandonment, lost belief in transcendent values or higher power/God

**Hyperthermia** r/t vigorous activity, hot environment

**Powerlessness** r/t lifestyle of helplessness

## Hematemesis

*See GI Bleed (Gastrointestinal Bleeding)*

## Hematological Disorder

Ineffective **Protection** r/t abnormal blood profile

*See cause of Hematological Disorder*

## Hematuria

Risk for deficient **Fluid** volume r/t excessive loss of blood through urinary system

## Hemianopia

**Anxiety** r/t change in vision

Disturbed **Sensory** perception r/t altered sensory reception, transmission, integration

Risk for **Injury** r/t disturbed sensory perception

Unilateral **Neglect** r/t effects of disturbed perceptual abilities

## Hemiplegia

**Anxiety** r/t change in health status

Disturbed **Body** image r/t functional loss of one side of body

Impaired physical **Mobility** r/t loss of neurological control of involved extremities

Impaired **Transfer** ability r/t partial paralysis

Impaired **Walking** r/t loss of neurological control of involved extremities

Risk for impaired **Skin** integrity r/t alteration in sensation, immobility

Risk for **Injury** r/t impaired mobility

Risk for unilateral **Neglect** r/t neurological impairment; loss of sensation, vision, movement

**Self-care** deficit: specify r/t neuromuscular impairment

Unilateral **Neglect** r/t effects of disturbed perceptual abilities

*See CVA (Cerebrovascular Accident)*

## Hemodialysis

Excess **Fluid** volume r/t renal disease with minimal urine output

Ineffective **Coping** r/t situational crisis

Ineffective **Health** maintenance r/t deficient knowledge regarding hemodialysis procedure, restrictions, blood access care

Interrupted **Family** processes r/t changes in role responsibilities as a result of therapy regimen

**Noncompliance**: dietary restrictions r/t denial of chronic illness

**Powerlessness** r/t treatment regimen

Risk for **Caregiver** role strain r/t complexity of care receiver treatment

Risk for deficient **Fluid** volume r/t excessive removal of fluid during dialysis

Risk for **Infection** r/t exposure to blood products, risk for developing hepatitis B or C

Risk for **Injury**: clotting of blood access r/t abnormal surface for blood flow

*See Renal Failure; Renal Failure, Acute/Chronic, Child*

## Hemodynamic Monitoring

Risk for **Infection** r/t invasive procedure

Risk for **Injury** r/t inadvertent wedging of catheter, dislodgement of catheter, disconnection of catheter with embolism

## Hemolytic Uremic Syndrome

Deficient **Fluid** volume r/t vomiting, diarrhea

Impaired **Comfort**: nausea/vomiting r/t effects of uremia

Risk for impaired **Skin** integrity r/t diarrhea

Risk for **Injury** r/t decreased platelet count, seizure activity

*See Hospitalized Child; Renal Failure, Acute/Chronic, Child*

## Hemophilia

Acute **Pain** r/t bleeding into body tissues

**Fear** r/t high risk for AIDS secondary to contaminated blood products

Impaired physical **Mobility** r/t pain from acute bleeds, imposed activity restrictions

Ineffective **Health** maintenance r/t knowledge and skill acquisition regarding home administration of intravenous clotting factors, protection from injury

Ineffective **Protection** r/t deficient clotting factors

Risk for **Injury** r/t deficient clotting factors, child's developmental level, age-appropriate play, inappropriate use of toys or sports equipment

*See Child with Chronic Condition; Hospitalized Child; Maturational Issues, Adolescent*

## Hemoptysis

**Fear** r/t serious threat to well-being

Risk for deficient **Fluid** volume r/t excessive loss of blood

Risk for ineffective **Airway** clearance r/t obstruction of airway with blood and mucus

## Hemorrhage

Deficient **Fluid** volume r/t massive blood loss

**Fear** r/t threat to well-being

*See cause of Hemorrhage; Hypovolemic Shock*

## Hemorrhoidectomy

Acute **Pain** r/t surgical procedure

**Anxiety** r/t embarrassment, need for privacy

**Constipation** r/t fear of pain with defecation

Ineffective **Health** maintenance r/t deficient knowledge regarding pain relief, use of stool softeners, dietary changes

Risk for deficient **Fluid** volume: hemorrhage r/t inadequate clotting

**Urinary** retention r/t pain, anesthetic effect

## Hemorrhoids

**Constipation** r/t painful defecation, poor bowel habits

Impaired **Comfort**: pruritus r/t inflammation of hemorrhoids

Ineffective **Health** maintenance r/t deficient knowledge regarding care of condition

## Hemothorax

Deficient **Fluid** volume r/t blood in pleural space

*See Pneumothorax*

## Hepatitis

**Activity** intolerance r/t weakness or fatigue secondary to infection

Acute **Pain** r/t edema of liver, bile irritating skin

Deficient **Diversional** activity r/t isolation

**Fatigue** r/t infectious process, altered body chemistry

Imbalanced **Nutrition**: less than body requirements r/t anorexia, impaired use of proteins and carbohydrates

Ineffective **Health** maintenance r/t deficient knowledge regarding disease process and home management

Risk for deficient **Fluid** volume r/t excessive loss of fluids via vomiting and diarrhea

**Social** isolation r/t treatment-imposed isolation

## Hernia

*See Hiatus Hernia; Inguinal Hernia Repair*

## Herniated Disk

*See Low Back Pain*

## Herniorrhaphy

*See Inguinal Hernia Repair*

## Herpes in Pregnancy

Acute **Pain** r/t active herpes lesion

**Fear** r/t threat to fetus, impending surgery

Impaired **Tissue** integrity r/t active herpes lesion

Impaired **Urinary** elimination r/t pain with urination

Ineffective **Health** maintenance r/t deficient knowledge regarding treatment of disease, protection of fetus

Risk for **Infection:** transmission r/t transplacental transfer during primary herpes, exposure to active herpes during birth process

Situational low **Self-esteem** r/t threat to fetus secondary to disease process

## Herpes Simplex I

Impaired **Dentition** r/t impaired oral mucous membranes

Impaired **Oral** mucous membranes r/t inflammatory changes in mouth

## Herpes Simplex II

Acute **Pain** r/t active herpes lesion

Impaired **Tissue** integrity r/t active herpes lesion

Impaired **Urinary** elimination r/t pain with urination

Ineffective **Health** maintenance r/t deficient knowledge regarding treatment, prevention of spread of disease

**Sexual** dysfunction r/t disease process

Situational low **Self-esteem** r/t expressions of shame or guilt

## Herpes Zoster

*See Shingles*

## HHNC (Hyperosmolar Hyperglycemic Nonketotic Coma)

*See Hyperosmolar Hyperglycemic Nonketotic Coma*

## Hiatus Hernia

Acute **Pain** r/t gastroesophageal reflux

Imbalanced **Nutrition**: less than body requirements r/t pain after eating

Ineffective **Health** maintenance r/t deficient knowledge regarding care of disease

**Nausea** r/t effects of gastric contents in esophagus

## Hip Fracture

Acute **Confusion** r/t sensory overload, sensory deprivation, medication side effects

Acute **Pain** r/t injury, surgical procedure

**Constipation** r/t immobility, narcotics, anesthesia

**Fear** r/t outcome of treatment, future mobility, present helplessness

Impaired physical **Mobility** r/t surgical incision, temporary absence of weight bearing

Impaired **Transfer** ability r/t immobilization of hip

Impaired **Walking** r/t temporary absence of weight bearing

**Powerlessness** r/t health care environment

Risk for deficient **Fluid** volume: hemorrhage r/t postoperative complication, surgical blood loss

Risk for impaired **Skin** integrity r/t immobility

Risk for **Infection** r/t invasive procedure

Risk for **Injury** r/t dislodged prosthesis, unsteadiness when ambulating

Risk for perioperative positioning **Injury** r/t immobilization, muscle weakness, emaciation

**Self-care** deficit: specify r/t musculoskeletal impairment

## Hip Replacement

*See Total Joint Replacement*

## Hirschsprung's Disease

Acute **Pain** r/t distended colon, incisional postoperative pain

**Constipation:** bowel obstruction r/t inhibited peristalsis secondary to congenital absence of parasympathetic ganglion cells in distal colon

**Grieving** r/t loss of perfect child, birth of child with congenital defect even though child expected to be normal within 2 years

Imbalanced **Nutrition**: less than body requirements r/t anorexia, pain from distended colon

Impaired **Skin** integrity r/t stoma, potential skin care problems associated with stoma

Ineffective **Health** maintenance r/t parental deficient knowledge regarding temporary stoma care, dietary management, treatment for constipation or diarrhea

*See Hospitalized Child*

## Hirsutism

Disturbed **Body** image r/t excessive hair

## Hitting Behavior

Acute **Confusion** r/t dementia, alcohol abuse, drug abuse, delirium

Impaired **Adjustment** r/t intense emotional state

Ineffective **Coping** r/t situational crises, maturational crises, personal vulnerability

Risk for other-directed **Violence** r/t history of violence, neurological impairment, cognitive impairment, history of childhood abuse, history of witnessing family violence, cruelty to animals, firesetting, history of alcohol/drug abuse, pathological intoxication, psychotic symptomatology, motor vehicle offenses, impulsivity, availability or possession of weapon, body language

## HIV (Human Immunodeficiency Virus)

**Fear** r/t possible death

Ineffective **Protection** r/t depressed immune system

*See AIDS (Acquired Immune Deficiency Syndrome)*

## Hodgkin's Disease

*See Anemia; Cancer; Chemotherapy*

## Home Maintenance Problems

Impaired **Home** maintenance r/t individual or family member disease or injury, insufficient family organization or planning, insufficient finances, unfamiliarity with neighborhood resources, impaired cognitive or emotional functioning, lack of knowledge, lack of role modeling, inadequate support systems

## Homelessness

Impaired **Home** maintenance r/t impaired cognitive or emotional functioning, inadequate support system, insufficient finances

**Powerlessness** r/t interpersonal interactions

Risk for **Trauma** r/t being in high-crime neighborhood

## Hopelessness

Chronic **Sorrow** r/t unresolved grief

**Hopelessness** r/t prolonged activity restriction creating isolation, failing or deteriorating physiological condition, long-term stress, abandonment, lost belief in transcendent values or higher power/God

**Powerlessness** r/t lifestyle of helplessness

## Hospitalized Child

**Activity** intolerance r/t fatigue associated with acute illness

Acute **Pain** r/t treatments, diagnostic or therapeutic procedures

**Anxiety**: separation (child) r/t familiar surroundings and separation from family and friends

Compromised family **Coping** r/t possible prolonged hospitalization that exhausts supportive capacity of significant people

Deficient **Diversional** activity r/t immobility, monotonous environment, frequent or lengthy treatments, reluctance to participate, therapeutic isolation, separation from peers

Delayed **Growth** and development r/t regression or lack of progression toward developmental milestones secondary to frequent or prolonged hospitalization, inadequate or inappropriate stimulation, cerebral insult, chronic illness, effects of physical disability, prescribed dependence

Disturbed **Sleep** pattern: child or parent r/t 24-hour care needs of hospitalization

**Fear** r/t deficient knowledge or maturational level with fear of unknown, mutilation, painful procedures, surgery

**Hopelessness**: child r/t prolonged activity restriction, uncertain prognosis

Ineffective **Coping**: parent r/t possible guilt regarding hospitalization of child, parental inadequacies

Interrupted **Family** processes r/t situational crisis of illness, disease, hospitalization

**Powerlessness**: child r/t health care environment, illness-related regimen

Readiness for enhanced family **Coping** r/t impact of crisis on family values, priorities, goals, relationships in family

Risk for impaired parent/child **Attachment** r/t separation

Risk for delayed **Growth** and development: regression r/t disruption of normal routine, unfamiliar environment or caregivers, developmental vulnerability of young children

Risk for imbalanced **Nutrition**: less than body requirements r/t anorexia, absence of familiar foods, cultural preferences

Risk for **Injury** r/t unfamiliar environment, developmental age, lack of parental knowledge regarding safety (e.g., side rails, IV site/pole)

## Hostile Behavior

Risk for other-directed **Violence** r/t antisocial personality disorder

## HTN (Hypertension)

Disturbed **Energy** field r/t pain, discomfort

Imbalanced **Nutrition**: more than body requirements r/t lack of knowledge of relationship between diet and disease process

Ineffective **Health** maintenance r/t deficient knowledge regarding treatment and control of disease process

**Noncompliance** r/t side effects of treatments, lack of understanding regarding importance of controlling hypertension

## Human Immunodeficiency Virus (HIV)

*See AIDS (Acquired Immune Deficiency Syndrome); HIV (Human Immunodeficiency Virus)*

## Huntington's Disease

Decisional **Conflict** r/t whether to have children

*See Neurological Disorders*

## Hydrocele

Acute **Pain** r/t severely enlarged hydrocele

Ineffective **Sexuality** pattern r/t recent surgery on area of scrotum

## Hydrocephalus

Decisional **Conflict** r/t unclear or conflicting values regarding selection of treatment modality

Delayed **Growth** and development r/t sequelae of increased intracranial pressure

Excess **Fluid** volume: cerebral ventricles r/t compromised regulatory mechanism

Imbalanced **Nutrition**: less than body requirements r/t inadequate intake secondary to anorexia, nausea, vomiting, feeding difficulties

Impaired **Skin** integrity r/t impaired physical mobility, mechanical irritation

Ineffective **Tissue** perfusion: cerebral r/t interrupted flow, hypervolemia of cerebral ventricles

Interrupted **Family** processes r/t situational crisis

Risk for delayed **Development** r/t sequelae of increased intracranial pressure

Risk for disproportionate **Growth** r/t sequelae of increased intracranial pressure

Risk for **Infection** r/t sequelae of invasive procedure (shunt placement)

*See Normal Pressure Hydrocephalous, Child with Chronic Condition; Hospitalized Child; Mental Retardation (if appropriate); Premature Infant (Child); Premature Infant (Parent)*

## Hygiene, Inability to Provide Own

Adult **Failure** to thrive r/t depression, apathy as evidenced by inability to perform self-care

**Self-care** deficit: bathing/hygiene r/t intolerance to activity, decreased strength and endurance, pain, discomfort, perceptual or cognitive impairment, neuromuscular impairment, musculoskeletal impairment, depression, severe anxiety

## Hyperactive Syndrome

Compromised family **Coping** r/t unsuccessful strategies to control excessive activity, behaviors, frustration, anger

Decisional **Conflict** r/t multiple or divergent sources of information regarding education, nutrition, medication regimens; willingness to change own food habits; limited resources

Impaired **Social** interaction r/t impulsive and overactive behaviors, concomitant emotional difficulties, distractibility and excitability

Ineffective **Role** performance: parent r/t stressors associated with dealing with hyperactive child, perceived or projected blame for causes of child's behavior, unmet needs for support or care, lack of energy to provide for those needs

Parental role **Conflict**: when siblings present r/t increased attention toward hyperactive child

Risk for delayed **Development** r/t behavior disorders

Risk for impaired **Parenting** r/t disruptive or uncontrollable behaviors of child

Risk for other-directed **Violence**: parent or child r/t frustration with disruptive behavior, anger, unsuccessful relationship(s)

**Self-esteem** disturbance r/t inability to achieve socially acceptable behaviors; frustration; frequent reprimands, punishment, or scoldings secondary to uncontrolled activity and behaviors; mood fluctuations and restlessness; inability to succeed academically; lack of peer support

## Hyperalimentation

*See TPN (Total Parenteral Nutrition)*

## Hyperbilirubinemia

**Anxiety**: parent r/t threat to infant, unknown future

Disturbed **Sensory** perception: visual (infant) r/t use of eye patches for protection of eyes during phototherapy

Imbalanced **Nutrition**: less than body requirements (infant) r/t disinterest in feeding because of jaundice-related lethargy

Parental role **Conflict** r/t interruption of family life because of care regimen

Risk for disproportionate **Growth**: infant r/t disinterest in feeding because of jaundice-related lethargy

Risk for **Imbalanced** body temperature: infant r/t phototherapy

Risk for **Injury**: infant r/t kernicterus, phototherapy lights

## Hypercalcemia

Decreased **Cardiac** output r/t bradydysrhythmia

Disturbed **Thought** processes r/t elevated calcium levels that cause paranoia, decreased level of consciousness

Imbalanced **Nutrition**: less than body requirements

r/t gastrointestinal manifestations of hypercalcemia (nausea, anorexia, ileus)

Impaired physical **Mobility** r/t decreased tone in smooth and striated muscle

Risk for **Trauma** r/t risk for fractures

## Hypercapnia

**Fear** r/t difficulty breathing

Impaired **Gas** exchange r/t ventilation perfusion imbalance

## Hyperemesis Gravidarum

**Anxiety** r/t threat to self and infant, hospitalization

Deficient **Fluid** volume r/t vomiting

Imbalanced **Nutrition**: less than body requirements r/t vomiting

Impaired **Home** maintenance r/t chronic nausea, inability to function

**Nausea** r/t hormonal changes of pregnancy

**Powerlessness** r/t health care regimen

**Social** isolation r/t hospitalization

## Hyperglycemia

Ineffective management of **Therapeutic** regimen r/t complexity of therapeutic regimen, decisional conflicts, economic difficulties, nonsupportive family, insufficient cues to action, deficient knowledge, mistrust, lack of acknowledgment of seriousness of condition

*See Diabetes Mellitus*

## Hyperkalemia

Risk for **Activity** intolerance r/t muscle weakness

Risk for decreased **Cardiac** output r/t possible dysrhythmia

Risk for excess **Fluid** volume r/t untreated renal failure

## Hypernatremia

Risk for deficient **Fluid** volume r/t abnormal water loss, inadequate water intake

## Hyperosmolar Hyperglycemic Nonketotic Coma (HHNC)

Deficient **Fluid** volume r/t polyuria, inadequate fluid intake

Disturbed **Thought** processes r/t dehydration, electrolyte imbalance

Risk for **Injury**: seizures r/t hyperosmolar state, electrolyte imbalance

*See Diabetes Mellitus; Diabetes Mellitus, Juvenile*

## Hyperphosphatemia

Deficient **Knowledge** r/t dietary changes needed to control phosphate levels

*See Renal Failure*

## Hypersensitivity to Slight Criticism

Defensive **Coping** r/t situational crisis, psychological impairment, substance abuse

## Hypertension

Imbalanced **Nutrition**: more than body requirements r/t lack of knowledge of relationship between diet and disease process

Ineffective **Health** maintenance r/t deficient knowledge regarding treatment and control of disease process

**Noncompliance** r/t side effects of treatment

## Hyperthermia

**Hyperthermia** r/t exposure to hot environment, vigorous activity, medications, anesthesia, inappropriate clothing, increased metabolic rate, illness, trauma, dehydration, inability or decreased ability to perspire

## Hyperthyroidism

**Activity** intolerance r/t increased oxygen demands from increased metabolic rate

**Anxiety** r/t increased stimulation, loss of control

**Diarrhea** r/t increased gastric motility

Disturbed **Sleep** pattern r/t anxiety, excessive sympathetic discharge

Imbalanced **Nutrition**: less than body requirements r/t increased metabolic rate, increased gastrointestinal activity

Ineffective **Health** maintenance r/t deficient knowledge regarding medications, methods of coping with stress

Risk for **Injury**: eye damage r/t exophthalmos

## Hyperventilation

Ineffective **Breathing** pattern r/t anxiety, acid-base imbalance

## Hypocalcemia

**Activity** intolerance r/t neuromuscular irritability

Imbalanced **Nutrition**: less than body requirements r/t effects of vitamin D deficiency, renal failure, malabsorption, laxative use

Ineffective **Breathing** pattern r/t laryngospasm

## Hypoglycemia

Disturbed **Thought** processes r/t insufficient blood glucose to brain

Imbalanced **Nutrition**: less than body requirements r/t imbalance of glucose and insulin level

Ineffective **Health** maintenance r/t deficient knowledge regarding disease process, self-care

*See Diabetes Mellitus; Diabetes Mellitus, Juvenile*

## Hypokalemia

**Activity** intolerance r/t muscle weakness

Decreased **Cardiac** output r/t possible dysrhythmia from electrolyte imbalance

## Hypomagnesemia

**Imbalanced Nutrition:** less than body requirements r/t deficient knowledge of nutrition, alcoholism

*See Alcoholism*

H

## Hypomania

Disturbed **Sleep** pattern r/t psychological stimulus

*See Manic Disorder, Bipolar I*

## Hyponatremia

Disturbed **Thought** processes r/t electrolyte imbalance

Excess **Fluid** volume r/t excessive intake of hypotonic fluids

Risk for **Injury** r/t seizures, new onset of confusion

## Hypoplastic Left Lung

*See Congenital Heart Disease/Cardiac Anomalies*

## Hypotension

Decreased **Cardiac** output r/t decreased preload, decreased contractility

Disturbed **Thought** processes r/t decreased oxygen supply to brain

Ineffective **Tissue** perfusion: cardiopulmonary/peripheral r/t hypovolemia, decreased contractility, decreased afterload

Risk for deficient **Fluid** volume r/t excessive fluid loss

*See cause of Hypotension*

## Hypothermia

**Hypothermia** r/t exposure to cold environment, illness, trauma, damage to hypothalamus, malnutrition, aging

## Hypothyroidism

**Activity** intolerance r/t muscular stiffness, shortness of breath on exertion

**Constipation** r/t decreased gastric motility

Disturbed **Thought** processes r/t altered metabolic process

Imbalanced **Nutrition**: more than body requirements r/t decreased metabolic process

Impaired **Gas** exchange r/t possible respiratory depression

Impaired **Skin** integrity r/t edema, dry or scaly skin

Ineffective **Health** maintenance r/t deficient knowledge regarding disease process and self-care

## Hypovolemic Shock

Deficient **Fluid** volume r/t trauma, third spacing, loss of fluid from body

*See Shock*

## Hypoxia

Acute **Confusion** r/t decreased oxygen supply to brain

Disturbed **Thought** processes r/t decreased oxygen supply to brain

**Fear** r/t breathlessness

Impaired **Gas** exchange r/t altered oxygen supply, inability to transport oxygen

## Hysterectomy

Acute **Pain** r/t surgical injury

Anticipatory **Grieving** r/t change in body image, loss of reproductive status

**Constipation** r/t opioids, anesthesia, bowel manipulation during surgery

Ineffective **Coping** r/t situational crisis of surgery

Ineffective **Health** maintenance r/t deficient knowledge regarding precautions and self-care following surgery

Risk for **Constipation** r/t narcotics, anesthesia, bowel manipulation during surgery

Risk for deficient **Fluid** volume r/t abnormal blood loss, hemorrhage

Risk for ineffective **Tissue** perfusion r/t thromboembolism

Risk for urge urinary **Incontinence** r/t edema in area, anesthesia, narcotics, pain

Risk for **Urinary** retention r/t edema in area, anesthesia, opioids, pain

**Sexual** dysfunction r/t disturbance in self-concept

*See Surgery, Perioperative; Surgery, Preoperative; Surgery, Postoperative*

# I

## IBS (Irritable Bowel Syndrome)

Chronic **Pain** r/t spasms, increased motility of bowel

**Constipation** r/t low-residue diet, stress

**Diarrhea** r/t increased motility of intestines associated with stress

Ineffective **Health** maintenance r/t deficient knowledge regarding self-care with IBS

Ineffective **Therapeutic** regimen management r/t deficient knowledge, powerlessness

Readiness for enhanced **Therapeutic** regimen management r/t an expressed desire to manage illness and prevent onset of symptoms

## ICD (Implantable Cardioverter/ Defibrillator)

Ineffective **Health** maintenance r/t deficient knowledge regarding self-care, action of internal cardiac defibrillator

Decreased **Cardiac** output r/t possible dysrhythmia

## IDDM (Insulin-Dependent Diabetes)

*See Diabetes Mellitus*

## Identity Disturbance

Disturbed personal **Identity** r/t situational crisis, psychological impairment, chronic illness, pain

Readiness for enhanced **Coping** r/t seeking social support

**Spiritual** distress r/t expression of alienation from others

## Idiopathic Thrombocytopenic Purpura

*See ITP (Idiopathic Thrombocytopenic Purpura)*

## Ileal Conduit

Deficient **Knowledge** r/t care of stoma

Disturbed **Body** image r/t presence of stoma

Ineffective **Sexuality** patterns r/t altered body function and structure

Ineffective **Therapeutic** regimen management r/t new skills required to care for appliance and self

Readiness for enhanced **Therapeutic** regimen management r/t expressed desire to care for stoma

Risk for impaired **Skin** integrity r/t difficulty obtaining tight seal of appliance

Risk for latex **Allergy** response r/t repeated exposures to latex associated with treatment and management of disease

**Social** isolation r/t alteration in physical appearance, fear of accidental spill of ostomy contents

## Ileostomy

Chronic **Sorrow** r/t physical changes associated with presence of stoma

**Constipation/Diarrhea** r/t dietary changes, change in intestinal motility

Deficient **Knowledge** r/t limited practice of stoma care, dietary modifications

Disturbed **Body** image r/t presence of stoma

Ineffective **Sexuality** patterns r/t altered body function and structure

Ineffective **Therapeutic** regimen management r/t new skills required to care for appliance and self

Risk for impaired **Skin** integrity r/t difficulty obtaining tight seal of appliance, caustic drainage

**Social** isolation r/t alteration in physical appearance, fear of accidental spill of ostomy contents

## Ileus

Acute **Pain** r/t pressure, abdominal distention

**Constipation** r/t decreased gastric motility

Deficient **Fluid** volume r/t loss of fluids from vomiting, fluids trapped in bowel

**Nausea** r/t gastrointestinal irritation

## Immobility

Adult **Failure** to thrive r/t limited physical mobility

**Constipation** r/t immobility

Disturbed **Thought** processes r/t sensory deprivation from immobility

Impaired physical **Mobility** r/t medically imposed bedrest

Impaired **Transfer** ability r/t limited physical mobility

Impaired **Walking** r/t limited physical mobility

Ineffective **Breathing** pattern r/t inability to deep breath in supine position

Ineffective **Tissue** perfusion: peripheral r/t interruption of venous flow

**Powerlessness** r/t forced immobility from health care environment

Risk for **Disuse** syndrome r/t immobilization

Risk for impaired **Skin** integrity r/t pressure on immobile parts, shearing forces when moved

## Immunosuppression

Ineffective **Protection** r/t medications, treatments or pathology suppressing immune system function

Risk for **Infection** r/t immunosuppression

## Impaction of Stool

**Constipation** r/t decreased fluid intake, less than adequate amounts of fiber and bulk-forming foods in diet, medication effect, or immobility

Readiness for enhanced **Therapeutic** regimen management r/t to appropriate nutritional choices to prevent constipation

## Imperforate Anus

**Anxiety** r/t ability to care for newborn

Deficient **Knowledge** r/t home care for newborn

Impaired **Skin** integrity r/t pruritus

Risk for impaired **Skin** integrity r/t presence of stool at surgical repair site

## Impetigo

Ineffective **Health** maintenance r/t parental deficient knowledge regarding care of impetigo

*See Communicable Diseases, Childhood*

## Implantable Cardioverter/ Defibrillator

*See ICD (Implantable Cardioverter/Defibrillator)*

## Impotence

Readiness for enhanced **Knowledge** of treatment information for erectile dysfunction

**Self-esteem** disturbance r/t physiological crisis, inability to practice usual sexual activity

**Sexual** dysfunction r/t altered body function

## Inactivity

**Activity** intolerance r/t imbalance between oxygen supply and demand, sedentary lifestyle, weakness, immobility

Impaired physical **Mobility** r/t intolerance to activity, decreased strength and endurance, depression, severe anxiety, musculoskeletal impairment, perceptual or cognitive impairment, neuromuscular impairment, pain, discomfort

Risk for **Constipation** r/t insufficient physical activity

## Incompetent Cervix

*See Premature Dilation of the Cervix*

## Incontinence of Stool

**Bowel** incontinence r/t decreased awareness of need to defecate, loss of sphincter control

Deficient **Knowledge** r/t lack of information on normal bowel elimination

Disturbed **Body** image r/t inability to control elimination of stool

Risk for impaired **Skin** integrity r/t presence of stool

Situational low **Self-esteem** r/t inability to control elimination of stool

Toileting **Self-care** deficit r/t toileting needs

## Incontinence of Urine

Functional **Incontinence** r/t altered environment; sensory, cognitive, or mobility deficits

Reflex **Incontinence** r/t neurological impairment

Risk for impaired **Skin** integrity r/t presence of urine

Risk for urge urinary **Incontinence** r/t effects of alcohol, caffeine, decreased bladder capacity, irritation of bladder stretch receptors causing spasm, increased urine concentration, overdistention of bladder

Toileting **Self-care** deficit r/t toileting needs

Situational low **Self-esteem** r/t inability to control passage of urine

Stress urinary **Incontinence** r/t degenerative change in pelvic muscles and structural supports associated with increased age, high intraabdominal pressure (e.g., from obesity, gravid uterus), incompetent bladder outlet, overdistention between voidings, weak pelvic muscles and structural supports

Total urinary **Incontinence** r/t neuropathy preventing transmission of reflex indicating bladder fullness, neurological dysfunction causing triggering of micturition at unpredictable times, independent contraction of detrusor reflex resulting from surgery, trauma or disease affecting spinal cord nerves, anatomical fistula

Urge urinary **Incontinence** r/t decreased bladder capacity (i.e., history of pelvic inflammatory disease, abdominal surgeries, indwelling urinary catheter), irritation of bladder stretch receptors causing spasm (e.g., bladder infection), alcohol, caffeine, increased fluids, increased urine concentration, overdistention of bladder

## Indigestion

Imbalanced **Nutrition**: less than body requirements r/t discomfort when eating

Impaired **Comfort** r/t burning, bloating, heaviness, unpleasant sensations experienced when eating

**Nausea** r/t gastrointestinal irritation

## Induction of Labor

**Anxiety** r/t medical interventions

Decisional **Conflict** r/t perceived threat to idealized birth

Ineffective **Coping** r/t situational crisis of medical intervention in birthing process

Readiness for enhanced **Family** processes r/t family support during induction of labor

Risk for imbalanced **Fluid** volume r/t intravenous fluid therapy

Risk for **Injury**: maternal and fetal r/t hypertonic uterus, potential prematurity of newborn

**Self-esteem** disturbance r/t inability to carry out normal labor

## Infant Apnea

*See Premature Infant; Respiratory Conditions of the Neonate; SIDS (Sudden Infant Death Syndrome)*

## Infant Behavior

Disorganized **Infant** behavior r/t pain, oral/motor problems, feeding intolerance, environmental overstimulation, lack of containment/boundaries, prematurity, invasive/painful procedures

Readiness for enhanced organized **Infant** behavior r/t prematurity, pain

Risk for disorganized **Infant** behavior r/t pain, oral/motor problems, environmental overstimulation, lack of containment/boundaries

## Infant Feeding Pattern, Ineffective

Disorganized **Infant** behavior r/t prematurity, immature neurological system

Impaired **Swallowing** r/t prematurity

Ineffective **Infant** feeding pattern r/t prematurity, neurological impairment or delay, oral hypersensitivity, prolonged NPO

Risk for imbalanced **Fluid** volume r/t intravenous fluid therapy, inadequate intake or absorption of fluids, regurgitation

## Infant of Diabetic Mother

Deficient **Fluid** volume r/t increased urinary excretion and osmotic diuresis

Delayed **Growth** and development r/t prolonged and severe postnatal hypoglycemia

Imbalanced **Nutrition**: less than body requirements r/t hypotonia, lethargy, poor sucking, postnatal metabolic changes from hyperglycemia to hypoglycemia and hyperinsulinism

Risk for decreased **Cardiac** output r/t increased incidence of cardiomegaly

Risk for delayed **Development** r/t prolonged and severe postnatal hypoglycemia

Risk for disproportionate **Growth** r/t prolonged and severe postnatal hypoglycemia

Risk for impaired **Gas** exchange r/t increased incidence of cardiomegaly, prematurity

*See Premature Infant; Respiratory Conditions of the Neonate*

## Infant of Substance-Abusing Mother (Fetal Alcohol Syndrome, Crack Baby, Other Drug Withdrawal Infants)

Delayed **Growth** and development r/t effects of maternal use of drugs, effects of neurological impairment, decreased attentiveness to environmental stimuli or inadequate stimuli

**Diarrhea** r/t effects of withdrawal, increased peristalsis secondary to hyperirritability

Disturbed **Sensory** perception r/t hypersensitivity to environmental stimuli

Disturbed **Sleep** pattern r/t hyperirritability/ hypersensitivity to environmental stimuli

Imbalanced **Nutrition**: less than body requirements r/t feeding problems; uncoordinated or ineffective suck and swallow; effects of diarrhea, vomiting, or colic associated with maternal substance abuse

Impaired **Parenting** r/t impaired or absent attachment behaviors, inadequate support systems

Ineffective **Airway** clearance r/t pooling of secretions secondary to lack of adequate cough reflex, effects of viral or bacterial lower airway infection secondary to altered protective state

Ineffective **Infant** feeding pattern r/t uncoordinated or ineffective sucking reflex

Ineffective **Protection** r/t effects of maternal substance abuse

Interrupted **Breastfeeding** r/t use of drugs or alcohol by mother

Risk for delayed **Development** r/t substance abuse

Risk for disproportionate **Growth** r/t substance abuse

Risk for **Infection**: skin, meningeal, respiratory r/t effects of withdrawal

*See Cerebral Palsy; Failure to Thrive, Nonorganic; Hospitalized Child; Hyperactive Syndrome; SIDS (Sudden Infant Death Syndrome)*

## Infantile Polyarteritis

*See Kawasaki Syndrome*

## Infantile Spasms

*See Seizure Disorders, Childhood*

## Infection

**Hyperthermia** r/t increased metabolic rate

Ineffective **Protection** r/t inadequate nutrition, abnormal blood profiles, drug therapies, treatments

## Infection, Potential for

Risk for **Infection** r/t inadequate primary defenses (e.g., broken skin, traumatized tissue, decrease in ciliary action, stasis of body fluids, change in pH secretions, altered peristalsis), inadequate secondary defenses (e.g., decreased hemoglobin, leukopenia suppressed inflammatory response), immunosuppression, inadequate acquired immunity, tissue destruction and increased environmental exposure, chronic disease, invasive procedures, malnutrition, pharmaceutical agents, trauma, rupture of amniotic membranes, insufficient knowledge to avoid exposure to pathogens

## Infertility

Chronic **Sorrow** r/t inability to conceive a child

Ineffective **Therapeutic** regimen management r/t deficient knowledge about infertility

**Powerlessness** r/t infertility

Risk for **Powerlessness** r/t inability to conceive a child

**Spiritual** distress r/t inability to conceive a child

## Inflammatory Bowel Disease (Child and Adult)

Acute **Pain** r/t abdominal cramping and anal irritation

Deficient **Fluid** volume r/t frequent and loose stools

**Diarrhea** r/t effects of inflammatory changes of the bowel

Imbalanced **Nutrition**: less than body requirements r/t anorexia, decreased absorption of nutrients from gastrointestinal tract

Impaired **Skin** integrity r/t frequent stools, development of anal fissures

Ineffective **Coping** r/t repeated episodes of diarrhea

**Social** isolation r/t diarrhea

*See Child with Chronic Condition; Crohn's Disease; Hospitalized Child; Maturational Issues, Adolescent*

## Influenza

Acute **Pain** r/t inflammatory changes in joints

Deficient **Fluid** volume r/t inadequate fluid intake

**Hyperthermia** r/t infectious process

Ineffective **Health** maintenance r/t deficient knowledge regarding self-care

Ineffective **Therapeutic** regimen management r/t lack of knowledge regarding preventive immunizations

Readiness for enhanced **Knowledge** of information to prevent influenza

## Inguinal Hernia Repair

Acute **Pain** r/t surgical procedure

Impaired physical **Mobility** r/t pain at surgical site and fear of causing hernia to "break open"

Risk for **Infection** r/t surgical procedure

**Urinary** retention r/t possible edema at surgical site

## Injury

Risk for **Falls** r/t orthostatic hypertension, impaired physical mobility, diminished mental status

Risk for **Injury** r/t environmental conditions interacting with client's adaptive and defensive resources

## Insomnia

**Anxiety** r/t actual or perceived loss of sleep

Disturbed **Sleep** pattern r/t sensory alterations, internal factors, external factors

**Sleep** deprivation r/t sustained inadequate sleep hygiene, prolonged use of pharmacological agents, aging-related sleep stage shifts

## Insulin Shock

*See Hypoglycemia*

## Intermittent Claudication

Acute **Pain** r/t decreased circulation to extremities with activity

Deficient **Knowledge** r/t lack of knowledge of cause and treatment of peripheral vascular diseases

Ineffective **Tissue** perfusion: peripheral r/t interruption of arterial flow

Readiness for enhanced **Knowledge** of prevention of pain and impaired circulation

Risk for **Injury** r/t tissue hypoxia

Risk for **Peripheral** neurovascular dysfunction r/t disruption in arterial flow

*See Peripheral Vascular Disease*

## Internal Cardioverter/Defibrillator

*See ICD (Implantable Cardioverter/Defibrillator)*

## Internal Fixation

Impaired **Walking** r/t repair of fracture

Risk for **Infection** r/t traumatized tissue, broken skin

*See Fracture*

## Interstitial Cystitis

Acute **Pain** r/t inflammatory process

Impaired **Urinary** elimination r/t inflammation of bladder

Risk for **Infection** r/t suppressed inflammatory response

Risk for urge urinary **Incontinence** r/t effects of alcohol, caffeine, decreased bladder capacity, irritation of bladder stretch receptors causing spasm, increased urine concentration, overdistention of bladder

## Intervertebral Disk Excision

*See Laminectomy*

## Intestinal Obstruction

*See Ileus*

## Intoxication

Acute **Confusion** r/t alcohol abuse

**Anxiety** r/t loss of control of actions

Disturbed **Sensory** perception r/t neurochemical imbalance in brain

Disturbed **Thought** processes r/t effect of substance on central nervous system

Impaired **Memory** r/t effects of alcohol on mind

Ineffective **Coping** r/t use of mind-altering substances as a means of coping

Risk for **Falls** r/t diminished mental status

Risk for other-directed **Violence** r/t inability to control thoughts and actions

## Intraaortic Balloon Counterpulsation

**Anxiety** r/t device providing cardiovascular assistance

Compromised family **Coping** r/t seriousness of significant other's medical condition

Decreased **Cardiac** output r/t failing heart needing counterpulsation

Impaired physical **Mobility** r/t restriction of movement because of mechanical device

Risk for **Peripheral** neurovascular dysfunction r/t vascular obstruction of balloon catheter, thrombus formation, emboli, edema

## Intracranial Pressure, Increased

Acute **Confusion** r/t increased intracranial pressure

Adult **Failure** to thrive r/t undetected changes from increased intracranial pressure

Decreased **Intracranial** adaptive capacity r/t sustained increase in intracranial pressure

Disturbed **Sensory** perception r/t pressure damage to sensory centers in brain

Disturbed **Thought** processes r/t pressure damage to brain

Impaired **Memory** r/t neurological disturbance

Ineffective **Breathing** pattern r/t pressure damage to breathing center in brain stem

Ineffective **Tissue** perfusion: cerebral r/t effects of increased intracranial pressure

*See cause of Increased Intracranial Pressure*

## Intrauterine Growth Retardation

**Anxiety**: maternal r/t threat to fetus

Delayed **Growth** and development r/t insufficient supply of oxygen and nutrients

Imbalanced **Nutrition**: less than body requirements r/t insufficient placenta

Impaired **Gas** exchange r/t insufficient placental perfusion

Ineffective **Coping**: maternal r/t situational crisis, threat to fetus

Risk for delayed **Development** r/t insufficient supply of oxygen and nutrients

Risk for disproportionate **Growth** r/t insufficient supply of oxygen and nutrients

Risk for **Injury** r/t insufficient supply of oxygen and nutrients

Risk for **Powerlessness** r/t unknown outcome of fetus

Situational low **Self-esteem**: maternal r/t guilt about threat to fetus

**Spiritual** distress r/t unknown outcome of fetus

## Intubation, Endotracheal or Nasogastric

Acute **Pain** r/t presence of tube

Disturbed **Body** image r/t altered appearance with mechanical devices

Imbalanced **Nutrition**: less than body requirements r/t inability to ingest food resulting from presence of tubes

Impaired **Oral** mucous membrane r/t presence of tubes

Impaired verbal **Communication** r/t endotracheal tube

## Irregular Pulse

*See Dysrhythmia*

## Irritable Bowel Syndrome

*See IBS (Irritable Bowel Syndrome)*

## Isolation

Adult **Failure** to thrive r/t depression

Risk for **Loneliness** r/t lack of affection, physical isolation, cathectic deprivation, social isolation

Risk for situational low **Self-esteem** r/t decreased power, control over environment

**Social** isolation r/t factors contributing to absence of satisfying personal relationships, such as delay in accomplishing developmental tasks, immature interests, alterations in mental status, unacceptable social behavior, unacceptable social values, altered state of wellness, inadequate personal resources, inability to engage in satisfying personal relationships

## Itching

Impaired **Comfort** r/t irritation of the skin

Risk for **Infection** r/t potential break in skin

## ITP (Idiopathic Thrombocytopenic Purpura)

Deficient **Diversional** activity r/t activity restrictions, safety precautions

Impaired **Home** health maintenance r/t parental lack of ability to follow through with safety precautions secondary to child's developmental stage (active toddler)

Ineffective **Protection** r/t decreased platelet count

Risk for **Injury** r/t decreased platelet count, developmental level, age-appropriate play

*See Hospitalized Child*

# J

## Jaundice

Disturbed **Thought** processes r/t toxic blood metabolites

Impaired **Comfort**: pruritus r/t toxic metabolites excreted in the skin

Risk for impaired **Skin** integrity r/t pruritus, itching

*See Cirrhosis; Hepatitis*

## Jaundice, Neonatal

Readiness for enhanced **Knowledge** of information on assessing jaundice when infant is discharged from the hospital, when to call the physician and possible preventive measures such as frequent breastfeeding

*See Hyperbilirubinemia*

## Jaw Pain and Heart Attacks

*See Chest Pain; MI (Myocardial Infarction)*

## Jaw Surgery

Acute **Pain** r/t surgical procedure

Deficient **Knowledge** r/t emergency care for wired jaws (e.g., cutting bands and wires), oral care

Imbalanced **Nutrition**: less than body requirements r/t jaws wired closed

Impaired **Swallowing** r/t edema from surgery

Risk for **Aspiration** r/t wired jaws

## Jet Lag Prevention

Readiness for enhanced **Knowledge** of getting adequate sleep prior to travel, drinking extra water and avoiding caffeine and alcohol, engaging in regular exercise but not at bedtime

## Jittery

**Anxiety** r/t unconscious conflict about essential values and goals, threat to or change in health status

Death **Anxiety** r/t unresolved issues relating to end of life

Risk for **Post-trauma** syndrome r/t occupation, survivor's role in event, inadequate social support

## Jock Itch

Impaired **Skin** integrity r/t moisture and irritating or tight-fitting clothing

Ineffective **Therapeutic** regimen management r/t prevention and treatment

*See Itching*

## Joint Inflammation

*See Arthritis*

## Joint Pain

*See Arthritis; Bursitis; JRA (Juvenile Rheumatoid Arthritis); Osteoarthritis; Rheumatoid Arthritis*

## Joint Replacement

Risk for **Peripheral** neurovascular dysfunction r/t orthopedic surgery

*See Total Joint Replacement*

## JRA (Juvenile Rheumatoid Arthritis)

Acute **Pain** r/t swollen or inflamed joints, restricted movement, physical therapy

Delayed **Growth** and development r/t effects of physical disability, chronic illness

**Fatigue** r/t chronic inflammatory disease

Impaired physical **Mobility** r/t pain, restricted joint movement

Risk for impaired **Skin** integrity r/t splints, adaptive devices

Risk for **Injury** r/t impaired physical mobility, splints, adaptive devices, increased bleeding potential secondary to antiinflammatory medications

Risk for situational low **Self-esteem** r/t disturbed body image

**Self-care** deficits: feeding, bathing/hygiene, dressing/grooming, toileting r/t restricted joint movement, pain

*See Child with Chronic Condition; Hospitalized Child*

## Juvenile Onset Diabetes

*See Diabetes Mellitus, Juvenile*

# K

## Kaposi's Sarcoma

Risk for dysfunctional **Grieving** r/t preloss psychological symptoms associated with unknown prognosis and outcome of disease

Risk for impaired **Religiosity** r/t illness/hospitalization

*See AIDS (Acquired Immune Deficiency Syndrome)*

## Kawasaki Syndrome (Formerly Mucocutaneous Lymph Node Syndrome)

Acute **Pain** r/t enlarged lymph nodes; erythematous skin rash that progresses to desquamation, peeling, denuding of skin

**Anxiety**: parental r/t progression of disease, complications of arthritis and cardiac involvement

**Hyperthermia** r/t inflammatory disease process

Imbalanced **Nutrition**: less than body requirements r/t impaired oral mucous membrane

Impaired **Oral** mucous membrane r/t inflamed mouth and pharynx; swollen lips that become dry, cracked, fissured

Impaired **Skin** integrity r/t inflammatory skin changes

*See Hospitalized Child*

## Kegel Exercise

**Health**-seeking behavior r/t desire for information to relieve incontinence

Risk for urge urinary **Incontinence** r/t effects of alcohol, caffeine, decreased bladder capacity, irritation of bladder stretch receptors causing spasm, increased urine concentration, overdistention of bladder

Stress urinary **Incontinence** r/t degenerative change in pelvic muscles

Urge urinary **Incontinence** r/t decreased bladder capacity

## Keloids

Disturbed **Body** image r/t presence of scar tissue at site of a healed skin injury

Readiness for enhanced **Therapeutic** regimen management r/t desire to have information to decrease discoloration of skin from sun exposure: covering the area and using sunblock at least 6 months after the injury or surgery for an adult and 18 months for a child

## Keratoconjunctivitis Sicca

Risk for **Infection** r/t dry eyes

*See Conjunctivitis*

## Keratoplasty

*See Corneal Transplant*

## Ketoacidosis, Diabetic

Deficient **Fluid** volume r/t excess excretion of urine, nausea, vomiting, increased respiration

Imbalanced **Nutrition**: less than body requirements r/t body's inability to use nutrients

Impaired **Memory** r/t fluid and electrolyte imbalance

Ineffective **Therapeutic** regimen management r/t denial of illness, lack of understanding of preventive measures and adequate blood sugar control

**Noncompliance**: diabetic regimen r/t ineffective coping with chronic disease

Risk for **Powerlessness** r/t illness-related regimen

*See Diabetes Mellitus*

## Ketoacidosis: Alcoholic

*See Alcohol Withdrawal; Alcoholism*

## Keyhole Heart Surgery

*See MIDCAB (Minimally Invasive Direct Coronary Bypass)*

## Kidney Failure

*See Renal Failure*

## Kidney Stone

Acute **Pain** r/t obstruction from renal calculi

Deficient **Knowledge** r/t fluid requirements and dietary restrictions

Impaired **Urinary** elimination: urgency and frequency r/t anatomical obstruction, irritation caused by stone

Risk for deficient **Fluid** volume r/t nausea, vomiting

Risk for **Infection** r/t obstruction of urinary tract with stasis of urine

## Kidney Tumor

*See Wilms' Tumor*

## Kidney Transplant

Decisional **Conflict** r/t acceptance of donor kidney

Ineffective **Protection** r/t immunosuppressive therapy

Readiness for enhanced **Family** processes r/t adapting to life without dialysis

Readiness for enhanced **Spiritual** well-being r/t heightened coping, living without dialysis

Readiness for enhanced **Therapeutic** regimen management r/t desire to manage the treatment and prevention of complications post transplant

*See Surgery, Perioperative Care; Surgery, Postoperative Care; Surgery, Preoperative Care*

## Kissing Disease

*See Mononucleosis*

## Knee Replacement

*See Total Joint Replacement*

L

## Knowledge

Readiness for enhanced **Knowledge** of (specify) r/t the following: expresses an interest in learning, explains knowledge of the topic, displays behaviors congruent with expressed knowledge, describes previous experiences pertaining to the topic

## Knowledge, Deficient

Deficient **Knowledge** r/t lack of exposure, lack of recall, information misinterpretation, cognitive limitation, lack of interest in learning, unfamiliarity with information resources

Ineffective **Health** maintenance r/t lack of or significant alteration in communication skills (written, verbal, and/or gestural)

Ineffective **Therapeutic** regimen management r/t complexity of therapeutic regimen

## Kock Pouch

*See Continent Ileostomy*

## Korsakoff's Syndrome

Acute **Confusion** r/t alcohol abuse

Dysfunctional **Family** processes: alcoholism r/t possible cause of syndrome

Impaired **Memory** r/t neurological changes

Risk for **Falls** r/t cognitive impairment

Risk for imbalanced **Nutrition**: less than body requirements r/t lack of adequate balanced intake

Risk for **Injury** r/t sensory dysfunction, lack of coordination when ambulating

# L

## Labor, Induction of

*See Induction of Labor*

## Labor, Normal

Acute **Pain** r/t uterine contractions, stretching of cervix and birth canal

**Anxiety** r/t fear of the unknown, situational crisis

Death **Anxiety** r/t threat of maternal mortality

Deficient **Knowledge** r/t lack of preparation for labor

**Fatigue** r/t childbirth

**Health**-seeking behaviors r/t healthy outcome of pregnancy, prenatal care, and childbirth education

Impaired **Tissue** integrity r/t passage of infant through birth canal, episiotomy

Readiness for enhanced family **Coping** r/t significant other providing support during labor

Risk for deficient **Fluid** volume r/t excessive loss of blood

Risk for **Infection** r/t multiple vaginal examinations, tissue trauma, prolonged rupture of membranes

Risk for **Injury**: fetal r/t hypoxia

Risk for **Post-trauma** syndrome r/t trauma or violence associated with labor pains, birth process, medical/surgical interventions, history of sexual abuse

Risk for **Powerlessness** r/t labor process

## Labyrinthitis

Risk for **Injury** r/t dizziness

Ineffective **Therapeutic** regimen management r/t delay in seeking treatment for respiratory and ear infections

Readiness for enhanced **Therapeutic** regimen management r/t management of episodes: keep still and rest during attacks, gradually resume activity, avoid sudden position changes, do not try to read during attacks, avoid bright lights.

## Lactation

*See Breastfeeding, Effective; Breastfeeding, Ineffective; Breastfeeding, Interrupted*

## Lactose Intolerance

Readiness for enhanced **Knowledge** r/t interest in identifying lactose intolerance, treatment, and substitutes for mild products

*See Abdominal Distention; Diarrhea*

## Laminectomy

Acute **Pain** r/t localized inflammation and edema

**Anxiety** r/t change in health status, surgical procedure

Deficient **Knowledge** r/t appropriate postoperative and postdischarge activities

Disturbed **Sensory** perception: tactile r/t possible edema or nerve injury

Impaired physical **Mobility** r/t neuromuscular impairment

Risk for impaired **Tissue** perfusion r/t edema, hemorrhage, or embolism

Risk for perioperative positioning **Injury** r/t prone position

**Urinary** retention r/t competing sensory impulses, effects of narcotics/anesthesia

*See Scoliosis; Surgery, Perioperative; Surgery, Postoperative; Surgery, Preoperative*

## Laparoscopic Laser Cholecystectomy

*See Cholecystectomy; Laser Surgery*

## Laparoscopy

Acute **Pain**: shoulder r/t gas irritating the diaphragm

Urge urinary **Incontinence** r/t pressure on the bladder from gas

## Laparotomy

*See Abdominal Surgery*

## Laryngectomy

Anticipatory **Grieving** r/t loss of voice, fear of death

Chronic **Sorrow** r/t change in body image

Death **Anxiety** r/t unknown results of surgery

Disturbed **Body** image r/t change in body structure and function

Imbalanced **Nutrition**: less than body requirements r/t absence of oral feeding, difficulty swallowing, increased need for fluids

Impaired **Oral** mucous membrane r/t absence of oral feeding

Impaired **Swallowing** r/t edema, laryngectomy tube

Impaired verbal **Communication** r/t removal of larynx

Ineffective **Airway** clearance r/t surgical removal of glottis, decreased humidification of air

Ineffective **Health** maintenance r/t deficient knowledge regarding self-care with laryngectomy

Interrupted **Family** processes r/t surgery, serious condition of family member, difficulty communicating

Risk for dysfunctional **Grieving** r/t loss and major life event

Risk for **Infection** r/t invasive procedure, surgery

Risk for **Powerlessness** r/t chronic illness, change in communication

Risk for situational low **Self-esteem** r/t disturbed body image

## Laser Surgery

Acute **Pain** r/t heat from laser

**Constipation** r/t laser intervention in vulval and perianal areas

Deficient **Knowledge** r/t preoperative and postoperative care associated with laser procedure

Risk for **Infection** r/t delayed heating reaction of tissue exposed to laser

Risk for **Injury** r/t accidental exposure to laser beam

## LASIK Eye Surgery (Laser-Assisted *In Situ* Keratomileusis)

Decisional **Conflict** r/t decision to have the surgery

Readiness for enhanced **Therapeutic** regimen management r/t preexamination preparation, contact lens wearing, surgical procedure pre- and postoperative teaching and expectations

## Latex Allergy

Latex **Allergy** r/t hypersensitivity to natural latex rubber

Readiness for enhanced **Knowledge** of prevention and treatment of exposure to latex products

Risk for latex **Allergy** response r/t multiple surgical procedures, especially from infancy (e.g., spina bifida); allergies to bananas, avocados, tropical fruits, kiwi fruit, chestnuts; professions with daily exposure to latex (e.g., medicine, nursing, dentistry); conditions needing continuous or intermittent catheterization; history of reactions to latex (e.g., balloons, condoms, gloves); allergies to poinsettia plants; history of allergies and asthma

## Laxative Abuse

Perceived **Constipation** r/t health belief, faulty appraisal, impaired thought processes

## Lead Poisoning

Impaired **Home** maintenance r/t presence of lead paint

Risk for delayed **Development** r/t lead poisoning

## Legionnaires' Disease

Ineffective community **Therapeutic** regimen management r/t contaminated air systems in large buildings

Risk for **Infection** r/t increased environmental exposure to pathogens (contaminated water in air-conditioning systems and sometimes showers)

*See Pneumonia*

## Lens Implant

*See Cataract Extraction; Vision Impairment*

## Lethargy/Listlessness

Adult **Failure** to thrive r/t apathy

Disturbed **Sleep** pattern r/t internal or external stressors

**Fatigue** r/t decreased metabolic energy production

Ineffective **Tissue** perfusion: cerebral r/t lack of oxygen supply to brain

*See cause of Lethargy/Listlessness*

## Leukemia

Ineffective **Protection** r/t abnormal blood profile

Risk for deficient **Fluid** volume r/t nausea, vomiting, bleeding, side effects of treatment

Risk for **Infection** r/t ineffective immune system

*See Cancer; Chemotherapy*

## Leukopenia

Ineffective **Protection** r/t leukopenia

Risk for **Infection** r/t low white blood cell count

## Level of Consciousness, Decreased

*See Confusion, Acute; Confusion, Chronic*

## Lice

Impaired **Comfort** r/t pruritis secondary to infestation

Impaired **Home** maintenance r/t close overcrowded conditions

Readiness for enhanced **Therapeutic** regimen management to prevent and treat infestation

*See Communicable Diseases, Childhood*

## Lightheadedness

*See Dizziness*

## Limb Reattachment Procedures

Anticipatory **Grieving** r/t unknown outcome of reattachment procedure

**Anxiety** r/t unknown outcome of reattachment procedure, use and appearance of limb

Disturbed **Body** image r/t unpredictability of function and appearance of reattached body part

Risk for deficient **Fluid** volume: hemorrhage r/t severed vessels

Risk for impaired **Religiosity** r/t pain, suffering, hospitalization

Risk for perioperative positioning **Injury** r/t immobilization

Risk for **Peripheral** neurovascular dysfunction r/t trauma, orthopedic and neurovascular surgery, compression of nerves and blood vessels

Risk for **Powerlessness** r/t unknown outcome of procedure

**Spiritual** distress r/t anxiety about condition

*See Surgery, Postoperative Care*

## Liposuction

Disturbed **Body** image r/t dissatisfaction with unwanted fat deposits in body

Readiness for enhanced **Self-concept** r/t satisfaction with new body image

*See Surgery, Perioperative Care; Surgery, Postoperative Care; Surgery, Preoperative Care*

## Lithotripsy

Readiness for enhanced **Therapeutic** regimen management r/t for desire for information related to procedure and after care and prevention of stones

*See Kidney Stone*

## Liver Biopsy

**Anxiety** r/t procedure and results

Risk for deficient **Fluid** volume r/t hemorrhage from biopsy site

Risk for **Powerlessness** r/t inability to control outcome of procedure

## Liver Disease

*See Cirrhosis; Hepatitis*

## Liver Transplant

Decisional **Conflict** r/t acceptance of donor liver

Readiness for enhanced **Family** processes: change in physical needs of family member

Ineffective **Protection** r/t immunosuppressive therapy

Readiness for enhanced **Spiritual** well-being r/t heightened coping

Readiness for enhanced **Therapeutic** regimen management r/t desire to manage the treatment and prevention of complications posttransplant

*See Surgery, Perioperative Care; Surgery, Postoperative Care; Surgery, Preoperative Care*

## Living Will

Readiness for enhanced **Religiosity** r/t request to meet with religious leaders/facilitators

Readiness for enhanced **Spiritual** well-being r/t acceptance of and preparation for end of life

*See Advance Directives*

## Lobectomy

*See Thoracotomy*

## Loneliness

Risk for impaired **Religiosity** r/t lack of social interaction

Risk for **Loneliness** r/t lack of affection, physical isolation, cathectic deprivation, social isolation

Risk for situational low **Self-esteem** r/t failure, rejection

**Spiritual** distress r/t loneliness/social alienation

## Loose Stools

**Diarrhea** r/t increased gastric motility

*See cause of Loose Stools*

## Lou Gehrig's Disease

*See ALS (Amyotrophic Lateral Sclerosis)*

## Low Back Pain

Chronic **Pain** r/t degenerative processes, musculotendinous strain, injury, inflammation, congenital deformities

Impaired physical **Mobility** r/t back pain

Ineffective **Health** maintenance r/t deficient knowledge regarding self-care with back pain

Readiness for enhanced **Therapeutic** regimen management r/t expressed desire for information to manage pain

Risk for **Powerlessness** r/t living with chronic pain

**Urinary** retention r/t possible spinal cord compression

## Lumbar Puncture

Acute **Pain**: headache r/t possible loss of cerebrospinal fluid

**Anxiety** r/t invasive procedure and unknown results

Deficient **Knowledge** r/t information about procedure

Risk for **Infection** r/t invasive procedure

## Lumpectomy

Decisional **Conflict** r/t treatment choices

Readiness for enhanced **Knowledge**: pre- and postoperative care

Readiness for enhanced **Spiritual** well-being r/t hope of benign diagnosis

*See Cancer*

## Lung Cancer

*See Cancer; Chemotherapy; Radiation Therapy; Thoracotomy*

## Lupus Erythematosus

Acute **Pain** r/t inflammatory process

Chronic **Sorrow** r/t presence of chronic illness

Disturbed **Body** image r/t change in skin, rash, lesions, ulcers, mottled erythema

**Fatigue** r/t increased metabolic requirements

Impaired **Religiosity** r/t ineffective coping with disease

Ineffective **Health** maintenance r/t deficient knowledge regarding medication, diet, and activity

**Powerlessness** r/t unpredictability of course of disease

Risk for impaired **Skin** integrity r/t chronic inflammation, edema, altered circulation

**Spiritual** distress r/t chronicity of disease, unknown etiology

## Lyme Disease

Acute **Pain** r/t inflammation of joints, urticaria, rash

Deficient **Knowledge** r/t lack of information concerning disease, prevention, treatment

**Fatigue** r/t increased energy requirements

Risk for decreased **Cardiac** output r/t dysrhythmia

Risk for **Powerlessness** r/t possible chronic condition

## Lymphedema

Deficient **Knowledge** r/t management of condition

Disturbed **Body** image r/t change in appearance of body part with edema

Excess **Fluid** volume r/t compromised regulatory system; inflammation, obstruction, or removal of lymph glands

Risk for situational low **Self-esteem** r/t disturbed body image

## Lymphoma

*See Cancer*

# M

## Macular Degeneration

Impaired **Adjustment** r/t deteriorating vision

Compromised **Family** coping r/t deteriorating vision of family member

Disturbed **Sensory** perception: visual r/t blurred, distorted, dim, or absent central vision

Effective management of **Therapeutic** regimen r/t practicing good nutrition, vitamin use; zinc, and abstaining from tobacco use

**Hopelessness** r/t deteriorating vision

Ineffective **Coping** r/t visual loss

Risk for **Falls** r/t visual difficulties

Risk for impaired **Religiosity** r/t possible lack of transportation

Risk for **Injury** r/t inability to distinguish traffic lights

Risk for **Powerlessness** r/t deteriorating vision

Sedentary **Lifestyle** r/t visual loss

**Social** isolation r/t inability to drive associated with visual changes

## Mad Cow Disease

Risk for dysfunctional **Grieving** r/t possible rapid fatal outcome of disease

*See CJD (Creutzfeldt-Jakob Disease)*

## Magnetic Resonance Imaging

*See MRI (Magnetic Resonance Imaging)*

## Major Depressive Disorder

M

Interrupted **Family** processes r/t change in health status of family member

Risk for **Loneliness** r/t social isolation associated with feelings of sadness, hopelessness

*See Depression*

## Malabsorption Syndrome

Deficient **Knowledge** r/t lack of information about diet and nutrition

**Diarrhea** r/t lactose intolerance, gluten sensitivity, resection of small bowel

Imbalanced **Nutrition**: less than body requirements r/t inability of body to absorb nutrients because of biological factors

Risk for deficient **Fluid** volume r/t diarrhea

Risk for disproportionate **Growth** r/t malnutrition from malabsorption

*See Abdominal Distention*

## Maladaptive Behavior

*See Crisis; Post-trauma Syndrome; Suicide Attempt*

## Malaise

*See Fatigue*

## Malaria

**Health seeking** behaviors r/t countries requiring malaria prophylaxis, appropriate malaria regimen, use of protective clothing and insecticides

Readiness for enhanced **Knowledge** r/t countries requiring malaria prophylaxis, appropriate malaria regimen, use of protective clothing and insecticides

Risk for **Infection** r/t increased environmental exposure (not wearing protective clothing, not using insecticide or repellant on skin and in room in areas where infected mosquitoes are present); inadequate defense mechanisms (inappropriate use of prophylactic regimen)

*See Anemia*

## Malignancy

*See Cancer*

## Malignant Hyperthermia

Effective **Therapeutic** regimen management r/t use of a general anesthetic: pretreatment with dantrolene sodium is recommended; if there is a family history of anesthesia-induced problems, it is imperative to alert the surgeon and anesthesiologist

**Hyperthermia** r/t anesthesia reaction associated with inherited condition

## Malnutrition

Adult **Failure** to thrive r/t undetected malnutrition

Deficient **Knowledge** r/t misinformation about normal nutrition, social isolation, lack of food-preparation facilities

Imbalanced **Nutrition**: less than body requirements r/t inability to ingest food, digest food, or absorb nutrients because of biological, psychological, or economic factors; institutionalization (i.e., lack of menu choices)

Ineffective **Protection** r/t inadequate nutrition

Ineffective **Therapeutic** regimen management r/t economic difficulties

Risk for disproportionate **Growth** r/t malnutrition

Risk for **Powerlessness** r/t possible inability to provide adequate nutrition

## Mammography

Effective **Therapeutic** regimen management r/t women schedule mammograms 1 to 2 years after age 40 or at earlier age based on family history of breast cancer or to evaluate a woman who has symptoms of a breast disease, such as a lump, nipple discharge, breast pain, dimpling of the skin on the breast, or retraction of the nipple

**Health-seeking** behaviors r/t information regarding mammograms: frequency and age recommendations; preparation; no deodorant, perfume, powders, or ointments under the arms or on the breasts on the day of the mammogram

## Manic Disorder, Bipolar I

**Anxiety** r/t change in role function

Deficient **Fluid** volume r/t decreased intake

Disturbed **Sleep** pattern r/t constant anxious thoughts

Disturbed **Thought** processes r/t mania

Imbalanced **Nutrition**: less than body requirements r/t lack of time and motivation to eat, constant movement

Impaired **Home** maintenance r/t altered psychological state, inability to concentrate

Ineffective **Coping** r/t situational crisis

Ineffective **Denial** r/t fear of inability to control behavior

Ineffective **Role** performance r/t impaired social interactions

Interrupted **Family** processes r/t family member's illness

Ineffective **Therapeutic** regimen management r/t lack of social supports

Ineffective **Therapeutic** regimen management: families r/t unpredictability of client, excessive demands on family, chronicity of condition

**Noncompliance** r/t denial of illness

Risk for **Caregiver** role strain r/t unpredictability of condition, mood swings

Risk for impaired **Religiosity** r/t depression

Risk for **Powerlessness** r/t inability to control changes in mood

Risk for self- or other-directed **Violence** r/t hallucinations, delusions

Risk for **Spiritual** distress r/t depression

Risk for **Suicide** r/t bipolar disorder

**Sleep** deprivation r/t hyperagitated state

## Manipulation of Organs, Surgical Incision

Deficient **Knowledge** r/t lack of exposure to information regarding care after surgery and at home

Risk for **Infection** r/t presence of urinary catheter

**Urinary** retention r/t swelling of urinary meatus

## Manipulative Behavior

Defensive **Coping** r/t superior attitude toward others

Impaired **Social** interaction r/t self-concept disturbance

Ineffective **Coping** r/t inappropriate use of defense mechanisms

Risk for **Loneliness** r/t inability to interact appropriately with others

Risk for **Self-mutilation** r/t inability to cope with increased psychological or physiological tension in healthy manner

Risk for situational low **Self-esteem** r/t history of learned helplessness

**Self-mutilation** r/t use of manipulation to obtain nurturing relationship with others

## Marasmus

*See Failure to Thrive, Nonorganic*

## Marfan Syndrome

Decreased **Cardiac** output r/t dilation of the aortic root, dissection or rupture of the aorta

Disturbed **Sensory** perception; visual r/t myopia associated with Marfan syndrome

Effective **Therapeutic** regimen management r/t medication to slow the heart rate (beta blockers) to help prevent stress on the aorta; not participating in competitive athletics and contact sports; yearly echocardiogram to assess the aortic root; surgical replacement of the aortic root and valve if needed

Readiness for enhanced **Therapeutic** regimen management r/t good oral health and routine dental evaluation; antibiotics before dental work or other procedures expected to contaminate the bloodstream with bacteria for all clients who have valvular heart disease, including a composite graft repair or placement of an artificial valve

*See Mitral Valve Prolapse; Scoliosis*

## Marshall-Marchetti-Krantz Operation

### PREOPERATIVE

Stress urinary **Incontinence** r/t weak pelvic muscles and pelvic supports

### POSTOPERATIVE

Acute **Pain** r/t manipulation of organs, surgical incision

Deficient **Knowledge** r/t lack of exposure to information regarding care after surgery and at home

Risk for **Infection** r/t presence of urinary catheter

**Urinary** retention r/t swelling of urinary meatus

## Mastectomy

Acute **Pain** r/t surgical procedure

Chronic **Sorrow** r/t disturbed body image, unknown long-term health status

Death **Anxiety** r/t threat of mortality associated with breast cancer

Deficient **Knowledge** r/t self-care activities

Disturbed **Body** image r/t loss of sexually significant body part

**Fear** r/t change in body image, prognosis

**Nausea** r/t chemotherapy

Risk for impaired physical **Mobility** r/t nerve or muscle damage, pain

Risk for **Post-trauma** syndrome r/t loss of body part, surgical wounds

Risk for **Powerlessness** r/t fear of unknown outcome of procedure

**Sexual** dysfunction r/t change in body image, fear of loss of femininity

**Spiritual** distress r/t change in body image

*See Cancer; Modified Radical Mastectomy; Surgery, Perioperative; Surgery, Postoperative; Surgery, Preoperative*

## Mastitis

Acute **Pain** r/t infectious disease process, swelling of breast tissue

**Anxiety** r/t threat to self, concern over safety of milk for infant

Deficient **Knowledge** r/t antibiotic regimen, comfort measures

Ineffective **Breastfeeding** r/t breast pain, conflicting advice from health care providers

Ineffective **Role** performance r/t change in capacity to function in expected role

## Maternal Infection

Ineffective **Protection** r/t invasive procedures, traumatized tissue, stress of recent childbirth

*See Postpartum, Normal Care*

## Maturational Issues, Adolescent

Deficient **Knowledge**: potential for enhanced health maintenance r/t information misinterpretation, lack of education regarding age-related factors

Impaired **Social** interaction r/t ineffective, unsuccessful, or dysfunctional interaction with peers

Ineffective **Coping** r/t maturational crises

Interrupted **Family** processes r/t developmental crises of adolescence secondary to challenge of parental authority and values, situational crises secondary to change in parental marital status

Readiness for enhanced **Communication** r/t expressing willingness to communicate with parental figures

Risk for **Injury/Trauma** r/t thrill-seeking behaviors

Risk for situational low **Self-esteem** r/t developmental changes

**Social** isolation r/t perceived alteration in physical appearance, social values not accepted by dominant peer group

*See Sexuality, Adolescent; Substance Abuse (if relevant)*

## Maze III Procedure

*See Open Heart Surgery; Dysrhythmia*

## Measles (Rubeola)

*See Communicable Diseases, Childhood*

## Meconium Aspiration

*See Respiratory Conditions of the Neonate*

## Melanoma

Acute **Pain** r/t surgical incision

Disturbed **Body** image r/t altered pigmentation, surgical incision

**Fear** r/t threat to well-being

Ineffective **Health** maintenance r/t deficient knowledge regarding self-care and treatment of melanoma

*See Cancer*

## Melena

**Fear** r/t presence of blood in feces

Risk for deficient **Fluid** volume r/t hemorrhage

*See GI Bleed (Gastrointestinal Bleeding)*

## Memory Deficit

Impaired **Memory** r/t acute or chronic hypoxia, anemia, decreased cardiac output, fluid and electrolyte imbalance, neurological disturbance, excessive environmental disturbances

Impaired environmental **Interpretation** syndrome r/t dementia

## Meniere's Disease

Effective management of **Therapeutic** regimen; prompt treatment of ear infection

Readiness for enhanced **Therapeutic** regimen management r/t avoiding sudden movements that may aggravate symptoms; help with walking due to loss of balance during attacks; rest during severe episodes, and gradually increase activity; during episodes, avoiding bright lights, television, and reading, which may make symptoms worse

Risk for **Injury** r/t symptoms from disease; avoiding hazardous activities such as driving, operating heavy machinery, climbing, and similar activities until one week after symptoms disappear

*See Dizziness*

## Meningitis/Encephalitis

Acute **Pain** r/t neck (nuchal) rigidity, inflammation of meninges, headache

Decreased **Intracranial** adaptive capacity r/t sustained increase in intracranial pressure (ICP) (10 to 15 mm Hg ICP)

Delayed **Growth** and development r/t brain damage secondary to infectious process, increased intracranial pressure

Disturbed **Sensory** perception: hearing r/t central nervous system infection, ear infection

Disturbed **Sensory** perception: kinesthetic r/t central nervous system infection

Disturbed **Sensory** perception: visual r/t photophobia secondary to central nervous system infection

Disturbed **Thought** processes r/t inflammation of brain, fever

Excess **Fluid** volume r/t increased intracranial pressure, syndrome of inappropriate secretion of antidiuretic hormone (SIADH)

Impaired **Comfort** r/t central nervous system inflammation

Impaired **Comfort**: photophobia r/t increased sensitivity to external stimuli secondary to central nervous system inflammation

Impaired **Mobility** r/t neuromuscular or central nervous system insult

Ineffective **Airway** clearance r/t seizure activity

Ineffective **Tissue** perfusion: cerebral r/t inflamed cerebral tissues and meninges, increased intracranial pressure

Risk for **Aspiration** r/t seizure activity

Risk for **Falls** r/t neuromuscular dysfunction

Risk for **Injury** r/t seizure activity

*See Hospitalized Child*

## Meningocele

*See Neurotube Defects*

## Menopause

**Health**-seeking behavior r/t menopause, therapies associated with change in hormonal levels

Impaired **Memory** r/t change in hormonal levels

Ineffective **Sexuality** patterns r/t altered body structure, lack of physiological lubrication, lack of knowledge of artificial lubrication

Ineffective **Thermoregulation** r/t changes in hormonal levels

Readiness for enhanced **Spiritual** well-being r/t desire for harmony of mind, body, and spirit

Readiness for enhanced **Therapeutic** regimen management r/t verbalized desire to manage menopause

Risk for imbalanced **Nutrition**: more than body requirements r/t change in metabolic rate caused by fluctuating hormone levels

Risk for **Powerlessness** r/t changes associated with menopause

Risk for situational low **Self-esteem** r/t developmental changes: menopause

Risk for urge urinary **Incontinence** r/t changes in hormonal levels affecting bladder function

## Menorrhagia

**Fear** r/t loss of large amounts of blood

Risk for deficient **Fluid** volume r/t excessive loss of menstrual blood

## Mental Illness

Chronic **Sorrow** r/t presence of mental illness

Compromised family **Coping** r/t lack of available support from client

Defensive **Coping** r/t psychological impairment, substance abuse

Disabled family **Coping** r/t chronically unexpressed feelings of guilt, anxiety, hostility, or despair

Disturbed **Thought** processes r/t head injury, mental disorder, personality disorder, organic mental disorder, substance abuse, severe interpersonal conflict, sleep deprivation, sensory deprivation or overload, impaired cerebral perfusion

Ineffective community **Therapeutic** regimen management r/t inadequate services to care for mentally ill clients, lack of information regarding how to access services

Ineffective **Coping** r/t situational crisis, coping with mental illness

Ineffective **Denial** r/t refusal to acknowledge abuse problem, fear of the social stigma of disease

Ineffective family **Therapeutic** regimen management r/t chronicity of condition, unpredictability of client, unknown prognosis

Risk for **Loneliness** r/t social isolation

Risk for **Powerlessness** r/t lifestyle of helplessness

## Mental Retardation

Chronic low **Self-esteem** r/t perceived differences

Delayed **Growth** and development r/t cognitive or perceptual impairment, developmental delay

**Grieving** r/t loss of perfect child, birth of child with congenital defect or subsequent head injury

Impaired **Home** maintenance r/t insufficient support systems

Impaired **Social** interaction r/t developmental lag or delay, perceived differences

Impaired **Swallowing** r/t neuromuscular impairment

Impaired verbal **Communication** r/t developmental delay

Interrupted **Family** processes r/t crisis of diagnosis and situational transition

Parental role **Conflict** r/t home care of child with special needs

Readiness for enhanced family **Coping** r/t adaptation and acceptance of child's condition and needs

Risk for delayed **Development** r/t cognitive or perceptual impairment

Risk for disproportionate **Growth** r/t mental retardation

Risk for impaired **Religiosity** r/t social isolation

Risk for **Self-mutilation** r/t separation anxiety, depersonalization

**Self-care** deficit: bathing/hygiene, dressing/grooming, feeding, toileting r/t perceptual or cognitive impairment

**Self-mutilation** r/t inability to express tension verbally

**Spiritual** distress r/t chronic condition of child with special needs

*See Child with Chronic Condition; Safety, Childhood*

## Metabolic Acidosis

*See Ketoacidosis, Diabetic; Ketoacidosis, Alcoholic*

## Metabolic Alkalosis

Deficient **Fluid** volume r/t fluid volume loss, vomiting, gastric suctioning, failure of regulatory mechanisms

## Metastasis

*See Cancer*

## MI (Myocardial Infarction)

Acute **Pain** r/t myocardial tissue damage from inadequate blood supply

**Anxiety** r/t threat of death, possible change in role status

**Constipation** r/t decreased peristalsis from decreased physical activity, medication effect, change in diet

Death **Anxiety** r/t seriousness of medical condition

Decreased **Cardiac** output r/t ventricular damage, ischemia, dysrhythmias

**Fear** r/t threat to well-being

Ineffective **Denial** r/t fear, deficient knowledge about heart disease

Ineffective family **Coping** r/t spouse or significant other's fear of partner loss

Ineffective **Health** maintenance r/t deficient knowledge regarding self-care and treatment

Ineffective **Sexuality** patterns r/t fear of chest pain, possibility of heart damage

Ineffective **Therapeutic** regimen management r/t knowledge deficit

Interrupted **Family** processes r/t crisis, role change

Readiness for enhanced **Knowledge** of heart problems and rehabilitation and prevention

Risk for **Powerlessness** r/t acute illness

Risk for **Spiritual** distress r/t physical illness: MI

Situational low **Self-esteem** r/t crisis of MI

## MIDCAB (Minimally Invasive Direct Coronary Bypass)

Readiness for enhanced **Therapeutic** regimen management r/t pre- and postoperative care associated with the surgery

Risk for **Infection** r/t large breasts on incision line

*See Angioplasty, Coronary; Coronary Artery Bypass Grafting*

## Midlife Crisis

Ineffective **Coping** r/t inability to deal with changes associated with aging

**Powerlessness** r/t lack of control over life situation

Readiness for enhanced **Spiritual** well-being r/t desire to find purpose and meaning to life

**Spiritual** distress r/t questioning belief/value system

## Migraine Headache

Acute **Pain**: headache r/t vasodilation of cerebral and extracerebral vessels

Disturbed **Energy** field r/t pain, disruption of normal flow of energy

Ineffective **Health** maintenance r/t deficient knowledge regarding prevention and treatment of headaches

Readiness for enhanced **Therapeutic** regimen

**management** r/t expressed desire to obtain information to prevent and treat pain associated with migraines

## Milk Intolerance

*See Lactose Intolerance*

## Minimally Invasive Heart Surgery

*See MIDCAB (Minimally Invasive Direct Coronary Bypass); OPCAB (Off-Pump Coronary Artery Bypass)*

## Miscarriage

*See Pregnancy Loss*

## Mitral Stenosis

**Activity** intolerance r/t imbalance between oxygen supply and demand

**Anxiety** r/t possible worsening of symptoms, activity intolerance, fatigue

Decreased **Cardiac** output r/t incompetent heart valves, abnormal forward or backward blood flow, flow into a dilated chamber, flow through an abnormal passage between chambers

**Fatigue** r/t reduced cardiac output

Ineffective **Health** maintenance r/t deficient knowledge regarding self-care with disorder

## Mitral Valve Prolapse

Acute **Pain** r/t mitral valve regurgitation

**Anxiety** r/t symptoms of condition: palpitations, chest pain

Effective management of **Therapeutic** regimen r/t prophylactic antibiotic therapy prior to invasive procedure such as dental work

**Fatigue** r/t abnormal catecholamine regulation, decreased intravascular volume

**Fear** r/t lack of knowledge about mitral valve prolapse, feelings of having a heart attack

Ineffective **Health** maintenance r/t deficient knowledge regarding methods to relieve pain and treat dysrhythmia and shortness of breath, need for prophylactic antibiotics before invasive procedures

Ineffective **Tissue** perfusion: cerebral r/t postural hypotension

Readiness for enhanced **Knowledge** of methods to treat and prevent symptoms associated with condition

Risk for **Infection** r/t invasive procedures

Risk for **Powerlessness** r/t unpredictability of onset of symptoms

## Mobility, Impaired Bed

Impaired bed **Mobility** r/t impaired ability to turn side to side; move from supine to sitting or sitting to supine; "scoot" or reposition self in bed; move from supine to prone or prone to supine; move from supine to long sitting or long sitting to supine

## Mobility, Impaired Physical

Impaired physical **Mobility** r/t intolerance to activity, decreased strength and endurance, pain, discomfort, perceptual or cognitive impairment, neuromuscular impairment, musculoskeletal impairment, depression, severe anxiety

Risk for **Falls** r/t impaired physical mobility

## Mobility, Impaired Wheelchair

Impaired wheelchair **Mobility** r/t impaired ability to operate manual or power wheelchair on even or uneven surface; impaired ability to operate manual or power wheelchair on an incline or decline; impaired ability to operate wheelchair on curbs

## Modified Radical Mastectomy

Decisional **Conflict** r/t treatment of choice

Readiness for enhanced **Communication** r/t to willingness to discuss options for treatment

*See Mastectomy*

## Mononucleosis

**Activity** intolerance r/t generalized weakness

Acute **Pain** r/t enlargement of lymph nodes, irritation of oropharyngeal cavity

**Fatigue** r/t disease state, stress

**Hyperthermia** r/t infectious process

Impaired **Swallowing** r/t irritation of oropharyngeal cavity

Ineffective **Health** maintenance r/t deficient knowledge concerning transmission and treatment of disease

Risk for **Injury** r/t possible rupture of spleen

## Mood Disorders

**Caregiver** role strain r/t symptoms associated with disorder of care receiver

Impaired **Adjustment** r/t hopelessness, altered locus of control

Readiness for enhanced **Communication** r/t willingness to communicate with others regarding problems associated with mood disorder

Risk for situational low **Self-esteem** r/t unpredictable changes in mood

**Social** isolation r/t alterations in mental status

*See specific disorder: Depression; Dysthymic Disorder; Hypomania; Manic Disorder, Bipolar I*

## Moon Face

Disturbed **Body** image r/t change in appearance from disease and medication

Risk for situational low **Self-esteem** r/t change in body image

*See Cushing's Syndrome*

## Moral/Ethical Dilemmas

Decisional **Conflict** r/t questioning personal values and belief, which alter decision

Readiness for enhanced **Religiosity** r/t requests assistance in expanding religious options

Readiness for enhanced **Spiritual** well-being r/t request for interaction with others regarding difficult decisions

Risk for **Powerlessness** r/t lack of knowledge to make a decision

Risk for **Spiritual** distress r/t moral or ethical crisis

## Mottling of Peripheral Skin

Ineffective **Tissue** perfusion: peripheral r/t interruption of arterial flow, decreased circulating blood volume

## Mourning

*See Grieving*

## Mouth Lesions

*See Mucous Membranes, Impaired Oral*

## MRI (Magnetic Resonance Imaging)

**Anxiety** r/t fear of being in closed spaces

Deficient **Knowledge** r/t preparation for examination, contraindications to test, especially presence of any metal in body

Readiness for enhanced **Knowledge** r/t appropriate preparation for examination

Readiness for enhanced **Therapeutic** regimen management r/t removing any metallic objects prior to the examination

## Mucocutaneous Lymph Node Syndrome

*See Kawasaki Syndrome*

## Mucous Membranes, Impaired Oral

Impaired **Oral** mucous membrane r/t chemotherapy; chemical irritants (e.g., alcohol, tobacco, acidic foods, drugs, regular use of inhalers or other noxious agents); depression; immunosuppression; aging-related loss of connective, adipose, or bone tissue; barriers to professional care; cleft lip or palate; medication side effects; lack of or decreased salivation; trauma; pathological conditions; oral cavity (radiation to head or neck); NPO for more than 24 hours; mouth breathing; malnutrition or vitamin deficiency; dehydration; infection; ineffective oral hygiene; mechanical (e.g., ill-fitting dentures, braces, tubes [endotracheal/nasogastric], surgery in oral cavity); decreased platelets; immunocompromised; radiation therapy; barriers to oral self-care; diminished hormone levels (women); stress; loss of supportive structures

## Multiinfarct Dementia

*See Dementia*

## Multiple Gestation

**Anxiety** r/t uncertain outcome of pregnancy

Death **Anxiety** r/t maternal complications associated with multiple gestation

Deficient **Knowledge** r/t caring for more than one infant

Disturbed **Sleep** pattern r/t discomforts of multiple gestation or care of infants

**Fatigue** r/t physiological demands of a multi-fetal pregnancy and/or care of more than one infant

Imbalanced **Nutrition**: less than body requirements r/t physiological demands of a multi-fetal pregnancy

Impaired **Home** maintenance r/t fatigue

Impaired physical **Mobility** r/t increased uterine size

Impaired **Transfer** ability r/t enlarged uterus

Readiness for enhanced **Family** processes r/t family adapting to change with more than one infant

Risk for **Constipation** r/t enlarged uterus

Risk for delayed **Development**: fetus r/t multiple gestation

Risk for disproportionate **Growth**: fetus r/t multiple gestation

Risk for ineffective **Breastfeeding** r/t lack of support, physical demands of feeding more than one infant

Stress urinary **Incontinence** r/t increased pelvic pressure

## Multiple Personality Disorder (Dissociative Identity Disorder)

**Anxiety** r/t loss of control of behavior and feelings

Chronic low **Self-esteem** r/t inability to deal with life events, history of abuse

Defensive **Coping** r/t unresolved past traumatic events, severe anxiety

Disturbed **Body** image r/t feelings of powerlessness with personality changes

Disturbed personal **Identity** r/t severe child abuse

**Hopelessness** r/t long-term stress

Ineffective **Coping** r/t history of abuse

Readiness for enhanced **Communication** r/t willingness to discuss problems associated with condition

Risk for **Self-mutilation** r/t need to act out to relieve stress

*See Dissociative Identity Disorder*

## Multiple Sclerosis (MS)

Chronic **Sorrow** r/t loss of physical ability

Disturbed **Energy** field r/t disruption in energy flow resulting from disharmony between mind and body

Disturbed **Sensory** perception: specify r/t pathology in sensory tracts

Impaired physical **Mobility** r/t neuromuscular impairment

Ineffective **Airway** clearance r/t decreased energy/fatigue

**Powerlessness** r/t progressive nature of disease

Readiness for enhanced **Spiritual** well-being r/t struggling with chronic debilitating condition

Readiness for enhanced **Therapeutic** regimen management r/t expressing a desire to manage condition

Risk for **Disuse** syndrome r/t physical immobility

Risk for imbalanced **Nutrition**: less than body requirements r/t impaired swallowing, depression

Risk for impaired **Religiosity** r/t illness

Risk for **Injury** r/t altered mobility, sensory dysfunction

Risk for natural rubber latex **Allergy** response r/t possible repeated exposures to latex associated with intermittent catheterizations

Risk for **Powerlessness** r/t chronic illness

**Self-care** deficit: specify r/t neuromuscular impairment

**Sexual** dysfunction r/t biopsychosocial alteration of sexuality

**Spiritual** distress r/t perceived hopelessness of diagnosis

**Urinary** retention r/t inhibition of the reflex arc

*See Neurological Disorders*

## Mumps

*See Communicable Diseases, Childhood*

## Murmurs

Decreased **Cardiac** output r/t incompetent heart valves, abnormal forward or backward blood flow, flow into a dilated chamber, flow through an abnormal passage between chambers

## Muscular Atrophy/Weakness

Risk for **Disuse** syndrome r/t impaired physical mobility

Risk for **Falls** r/t impaired physical mobility

## Muscular Dystrophy (MD)

**Activity** intolerance r/t fatigue

**Constipation** r/t immobility

Decreased **Cardiac** output r/t effects of CHF

Disturbed **Energy** field r/t illness

**Fatigue** r/t increased energy requirements to perform activities of daily living

Imbalanced **Nutrition**: less than body requirements r/t impaired swallowing or chewing

Imbalanced **Nutrition**: more than body requirements r/t inactivity

Impaired **Mobility** r/t muscle weakness and development of contractures

Impaired **Transfer** ability r/t muscle weakness

Impaired **Walking** r/t muscle weakness

Ineffective **Airway** clearance r/t muscle weakness and decreased ability to cough

Readiness for enhanced **Self-concept** r/t acceptance of strength and abilities

Risk for **Aspiration** r/t impaired swallowing

Risk for **Disuse** syndrome r/t complications of immobility

Risk for **Falls** r/t muscle weakness

Risk for impaired **Gas** exchange r/t ineffective airway clearance and ineffective breathing pattern secondary to muscle weakness

Risk for impaired **Religiosity** r/t illness

Risk for impaired **Skin** integrity r/t immobility, braces, or adaptive devices

Risk for ineffective **Breathing** pattern r/t muscle weakness

Risk for **Infection** r/t pooling of pulmonary secretions secondary to immobility and muscle weakness

Risk for **Injury** r/t muscle weakness and unsteady gait

Risk for **Powerlessness** r/t chronic condition

Risk for situational low **Self-esteem** r/t presence of chronic condition

**Self-care** deficits: feeding, bathing, dressing, toileting r/t muscle weakness and fatigue

*See Child with Chronic Condition; Hospitalized Child*

## MVA (Motor Vehicle Accident)

*See Fracture; Head Injury; Injury; Pneumothorax*

## Myasthenia Gravis

**Fatigue** r/t paresthesia, aching muscles

Imbalanced **Nutrition**: less than body requirements r/t difficulty eating and swallowing

Impaired physical **Mobility** r/t defective transmission of nerve impulses at the neuromuscular junction

Impaired **Swallowing** r/t neuromuscular impairment

Ineffective **Airway** clearance r/t decreased ability to cough and swallow

Ineffective **Therapeutic** regimen management r/t lack of knowledge of treatment, uncertainty of outcome

Interrupted **Family** processes r/t crisis of dealing with diagnosis

Readiness for enhanced **Spiritual** well-being r/t heightened coping with serious illness

Risk for **Caregiver** role strain r/t severity of illness of client

Risk for impaired **Religiosity** r/t illness

*See Neurological Disorders*

## Mycoplasma Pneumonia

*See Pneumonia*

## Myelocele

*See Neurotube Defects*

## Myelogram, Contrast

Acute **Pain** r/t irritation of nerve roots

Risk for deficient **Fluid** volume r/t possible dehydration, loss of cerebrospinal fluid

Risk for ineffective **Tissue** perfusion: cerebral r/t hypotension, loss of cerebrospinal fluid

**Urinary** retention r/t pressure on spinal nerve roots

## Myelomeningocele

*See Neurotube Defects*

## Myocardial Infarction

*See MI (Myocardial Infarction)*

## Myocarditis

**Activity** intolerance r/t reduced cardiac reserve and prescribed bed rest

Decreased **Cardiac** output r/t impaired contractility of ventricles

Deficient **Knowledge** r/t treatment of disease

Readiness for enhanced **Knowledge** of treatment of disease

*See CHF (Congestive Heart Failure), if appropriate*

## Myringotomy

Acute **Pain** r/t surgical procedure

Disturbed **Sensory** perception r/t possible hearing impairment

**Fear** r/t hospitalization, surgical procedure

Ineffective **Health** maintenance r/t deficient knowledge regarding self-care following surgery

Risk for **Infection** r/t invasive procedure

## Myxedema

*See Hypothyroidism*

# N

## Narcissistic Personality Disorder

Decisional **Conflict** r/t lack of realistic problem-solving skills

Defensive **Coping** r/t grandiose sense of self

Disturbed **Personal** identity r/t psychological impairment

Impaired **Social** interaction r/t self-concept disturbance

Interrupted **Family** processes r/t taking advantage of others to achieve own goals

Risk for **Loneliness** r/t inability to interact appropriately with others

Risk for **Self-mutilation** r/t inadequate coping

## Narcolepsy

**Anxiety** r/t fear of lack of control over falling asleep

Disturbed **Sleep** pattern r/t uncontrollable desire to sleep

Readiness for enhanced **Sleep** r/t expression of willingness to enhance sleep

Risk for **Trauma** r/t falling asleep during potentially dangerous activity

## Narcotic Use

Risk for **Constipation** r/t effects of opioids on peristalsis

*See Substance Abuse (if relevant)*

## Nasogastric Suction

Impaired **Comfort** r/t presence of nasogastric tube

Impaired **Oral** mucous membrane r/t presence of nasogastric tube

Risk for deficient **Fluid** volume r/t loss of gastrointestinal fluids without adequate replacement

## Nausea

### TREATMENT RELATED

**Nausea** r/t gastric irritation: pharmaceuticals (e.g., aspirin, nonsteroidal antiinflammatory drugs, steroids, antibiotics), alcohol, iron, blood; gastric distention: delayed gastric emptying caused by pharmacological interventions (e.g., narcotics administration, anesthesia agents); pharmaceuticals (e.g., analgesics, antiviral agents for HIV, aspirin, opioids, chemotherapeutic agents); toxins (e.g., radiotherapy)

### BIOPHYSICAL

**Nausea** r/t biochemical disorders (e.g., uremia, diabetic ketoacidosis, pregnancy), cardiac pain, cancer of the stomach or intraabdominal tumors (e.g., pelvic or colorectal cancers), esophageal or pancreatic disease, gastric distention due to delayed gastric emptying, pyloric intestinal obstruction, genitourinary and biliary distension, upper bowel stasis, external compression of the stomach (liver, spleen, or other organ), enlargement that slows the stomach functioning (squashed stomach syndrome), excess food intake, gastric irritation due to pharyngeal and/or peritoneal inflammation, liver or splenetic capsule stretch, local tumors (e.g., acoustic neuroma, primary or secondary brain tumors, bone metastases at base of skull), motion sickness, Meniere's disease or labyrinthitis, physical factors (e.g., increased intracranial pressure, meningitis), toxins (e.g., tumor-produced peptides, abnormal metabolites due to cancer)

### SITUATIONAL

**Nausea** r/t psychological factors (e.g., pain, fear, anxiety, noxious odors, taste, unpleasant visual stimulation)

## Near-Drowning

Anticipatory/dysfunctional **Grieving** r/t potential death of child, unknown sequelae, guilt about accident

**Aspiration** r/t aspiration of fluid into the lungs

**Fear**: parental r/t possible death of child, possible permanent and debilitating sequelae

**Hypothermia** r/t central nervous system injury, prolonged submersion in cold water

Impaired **Gas** exchange r/t laryngospasm, holding breath, aspiration

Ineffective **Airway** clearance r/t aspiration, impaired gas exchange

Ineffective **Health** maintenance r/t parental deficient knowledge regarding safety measures appropriate for age

Readiness for enhanced **Spiritual** well-being r/t struggle with survival of life-threatening situation

Risk for delayed **Development** and disproportionate growth r/t hypoxemia, cerebral anoxia

Risk for **Infection** r/t aspiration, invasive monitoring

*See Child with Chronic Condition; Hospitalized Child; Safety, Childhood; Terminally Ill Child/Death of Child, Parent*

## Nearsightedness

Effective management of **Therapeutic** regimen r/t early diagnosis and appropriate referral for eyeglasses or contact lenses when nearsightedness is suspected; signs, which may indicate a vision problem: sitting close to television, holding books very close when reading, or having difficulty reading the blackboard in school or signs on a wall.

## Near Sightedness; Corneal Surgery

*See LASIK Eye Surgery (Laser-Assisted* In Situ *Keratomileusis)*

## Neck Vein Distention

Decreased **Cardiac** output r/t decreased contractility of heart and resulting increased preload

Excess **Fluid** volume r/t excess fluid intake, compromised regulatory mechanisms

*See CHF (Congestive Heart Failure)*

## Necrosis, Renal Tubular; ATN (Acute Tubular Necrosis); Necrosis, Acute Tubular

*See Renal Failure*

## Necrotizing Enterocolitis (NEC)

Deficient **Fluid** volume r/t vomiting, gastrointestinal bleeding

Disturbed **Energy** field r/t illness

Imbalanced **Nutrition**: less than body requirements r/t decreased ability to absorb nutrients, decreased perfusion to gastrointestinal tract

Ineffective **Breathing** pattern r/t abdominal distention, hypoxia

Ineffective **Tissue** perfusion: gastrointestinal r/t shunting of blood away from mesenteric circulation and toward vital organs secondary to perinatal stress, hypoxia

N

Risk for **Infection** r/t bacterial invasion of gastrointestinal tract, invasive procedures

*See Hospitalized Child; Premature Infant (Child)*

## Necrotizing Fasciitis (Flesh-Eating Bacteria)

Acute **Pain** r/t toxins interfering with blood flow

Anticipatory **Grieving** r/t poor prognosis associated with disease

Decreased **Cardiac** output r/t tachycardia and hypotension

**Fear** r/t possible fatal outcome of disease

**Hyperthermia** r/t presence of infection

Ineffective **Protection** r/t cellulites resistant to treatment

Ineffective **Tissue** perfusion: peripheral r/t thrombosis of the subcutaneous blood vessels, leading to necrosis of nerve fibers.

*See Renal Failure; Septicemia*

## Negative Feelings About Self

Chronic low **Self-esteem** r/t long-standing negative self-evaluation

Readiness for enhanced **Self-concept** r/t expressed willingness to enhance self-concept

**Self-esteem** disturbance r/t inappropriate learned negative feelings about self

## Neglect, Unilateral

*See Unilateral Neglect of One Side of Body*

## Neglectful Care of Family Member

**Caregiver** role strain r/t care demands of family member, lack of social or financial support

Deficient **Knowledge** r/t care needs

Disabled family **Coping** r/t highly ambivalent family relationships, lack of respite care

Ineffective community **Therapeutic** regimen management r/t deficits in community for support of caregivers, detection of client neglect

Interrupted **Family** processes r/t situational transition or crisis

## Neonate

*See Newborn, Normal, Postmature, Small for Gestational Age*

## Neoplasm

**Fear** r/t possible malignancy

*See Cancer*

N

## Nephrectomy

Acute **Pain** r/t incisional discomfort

**Anxiety** r/t surgical recovery, prognosis

**Constipation** r/t lack of return of peristalsis

Impaired **Urinary** elimination r/t loss of kidney

Ineffective **Breathing** pattern r/t location of surgical incision

Risk for deficient **Fluid** volume r/t vascular losses, decreased intake

Risk for **Infection** r/t invasive procedure, lack of deep breathing because of location of surgical incision

**Spiritual** distress r/t chronic illness

## Nephrostomy, Percutaneous

Acute **Pain** r/t invasive procedure

Impaired **Urinary** elimination r/t nephrostomy tube

Risk for **Infection** r/t invasive procedure

## Nephrotic Syndrome

**Activity** intolerance r/t generalized edema

Disturbed **Body** image r/t edematous appearance and side effects of steroid therapy

Excess **Fluid** volume r/t edema secondary to oncotic fluid shift resulting from serum protein loss and renal retention of salt and water

Imbalanced **Nutrition**: less than body requirements r/t anorexia, protein loss

Imbalanced **Nutrition**: more than body requirements r/t increased appetite secondary to steroid therapy

Impaired **Comfort** r/t edema

Risk for impaired **Skin** integrity r/t edema

Risk for **Infection** r/t altered immune mechanisms secondary to disease and effects of steroids

Risk for **Noncompliance** r/t side effects of home steroid therapy

**Social** isolation r/t edematous appearance

*See Child with Chronic Condition; Hospitalized Child*

## Nerve Entrapment

*See Carpal Tunnel Syndrome*

## Neuritis

**Activity** intolerance r/t pain with movement

Acute **Pain** r/t stimulation of affected nerve endings, inflammation of sensory nerves

Ineffective **Health** maintenance r/t deficient knowledge regarding self-care with neuritis

## Neurofibromatosis

Compromised **Family** coping r/t cost and emotional needs of disease

Disturbed **Energy** field r/t disease

Disturbed **Sensory** perception r/t optic nerve gliomas associated with disease

Effective **Therapeutic** regimen management r/t evaluate visual disturbances associated with NF1 optic pathway tumors: dimness of vision, headache, visual field defects, nystagmus and distortion of binocular fixation, decreased visual acuity, proptosis or a droopy eyelid

Impaired **Skin** integrity r/t café-au-lait spots

Readiness for enhanced **Therapeutic** regimen management r/t seek cancer screening, education and genetic counseling

Risk for delayed **Development:** learning disorders including attention deficit/hyperactivity disorder (ADHD), low intelligent quotient (IQ) scores, and developmental delay r/t genetic disorder

Risk for decreased **Cardiac** output r/t hypertension associated with condition

Risk for **Constipation** r/t intestinal neurofibromas

Risk for disproportionate **Growth**: short stature, precocious puberty, delayed maturation, thyroid disorders r/t genetic disorder

Risk for **Injury** r/t possible problems with balance

Risk for **Spiritual** distress r/t possible severity of disease

*See Abdominal Distension; Surgery, Perioperative; Surgery, Postoperative; Surgery, Preoperative*

## Neurogenic Bladder

Reflex **Incontinence** r/t neurological impairment

Risk for latex **Allergy** response r/t repeated exposures to latex associated with possible repeated catheterizations

**Urinary** retention r/t interruption in the lateral spinal tracts

## Neurological Disorders

Acute **Confusion** r/t dementia, alcohol abuse, drug abuse, delirium

Anticipatory **Grieving** r/t loss of usual body functioning

Disturbed **Energy** field r/t illness

Imbalanced **Nutrition**: less than body requirements r/t impaired swallowing, depression, difficulty feeding self

Impaired **Home** maintenance r/t client's or family member's disease

Impaired **Memory** r/t neurological disturbance

Impaired physical **Mobility** r/t neuromuscular impairment

Impaired **Swallowing** r/t neuromuscular dysfunction

Ineffective **Airway** clearance r/t perceptual or cognitive impairment, decreased energy, fatigue

Ineffective **Coping** r/t disability requiring change in lifestyle

Interrupted **Family** processes r/t situational crisis, illness, or disability of family member

**Powerlessness** r/t progressive nature of disease

Risk for **Disuse** syndrome r/t physical immobility, neuromuscular dysfunction

Risk for impaired **Religiosity** r/t life transition

Risk for impaired **Skin** integrity r/t altered sensation, altered mental status, paralysis

Risk for **Injury** r/t altered mobility, sensory dysfunction, cognitive impairment

**Self-care** deficit: specify r/t neuromuscular dysfunction

**Sexual** dysfunction r/t biopsychosocial alteration of sexuality

**Social** isolation r/t altered state of wellness

**Wandering** r/t cognitive impairment

## Neuropathy, Peripheral

Chronic **Pain** r/t damage to nerves in the peripheral nervous system secondary to medication side effects, vitamin deficiency or diabetes

Ineffective **Thermoregulation** r/t decreased ability to regulate body temperature

Risk for **Injury** r/t lack of muscle control and decreased sensation

Risk for **Peripheral** neurovascular dysfunction r/t compression, entrapment

*See Peripheral Vascular Disease*

## Neurosurgery

*See Crainiectomy/Craniotomy*

## Neurotube Defects (Meningocele, Myelomeningocele, Spina Bifida, Anencephaly)

Chronic low **Self-esteem** r/t perceived differences, decreased ability to participate in physical and social activities at school

**Constipation** r/t immobility or less than adequate mobility

Delayed **Growth** and development r/t physical impairments, possible cognitive impairment

Disturbed **Sensory** perception: visual r/t altered reception secondary to strabismus

**Grieving** r/t loss of perfect child, birth of child with congenital defect

Impaired **Mobility** r/t neuromuscular impairment

Impaired **Skin** integrity r/t incontinence

Readiness for enhanced family **Coping** r/t effective adaptive response by family members

Readiness for enhanced **Family** processes r/t family supporting each other

Reflex **Incontinence** r/t neurogenic impairment

Risk for delayed **Development** r/t chronic illness

Risk for disproportionate **Growth** r/t chronic illness

Risk for imbalanced **Nutrition**: more than body requirements r/t diminished, limited, or impaired physical activity

Risk for impaired **Skin** integrity: lower extremities r/t decreased sensory perception

Risk for latex **Allergy** response r/t multiple exposures to latex products

Risk for **Powerlessness** r/t debilitating disease

Total urinary **Incontinence** r/t neurogenic impairment

Urge urinary **Incontinence** r/t neurogenic impairment

*See Child with Chronic Condition; Premature Infant (Child)*

## Newborn, Normal

Effective **Breastfeeding** r/t normal oral structure and gestational age >34 weeks

Ineffective **Protection** r/t immature immune system

Ineffective **Thermoregulation** r/t immaturity of neuroendocrine system

Readiness for enhanced organized **Infant** behavior r/t appropriate environmental stimuli

Readiness for enhanced **Parenting** r/t providing emotional and physical needs of infant

Risk for **Infection** r/t open umbilical stump

Risk for **Injury** r/t immaturity, need for caretaking

Risk for sudden infant **Death** syndrome r/t lack of knowledge regarding infant sleeping in prone or side-lying position, prenatal or postnatal infant smoke exposure, infant overheating/overwrapping, soft underlayment/loose articles in the sleep environment

## Newborn, Postmature

**Hypothermia** r/t depleted stores of subcutaneous fat

Impaired **Skin** integrity r/t cracked and peeling skin secondary to decreased vernix

Risk for ineffective **Airway** clearance r/t meconium aspiration

Risk for **Injury** r/t hypoglycemia secondary to depleted glycogen stores

## Newborn, Small for Gestational Age (SGA)

Imbalanced **Nutrition**: less than body requirements r/t history of placental insufficiency

Ineffective **Thermoregulation** r/t decreased brown fat, subcutaneous fat

Risk for delayed **Development** r/t history of placental insufficiency

Risk for disproportionate **Growth** r/t history of placental insufficiency

Risk for **Injury** r/t hypoglycemia, perinatal asphyxia, meconium aspiration

Risk for sudden infant **Death** syndrome r/t low birth weight

## Nicotine Addiction

Ineffective **Health** maintenance r/t lack of ability to make a judgment about smoking cessation

**Powerlessness** r/t perceived lack of control over ability to give up nicotine

Readiness for enhanced **Therapeutic** regimen management r/t expresses desire to learn measures to stop smoking

## NIDDM (Non–Insulin-Dependent Diabetes Mellitus)

**Health**-seeking behaviors r/t desiring information on exercise and diet to manage diabetes

*See Diabetes Mellitus*

## Nightmares

Disturbed **Energy** field r/t disharmony of body and mind

**Post-trauma** response r/t disaster, war, epidemic, rape, assault, torture, catastrophic illness, or accident

**Rape-trauma** syndrome: compound reaction/silent reaction r/t forced violent sexual penetration against the victim's will and consent

## Nipple Soreness

Acute **Pain** r/t injury to nipples

*See Painful Breasts, Sore Nipples*

## Nocturia

Impaired **Urinary** elimination r/t sensory motor impairment, urinary tract infection

Risk for **Powerlessness** r/t to inability to control nighttime voidings

Total **Urinary** incontinence r/t neuropathy preventing transmission of reflex indicating bladder fullness, neurological dysfunction causing triggering of micturition at unpredictable times, independent contraction of detrusor reflex as result of surgery, trauma or disease affecting spinal cord nerves, anatomical fistula

Urge urinary **Incontinence** r/t decreased bladder capacity, irritation of bladder stretch receptors causing spasm, alcohol, caffeine, increased fluids, increased urine concentration, overdistention of bladder

## Nocturnal Myoclonus

*See Restless Leg Syndrome; Stress*

## Nocturnal Paroxysmal Dyspnea

*See PND (Paroxysmal Nocturnal Dyspnea)*

## Noncompliance

**Noncompliance** r/t *Healthcare Plan:* Duration, significant others, cost, intensity, complexity; *Individual Factors*: Personal and developmental abilities, health beliefs, cultural influences, spiritual values, knowledge and skill relevant to the regimen behavior, motivational forces; *Health System:* Satisfaction with care, credibility of provider, access and convenience of care, financial flexibility of plan, client-provider relationships, provider reimbursement of teaching and follow-up, provider continuity and regular follow-up, individual health coverage, communication and teaching skills of the provider; *Network:* Involvement of members in health plan, social value regarding plan, perceived belief of significant others

## Non–Insulin-Dependent Diabetes Mellitus (NIDDM)

*See Diabetes Mellitus*

## Normal Pressure Hydrocephalus (NPH)

Acute **Confusion** r/t dementia secondary to obstruction to flow of cerebrospinal fluid (CSF)

Impaired **Memory** r/t neurological disturbance

Impaired verbal **Communication** r/t obstruction of flow of CSF

Ineffective **Tissue** perfusion: cerebral r/t obstruction to flow of CSF secondary to closed head injury, craniotomy, meningitis or subarachnoid hemorrhage

Risk for **Falls** r/t unsteady gait secondary to obstruction of CSF

## Norwalk Virus

*See Viral Gastroenteritis*

## Nursing

*See Breastfeeding, Effective; Breastfeeding, Ineffective; Breastfeeding, Interrupted*

## Nutrition

Readiness for enhanced **Nutrition** r/t expresses willingness to enhance nutrition, eats regularly, consumes adequate food and fluid, expresses knowledge of healthy food and fluid choices, follows an appropriate standard for intake (e.g., the food guide pyramid or America Diabetic Association guidelines), safe preparation and storage for food and fluids, attitude toward eating and drinking is congruent with health goals

## Nutrition, Imbalanced

Imbalanced **Nutrition**: less than body requirements r/t inability to ingest or digest food or absorb nutrients because of biological, psychological, economic factors

Imbalanced **Nutrition**: more than body requirements r/t excessive intake in relation to metabolic need

Risk for imbalanced **Nutrition**: more than body requirements r/t reported use of solid food as major food source before 5 months of age; concentrating food intake at end of day; reported or observed obesity in one or both parents; rapid transition across growth percentiles in infants or children; pairing food with other activities; observed use of food as reward or comfort measure; eating in response to external cues (e.g., time of day, social situation); dysfunctional eating patterns

## Obesity

Chronic low **Self-esteem** r/t ineffective coping, overeating

Disturbed **Body** image r/t eating disorder, excess weight

Imbalanced **Nutrition**: more than body requirements r/t caloric intake exceeding energy expenditure

Readiness for enhanced **Nutrition** r/t expressing willingness to enhance nutrition

O

## OBS (Organic Brain Syndrome)

*See Organic Mental Disorders*

## Obsessive-Compulsive Disorder

**Anxiety** r/t threat to self-concept, unmet needs

Decisional **Conflict** r/t inability to make a decision for fear of reprisal

Disabled family **Coping** r/t family process being disrupted by client's ritualistic activities

Disturbed **Thought** processes r/t persistent thoughts, ideas, impulses that seem irrelevant and will not relent

Ineffective **Coping** r/t expression of feelings in an unacceptable way, ritualistic behavior

**Powerlessness** r/t unrelenting repetitive thoughts to perform irrational activities

Risk for situational low **Self-esteem** r/t inability to control repetitive thoughts and actions

## Obstruction, Bowel

*See Bowel Obstruction*

## Obstructive Sleep Apnea

Disturbed **Sleep** pattern r/t blocked airway

**Health-seeking** behaviors r/t seeking nutritional information to control weight that may be contributing to sleep apnea

Imbalanced **Nutrition**: more than body requirements r/t excessive intake related to metabolic need

*See PND (Paroxysmal Nocturnal Dyspnea)*

## ODD

*See Oppositional Defiant Disorder (ODD)*

## Older Adult

*See Aging*

## Oligohydramnios

**Anxiety**: maternal r/t fear of unknown, threat to fetus

Risk for **Injury**: fetal r/t decreased umbilical cord blood flow secondary to compression

## Oliguria

Deficient **Fluid** volume r/t active fluid loss, failure of regulatory mechanism

*See Cardiac Output Decrease; Renal Failure; Shock*

## Omphalocele

*See Gastroschisis/Omphalocele*

## Onychomycosis

*See Ringworm of Nails*

## Oophorectomy

Risk for ineffective **Sexuality** patterns r/t altered body function

*See Surgery, Perioperative; Surgery, Postoperative; Surgery, Preoperative*

## OPCAB (Off-Pump Coronary Artery Bypass)

Acute **Confusion** r/t possible decreased cerebral tissue perfusion

Acute **Pain** r/t possible gastrointestinal dysfunction

Decreased **Cardiac** output r/t increased vasodilation

Impaired **Gas** exchange r/t alveolar-capillary membrane changes

Impaired **Memory** r/t possible decreased cerebral tissue perfusion

Readiness for enhanced **Therapeutic** regimen management r/t pre- and postoperative care associated with the surgery

Risk for deficient **Fluid** volume r/t bleeding associated with anticoagulant therapy

*See Angioplasty, Coronary; Coronary Artery Bypass Grafting*

## Open Heart Surgery

Decreased **Cardiac** output r/t altered preload or afterload

Impaired **Gas** exchange r/t cardiac surgery

*See Coronary Artery Bypass Grafting; Dysrhythmia*

## Open Reduction of Fracture with Internal Fixation (Femur)

**Anxiety** r/t outcome of corrective procedure

Impaired physical **Mobility** r/t postoperative position, abduction of leg, avoidance of acute flexion

**Powerlessness** r/t loss of control, unanticipated change in lifestyle

Risk for perioperative positioning **Injury** r/t immobilization

Risk for **Peripheral** neurovascular dysfunction r/t mechanical compression, orthopedic surgery, immobilization

*See Surgery, Postoperative Care*

## Opiate Use

Risk for **Constipation** r/t effects of opiates on peristalsis.

*See Drug Abuse; Drug Withdrawal*

## Opportunistic Infection

Delayed **Surgical** recovery r/t abnormal blood profiles, impaired healing

Risk for **Infection** r/t abnormal blood profiles

*See AIDS (Acquired Immune Deficiency Syndrome); HIV (Human Immunodeficiency Virus)*

## Oppositional Defiant Disorder (ODD)

**Anxiety** r/t feelings of anger and hostility towards authority figures

Chronic or situational low **Self-esteem** r/t poor self-control and disruptive behaviors

Disabled **Family** coping r/t feelings of anger, hostility; defiant behavior toward authority figures

Disturbed **Thought** processes r/t difficulty thinking, making appropriate decisions

Impaired **Adjustment** r/t multiple stressors associated with condition

Impaired **Social** interaction r/t being touchy or easily annoyed, blaming others for own mistakes, constant trouble in school

Ineffective **Coping** r/t lack of self control or perceived lack of self-control

Ineffective family **Therapeutic** regimen management r/t difficulty in limit setting and managing oppositional behaviors

Risk for impaired **Parenting** r/t childrens' difficult behaviors and inability to set limits

Risk for other-directed **Violence** r/t history of violence, threats of violence against others; history of antisocial behavior; history of indirect violence

Risk for **Powerlessness** r/t inability to deal with difficulty behaviors

Risk for **Spiritual** distress r/t anxiety and stress in dealing with difficulty behaviors

**Social** isolation r/t unaccepted social behavior

## Oral Mucous Membrane, Impaired

Impaired **Oral** mucous membrane r/t pathological conditions—oral cavity (radiation to head or neck), dehydration, chemical trauma (e.g., acidic foods, drugs, noxious agents, alcohol), mechanical trauma (e.g., ill-fitting dentures, braces, endotracheal and nasogastric tubes, surgery in oral cavity), NPO for more than 24 hours, ineffective oral hygiene, mouth breathing, malnutrition, infection, lack of or decreased salivation, medication

## Oral Thrush

*See Candidiasis, Oral*

## Orchitis

Readiness for enhanced **Therapeutic** regimen management r/t follows recommendations for mumps vaccination

*See Epididymitis*

## Organic Mental Disorders

Adult **Failure** to thrive r/t undetected organic mental disorder

Impaired **Social** interaction r/t disturbed thought processes

Risk for **Injury** r/t disorientation to time, place, person

*See Dementia*

## Orthopedic Traction

Impaired **Social** interaction r/t limited physical mobility

Impaired **Transfer** ability r/t limited physical mobility

Ineffective **Role** performance r/t limited physical mobility

Risk for impaired **Religiosity** r/t immobility

*See Traction and Casts*

## Orthopnea

Decreased **Cardiac** output r/t inability of heart to meet demands of body

Ineffective **Breathing** pattern r/t inability to breathe with head of bed flat

## Orthostatic Hypotension

*See Dizziness*

## Osteoarthritis

**Activity** intolerance r/t pain after exercise or use of joint

Acute **Pain** r/t movement

Impaired **Transfer** ability r/t pain

*See Arthritis*

## Osteomyelitis

Acute **Pain** r/t inflammation in affected extremity

Deficient **Diversional** activity r/t prolonged immobilization, hospitalization

**Fear**: parental r/t concern regarding possible growth plate damage secondary to infection, concern that infection may become chronic

**Hyperthermia** r/t infectious process

Impaired physical **Mobility** r/t imposed immobility secondary to infected area

Ineffective **Health** maintenance r/t continued immobility at home, possible extensive casts, continued antibiotics

Risk for **Constipation** r/t immobility

Risk for impaired **Skin** integrity r/t irritation from splint/cast

Risk for **Infection** r/t inadequate primary and secondary defenses

*See Hospitalized Child*

## Osteoporosis

Acute **Pain** r/t fracture, muscle spasms

Deficient **Knowledge** r/t diet, exercise, need to abstain from alcohol and nicotine

Effective **Therapeutic** regimen management: individual r/t appropriate choices for diet and exercise to prevent and manage condition

Imbalanced **Nutrition**: less than body requirements r/t inadequate intake of calcium and vitamin D

Impaired physical **Mobility** r/t pain, skeletal changes

Readiness for enhanced **Therapeutic** regimen management r/t expressing desire to manage the treatment of illness and prevention of complications

Risk for **Injury**: fracture r/t lack of activity, risk of falling resulting from environmental hazards, neuromuscular disorders, diminished senses, cardiovascular responses, responses to drugs

Risk for **Powerlessness** r/t debilitating disease

## Ostomy

*See Child with Chronic Condition; Colostomy; Ileal Conduit; Ileostomy*

P

## Otitis Media

Acute **Pain** r/t inflammation, infectious process

Disturbed **Sensory** perception: auditory r/t incomplete resolution of otitis media, presence of excess drainage in middle ear

Readiness for enhanced **Knowledge** of information relating to treatment and prevent of disease

Risk for delayed **Development** r/t frequent otitis media

Risk for **Infection** r/t eustachian tube obstruction, traumatic eardrum perforation, infectious disease process

## Ovarian Carcinoma

Death **Anxiety** r/t unknown outcome, possible poor prognosis

**Fear** r/t unknown outcome, possible poor prognosis

Ineffective **Health** maintenance r/t deficient knowledge regarding self-care, treatment of condition

*See Chemotherapy; Hysterectomy; Radiation Therapy*

## Oxyuriasis

*See Pinworms*

# P

## Pacemaker

Acute **Pain** r/t surgical procedure

**Anxiety** r/t change in health status, presence of pacemaker

Death **Anxiety** r/t worry over possible malfunction of pacemaker

Deficient **Knowledge** r/t self-care program, when to seek medical attention

Readiness for enhanced **Therapeutic** regimen management r/t appropriate health care management of pacemaker

Risk for decreased **Cardiac** output r/t malfunction of pacemaker

Risk for **Infection** r/t invasive procedure, presence of foreign body (catheter and generator)

Risk for **Powerlessness** r/t presence of electronic device to stimulate heart

## Paget's Disease

Chronic **Sorrow** r/t chronic condition with altered body image

Deficient **Knowledge** r/t appropriate diet high in protein and calcium, mild exercise

Disturbed **Body** image r/t possible enlarged head, bowed tibias, kyphosis

Risk for **Trauma**: fracture r/t excessive bone destruction

## Pain, Acute

Acute **Pain** r/t injury agents (biological, chemical, physical, psychological)

Disturbed **Energy** field r/t unbalanced energy field

## Pain, Chronic

Chronic **Pain** r/t chronic physical or psychosocial disability

Disturbed **Energy** field r/t unbalanced energy field

## Painful Breasts, Engorgement

Acute **Pain** r/t distention of breast tissue

Impaired **Tissue** integrity r/t excessive fluid in breast tissues

Ineffective **Role** performance r/t change in physical capacity to assume role of breastfeeding mother

Risk for ineffective **Breastfeeding** r/t pain, infant's inability to latch on to engorged breast

Risk for **Infection** r/t milk stasis

## Painful Breasts, Sore Nipples

Acute **Pain** r/t cracked nipples

Impaired **Skin** integrity r/t mechanical factors involved in suckling, breastfeeding management

Ineffective **Breastfeeding** r/t pain

Ineffective **Role** performance r/t change in physical capacity to assume role of breastfeeding mother

Risk for **Infection** r/t break in skin

## Pallor of Extremities

Ineffective **Tissue** perfusion: peripheral r/t interruption of vascular flow

## Palpitations (Heart Palpitations)

*See Dysrhythmia*

## Pancreatic Cancer

Anticipatory **Grieving** r/t shortened life span

Death **Anxiety** r/t possible poor prognosis of disease process

Deficient **Knowledge** r/t disease-induced diabetes, home management

**Fear** r/t poor prognosis of the disease

Ineffective family **Coping** r/t poor prognosis

**Spiritual** distress r/t poor prognosis

*See Cancer; Chemotherapy; Radiation Therapy; Surgery, Perioperative; Surgery, Postoperative; Surgery, Preoperative*

## Pancreatitis

Acute **Pain** r/t irritation and edema of the inflamed pancreas

Chronic **Sorrow** r/t chronic illness

**Diarrhea** r/t decrease in pancreatic secretions resulting in steatorrhea

Deficient **Fluid** volume r/t vomiting, decreased fluid intake, fever, diaphoresis, fluid shifts

Imbalanced **Nutrition**: less than body requirements r/t inadequate dietary intake, increased nutritional needs secondary to acute illness, increased metabolic needs caused by increased body temperature

Ineffective **Breathing** pattern r/t splinting from severe pain

Ineffective **Denial** r/t ineffective coping, alcohol use

Ineffective **Health** maintenance r/t deficient knowledge concerning diet, alcohol use, medication

**Nausea** r/t irritation of gastrointestinal system

## Panic Disorder

**Anxiety** r/t situational crisis

Ineffective **Coping** r/t personal vulnerability

**Post-trauma** syndrome r/t previous catastrophic event

Readiness for enhanced **Coping** r/t seeking problem-oriented and emotion-oriented strategies to manage condition

Risk for **Loneliness** r/t inability to socially interact because of fear of losing control

Risk for **Post-trauma** syndrome r/t perception of the event, diminished ego strength

Risk for **Powerlessness** r/t ineffective coping skills

**Social** isolation r/t fear of lack of control

*See Anxiety; Anxiety Disorder*

## Paralysis

Acute **Pain** r/t prolonged immobility

Chronic **Sorrow** r/t loss of physical mobility

**Constipation** r/t effects of spinal cord disruption, inadequate fiber in diet

Disturbed **Body** image r/t biophysical changes, loss of movement, immobility

Impaired **Home** maintenance r/t physical disability

Impaired physical **Mobility** r/t neuromuscular impairment

Impaired **Transfer** ability r/t paralysis

Ineffective **Health** maintenance r/t deficient knowledge regarding self-care with paralysis

**Powerlessness** r/t illness-related regimen

Reflex **Incontinence** r/t neurological impairment

Risk for **Disuse** syndrome r/t paralysis

Risk for **Falls** r/t to paralysis

Risk for impaired **Religiosity** r/t immobility, possible lack of transportation

Risk for impaired **Skin** integrity r/t altered circulation, altered sensation, immobility

Risk for **Injury** r/t altered mobility, sensory dysfunction

Risk for natural rubber latex **Allergy** response r/t possible repeated urinary catheterizations

Risk for **Post-trauma** syndrome r/t event causing paralysis

Risk for situational low **Self-esteem** r/t change in body image and function

**Self-care** deficit: specify r/t neuromuscular impairment

**Sexual** dysfunction r/t loss of sensation, biopsychosocial alteration

*See Child with Chronic Condition; Hemiplegia; Hospitalized Child; Neurotube Defects; Spinal Cord Injury*

## Paralytic Ileus

Acute **Pain** r/t pressure, abdominal distention

**Constipation** r/t decreased gastric motility

Deficient **Fluid** volume r/t loss of fluids from vomiting, retention of fluid in bowel

Impaired **Oral** mucous membrane r/t presence of nasogastric tube

**Nausea** r/t gastrointestinal irritation

## Paranoid Personality Disorder

**Anxiety** r/t uncontrollable intrusive, suspicious thoughts

Chronic low **Self-esteem** r/t inability to trust others

Disturbed personal **Identity** r/t difficulty with reality testing

Disturbed **Sensory** perception: specify r/t psychological dysfunction, suspicious thoughts

Disturbed **Thought** processes r/t psychological conflicts

Impaired **Adjustment** r/t intense emotional state

Risk for **Loneliness** r/t social isolation

Risk for other-directed **Violence** r/t being suspicious of others and others' actions

Risk for **Post-trauma** syndrome r/t exaggerated sense of responsibility

Risk for **Suicide** r/t psychiatric illness

**Social** isolation r/t inappropriate social skills

## Paraplegia

*See Spinal Cord Injury*

## Parathyroidectomy

**Anxiety** r/t surgery

Risk for impaired verbal **Communication** r/t possible laryngeal damage, edema

Risk for ineffective **Airway** clearance r/t edema or hematoma formation, airway obstruction

Risk for **Infection** r/t surgical procedure

*See Hypocalcemia*

P

## Parent Attachment

Chronic **Sorrow** r/t difficult parent-child relationship

Risk for impaired parent/infant/child **Attachment** r/t physical barriers; anxiety associated with parental role; substance abuse; premature infant; ill infant/child who is unable to effectively initiate parental contact as a result of altered behavioral organization; lack of privacy; inability of parents to meet personal needs; separation

Risk for **Spiritual** distress r/t altered relationships

## Parental Role Conflict

Chronic **Sorrow** r/t difficult parent-child relationship

Parental role **Conflict** r/t change in marital status; home care of a child with special needs (e.g., apnea monitoring, postural drainage, hyperalimentation); interruptions of family life because of home care regimen (e.g., treatments, caregivers, lack of respite); specialized care center policies; separation from child because of chronic illness; intimidation with invasive or restrictive modalities (e.g., isolation, intubation)

Readiness for enhanced **Parenting** r/t willingness to enhance parenting

Risk for **Spiritual** distress r/t altered relationships

## Parenting

Readiness for enhanced **Parenting** r/t expresses willingness to enhance parenting; children or other dependent person(s) express satisfaction with home, environment; emotional and tacit support of children or dependent person(s) evident; bonding or attachment evident; physical and emotional needs of children/dependent person(s) are met; realistic expectations of children/dependent person(s) exhibited

## Parenting, Impaired

Chronic **Sorrow** r/t difficult parent-child relationship

Impaired **Parenting** r/t *Social:* Lack of access to resources; social isolation; lack of resources; poor home environment; lack of family cohesiveness; inadequate child care arrangements; lack of transportation; unemployment or job problems; role strain or overload; marital conflict, declining satisfaction; lack of value of parenthood; change in family unit; low socioeconomic class; unplanned or unwanted pregnancy; presence of stress (e.g., financial, legal, recent cresis, cultural move); lack of, or poor, parental role model; single parent; lack of social support networks; father of child not involved; history of being abusive; history of being abused; financial difficulties; maladaptive coping strategies; poverty; poor problem-solving skills; inability to put child's needs before own; low self-esteem; relocations; legal difficulties. *Knowledge:* Lack of knowledge about child health maintenance; lack of knowledge about parenting skills; unrealistic expectation for self, infant, partner; limited cognitive functioning; lack of knowledge about child development; inability to recognize and act on infant cues; low educational level or attainment; poor communication skills; Lack of cognitive readiness for parenthood; preference for physical punishment. *Physiological:* Physical illness. *Infant or Child:* Premature birth; illness; prolonged separation from parent; not desired gender; attention deficit/hyperactivity disorder; difficult temperament; separation from parent at birth; lack of goodness of fit (temperament) with parental expectations; unplanned or unwanted child; handicapping condition or developmental delay; multiple births; altered perceptual abilities. *Psychological:* History of substance abuse or dependencies; disability; depression; difficult labor and/or delivery; young age, especially adolescent; history of mental illness; high number or closely spaced pregnancies; sleep deprivation or disruption; lack of, or late, prenatal care; separation from infant/child

Risk for **Spiritual** distress r/t altered relationships

## Parenting, Risk for Impaired

Chronic **Sorrow** r/t difficult parent-child relationship

Risk for impaired **Parenting** r/t *Social:* Marital conflict, declining satisfaction; history of being abused; poor problem-solving skills; role strain/overload; social isolation; legal difficulties; lack of access to resources; lack of value of parenthood; relocation; poverty; poor home environment; lack of family cohesiveness; lack of or poor parental role model; father of child not involved; history of being abusive; financial difficulties; low self-esteem; lack of resources; unplanned or unwanted pregnancy; inadequate child care arrangements; maladaptive coping strategies; low socioeconomic class; lack of transportation; change in family unit; unemployment or job problems; single parent; lack of social support network; inability to put child's needs before own; stress. *Knowledge:* Low educational level or attainment; unrealistic expectations of child; lack of knowledge about parenting skills; poor communication skills; preference for physical punishment; inability to recognize and act on infant cues functioning; lack of knowledge about child health maintenance; lack of knowledge about child development; lack of cognitive readiness for parenthood. *Physiological:* Physical illness. *Infant or Child:* Multiple births; jandicapping condition or developmental delay; illness; altered perceptual abilities; lack of goodness of fit (temperament) with parental expectations; unplanned or unwanted child; premature birth; not gender desired; difficult temperament; attention deficit/hyperactivity disorder; prolonged separation from parent; separation from parent at birth. *Psychological:* Separation from infant/child; high number or closely spaced children; disability; sleep deprivation or disruption; difficult labor and/or delivery; young age, especially adolescent; depression; history of mental illness; lack of, or late, prenatal care; history of substance abuse or dependence

Risk for **Spiritual** distress r/t altered relationships

## Paresthesia

Disturbed **Sensory** perception: tactile r/t altered sensory reception, transmission, integration

Risk for **Injury** r/t inability to feel temperature changes, pain

## Parkinson's Disease

Chronic **Sorrow** r/t loss of physical capacity

**Constipation** r/t weakness of defecation muscles, lack of exercise, inadequate fluid intake, decreased autonomic nervous system activity

Imbalanced **Nutrition**: less than body requirements r/t tremor, slowness in eating, difficulty in chewing and swallowing

Impaired verbal **Communication** r/t decreased speech volume, slowness of speech, impaired facial muscles

Risk for **Injury** r/t tremors, slow reactions, altered gait

*See Neurological Disorders*

## Paroxysmal Nocturnal Dyspnea

*See PND (Paroxysmal Nocturnal Dyspnea)*

## Patent Ductus Arteriosus (PDA)

*See Congenital Heart Disease/Cardiac Anomalies*

## Patient-Controlled Analgesia

*See PCA (Patient-Controlled Analgesia)*

## Patient Education

Deficient **Knowledge** r/t lack of exposure to information, information misinterpretation, unfamiliarity with information resources

Effective **Therapeutic** regimen management r/t verbalized desire to manage illness, prevent complications

**Health-seeking** behaviors r/t expressed or observed desire to seek a higher level of wellness, control of health practices

Readiness for enhanced **Knowledge** of (specify) r/t interest in learning, knowledge of the topic, behaviors congruent with expressed knowledge, previous experiences pertaining to the topic

Readiness for enhanced **Spiritual** well-being r/t desire to reach harmony with self, others, higher power/God

Readiness for enhanced **Therapeutic** regimen management r/t the following: expresses a desire to manage the treatment of illness and prevent sequelae, makes choices of daily living that are appropriate for meeting the goals of treatment or prevention, expresses little to no difficulty with regulation/integration of one or more prescribed regimens for treatment of illness or prevention of complications, describes reduction of risk factors for progression of illness and sequelae, shows no unexpected acceleration of illness symptoms

## PCA (Patient-Controlled Analgesia)

Deficient **Knowledge** r/t self-care of pain control

Effective **Therapeutic** regimen management r/t ability to manage pain with appropriate use of PCA

Impaired **Comfort**: pruritus, nausea, vomiting r/t side effects of medication

Readiness for enhanced **Knowledge** of appropriate management of PCA

Risk for **Injury** r/t possible complications associated with PCA

## Pediculosis

*See Lice*

## Pelvic Inflammatory Disease

*See PID (Pelvic Inflammatory Disease)*

## Penile Prosthesis

**Health-seeking** behaviors r/t information regarding use and care of prosthesis

Ineffective **Sexuality** pattern r/t use of penile prosthesis

Risk for **Infection** r/t invasive surgical procedure

Risk for situational low **Self-esteem** r/t ineffective Sexuality patterns

*See Impotence*

## Peptic Ulcer

*See Ulcer, Peptic*

## Percutaneous Transluminal Coronary Angioplasty (PTCA)

*See Angioplasty, Coronary*

## Pericardial Friction Rub

Acute **Pain** r/t inflammation, effusion

Decreased **Cardiac** output r/t inflammation in pericardial sac, fluid accumulation compressing heart

Delayed **Surgical** recovery r/t complications associated with cardiac problems

## Pericarditis

**Activity** intolerance r/t reduced cardiac reserve, prescribed bed rest

Acute **Pain** r/t biological injury, inflammation

Delayed **Surgical** recovery r/t complications associated with cardiac problems

Deficient **Knowledge** r/t unfamiliarity with information sources

Ineffective **Tissue** perfusion: cardiopulmonary/peripheral r/t risk for development of emboli

Risk for decreased **Cardiac** output r/t inflammation in pericardial sac, fluid accumulation compressing heart function

Risk for imbalanced **Nutrition**: less than body requirements r/t fever, hypermetabolic state associated with fever

## Perioperative Positioning

Risk for perioperative positioning **Injury** r/t disorientation, edema, emaciation, immobilization; muscle weakness, obesity, sensory/perceptual disturbances resulting from anesthesia

## Peripheral Neuropathy

*See Neuropathy, Peripheral*

## Peripheral Neurovascular Dysfunction

Risk for **Peripheral** neurovascular dysfunction r/t trauma; vascular obstruction; orthopedic surgery; fractures; burns; mechanical compression (e.g., tourniquet, cane, cast, brace, dressing, restraint); immobilization

*See Neuropathy, Peripheral; Peripheral Vascular Disease*

## Peripheral Vascular Disease

**Activity** intolerance r/t imbalance between peripheral oxygen supply and demand

Chronic **Pain**: intermittent claudication r/t ischemia

Ineffective **Health** maintenance r/t deficient knowledge regarding self-care and treatment of disease

Ineffective **Tissue** perfusion: peripheral r/t interruption of vascular flow

Readiness for enhanced **Therapeutic** regimen management r/t self-care and treatment of disease

Risk for **Falls** r/t altered mobility

Risk for impaired **Skin** integrity r/t altered circulation or sensation

Risk for **Injury** r/t tissue hypoxia, altered mobility, altered sensation

Risk for **Peripheral** neurovascular dysfunction r/t possible vascular obstruction

*See Neuropathy, Peripheral; Peripheral Neurovascular Dysfunction*

## Peritoneal Dialysis

Acute **Pain** r/t instillation of dialysate, temperature of dialysate

Chronic **Sorrow** r/t chronic disability

Deficient **Knowledge** r/t treatment procedure, self-care with peritoneal dialysis

Impaired **Home** maintenance r/t complex home treatment of client

Risk for **Fluid** volume excess r/t retention of dialysate

Risk for ineffective **Breathing** pattern r/t pressure from dialysate

Risk for ineffective **Coping** r/t disability requiring change in lifestyle

Risk for **Infection**: peritoneal r/t invasive procedure, presence of catheter, dialysate

Risk for **Powerlessness** r/t chronic condition and care involved

*See Child with Chronic Condition; Hospitalized Child; Renal Failure; Renal Failure, Acute/Chronic, Child*

## Peritonitis

Acute **Pain** r/t inflammation, stimulation of somatic nerves

**Constipation** r/t decreased oral intake, decrease of peristalsis

Deficient **Fluid** volume r/t retention of fluid in bowel with loss of circulating blood volume

Imbalanced **Nutrition**: less than body requirements r/t nausea, vomiting

Ineffective **Breathing** pattern r/t pain, increased abdominal pressure

**Nausea** r/t gastrointestinal irritation

## Pernicious Anemia

**Diarrhea** r/t malabsorption of nutrients

Effective **Therapeutic** regimen management r/t follows treatment plan; lifelong replacement of vitamin $B_{12}$

**Fatigue** r/t imbalanced nutrition: less than body requirements

Imbalanced **Nutrition**: less than body requirements r/t lack of appetite associated with nausea and altered oral mucous membrane

Impaired **Memory** r/t anemia; lack of adequate red blood cells

Impaired **Oral** mucous membranes r/t vitamin deficiency; inability to absorb vitamin $B_{12}$ associated with lack of intrinsic factor

**Nausea** r/t altered oral mucous membrane; sore tongue, bleeding gums

Risk for **Peripheral** neurovascular dysfunction r/t anemia

Risk for **Falls** r/t dizziness, lightheadedness

## Persistent Fetal Circulation

*See Congenital Heart Disease/Cardiac Anomalies*

## Personal Identity Problems

Disturbed personal **Identity** r/t situational crisis, psychological impairment, chronic illness, pain

## Personality Disorder

Chronic low **Self-esteem** r/t inability to set and achieve goals

Compromised family **Coping** r/t inability of client to provide positive feedback to family, chronicity exhausting family

Decisional **Conflict** r/t low self-esteem, feelings that choices will always be wrong

Disturbed personal **Identity** r/t lack of consistent positive self-image

Impaired **Adjustment** r/t ambivalent behavior toward others, testing of others' loyalty

Impaired **Social** interaction r/t knowledge or skill deficit regarding ways to interact effectively with others, self-concept disturbances

Readiness for enhanced **Self-concept** r/t expressing willingness to enhance self-concept

Risk for **Loneliness** r/t inability to interact appropriately with others

Risk for **Self-mutilation** r/t disturbed interpersonal relationships, borderline personality disorders

Risk for situational low **Self-esteem** r/t history of learned helplessness

**Spiritual** distress r/t lack of identifiable values, lack of meaning to life

*See Antisocial Personality Disorder; Borderline Personality Disorder; Obsessive-Compulsive Disorder; Paranoid Personality Disorder*

## Pertussis (Whooping Cough)

*See Respiratory Infections, Acute Childhood*

## Pesticide Contamination

Effective **Therapeutic** regimen management r/t verbalizes intent to reduce risk factors associated with environmental toxins; meticulous hand hygiene

**Health-seeking** behaviors r/t expression of concern about environmental conditions

Risk for disproportionate **Growth** r/t environmental contamination

## Petechiae

*See Clotting Disorder; Anticoagulant Therapy; DIC (Disseminated Intravascular Coagulation); Hemophilia*

## Petit Mal Seizure

Effective **Therapeutic** regimen management r/t follows prescribed medication regimen

Readiness for enhanced **Therapeutic** regimen management r/t wears medical alert bracelet; limits hazardous activities such as driving, swimming, skiing, working at heights, operating equipment

*See Epilepsy*

## Pharyngitis

*See Sore Throat*

## Phenylketonuria

*See PKU (Phenylketonuria)*

## Pheochromocytoma

**Anxiety** r/t symptoms from increased catecholamines—headache, palpitations, sweating, nervousness, nausea, vomiting, syncope

Disturbed **Sleep** pattern r/t high levels of catecholamines

Ineffective **Health** maintenance r/t deficient knowledge regarding treatment and self-care

**Nausea** r/t increased catecholamines

Risk for ineffective **Tissue** perfusion: cardiopulmonary and renal r/t episodes of hypertension

*See Surgery, Perioperative; Surgery, Postoperative; Surgery, Preoperative*

## Phlebitis

*See Thrombophlebitis*

## Phobia (Specific)

**Anxiety** r/t inability to control emotions when dreaded object or situation is encountered

**Fear** r/t presence or anticipation of specific object or situation

Ineffective **Coping** r/t transfer of fears from self to dreaded object situation

**Powerlessness** r/t anxiety about encountering unknown or known entity

Readiness for enhanced **Communication** r/t willingness to discuss situation

Risk for **Post-trauma** syndrome r/t exposure to dreaded object or situation

Risk for **Powerlessness** r/t inadequate coping patterns

Risk for situational low **Self-esteem** r/t decreased power/control over fears

*See Anxiety; Anxiety Disorder; Panic Disorder*

## Photosensitivity

Ineffective **Health** maintenance r/t deficient knowledge regarding medications inducing photosensitivity

Risk for impaired **Skin** integrity r/t exposure to sun

## Physical Abuse

*See Abuse, Child; Abuse, Spouse, Parent, or Significant Other*

## Pica

**Anxiety** r/t stress from urge to eat nonnutritive substances

Imbalanced **Nutrition**: less than body requirements r/t eating nonnutritive substances

Impaired **Parenting** r/t lack of supervision, food deprivation

Risk for **Constipation** r/t presence of undigestible materials in gastrointestinal tract

Risk for **Infection** r/t ingestion of infectious agents via contaminated substances

Risk for **Poisoning** r/t ingestion of substances containing lead

## PID (Pelvic Inflammatory Disease)

Acute **Pain** r/t biological injury; inflammation, edema, congestion of pelvic tissues

Ineffective **Health** maintenance r/t deficient knowledge regarding self-care, treatment of disease

Ineffective **Sexuality** patterns r/t medically imposed abstinence from sexual activities until acute infection subsides, change in reproductive potential

Risk for **Infection** r/t insufficient knowledge to avoid exposure to pathogens; proper hygiene, nutrition, other health habits

Risk for urge urinary **Incontinence** r/t inflammation, edema, congestion of pelvic tissues

*See Maturational Issues, Adolescent*

## PIH (Pregnancy-Induced Hypertension/Preeclampsia)

**Anxiety** r/t fear of the unknown, threat to self and infant, change in role functioning

Death **Anxiety** r/t threat of preeclampsia

Deficient **Diversional** activity r/t bed rest

Deficient **Knowledge** r/t lack of experience with situation

Excess **Fluid** volume r/t decreased renal function

Impaired **Home** maintenance r/t bed rest

Impaired **Parenting** r/t bed rest

Impaired physical **Mobility** r/t medically prescribed limitations

Impaired **Social** interaction r/t imposed bed rest

Ineffective **Role** performance r/t change in physical capacity to assume role of pregnant woman or resume other roles

Interrupted **Family** processes r/t situational crisis

**Powerlessness** r/t complication threatening pregnancy, medically prescribed limitations

Readiness for enhanced **Knowledge** r/t desire for information on managing condition

Risk for imbalanced **Fluid** volume r/t hypertension, altered renal function

Risk for **Injury**: fetal r/t decreased uteroplacental perfusion, seizures

Risk for **Injury**: maternal r/t vasospasm, high blood pressure

Situational low **Self-esteem** r/t loss of idealized pregnancy

## Piloerection

**Hypothermia** r/t exposure to cold environment

## Pimples

*See Acne*

## Pinworms

Impaired **Comfort**: itching r/t worms and eggs in the anal area

Disturbed **Sleep** pattern r/t discomfort

Effective **Therapeutic** regimen management r/t adheres to guidelines for antiparasitic medication for infected person and members of household; check for pinworms with flashlight; check for eggs; place tape over anal area in the morning (tape is placed on slide and taken to health care provider to look for eggs)

Impaired **Home** maintenance r/t inadequate cleaning of bed linen and toilet seats

Readiness for enhanced **Therapeutic** regimen r/t proper hand washing; short clean fingernails; avoiding hand, mouth, nose contact with unwashed hands; appropriate cleaning of bed linen and toilet seats

## Pituitary Cushing's

*See Cushing's Syndrome*

## PKU (Phenylketonuria)

Effective management of **Therapeutic** regimen r/t testing of newborn for PKU and following prescribed dietary regimen if test is positive

Risk for delayed **Development** r/t not following strict dietary program; eating foods extremely low in phenylalanine; avoiding eggs, milk, any foods containing aspartame (Nutrasweet)

## Placenta Abruptio

Acute **Pain**: abdominal/back r/t premature separation of placenta before delivery

Death **Anxiety** r/t threat of mortality associated with bleeding

**Fear** r/t threat to self and fetus

Ineffective **Health** maintenance r/t deficient knowledge regarding treatment and control of hypertension associated with placenta abruptio

Risk for deficient **Fluid** volume r/t maternal blood loss

Risk for **Powerlessness** r/t complications of pregnancy and unknown outcome

Risk for **Spiritual** distress r/t fear from unknown outcome of pregnancy

## Placenta Previa

Death **Anxiety** r/t threat of mortality associated with bleeding

Deficient **Diversional** activity r/t long-term hospitalization

Disturbed **Body** image r/t negative feelings about body and reproductive ability, feelings of helplessness

**Fear** r/t threat to self and fetus, unknown future

Impaired **Home** maintenance r/t maternal bed rest, hospitalization

Impaired physical **Mobility** r/t medical protocol, maternal bed rest

Ineffective **Coping** r/t threat to self and fetus

Ineffective **Role** performance r/t maternal bed rest, hospitalization

Ineffective **Tissue** perfusion: placental r/t dilation of cervix, loss of placental implantation site

Interrupted **Family** processes r/t maternal bed rest, hospitalization

Risk for **Constipation** r/t bed rest, pregnancy

Risk for deficient **Fluid** volume r/t maternal blood loss

Risk for imbalanced **Fluid** volume r/t maternal blood loss

Risk for impaired **Parenting** r/t maternal bed rest, hospitalization

Risk for **Injury**: fetal and maternal r/t threat to uteroplacental perfusion, hemorrhage

Risk for **Powerlessness** r/t complications of pregnancy and unknown outcome

Situational low **Self-esteem** r/t situational crisis

**Spiritual** distress r/t inability to participate in usual religious rituals, situational crisis

## Pleural Effusion

Acute **Pain** r/t inflammation, fluid accumulation

Excess **Fluid** volume r/t compromised regulatory mechanisms; heart, liver, or kidney failure

**Hyperthermia** r/t increased metabolic rate secondary to infection

Ineffective **Breathing** pattern r/t pain

## Pleural Friction Rub

Acute **Pain** r/t inflammation, fluid accumulation

Ineffective **Breathing** pattern r/t pain

*See cause of Pleural Friction Rub*

## Pleural Tap

*See Pleural Effusion*

## Pleurisy

Acute **Pain** r/t pressure on pleural nerve endings associated with fluid accumulation or inflammation

Ineffective **Breathing** pattern r/t pain

Risk for impaired **Gas** exchange r/t ventilation perfusion imbalance

Risk for impaired physical **Mobility** r/t activity intolerance, inability to "catch breath"

Risk for ineffective **Airway** clearance r/t increased secretions, ineffective cough because of pain

## PMS (Premenstrual Tension Syndrome)

Acute **Pain** r/t hormonal stimulation of gastrointestinal structures

Deficient **Knowledge** r/t methods to deal with and prevent syndrome

Excess **Fluid** volume r/t alterations of hormonal levels inducing fluid retention

**Fatigue** r/t hormonal changes

Readiness for enhanced **Communication** r/t willingness to express thoughts and feelings about PMS

Readiness for enhanced **Therapeutic** regimen management r/t desire for information to manage and prevent symptoms

Risk for **Powerlessness** r/t lack of knowledge and ability to deal with symptoms

## PND (Paroxysmal Nocturnal Dyspnea)

**Anxiety** r/t inability to breathe during sleep

Decreased **Cardiac** output r/t failure of the left ventricle

Disturbed **Sleep** pattern r/t suffocating feeling from fluid in lungs on awakening from sleep

Ineffective **Breathing** pattern r/t increase in carbon dioxide levels, decrease in oxygen levels

Readiness for enhanced **Sleep** r/t expressing willingness to learn measures to enhance sleep

Risk for **Powerlessness** r/t inability to control nocturnal dyspnea

**Sleep** deprivation r/t inability to breathe during sleep

## Pneumonia

**Activity** intolerance r/t imbalance between oxygen supply and demand

Deficient **Knowledge** r/t risk factors predisposing person to pneumonia, treatment

**Hyperthermia** r/t dehydration, increased metabolic rate, illness

Imbalanced **Nutrition**: less than body requirements r/t loss of appetite

Impaired **Gas** exchange r/t decreased functional lung tissue

Impaired **Oral** mucous membrane r/t dry mouth from mouth breathing, decreased fluid intake

Ineffective **Airway** clearance r/t inflammation and presence of secretions

Ineffective **Health** maintenance r/t deficient knowledge regarding self-care and treatment of disease

Risk for deficient **Fluid** volume r/t inadequate intake of fluids

*See Respiratory Infections, Acute Childhood*

## Pneumothorax

Acute **Pain** r/t recent injury, coughing, deep breathing

**Fear** r/t threat to own well-being, difficulty breathing

Impaired **Gas** exchange r/t ventilation-perfusion imbalance

Risk for **Injury** r/t possible complications associated with closed chest drainage system

## Poisoning, Risk for

**EXTERNAL**

Risk for **Poisoning** r/t unprotected contact with heavy metals or chemicals; medicine stored in unlocked cabinets accessible to children or confused people; presence of poisonous vegetation; presence of atmospheric pollutants; paint or lacquer used in poorly ventilated areas or without effective protection; flaking or peeling paint or plaster in presence of young children; chemical contamination of food and water; availability of illicit drugs potentially contaminated by poisonous additives; large supplies of drugs in house, dangerous products placed or stored within the reach of children or confused persons

**INTERNAL**

Risk for **Poisoning** r/t reduced vision, verbalization of occupational settings without adequate safeguards; reduced vision; lack of safety or drug education, lack of proper precaution; insufficient finances; cognitive or emotional difficulties

## Polydipsia

Readiness for enhanced **Fluid** balance r/t no excessive thirst when diabetes is controlled

*See Diabetes Mellitus*

## Polyphagia

Readiness for enhanced **Nutrition** r/t knowledge of appropriate diet for diabetes

*See Diabetes Mellitus*

## Polyuria

Readiness for enhanced **Urinary** elimination r/t willingness to learn measures to enhance urinary elimination

*See Diabetes Mellitus*

## Postoperative Care

*See Surgery, Postoperative*

## Postpartum Blues

**Anxiety** r/t new responsibilities of parenting

Chronic **Sorrow** r/t loss of ideal postpartum experience or ideal parent-infant relationship

Deficient **Knowledge** r/t lifestyle changes

Disturbed **Body** image r/t normal postpartum recovery

Disturbed **Sleep** pattern r/t new responsibilities of parenting

**Fatigue** r/t childbirth, postpartum state

Impaired **Adjustment** r/t lack of support systems

Impaired **Home** maintenance r/t fatigue, care of newborn

Impaired **Parenting** r/t hormone-induced depression

Impaired **Social** interaction r/t change in role functioning

Ineffective **Coping** r/t hormonal changes, maturational crisis

Ineffective **Role** performance r/t new responsibilities of parenting

Risk for **Post-trauma** syndrome r/t trauma or violence associated with labor and birth process, medical/surgical interventions, history of sexual abuse

Risk for situational low **Self-esteem** r/t decreased power over feelings of sadness

Risk for **Spiritual** distress r/t altered relationships, social isolation

**Sexual** dysfunction r/t fear of another pregnancy, postpartum pain, lochia flow

## Postpartum Hemorrhage

**Activity** intolerance r/t anemia from loss of blood

Acute **Pain** r/t nursing and medical interventions to control bleeding

Death **Anxiety** r/t threat of mortality associated with bleeding

Decreased **Cardiac** output r/t hypovolemia

Deficient **Fluid** volume r/t uterine atony, loss of blood

Deficient **Knowledge** r/t lack of exposure to situation

Disturbed **Body** image r/t loss of ideal childbirth

**Fear** r/t threat to self, unknown future

Impaired **Home** maintenance r/t lack of stamina

Ineffective **Tissue** perfusion r/t hypovolemia

Interrupted **Breastfeeding** r/t separation from infant for medical treatment

Risk for imbalanced **Fluid** volume r/t maternal blood loss

Risk for **Infection** r/t loss of blood, depressed immunity

Risk for impaired **Parenting** r/t weakened maternal condition

Risk for **Powerlessness** r/t acute illness

## Postpartum, Normal Care

Acute **Pain** r/t episiotomy, lacerations, bruising, breast engorgement, headache, sore nipples, epidural or intravenous (IV) site, hemorrhoids

**Anxiety** r/t change in role functioning, parenting

**Constipation** r/t hormonal effects on smooth

muscles, fear of straining with defecation, effects of anesthesia

Deficient **Knowledge**: infant care r/t lack of preparation for parenting

Disturbed **Sleep** pattern r/t care of infant

Effective **Breastfeeding** r/t basic breastfeeding knowledge, support of partner and health care provider

**Fatigue** r/t childbirth, new responsibilities of parenting, body changes

**Health-seeking** behaviors r/t postpartum recovery and adaptation

Impaired **Skin** integrity r/t episiotomy, lacerations

Impaired **Urinary** elimination r/t effects of anesthesia, tissue trauma

Ineffective **Breastfeeding** r/t lack of knowledge, lack of support, lack of motivation

Ineffective **Role** performance r/t new responsibilities of parenting

Readiness for enhanced family **Coping** r/t adaptation to new family member

Readiness for enhanced **Parenting** r/t expressing willingness to enhance parenting skills

Risk for **Constipation** r/t hormonal effects on smooth muscles, fear of straining with defecation, effects of anesthesia

Risk for imbalanced **Fluid** volume r/t shift in blood volume, edema



Risk for impaired **Parenting** r/t lack of role models, deficient knowledge

Risk for **Infection** r/t tissue trauma, blood loss

Risk for **Post-trauma** syndrome r/t trauma or violence associated with labor and birth process, medical/surgical interventions, history of sexual abuse

Risk for urge urinary **Incontinence** r/t effects of anesthesia or tissue trauma

**Sexual** dysfunction r/t fear of pain or pregnancy

## Post-Trauma Syndrome

**Post-trauma** syndrome r/t events outside the range of the usual human experience; physical and psychosocial abuse; tragic occurrence involving multiple deaths; epidemics; sudden destruction of one's home or community; being held as a prisoner of war or enduring criminal victimization (torture); wars; rape; natural or produced disasters; serious accidents; assault; witnessing mutilation, violent death, other horrors; serious threat or injury to self or loved ones; industrial and motor vehicle accidents; military combat

## Post-Trauma Syndrome, Risk for

Risk for **Post-trauma** syndrome r/t exaggerated sense of responsibility; perception of event; survivor's role in the event; occupation (e.g., police, fire, rescue, corrections, emergency room staff, mental health worker); displacement from home; inadequate social support, nonsupportive environment; diminished ego strength; duration of the event

## Post-Traumatic Stress Disorder

**Anxiety** r/t exposure to internal or external cues that symbolize or resemble an aspect of the traumatic event

Death **Anxiety** r/t psychological stress associated with traumatic event

Disturbed **Energy** field r/t disharmony of mind, body, spirit

Disturbed **Sensory** perception r/t psychological stress

Disturbed **Sleep** pattern r/t recurring nightmares

Disturbed **Thought** processes r/t sense of reliving the experience (flashbacks)

Ineffective **Breathing** pattern r/t hyperventilation associated with anxiety

Ineffective **Coping** r/t extreme anxiety

**Post-trauma** syndrome r/t exposure to a traumatic event

Readiness for enhanced **Communication** r/t willingness to express feelings and thoughts

Readiness for enhanced **Spiritual** well-being r/t desire for harmony after stressful event

Risk for **Powerlessness** r/t flashbacks, reliving event

Risk for self- or other-directed **Violence** r/t fear of self or others

**Sleep** deprivation r/t nightmares associated with traumatic event

**Spiritual** distress r/t feelings of detachment or estrangement from others

## Potassium, Increase/Decrease

*See Hyperkalemia; Hypokalemia*

## Powerlessness

**Powerlessness** r/t health care environment, illness-related regimen, interpersonal interaction, lifestyle of helplessness

Risk for **Powerlessness** r/t *Physiological:* Chronic or acute illness (hospitalization, intubation, ventilator, suctioning); acute injury or progressive debilitating disease process (e.g., spinal cord injury, multiple sclerosis); aging (decreased physical strength, decreased mobility); dying. *Psychological:* Lack of knowledge of illness or health care style, lifestyle of dependency with inadequate coping patterns, absence of integrality, decreased self-esteem, low or unstable body image

## Preeclampsia

*See PIH (Pregnancy-Induced Hypertension/Preeclampsia)*

## Pregnancy, Cardiac Disorders

*See Cardiac Disorders in Pregnancy*

## Pregnancy Loss

Acute **Pain** r/t surgical intervention

**Anxiety** r/t threat to role functioning, health status, situational crisis

Chronic **Sorrow** r/t loss of a fetus or child

Compromised family **Coping** r/t lack of support by significant other because of personal suffering

Ineffective **Coping** r/t situational crisis

Ineffective **Role** performance r/t inability to assume parenting role

Ineffective **Sexuality** patterns r/t self-esteem disturbance resulting from pregnancy loss and anxiety about future pregnancies

Readiness for enhanced **Communication** r/t willingness to express feelings and thoughts about loss

Readiness for enhanced **Spiritual** well-being r/t desire for acceptance of loss

Risk for deficient **Fluid** volume r/t blood loss

Risk for dysfunctional **Grieving** r/t loss of pregnancy

Risk for ineffective **Sexuality** patterns r/t self-esteem disturbance, anxiety, grief

Risk for **Infection** r/t retained products of conception

Risk for **Powerlessness** r/t situational crisis

Risk for **Spiritual** distress r/t intense suffering

**Spiritual** distress r/t intense suffering

## Pregnancy, Normal

Deficient **Knowledge** r/t primiparity

Disturbed **Body** image r/t altered body function and appearance

Disturbed **Sleep** pattern r/t sleep deprivation secondary to uncomfortable pregnancy state

**Fear** r/t labor and delivery

**Health-seeking** behaviors r/t desire to promote optimal fetal and maternal health

Imbalanced **Nutrition**: less than body requirements r/t growing fetus, nausea

Imbalanced **Nutrition**: more than body requirements r/t deficient knowledge regarding nutritional needs of pregnancy

Ineffective **Coping** r/t personal vulnerability, situational crisis

Interrupted **Family** processes r/t developmental transition of pregnancy

**Nausea** r/t hormonal changes of pregnancy

Readiness for enhanced family **Coping** r/t satisfying partner relationship, attention to gratification of needs, effective adaptation to developmental tasks of pregnancy

Readiness for enhanced **Parenting** r/t expressing willingness to enhance parenting skills

**Sexual** dysfunction r/t altered body function, self-concept, body image with pregnancy

*See Discomforts of Pregnancy*

## Pregnancy-Induced Hypertension/ Preeclampsia

*See PIH (Pregnancy-Induced Hypertension/Preeclampsia)*

## Premature Dilation of the Cervix (Incompetent Cervix)

Anticipatory **Grieving** r/t potential loss of infant

Deficient **Diversional** activity r/t bed rest

Deficient **Knowledge** r/t treatment regimen, prognosis for pregnancy

**Fear** r/t potential loss of infant

Ineffective **Coping** r/t bed rest, threat to fetus

Ineffective **Role** performance r/t inability to continue usual patterns of responsibility

Impaired physical **Mobility** r/t imposed bed rest to prevent preterm birth

Impaired **Social** interaction r/t bed rest

**Powerlessness** r/t inability to control outcome of pregnancy

Risk for **Infection** r/t invasive procedures to prevent preterm birth

Risk for **Injury**: fetal r/t preterm birth, use of anesthetics

Risk for **Injury**: maternal r/t surgical procedures to prevent preterm birth (e.g., cerclage)

Risk for **Spiritual** distress r/t physical/psychological stress

**Sexual** dysfunction r/t fear of harm to fetus

Situational low **Self-esteem** r/t inability to complete normal pregnancy

P

## Premature Infant (Child)

Delayed **Growth** and development: developmental lag r/t prematurity, environmental and stimulation deficiencies, multiple caretakers

Disorganized **Infant** behavior r/t prematurity

Disturbed **Sensory** perception r/t noxious stimuli, noisy environment

Disturbed **Sleep** pattern r/t noisy and noxious intensive care environment

Imbalanced **Nutrition**: less than body requirements r/t delayed or understimulated rooting reflex, easy fatigue during feeding, diminished endurance

Impaired **Gas** exchange r/t effects of cardiopulmonary insufficiency

Impaired **Swallowing** r/t decreased or absent gag reflex, fatigue

Ineffective **Thermoregulation** r/t large body surface/weight ratio, immaturity of thermal regulation, state of prematurity

Readiness for enhanced organized **Infant** behavior r/t prematurity

Risk for delayed **Development** r/t prematurity

Risk for disproportionate **Growth** r/t prematurity

Risk for **Infection** r/t inadequate, immature, or undeveloped acquired immune response

Risk for **Injury** r/t prolonged mechanical ventilation, retinopathy of prematurely (ROP) secondary to 100% oxygen environment

P

## Premature Infant (Parent)

Anticipatory **Grieving** r/t loss of perfect child possibly leading to dysfunctional grieving

Chronic **Sorrow** r/t threat of loss of a child, prolonged hospitalization

Compromised family **Coping** r/t disrupted family roles and disorganization, prolonged condition exhausting supportive capacity of significant persons

Decisional **Conflict** r/t support system deficit, multiple sources of information

Dysfunctional **Grieving** (prolonged) r/t unresolved conflicts

Ineffective **Breastfeeding** r/t disrupted establishment of effective pattern secondary to prematurity or insufficient opportunities

Parental role **Conflict** r/t expressed concerns, expressed inability to care for child's physical, emotional, or developmental needs

Readiness for enhanced **Family** process r/t adaptation to change associated with premature infant

Risk for impaired parent/infant/child **Attachment** r/t separation, physical barriers, lack of privacy

Risk for **Powerlessness** r/t inability to control situation

Risk for **Spiritual** distress r/t challenged belief or value systems regarding moral or ethical implications of treatment plans

**Spiritual** distress r/t challenged belief or value systems regarding moral or ethical implications of treatment plans

*See Child with Chronic Condition; Hospitalized Child*

## Premature Rupture of Membranes

Anticipatory **Grieving** r/t potential loss of infant

**Anxiety** r/t threat to infant's health status

Disturbed **Body** image r/t inability to carry pregnancy to term

Ineffective **Coping** r/t situational crisis

Risk for **Infection** r/t rupture of membranes

Risk for **Injury**: fetal r/t risk of premature birth

Situational low **Self-esteem** r/t inability to carry pregnancy to term

## Premenstrual Tension Syndrome

*See PMS (Premenstrual Tension Syndrome)*

## Prenatal Care, Normal

**Anxiety** r/t unknown future, threat to self secondary to pain of labor

**Constipation** r/t decreased gastrointestinal motility secondary to hormonal stimulation

Deficient **Knowledge** r/t lack of experience with pregnancy and care

Disturbed **Sleep** pattern r/t discomforts of pregnancy and fetal activity

**Fatigue** r/t increased energy demands

**Health-seeking** behaviors r/t consistent prenatal care and education

Imbalanced **Nutrition**: less than body requirements r/t nausea from normal hormonal changes

Impaired **Urinary** elimination r/t frequency caused by increased pelvic pressure and hormonal stimulation

Ineffective **Breathing** pattern r/t increased intrathoracic pressure and decreased energy secondary to enlarged uterus

Interrupted **Family** processes r/t developmental transition

Readiness for enhanced **Knowledge** of appropriate prenatal care

Readiness for enhanced **Nutrition** r/t desire for knowledge of appropriate nutrition during pregnancy

Readiness for enhanced **Parenting** r/t realistic expectations of new role as parent

Readiness for enhanced **Spiritual** well-being r/t oncoming new role as parent

Risk for **Activity** intolerance r/t enlarged abdomen, increased cardiac workload

Risk for **Constipation** r/t decreased gastrointestinal motility secondary to hormonal stimulation

Risk for **Injury**: maternal r/t change in balance and center of gravity secondary to enlarged abdomen

Risk for **Sexual** dysfunction r/t enlarged abdomen, fear of harm to infant

## Prenatal Testing

Acute **Pain** r/t invasive procedures

**Anxiety** r/t unknown outcome, delayed test results

**Health-seeking** behaviors r/t desire to have information regarding prenatal testing

Risk for **Infection** r/t invasive procedures during amniocentesis or chorionic villi sampling

Risk for **Injury**: fetal r/t invasive procedures

## Preoperative Teaching

**Health-seeking** behaviors r/t preoperative regimens, postoperative precautions, expectations of role of client during preoperative or postoperative time

*See Surgery, Preoperative Care*

## Pressure Ulcer

Acute **Pain** r/t tissue destruction, exposure of nerves

Imbalanced **Nutrition**: less than body requirements r/t limited access to food, inability to absorb nutrients because of biological factors, anorexia

Impaired bed **Mobility** r/t intolerance to activity, pain, cognitive impairment, depression, severe anxiety

Impaired **Skin** integrity: stage I or II pressure ulcer r/t physical immobility, mechanical factors, altered circulation, skin irritants

Impaired **Tissue** integrity: stage III or IV pressure ulcer r/t altered circulation, impaired physical mobility

Risk for **Infection** r/t physical immobility, mechanical factors (shearing forces, pressure, restraint, altered circulation, skin irritants)

Total urinary **Incontinence** r/t neurological dysfunction

## Preterm Labor

Anticipatory **Grieving** r/t loss of idealized pregnancy, potential loss of fetus

**Anxiety** r/t threat to fetus, change in role functioning, change in environment and interaction patterns, use of tocolytic drugs

Deficient **Diversional** activity r/t long-term hospitalization

Disturbed **Sleep** pattern r/t change in usual pattern secondary to contractions, hospitalization, treatment regimen

Impaired **Home** maintenance r/t medical restrictions

Impaired physical **Mobility** r/t medically imposed restrictions

Impaired **Social** interaction r/t prolonged bed rest or hospitalization

Ineffective **Coping** r/t situational crisis, preterm labor

Ineffective **Role** performance r/t inability to carry out normal roles secondary to bed rest or hospitalization, change in expected course of pregnancy

Readiness for enhanced **Communication** r/t willingness to discuss thoughts and feelings about situation

Risk for **Injury**: fetal r/t premature birth, immature body systems

Risk for **Injury**: maternal r/t use of tocolytic drugs

Risk for **Powerlessness** r/t lack of control over preterm labor

**Sexual** dysfunction r/t actual or perceived limitation imposed by preterm labor and/or prescribed treatment, separation from partner because of hospitalization

Situational low **Self-esteem** r/t threatened ability to carry pregnancy to term

## Problem-Solving Ability

Defensive **Coping** r/t situational crisis

Impaired **Adjustment** r/t altered locus of control

Ineffective **Coping** r/t situational crisis

Readiness for enhanced **Communication** r/t willingness to share ideas with others

Readiness for enhanced **Spiritual** well-being r/t desire to draw on inner strength and find meaning and purpose to life

## Projection

**Anxiety** r/t threat to self-concept

Chronic low **Self-esteem** r/t failure

Defensive **Coping** r/t inability to acknowledge that own behavior may be a problem, blaming others

Impaired **Social** interaction r/t self-concept disturbance, confrontational communication style

Risk for **Loneliness** r/t blaming others for problems

Risk for **Post-trauma** syndrome r/t diminished ego strength

## Prolapsed Umbilical Cord

**Fear** r/t threat to fetus, impending surgery

Ineffective **Tissue** perfusion: fetal r/t interruption in umbilical blood flow

Risk for **Injury**: fetal r/t cord compression, ineffective tissue perfusion

Risk for **Injury**: maternal r/t emergency surgery

## Prolonged Gestation

**Anxiety** r/t potential change in birthing plans, need for increased medical intervention, unknown outcome for fetus

Defensive **Coping** r/t underlying feeling of inadequacy regarding ability to give birth normally

Imbalanced **Nutrition**: less than body requirements (fetal) r/t aging of placenta

**Powerlessness** r/t perceived lack of control over outcome of pregnancy

Situational low **Self-esteem** r/t perceived inadequacy of body functioning

## Prostatectomy

*See TURP (Transurethral Resection of the Prostate)*

## Prostatic Hypertrophy

Disturbed **Sleep** pattern r/t nocturia

Ineffective **Health** maintenance r/t deficient knowledge regarding self-care and prevention of complications

Risk for **Infection** r/t urinary residual after voiding, bacterial invasion of bladder

Risk for urge urinary **Incontinence** r/t small bladder capacity

**Urinary** retention r/t obstruction

*See BPH (Benign Prostatic Hypertrophy)*

## Prostatitis

Ineffective **Health** maintenance r/t deficient knowledge regarding treatment

Ineffective **Protection** r/t depressed immune system

Risk for urge **Incontinence** r/t irritation of bladder

## Protection, Altered

Ineffective **Protection** r/t abnormal blood profiles (e.g., leukopenia, thrombocytopenia, anemia, coagulation), inadequate nutrition, extremes of age; drug therapies (e.g., antineoplastic, corticosteroid, immune, anticoagulant, thrombolytic); alcohol abuse; treatments (e.g. surgery, radiation); diseases such as cancer, immune disorders

## Pruritus

Deficient **Knowledge** r/t methods to treat and prevent itching

Impaired **Comfort**: pruritus r/t inflammation in tissues

Risk for impaired **Skin** integrity r/t scratching from pruritus

## Psoriasis

Disturbed **Body** image r/t lesions on body

Impaired **Skin** integrity r/t lesions on body

Ineffective **Health** maintenance r/t deficient knowledge regarding treatment modalities

**Powerlessness** r/t lack of control over condition with frequent exacerbations and remissions

## Psychosis

**Anxiety** r/t unconscious conflict with reality

Chronic **Sorrow** r/t chronic mental illness

Disturbed **Sleep** pattern r/t sensory alterations contributing to fear and anxiety

Disturbed **Thought** processes r/t inaccurate interpretations of environment

**Fear** r/t altered contact with reality

Imbalanced **Nutrition**: less than body requirements r/t lack of awareness of hunger, disinterest toward food

Impaired **Home** maintenance r/t impaired cognitive or emotional functioning, inadequate support systems

Impaired **Social** interaction r/t impaired communication patterns, self-concept disturbance, disturbed thought processes

Impaired verbal **Communication** r/t psychosis, inaccurate perceptions, hallucinations, delusions

Ineffective **Coping** r/t inadequate support systems, unrealistic perceptions, disturbed thought processes, impaired communication

Ineffective **Health** maintenance r/t cognitive impairment, ineffective individual and family coping

Interrupted **Family** processes r/t inability to express feelings, impaired communication

Risk for **Post-trauma** syndrome r/t diminished ego strength

Risk for self- or other-directed **Violence** r/t lack of trust, panic, hallucinations, delusional thinking

Risk for **Suicide** r/t psychiatric illness/disorder

**Self-care** deficit r/t loss of contact with reality, impairment of perception

**Self-esteem** disturbance r/t excessive use of defense mechanisms (e.g., projection, denial, rationalization)

**Social** isolation r/t lack of trust, regression, delusional thinking, repressed fears

*See Schizophrenia*

## PTCA (Percutaneous Transluminal Coronary Angioplasty)

*See Angioplasty, Coronary*

## Pulmonary Edema

**Anxiety** r/t fear of suffocation

Impaired **Gas** exchange r/t extravasation of extravascular fluid in lung tissues and alveoli

Ineffective **Breathing** pattern r/t presence of tracheobronchial secretions

Ineffective **Health** maintenance r/t deficient knowledge regarding treatment regimen

**Sleep** deprivation r/t inability to breathe

*See CHF (Congestive Heart Failure)*

## Pulmonary Embolism

Acute **Pain** r/t biological injury, lack of oxygen to cells

Deficient **Knowledge** r/t activities to prevent embolism, self-care after diagnosis of embolism

Delayed **Surgical** recovery r/t complications associated with respiratory difficulty

**Fear** r/t severe pain, possible death

Impaired **Gas** exchange r/t altered blood flow to alveoli secondary to lodged embolus

Ineffective **Tissue** perfusion: pulmonary r/t interruption of pulmonary blood flow secondary to lodged embolus

Risk for altered **Cardiac** output r/t right ventricular failure secondary to obstructed pulmonary artery

*See Anticoagulant Therapy*

## Pulmonary Stenosis

*See Congenital Heart Disease/Cardiac Anomalies*

## Pulse Deficit

Decreased **Cardiac** output r/t dysrhythmia

*See Dysrhythmia*

## Pulse Oximetry

Readiness for enhanced **Knowledge** r/t treatment regimen

*See Hypoxia*

## Pulse Pressure, Increased

*See Intracranial Pressure, Increased*

## Pulse Pressure, Narrowed

*See Shock*

## Pulses, Absent or Diminished Peripheral

Ineffective **Tissue** perfusion: peripheral r/t interruption of arterial flow

Risk for **Peripheral** neurovascular dysfunction r/t fractures, mechanical compression, orthopedic surgery trauma, immobilization, burns, vascular obstruction

*See cause of Absent or Diminished Peripheral Pulses*

## Purpura

*See Clotting Disorder*

## Pyelonephritis

Acute **Pain** r/t inflammation and irritation of urinary tract

Disturbed **Sleep** pattern r/t urinary frequency

Impaired **Comfort** r/t chills and fever

Impaired **Urinary** elimination r/t irritation of urinary tract

Ineffective **Health** maintenance r/t deficient knowledge regarding self-care, treatment of disease, prevention of further urinary tract infections

Risk for urge urinary **Incontinence** r/t irritation of urinary tract

## Pyloric Stenosis

Acute **Pain** r/t surgical incision

Deficient **Fluid** volume r/t vomiting, dehydration

Imbalanced **Nutrition**: less than body requirements r/t vomiting secondary to pyloric sphincter obstruction

Ineffective **Health** maintenance r/t parental deficient knowledge regarding home care feeding regimen, wound care

*See Hospitalized Child*

## Quadriplegia

Anticipatory **Grieving** r/t loss of normal lifestyle, severity of disability

Disturbed **Energy** field r/t illness, grieving of loss of normal function

Impaired **Transfer** ability r/t quadriplegia

Impaired wheelchair **Mobility** r/t quadriplegia

Ineffective **Breathing** pattern r/t inability to use intercostal muscles

Readiness for enhanced **Spiritual** well being r/t heightened coping associated with disability

Risk for **Autonomic** dysreflexia r/t bladder distention, bowel distention, skin irritation, lack of client and caregiver knowledge

Risk for impaired **Religiosity** r/t immobility and possible lack of transportation

*See Spinal Cord Injury*

# R

## RA

*See Rheumatoid Arthritis*

## Rabies

Acute **Pain** r/t multiple immunization injections

**Health**-seeking behaviors r/t prophylactic immunization of domestic animals, avoidance of contact with wild animals

**Hopelessness** r/t poor prognosis

Ineffective **Health** maintenance r/t deficient knowledge regarding care of wound, isolation and observation of infected animal

## Radial Nerve Dysfunction

Acute **Pain** r/t trauma to hand/arm

*See Neuropathy, Peripheral*

## Radiation Therapy

**Activity** intolerance r/t fatigue from possible anemia

Deficient **Knowledge** r/t what to expect with radiation therapy

**Diarrhea** r/t irradiation effects

Disturbed **Body** image r/t change in appearance, hair loss

Imbalanced **Nutrition**: less than body requirements r/t anorexia, nausea, vomiting, irradiation of areas of pharynx and esophagus

Impaired **Oral** mucous membrane r/t irradiation effects

Ineffective **Protection** r/t suppression of bone marrow

**Nausea** r/t side effects of radiation

Risk for impaired **Skin** integrity r/t irradiation effects

Risk for **Powerlessness** r/t medical treatment and possible side effects

Risk for **Spiritual** distress r/t radiation treatment, prognosis

## Radical Neck Dissection

*See Laryngectomy*

## Rage

Risk for other-directed **Violence** r/t panic state, manic excitement, organic brain syndrome

Risk for **Self-mutilation** r/t command hallucinations

Risk for **Suicide** r/t desire to kill oneself

## Rape-Trauma Syndrome

Chronic **Sorrow** r/t forced loss of virginity

**Rape-trauma** syndrome r/t forced, violent sexual penetration against victim's will and consent

**Rape-trauma** syndrome: compound reaction r/t forced and violent sexual penetration against victim's will and consent, activation of previous health disruptions (e.g., physical illness, psychiatric illness, substance abuse)

**Rape-trauma** syndrome: silent reaction r/t forced and violent sexual penetration against victim's will and consent, demonstration of repression of incident

Risk for **Post-trauma** syndrome r/t trauma or violence associated with rape

Risk for **Powerlessness** r/t inability to control thoughts about incident

Risk for **Spiritual** distress r/t forced loss of virginity

## Rash

Impaired **Comfort**: pruritus r/t inflammation in skin

Impaired **Skin** integrity r/t mechanical trauma

Risk for **Infection** r/t traumatized tissue, broken skin

Risk for latex **Allergy** r/t multiple surgical procedures, allergies to products associated with latex allergy, professions with daily associations with latex, history of reactions to latex

## Rationalization

Defensive **Coping** r/t situational crisis, inability to accept blame for consequences of own behavior

Ineffective **Denial** r/t fear of consequences, actual or perceived loss

Readiness for enhanced **Communication** r/t expressing desire to share thoughts and feelings

Readiness for enhanced **Spiritual** well-being r/t possibility of seeking harmony with self, others, higher power/God

Risk for **Post-trauma** syndrome r/t survivor's role in event

## Rats, Rodents in the Home

Impaired **Home** maintenance r/t lack of knowledge, insufficient finances

*See Filthy Home Environment*

## Raynaud's Disease

Deficient **Knowledge** r/t lack of information about disease process, possible complications, self-care needs regarding disease process and medication

Ineffective **Tissue** perfusion: peripheral r/t transient reduction of blood flow

## RDS (Respiratory Distress Syndrome)

*See Respiratory Conditions of the Neonate*

## Rectal Fullness

**Constipation** r/t decreased activity level, decreased fluid intake, inadequate fiber in diet, decreased peristalsis, side effects from antidepressant or antipsychotic therapy

Risk for **Constipation** r/t habitual denial/ignoring of urge to defecate

## Rectal Pain/Bleeding

Acute **Pain** r/t pressure of defecation

**Constipation** r/t pain on defecation

Deficient **Knowledge** r/t possible causes of rectal bleeding, pain, treatment modalities

Risk for deficient **Fluid** volume: bleeding r/t untreated rectal bleeding

## Rectal Lump

*See Hemorrhoids*

## Rectal Surgery

*See Hemorrhoidectomy*

## Rectocele Repair

Acute **Pain** r/t surgical procedure

**Constipation** r/t painful defecation

Ineffective **Health** maintenance r/t deficient knowledge of postoperative care of surgical site, dietary measures, exercise to prevent constipation

Risk for **Infection** r/t surgical procedure, possible contamination of site with feces

Risk for urge urinary **Incontinence** r/t edema from surgery

**Urinary** retention r/t edema from surgery

## Reflex Incontinence

Reflex **Incontinence** r/t neurological impairment

## Regression

**Anxiety** r/t threat to or change in health status

Defensive **Coping** r/t denial of obvious problems, weaknesses

Ineffective **Role** performance r/t powerlessness over health status

**Powerlessness** r/t health care environment

*See Hospitalized Child; Separation Anxiety*

## Regretful

**Anxiety** r/t situational or maturational crises

Death **Anxiety** r/t feelings of not having accomplished goals in life

Risk for **Spiritual** distress r/t inability to forgive

## Rehabilitation

Impaired **Comfort** r/t difficulty in performing rehabilitation tasks

Impaired physical **Mobility** r/t injury, surgery, psychosocial condition warranting rehabilitation

Ineffective **Coping** r/t loss of normal function

Readiness for enhanced **Self-concept** r/t accepts strengths and limitations

Readiness for enhanced **Therapeutic** regimen management r/t expression of desire to manage rehabilitation

**Self-care** deficit r/t impaired physical mobility

## Relaxation Techniques

**Anxiety** r/t disturbed energy field

**Health-seeking** behaviors r/t requesting information about ways to relieve stress

Readiness for enhanced **Religiosity** r/t requests religious materials and/or experiences

Readiness for enhanced **Self-concept** r/t willingness to enhance self-concept

Readiness for enhanced **Spiritual** well-being r/t seeking comfort from higher power

## Religiosity

Impaired **Religiosity** r/t *Physical:* Sickness/illness, pain. *Psychological:* Ineffective support/coping, personal disaster/crisis, lack of security, anxiety, fear of death, ineffective coping with disease, use of religion to manipulate. *Sociocultural:* Barriers to practicing religion (cultural and environmental), lack of social integration, lack of social/cultural interaction. *Spiritual:* Spiritual crises, suffering. *Developmental and Situational:* End-stage life crises, life transitions, aging

Readiness for enhanced **Religiosity** r/t expresses

desire to strengthen religious belief patterns and customs that had provided comfort/religion in the past; request for assistance to increase participation in prescribed religious beliefs through: religious ceremonies, dietary regulations/rituals, clothing, prayer, worship/religious services, private religious behaviors/ reading religious materials/media, holiday observances; requests assistance expanding religious options; requests meeting with religious leaders/facilitators; requests forgiveness, reconciliation; requests religious material and/or experiences; questions or rejects belief patterns and customs that are harmful

Risk for impaired **Religiosity** r/t *Physical:* Illness/ hospitalization, pain. *Psychological:* Ineffective support/ coping/caregiving, depression; lack of security. *Sociocultural:* Lack of social interaction, cultural barrier to practing religion, social isolation. *Spiritual:* Suffering. *Environmental:* Lack of transportation, environmental barriers to practicing religion. *Developmental:* Life transitions

## Religious Concerns

Readiness for enhanced **Spiritual** well-being r/t desire for increased spirituality

Risk for impaired **Religiosity** r/t ineffective support/ coping/caregiving

Risk for **Spiritual** distress r/t physical or psychological stress

**Spiritual** distress r/t separation from religious or cultural ties

## Relocation Stress Syndrome

**Relocation** stress syndrome r/t unpredictability of experience; isolation from family/friends; past, concurrent, recent losses; feeling of powerlessness; lack of adequate support system; lack of predeparture counseling; passive coping; impaired psychosocial health; language barrier; decreased health status

## Renal Failure

**Activity** intolerance r/t effects of anemia, CHF

Chronic **Sorrow** r/t chronic illness

Death **Anxiety** r/t unknown outcome of disease

Decreased **Cardiac** output r/t effects of congestive heart failure, elevated potassium levels interfering with conduction system

Excess **Fluid** volume r/t decreased urine output, sodium retention, inappropriate fluid intake

**Fatigue** r/t effects of chronic uremia and anemia

Imbalanced **Nutrition**: less than body requirements r/t anorexia, nausea, vomiting, altered taste sensation, dietary restrictions

Impaired **Comfort**: pruritus r/t effects of uremia

Impaired **Oral** mucous membrane r/t irritation from nitrogenous waste products

Impaired **Urinary** elimination r/t effects of disease, need for dialysis

Ineffective **Coping** r/t depression secondary to chronic disease

Risk for impaired **Oral** mucous membrane r/t dehydration, effects of uremia

Risk for **Infection** r/t altered immune functioning

Risk for **Injury** r/t bone changes, neuropathy, muscle weakness

Risk for **Noncompliance** r/t complex medical therapy

Risk for **Powerlessness** r/t chronic illness

**Spiritual** distress r/t dealing with chronic illness

## Renal Failure, Acute/Chronic, Child

Deficient **Diversional** activity r/t immobility during dialysis

Disturbed **Body** image r/t growth retardation, bone changes, visibility of dialysis access devices (shunt, fistula), edema

*See Child with Chronic Condition; Hospitalized Child; Renal Failure*

## Renal Failure, Nonoliguric

**Anxiety** r/t change in health status

Risk for deficient **Fluid** volume r/t loss of large volumes of urine

*See Renal Failure*

## Renal Transplantation, Donor

Decisional **Conflict** r/t harvesting of kidney from traumatized donor

Readiness for enhanced **Communication** r/t expressing thoughts and feelings about situation

Readiness for enhanced family **Coping** r/t decision to allow organ donation

Readiness for enhanced **Spirituality** r/t inner peace resulting from allowance of organ donation

**Spiritual** distress r/t anticipatory grieving from loss of significant person

*See Nephrectomy*

## Renal Transplantation, Recipient

**Anxiety** r/t possible rejection, procedure

Deficient **Knowledge** r/t specific nutritional needs, possible paralytic ileus, fluid or sodium restrictions

Impaired **Health** maintenance r/t long-term home

treatment after transplantation, diet, signs of rejection, use of medications

Impaired **Urinary** elimination r/t possible impaired renal function

Ineffective **Protection** r/t immunosuppression therapy

Readiness for enhanced **Spiritual** well-being r/t acceptance of situation

Risk for **Infection** r/t use of immunosuppressive therapy to control rejection

Risk for **Spiritual** distress r/t obtaining transplanted kidney from someone's traumatic loss

## Respiratory Acidosis

*See Acidosis, Respiratory*

## Respiratory Conditions of the Neonate (Respiratory Distress Syndrome [RDS], Meconium Aspiration, Diaphragmatic Hernia)

**Fatigue** r/t increased energy requirements and metabolic demands

Impaired **Gas** exchange r/t decreased surfactant, immature lung tissue

Ineffective **Airway** clearance r/t sequelae of attempts to breathe in utero resulting in meconium aspiration

Ineffective **Breathing** pattern r/t prolonged ventilator dependence

Risk for **Infection** r/t tissue destruction or irritation secondary to aspiration of meconium fluid

*See Bronchopulmonary Dysplasia; Hospitalized Child; Premature Infant, Child*

## Respiratory Distress

*See Dyspnea*

## Respiratory Distress Syndrome (RDS)

*See Respiratory Conditions of the Neonate*

## Respiratory Infections, Acute Childhood (Croup, Epiglottitis, Pertussis, Pneumonia, Respiratory Syncytial Virus)

**Activity** intolerance r/t generalized weakness, dyspnea, fatigue, poor oxygenation

**Anxiety**/fear r/t oxygen deprivation, difficulty breathing

Deficient **Fluid** volume r/t insensible losses (fever, diaphoresis), inadequate oral fluid intake

**Hyperthermia** r/t infectious process

Imbalanced **Nutrition**: less than body requirements r/t anorexia, fatigue, generalized weakness, poor sucking and breathing coordination, dyspnea

Impaired **Gas** exchange r/t insufficient oxygenation secondary to inflammation or edema of epiglottis, larynx, bronchial passages

Ineffective **Airway** clearance r/t excess tracheobronchial secretions

Ineffective **Breathing** pattern r/t inflamed bronchial passages, coughing

Risk for **Aspiration** r/t inability to coordinate breathing, coughing, sucking

Risk for **Infection**: transmission to others r/t virulent infectious organisms

Risk for **Injury** (to pregnant others) r/t exposure to aerosolized medications (e.g., ribavirin, pentamidine), resultant potential fetal toxicity

Risk for **Suffocation** r/t inflammation of larynx, epiglottis

*See Hospitalized Child*

## Respiratory Syncytial Virus

*See Respiratory Infections, Acute Childhood*

## Restless Leg Syndrome

Disturbed **Sleep** pattern r/t leg discomfort during sleep relieved by frequent leg movement

**Sleep** deprivation r/t frequent leg movements

*See Stress*

## Retarded Growth and Development

*See Growth and Development Lag*

## Retching

Imbalanced **Nutrition**: less than body requirements r/t inability to ingest food

**Nausea** r/t chemotherapy, postsurgical anesthesia, irritation to gastrointestinal system, stimulation of neuropharmacological mechanisms

## Retinal Detachment

**Anxiety** r/t change in vision, threat of loss of vision

Deficient **Knowledge** r/t symptoms, need for early intervention to prevent permanent damage

Disturbed **Sensory** perception: visual r/t changes in vision, sudden flashes of light, floating spots, blurring of vision

Risk for impaired **Home** maintenance r/t postoperative care, activity limitations, care of affected eye

*See Vision Impairment*

## Retinopathy, Diabetic

*See Diabetic Retinopathy*

## Retinopathy of Prematurity (ROP)

Effective **Therapeutic** regimen management r/t at least two eye examinations, by a qualified ophthalmologist, for very-low-birth-weight or premature babies (less than 28 weeks gestational age), as well as other premature or low-birth-weight babies who have unstable conditions; follow-up examinations at appropriate times.

Risk for **Injury** r/t prolonged mechanical ventilation, retinopathy of prematurely (ROP) secondary to 100% oxygen environment

*See Retinal Detachment*

## Reye's Syndrome

Anticipatory **Grieving** r/t uncertain prognosis and sequelae

Compromised family **Coping** r/t acute situational crisis

Deficient **Fluid** volume r/t vomiting, hyperventilation

Disturbed **Sensory** perception r/t cerebral edema

Disturbed **Thought** processes r/t degenerative changes in fatty brain tissue

Excess **Fluid** volume: cerebral r/t cerebral edema

Imbalanced **Nutrition**: less than body requirements r/t effects of liver dysfunction, vomiting

Impaired **Gas** exchange r/t hyperventilation, sequelae of increased intracranial pressure

Impaired **Skin** integrity r/t effects of decorticate or decerebrate posturing, seizure activity

Ineffective **Breathing** pattern r/t neuromuscular impairment

Ineffective **Health** maintenance r/t deficient knowledge regarding use of salicylates during viral illness of child

Risk for **Injury** r/t combative behavior, seizure activity

Situational low **Self-esteem**: family r/t negative perceptions of self, perceived inability to manage family situation, expressions of guilt

*See Hospitalized Child*

## Rh Factor Incompatibility

**Anxiety** r/t unknown outcome of pregnancy

Deficient **Knowledge** r/t treatment regimen from lack of experience with situation

Effective **Therapeutic** regimen management r/t following recommended protocol; if the father of the infant is Rh-positive, and the mother Rh-negative, the mother is given a midterm injection of RhoGAM and a second injection within a few days of delivery.

**Health-seeking** behaviors r/t prenatal care, compliance with diagnostic and treatment regimen

**Powerlessness** r/t perceived lack of control over outcome of pregnancy

Risk for fetal **Injury** r/t intrauterine destruction of red blood cells, transfusions

## Rhabdomyolyis

Impaired physical **Mobility** r/t myalgia and muscle weakness

Impaired **Urinary** elimination r/t presence of myoglobin in the kidneys

Ineffective **Coping** r/t serious of condition

Readiness for enhanced **Therapeutic** regimen management r/t seeks information to avoid condition

Risk for deficient **Fluid** volume r/t reduced blood flow to kidneys

*See Renal Failure*

## Rheumatic Fever

*See Endocarditis*

## Rheumatoid Arthritis

Chronic **Pain** r/t swollen or inflamed joints, restricted movement, physical therapy

Effective **Therapeutic** regimen management r/t following prescribed medication and adhering to exercise program; physical therapy

**Fatigue** r/t chronic inflammatory disease

Impaired physical **Mobility** r/t pain, limited range of motion

Imbalanced **Nutrition**: less than body requirements r/t loss of appetite

Risk for impaired **Skin** integrity r/t splints, adaptive devices

Risk for **Injury** r/t impaired physical mobility, splints, adaptive devices, increased bleeding potential secondary to antiinflammatory medications

Risk for situational low **Self-esteem** r/t disturbed body image

**Self-care** deficits: feeding, bathing/hygiene, dressing/grooming, toileting r/t restricted joint movement, pain

*See Arthritis; JRA (Juvenile Rheumatoid Arthritis)*

## Rib Fracture

Acute **Pain** r/t movement, deep breathing

Ineffective **Breathing** pattern r/t fractured ribs

*See Ventilator Client (if relevant)*

## Ridicule of Others

Defensive **Coping** r/t situational crisis, psychological impairment, substance abuse

Risk for **Post-trauma** syndrome r/t perception of the event

## Ringworm of Body

Impaired **Skin** integrity r/t presence of macules associated with fungus

Ineffective **Therapeutic** regimen management r/t deficient knowledge of prevention, treatment

*See Itching*

## Ringworm of Nails

Disturbed **Body** image r/t appearance of nails, removed nails

Ineffective **Therapeutic** regimen management r/t deficient knowledge of prevention, treatment

## Ringworm of Scalp

Disturbed **Body** image r/t possible hair loss (alopecia)

Ineffective **Therapeutic** regimen management r/t deficient knowledge of prevention, treatment

*See Itching*

## Risk for Relocation Stress Syndrome

*See Relocation Stress Syndrome*

## Roaches, Invasion of Home with

Impaired **Home** maintenance r/t lack of knowledge, insufficient finances

*See Filthy Home Environment*

## Role Performance, Altered

Ineffective **Role** performance r/t *Social:* Inadequate or inappropriate linkage with the health care system; job schedule demands; young age; developmental level; lack of rewards; poverty; family conflict; inadequate support system; inadequate role socialization (e.g., role model, expectations, responsibilities); *Knowledge:* Inadequate role preparation (e.g., role transition, skill rehearsal, validation); lack of knowledge about role, role skills, role transition, lack of opportunity for role rehearsal; developmental transitions; unrealistic role expectations education attainment level; lack of or inadequate role model; *Physiological:* Inadequate/ inappropriate linkage with health care system; substance abuse; mental illness; body image alteration' physical illness; cognitive deficits; health alterations (e.g., physical health, body image, self-esteem, mental health, psychosocial health, cognition, learning style, neurological health); depression; low self-esteem; pain; fatigue

## ROP

*See Retinopathy of Prematurity (ROP)*

## RSV (Respiratory Syncytial Virus)

*See Respiratory Infection, Acute Childhood*

## Rubella

*See Communicable Diseases, Childhood*

## Rubor of Extremities

Ineffective **Tissue** perfusion: peripheral r/t interruption of arterial flow

*See Peripheral Vascular Disease*

## Ruptured Disk

*See Low Back Pain*

# S

## SAD (Seasonal Affective Disorder)

Effective **Therapeutic** regimen management r/t uses SAD lights during winter months

*See Depression*

## Sadness

Adult **Failure** to thrive r/t depression, apathy

Dysfunctional **Grieving** r/t actual or perceived loss

Readiness for enhanced **Communication** r/t willingness to share feelings and thoughts

Readiness for enhanced **Spiritual** well-being r/t desire for harmony following actual or perceived loss

Risk for **Powerlessness** r/t actual or perceived loss

Risk for **Spiritual** distress r/t loss of loved one

**Spiritual** distress r/t intense suffering

*See Depression*

## Safe Sex

Effective **Therapeutic** regimen management r/t taking appropriate precautions sexual activity to keep from contacting a sexually transmitted disease

*See Sexuality, Adolescent; STD (Sexually Transmitted Disease)*

## Safety, Childhood

Deficient **Knowledge**: potential for enhanced health maintenance r/t parental knowledge and skill acquisition regarding appropriate safety measures

**Health-seeking** behaviors: enhanced parenting r/t adequate support systems, appropriate requests for help, desire and request for safety information, requests for information or assistance regarding parenting skills

Risk for altered **Health** maintenance r/t parental deficient knowledge regarding appropriate safety needs per developmental stage, childproofing house, infant and child car restraints, water safety, teaching child ways to avoid molestation

Risk for **Aspiration** and/or **Suffocation** r/t pillow or propped bottle placed in infant's crib; sides of playpen/crib being wide enough for child to get head through; child left in car with engine running; enclosed areas; plastic bags or small objects used as toys; toys with small, breakaway parts; refrigerators or freezers with doors accessible as play areas; child left unattended in or near bathtub, pool, spa; low clotheslines; electric garage doors without automatic stop/reopen; pacifier hung around infant's neck; food not cut into small, bite-size, age-appropriate pieces; balloons, hot dogs, nuts, or popcorn given to infant or young child, especially <1 year of age; use of baby powder

Risk for impaired **Parenting** r/t lack of available and effective role model, lack of knowledge; misinformation from other family members (old wives' tales)

Risk for **Injury/Trauma** r/t developmental age, altered home maintenance management (house not childproofed); impaired parenting; hot liquids within child's reach, no infant or child car restraints, no gate at top of stairs, lack of immunization; no fences or pool or spa covers; child left unattended in car with closed windows in hot weather; firearms loaded and within child's reach

Risk for **Poisoning** r/t use of lead-based paint; presence of asbestos or radon gas; drugs not locked in cabinet; household products left in accessible area (bleach, detergent, drain cleaners, household cleaners); alcohol and perfume within reach of child; presence of poisonous plants; atmospheric pollutants

## Salmonella

S

Readiness for enhanced **Therapeutic** regimen management r/t avoiding improperly prepared or stored food, wearing gloves when handling pet reptiles or its feces

Impaired **Home** maintenance r/t improper preparation or storage of food, lack of safety measures when caring for pet reptile

*See Gastroenteritis; Gastroenteritis, Child*

## Salpingectomy

Anticipatory **Grieving** r/t possible loss due to tubal pregnancy

Decisional **Conflict** r/t sterilization procedure

Risk for impaired **Urinary** elimination r/t trauma to ureter during surgery

*See Hysterectomy; Surgery, Perioperative Care; Surgery, Postoperative Care; Surgery, Preoperative Care*

## Sarcoidosis

Acute **Pain** r/t possible disease affecting joints

**Anxiety** r/t change in health status

Impaired **Gas** exchange r/t ventilation-perfusion imbalance

Ineffective **Health** maintenance r/t deficient knowledge regarding home care and medication regimen

Risk for decreased **Cardiac** output r/t dysrhythmias

## SARS (Severe Acute Respiratory Syndrome)

Risk for **Infection** r/t increased environmental exposure (travelers in close proximity to infected persons, traveling when a fever is present)

Readiness for enhanced **Knowledge** of information regarding travel and precautions to avoid exposure to SARS

Effective **Therapeutic** regimen management r/t uses appropriate hand hygiene

*See Pneumonia*

## SBE (Self-Breast Examination)

Effective **Therapeutic** regimen management r/t practices self-breast examination per recommended protocol

**Health-seeking** behaviors r/t desire to have information about self-breast examination

Readiness for enhanced **Knowledge** of self-breast examination

## Scabies

*See Communicable Diseases, Childhood*

## Scared

**Anxiety** r/t threat of death, threat to or change in health status

Death **Anxiety** r/t unresolved issues surrounding end-of-life decisions

**Fear** r/t hospitalization, real or imagined threat to own well-being

Readiness for enhanced **Communication** r/t willingness to share thoughts and feelings

## Schizophrenia

**Anxiety** r/t unconscious conflict with reality

Chronic **Sorrow** r/t chronic mental illness

Deficient **Diversional** activity r/t social isolation, possible regression

Disturbed **Sleep** pattern r/t sensory alterations contributing to fear and anxiety

Disturbed **Sensory** perception r/t biochemical imbalances for sensory distortion (illusions, hallucinations)

Disturbed **Thought** processes r/t inaccurate interpretations of environment

**Fear** r/t altered contact with reality

Imbalanced **Nutrition**: less than body requirements r/t fear of eating, lack of awareness of hunger, disinterest toward food

Impaired **Home** maintenance r/t impaired cognitive or emotional functioning, insufficient finances, inadequate support systems

Impaired **Social** interaction r/t impaired communication patterns, self-concept disturbance, disturbed thought processes

Impaired verbal **Communication** r/t psychosis, disorientation, inaccurate perception, hallucinations, delusions

Ineffective **Coping** r/t inadequate support systems, unrealistic perceptions, inadequate coping skills, disturbed thought processes, impaired communication

Ineffective **Health** maintenance r/t cognitive impairment, ineffective individual and family coping, lack of material resources

Ineffective family **Therapeutic** regimen management r/t chronicity and unpredictability of condition

Interrupted **Family** processes r/t inability to express feelings, impaired communication

Risk for **Caregiver** role strain r/t bizarre behavior of client, chronicity of condition

Risk for impaired **Religiosity** r/t ineffective coping; lack of security

Risk for **Loneliness** r/t inability to interact socially

Risk for **Post-trauma** syndrome r/t diminished ego strength

Risk for **Powerlessness** r/t intrusive, distorted thinking

Risk for self- and other-directed **Violence** r/t lack of trust, panic, hallucinations, delusional thinking

Risk for **Suicide** r/t psychiatric illness

**Self-care** deficit r/t loss of contact with reality, impairment of perception

**Self-esteem** disturbance r/t excessive use of defense mechanisms (e.g., projection, denial, rationalization)

**Sleep** deprivation r/t intrusive thoughts, nightmares

**Social** isolation r/t lack of trust, regression, delusional thinking, repressed fears

**Spiritual** distress r/t loneliness/social alienation

## Sciatica

*See Neuropathy, Peripheral*

## Scoliosis

Acute **Pain** r/t musculoskeletal restrictions, surgery, reambulation with cast or spinal rod

Chronic **Sorrow** r/t chronic disability

Disturbed **Body** image r/t use of therapeutic braces, postsurgery scars, restricted physical activity

Impaired **Adjustment** r/t lack of developmental maturity to comprehend long-term consequences of noncompliance with treatment procedures

Impaired **Gas** exchange r/t restricted lung expansion secondary to severe presurgery curvature of spine, immobilization

Impaired physical **Mobility** r/t restricted movement, dyspnea secondary to severe curvature of spine

Impaired **Skin** integrity r/t braces, casts, surgical correction

Ineffective **Breathing** pattern r/t restricted lung expansion secondary to severe curvature of spine

Ineffective **Health** maintenance r/t deficient knowledge regarding treatment modalities, restrictions, home care, postoperative activities

Readiness for enhanced **Therapeutic** regimen management r/t desire for knowledge regarding treatment for condition

Risk for **Infection** r/t surgical incision

Risk for perioperative positioning **Injury** r/t prone position

*See Hospitalized Child; Maturational Issues, Adolescent*

## Sedentary Lifestyle

**Activity** intolerance r/t sedentary lifestyle

Readiness for enhanced **Coping** r/t seeking knowledge of new strategies to adjust to sedentary lifestyle

**Sedentary** lifestyle r/t deficient knowledge of health benefits of physical exercise; lack of motivation, interest, training for accomplishment of physical exercise, lack of resources: time, money, companionship, facilities

## Seizure Disorders, Adult

Acute **Confusion** r/t postseizure state

Impaired **Memory** r/t seizure activity

Ineffective **Health** maintenance r/t lack of knowledge regarding anticonvulsive therapy

Readiness for enhanced **Knowledge** of anticonvulsive therapy

Risk for disturbed **Thought** processes r/t effects of anticonvulsant medications

Risk for **Falls** r/t uncontrolled seizure activity

Risk for ineffective **Airway** clearance r/t accumulation of secretions during seizure

Risk for **Injury** r/t uncontrolled movements during seizure, falls, drowsiness secondary to anticonvulsants

Risk for **Powerlessness** r/t possible seizure

**Social** isolation r/t unpredictability of seizures, community-imposed stigma

*See Epilepsy*

## Seizure Disorders, Childhood (Epilepsy, Febrile Seizures, Infantile Spasms)

Ineffective **Health** maintenance r/t lack of knowledge regarding anticonvulsive therapy, fever reduction (febrile seizures)

Risk for delayed **Development** and disproportionate growth r/t effects of seizure disorder, parental overprotection

Risk for disturbed **Thought** processes r/t effects of anticonvulsant medications

Risk for **Falls** r/t possible seizure

Risk for ineffective **Airway** clearance r/t accumulation of secretions during seizure

Risk for **Injury** r/t uncontrolled movements during seizure, falls, drowsiness secondary to anticonvulsants

**Social** isolation r/t unpredictability of seizures, community-imposed stigma

*See Epilepsy*

S

## Self-Breast Examination

*See SBE (Self-Breast Examination)*

## Self-Care Deficit, Bathing/Hygiene

Bathing/hygiene **Self-care** deficit r/t decreased or lack of motivation; weakness and tiredness; severe anxiety; inability to perceive body part or spatial relationship; perceptual or cognitive impairment; pain; neuromuscular, musculoskeletal impairment; environmental barriers

## Self-Care Deficit, Dressing/Grooming

Dressing/grooming **Self-care** deficit r/t decreased or lack of motivation; pain; severe anxiety; perceptual or cognitive impairment; weakness or tiredness; neuromuscular, musculoskeletal impairment; discomfort; environmental barriers

## Self-Care Deficit, Feeding Discomfort

Feeding **Self-care** deficit r/t weakness or tiredness, severe anxiety, neuromuscular impairment, pain, perceptual or cognitive impairment, discomfort, environmental barriers, decreased or lack of motivation, musculoskeletal impairment

## Self-Care Deficit, Toileting

Toileting **Self-care** deficit r/t environmental barriers, weakness or tiredness, decreased or lack of motivation, severe anxiety, impaired mobility status, impaired transfer ability, musculoskeletal impairment, neuromuscular impairment, pain, perceptual or cognitive impairment

## Self-Concept

Readiness for enhanced **Self-concept** r/t expresses willingness to enhance self-concept; expresses satisfaction with thoughts about self, sense of worthiness, role performance, body image, personal identity; actions are congruent with expressed feelings and thoughts; expresses confidence in abilities; accepts strengths and limitations

## Self-Destructive Behavior

**Post-trauma** response r/t unresolved feelings from traumatic event

Risk for self-directed **Violence** r/t panic state, history of child abuse, toxic reaction to medication

Risk for **Self-mutilation** r/t feelings of depression, rejection, self-hatred, depersonalization; command hallucinations

Risk for **Suicide** r/t history of self-destructive behavior

## Self-Esteem, Chronic Low

Chronic low **Self-esteem** r/t long-standing negative self-evaluation

## Self-Esteem, Situational Low

Risk for situational low **Self-esteem** r/t developmental changes (specify); disturbed body image; functional impairment (specify); loss (specify); social role changes (specify); history of learned helplessness; history of abuse, neglect, or abandonment; unrealistic self-expectations; behavior inconsistent with values; lack of recognition/rewards; failures/rejections; decreased power; control over environment; physical illness (specify)

**Self-esteem** disturbance r/t inappropriate and learned negative feelings about self

Situational low **Self-esteem** r/t developmental changes (specify); disturbed body image; functional impairment (specify); loss (specify); social role changes (specify); lack of recognition/rewards; behavior inconsistent with values; failures/rejections

## Self-Mutilation, Risk for

Risk for **Self-mutilation**: psychotic state (command hallucinations) r/t inability to express tension verbally; childhood sexual abuse; violence between parental figures; family divorce, alcoholism; family history of self-destructive behaviors; adolescence; peers who self-mutilate; isolation from peers; perfectionism; substance abuse; eating disorders; sexual identity crisis; low or unstable self-esteem; low or unstable body image; labile behavior (mood swings); history of inability to plan solutions or see long-term consequences; use of manipulation to obtain nurturing relationship with others; chaotic/disturbed interpersonal relationships; emotionally disturbed and/or battered children; feels threatened with actual or potential loss of significant relationship; loss of parent/parental relationships; experiences dissociation or depersonalization; experiences mounting tension that is intolerable; impulsivity; inadequate coping; experiences irresistible urge to cut/damage self; needs quick reduction of stress; childhood illness or surgery; foster, group, or institutional care; incarceration; character disorders; borderline personality disorders; loss of control over problem-solving situations; developmentally delayed or autistic individuals; history of self-injurious behavior; feelings of depression, rejection, self-hatred, separation anxiety, guilt, depersonalization

**Self-mutilation** r/t psychotic state (command hallucinations); inability to express tension verbally; childhood sexual abuse; violence between parental figures; family divorce; family alcoholism; family history of self-destructive behaviors; adolescence; peers who self-mutilate; isolation from peers; perfectionism; substance abuse; eating disorders; sexual identity crisis; low or unstable self-esteem; low or unstable body image; labile behavior (mood swings); history of inability to plan solutions or see long-term consequences; use of manipulation to obtain nurturing relationship with others; chaotic/disturbed interpersonal relationships; emotionally disturbed; battered child; feels threatened with actual or potential loss of significant relationship (e.g., loss of parent, parental relationship); experiences dissociation or depersonalization; mounting tension that is intolerable; impulsivity; inadequate coping; irresistible urge to cut/damage self; needs quick reduction of stress; childhood illness or surgery; foster, group, or institutional care; incarceration; character disorders; borderline personality disorders; developmentally delayed or autistic individual; history of self-injurious behavior; feelings of depression, rejection, self-hatred, separation anxiety, guilt, depersonalization; poor parent adolescent communication; lack of family confidant

## Senile Dementia

**Sedentary** lifestyle r/t lack of interest

*See Dementia*

## Sensory/Perceptual Alterations

Disturbed **Sensory** perception: visual, auditory, kinesthetic, gustatory, tactile, olfactory r/t altered sensory perception; excessive environmental stimuli; psychological stress; altered sensory reception, transmission, and/or integration; insufficient environmental stimuli; biochemical imbalances for sensory distortion (e.g., illusions, hallucinations); electrolyte imbalance; biochemical imbalance

## Separation Anxiety

Disturbed **Sleep** patterns r/t separation for significant others

Ineffective **Coping** r/t maturational and situational crises, vulnerability secondary to developmental age, hospitalization, separation from family and familiar surroundings, multiple caregivers

Risk for impaired parent/infant/child **Attachment** r/t separation

*See Hospitalized Child*

## Sepsis, Child

Delayed **Surgical** recovery r/t presence of infection

Imbalanced **Nutrition**: less than body requirements r/t anorexia, generalized weakness, poor sucking reflex

Impaired **Comfort**: increased sensitivity to environmental stimuli r/t disturbed sensory perceptions: visual, auditory, kinesthetic

Ineffective **Thermoregulation** r/t infectious process, septic shock

Ineffective **Tissue** perfusion: cardiopulmonary, peripheral r/t arterial or venous blood flow exchange problems, septic shock

Risk for impaired **Skin** integrity r/t desquamation secondary to disseminated intravascular coagulation (DIC)

*See Hospitalized Child; Premature Infant, Child*

## Septicemia

Deficient **Fluid** volume r/t vasodilation of peripheral vessels, leaking of capillaries

Imbalanced **Nutrition**: less than body requirements r/t anorexia, generalized weakness

Ineffective **Tissue** perfusion r/t decreased systemic vascular resistance

*See Sepsis, Child; Shock; Shock, Septic*

## Severe Acute Respiratory Syndrome

*See SARS (Severe Acute Respiratory Syndrome); Pneumonia*

## Sexual Dysfunction

Chronic **Sorrow** r/t loss of ideal sexual experience, altered relationships

**Sexual** dysfunction r/t misinformation or lack of knowledge; vulnerability; values conflict; psychosocial abuse (e.g., harmful relationships); physical abuse; lack of privacy; ineffectual or absent role models; altered body structure or function (e.g., pregnancy, recent childbirth, drugs, surgery, anomalies, disease process, trauma, radiation); lack of significant other; biopsychosocial alteration of sexuality

*See Erectile Dysfunction*

## Sexuality, Adolescent

Decisional **Conflict**: sexual activity r/t undefined personal values or beliefs, multiple or divergent sources of information, lack of relevant information

Deficient **Knowledge**: potential for enhanced health maintenance r/t multiple or divergent sources of information or lack of relevant information regarding sexual transmission of disease, contraception, prevention of toxic shock syndrome

Disturbed **Body** image r/t anxiety secondary to unachieved developmental milestone (puberty) or deficient knowledge regarding reproductive maturation as manifested by amenorrhea or expressed concerns regarding lack of growth of secondary sex characteristics

Risk for **Rape-trauma** syndrome r/t date rape, campus rape, insufficient knowledge regarding self-protection mechanisms

*See Maturational Issues, Adolescent*

S

## Sexuality Patterns, Ineffective

Ineffective **Sexuality** patterns r/t lack of significant other; conflicts with sexual orientation or variant preferences; fear of pregnancy or acquiring a sexually transmitted disease; impaired relationship with a significant other; ineffective or absent role models; knowledge skill deficit regarding alternative responses to health-related transitions, altered body function or structure, illness or medical treatment; lack of privacy

## Sexually Transmitted Disease

*See STD (Sexually Transmitted Disease)*

## Shaken Baby Syndrome

Decreased **Intracranial** adaptive capacity r/t brain injury

Impaired **Parenting** r/t stress, history of being abusive

Risk for other-directed **Violence** r/t history of violence against others; perinatal complications

*See Child Abuse; Suspected Child Abuse and Neglect (SCAN), Child; Suspected Child Abuse and Neglect (SCAN), Parent*

## Shakiness

**Anxiety** r/t situational or maturational crisis, threat of death

## Shame

**Self-esteem** disturbance r/t inability to deal with past traumatic events, blaming of self for events not under one's control

## Shingles

Acute **Pain** r/t vesicular eruption along the nerves

Ineffective **Protection** r/t abnormal blood profiles

Risk for **Infection** r/t tissue destruction

**Social** isolation r/t altered state of wellness, contagiousness of disease

*See Itching*

## Shivering

Hypothermia r/t exposure to cool environment

## Shock

**Fear** r/t serious threat to health status

Ineffective **Tissue** perfusion: cardiopulmonary; peripheral r/t arterial/venous blood flow exchange problems

Risk for **Injury** r/t prolonged shock resulting in multiple organ failure, death

*See Shock, Cardiogenic; Shock, Hypovolemic; Shock, Septic*

## Shock, Cardiogenic

Decreased **Cardiac** output r/t decreased myocardial contractility, dysrhythmia

*See Shock*

## Shock, Hypovolemic

Deficient **Fluid** volume r/t abnormal loss of fluid

*See Shock*

## Shock, Septic

Deficient **Fluid** volume r/t abnormal loss of fluid through capillaries, pooling of blood in peripheral circulation

Ineffective **Protection** r/t inadequately functioning immune system

*See Sepsis, Child; Septicemia; Shock*

## Shoulder Repair

Risk for perioperative positioning **Injury** r/t immobility

**Self-care** deficit: bathing/hygiene, dressing/grooming, feeding r/t immobilization of affected shoulder

*See Surgery, Preoperative; Surgery, Perioperative; Surgery, Postoperative; Total Joint Replacement*

## Sickle Cell Anemia/Crisis

**Activity** intolerance r/t fatigue, effects of chronic anemia

Acute **Pain** r/t viscous blood, tissue hypoxia

Deficient **Fluid** volume r/t decreased intake, increased fluid requirements during sickle cell crisis, decreased ability of kidneys to concentrate urine

Impaired physical **Mobility** r/t pain, fatigue

Risk for ineffective **Tissue** perfusion: renal, cerebral, cardiac, gastrointestinal, peripheral r/t effects of red cell sickling; infarction of tissues

Risk for **Infection** r/t alterations in splenic function

*See Child with Chronic Condition; Hospitalized Child*

## SIDS (Sudden Infant Death Syndrome)

Anticipatory **Grieving** r/t potential loss of infant

**Anxiety/Fear**: parental r/t life-threatening event

Deficient **Knowledge**: potential for enhanced health maintenance r/t knowledge or skill acquisition of cardiopulmonary resuscitation (CPR) and home apnea monitoring

Disturbed **Sleep** pattern: parental/infant r/t home apnea monitoring

Interrupted **Family** processes r/t stress secondary to special care needs of infant with apnea

Risk for **Powerlessness** r/t unanticipated life-threatening event

Risk for sudden infant **Death** syndrome r/t modifiable risk factors such as infants placed to sleep in the prone or side-lying position, prenatal and/or postnatal infant smoke exposure, infant overheating/overwrapping, soft underlayment/loose articles in the sleep environment, delayed or nonattendance of prenatal care; potentially modifiable risk factors such as low birth weight, prematurity, young maternal age; nonmodifiable risk factors such as male gender, ethnicity (e.g., African-American, Native-American race of mother), seasonality of SIDS deaths (higher in winter and fall months); peaking of SIDS mortality between infant ages of 2 and 4 months

*See Terminally Ill Child/Death of Child, Parent*

## Situational Crisis

Ineffective **Coping** r/t situational crisis

Interrupted **Family** processes r/t situational crisis

Readiness for enhanced **Communication** r/t willingness to share feelings and thoughts

Readiness for enhanced **Religiosity** r/t requests religious material and/or experiences

Readiness for enhanced **Spiritual** well-being r/t desire for harmony following crisis

## Skin Cancer

Impaired **Skin** integrity r/t abnormal cell growth in skin, treatment of skin cancer

Ineffective **Health** maintenance r/t deficient knowledge regarding self-care with skin cancer

Readiness for enhanced **Knowledge** of self-care to prevent and treat skin cancer

## Skin Disorders

### INTERNAL

Impaired **Skin** integrity r/t altered metabolic state, skeletal prominence; immunological deficit; developmental factors; altered sensation; altered nutritional state (e.g., obesity, emaciation); altered pigmentation; altered circulation; alterations in turgor (change in elasticity); altered fluid status

### EXTERNAL

Impaired **Skin** integrity r/t hyperthermia; hypothermia; chemical substances; humidity mechanical factors (e.g., shearing forces, pressure, restraint); physical immobilization; radiation; extremes in age, moisture, medication

## Skin Integrity, Risk for Impaired

### INTERNAL

Risk for impaired **Skin** integrity r/t medication; skeletal prominence; immunologic factors; developmental factors; altered sensation; altered pigmentation; altered metabolic state; altered circulation; alterations to skin turgor (changes in elasticity); alterations in nutritional state (e.g., obesity, emaciation); psychogenetic

### EXTERNAL

Risk for impaired **Skin** integrity r/t radiation, physical immobilization, mechanical factors (e.g., shearing forces, pressure, restraint); hypothermia or hyperthermia; humidity; chemical substance; excretions and/or secretions; moisture; extremes of age

## Skin Turgor, Change in Elasticity

Deficient **Fluid** volume r/t active fluid loss (decreased skin turgor can be a normal finding in the elderly)

## Sleep

Readiness for enhanced **Sleep** r/t expresses willingness to enhance sleep, amount of sleep and rapid eye movement (REM) sleep is congruent with developmental needs, expressed feeling of being rested after sleep, following sleep routines that promote sleep habits, occasional or infrequent use of medications to induce sleep

## Sleep Apnea

*See PND (Paroxysmal Nocturnal Dyspnea)*

## Sleep Deprivation

Disturbed **Sensory** perception r/t lack of sleep

**Fatigue** r/t lack of sleep

**Sleep** deprivation r/t prolonged physical discomfort; prolonged psychological discomfort; sustained inadequate sleep hygiene; prolonged use of pharmacological or dietary antisoporifics; aging-related sleep stage shifts; sustained circadian asynchrony; inadequate daytime activity; sustained environmental stimulation; sustained unfamiliar or uncomfortable sleep environment; non–sleep-inducing parenting practices; sleep apnea; periodic limb movement (e.g., restless leg syndrome, nocturnal myoclonus); sundown syndrome; narcolepsy; idiopathic central nervous system hypersomnolence; sleep walking; sleep terror; sleep-related enuresis; nightmares; familial sleep paralysis; sleep-related painful erections; dementia

## Sleep Pattern Disorders

Disturbed **Sleep** pattern r/t *Psychological:* Ruminative presleep thought; daytime activity pattern; thinking about home; body temperature; temperament; dietary; childhood onset; inadequate sleep hygiene; sustained use of antisleep agents; circadian asynchrony; frequently changing sleep-wake schedule; depression; loneliness; frequent travel across time zones; daylight/darkness exposure; grief; anticipation; shift work; delayed or advance sleep phase syndrome; loss of sleep partner; life change; preoccupation with trying to sleep; periodic gender related hormonal shifts; biochemical agents; fear; separation from significant others; social schedule inconsistent with chronotype; aging-related sleep shifts; anxiety; medications; fear of insomnia; maladaptive conditioned wakefulness; fatigue; boredom; *Environmental:* Noise; lighting; unfamiliar sleep furnishings; ambient temperature, humidity; other-generated awakening; excessive stimulation; physical restraint; lack of sleep privacy/control; interruptions for therapeutics, monitoring, lab tests; sleep partner; noxious odors; *Parental:* Mother's sleep-wake pattern; parent-infant interaction; mother's emotional support; *Physiological:* Urinary urgency, incontinence; fever; nausea; stasis of secretions; shortness of breath; position; gastroesophageal reflux

## Sleep Pattern, Disturbed, Parent/Child

Disturbed **Sleep** pattern: child r/t anxiety or apprehension secondary to parental deprivation, fear, night terrors, enuresis, inconsistent parental responses to child's requests to alter bedtime rules, frequent nighttime awakening, inability to wean from parents' bed, hypervigilance

Disturbed **Sleep** pattern: parent r/t time-intensive home treatments, increased caretaker demands

*See Suspected Child Abuse and Neglect*

## Slurring of Speech

Impaired verbal **Communication** r/t decrease in circulation to brain, brain tumor, anatomical defect, cleft palate

Situational low **Self-esteem** r/t speech impairment

*See Communication Problems*

## Small Bowel Resection

*See Abdominal Surgery*

## Smell, Loss of Ability to

Risk for **Injury** r/t inability to detect gas fumes, smoke smells

*See Anosmia*

## Smoking Behavior

Altered **Health** maintenance r/t denial of effects of smoking, lack of effective support for smoking withdrawal

Readiness for enhanced **Knowledge** of smoking cessation

## Social Interaction, Impaired

Impaired **Social** interaction r/t knowledge/skill deficit regarding ways to enhance mutuality; therapeutic isolation; sociocultural dissonance; limited physical mobility; environmental barriers; communication barriers; altered thought processes; absence of available significant others or peers; self-concept disturbance

## Social Isolation

**Social** isolation r/t alterations in mental status; inability to engage in satisfying personal relationships; unacceptable social values; unacceptable social behavior; inadequate personal resources; immature interests; factors contributing to absence of satisfying personal relationships (e.g., delay in accomplishing developmental tasks); alterations in physical appearance; altered state of wellness

## Sociopathic Personality

*See Antisocial Personality Disorder*

## Sodium, Decrease/Increase

*See Hyponatremia/Hypernatremia*

## Somatization Disorder

**Anxiety** r/t unresolved conflicts channeled into physical complaints or conditions

Chronic **Pain** r/t unexpressed anger, multiple physical disorders, depression

Ineffective **Coping** r/t lack of insight into underlying conflicts

Ineffective **Denial** r/t displaces psychological stress to physical symptoms

## Sore Nipples, Breastfeeding

Ineffective **Breastfeeding** r/t deficient knowledge regarding correct feeding procedure

*See Painful Breasts, Sore Nipples*

## Sore Throat

Acute **Pain** r/t inflammation, irritation, dryness

Deficient **Knowledge** r/t treatment, relief of discomfort

Impaired **Oral** mucous membrane r/t inflammation or infection of oral cavity

Impaired **Swallowing** r/t irritation of oropharyngeal cavity

## Sorrow

Anticipatory **Grieving** r/t impending loss of significant person or object

Chronic **Sorrow** r/t unresolved grief

**Grieving** r/t loss of significant person, object, or role

Readiness for enhanced **Communication** r/t expresses thoughts and feelings

Readiness for enhanced **Spiritual** well-being r/t desire to find purpose and meaning of loss

## Spastic Colon

*See IBS (Irritable Bowel Syndrome)*

## Speech Disorders

**Anxiety** r/t difficulty with communication

Delayed **Growth** and development r/t effects of physical/mental disability

Disturbed **Sensory** perception (auditory) r/t altered sensory reception, transmission, and/or integration

Impaired verbal **Communication** r/t anatomical defect, cleft palate, psychological barriers, decrease in circulation to brain

## Spina Bifida

Risk for latex **Allergy** response r/t multiple exposures to latex products

*See Neurotube Defects*

## Spinal Cord Injury

Chronic **Sorrow** r/t immobility, change in body function

**Constipation** r/t immobility, loss of sensation

Deficient **Diversional** activity r/t long-term hospitalization, frequent lengthy treatments

Disturbed **Body** image r/t change in body function

Dysfunctional **Grieving** r/t loss of usual body function

**Fear** r/t powerlessness over loss of body function

Impaired **Home** maintenance r/t change in health status, insufficient family planning or finances, deficient knowledge, inadequate support systems

Impaired physical **Mobility** r/t neuromuscular impairment

Ineffective **Health** maintenance r/t deficient knowledge regarding self-care with spinal cord injury

Reflex **Incontinence** r/t spinal cord lesion interfering with conduction of cerebral messages

Risk for **Autonomic** dysreflexia r/t bladder or bowel distention, skin irritation, deficient knowledge of patient and caregiver

Risk for **Disuse** syndrome r/t paralysis

Risk for impaired **Skin** integrity r/t immobility, paralysis

Risk for ineffective **Breathing** pattern r/t neuromuscular impairment

Risk for **Infection** r/t chronic disease, stasis of body fluids

Risk for latex **Allergy** response r/t continuous or intermittent catherization

Risk for **Loneliness** r/t physical immobility

Risk for **Powerlessness** r/t loss of function

**Self-care** deficit r/t neuromuscular impairment

**Sedentary** lifestyle r/t lack of resources/interest

**Sexual** dysfunction r/t altered body function

**Urinary** retention r/t inhibition of reflex arc

*See Child with Chronic Condition; Hospitalized Child; Neurotube Defects*

## Spinal Fusion

Impaired bed **Mobility** r/t impaired ability to turn side-to-side keeping spine in proper alignment

Impaired physical **Mobility** r/t musculoskeletal impairment associated with surgery, possible back brace

Readiness for enhanced **Knowledge**: expresses interest in information associated with surgery

*See Acute Back; Back Pain; Scoliosis; Surgery, Preoperative Care; Surgery, Perioperative Care; Surgery, Postoperative Care*

## Spiritual Distress

Risk for **Spiritual** distress r/t *Physical:* Physical illness, substance abuse/excessive drinking, chronic illness; *Psychosocial:* Low self-esteem, depression, anxiety, stress, poor relationships, separate from support systems, blocks to experiencing love, inability to forgive, loss; *Sociocultural:* Racial/cultural conflict, change in religious rituals; *Spiritual:* Change in spiritual practices; *Developmental:* Life transitions; *Environmental:* Environmental changes, natural disasters

**Spiritual** distress r/t self-alienation, loneliness/social isolation, anxiety, sociocultural deprivation, death and dying of self or others, pain, life change, chronic illness of self or others

## Spiritual Well-Being

Readiness for enhanced **Spiritual** well-being r/t health-seeking behaviors, empathy, self-care, self-awareness, desire for harmonious interconnectedness, desire to find meaning and purpose in life

## Splenectomy

*See Abdominal Surgery*

S

## Sprains

Acute **Pain** r/t physical injury

Effective **Therapeutic** regimen management r/t not exercising when tired or in pain; maintaining healthy weight; wearing properly fitting shoes; appropriate warm up, stretching and cool down exercises; wearing protective equipment; running on even surfaces; staying physically fit

Impaired physical **Mobility** r/t injury

## Stapedectomy

Acute **Pain** r/t headache

Disturbed **Sensory** perception: auditory r/t hearing loss caused by edema from surgery

Risk for **Falls** r/t dizziness

Risk for **Infection** r/t invasive procedure

Risk for **Injury**: falls r/t dizziness

## Stasis Ulcer

Impaired **Tissue** integrity r/t chronic venous congestion

*See CHF (Congestive Heart Failure); Varicose Veins*

## STD (Sexually Transmitted Disease)

Acute **Pain** r/t biological or psychological injury

**Fear** r/t altered body function, risk for social isolation, fear of incurable illness

Ineffective **Health** maintenance r/t deficient knowledge regarding transmission, symptoms, treatment of STD

Ineffective **Sexuality** patterns r/t illness, altered body function

Readiness for enhanced **Knowledge** of prevention and treatment of STDs

Risk for **Infection**/spread of infection r/t lack of knowledge concerning transmission of disease

**Social** isolation r/t fear of contracting or spreading disease

*See Maturational Issues, Adolescent*

## Sterilization Surgery

Decisional **Conflict** r/t multiple or divergent sources of information; unclear personal values/beliefs

*See Surgery, Preoperative Care; Surgery, Perioperative Care; Surgery, Postoperative Care; Tubal Ligation; Vasectomy*

## Stertorous Respirations

Ineffective **Airway** clearance r/t pharyngeal obstruction

## Stillbirth

*See Pregnancy Loss*

## Stoma

*See Colostomy; Ileostomy*

## Stomatitis

Impaired **Oral** mucous membrane r/t pathological conditions of oral cavity

## Stone, Kidney

*See Kidney Stone*

## Stool, Hard/Dry

**Constipation** r/t inadequate fluid intake, inadequate fiber intake, decreased activity level, decreased gastric motility

## Straining with Defecation

**Constipation** r/t less than adequate fluid intake, less than adequate dietary intake

Risk for decreased **Cardiac** output r/t vagal stimulation with dysrhythmia secondary to Valsalva maneuver

## Stress

**Anxiety** r/t feelings of helplessness, feelings of being threatened

Disturbed **Energy** field r/t low energy level, feelings of hopelessness

**Fear** r/t powerlessness over feelings

Ineffective **Coping** r/t ineffective use of problem-solving process, feelings of apprehension or helplessness

Readiness for enhanced **Communication** r/t willingness to share thoughts and feelings

Readiness for enhanced **Spiritual** well-being r/t desire for harmony and peace in stressful situation

Risk for **Post-trauma** syndrome r/t perception of event, survivor's role in event

**Self-esteem** disturbance r/t inability to deal with life events

## Stress Urinary Incontinence

Risk for urge urinary **Incontinence** r/t involuntary sphincter relaxation

Stress urinary **Incontinence** r/t degenerative change in pelvic muscles

*See Incontinence of Urine*

## Stridor

Ineffective **Airway** clearance r/t obstruction, tracheobronchial infection, trauma

## Stroke

*See CVA (Cerebrovascular Accident)*

## Stuttering

**Anxiety** r/t impaired verbal communication

Impaired verbal **Communication** r/t anxiety, psychological problems

## Subarachnoid Hemorrhage

Acute **Pain**: headache r/t irritation of meninges from blood, increased intracranial pressure

Ineffective **Tissue** perfusion: cerebral r/t bleeding from cerebral vessel

*See Intracranial Pressure, Increased*

## Substance Abuse

**Anxiety** r/t loss of control

Compromised/disabled family **Coping** r/t codependency issues

Defensive **Coping** r/t substance abuse

Disturbed **Sleep** pattern r/t irritability, nightmares, tremors

Dysfunctional **Family** processes: alcohol r/t inadequate coping skills

Imbalanced **Nutrition**: less than body requirements r/t anorexia

Ineffective **Coping** r/t use of substances to cope with life events

Ineffective **Denial** r/t refusal to acknowledge substance abuse problem

Ineffective **Protection** r/t malnutrition, sleep deprivation

**Powerlessness** r/t substance addiction

Readiness for enhanced **Coping** r/t seeking social support and seeking knowledge of new strategies

Readiness for enhanced **Self-concept** r/t accepting strengths and limitations

Risk for impaired parent/infant/child **Attachment** r/t substance abuse

Risk for **Injury** r/t alteration in sensory perception

Risk for self- or other-directed **Violence** r/t reactions to substances used, impulsive behavior, disorientation, impaired judgment

Risk for **Suicide** r/t substance abuse

**Self-esteem** disturbance r/t failure at life events

**Social** isolation r/t unacceptable social behavior or values

*See Maturational Issues, Adolescent*

## Substance Abuse, Adolescent

*See Alcohol Withdrawal; Maturational Issues, Adolescent; Substance Abuse*

## Substance Abuse in Pregnancy

Altered **Health** maintenance r/t addiction

Defensive **Coping** r/t denial of situation, differing value system

Deficient **Knowledge** r/t lack of exposure to information regarding effects of substance abuse in pregnancy

**Health-seeking** behaviors (substance abuse counseling) r/t desire to provide child with substance-free perinatal period

**Noncompliance** r/t differing value system, cultural influences, addiction

Risk for fetal **Injury** r/t effects of drugs on fetal growth and development

Risk for impaired parent-infant **Attachment** r/t substance abuse, inability of parent to meet infant's/own personal needs

Risk for impaired **Parenting** r/t lack of ability to meet infant's needs

Risk for **Infection** r/t intravenous drug use, lifestyle

Risk for maternal **Injury** r/t drug use

*See Substance Abuse*

## Sucking Reflex

Effective **Breastfeeding** r/t regular and sustained suckling and swallowing at breast

## Sudden Infant Death Syndrome

*See SIDS (Sudden Infant Death Syndrome)*

## Suffocation, Risk for

### INTERNAL

Risk for **Suffocation** r/t reduced olfactory sensation, reduced motor abilities; cognitive or emotional difficulties, disease or injury process, lack of safety education, lack of safety precautions

### EXTERNAL

Risk for **Suffocation** r/t vehicle running in closed garage, use of fuel-burning heaters not vented to outside, smoking in bed, children playing with plastic bags or inserting small objects into mouth or nose, propped bottle placed in infant's crib, pillow placed in an infant's crib, person who eats large mouthfuls of food, discarded or unused refrigerators or freezers without removed doors, children left unattended in bathtubs or pools, household gas leaks, low-strung clothesline, pacifier hung around infant's neck

S

## Suicide Attempt

**Hopelessness** r/t perceived or actual loss, substance abuse, low self-concept, inadequate support systems

Ineffective **Coping** r/t anger, dysfunctional grieving

**Post-trauma** response r/t history of traumatic events, abuse, rape, incest, war, torture

Readiness for enhanced **Communication** r/t willingness to share thoughts and feelings

Readiness for enhanced **Spiritual** well-being r/t desire for harmony and inner strength to help redefine purpose for life

Risk for **Post-trauma** syndrome r/t survivor's role in suicide attempt

Risk for **Suicide** r/t *Behavioral:* History of prior suicide attempt; impulsiveness; buying a gun; stockpiling medicines; making or changing a will; giving away possessions; sudden euphoric recovery from major depression; marked changes in behavior, attitude, or school performance; *Verbal:* Threats of killing oneself; states desire to die/end it all; *Situational:* Living alone; retirement; relocation, institutionalization; economic instability; loss of autonomy/independence; presence of gun in home; adolescents living in nontraditional setting (e.g., juvenile detention center, prison, half-way house, group home); *Psychological:* Family history of suicide; alcohol and substance use/abuse; psychiatric illness/disorder (e.g., depression, schizophrenia, bipolar disorder); abuse in childhood; guilt; gay or lesbian orientation in youth; *Demographic:* Age: elderly, young adult male, adolescents; Race: Caucasian, Native American; Gender: male; Marital status: divorced, widowed; *Physical:* Physical illness; terminal illness; chronic pain; *Social:* Loss of important relationship; disrupted family life; grief, bereavement; poor support systems; loneliness; hopelessness; helplessness; social isolation; legal or disciplinary problems; cluster suicides

**Self-esteem** disturbance r/t guilt, inability to trust, feelings of worthlessness or rejection

**Social** isolation r/t inability to engage in satisfying personal relationships

**Spiritual** distress r/t hopelessness, despair

*See Violent Behavior*

## Support System

Readiness for enhanced family **Coping** r/t ability to adapt to tasks associated with care, support of significant other during health crisis

Readiness for enhanced **Family** processes r/t activities support the growth of family members

Readiness for enhanced **Parenting** r/t children or other dependent person(s) expressing satisfaction with home environment

## Suppression of Labor

*See Preterm Labor; Tocolytic Therapy*

## Surgery, Perioperative Care

Risk for imbalanced **Fluid** volume r/t surgery

Risk for perioperative positioning **Injury** r/t predisposing condition, prolonged surgery

## Surgery, Postoperative Care

**Activity** intolerance r/t pain, surgical procedure

Acute **Pain** r/t inflammation or injury in surgical area

**Anxiety** r/t change in health status, hospital environment

Deficient **Knowledge** r/t postoperative expectations, lifestyle changes

Imbalanced **Nutrition**: less than body requirements r/t anorexia, nausea, vomiting, decreased peristalsis

**Nausea** r/t manipulation of gastrointestinal tract, postsurgical anesthesia

Risk for **Constipation** r/t decreased activity, decreased food or fluid intake, anesthesia, pain medication

Risk for deficient **Fluid** volume r/t hypermetabolic state, fluid loss during surgery, presence of indwelling tubes

Risk for ineffective **Breathing** pattern r/t pain, location of incision, effects of anesthesia/narcotics

Risk for ineffective **Tissue** perfusion: peripheral r/t hypovolemia, circulatory stasis, obesity, prolonged immobility, decreased coughing, decreased deep breathing

Risk for **Infection** r/t invasive procedure, pain, anesthesia, location of incision, weakened cough as a result of aging

**Urinary** retention r/t anesthesia, pain, fear, unfamiliar surroundings, client's position

## Surgery, Preoperative Care

**Anxiety** r/t threat to or change in health status, situational crisis, fear of the unknown

Deficient **Knowledge** r/t preoperative procedures, postoperative expectations

Disturbed **Sleep** pattern r/t anxiety about upcoming surgery

Readiness for enhanced **Knowledge** of preoperative and postoperative expectations for self-care

## Suspected Child Abuse and Neglect (SCAN), Child

Acute **Pain** r/t physical injuries

**Anxiety/Fear**: child r/t threat of punishment for perceived wrongdoing

Chronic low **Self-esteem** r/t lack of positive feedback, excessive negative feedback

Deficient **Diversional** activity r/t diminished or absent environmental or personal stimuli

Delayed **Growth** and development: regression versus delayed r/t diminished or absent environmental stimuli, inadequate caretaking, inconsistent responsiveness by caretaker

Disturbed **Sleep** pattern r/t hypervigilance, anxiety

Imbalanced **Nutrition**: less than body requirements r/t inadequate caretaking

Impaired **Skin** integrity r/t altered nutritional state, physical abuse

**Post-trauma** response r/t physical abuse, incest, rape, molestation

**Rape-trauma** syndrome: compound/silent reaction r/t altered lifestyle secondary to abuse, changes in residence

Readiness for enhanced community **Coping** r/t obtaining resources to prevent child abuse, neglect

Risk for **Poisoning** r/t inadequate safeguards, lack of proper safety precautions, accessibility of illicit substances secondary to impaired home maintenance

Risk for **Suffocation**: secondary to aspiration r/t propped bottle, unattended child

Risk for **Trauma** r/t inadequate precautions, cognitive or emotional difficulties

**Social** isolation: family-imposed r/t fear of disclosure of family dysfunction and abuse

*See Hospitalized Child; Maturational Issues, Adolescent*

## Suspected Child Abuse and Neglect (SCAN), Parent

Chronic low **Self-esteem** r/t lack of successful parenting experiences

Disabled family **Coping** r/t dysfunctional family, underdeveloped nurturing parental role, lack of parental support systems or role models

Dysfunctional **Family** processes: alcoholism r/t inadequate coping skills

Impaired **Home** maintenance r/t disorganization, parental dysfunction, neglect of safe and nurturing environment

Impaired **Parenting** r/t unrealistic expectations of child; lack of effective role model; unmet social, emotional, or maturational needs of parents; interruption in bonding process

Ineffective **Health** maintenance r/t deficient knowledge of parenting skills secondary to unachieved developmental tasks

**Powerlessness** r/t inability to perform parental role responsibilities

Risk for **Violence** toward child r/t inadequate coping mechanisms, unresolved stressors, unachieved maturational level by parent

## Suspicion

Impaired **Social** interaction r/t disturbed thought processes, paranoid delusions, hallucinations

**Powerlessness** r/t repetitive paranoid thinking

Risk for self- or other-directed **Violence** r/t inability to trust

## Swallowing Difficulties

Impaired **Swallowing** r/t *Congenital Defects:* Upper airway anomalies; failure to thrive or protein energy malnutrition; conditions with severe hyptonia; respiratory disorders; history of tube feeding; behavioral problems; self-injurious behavior; neuromuscular impairment (e.g., decreased or absent gag reflex, decreased strength or excursion of muscles involved in mastication, perceptual impairment, facial paralysis); mechanical obstruction (e.g., edema, tracheostomy tube, tumor); congenital heart disease; cranial nerve involvement; *Neurological:* Upper airway anomalies; laryngeal abnormalities; achalasia; gastrointestinal reflux disease; acquired anatomic defects; cerebral palsy; internal or external traumas; tracheal, laryngeal, esophageal defects; traumatic head injury; developmental delay; nasal or nasopharyngeal cavity defects; oral cavity or oropharynx abnormalities; premature infants

## Syncope

**Anxiety** r/t fear of falling

Decreased **Cardiac** output r/t dysrhythmia

Impaired physical **Mobility** r/t fear of falling

Ineffective **Tissue** perfusion: cerebral r/t interruption of blood flow

Risk for **Falls** r/t syncope

Risk for **Injury** r/t altered sensory perception, transient loss of consciousness, risk for falls

**Social** isolation r/t fear of falling

## Syphilis

*See STD (Sexually Transmitted Disease)*

## Systemic Lupus Erythematosus

*See Lupus Erythematosus*

T

# T

## T & A (Tonsillectomy and Adenoidectomy)

Acute **Pain** r/t surgical incision

Deficient **Knowledge**: potential for enhanced health maintenance r/t insufficient knowledge regarding postoperative nutritional and rest requirements, signs and symptoms of complications, positioning

Impaired **Comfort** r/t effects of anesthesia (nausea and vomiting)

Ineffective **Airway** clearance r/t hesitation or reluctance to cough secondary to pain

Risk for **Aspiration/Suffocation** r/t postoperative drainage and impaired swallowing

Risk for deficient **Fluid** volume r/t decreased intake secondary to painful swallowing, effects of anesthesia (nausea, vomiting), hemorrhage

Risk for imbalanced **Nutrition**: less than body requirements r/t hesitation or reluctance to swallow

## Tachycardia

*See Dysrhythmia*

## Tachypnea

Ineffective **Breathing** pattern r/t pain, anxiety

*See cause of Tachypnea*

## Tardive Dyskinesia

Deficient **Knowledge** r/t cognitive limitation in assimilating information relating to side effects associated with neuroleptic medications

Disturbed sensory **Perception** r/t tardive dyskinesia

Risk for **Injury** r/t drug induced abnormal body movements

## Taste Abnormality

Adult **Failure** to thrive r/t imbalanced nutrition: less than body requirements associated with taste abnormality

Disturbed **Sensory** perception: gustatory r/t medication side effects; altered sensory reception, transmission, integration; aging changes

## TB (Pulmonary Tuberculosis)

**Fatigue** r/t disease state (TB)

**Hyperthermia** r/t infection

Impaired **Gas** exchange r/t disease process

Impaired **Home** maintenance management r/t client/family member with disease

Ineffective **Airway** clearance r/t increased secretions, excessive mucus

Ineffective **Breathing** pattern r/t decreased energy/fatigue

Ineffective **Therapeutic** regimen management r/t deficient knowledge of prevention and treatment regimen

Readiness for enhanced **Therapeutic** regimen management r/t taking medications according to prescribed protocol for prevention and treatment

Risk for **Infection** r/t insufficient knowledge regarding avoidance of exposure to pathogens

## TBI (Traumatic Brain Injury)

Acute **Confusion** r/t brain injury

Chronic **Sorrow** r/t change in person's health status and functional ability

Decreased **Intracranial** adaptive capacity r/t brain injury

Disturbed **Sensory** perception: specify r/t pressure damage to sensory centers in brain

Disturbed **Thought** processes r/t pressure damage to brain

Impaired **Memory** r/t neurological disturbances

Ineffective **Tissue** perfusion: cerebral r/t effects of increased intracranial pressure

Ineffective **Breathing** pattern r/t pressure damage to breathing center in brain stem

Interrupted **Family** processes r/t traumatic injury to family member

Risk for impaired **Religiosity** r/t impaired physical mobility

Risk for **Post-trauma** syndrome r/t perception of event causing traumatic brain injury

## TD (Traveler's Diarrhea)

Risk for deficient **Fluid** volume r/t excessive loss of fluids; diarrhea

Risk for **Infection** r/t insufficient knowledge regarding avoidance of exposure to pathogens (water supply, iced drinks, local cheeses, ice cream, undercooked meat, fish and shellfish, uncooked vegetables, unclean eating utensils, improper hand washing)

## Temperature, Decreased

**Hypothermia** r/t exposure to cold environment

## Temperature, Increased

**Hyperthermia** r/t dehydration, illness, trauma

## Temperature Regulation, Impaired

Ineffective **Thermoregulation** r/t trauma, illness

## Tension

**Anxiety** r/t threat to or change in health status, situational crisis

Disturbed **Energy** field r/t change in health status, discouragement, pain

Readiness for enhanced **Communication** r/t willingness to share feelings and thoughts

*See Stress*

## Terminally Ill Adult

Anticipatory **Grieving** r/t loss of self or significant other

Compromised family **Coping** r/t inability to discuss impending death

Death **Anxiety** r/t unresolved issues relating to death and dying

Decisional **Conflict** r/t planning for advance directives

Disturbed **Energy** field r/t impending disharmony of mind, body, spirit

Readiness for enhanced **Religiosity** r/t requests religious material and or/experiences

Readiness for enhanced **Spiritual** well-being r/t desire to achieve harmony of mind, body, spirit

Risk for **Spiritual** distress r/t impending death

**Spiritual** distress r/t suffering before death

## Terminally Ill Child, Adolescent

Disturbed **Body** image r/t effects of terminal disease, already critical feelings of group identity and self-image

Impaired **Social** interaction/social isolation r/t forced separation from peers

Ineffective **Coping** r/t inability to establish personal and peer identity secondary to threat of being different or not being, inability to achieve maturational tasks

*See Child with Chronic Condition; Hospitalized Child*

## Terminally Ill Child, Infant/Toddler

Ineffective **Coping** r/t separation from parents and familiar environment secondary to inability to understand dying process

*See Child with Chronic Condition*

## Terminally Ill Child, Preschool Child

**Fear** r/t perceived punishment, bodily harm, feelings of guilt secondary to magical thinking (i.e., believing that thoughts cause events)

*See Child with Chronic Condition*

## Terminally Ill Child, School-Age Child/Preadolescent

**Fear** r/t perceived punishment, body mutilation, feelings of guilt

*See Child with Chronic Condition*

## Terminally Ill Child/Death of Child, Parent

Anticipatory **Grieving** r/t possible, expected, or imminent death of child

Compromised family **Coping** r/t inability or unwillingness to discuss impending death and feelings with child or to support child through terminal stages of illness

Decisional **Conflict** r/t continuation or discontinuation of treatment, do not resuscitate decision, ethical issues regarding organ donation

Disturbed **Sleep** pattern r/t grieving process

**Grieving** r/t death of child

**Hopelessness** r/t overwhelming stresses secondary to terminal illness

Impaired **Parenting** r/t risk for overprotection of surviving siblings

Impaired **Social** interaction r/t dysfunctional grieving

Ineffective **Denial** r/t dysfunctional grieving

Interrupted **Family** processes r/t situational crisis

**Powerlessness** r/t inability to alter course of events

Readiness for enhanced family **Coping** r/t impact of crisis on family values, priorities, goals, or relationships; expressed interest or desire to attach meaning to child's life and death

Risk for dysfunctional **Grieving** r/t prolonged, unresolved, obstructed progression through stages of grief and mourning

**Social** isolation: imposed by others r/t feelings of inadequacy in providing support to grieving parents

**Social** isolation: self-imposed r/t unresolved grief, perceived inadequate parenting skills

**Spiritual** distress r/t sudden and unexpected death, prolonged suffering before death, questioning the death of youth, questioning the meaning of one's own existence

## Tetralogy of Fallot

*See Congenital Heart Disease/Cardiac Anomalies*

## Therapeutic Regimen, Effective Management

Effective **Therapeutic** regimen management r/t appropriate choices of daily activities for meeting goals of a treatment or prevention program, illness symptoms within normal range of expectation, verbalization of desire to manage treatment of illness and prevention of sequelae, verbalization of intent to reduce risk factors for progression of illness and sequelae

## Therapeutic Regimen, Ineffective Management

Ineffective **Therapeutic** regimen management r/t perceived barriers, social support deficits, powerlessness; perceived susceptibility, perceived benefits; mistrust of regimen and/or health care personnel, knowledge deficit, family patterns of health care, family conflict, excessive demands made on individual or family, economic difficulties; decisional conflicts, complexity of therapeutic regimen, complexity of health care system, faulty perception of illness seriousness, inadequate number and types of cues to action

## Therapeutic Regimen, Ineffective Management: Community

Ineffective community **Therapeutic** regimen management r/t illness symptoms above the norm expected for the number and type of population, unexpected acceleration of illness(es), number of health care resources insufficient for the incidence or prevalence of illness(es), deficits in advocates for aggregates, deficits in people and programs to be accountable for illness care of aggregates, deficits in community activities for secondary and tertiary prevention, unavailable health care resources for illness care

## Therapeutic Regimen, Ineffective Management: Family

Ineffective family **Therapeutic** regimen management r/t complexity of health care system, complexity of therapeutic regimen, decisional conflicts, economic difficulties, excessive demands on individual or family, family conflict

## Therapeutic Regimen Management, Readiness for Enhanced

Readiness for enhanced **Therapeutic** regimen management r/t the following: expresses desire to manage the treatment of illness and prevention of sequelae, makes choices of daily living that are appropriate for meeting the goals of treatment or prevention, expresses little to no difficulty with regulation/integration of one or more prescribed regimens for treatment of illness or prevention of complications, describes reduction of risk factors for progression of illness and sequelae, shows no unexpected acceleration of illness symptoms

## Therapeutic Touch

Disturbed **Energy** field r/t low energy levels, disturbance in energy fields, pain, depression, fatigue

## Thermoregulation, Ineffective

Ineffective **Thermoregulation** r/t aging, fluctuating environmental temperature, immaturity trauma or illness

## Thoracentesis

*See Pleural Effusion*

## Thoracotomy

**Activity** intolerance r/t pain, imbalance between oxygen supply and demand, presence of chest tubes

Acute **Pain** r/t surgical procedure, coughing, deep breathing

Deficient **Knowledge** r/t self-care, effective breathing exercises, pain relief

Ineffective **Airway** clearance r/t drowsiness, pain with breathing and coughing

Ineffective **Breathing** pattern r/t decreased energy, fatigue, pain

Risk for **Infection** r/t invasive procedure

Risk for **Injury** r/t disruption of closed-chest drainage system

Risk for perioperative positioning **Injury** r/t lateral positioning, immobility

## Thought Disorders

Disturbed **Thought** processes r/t disruption in cognitive thinking, processing

*See Schizophrenia*

## Thought Processes, Disturbed

Disturbed **Thought** processes r/t head injury, mental disorder, personality disorder, organic mental disorder, substance abuse, severe interpersonal conflict, sleep deprivation, sensory deprivation or overload, impaired cerebral perfusion

## Thrombocytopenic Purpura

*See ITP (Idiopathic Thrombocytopenic Purpura)*

## Thrombophlebitis

Acute **Pain** r/t vascular inflammation, edema

**Constipation** r/t inactivity, bed rest

Deficient **Diversional** activity r/t bed rest

Deficient **Knowledge** r/t pathophysiology of condition, self-care needs, treatment regimen and outcome

Delayed **Surgical** recovery r/t complication associated with inactivity

Impaired physical **Mobility** r/t pain in extremity, forced bedrest

Ineffective **Tissue** perfusion: peripheral r/t interruption of venous blood flow

Risk for **Injury** r/t possible embolus

Sedentary lifestyle r/t deficient knowledge of benefits of physical exercise

*See Anticoagulant Therapy*

## Thyroidectomy

Risk for altered verbal **Communication** r/t edema, pain, vocal cord of laryngeal nerve damage

Risk for ineffective **Airway** clearance r/t edema or hematoma formation, airway obstruction

Risk for **Injury** r/t possible parathyroid damage or removal

*See Surgery, Preoperative Care; Surgery, Perioperative Care; Surgery, Postoperative Care*

## TIA (Transient Ischemic Attack)

Acute **Confusion** r/t hypoxia

**Health-seeking** behaviors r/t obtaining knowledge regarding treatment, prevention of inadequate oxygenation

Ineffective **Tissue** perfusion: cerebral r/t lack of adequate oxygen supply to brain

Risk for decreased **Cardiac** output r/t dysrhythmia contributing to inadequate oxygen supply to brain

Risk for **Falls** r/t hypoxia

Risk for **Injury** r/t possible syncope

*See Syncope*

## Tic Disorder

*See Tourette's Syndrome (TS)*

## Tinea Capitis

*See Ringworm of Scalp*

## Tinea Corporis

*See Ringworm of Body*

## Tinea Cruris

*See Jock Itch; Itching*

## Tinea Pedis

*See Athlete's Foot; Itching*

## Tinea Unguium (Onychomycosis)

*See Ringworm of Nails*

## Tinnitus

Disturbed **Sensory** perception: auditory r/t altered sensory reception, transmission, integration

Ineffective **Health** maintenance r/t deficient knowledge regarding self-care with tinnitus

## Tissue Damage, Corneal, Integumentary, or Subcutaneous

Impaired **Tissue** integrity r/t mechanical irritants (pressure, shear, friction); radiation (including therapeutic radiation); nutritional deficit or excess; thermal irritants (temperature extremes); knowledge deficit;

irritants; chemical (including body excretions; secretions, medications); impaired physical mobility; altered circulation; fluid deficit or excess

## Tissue Perfusion, Decreased

Ineffective **Tissue** perfusion r/t hypovolemia, hypervolemia; interruption of flow, arterial; exchange problems; interruption of flow, venous; mechanical reduction of venous and/or arterial blood flow; hypoventilation; impaired transport of oxygen across alveolar and/or capillary membrane; mismatch of ventilation with blood flow; decreased hemoglobin concentration in blood; enzyme poisoning; altered affinity of hemoglobin for oxygen

## Tocolytic Therapy

Ineffective **Health** maintenance r/t deficient knowledge regarding management of preterm labor, treatment regimen

Risk for **Fluid** volume excess r/t effects of tocolytic drugs

*See Preterm Labor*

## Toilet Training

**Health-seeking** behaviors: bladder/bowel training r/t achievement of developmental milestone secondary to enhanced parenting skills

## Toileting Problems

Impaired **Transfer** ability r/t neuromuscular deficits

**Self-care** deficit: toileting r/t impaired transfer ability, impaired mobility status, intolerance of activity, neuromuscular impairment, cognitive impairment

## Tonsillectomy and Adenoidectomy

*See T & A (Tonsillectomy and Adenoidectomy)*

## Toothache

Acute **Pain** r/t inflammation/infection

Impaired **Dentition** r/t ineffective oral hygiene, barriers to self-care, economic barriers to professional care, nutritional deficits, lack of knowledge regarding dental health

T

## Total Anomalous Pulmonary Venous Return

*See Congenital Heart Disease/Cardiac Anomalies*

## Total Joint Replacement (Total Hip/ Total Knee/Shoulder)

Acute **Pain** r/t possible edema, physical injury, surgery

Deficient **Knowledge** r/t self-care, treatment regimen, outcomes

Disturbed **Body** image r/t large scar, presence of prosthesis

Impaired physical **Mobility** r/t musculoskeletal impairment, surgery, prosthesis

Risk for **Infection** r/t invasive procedure, anesthesia, immobility

Risk for **Injury:** neurovascular r/t altered peripheral tissue perfusion, altered mobility, prosthesis

*See Surgery, Preoperative Care; Surgery, Perioperative Care; Surgery, Postoperative Care*

## Total Parenteral Nutrition

*See TPN (Total Perenteral Nutrition)*

## Total Urinary Incontinence

Total urinary **Incontinence** r/t neuropathy preventing transmission of reflex indication bladder fullness; trauma or disease affecting spinal cord nerves; anatomic (fistula); independent contraction of detrusor reflex due to surgery; neurological dysfunction causing triggering of micturition at unpredictable times

## Tourette's Syndrome (TS)

**Hopelessness** r/t inability to control behavior

Risk for situational low **Self-esteem** r/t uncontrollable behavior, motor/phonic tics

*See Attention Deficit Disorder*

## Toxemia

*See PIH (Pregnancy-Induced Hypertension/Preeclampsia)*

## TPN (Total Parenteral Nutrition)

Imbalanced **Nutrition**: less than body requirements r/t inability to ingest or digest food or absorb nutrients as a result of biological or psychological factors

Risk for **Fluid** volume excess r/t rapid administration of TPN

Risk for **Infection** r/t concentrated glucose solution, invasive administration of fluids

## Tracheoesophageal Fistula

Imbalanced **Nutrition**: less than body requirements r/t difficulties in swallowing

Ineffective **Airway** clearance r/t aspiration of feeding secondary to inability to swallow

Risk for **Aspiration** r/t common passage of air and food

*See Respiratory Conditions of the Neonate; Hospitalized Child*

## Tracheostomy

Acute **Pain** r/t edema, surgical procedure

**Anxiety** r/t impaired verbal communication, ineffective airway clearance

Deficient **Knowledge** r/t self-care, home maintenance management

Disturbed **Body** image r/t abnormal opening in neck

Impaired verbal **Communication** r/t presence of mechanical airway

Risk for **Aspiration** r/t presence of tracheostomy

Risk for ineffective **Airway** clearance r/t increased secretions, mucous plugs

Risk for **Infection** r/t invasive procedure, pooling of secretions

## Traction and Casts

Acute **Pain** r/t immobility, injury, or disease

**Constipation** r/t immobility

Deficient **Diversional** activity r/t immobility

Impaired physical **Mobility** r/t imposed restrictions on activity secondary to bone or joint disease injury

Impaired **Transfer** ability r/t presence of traction, casts

Risk for **Disuse** syndrome r/t mechanical immobilization

Risk for impaired **Skin** integrity r/t contact of traction or cast with skin

Risk for **Peripheral** neurovascular dysfunction r/t mechanical compression

**Self-care** deficit: feeding, dressing/grooming, bathing/hygiene, toileting r/t degree of impaired physical mobility, body area affected by traction or cast

## Transfer Ability

Impaired **Transfer** ability r/t intolerance of activity, decreased strength and endurance, pain or discomfort, perceptual or cognitive impairment, neuromuscular impairment, musculoskeletal impairment, depression, severe anxiety

## Transient Ischemic Attack

*See TIA (Transient Ischemic Attack)*

## Transposition of Great Vessels

*See Congenital Heart Disease/Cardiac Anomalies*

## Transurethral Resection of the Prostate

*See TURP (Transurethral Resection of the Prostate)*

## Trauma in Pregnancy

Acute **Pain** r/t trauma

**Anxiety** r/t threat to self or fetus, unknown outcome

Deficient **Knowledge** r/t lack of exposure to situation

Impaired **Skin** integrity r/t trauma

Risk for deficient **Fluid** volume r/t blood loss

Risk for fetal **Injury** r/t premature separation of placenta

Risk for **Infection** r/t traumatized tissue

## Trauma, Risk for

### INTERNAL

Risk for **Trauma** r/t lack of safety education, insufficient finances to purchase safety equipment or effect repairs, history of previous trauma, lack of safety precautions, poor vision, reduced temperature and/or tactile sensation, balancing difficulties, cognitive or emotional difficulties, reduced large or small muscle coordination, weakness, reduced hand-eye coordination

### EXTERNAL

Risk for **Trauma** r/t high-crime neighborhood and vulnerable clients; pot handles facing toward front of stove; knives stored uncovered; inappropriate call-for-aid mechanisms for bed-resting client; inadequately stored combustibles or corrosives (e.g., matches, oily rags, lye); highly flammable children's toys or clothing; obstructed passageways; high beds; large icicles hanging from the roof; nonuse or misuse of seat restraints; overexposure to sun, sun lamps, radiotherapy; overloaded electrical outlets; overloaded fuse boxes; play or work near vehicle pathways (e.g., driveways, lanes, railroad tracks); playing with fireworks of gunpowder; guns or ammunition stored unlocked; contact with rapidly moving machinery, industrial belts, or pulleys; litter of liquid spills on floor or stairways; defective appliances; bathing in very hot water (e.g., unsupervised bathing of young children); bathtub without hand grip or antislip equipment; children playing with matches, candles, cigarettes, sharp-edged toys; children playing without gates at top of stairs; children riding in the front seat in car; delayed lighting of gas burner or oven; contact with intense cold; grease waste collected on stoves; driving a mechanically unsafe vehicle; driving after partaking of alcoholic beverages or drugs; driving at excessive speeds; entering unlighted rooms; experimenting with chemical or gasoline; exposure to dangerous machinery; faulty electrical plugs; frayed wires; contact with acids or alkalis; unsturdy or absent stair rails; use of unsteady ladders or chairs; use of cracked dishware or glasses; wearing plastic apron or flowing clothes around open flame; unscreened fires or heaters; unsafe window protection in homes with young children; sliding on coarse bed linen or struggling within bed restraints; use of thin or worn potholders; unanchored electric wires; misuse of necessary headgear for motorized cyclists or young children carried on adult bicycles; potential igniting of gas leaks; unsafe road or road crossing conditions; slippery floors (e.g., wet or highly waxed); smoking in

T

bed or near oxygen; snow or ice collected on stairs, walkways; unanchored rugs; driving without necessary visual aids

## Traumatic Brain Injury (TBI)

*See TBI (Traumatic Brain Injury); Intracranial Pressure, Increased*

## Traumatic Event

**Post-trauma** syndrome r/t previously experienced trauma

## Traveler's Diarrhea

*See TD (Traveler's Diarrhea)*

## Trembling of Hands

**Anxiety/Fear** r/t threat to or change in health status, threat of death, situational crisis

## Tricuspid Atresia

*See Congenital Heart Disease/Cardiac Anomalies*

## Trigeminal Neuralgia

Acute **Pain** r/t irritation of trigeminal nerve

Imbalanced **Nutrition**: less than body requirements r/t pain when chewing

Ineffective **Therapeutic** regimen management r/t deficient knowledge regarding prevention of stimuli that trigger pain

Risk for **Injury** (eye) r/t possible decreased corneal sensation

## Truncus Arteriosus

*See Congenital Heart Disease/Cardiac Anomalies*

## TS (Tourette's Syndrome)

*See Tourette's Syndrome (TS)*

## TSE (Testicular Self-Examination)

**Health-seeking** behavior r/t procedure for doing testicular self-examinations

T

## Tubal Ligation

Decisional **Conflict** r/t tubal sterilization

*See Laparoscopy*

## Tube Feeding

Risk for **Aspiration** r/t improperly administered feeding, improper placement of tube, improper positioning of client during and after feeding, excessive residual feeding or lack of digestion, altered gag reflex

Risk for deficient **Fluid** volume r/t inadequate water administration with concentrated feeding

Risk for imbalanced **Nutrition**: less than body requirements r/t intolerance to tube feeding, inadequate calorie replacement to meet metabolic needs

## Tuberculosis

*See TB (Pulmonary Tuberculosis)*

## TURP (Transurethral Resection of the Prostate)

Acute **Pain** r/t incision, irritation from catheter, bladder spasms, kidney infection

Deficient **Knowledge** r/t postoperative self-care, home maintenance management

Risk for deficient **Fluid** volume r/t fluid loss, possible bleeding

Risk for **Infection** r/t invasive procedure, route for bacteria entry

Risk for urge urinary **Incontinence** r/t edema from surgical procedure

Risk for **Urinary** retention r/t obstruction of urethra or catheter with clots

# U

## Ulcer, Peptic (Duodenal or Gastric)

Acute **Pain** r/t irritated mucosa from acid secretion

**Fatigue** r/t loss of blood, chronic illness

Ineffective **Health** maintenance r/t lack of knowledge regarding health practices to prevent ulcer formation

**Nausea** r/t gastrointestinal irritation

*See GI Bleed (Gastrointestinal Bleeding)*

## Ulcerative Colitis

*See Inflammatory Bowel Disease (Child and Adult)*

## Ulcers, Stasis

*See Stasis Ulcer*

## Unilateral Neglect of One Side of Body

Unilateral **Neglect** r/t effects of disturbed perceptual abilities (e.g., hemianopia); neurological illness or trauma; one-sided blindness

## Unsanitary Living Conditions

Impaired **Home** maintenance r/t impaired cognitive or emotional functioning, lack of knowledge, insufficient finances

## Urgency to Urinate

Risk for urge urinary **Incontinence** r/t effects of alcohol, caffeine, decreased bladder capacity, irritation of bladder stretch receptors causing spasm, increased urine concentration, overdistention of bladder

Urge urinary **Incontinence** r/t decreased bladder capacity, irritation of bladder stretch receptors causing spasm, alcohol, caffeine, increased fluids, increased urine concentration, overdistention of bladder

## Urinary Diversion

*See Ileal Conduit*

## Urinary Elimination, Altered

Impaired **Urinary** elimination r/t anatomical obstruction, sensory motor impairment, urinary tract infection

## Urinary Incontinence

*See Incontinence of Urine*

## Urinary Readiness

Readiness for enhanced **Urinary** elimination

## Urinary Retention

**Urinary** retention r/t high urethral pressure caused by weak detrusor, inhibition of reflex arc, strong sphincter, blockage

## Urinary Tract Infection (UTI)

*See UTI (Urinary Tract Infection)*

## Urolithiasis

*See Kidney Stone*

## Uterine Atony in Labor

*See Dystocia*

## Uterine Atony in Postpartum

*See Postpartum Hemorrhage*

## Uterine Bleeding

*See Hemorrhage; Postpartum Hemorrhage; Shock*

## UTI (Urinary Tract Infection)

Acute **Pain**: dysuria r/t inflammatory process in bladder

Impaired **Urinary** elimination: frequency r/t urinary tract infection

Ineffective **Health** maintenance r/t deficient knowledge regarding methods to treat and prevent UTIs

Risk for urge urinary **Incontinence** r/t hyperreflexia from cystitis

# V

## Vaginal Hysterectomy

Risk for **Infection** r/t surgical site

Risk for **Perioperative** positioning injury r/t lithotomy position

Risk for urge urinary **Incontinence** r/t edema, congestion of pelvic tissues

**Urinary** retention r/t edema at surgical site

*See Postpartum Hemorrhage*

## Vaginitis

Acute **Pain**: pruritus r/t inflamed tissues, edema

Ineffective **Health** maintenance r/t deficient knowledge regarding self-care with vaginitis

Ineffective **Sexuality** patterns r/t abstinence during acute stage, pain

Risk for **Infection** r/t spread of infection, risk of reinfection

## Vagotomy

*See Abdominal Surgery*

## Value System Conflict

Decisional **Conflict** r/t unclear personal values/beliefs

Readiness for enhanced **Spiritual** well-being r/t desire for harmony with self, others, higher power/God

**Spiritual** distress r/t challenged value system

## Varicose Veins

Chronic **Pain** r/t impaired circulation

Ineffective **Health** maintenance r/t deficient knowledge regarding health care practices, prevention, treatment regimen

Ineffective **Tissue** perfusion: peripheral r/t venous stasis

Risk for impaired **Skin** integrity r/t altered peripheral tissue perfusion

## Vascular Dementia (Formerly Called *Multiinfarct Dementia*)

*See Dementia*

## Vascular Obstruction—Peripheral

Acute **Pain** r/t vascular obstruction

**Anxiety** r/t lack of circulation to body part

Ineffective **Tissue** perfusion: peripheral r/t interruption of circulatory flow

Risk for **Peripheral** neurovascular dysfunction r/t vascular obstruction

## Vasectomy

Decisional **Conflict** r/t surgery as method of permanent sterilization

Effective **Therapeutic** regimen management r/t practices alternate forms of contraception until two to three sperm counts are negative

## Vasocognopathy

*See Alzheimer's Type Dementia*

## Venereal Disease

*See STD (Sexually Transmitted Disease)*

## Ventilation, Inability to Sustain Spontaneous

Impaired spontaneous **Ventilation** r/t respiratory muscle fatigue, metabolic factors

## Ventilator Client

Dysfunctional **Ventilatory** weaning response r/t psychological, situational, physiological factors

**Fear** r/t inability to breathe on own, difficulty communicating

Impaired **Gas** exchange r/t ventilation-perfusion imbalance

Impaired spontaneous **Ventilation** r/t metabolic factors, respiratory muscle fatigue

Impaired verbal **Communication** r/t presence of endotracheal tube, decreased mentation

Ineffective **Airway** clearance r/t increased secretions, decreased cough and gag reflex

Ineffective **Breathing** pattern r/t decreased energy and fatigue secondary to possible altered nutrition: less than body requirements

**Powerlessness** r/t health treatment regimen

Risk for **Infection** r/t presence of endotracheal tube, pooled secretions

Risk for latex **Allergy** r/t repeated exposure to latex products

**Social** isolation r/t impaired mobility, ventilator dependence

*See Child with Chronic Condition; Hospitalized Child; Respiratory Conditions of the Neonate*

## Ventilatory, Dysfunctional Weaning Response (DVWR)

Dysfunctional **Ventilatory** weaning response r/t *Psychological:* Patient perceived inefficacy about the ability to wean; powerlessness; anxiety: moderate, severe; knowledge deficit of the weaning process, patient role; hopelessness; fear; decreased motivation; decreased self-esteem; insufficient trust in the nurse. *Situational:* Uncontrolled episodic energy demands or problems; history of multiple unsuccessful weaning attempts; adverse environment (e.g., noisy, active environment, negative events in the room, low nurse-patient ratio, extended nurse absence from bedside, unfamiliar nursing staff); history of ventilator dependence >4 days to 1 week; inappropriate pacing of diminished ventilator support; inadequate social support. *Physiological:* Inadequate nutrition, sleep pattern disturbance, uncontrolled pain or discomfort, ineffective airway clearance

V

## Ventricular Fibrillation

*See Dysrhythmia*

## Vertigo

Disturbed **Sensory** perception: kinesthetic r/t altered sensory reception, transmission, integration; medications

Ineffective **Tissue** perfusion: cerebral r/t decreased blood supply to brain

Risk for **Falls** r/t vertigo

Risk for **Injury** r/t disturbed sensory perception

## Violent Behavior

Risk for other-directed **Violence** r/t body language (e.g., rigid posture, clenching of fists and jaw, hyperactivity, pacing, breathlessness, threatening stances); history of violence against others (e.g., hitting someone, kicking someone, spitting at someone, scratching someone, throwing objects at someone, biting someone, attempted rape, rape, sexual molestation, urinating/defecating on a person); history of threats of violence (e.g., verbal threats against property, verbal threats against person, social threats, cursing, threatening notes/letters, threatening gestures, sexual threats); history of violent antisocial behavior (e.g., stealing, insistent borrowing, insistent demands for privileges, insistent interruption of meetings, refusal to eat, refusal to take medication, ignoring instructions); history of violence, indirect (e.g., tearing of clothes, ripping objects off walls, writing on walls, urinating on floor, defecating on floor, stamping feet, temper tantrum, running in corridors, yelling, throwing objects, breaking a window, slamming doors, sexual advances); neurological impairment (e.g., positive EEG, CAT, MRI, neurological findings; head trauma; seizure disorders); cognitive impairment (e.g., learning disabilities, attention deficit/hyperactivity disorder, decreased intellectual functioning); history of childhood abuse; history of witnessing family violence; cruelty to animals, fire setting; pre/perinatal complications/abnormalities; history of drug/alcohol abuse/pathological intoxication; psychotic symptomatology (e.g., auditory, visual, command hallucinations; paranoid delusions; loose, rambling, or illogical thought processes); motor vehicle offenses (e.g., frequent traffic violations, use of a motor vehicle to release anger); suicidal behavior; impulsivity; availability/possession of weapon(s)

Risk for self-directed **Violence** r/t suicidal ideation (frequent, intense prolonged); suicidal plan (clear and specific lethality; method and availability of destructive means); history of multiple suicide attempts; behavioral clues (e.g., writing forlorn love notes, directing angry messages at a significant other who has rejected the person, giving away personal items, taking out a large life insurance policy); verbal clues (e.g., talking about death, "better off without me," asking questions about lethal dosages of drugs); emotional status (hopelessness, despair, increased anxiety, panic, anger, hostility); mental health (severe depression, psychosis, severe personality disorder, alcoholism or drug abuse); physical health (hypochondriasis, chronic or terminal illness); employment (unemployed, recent job loss/failure; age 15 to 19; age over 45; marital status (single, widowed, divorced); occupation (executive, administrator/owner of business, professional, semiskilled worker); conflicting interpersonal relationships; family background (chaotic or conflicting, history of suicide); sexual orientation (bisexual [active], homosexual [inactive]); personal resources (poor insight, affect unavailable and poorly controlled); social resources (poor rapport, social isolated, unresponsive family); people who engage in autoerotic sexual acts

## Viral Gastroenteritis

**Diarrhea** r/t infectious process, rotavirus, Norwalk virus

Ineffective **Therapeutic** regimen management r/t inadequate hand washing

Ineffective community **Therapeutic** regimen management r/t contaminated food and/or water

*See Gastroenteritis, Child*

## Vision Impairment

Disturbed **Sensory** perception r/t altered sensory reception associated with impaired vision

**Fear** r/t loss of sight

Risk for **Injury** r/t disturbed sensory perception

**Self-care** deficit: specify r/t perceptual impairment

**Social** isolation r/t altered state of wellness, inability to see

*See Blindness*

## Vomiting

**Nausea** r/t chemotherapy, postsurgical anesthesia, irritation to the gastrointestinal system, stimulation of neuropharmacological mechanisms

Risk for deficient **Fluid** volume r/t decreased intake, loss of fluids with vomiting

Risk for imbalanced **Nutrition**: less than body requirements r/t inability to ingest food

## von Recklinghause's Disease

*See Neurofibromatosis*

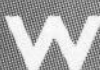

# W

## Walking Impairment

Impaired **Walking** r/t intolerance to activity, decreased strength and endurance, pain or discomfort, perceptual or cognitive impairment, neuromuscular impairment, musculoskeletal impairment, depression, severe anxiety, lower extremity amputation

## Wandering

**Wandering** r/t cognitive impairment, specifically memory and recall deficits, disorientation, poor visuoconstructive (or visuospatial) ability, language (primarily expressive) defects; cortical atrophy; premorbid behavior (e.g., outgoing, sociable personality; premorbid dementia); separation from familiar people and places; sedation; emotional state, especially frustration, anxiety, boredom, or depression (agitation); overstimulating/understimulating social or physical environment; physiological state or need (e.g., hunger/thirst, pain, urination, constipation); time of day

## Weakness

**Fatigue** r/t decreased or increased metabolic energy production

Risk for **Falls** r/t weakness

## Weight Gain

Imbalanced **Nutrition**: more than body requirements r/t excessive intake in relation to metabolic need

## Weight Loss

Imbalanced **Nutrition**: less than body requirements r/t inability to ingest food because of biological, psychological, economic factors

## Wellness-Seeking Behavior

**Health-seeking** behaviors r/t expressed desire for increased control of health practice

## Wernicke Korsakoff Syndrome

*See Korsakoff's Syndrome*

## West Nile Virus

Effective **Therapeutic** regimen management r/t avoid mosquito bites, use mosquito-repellant products containing DEET and wear long sleeves and pants, mosquito-proof the home, community spraying for mosquitos

*See Meningitis/Encephalitis*

## Wheelchair Use Problems

Impaired wheelchair **Mobility** r/t intolerance to activity, decreased strength and endurance, pain or discomfort, perceptual or cognitive impairment, neuromuscular impairment, musculoskeletal impairment, depression, severe anxiety, amputation

## Wheezing

Ineffective **Airway** clearance r/t tracheobronchial obstructions, secretions

## Wilms' Tumor

Acute **Pain** r/t pressure from tumor

**Constipation** r/t obstruction associated with presence of tumor

*See Chemotherapy; Hospitalized Child; Radiation Therapy; Surgery, Preoperative Care; Surgery, Perioperative Care; Surgery, Postoperative Care*

## Withdrawal from Alcohol

*See Alcohol Withdrawal*

## Withdrawal from Drugs

*See Drug Withdrawal*

## Wound Débridement

Acute **Pain** r/t debridement of wound

Impaired **Tissue** integrity r/t debridement, open wound

Risk for **Infection** r/t open wound, presence of bacteria

## Wound Dehiscence, Evisceration

**Fear** r/t client fear of body parts falling out, surgical procedure not going as planned

Imbalanced **Nutrition**: less than body requirements r/t inability to digest nutrients, need for increased protein for healing

Risk for deficient **Fluid** volume r/t inability to ingest nutrients, obstruction, fluid loss

Risk for delayed **Surgical** recovery r/t separation of wound, exposure of abdominal contents

Risk for **Injury** r/t exposed abdominal contents

## Wound Infection

Disturbed **Body** image r/t dysfunctional open wound

**Hyperthermia** r/t increased metabolic rate, illness, infection

Imbalanced **Nutrition**: less than body requirements r/t biological factors, infection, hyperthermia

Impaired **Tissue** integrity r/t wound, presence of infection

Risk for deficient **Fluid** volume r/t increased metabolic rate

Risk for delayed **Surgical** recovery r/t presence of infection

Risk for **Infection**: spread of r/t imbalanced nutrition: less than body requirements

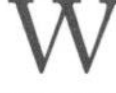

SECTION

# III Guide to Planning Care

Section III is a listing of nursing diagnosis care plans according to NANDA-I. The care plans are arranged alphabetically by diagnostic concept.

## MAKING AN ACCURATE NURSING DIAGNOSIS

Verify the accuracy of the previously suggested nursing diagnoses (from Section II) for the client. To do this:

- Read the definition for the suggested nursing diagnosis and determine if it sounds appropriate
- Compare the Defining Characteristics with the client data collected

or

- Compare the Risk Factors with the client data collected (if it is a "Risk for" Nursing Diagnosis, they do not have defining characteristics)

## WRITING OUTCOMES STATEMENTS AND NURSING INTERVENTIONS

After selecting the appropriate nursing diagnosis, use this section to write outcomes and interventions:

- Use the NOC/NIC outcomes and interventions with the associated rating scales

or

- Use the Client Outcomes/Nursing Interventions as written by the authors and contributors
- Read the rationales, many of them based on nursing or clinical research that validate the efficacy of the interventions.

Following these steps, you will be able to write a nursing care plan, which should be implemented and then evaluated after using the interventions to give care to the client.

# Activity intolerance

evolve

*Terri Ellis and Betty J. Ackley*

## NANDA

### Definition

Insufficient physiological or psychological energy to endure or complete required or desired daily activities

### Defining Characteristics

Verbal report of fatigue or weakness, abnormal heart rate or blood pressure response to activity, exertional discomfort or dyspnea, electrocardiographic changes reflecting arrhythmias or ischemia

### Related Factors (r/t)

Bed rest or immobility, generalized weakness, sedentary lifestyle, imbalance between oxygen supply and demand

## NOC

### Outcomes (Nursing Outcomes Classification)

#### Suggested NOC Outcomes

Activity Tolerance, Endurance, Energy Conservation, Self-Care: Instrumental Activities of Daily Living (IADLs)

**Example NOC Outcome with Indicators**

**Endurance** as evidenced by the following indicators: Performance of usual routine/Activity/Rested appearance/Concentration/Interest in surroundings/Muscle endurance/Eating pattern/Libido/Energy restored after rest/Blood oxygen level/Hemoglobin/Hematocrit/Blood glucose/Serum electrolytes (Rate each indicator of **Endurance:** 1 = severely compromised, 2 = substantially compromised, 3 = moderately compromised, 4 = mildly compromised, 5 = not compromised [see Section I].)

### Client Outcomes

**Client Will (Specify Time Frame):**

- Participate in prescribed physical activity with appropriate increases in heart rate, blood pressure, and breathing rate; maintains monitor patterns (rhythm and ST segment) within normal limits
- State symptoms of adverse effects of exercise and report onset of symptoms immediately
- Maintain normal skin color and skin is warm and dry with activity

A

- Verbalize an understanding of the need to gradually increase activity based on testing, tolerance, and symptoms
- Express an understanding of the need to balance rest and activity
- Demonstrate increased activity tolerance

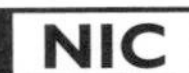

## Interventions (Nursing Interventions Classification)

### Suggested NIC Interventions

Activity Therapy, Energy Management

**Example NIC Activities—Energy Management**

Monitor cardiorespiratory response to activity; monitor location and nature of discomfort or pain during movement/activity

## Nursing Interventions and Rationales

- Determine cause of activity intolerance (see Related Factors) and determine whether cause is physical, psychological, or motivational. *Determining the cause of a disease can help direct appropriate interventions.*
- Assess the client daily for appropriateness of activity and bed rest orders. *Inappropriate prolonged bed rest orders may contribute to activity intolerance (Kasper, Braunwald, & Fauci, 2005).* **EB:** *A review of 39 studies on bed rest resulting from 15 disorders demonstrated that bed rest for treatment of medical conditions is associated with worse outcomes than early mobilization (Allen et al, 1999).*
- If mainly on bed rest, minimize cardiovascular deconditioning by positioning the client in an upright position several times daily. *Deconditioning of the cardiovascular system occurs within days and involves fluid shifts, fluid loss, decreased cardiac output, decreased peak oxygen uptake, and increased resting heart rate (Resnick, 1998; Fletcher, 2005; Kasper, Braunwald, & Fauci, 2005).*
- If client is mostly immobile, consider use of a transfer chair, a chair that becomes a stretcher. *Using a transfer chair where the client is pulled onto a flat surface and then seated upright in the chair can help previously immobile clients get out of bed (Nelson et al, 2003).*
- When appropriate, gradually increase activity, allowing the client to assist with positioning, transferring, and self-care as possible. Progress from sitting in bed to dangling, to standing, to ambulation. *Always have the client dangle at the bedside before trying standing to evaluate for postural hypotension. Watch the client closely for dizziness during increased activity (Fried & Fried, 2001). Postural hypotension can be detected in up to 30% of elderly clients. These methods can help prevent falls (Tinetti, 2003).*
- When getting a client up, observe for symptoms of intolerance such as nausea, pallor, dizziness, visual dimming, and impaired consciousness, as well as changes in vital signs. *When an adult rises to the standing position, 300 to 800 mL of blood pools in the*

*lower extremities. Maintenance of blood pressure during position change is quite complex; many sensitive cardiac, vascular, neurologic, muscular, and neurohumoral responses must occur quickly. If any of these responses are abnormal, blood pressure and organ perfusion can be reduced. As a result, symptoms of central nervous system hypoperfusion may occur, including feelings of weakness, nausea, headache, neck ache, lightheadedness, dizziness, blurred vision, fatigue, tremulousness, palpitations, and impaired cognition (Bradley & Davis, 2003).*

- ▲ If a client experiences syncope with activity, refer for evaluation by a physician. *Syncope has many causes, including benign vasovagal, but can also be due to serious cardiac disease, resulting in death (Hauer, 2003).*
- • Perform range-of-motion (ROM) exercises if the client is unable to tolerate activity or is mostly immobile. *Inactivity rapidly contributes to muscle shortening and changes in periarticular and cartilaginous joint structure. These factors contribute to contracture and limitation of motion (Fried & Fried, 2001).*
- • Monitor and record the client's ability to tolerate activity: note pulse rate, blood pressure, monitor pattern, dyspnea, use of accessory muscles, and skin color before and after activity. If the following signs and symptoms of cardiac decompensation develop, activity should be stopped immediately (Wenger, 2001):
  - Onset of chest discomfort
  - Dyspnea
  - Palpitations
  - Excessive fatigue
  - Lightheadedness, confusion, ataxia, pallor, cyanosis, dyspnea, nausea, or any peripheral circulatory insufficiency
  - Dysrhythmia (symptomatic supraventricular tachycardia, ventricular tachycardia, exercise-induced intraventricular conduction defect, second- or third-degree atrioventricular block, frequent premature ventricular contractions)
  - Exercise hypotension (drop in systolic blood pressure of 10 mm Hg from baseline blood pressure despite an increase in workload)
  - Excessive rise in blood pressure (systolic >180 mm Hg or diastolic >110 mm Hg) NOTE: These are upper limits; activity may be stopped before reaching these values
  - Inappropriate bradycardia (drop in heart rate >10 beats/min or < 50 beats/min)
  - Increased heart rate above 100 beats/min
- • Instruct the client to stop the activity immediately and report to the physician if the client is experiencing the following symptoms: new or worsened intensity or increased frequency of discomfort; tightness or pressure in chest, back, neck, jaw, shoulders, and/or arms; palpitations; dizziness; weakness; unusual and extreme fatigue; excessive air hunger. *These are common symptoms of angina and are caused by a temporary insufficiency of coronary blood supply. Symptoms typically last for minutes as opposed to momentary twinges. If symptoms last longer than 5 to 10 minutes, the client should be evaluated by a physician. The client should be evaluated before resuming activity.*
- • Observe and document skin integrity several times a day. *Activity intolerance may lead to pressure ulcers. Mechanical pressure, moisture, friction, and shearing forces all predispose to their development (Resnick, 1998; Kasper, Braunwald, & Fauci, 2005).*

- Assess for constipation. If present, refer to care plan for **Constipation**. *Impaired mobility is associated with increased risk of constipation.*
- ▲ Refer the client to physical therapy to help increase activity levels and strength.
- ▲ Consider dietitian referral to assess nutritional needs related to activity intolerance. Recognize that undernutrition causes significant morbidity due to the loss of lean body mass. *The decline in body mass, with physical weakness, inhibits mobility, increasing liability to deep vein thrombosis and pressure sores. Respiratory muscle weakness causes difficulty in expectorating, increasing susceptibility to chest infection. Immunocompetence declines, increasing the risk of infection, which in turn reduces nutritional status (Holmes, 2003).*
- Identify the factors that contribute to undernutrition in hospital patients. *There are two main ways in which undernutrition develops. The first, protein-energy malnutrition arises during acute injury or illness when increased nutrient requirements and loss of body protein are common. The second is inadequate nutrient intake during a time of increased nutritional demand or over a prolonged period of reduced dietary consumption. This is particularly common in older people and those with disabilities and chronic or mental illness (Holmes, 2003).*
- Provide emotional support and encouragement to the client to gradually increase activity. *Fear of breathlessness, pain, or falling may decrease willingness to increase activity.*
- Observe for pain before activity. If possible, treat pain before activity and ensure that the client is not heavily sedated. *Pain restricts the client from achieving a maximal activity level and is often exacerbated by movement.*
- Obtain any necessary assistive devices or equipment needed before ambulating the client (e.g., walkers, canes, crutches, portable oxygen). *Assistive devices can increase mobility by helping the client overcome limitations.*
- Use a gait walking belt when ambulating the client. *Gait belts help improve the caregiver's grasp, reducing the incidence of injuries (Nelson, 2003).*
- Work with the client to set mutual goals that increase activity levels.
- ▲ If the client is scheduled for a surgical intervention that will result in bed rest in intensive care, consider referring to physical therapy for a prehabilitation program including warm-up, aerobic conditioning, strength building, and flexibility enhancement. **EBN**: *Increasing a client's functional capacity before hospitalization can be a helpful means of modifying the predictable deconditioning that happens with intensive care unit (ICU) admission (Topp et al, 2002).*

### Activity Intolerance Due to Respiratory Disease

- If the client is able to walk and has chronic obstructive pulmonary disease (COPD), consider the use of an accelerometer to assess walking ability or use the traditional 6-minute walk distance. **EBN and EB:** *Use of the accelerometer was very predictive of maximum distance walked during a 6-minute walk test (Belza et al, 2001). The 6-minute walk test predicted mortality in COPD clients (Pinto-Plata et al, 2004).*
- Ensure that the chronic pulmonary client has oxygen saturation testing with exercise. Use supplemental oxygen to keep oxygen saturation 90% or above or as prescribed with activity. *Clients with COPD may suffer from inadequate gas exchange, cor pulmonale, and other factors limiting oxygen transport. The use of oxygen increases survival, lowers*

*pulmonary artery pressure and pulmonary vascular resistance, and improves cardiac function, exercise capacity, and tolerance of ADLs (Garvey, 2001).*

- Monitor a COPD client's response to activity by observing for symptoms of respiratory intolerance such as increased dyspnea, loss of ability to control breathing rhythmically, use of accessory muscles, and skin tone changes such as pallor and cyanosis.
- Instruct and assist a COPD client in using conscious, controlled breathing techniques, including pursed-lip breathing and diaphragmatic breathing. *Training a client with COPD to slow his or her respiratory rate with a prolonged exhalation with pursed lips helps control dyspnea and results in improved ventilation, increased tidal volume, decreased respiratory rate, and a reduced alveolar-arterial oxygen difference.* **EB:** *Pursed-lip breathing reduces end expiratory volume and breathlessness (Bianchi et al, 2004).*
- Refer the COPD client to a pulmonary rehabilitation program. **EB:** *Pulmonary rehabilitation has been shown to relieve dyspnea and fatigue, and enhance clients' sense of control over their disease. It also causes a modest increase in ability to exercise (Lacasse et al, 2002). Pulmonary rehabilitation was effective in reducing the utilization of health care resources (California Pulmonary Rehabilitation Collaborative Group, 2004).*

## Activity Intolerance Due to Cardiovascular Disease

- If the client is able to walk and has heart failure, consider use of the 6-minute walk test to determine physical ability. **EBN and EB:** *The distance walked in 6 minutes was useful in patients with left ventricular dysfunction, as well as those with preserved function, and that distance walked was directly related to rates of rehospitalization and death for 100 patients with dilated cardiomyopathy (Ford et al, 2004) The 6-minute walk test was shown to be highly reproducible in determining ability to ambulate in a client in heart failure (Demers et al, 2001).*
- Allow for periods of rest before and after planned exertion periods such as meals, baths, treatments, and physical activity. *Both physical and emotional rest helps lower arterial pressure and reduce the workload of the myocardium (Kasper, Braunwald, & Fauci, 2005).* **EB:** *Limited exercise tolerance in heart failure is often the first and central clinical feature, reflecting both decreased cardiac and peripheral responses (Lucas et al, 1999).*
- ▲ Refer to heart failure program or cardiac rehabilitation program for education, evaluation, and guided support to increase activity and rebuild life. **EB:** *Exercise can help many clients with heart failure. Whereas rest was commonly recommended a few years ago, it has become clear that inactivity can worsen the skeletal muscle myopathy in these clients. A carefully monitored exercise program can improve both exercise capacity and quality of life in mild to moderate heart failure clients (Rees et al, 2004). Exercise-based cardiac rehabilitation is effective in reducing the number of cardiac deaths, also decreasing cholesterol levels, systolic blood pressure, and self-reported smoking (Jolliffe, 2001; Taylor et al, 2004).*

## Geriatric

- Slow the pace of care. Allow the client extra time to carry out activities.
- Encourage families to help/allow an elderly client to be independent in whatever activities possible. S*ometimes families believe they are assisting by allowing clients to be sedentary. Encouraging activity not only enhances good functioning of the body's systems*

*but also promotes a sense of worth (Eliopoulous, 1997; Kasper, Braunwald, & Fauci, 2005).*

- ▲ If the client has heart disease causing activity intolerance, refer for cardiac rehabilitation. **EB:** *Elderly clients with coronary artery disease in exercise regimens after hospitalization have exercise trainability comparable with that of younger clients participating in similar experiences (Williams et al, 1985; Shepard, 1990).*
- ▲ Refer the client to physical therapy for resistance exercise training as able, including abdominal crunch, leg press, leg extension, leg curl, calf press, and more. **EB:** *A study demonstrated that 6 months of resistance exercise for the elderly greatly increased their aerobic capacity, possibly from increased skeletal muscle strength (Vincent et al, 2002).*
- • When mobilizing the elderly client, watch for orthostatic hypotension accompanied by dizziness and fainting. *Postural hypotension can be detected in up to 30% of elderly clients. These methods can help prevent falls (Tinetti, 2003).*
- • Once the client is able to walk independently and needs an exercise program, suggest the client enter an exercise program with a friend. **EBN:** *Findings from a study of exercise behavior found that friends have the strongest influence to keep on an exercise program, more than family members or experts (Resnick et al, 2002).*

## Home Care

- ▲ Begin discharge planning as soon as possible with case manager or social worker to assess need for home support systems and the need for community or home health services.
- ▲ Assess the home environment for factors that precipitate or contribute to decreased activity tolerance: stairs; lack of assistive bed or bathroom devices; distance to bathroom; presence of allergens such as dust, smoke, and those associated with pets; temperature; energy-intensive activity patterns; and furniture placement. Refer to occupational therapy if needed to assist the client in restructuring the home and ADL patterns. *During hospitalization, clients and families often estimate energy requirements at home inaccurately because the hospital's availability of staff support distorts the level of care that will be needed.*
- ▲ Refer to physical therapy for strength training and possible weight training. Physical therapists can initiate a program of exercise for the client, with family assistance, to regain strength, increase endurance, and improve balance. Use of hand weights or stretch bands can be used to increase muscle strength. If the client is homebound, the physical therapist can also initiate cardiac rehabilitation.
- ▲ Support strength training program prescribed by physical therapist. A client may resist exercise in light of low energy level; reminders and positive feedback by other care providers will help the client maintain prescribed exercises.
- • Normalize the client's activity intolerance; encourage progress with positive feedback. The client's experience should be validated as within expected norms. Recognition of progress enhances motivation. **EBN:** *In qualitative studies, fatigued women reported that they felt distressed when health care providers invalidated their experiences of fatigue (Patusky, 2002; Asbring & Narvanen, 2004).*
- • Teach the client/family the importance of and methods for setting priorities for activities, especially those having a high energy demand (e.g., home/family events). In-

struct in realistic expectations. *The client and/or family may assume a more rapid rate of energy recovery than actually occurs. Assistance may be needed to ensure accuracy of expectations for the client.* **EBN:** *Unrealistic expectations provoke guilt feelings in the client, leading to efforts that can exceed the client's energy capacity (Patusky, 2002).*

- • Provide the client/family with resources such as senior centers, exercise classes, educational and recreational programs, and volunteer opportunities that can aid in promoting socialization and appropriate activity. *Social isolation can be an outcome of and contribute to activity intolerance.*
- • Discuss the importance of sexual activity as part of daily living. Instruct the client in adaptive techniques to conserve energy during sexual interactions. *Families may make unsafe choices for sexual activity or place added stress on themselves trying to cope with this issue without proper support or teaching.*
- • Instruct the client and family in the importance of maintaining proper nutrition, rest, and behavioral pacing for energy conservation and rehabilitation. Instruct in use of dietary supplements as indicated. *Illness may suppress appetite, leading to inadequate nutrition. Pacing activities to energy capacity and need for rest are important to ensure the client does not overdo his or her capability.*
- ▲ Refer to medical social services as necessary to assist the family in adjusting to major changes in patterns of living.
- • Assess the need for long-term supports for optimal activity tolerance of priority activities (e.g., assistive devices, oxygen, medication, catheters, massage), especially for a hospice client. Evaluate intermittently. *Assessments ensure the safety and appropriate use of these supports.*
- ▲ Refer to home health aide services to support the client and family through changing levels of activity tolerance. Introduce aide support early. Instruct the aide to promote independence in activity as tolerated. *Home health aides provide initial assistance with ADLs that may involve experience with safe body mechanics. Changes in the amount of support necessary as the client progresses are important because providing unnecessary assistance with transfers and bathing activities may promote dependence and a loss of mobility.*
- • Be aware of increased risk of bone fracture even after muscle strength is normalized, especially in osteoporosis-prone individuals such as estrogen-deficient women and the elderly. *Reduction in weight-bearing muscle activity during bed rest invariably produces significant changes in calcium balance and, in weeks, changes in bone mass (Bloomfield, 1997).*
- • Allow terminally ill clients and their families to guide care. *Control by the client or family respects their autonomy and promotes effective coping.*
- • Provide increased attention to comfort and dignity of the terminally ill client in care planning. *Interventions should be provided as much for psychological effect as for physiological support. For example, oxygen may be more valuable as a support to the client's psychological comfort than as a booster of oxygen saturation.*
- • Institute case management of frail elderly to support continued independent living. *Difficulties with activity intolerance can lead to increasing needs for assistance in using the health care system effectively. Case management combines nursing activities of the client and family assessment, planning and coordination of care among all health care providers, de-*

*livery of direct nursing care, and monitoring of care and outcomes. These activities are able to address continuity of care, mutual goal setting, behavior management, and prevention of worsening health problems (Guttman, 1999).*

- In the presence of psychiatric illness, refer for psychiatric home health care services for client reassurance and implementation of a therapeutic regimen. **EBN:** *Psychiatric home care nurses can address issues relating to the client's depression with activity intolerance. Behavioral interventions in the home can assist the client to participate more effectively in treatment plan (Patusky et al, 1996).*

## Client/Family Teaching

- Instruct the client on rationale and techniques for avoiding activity intolerance.
- Teach the client to use controlled breathing techniques with activity.
- Teach the client the importance and method of coughing, clearing secretions.
- Instruct the client in the use of relaxation techniques during activity.
- Help client with energy conservation and work simplification techniques in ADLs.
- Teach the client the importance of proper nutrition.
- Describe to the client the symptoms of activity intolerance, including which symptoms to report to the physician.
- Explain to the client how to use assistive devices or medications before or during activity.
- Help client set up an activity log to record exercise and exercise tolerance.

## evolve WEBSITES FOR EDUCATION

See the EVOLVE website for World Wide Web resources for client education.

## REFERENCES

Allen C, Glasziou P, Del Mar C: Bed rest: a potentially harmful treatment needing more careful evaluation, *Lancet* 354(9186): 1229, 1999.

Asbring P, Narvanen A: Patient power and control: a study of women with uncertain illness trajectories, *Qual Health Res* 14(2): 226, 2004.

Belza B, Steele BG, Hunziker J et al: Correlates of physical activity in chronic obstructive pulmonary disease, *Nurs Res* 50(4):195, 2001.

Bianchi R, Gigliotti F, Romagnoli I et al: Chest wall kinematics and breathlessness during pursed-lip breathing in patients with COPD, *Chest* 125(2):459, 2004.

Bloomfield SA: Changes in musculoskeletal structure and function with prolonged bed rest, *Med Sci Sports Exerc* 29(2):197, 1997.

Bradley JG, Davis KA: Orthostatic hypotension, *Am Fam Physician* 68(12):2393, 2003.

California Pulmonary Rehabilitation Collaborative Group: Effects of pulmonary rehabilitation on dyspnea, quality of life and healthcare costs in California, *J Cardiopulm Rehabil* 24(1):52, 2004.

Demers C, McKelvie RS, Negassa A et al: Reliability, validity, and responsiveness of the six-minute walk test in patients with heart failure, *Am Heart J* 142(4):698, 2001.

Eliopoulous C: *Gerontological nursing,* ed 4, Philadelphia, 1997, Lippincott.

Fletcher K: Immobility: geriatric self-learning module, *Medsurg Nurs* 14(1):35, 2005.

Ford CM, Pruitt R, Parker V et al: CHF: effects of cardiac rehabilitation and brain natriuretic peptide, *Nurse Pract* 29(3):36, 2004.

Fried KM, Fried GW: Immobility. In Derstine JB, Hargrove SD, editors: *Comprehensive rehabilitation nursing,* Philadelphia, 2001, WB Saunders.

Garvey C: Pulmonary rehabilitation for the elderly client, *Topics Adv Prac Nurs eJournal* 1(2), 2001. Available at www.medscape.com/viewarticle/408409, accessed on April 5, 2005.
Guttman R: Case management of the frail elderly in the community, *Clin Nurs Spec* 13(4):174, 1999.
Hauer KE: Discovering the cause of syncope, *Postgrad Med* 113(1):31, 2003.
Holmes S: Undernutrition in hospital patients, *Nurs Stand* 17(19):45, 2003.
Jolliffe JA, Rees K, Taylor RS et al: Exercise-based rehabilitation for coronary heart disease, *Cochrane Library* (1):CD001800, 2001.
Kasper DL, Braunwald E, Fauci AS et al: *Harrison's principles of internal medicine*, ed 16, New York, 2005, McGraw-Hill.
Lacasse Y, Brosseau L, Milne S et al: Pulmonary rehabilitation for chronic obstructive pulmonary disease, *Cochrane Database Syst Rev* (3):CD003793, 2002.
Lucas C, Stevenson LW, Johnson W et al: The 6-min walk and peak oxygen consumption in advanced heart failure: aerobic capacity and survival, *Am Heart J* 138(4 Pt 1):618, 1999.
Nelson A, Owen B, Lloyd JD et al: Safe patient handling and movement, *Am J Nurs* 103(3):32, 2003.
Patusky KL: Relatedness theory as a framework for the treatment of fatigued women, *Arch Psychiatr Nurs* 5:224, 2002.
Patusky KL, Rodning C, Martinez-Kratz M: Clinical lessons in psychiatric home care: a case study approach, *J Home Health Case Manage* 9:18, 1996.
Pinto-Plata VM, Cote C, Cabral H et al: The 6-min walk distance: change over time and value as a predictor of survival in severe COPD, *Eur Respir J* 23(1):23, 2004.
Rees K, Taylor RS, Singh S et al: Exercise based rehabilitation for heart failure, *Cochrane Database Syst Rev* (3):CD003331, 2004.
Resnick B, Orwig D, Magaziner J: The effect of social support on exercise behavior in older adults, *Clin Nurs Res* 11(1):52, 2002.
Resnick N: Geriatric medicine. In Tierney L Jr, McPhee S, Papadakis M, editors: *Current medical diagnosis and treatment,* ed 37, Stamford, Conn, 1998, Appleton and Lange.
Shepard RJ: The scientific basis of exercise prescribing for the very old, *J Am Geriatr Soc* 38:62, 1990.
Taylor RS, Brown A, Ebrahim S et al: Exercise-based rehabilitation for patients with coronary heart disease: systematic review and meta-anlysis of randomized controlled trials, *Am J Med* 116(10):682, 2004.
Tinetti ME: Preventing falls in elderly persons, *N Engl J Med* 348(1):421, 2003.
Topp R, Ditmyer M, King K et al: The effect of bed rest and potential of prehabilitation on patients in the intensive care unit, *AACN Clin Issues* 13(2):263, 2002.
Vincent KR, Braith RW, Feldman RA et al: Improved cardiorespiratory endurance following 6 months of resistance exercise in elderly men and women, *Arch Intern Med* 162(6):673, 2002.
Wenger NK: Rehabilitation of the patient with coronary heart disease. In Fuster V et al, editors: *Hurst's the heart,* ed 10, New York, 2001, McGraw-Hill.
Williams MA, Maresh CM, Esterbrooks DJ et al: Early exercise training in patients older than age 65 years compared with that in younger patients after acute myocardial infarction or coronary artery bypass grafting, *Am J Cardiol* 55(4):263, 1985.

# Risk for Activity intolerance

*Betty J. Ackley*

**NANDA**

## Definition

At risk for experiencing insufficient physiological or psychological energy to endure or complete required or desired daily activities

## Risk Factors

History of previous intolerance, deconditioned status, presence of circulatory or respiratory problems, inexperience with activity

• = Independent; ▲ = Collaborative; EBN = Evidence-Based Nursing; EB = Evidence-Based

**Related Factors (r/t)**

See Risk Factors

**NOC**

**Outcomes (Nursing Outcomes Classification)**

**Suggested NOC Outcomes**

Activity Tolerance, Endurance, Energy Conservation

**Example NOC Outcome with Indicators**

**Endurance** as evidenced by the following indicators: Performance of usual routine/Activity/Rested appearance/Blood oxygen level within normal limits/Concentration/Interest in surroundings/Muscle endurance/ Eating pattern/Libido/Energy restored after rest/Blood oxygen level/Hemoglobin/Hematocrit/Blood glucose/Serum electrolytes (Rate each indicator of **Endurance:** 1 = severely compromised, 2 = substantially compromised, 3 = moderately compromised, 4 = mildly compromised, 5 = not compromised [see Section I].)

**NIC**

**Interventions (Nursing Interventions Classification)**

**Suggested NIC Interventions**

Energy Management, Exercise Promotion: Strength Training, Activity Therapy

**Example NIC Activities—Energy Management**

Monitor cardiorespiratory response to activity; monitor location and nature of discomfort or pain during movement/activity

**Client Outcomes, Nursing Interventions and Rationales, and Client/Family Teaching**

See care plan for **Activity intolerance**.

## Impaired Adjustment

*Ann Keeley*

**NANDA**

**Definition**

Inability to modify lifestyle/behavior in a manner consistent with a change in health status

## Defining Characteristics

Denial of health status change; failure to take actions that would prevent further health problems, failure to achieve optimal sense of control, demonstration of nonacceptance of health status change

## Related Factors (r/t)

Low state of optimism, intense emotional state, negative attitudes toward health behavior, absence of intent to change behavior, multiple stressors, absence of social support for changed beliefs and practices, disability or health status change requiring change in lifestyle, lack of motivation to change behaviors

NOC

## Outcomes (Nursing Outcomes Classification)

### Suggested NOC Outcomes

Acceptance: Health Status, Coping, Grief Resolution, Health-Seeking Behavior, Participation in Health Care Decisions, Psychosocial Adjustment: Life Change, Treatment Behavior: Illness or Injury

**Example NOC Outcome with Indicators**

**Acceptance: Health Status** as evidenced by the following indicators: Peacefulness/Relinquishment of previous concept of health/Expressed reactions to health status/Recognition of reality of health situation/Coping with health status (Rate each indicator of **Acceptance: Health Status:** 1 = never demonstrated, 2 = rarely demonstrated, 3 = sometimes demonstrated, 4 = often demonstrated, 5 = consistently demonstrated [see Section I].)

## Client Outcomes

**Client Will (Specify Time Frame):**

- State acceptance of change in health status
- Request assistance in altering behaviors to adapt to change
- State personal goals for dealing with change in health status and means to prevent further health problems
- State experience of a period of grief that is proportional to the actual or perceived effect of the loss
- Report and/or demonstrate behavior changes mutually agreed upon with nurse as evidence of positive adaptation

NIC

## Interventions (Nursing Interventions Classification)

### Suggested NIC Intervention

Coping Enhancement

**Example NIC Activities—Coping Enhancement**

Assist the client with developing an objective appraisal of the event; explore with the client previous methods of dealing with life problems

## Nursing Interventions and Rationales

- Assess the client's perception about the illness/event. Ask the client to state feelings related to the change in health status. **EBN:** *Negative responses to a need for change in behavior related to an alteration in health status can be understood only following a thorough assessment of the client's appraisal framework (Dudley-Brown, 2002).*
- Assess the client and family for the presence of additional stressors (e.g., financial difficulty, health of other family members, occupational changes). *Additional stressors have been found to hinder the client's and/or family's adjustment (Dibartolo, 2002).*
- Assess the client's feelings about whether change in health status is personally being dealt with effectively. **EBN:** *Psychological distress can negatively affect positive adaptation (Dudley-Brown, 2002).*
- Assess for negative affect and internalization of problems. **EBN:** *Exploring the meaning of health status change and the adjustments required for a successful adaptation within the client's life experience fosters positive growth (Norris & Spelic, 2002; Richer & Ezer, 2002).*
- Assess the socioeconomic status of all clients.
- Allow the client adequate time to express feelings about the change in health status. **EBN:** *Nurses need to provide an opportunity for clients to address all aspects of the impact of a health status change on their lives (Richer & Ezer, 2002).*
- Help the client work through the stages of grief. Denial is usually the initial response. Acknowledge that grief takes time, and give the client permission to grieve; accept crying. *The process of grieving is integral to adaptation to a disruption of health status (Norris & Spelic, 2002).* **EBN:** *Cognitive dysfunction is a manifestation of grieving a change in health status (Wassem et al, 2001).*
- Recognize that denial may be adaptive at certain stages of a threatening encounter. *Denial is the initial phase of the grieving response and would be expected when a client is told of a significant change in health status (Norris & Spelic, 2002).*
- Discuss resources (e.g., the client's support system) that have worked previously when dealing with changes in lifestyle or health status. *As a client adjusts to a change in health status, he or she will call on previous behaviors that proved successful in a crisis situation (Norris & Spelic, 2002).* **EBN:** *Integration of a client's repertoire of coping strategies into an intervention program to facilitate adaptation to a change in health status will facilitate positive coping (Wassem et al, 2001).*

▲ Refer to community resources. Provide general and contact information for ease of use. *Available resources should be integrated into any intervention aimed at facilitating a positive adjustment to a change in health status (Norris & Spelic, 2002).* **EBN:** *Social support is necessary to coordinate all possible resources that may assist the client and/or family in their adjustment to a change in health status (Wassem et al, 2001).*

- Use open-ended questions to allow the client free expression (e.g., "Tell me about your last hospitalization" or "How does this time compare?"). **EBN:** *Active listening aimed* *at clarifying family concerns regarding the change in health status will facilitate nursing interventions that promote positive coping behaviors (Weiss & Chan, 2002).*

- Discuss the client's current goals. If appropriate, have the client list goals so that they can be referred to and steps can be taken to accomplish them. **EBN:** *Clarification of the client/family goals and expectations will allow the nurse to clarify what is possible and to identify measures that can facilitate achievement of the goals (Northouse et al, 2002).*
- List the client activities that may require assistance and those that can be performed independently. **EBN:** *Clarification of behaviors conducive to a positive adjustment to a change in health status and the resources available to the client facilitates positive coping behaviors toward adaptation (Northouse et al, 2002).*
- Allow the client choices in daily care, particularly choices that result from the change in health status. **EBN:** *A client will demonstrate a more positive adaptation if the resources, and interventions offered by the nurse are adapted to the client's perceived circumstances and needs (LeClere et al, 2002).*
- Allow the client time to adjust to new situations. Introduce new material gradually to prevent overload. Ask for frequent feedback. *The stress of changes in health care can be overwhelming. New material takes longer to learn and absorb; thus, clarification of information and frequent repetition may be necessary.*
- Give the client positive feedback for accomplishments, no matter how small. **EBN:** *The nurse's provision of a climate of acceptance and encouragement facilitates a positive adaptation (Riche & Ezer, 2002).*
- Manipulate the environment to decrease stress; allow the client to display personal items that have meaning. **EBN:** *Appraisal uncertainty is a risk factor for a negative adaptation to health change (Dudley-Brown, 2002).*
- Maintain consistency and continuity in daily schedule. When possible, provide the same caregiver. **EBN:** *The predictability of interaction with the same nurses as a part of treatment facilitates trust, confidence, and positive adaptation (Riche & Ezer, 2002).*
- Foster communication between the client/family and medical staff. **EBN:** *Perceived ability to access a variety of resources promotes self-efficacy and positive adaptation to health status changes (Czuchta & McCay, 2001).* **EBN:** *Family members of individuals undergoing cardiopulmonary resuscitation expressed a need to be involved and present or informed at all times during the process (Wagner, 2004).*
- Promote use of positive spiritual influences. *Spiritual coping strategies may facilitate a positive adaptation to a change in health status (Baldacchino & Draper, 2001).*

## Geriatric

- ▲ Assess for signs of depression resulting from illness-associated changes and make appropriate referral. **EBN:** *Signs and symptoms of depression when evident would assist the nurse in the individualization of interventions to a particular client (Reynaud & Meeker, 2002).*
- Monitor the client for agitation. *The elderly often use agitation to express an inability to accept change.*
- Increase and mobilize support available to the elderly client. Encourage interaction with family and friends. **EBN:** *Relationships are pivotal in supporting coping of older*

*adults (Cutcliff & Grant, 2001). Maintain continuity of care by keeping the number of caregivers to a minimum.*

### Multicultural

- Assess for the influence of cultural beliefs, norms, and values on the client's ability to modify health behavior. **EBN:** *What the client considers normal and abnormal health behavior may be based on cultural perceptions (Cochran, 1998; Doswell & Erlen, 1998; Leininger & McFarland, 2002).*
- Encourage spirituality as a source of support for coping. **EBN:** *Many African Americans and Latinos identify spirituality, religiousness, prayer, and church-based approaches as coping resources (Samuel-Hodge et al, 2000).*
- Discuss with the client those aspects of his or her health behavior/lifestyle that will remain unchanged by their health status.
- Negotiate with the client regarding the aspects of health behavior that will need to be modified. **EBN:** *Give-and-take with the client will lead to culturally congruent care (Leininger & McFarland, 2002).*
- Assess the role of fatalism on the client's ability to modify health behavior. **EB:** *Fatalistic perspectives, which involve the belief that you cannot control your own fate, may influence health behaviors in some African-American, Asian, and Latino populations (Phillips et al, 1999; Powe & Finnie, 2003 ).*
- Identify which family members the client can rely on for support. **EBN:** *A variety of different cultures rely on family members to cope with stress (Aziz & Rowland, 2002; Donnelly, 2002; Gleeson-Kreig et al, 2002; White et al, 2002).*
- Validate the client's feelings regarding the impact of health status on current lifestyle. *Validation lets the client know that the nurse has heard and understands what was said, thus promoting the nurse-client relationship (Stuart & Laraia, 2001).*
- ▲ Assess for signs of depression and level of social support and make appropriate referrals. **EB:** *Increased depressed feelings and lower levels of available social support were reported by minority following injury (Brown et al, 2004).*

### Home Care

- Include a spiritual assessment in overall assessment of client and family resources. **EBN:** *Many African Americans and Latinos identify spirituality, religiousness, prayer, and church-based approaches as coping resources (Samuel-Hodge et al, 2000).*
- ▲ Refer to medical social services to facilitate the listed interventions and support client care goals. *Support for transition to the home setting can facilitate acceptance of the changes required to maintain the client in the home setting.*
- Assess affective climate within family and family support system. *Positive family affective climate and family support have been found to enhance social adjustment (Langfitt et al, 1999).*
- ▲ Observe for signs of caregiver stress on an ongoing basis. Refer to necessary support services. **EBN:** *Support groups provide an essential resource to clients and their families when adapting to health status change (Fung & Chien, 2002).*
- ▲ Refer the client to counselor or therapist for follow-up care. Initiate community refer-

rals as needed (e.g., grief counseling, self-help groups). **EBN:** *Families need assistance in coping with health changes. The nurse is often perceived as the individual who can help them obtain necessary social support (Northouse et al, 2002; Tak & McCubbin, 2002). Support groups can provide families with a close setting that allows for minor problems and fears to be resolved readily (Herranz & Gavilan, 1999).*

- Assist client to recognize and exercise power in using self-care management to adjust to health change. **EBN:** *Women post myocardial infarction reported that not participating in their health process increased their suffering and left them feeling powerless (Johansson, Dahlberg, & Ekebergh, 2003).* Refer to care plan for **Powerlessness**.
- Take the client's perspective into consideration, and use a holistic approach in assessing and responding to client planning for the future. **EBN:** *A study of women recovering from myocardial infarction revealed that these women lived with a feeling of insecurity, based on a new inability to trust their bodies. Caring for women post–myocardial infarction (MI), researchers concluded, must approach health as being more than the absence of illness (Johansson et al, 2003).*

## Client/Family Teaching

- Assess family/caregivers for coping and teaching/learning styles. **EBN:** *The degree of optimism and pessimism influences the coping and health outcomes of caregivers of patients with Parkinson's desease (Lyons et al, 2004).*
- Teach the client to maintain a positive outlook by listing current strengths. *Successful adaptation requires a coordination of efforts to fit the nursing interventions to the client's perception of the threat, personal values and beliefs, and recognition of personal strengths (Norris & Spelic, 2002). Parents of critically ill children demonstrated fewer complications following their participation in a structured hospital based intervention (Melnyk et al, 2004).*
- Teach a client and his or her family relaxation techniques (controlled breathing, guided imagery) and help them practice. **EBN:** *Relaxation training has been demonstrated to improve self-efficacy in Alzheimer family caregivers (Fisher & Laschinger, 2001).*
- Allow the client to proceed at own pace in learning; provide time for return demonstrations (e.g., self-injection of insulin). **EBN:** *Use clear and distinct language free of medical jargon and meaningless values. Family members of individuals undergoing cardiopulmonary resuscitation expressed a need to be involved and present or informed at all times during the process (Wagner, 2004). Successful adaptation requires a coordination of efforts to fit the nursing interventions to the client's perception of the threat, personal values and beliefs, and recognition of personal strengths (Norris & Spelic, 2002).*
- Involve significant others in planning and teaching. **EBN:** *Client's ability to cognitively absorb new information will vary according to his or her perceived threat, prior coping successes, and support (Northouse et al, 2002). Parents of critically ill children demonstrated fewer complications following their participation in a structured hospital based intervention (Melnyk et al, 2004). Successful adaptation requires a coordination of efforts to fit the nursing interventions to the client's perception of the threat, personal values and beliefs, and recognition of personal strengths (Norris & Spelic, 2002).*
- If long-term deficits are expected, inform the family as soon as possible. **EBN:** *An honest assessment shared by the nurse of a particular situation is important to the family's*

*sense of what is expected of them in adapting to a health care change (Weiss & Chen, 2002). Successful adaptation requires a coordination of efforts to fit the nursing interventions to the client's perception of the threat, personal values and beliefs, and recognition of personal strengths (Norris & Spelic, 2002).*

- Teach families intervention techniques for family members such as setting limits, communicating acceptable behavior, and having time-outs. *Psychological, social, and behavioral interventions are effective in mediating aggressive behavior (Harper-Jaques & Reimer, 2002). Parents of critically ill children demonstrated fewer complications following their participation in a structured hospital based intervention (Melnyk et al, 2004).*
- Educate and prepare families regarding the appearance of the client and the environment before initial exposure. *Successful adaptation requires a coordination of efforts to fit the nursing interventions to the client's perception of the threat, personal values and beliefs and recognition of personal strengths (Norris & Spelic, 2002).*

## evolve WEBSITES FOR EDUCATION

See the EVOLVE website for World Wide Web resources for client education.

## REFERENCES


Baldacchino D, Draper P: Spiritual coping strategies: a review of the EBN literature, *J Adv Nurs* 34(6):833, 2001.

Brown SA, McCauley SR, Levin HS et al: Perception of health and quality of life in minorities after mild-to-moderate traumatic brain injury, *Appl Neuropsychol* 11(1):54-64, 2004.

Czuchta DM, McCay E: Help-seeking for parents of individuals experiencing a first episode of schizophrenia, *Arch Psychiatr Nurs* 15(4):159, 2001.

Dudley-Brown S: Prevention of psychological distress in persons with inflammatory bowel disease, *Issues Ment Health Nurs* 23:403, 2002.

Harper-Jaques S, Reimer M: Management of aggression. In Boyd MA, editor: *Psychiatric nursing in contemporary practice,* ed 2, Philadelphia, 2002, Lippincott.

Johansson A, Dahlberg K, Ekebergh M: Living with experiences following a myocardial infarction, *Euro J Cardiovasc Nurs* 2:229, 2003.

Kuo TT, Ma FC: Symptom distresses and coping strategies in patients with non-small cell lung cancer, *Cancer Nurs* 25(4):309-317, 2002.

LeClerc CM, Wells DL, Craig D et al: Falling short of the mark, *Clin Nurs Res* 11(3):242-263, 2002.

Leininger MM, McFarland MR: *Transcultural nursing: concepts, theories, research and practices,* ed 3, New York, 2002, McGraw-Hill.

Lyons KS, Stewart BJ, Archbold PG et al: Pessimism and optimism as early warning signs for compromised health for caregivers of patients with Parkinson's disease, *Nurs Res* 53(6):354-362, 2004.

Melnyk BM, Alpert-Gillis L, Feinstein NF et ak: Creating opportunities for parent empowerment: program effects on the mental health/coping outcomes of critically ill young children and their mothers, *Pediatrics* 113(6):e597-607, 2004.

Miles MS, Holditch-Davis, D, Eron J et al: An HIV self-care symptom management intervention for African American mothers, *Nurs Res,* 52(6):350-60, 2003.

Norris J, Spelic SS: Supporting adaption to body image disruption, *Rehabil Nurs* 27(1):8-12, 2002.

Northouse L, Walker J, Schafenacker A et al: A family-based program of care for women with recurrent breast cancer and their family members, *Oncol Nurs Forum* 29(10):1411-1419, 2002.

Overcash JA: Using narrative research to understand the quality of life of older women with breast cancer, *Oncol Nurs Forum* 31(6):1153-1159, 2004.

Phillips JM, Cohen MZ, Moses G: Breast cancer screening and African American women: fear, fatalism, and silence, *Oncol Nurs Forum* 26(3):561, 1999.

Powe BD, Finnie R: Cancer fatalism: the state of the science, *Cancer Nurs* 26(6):454-465, 2003.
Purnell LD, Pualanka BJ: *Guide to culturally competent health care,* Philadelphia, 2005, FA Davis Company.
Reynaud SN, Meeker BJ: Coping styles of older adults with ostomies, *J Gerontol Nurs* 28(5):30-36, 2002.
Richer MC, Ezer H: Living in it, living with it, and moving on: dimensions of meaning during chemotherapy, *Oncol Nurs Forum* 29(1):113-119, 2002.
Rittman M, Faircloth C, Boylestein C et al: The experience of time in the transition from hospital to home following stroke, *J Rehabil Res Dev* 41(3A):259-268, 2004.
Stuart GW, Laraia MT: Therapeutic nurse-client relationship. In Stuart GW, Laraia MT, editors: *Principles and practice of psychiatric nursing,* St Louis, 2001, Mosby.
Wagner JM: Lived experience of critically ill patients' family members during cardiopulmonary resuscitation: *Am J Crit Care* 13(5): 416-420, 2004.

# Ineffective Airway clearance

evolve

*Betty J. Ackley*

**NANDA**

## Definition

Inability to clear secretions or obstructions from the respiratory tract to maintain a clear airway

## Defining Characteristics

Dyspnea; diminished breath sounds; orthopnea; adventitious breath sounds (rales, crackles, rhonchi, wheezes); cough, ineffective or absent; sputum production; cyanosis; difficulty vocalizing; wide-eyed; changes in respiratory rate and rhythm; restlessness

## Related Factors (r/t)

### Environmental

Smoking, smoke inhalation, second-hand smoke

### Obstructed Airway

Airway spasm, retained secretions, excessive mucus, presence of artificial airway, foreign body in airway, secretions in bronchi, exudate in alveoli

### Physiological

Neuromuscular dysfunction, hyperplasia of bronchial walls, COPD, infection, asthma, allergic airways

**NOC**

## Outcomes (Nursing Outcomes Classification)

### Suggested NOC Outcomes

Aspiration Prevention; Respiratory Status: Airway Patency, Gas Exchange, Ventilation

**Example NOC Outcome with Indicators**

**Respiratory Status: Ventilation** as evidenced by the following indicators: Respiratory rate/Moves sputum out of airway/Adventitious breath sounds not present/SOB not present/Auscultated breath sounds IER/ Auscultated vocalization IER/Chest x-ray findings IER (Rate each indicator of **Respiratory Status: Ventilation:** 1 = severely compromised, 2 = substantially compromised, 3 = moderately compromised, 4 = mildly compromised, 5 = not compromised [see Section I].)

IER, In expected range; SOB, shortness of breath.

## Client Outcomes

### Client Will (Specify Time Frame):

- Demonstrate effective coughing and clear breath sounds; is free of cyanosis and dyspnea
- Maintain a patent airway at all times
- Relate methods to enhance secretion removal
- Relate the significance of changes in sputum to include color, character, amount, and odor
- Identify and avoid specific factors that inhibit effective airway clearance

**NIC**

## Interventions (Nursing Interventions Classification)

### Suggested NIC Interventions

Airway Management, Airway Suctioning, Cough Enhancement

**Example NIC Activities—Airway Management**

Instruct how to cough effectively; auscultate breath sounds, noting areas of decreased or absent ventilation and presence of adventitious sounds

## Nursing Interventions and Rationales

- Auscultate breath sounds q1 to 4 hours. Breath sounds are normally clear or scattered fine crackles at bases, which clear with deep breathing. *The presence of coarse crackles during late inspiration indicates fluid in the airway; wheezing indicates an airway obstruction (Kasper et al, 2005).*
- Monitor respiratory patterns, including rate, depth, and effort. A normal respiratory rate for an adult without dyspnea is 12 to 16. *With secretions in the airway, the respiratory rate will increase.*
- Monitor blood gas values and pulse oxygen saturation levels as available. *An oxygen saturation of less than 90% (normal: 95% to 100%) or a partial pressure of oxygen of less than 80 (normal: 80 to 100) indicates significant oxygenation problems (Grap, 2002; Berry & Pinard, 2002).*

- Position the client to optimize respiration (e.g., head of bed elevated 45 degrees and repositioned at least every 2 hours). *An upright position allows for maximal lung expansion; lying flat causes abdominal organs to shift toward the chest, which crowds the lungs and makes it more difficult to breathe.* **EB:** *Studies have shown that in a mechanically ventilated client, there is a decreased incidence of pneumonia if the client is positioned at a 45-degree semirecumbent position as opposed to a supine position (Collard et al, 2003; Drakulovic et al, 1999).*
- If the client has unilateral lung disease, alternate a semi-Fowler's position with a lateral position (with a 10- to 15-degree elevation and "good lung down") for 60 to 90 minutes. This method is contraindicated for a client with a pulmonary abscess or hemorrhage or with interstitial emphysema. *Gravity and hydrostatic pressure allow the dependent lung to become better ventilated and perfused, which increases oxygenation (Smith-Sims, 2001).*
- Help the client deep breathe and perform controlled coughing. Have the client inhale deeply, hold breath for several seconds, and cough two or three times with mouth open while tightening the upper abdominal muscles. *This technique can help increase sputum clearance and decrease cough spasms (Donahue, 2002). Controlled coughing uses the diaphragmatic muscles, making the cough more forceful and effective.*
- If the client has COPD, cystic fibrosis, or bronchiectasis, consider helping the client use the forced expiratory technique, the "huff cough." The client does a series of coughs while saying the word "huff." *This technique prevents the glottis from closing during the cough and is effective in clearing secretions in the central airways (Goodman & Jones, 2002; Hess, 2001).*
- Encourage the client to use an incentive spirometer. *The incentive spirometer is an effective tool that can help prevent atelectasis and retention of bronchial secretions (Smith-Sims, 2001).* **EB:** *A study of postoperative abdominal surgery clients demonstrated that coughing and deep breathing clients vs. use of an incentive spirometer resulted in no significant difference in oxygenation (Genc et al, 2004).*
- Assist with clearing secretions from pharynx by offering tissues and gentle suction of the oral pharynx if necessary. *In the debilitated client, gentle suctioning of the posterior pharynx may stimulate coughing and remove secretions.*
- Observe sputum, noting color, odor, and volume. *Normal sputum is clear or gray and minimal; abnormal sputum is green, yellow, or bloody; malodorous; and often copious.*
- When suctioning an endotracheal tube or tracheostomy tube for a client on a ventilator, do the following:
  - Explain the process of suctioning before and ensure the client is not in pain or overly anxious. *Suctioning can be a frightening experience; an explanation along with adequate pain relief or needed sedation can reduce stress, anxiety, and pain (Day, Farnell, & Wilson-Barnett, 2002).*
  - Hyperoxygenate before and between endotracheal suction sessions. **EBN:** *Studies have demonstrated that hyperoxygenation helps prevent oxygen desaturation in a suctioned client (Adlkofer & Powaser, 1978; Harshbarger et al, 1992). One study demonstrated that oxygen saturation was higher when the client was hyperoxygenated with the ventilator versus use of a manual resuscitation bad with oxygen (Grap, 1996).*

- ■ Use a closed, in-line suction system. **EB:** *The closed, in-line suction system is associated with a decrease in nosocomial pneumonia (Deppe et al, 1990; Johnson et al, 1994). An additional study demonstrated that endotracheal suctioning using a closed system resulted in less deoxygenation of the client than when disconnecting the tubing for suctioning (Maggiore et al, 2003). A study demonstrated that using a closed system for suctioning, using pressure support as a recruitment measure and avoiding disconnecting the tubing resulted in decreased collapse of alveoli with suctioning and increased oxygenation (Maggiore, 2003).*
- ■ Avoid saline instillation during suctioning. **EBN:** *Repeated studies have demonstrated that saline instillation before suctioning has an adverse effect on oxygen saturation in both adults and children (Ackerman, 1993; Ackerman & Mick, 1998; Kinloch & Rock, 1999; Ridling, Martin, & Bratton, 2003).* **EB:** *A study demonstrated that instillation of a small amount of saline into the endotracheal tube increased greatly the number of colonies of bacteria dislodged from the tube to enter the lower airways, which can result in pneumonia (Hagler & Traver, 1994).*
- ■ Document results of coughing and suctioning, particularly client tolerance and secretion characteristics such as color, odor, and volume.

- • Provide oral care every 4 hours using a tooth brush. **EBN and EB:** *The toothbrush is the most important tool for oral care. Brushing the teeth is the most effective method for reducing plaque and controlling periodontal disease (Pearson & Hutton, 2002; Stiefel, 2000; ADA, 2004).*
- • Encourage activity and ambulation as tolerated. If unable to ambulate the client, turn the client from side to side at least every 2 hours. *Body movement helps mobilize secretions and can be a powerful means to maintain lung health (Fink, 2002).* **EB:** *Changes of postoperative position from sitting to standing are very important to improve outcomes, and the supine position should be avoided (Nielsen, Holte, & Kehlet, 2003).* See interventions for **Impaired Gas exchange** for further information on positioning a respiratory client.
- • If client is intubated, consider use of kinetic therapy, using a kinetic bed that slowly moves the client with 40-degree turns. **EBN:** *A study demonstrated that use of the kinetic bed versus turning patients every 2 hours resulted in decreased ventilator-associated pneumonia and atelectasis (Ahrens et al, 2004).*
- • Encourage fluid intake of up to 2500 mL/day within cardiac or renal reserve. *Fluids help minimize mucosal drying and maximize ciliary action to move secretions (Smith-Sims, 2001). Some clients cannot tolerate increased fluids because of underlying disease.*
- • Administer oxygen as ordered. *Oxygen has been shown to correct hypoxemia, which can be caused by retained respiratory secretions.*
- ▲ Administer medications such as bronchodilators or inhaled steroids as ordered. Watch for side effects such as tachycardia or anxiety with bronchodilators, or inflamed pharynx with inhaled steroids. *Bronchodilators decrease airway resistance secondary to bronchoconstriction.*
- ▲ Provide postural drainage, percussion, and vibration only as ordered. **EB:** *Chest physiotherapy has short-term effects of increasing mucous transport in the cystic fibrosis client, and insufficient evidence shows that it has long-term effects in this population (van der Schans,*

*Prasad, & Main, 2000). A Cochrane review of studies demonstrated that there is no advantage of chest physiotherapy over other airway clearance techniques for cystic fibrosis clients (Main, Prasad, & van der Schans, 2005). In most clinical trials, there is not enough evidence to support or refute the use of bronchial hygiene physical therapy in COPD or bronchiectasis clients (Jones & Rowe, 2000).*

▲ Refer for physical therapy or respiratory therapy for further treatment.

## Geriatric

- Encourage ambulation as tolerated without causing exhaustion. *Immobility is often harmful to the elderly because it decreases ventilation and increases stasis of secretions, leading to atelectasis or pneumonia (Fletcher, 2005).*
- Actively encourage the elderly to deep breathe and cough. *Cough reflexes are blunted, and coughing is decreased in the elderly (Miller, 2004).*
- Ensure adequate hydration within cardiac and renal reserves. *The elderly are prone to dehydration and therefore more viscous secretions because they frequently use diuretics or laxatives and forget to drink adequate amounts of water (Miller, 2004).*

## Home Care

- Some of the above interventions may be adapted for home care use.

▲ Begin discharge planning as soon as possible with case manager or social worker to assess need for home support systems, assistive devices, and community or home health services.

- Assess home environment for factors that exacerbate airway clearance problems (e.g., presence of allergens, lack of adequate humidity in air, poor air flow, stressful family relationships). **EBN:** *Home environmental triggers of asthma have been found to include dust/dust mites, animal dander, mold, perfumes/detergents, and cigarette smoke. Psychosocial triggers included family tensions, physical activity, anxiety/stress, and friends/peer pressure (Navaie-Waliser et al, 2004).*
- Assess affective climate within family and family support system. *Problems with respiratory function and resulting anxiety can provoke anger and frustration in the client. Feelings may be displaced onto caregiver and require intervention to ensure continued caregiver support.* Refer to care plan for **Caregiver role strain.**
- Refer to GOLD and ACP-ASIM/ACCP guidelines for management of home care and indications of hospital admission criteria (Chojnowski, 2003).
- Provide the client with emotional support in dealing with symptoms of respiratory distress. **EBN:** *Social support helped asthma sufferers fight the sense of powerlessness caused by their illness (Makinen, Suominen, & Lauri, 2000).*
- When respiratory procedures (e.g., apneic monitoring for an infant) are being implemented, explain equipment and procedures to family members, and provide needed emotional support. *Family members assuming responsibility for respiratory monitoring often find this stressful. They may not have been able to assimilate fully any instructions provided by hospital staff (McNeal, 2000).*
- When electrically based equipment for respiratory support is being implemented, evaluate home environment for electrical safety, proper grounding, and so on. Ensure that notification is sent to the local utility company, the emergency medical team, and

police and fire departments. *Notification is important to provide for priority service (McNeal, 2000).*

- Support clients' efforts at self-care. Ensure they have all the information they need to participate in care. **EBN:** *Self-care study participants showed competence at managing care of their own asthma (Makinen et al, 2000).* **EB:** *In another study of asthma clients, less self-efficacy, more depressive symptoms, expectation to be cured of asthma, having difficult access to care, and being Hispanic or African American predicted lower scores on quality-of-life questionnaires (Mancuso et al, 2001).*
- Provide family with support for care of a client with chronic or terminal illness. *Breathing difficulty can provoke extreme anxiety, which can interfere with the client's ability or willingness to adhere to the treatment plan.* Refer to care plan for **Anxiety.** *Witnessing breathing difficulties and facing concerns of dealing with chronic or terminal illness can create fear in caregiver. Fear inhibits effective coping.* **EBN:** *Parents of a child with cystic fibrosis particularly benefit from nursing support. Parents deal with devastation upon receiving the diagnosis, a sense of fear and isolation, an overwhelming sense of guilt and powerlessness, vigilance, and returning to normalcy (Carpenter & Narsavage, 2004).* Refer to care plan for **Powerlessness.**
- Instruct the client to avoid exposure to persons with upper respiratory infections.

▲ Provide/teach percussion and postural drainage per physician orders. Teach adaptive breathing techniques. *Adaptive breathing, percussion, and postural drainage loosen secretions and allow more effective oxygenation.*

- Determine client adherence to medical regimen. Instruct the client and family in importance of reporting effectiveness of current medications to physician. *Inappropriate use of medications (too much or too little) can influence amount of respiratory secretions.*
- Teach the client when and how to use inhalant or nebulizer treatments at home.
- Teach the client/family importance of maintaining regimen and having PRN drugs easily accessible at all times. *Success in avoiding emergency or institutional care may rest solely on medication compliance or availability.* **EBN:** *Parents/family have been found to have inadequate knowledge about recognition of asthma attacks, triggers, and management (Navaie-Waliser et al, 2004).*
- Teach the client/family the importance of and methods for setting priorities for activities, especially those having a high energy demand (e.g., home/family events). Instruct in realistic expectations. **EBN:** *Client and/or family may assume a higher degree of energy than is actually present. Assistance may be needed to ensure accuracy of expectations for the client. Unrealistic expectations provoke guilt feelings in the client, leading to efforts that can exceed the client's energy capacity (Patusky, 2002).*
- Instruct the client and family in the importance of maintaining proper nutrition, adequate fluids, rest, and behavioral pacing for energy conservation and rehabilitation.
- Instruct in use of dietary supplements as indicated. *Illness may suppress appetite, leading to inadequate nutrition. Pacing activities to energy capacity and rest are important to ensure the client does not overdo his or her capability. Low fluid intake can increase the thickness of respiratory secretions.*
- Identify an emergency plan, including criteria for use. *Ineffective airway clearance can be life-threatening.*

▲ Refer for home health aide services for assist with ADLs. *Clients with decreased oxy-*

*genation and copious respiratory secretions are often unable to maintain energy for ADLs.*

- ▲ Assess family for role changes and coping skills. Refer to medical social services as necessary. *Clients with decreased oxygenation are unable to maintain role activities and therefore experience frustration and anger, which may pose a threat to family integrity. Family counseling to adapt to role changes may be needed.*
- ▲ Institute case management of frail elderly to support continued independent living. *Respiratory difficulties represent and can lead to increasing needs for assistance in using the health care system effectively. Case management combines nursing activities of the client and family assessment, planning and coordination of care among all health care providers, delivery of direct nursing care, and monitoring of care and outcomes. These activities are able to address continuity of care, mutual goal setting, behavior management, and prevention of worsening health problems (Guttman, 1999).*

## Client/Family Teaching

- ▲ Teach importance of not smoking. Be aggressive in approach, ask to set a date for smoking cessation, and recommend nicotine replacement therapy (nicotine patch or gum). Refer to smoking cessation programs, and encourage clients who relapse to keep trying to quit. *All health care clinicians should be aggressive in helping smokers quit (AHCPR Guidelines, 1996).* **EB:** *A systemic review of research demonstrated that the combination of nicotine therapy and an intensive, prolonged relapse prevention program are effective in promoting long term abstinence from smoking (Wagena et al, 2004).*
- • Teach the client how to use a flutter clearance device if ordered, which vibrates to loosen mucus and gives positive pressure to keep airways open. **EB:** *This device has been shown to effectively decrease mucous viscosity and elasticity (App et al, 1998), increase amount of sputum expectorated (Bellone et al, 2000), and increase peak expiratory flow rate (Burioka et al, 1998). Daily use of the flutter device was shown to be as effective as the active cycle of breathing technique and was a preferred technique by clients (Thompson et al, 2002). A study demonstrated that use of the mucus clearance device had improved exercise performance compared with COPD clients who use a sham device (Wolkove et al, 2004).*
- ▲ Teach the client how to use peak expiratory flow rate (PEFR) meter if ordered and when to seek medical attention if PEFR reading drops. Also teach how to use metered dose inhalers and self-administer inhaled corticosteroids following precautions to decrease side effects (Owen, 1999).
- • Teach the client how to deep breathe and cough effectively. **EB:** *Controlled coughing uses the diaphragmatic muscles, making the cough more forceful and effective (Bellone et al, 2000).*
- • Teach the client/family to identify and avoid specific factors that exacerbate ineffective airway clearance, including known allergens and especially smoking (if relevant) or exposure to second-hand smoke.
- • Educate the client and family about the significance of changes in sputum characteristics, including color, character, amount, and odor. *With this knowledge, the client and family can identify early the signs of infection and seek treatment before acute illness occurs.*

A

- Teach the client/family need to take antibiotics until the prescription has run out. *Taking the entire course of antibiotics helps to eradicate bacterial infection, which decreases lingering, chronic infection.*

## evolve WEBSITES FOR EDUCATION

See the EVOLVE website for World Wide Web resources for client education.

## REFERENCES


Ackerman MH: The effect of saline lavage prior to suctioning, *Am J Crit Care* 2(4):326, 1993.

Ackerman MH, Mick DJ: Instillation of normal saline before suctioning in patients with pulmonary infections: a prospective randomized controlled trial, *Am J Crit Care* 7(4):261, 1998.

Adlkofer R, Powaser M: The effect of endotracheal suctioning on arterial blood gases in patients after cardiac surgery, *Heart Lung* 7(6):1011, 1978.

Agency for Health Care Policy and Research: *Smoking cessation, clinical practice guideline,* Washington, DC, 1996, U.S. Government Printing Office.

Ahrens T, Kollef M, Stewart J et al: Effect of kinetic therapy on pulmonary complications, *Am J Crit Care* 13(5):376, 2004.

American Dental Association: *Cleaning your teeth and gums.* Available at www.ada.org/public/faq/cleaning.html, accessed December 22, 2004.

App EM, Kieselmann R, Reinhardt D et al: Sputum rheology changes in cystic fibrosis lung disease following two different types of physiotherapy: flutter vs. autogenic drainage, *Chest* 114(1):171, 1998.

Bellone A, Lascioli R, Raschi S et al: Chest physical therapy in patients with acute exacerbation of chronic bronchitis: effectiveness of three modes, *Arch Phys Med Rehabil* 81(5):558, 2000.

Berry BE, Pinard AE: Assessing tissue oxygenation, *Crit Care Nurs* 22(3):22, 2002.

Burioka N, Sugimoto Y, Suyama H et al: Clinical efficacy of the FLUTTER device for airway mucus clearance in patients with diffuse panbronchiolitis, *Respirology* 3(3):183, 1998.

Carpenter DR, Narsavage GL: One breath at a time: living with cystic fibrosis, *J Pediatr Nurs* 19(1):25, 2004.

Chojnowski D: "GOLD" standards for acute exacerbation in COPD, *Nurs Pract* 28(5):26, 2003.

Collard HR, Saint S, Matthay MA: Prevention of ventilator-associated pneumonia: an evidenced-based systemic review, *Ann Intern Med* 138(6):494, 2003.

Day T, Farnell S, Wilson-Barnett J: Suctioning: a review of current research recommendations, *Int Crit Care Nurs* 18(2):79, 2002.

Deppe SA, Kelly JW, Thoi LL et al: Incidence of colonization, nosocomial pneumonia, and mortality in critically ill patients using a Trach Care closed-suction system: prospective, randomized study, *Crit Care Med* 18:1389, 1990.

Donahue M: "Spare the cough, spoil the airway": back to the basics in airway clearance, *Pediatr Nurs* 28(2):119, 2002.

Drakulovic MB, Torres A, Bauer TT et al: Supine body position as a risk factor for nosocomial pneumonia in mechanically ventilated patients: a randomised trial, *Lancet* 354(9193):1851, 1999.

Fink JB: Positioning versus postural drainage, *Respir Care* 47(7):769, 2002.

Fletcher K: Immobility: geriatric self-learning module, *Medsurg Nurs* 14(1):35, 2005.

Genc A, Yildirim Y, Gnerli A: Researching of the effectiveness of deep breathing and incentive spirometry in postoperative early stage, *Fizyoterapi Rehabil* 15(1), 2004.

Goodman LT, Jones M: Bronchial hygiene therapy, *Am J Nurs* 102(1):37, 2002.

Grap MJ: Protocols for practice: applying research at the bedside: pulse oximetry, *Crit Care Nurs* 22(3):69, 2002.

Grap MJ, Glass C, Corley M et al: Endotracheal suctioning: ventilator versus manual delivery of hyperoxygenation breaths, *Am J Crit Care* 5:192, 1996.

Guttman R: Case management of the frail elderly in the community, *Clin Nurs Spec* 13(4):174, 1999.

Hagler DA, Traver GA: Endotracheal saline and suction catheters: sources of lower airway contamination, *Am J Crit Care* 3(6):444, 1994.

Harshbarger SA, Hoffman LA, Zullo TG et al: Effects of a closed tracheal suction system on ventilatory and cardiovascular parameters, *Am J Crit Care* 1(3):57, 1992

Hess DR: The evidence for secretion clearance techniques. *Respir Care* 46(11):1276, 2001.

Hoyt MM: Impaired gas exchange in the elderly, *Geriatr Nurs* 13:262, 1992.

A

Johnson KL, Kearney PA, Johnson SB et al: Closed versus open endotracheal suctioning: costs and physiologic consequences, *Crit Care Med* 22(4):658, 1994.
Jones AP, Rowe BH: Bronchopulmonary hygiene physical therapy for chronic obstructive pulmonary disease and bronchiectasis, *Cochrane Database Syst Rev* (2):CD000045, 2000.
Kasper DL: *Harrison's principles of internal medicine*, 16th ed, New York, 2005, McGraw-Hill.
Kinloch D, Rock L: Instillation of normal saline during endotracheal suctioning; effects on mixed venous oxygen saturation, *Am J Crit Care* 8(4):231, 1999.
Maggiore SM, Lellouche F, Pigeot J et al: Prevention of endotracheal suctioning-induced alveolar decruitement in acute lung injury, *Am J Respir Crit Care Med* 167(9):1215, 2003.
Makinen S, Suominen T, Lauri S: Self-care in adults with asthma: how they cope, *J Clin Nurs* 9:557, 2000.
Main E, Prasad A, Schans C: Conventional chest physiotherapy compared to other airway clearance techniques for cystic fibrosis, *Cochrane Database Syst Rev*, (1):CD002011, 2005.
Mancuso CA, Rincon M, McCulloch CE et al: Self-efficacy, depressive symptoms, and patients' expectations predict outcomes in asthma, *Med Care* 39(12):1326, 2001.
Mathews PJ, Mathews LM: Reducing the risks of ventilator-associated infections, *Dimens Crit Care Nurs* 19(1):17, 2000.
McNeal GJ: *AACN guide to acute care procedures in the home,* Philadelphia, 2000, Lippincott.
Miller CA: *Nursing for wellness in older adults*, 4th ed. Philadelphia, 2004, Lippincott.
Navaie-Waliser M, Misener M, Mersman C et al: Evaluating the needs of children with asthma in home care: the vital role of nurses as caregivers and educators, *Public Health Nurs* 21(4):306, 2004.
Nielsen KG, Holte K, Kehlet H: Effects of posture on postoperative pulmonary function, *Acta Anaesthesiol Scand* 47(10):1270, 2003.
Owen CL: New directions in asthma management, *Am J Nurs* 99(3):27, 1999.
Patusky KL: Relatedness theory as a framework for the treatment of fatigued women, *Arch Psychiatr Nurs* 5:224, 2002.
Pearson LS, Hutton JL: A controlled trial to compare the ability of foam swabs and toothbrushes to remove dental plaque, *J Adv Nurs* 39(5):480, 2002
Ridling DA, Martin LD, Bratton SL: Endotracheal suctioning with or without instillation of isotonic sodium chloride solution in critically ill children, *Am J Crit Care* 12(3):212, 2003.
Smith-Sims K: Hospital-acquired pneumonia, *Am J Nurs* 101(1):24AA, 2001.
Sparrow D, Weiss S: Pulmonary system. In Rose JW, Besdine RS, editors: *Geriatric medicine,* Boston, 1988, Little, Brown.
Stiefel KA, Damron S, Sowers NJ et al: Improving oral hygiene for the seriously ill patient: implementing research-based practice, *Medsurg Nurs* 9(1):40, 2000.
Thompson CS, Harrison S, Ashley J: Randomised crossover study of the flutter device and the active cycle of breathing technique in noncystic fibrosis bronchiectasis, *Thorax* 57:446, 2002.
Van der Schans C, Prasad A, Main E: Chest physiotherapy compared to no chest physioitherapy for cystic fibrosis, *Cochrane Database Syst Rev*(2):CD001401, 2000.
Wagena EJ, van der Meer RM, Ostelo RJ et al: The efficacy of smoking cessation strategies in people with chronic obstructive pulmonary disease: results from a systematic review, *Respir Med* 98(9):805, 2004.
Wolkove N, Baltzan MA Jr, Kamel H et al: A randomized trial to evaluate the sustained efficacy of a mucus clearance device in ambulatory patients with chronic obstructive pulmonary disease, *Can Respir J* 11(8):567, 2004.

## Latex Allergy response

evolve

*Leslie H. Nicoll*

**NANDA**

### Definition

An allergic response to natural latex rubber products

• = Independent; ▲ = Collaborative; EBN = Evidence-Based Nursing; EB = Evidence-Based

## Defining Characteristics

**Type I reactions:** Immediate reactions (<1 hour) to latex proteins (can be life-threatening); contact urticaria progressing to generalized symptoms; edema of the lips, tongue, uvula, and/or throat; shortness of breath, tightness in chest, wheezing, bronchospasm leading to respiratory arrest; hypotension, syncope, cardiac arrest

**May also include:** Orofacial characteristics: edema of sclera or eyelids, erythema and/or itching of the eyes, tearing of the eyes, nasal congestion, itching and/or erythema, rhinorrhea, facial erythema, facial itching, oral itching; gastrointestinal characteristics: abdominal pain, nausea; generalized characteristics: flushing, general discomfort, generalized edema, increasing complaint of total body warmth, restlessness

**Type IV reactions:** Delayed onset (hours); eczema; irritation; reaction to additives (e.g., thiurams, carbamates) causes discomfort; redness

**Irritant Reactions:** Erythema, chapped or cracked skin, blisters

## Related Factors (r/t)

No immune mechanism response

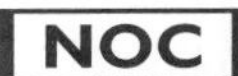

## Outcomes (Nursing Outcomes Classification)

### Suggested NOC Outcomes

Allergic Response: Localized, Systemic; Immune Hypersensitivity Response; Symptom Severity; Tissue Integrity: Skin and Mucous Membranes

**Example NOC Outcome with Indicators**

**Immune Hypersensitivity Response** as evidenced by the following indicators: Respiratory, cardiac, gastrointestinal, renal, and neurological function status IER/Free of allergic reactions (Rate each indicator of **Immune Hypersensitivity Response:** 1 = severely compromised, 2 = substantially compromised, 3 = moderately compromised, 4 = mildly compromised, 5 = not compromised N/A [see Section I].)

IER, In expected range.

## Client Outcomes

### Client Will (Specify Time Frame):

- Identify presence of natural rubber latex (NRL) allergy
- List history of risk factors
- Identify type of reaction
- State reasons not to use or to have anyone use latex products
- Experience a latex-safe environment for all healthcare procedures
- Avoid areas where there is powder from NRL gloves
- State the importance of wearing a Medic-Alert bracelet and wear one
- State the importance of carrying an emergency kit with a supply of nonlatex gloves, antihistamines, and an autoinjectable epinephrine syringe (Epi-pen), and carry one

NIC

## Interventions (Nursing Interventions Classification)

### Suggested NIC Interventions

Allergy Management; Latex Precautions

**Example NIC Activities—Latex Precautions**

Question client or appropriate other about history of systemic reaction or sensitization to NRL (e.g., facial or scleral edema, tearing eyes, urticaria, rhinitis, and wheezing); place an allergy band on client

## Nursing Interventions and Rationales

- Identify clients at risk: those persons who are most likely to exhibit a sensitivity to NRL that may result in varying degrees of reactivity. Consider the following client groups:
  - Persons with neural tube defects including spina bifida, myelomeningocele/meningocele. **EB:** *Patients with spina bifida represent the highest-risk group for developing NRL hypersensitivity.* **EB:** *Recognized risk factors for these clients are repeated surgeries and an atopic disposition (Buck et al, 2000).* **EB:** *Incidence of latex allergy in patients with spina bifida varies between 28% and 67% (Gulbahar et al, 2004).* **EB:** *Spina bifida, even in the absence of multiple surgeries, seems to be an independent risk factor for latex sensitization (Hochleitner et al, 2001).*
  - Children who have experienced three or more surgeries, particularly as a neonate. **EB:** *A significant correlation between the total number of surgeries, particularly during the first year of life, and degree of sensitization has been established (Degenhardt et al, 2001; Sparta et al, 2004).*
  - Children with chronic renal failure. **EB:** *Children with chronic renal failure are at risk because of their intense exposure to latex through catheters, gloves, and anesthetic equipment during frequent hospitalizations from early life on (Dehlink et al, 2004).*
  - Atopic individuals (persons with a tendency to have multiple allergic conditions), including allergies to food products. Particular allergies to fruits and vegetables including bananas, avocado, celery, fig, chestnut, papaya, potato, tomato, melon, and passion fruit are significant. **EB:** *Children with atopic dermatitis are a high-risk group for NRL sensitization and latex-associated foods (Taylor & Erkek, 2004).* **EB:** *Class I chitinases, related to plant defense, are the panallergens in these foods and are associated with latex-fruit syndrome (Perkin, 2000; Salcedo, Diaz-Perales, & Sanchez-Monge 2001; Sanchez-Monge, Blanco, Perales et al, 2000).*
  - Persons who possess a known or suspected NRL allergy by having exhibited an allergic or anaphylactic reaction, positive skin testing, or positive IgE antibodies against latex. **EB:** *Persons who are sensitized or have demonstrated an NRL allergy are at risk, even when a latex-free environment is adopted (Mazon et al, 2000; Taylor & Erkek, 2004).*

- Persons who have had an ongoing occupational exposure to NRL, including health care workers, rubber industry workers, bakers, laboratory personnel, food handlers, hairdressers, janitors, policemen, and firefighters. **EB:** *The predominant pattern of allergen reactivity in health care workers and others with occupational exposure is different from that among children with spina bifida; it has been suggested that occupational exposure is from NRL glove proteins inhaled through powders as opposed to particle bound latex proteins in urinary catheters (Sutherland et al, 2002; Barbara et al, 2004).* **EB:** *Ongoing exposure by health care workers has been shown to be associated with an increased risk of IgE sensitization to NRL (Galobardes et al, 2001; Weissman & Lewis, 2002).* **EB:** *Atopic persons with increasing years of occupational exposure have an increased risk of developing NRL allergy (Galobardes et al, 2001). Estimates of prevalence in health care workers range from 2% to 17% (Ahmed, Aw, & Adisesh, 2004).* **EB:** *Allergic reactions to NRL have increased during the past 10 years, especially in healthcare workers who have high exposure to latex allergens both by direct skin contact and by inhalation of latex particles from powdered gloves (Jones et al, 2004).* **EB:** *While many argue that the implementation of universal precautions is a driving factor behind the increase of latex allergy in health care workers, researchers at the University of Minnesota dispute that claim (McCall, Horwitz, & Kammeyer-Mueller, 2003).*

- Take a thorough history of the client at risk. **EB:** *A complete and thorough history remains as the most reliable screening test to predict the likelihood of an anaphylactic reaction (Hepner & Castells, 2003).* **EB:** *Skin prick tests and serum IgE are of limited value in epidemiological studies of NRL allergy; questionnaires about local symptoms are more relevant (Galobardes et al, 2001).* **EB:** *It is possible to make a diagnosis of type I NRL allergy by taking an accurate history, including questions on atopic status, food allergy, and possible reactions to latex devices (Toraason et al, 2000).*
- Question the client about associated symptoms of itching, swelling, and redness after contact with rubber products such as rubber gloves, balloons, and barrier contraceptives, or swelling of the tongue and lips after dental examinations. **EB:** *Dermatitis, itching, erythema, contact urticaria, asthma and/or rhinitis were significantly related to skin prick tests that were positive for latex (Larese Filon et al, 2001; Ylitalo et al, 2000).*
- Consider a skin prick test with NRL extracts to identify IgE-mediated immunity. **EB:** *Skin prick tests with well-characterized latex extracts are highly sensitive and specific predictors of latex-specific IgE antibodies (Ownby, 2003).*
- All latex-sensitive clients are treated as if they have NRL allergy. **EB:** *Even if a person has not experienced an NRL reaction, if it can be documented that he or she has been sensitized, then he or she should be treated as if he or she has an NRL allergy. Every hospital and scientific research facility should institute a comprehensive emergency treatment program for NRL allergic patients and workers, latex-safe areas in their facilties, and a prevention program that includes the wide use of latex-free gloves and absence of powdered gloves throughout these facilties (Edlich et al, 2003).* **EB:** *Reducing exposure to latex is a safe and more economical alternative to complete removal of the individual from the place of employment (Ranta & Ownby, 2004).*

- Patients with spina bifida and others with a positive history of NRL sensitivity or NRL allergy should have all medical/surgical/dental procedures performed in a latex-controlled environment. **EB:** *A latex-controlled environment is defined as one in which no latex gloves are used in the room or surgical suite and no latex accessories (catheters, adhesives, tourniquet, and anesthesia equipment) come in contact with the client (Joint Task Force on Practice Parameters, 1998).* **EB:** *The American Society of Anesthesiologists Task Force of Latex Sensitivity recommends that patients who are latex allergic have a surgical procedure performed as the first case in the morning, when the levels of latex aeroallergens are the smallest (Berry et al, 1999).*
- The most effective approach to preventing NRL anaphylaxis is complete latex avoidance. Medications may reduce certain symptoms. **EB:** *Safe and readily available immunotherapy for NRL allergy is currently lacking (Brehler & Kutting, 2001; Sutherland et al, 2002).* **EB:** *Prevention is the cornerstone in the management of latex sensitization (Hepner & Castells, 2003).*
- Materials and items that contain NRL must be identified, and latex-free alternatives must be found. **EB:** *A wide variety of products contain NRL: medical supplies, personal protective equipment, and numerous household objects (Hepner & Castells, 2003; National Institute for Occupational Safety and Health, 1998).* **EB:** *Effective September 1998, all medical devices must be labeled regarding their latex content (Hubbard, 1997).*
- In health care settings, general use of latex gloves having negligible allergen content, powder-free latex gloves, and nonlatex gloves and medical articles should be considered in an effort to minimize exposure to latex allergen. **EB:** *The risk of NRL allergy appears to be largely linked to occupational exposure and NRL-associated occupational asthma is due almost solely to powdered glove use. Airborne NRL is dependent on the use of powdered NRL gloves; conversion to non-NRL or nonpowdered NRL substitutes results in predictable rapid disappearance of detectable levels of aeroallergen (Charous et al, 2002).*
- ▲ If latex gloves are chosen for protection from blood or body fluids, a reduced-protein, powder-free glove should be selected. **EB:** *Until well-accepted standardized tests are available, total protein serves as a useful indicator of the exposure of concern. Protein levels below 50 mg/g are considered the least allergenic (Muller, 2003).*
- See Box III-1 for examples of products that may contain NRL and safe alternatives that are available. **EB:** *Anaphylaxis from NRL allergy is a medical emergency and must be treated as such. Latex is a potent allergen and a type I anaphylactic reaction may be immediate in sensitized individuals. Acute treatment must be carried out in a latex-free environment (Hepner & Castells, 2003).*

## Home Care

- Assess the home environment for presence of NRL products (e.g., balloons, condoms, gloves, and products of related allergies, such as bananas, avocados, and poinsettia plants). **EB:** *Latex avoidance measures in the home setting are the key to prevention (Mazon et al, 2000).*
- At onset of care, assess client history and current status of NRL allergy response. *A complete and thorough history remains as the most reliable screening test to predict*

## BOX III-1 PRODUCTS THAT MAY CONTAIN LATEX AND LATEX-FREE ALTERNATIVES USED IN HEALTH CARE SETTINGS

| Frequently Contain Latex | Latex-Free Alternative |
|---|---|
| Ace wraps | Teds, pneumatic boots |
| Airways | Hudson airways, oxygen masks |
| Ambu (bag-valve) masks (black or blue reusable) | Clear, disposable ambu-bags |
| Bandaids | Sterile dressing with plastic tape or tegaderm |
| Blood pressure cuffs | Dura-Cuf® Critikon Vital Answers or use over gown or stockinetter |
| Catheter, indwelling | Silocone foley (Kendall, Argyle, Baxter) |
| Catheter, straight | Plastic (Mentor, Bard)<br>Double, triple lumen (Bard, Rusch) |
| Chux | Disposable underpads |
| Disposable gloves, latex, non-sterile | Sensicare gloves |
| Dressings: Moleskin, Micropore, Coban (3M) | Tegaderm (3M), Steri-strips |
| Electrode pads | 3M, Baxter electrocardiogram pads<br>Dantec surface electrocardiogram pads |
| Endotracheal tubes | Mallinckrodt, Sheridan, Portex tube styletes<br>Laryngeal mask airway |
| Gloves, sterile and exam, surgical and medical | Vinyl, neoprene gloves (Neolon, Tachylon, Tru-touch, Elastryn |
| Heplock-PRN adapter | Use stopcock to inject medications |
| IV solutions and tubing systems | Baxter, Abbott, Walrus tubing<br>Walrus anesthesia sets are latex-free<br>Abbott IV fluid |
| Medication syringes | Becton Dickinson angiocaths and syringes<br>Concord Portex, Bard syringes |
| Medication vial | Remove latex stopper |
| Oral and nasal airways | Hudson airways, oxygen masks |
| OR caps with elastic (bouffant) | Caps with ties |
| Oxygen tubing | Nasal, face mask |
| Stethoscope tubing | Do not let tubing touch patient, cover with web roll |
| Suction tubing | Mallinckrodt, Yankauer, Davol suction catheters |
| Tape: cloth, adhesive, paper | Plastic, silk, 3M Microfoam Blenderm, Durapore |
| Tourniquets | Latex-free tourniquet (blue) |

Data from American Association of Nurse Anesthetists: *AANA latex protocol,* Park Ridge, Ill, 1998, The Association, pp 1-9; National Institute for Occupational Safety and Health: *Preventing allergic reactions to natural rubber latex in the workplace,* Cincinnati, July 1998, The Institute; Hepner DL, Castells MC: Latex allergy: an update, *Anesth Analg* 96(4):1219-1229, 2003.

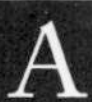

*the likelihood of an anaphylactic reaction (American Association of Nurse Anesthetists [AANA], 1998).*

- ▲ Seek medical care as necessary.
- • Do not use NRL products in caregiving.
- • Assist the client in identifying and obtaining alternatives to NRL products. **EBN:** *Preventing exposure to latex is the key to managing and preventing this allergy. Providing a safe environment for clients with NRL allergy is the responsibility of all health care professionals (AANA, 1998).* **EB:** *Avoidance management should be individualized, taking into consideration factors such as age, activity, occupation, hobbies, residential conditions, and the client's level of personal anxiety (Joint Task Force on Practice Parameters, 1998).*

## Client/Family Teaching

- • Provide written information about NRL allergy and sensitivity. **EB:** *Patient education is the most important preventive strategy. Patients should be carefully instructed about "hidden" latex, cross reactions, particularly foods, and unforeseen risks during medical procedures (Joint Task Force on Practice Parameters, 1998).*
- • Instruct the client to inform healthcare professionals if he or she has an NRL allergy, particularly if they are scheduled for surgery. **EB:** *It is essential to recognize which patients and colleagues are sensitized to latex to provide appropriate treatment and to establish adequate prevention (Hepner & Castells, 2003).*
- • Teach the client what products contain NRL and to avoid direct contact with all latex products and foods that trigger allergic reactions. **EBN:** *Once an individual becomes allergic to latex, special precautions are needed to prevent exposures. Teaching is an effective strategy (Society of Gastroenterology Nurses and Associates, Inc., 2004).*
- • See Box III-2 for examples of products found in the community that may contain NRL and safe alternatives that are available.
- • Teach the client to avoid areas where powdered latex gloves are used, as well as where latex balloons are inflated or deflated. **EB:** *Powder from gloves acts as a carrier for latex protein (Hepner & Castells, 2003).*
- • Instruct the client with NRL allergy to wear a medical identification bracelet and/or carry a medical identification card. **EB:** *Identification of the client with NRL allergy is critical for preventing problems and for early intervention with appropriate treatment if an exposure occurs (Joint Task Force on Practice Parameters, 1998; Hepner & Castells, 2003).*
- • Instruct the client to carry an emergency kit with a supply of nonlatex gloves, antihistamines, and an autoinjectable epinephrine syringe (Epi-Pen). **EB:** *An autoinjectable epinephrine syringe should be prescribed to sensitized clients who are at risk for an anaphylactic episode with accidental latex exposure (Joint Task Force on Practice Parameters, 1998; National Institute for Occupational Safety and Health, 1998; Tarlo, 1998).*

## evolve WEBSITES FOR EDUCATION

See the EVOLVE website for World Wide Web resources for client education.

**BOX III-2 LATEX PRODUCTS AND SAFE ALTERNATIVES OUTSIDE OF THE HEALTH CARE SETTING**

| Containing Latex | Latex-Free Alternative |
|---|---|
| Balloons | Mylar balloons |
| Balls, koosh ball | Vinyl, thornton sport ball |
| Belt for clothing | Leather or cloth belts |
| Beach shoes | Cotton socks |
| Bungee cords | Rope or twine |
| Cleaning/kitchen gloves | Vinyl gloves |
| Condoms | Polyurethane avanti for males<br>Polyurethane reality for femles |
| Crib mattress pads | Heavy cotton pads |
| Elastic bands | Paper clips, staples, twine |
| Elastic on legs, waist of clothing, disposable diapers, rubber pants | Velcro closures<br>Cloth diapers |
| Halloween rubber masks | Plastic mask or water based paints |
| Pacifiers | Plastic pacifier "The First Years"<br>Silicone: Pur, Gerber, Soft-Flex |
| Raquet handles | Leather handles |
| Raincoats/slickers | Nylon or synthetic waterproof coats |
| Swim fins | Clear plastic fins |
| Telephone cords | Clear cords |

Data from American Association of Nurse Anesthetists: *AANA latex protocol,* Park Ridge, Ill, 1998, The Association, pp 1-9; National Institute for Occupational Safety and Health: *Preventing allergic reactions to natural rubber latex in the workplace,* Cincinnati, July 1998, The Institute; Hepner DL, Castells MC: Latex allergy: an update, *Anesth Analg* 96(4):1219-1229, 2003.

## REFERENCES

Ahmed SM, Aw TC, Adisesh A: Toxicological and immunological aspects of occupational latex allergy, *Toxicol Rev*, 23(2):123-134, 2004.

American Association of Nurse Anesthetists: *AANA latex protocol,* Park Ridge, Ill, 1998, The Association.

Barbara J, Santais MC, Levy DA et al: Inhaled cornstarch glove powder increases latex-induced airway hyper-sensitivity in guinea pigs, *Clin Exp Allergy* 34(6):978-983, 2004.

Berry AJ, Katz JD, Brown RH et al: *Natural rubber latex allergy: considerations for anesthesiologists*, Park Ridge, Ill, 1999, American Society of Anesthesiologists, 1-34.

Brehler R, Kutting B: Natural rubber latex allergy: a problem of interdisciplinary concern in medicine, *Arch Intern Med* 161(8): 1057-1064, 2001.

Buck D, Michael T, Wahn U et al: Ventricular shunts and the prevalence of sensitization and clinically relevant allergy to latex in patients with spina bifida, *Pediatr Allergy Immunol* 11(2):111-115, 2000.

Charous BL, Blanco C, Tarlo S et al: Natural rubber latex allergy after 12 years: recommendations and perspectives, *J Allergy Clin Immunol* 109(1):31-34, 2002.

Degenhardt P, Golla S, Wahn F et al: Latex allergy in pediatric surgery is dependent on repeated operations in the first year of life, *J Pediatr Surg* 36(10):1535-1539, 2001.

Dehlink E, Prandstetter C, Eiwegger T et al: Increased prevalence of latex-sensitization among children with chronic renal failure, *Allergy* 59(7):734-738, 2004.

A

Edlich RF, Woodard CR, Hill LG et al: Latex allergy: a life-threatening epidemic for scientists, healthcare personnel, and their patients, *J Long Term Eff Med Implants* 13(1):11-19, 2003.

Galobardes B, Quiliquini AM, Roux N et al: Influence of occupational exposure to latex on the prevalence of sensitization and allergy to latex in a Swiss hospital, *Dermatology* 203(3):226-232, 2001.

Gulbahar O, Demir F, Mete N et al: Latex allergy and associated risk factors in a group of Turkish patients with spina bifida, *Turk J Pediatr* 46(3):226-231, 2004.

Hepner DL, Castells MC: Latex allergy: an update, *Anesth Analg* 96(4):1219-1229, 2003.

Hochleitner BW, Menardi G, Haussler B et al: Spina bifida as an independent risk factor for sensitization to latex, *J Urol* 166(6): 2370-2373, 2001.

Hubbard WK: Department of Health and Human Services. Food and Drug Administration: natural rubber-containing medical devices–user labeling, *Federal Register* 62:189, 1997.

Joint Task Force on Practice Parameters; American Academy of Allergy, Asthma and Immunology; American College of Allergy, Asthma and Immunology; and the Joint Council of Allergy, Asthma and Immunology: The diagnosis and management of anaphylaxis, *J Allergy Clin Immunol* 101(6 Pt 2):S465, 1998.

Jones KP, Rolf S, Stingl C et al: Longitudinal study of sensitization to natural rubber latex among dental school students using powder-free gloves, *Ann Occup Hyg* 48(5):455-457, 2004.

Larese Filon F, Bosco A, Fiorito A et al: Latex symptoms and sensitisation in healthcare workers, *Int Arch Occup Environ Health* 74(3):219-223, 2001.

Mazon A, Nieto A, Linana JJ et al: Latex sensitization in children with spina bifida: follow-up comparative study after two years, *Ann Allergy Asthma Immunol* 84(2):207, 2000.

McCall BP, Horwitz IB, Kammeyer-Mueller JD: Have health conditions associated with latex increased since the issuance of universal precautions? *Am J Public Health* 93(4):599-604, 2003.

Muller BA: Minimizing latex exposure and allergy: how to avoid or reduce sensitization in the healthcare setting, *Postgrad Med* 113(4):91-96, 2003.

National Institute for Occupational Safety and Health: *Preventing allergic reactions to natural rubber latex in the workplace,* Cincinnati, 1998, The Institute.

Ownby DR: Strategies for distinguishing asymptomatic latex sensitization from true occupational allergy or asthma, *Ann Allergy Asthma Immunol* 90(5 Suppl 2):42-46, 2003.

Perkin JE: The latex and food allergy connection, *J Am Diet Assoc* 100(11):1381-1384, 2000.

Ranta PM, Ownby DR: A review of natural-rubber latex allergy in healthcare workers, *Clin Infect Dis* 38(2):252-256, 2004.

Salcedo G, Diaz-Perales A, Sanchez-Monge R: The role of plant panallergens in sensitization to natural rubber latex, *Curr Opin Allergy Clin Immunol* 1(2):177-183, 2001.

Sanchez-Monge R, Blanco C, Perales AD et al: Class I chitinases, the panallergens responsible for the latex-fruit syndrome, are induced by ethylene treatment and inactivated by heating, *J Allergy Clin Immunol* 106(1 Pt 1):190-195, 2000.

Society for Gastroenterology Nurses and Associates, Inc: SGNA guidelines for preventing sensitivity and allergic reactions to natural rubber latex in the workplace, *Gastroenterol Nurs* 27(4):191-197, 2004.

Sparta G, Kemper MJ, Gerber AC et al: Latex allergy in children with urological malformation and chronic renal failure, *J Urol* 171(4):1647-1649, 2004.

Sutherland MF, Suphioglu C, Rolland JM et al: Latex allergy: towards immunotherapy for healthcare workers, *Clin Exp Allergy* 32(5):667-673, 2002.

Tarlo SM: Latex allergy: a problem for both healthcare professionals and patients, *Ostomy Wound Manage* 44(8):80-88, 1998.

Taylor JS, Erkek E: Latex allergy: diagnosis and management, *Dermatol Ther* 17(4):289-301, 2004.

Toraason M, Sussman G, Biagini R et al: Latex allergy in the workplace, *Toxicol Sci* 58(1):5-14, 2000.

Weissman DN, Lewis DM: Allergic and latex-specific sensitization: route, frequency, and amount of exposure that are required to initiate IgE production, *J Allergy Clin Immunol* 110(2 suppl):S57-S63, 2002.

Ylitalo L, Alenius H, Turjanmaa K et al: Natural rubber latex allergy in children: a follow-up study, *Clin Exp Allergy* 30(11):1611-1617, 2000.

# Risk for latex Allergy response

evolve

*Leslie H. Nicoll*

## NANDA

### Definition

At risk for allergic response to natural latex rubber products

### Risk Factors

Multiple surgical procedures, especially from infancy (e.g., spina bifida); allergies to bananas, avocados, tropical fruits, kiwi, chestnuts; professions with daily exposure to latex (e.g., medicine, nursing, dentistry); conditions associated with continuous or intermittent catheterization; history of reactions to latex (e.g., balloons, condoms, gloves); allergies to poinsettia plants; history of allergies and asthma

## NOC

### Outcomes (Nursing Outcomes Classification)

#### Suggested NOC Outcomes

Allergic Response: Systemic, Immune Hypersensitivity Response, Knowledge: Health Behavior, Risk Control, Risk Detection, Tissue Integrity, Skin and Mucous Membranes

**Example NOC Outcome with Indicators**

**Immune Hypersensitivity Response** as evidenced by the following indicators: Respiratory, cardiac, gastrointestinal, renal and neurological function status IER/Free of allergic reactions (Rate each indicator of **Immune Hypersensitivity Response:** 1 = severely compromised, 2 = substantially compromised, 3 = moderately compromised, 4 = mildly compromised, 5 = not compromised N/A [see Section I].)

IER, In expected range.

### Client Outcomes

**Client Will (Specify Time Frame):**

- State risk factors for NRL allergy
- Request latex-free environment
- Demonstrate knowledge of plan to treat NRL allergic reaction

## NIC

### Interventions (Nursing Interventions Classification)

#### Suggested NIC Interventions

Allergy Management; Latex Precautions

A

**Example NIC Activities—Latex Precautions**

Question client or appropriate other about history of systemic reaction to NRL (e.g., facial or scleral edema, tearing eyes, urticaria, rhinitis, and wheezing); place an allergy band on client

## Nursing Interventions and Rationales

- Clients at high risk need to be identified, such as those with frequent bladder catheterizations, occupational exposure to latex, past history of atopy (e.g., hay fever, asthma, dermatitis, or food allergy to fruits such as bananas, avocados, papaya, chestnut, or kiwi fruit); those with a history of anaphylaxis of uncertain etiology, especially if associated with surgery; health care workers; and females exposed to barrier contraceptives and routine examinations during gynecological and obstetric procedures. **EB:** *Latex allergy is an increasingly common condition because the use of latex products is widespread (Eustachio et al, 2003).* **EB:** *Health care professionals, hospital patients, and rubber industry workers have noted a marked increase in allergic reactions to NRL in the past 10 years (Ranta & Ownby, 2004).* **EB:** *Recent studies have shown that allergy to NRL is significantly associated with hypersensitivity to certain foods, including avocados, chestnuts, papayas, kiwis, potatoes, tomatoes, and bananas (Isola et al, 2003).* **EBN:** *A latex-directed history is the primary method of identifying latex sensitivity, although both skin and serum testing are available and are increasingly accurate (American Association of Nurse Anesthetists, 1998; Hepner & Castells, 2003; Society of Gastroenterology Nurses and Associates, Inc., 2004).*
- Clients with spina bifida are a high-risk group for NRL allergy and should remain latex free from the first day of life. **EB:** *Spina bifida, even in the absence of multiple surgical procedures, seems to be an independent risk factor for latex sensitization (Hochleitner et al, 2001).* **EB:** *Clients with spina bifida represent the highest risk group for developing NRL hypersensitivity. Recognized risk factors for these clients are repeated surgeries and an atopic disposition (Buck et al, 2000).* **EB:** *Latex-free precautions from birth in children with spina bifida are more effective in preventing latex sensitization than the same precautions instituted in later life (Nieto et al, 2002).*
- Children who are on home ventilation should be assessed for NRL allergy. **EB:** *This study showed a high incidence of NRL allergy in children on home ventilation. All children on home ventilation should be screened for NRL allergy to prevent untoward reactions from exposure to latex (Nakamura et al, 2000).*
- Children with chronic renal failure should be assessed for NRL allergy. **EB:** *This study demonstrated a high incidence of NRL in children with chronic renal failure. Children with chronic renal failure are at risk because of their intense exposure to latex through catheters, gloves, and anesthetic equipment during frequent hospitalizations from early life on (Dehlink et al, 2004).*
- Assess for NRL allergy in clients who are exposed to "hidden" latex. **EB:** *Case studies have reported on serious complications in clients exposed to latex through hair glue (Cogen & Beezhold, 2002) and microdermabrasion (Farris & Rietschel, 2002).*
- See care plan for **Latex Allergy response**.

### Home Care

- ▲ Ensure that the client has a medical plan if a response develops. Prompt treatment decreases potential severity of response.
- • See care plan for **Latex Allergy response**. NOTE: client history and environmental assessment.

## Client/Family Teaching

- ▲ A client who has had symptoms of NRL allergy or who suspects he or she is allergic to latex should tell his or her employer and contact his or her institution's occupational health services. **EB:** *Occupational health services can arrange testing by an allergist. If an allergy is present, measures to protect the client's well-being in the workplace should be instituted (National Institute for Occupational Safety and Health, 1998).*
- • Provide written information about latex allergy and sensitivity. **EB:** *Patient education is the most important preventive strategy. Patients should be carefully instructed about "hidden" latex; cross reactions, particularly foods; and unforeseen risks during medical procedures (Joint Task Force on Practice Parameters, 1998).*
- • Health care workers should avoid the use of latex gloves and seek alternatives such as gloves made from nitrile. **EB:** *The risk of NRL allergy appears to be largely linked to occupational exposure and NRL-associated occupational asthma is due almost solely to powdered glove use. Airborne NRL is dependent on the use of powdered NRL gloves; conversion to non-NRL or nonpowdered NRL substitutes results in predictable rapid disappearance of detectable levels of aeroallergen (Brown et al, 2004; Charous et al, 2002).* **EB:** *Preliminary reports of primary preventive strategies suggest that avoidance of high-protein, powdered gloves in health care facilities can be cost-effective and is associated with a decline in sensitized workers (Tarlo et al, 2001).* **EB:** *A case study report of two nurses indicated worsening symptoms when they worked in an environment with powdered gloves, even though they avoided direct skin contact with latex (Amr & Suk, 2004).* **EBN:** *Nitrile examination gloves offer better protection than latex types when handling lipid-soluble substances and chemicals (Russell-Fell, 2000).*
- • Health care institutions should develop prevention programs for the use of latex-free gloves and the absence of powdered gloves; they should also establish latex-safe areas in their facilities. **EB:** *Latex allergy has become a global epidemic, affecting patients, health care workers, and scientific personnel (Edlich et al, 2003).*

## REFERENCES


American Association of Nurse Anesthetists: *AANA latex protocol,* Park Ridge, Ill, 1998, The Association.

Amr S, Suk WA: Latex allergy and occupational asthma in healthcare workers: adverse outcomes, *Environ Health Perspect* 112(3):378-381, 2004.

Brown RH, Taenkhum K, Buckley TJ et al: Different latex aeroallergen size distributions between powdered surgical and examination gloves: significance for environmental avoidance, *J Allergy Clin Immunol* 114(2):358-363, 2004.

Buck D, Michael T, Wahn U et al: Ventricular shunts and the prevalence of sensitization and clinically relevant allergy to latex in patients with spina bifida, *Pediatr Allergy Immunol* 11(2):111-115, 2000.

Charous BL, Blanco C, Tarlo S et al: Natural rubber latex allergy after 12 years: recommendations and perspectives, *J Allergy Clin Immunol* 109(1):31-34, 2002.

Cogen FC, Beezhold DH: Hair glue anaphylaxis: a hidden latex allergy, *Ann Allergy Asthma Immunol* 88(1):61-63, 2002.

A

Dehlink E, Prandstetter C, Eiwegger T et al: Increased prevalence of latex-sensitization among children with chronic renal failure, *Allergy* 59(7):734-738, 2004.
Eustachio N, Cristina CM, Antonio F et al: A discussion of natural rubber latex allergy with special reference to children: clinical considerations, *Curr Drug Targets Immune Endocr Metabol Disord* 3(3):171-180, 2003.
Farris PK, Rietschel RL: An unusual acute urticarial response following microdermabrasion, *Dermatol Surg* 28(7):606-608, 2002.
Hepner DL, Castells MC: Latex allergy: An update, *Anesth Analg* 96(4):1219-1229, 2003.
Hochleitner BW, Menardi G, Haussler B et al: Spina bifida as an independent risk factor for sensitization to latex, *J Urol* 166(6): 2370-2373, 2001.
Isola S, Ricciardi L, Saitta S et al: Latex allergy and fruit cross-reaction in subjects who are nonatopic, *Allergy Asthma Proc* 24(3): 193-197, 2003.
Joint Task Force on Practice Parameters; American Academy of Allergy, Asthma and Immunology; American College of Allergy, Asthma and Immunology; and the Joint Council of Allergy, Asthma and Immunology: The diagnosis and management of anaphylaxis, *J Allergy Clin Immunol* 101(6 Pt 2):S465, 1998.
Nakamura CT, Ferdman RM, Keens TG et al: Latex allergy in children on home mechanical ventilation, *Chest* 118(4):1000-1003, 2000.
National Institute for Occupational Safety and Health: *Preventing allergic reactions to natural rubber latex in the workplace,* Cincinnati, 1998, The Institute.
Nieto A, Mazon A, Pamies R et al: Efficacy of latex avoidance for primary prevention of latex sensitization in children with spina bifida, *J Pediatr* 140(3):370-372, 2002.
Perkin JE: The latex and food allergy connection, *J Am Diet Assoc* 100(11):1381-1384, 2000.
Russell-Fell R: Avoiding problems: evidence-based selection of medical gloves, *Br J Nurs* 9(3):139-142, 144-146, 2000.
Ranta PM, Ownby DR: A review of natural-rubber latex allergy in healthcare workers, *Clin Infect Dis* 38(2):252-256, 2004.
Salcedo G, Diaz-Perales A, Sanchez-Monge R: The role of plant panallergens in sensitization to natural rubber latex, *Curr Opin Allergy Clin Immunol* 1(2):177-183, 2001.
Sanchez-Monge R, Blanco C, Perales AD et al: Class I chitinases, the panallergens responsible for the latex-fruit syndrome, are induced by ethylene treatment and inactivated by heating, *J Allergy Clin Immunol* 106(1 Pt 1):190-195, 2000.
Society for Gastroenterology Nurses and Associates, Inc: SGNA guidelines for preventing sensitivity and allergic reactions to natural rubber latex in the workplace, *Gastroenterol Nurs* 27(4):191-197, 2004.
Tarlo SM, Easty A, Eubanks K et al: Outcomes of a natural rubber latex control program in an Ontario teaching hospital, *J Allergy Clin Immunol* 108(4):628-633, 2001.

# Anxiety

evolve

*Teresa Howell*

**NANDA**

## Definition

A vague, uneasy feeling of discomfort or dread accompanied by an autonomic response, with the source often nonspecific or unknown to the individual; a feeling of apprehension caused by anticipation of danger. Anxiety is an alerting signal that warns of impending danger and enables the individual to take measures to deal with threat

## Defining Characteristics

### Behavioral

Diminished productivity; scanning and vigilance; poor eye contact; restlessness; glancing about; extraneous movement (e.g., foot shuffling, hand/arm movements); expressed concerns due to change in life events; insomnia; fidgeting

### Affective

Regretful, irritability, anguish, scared, jittery, overexcited, increased helplessness, rattled, uncertainty, increased wariness, focus on self, feelings of inadequacy, fearful, distressed, worried or apprehensive, anxious

### Physiological

Voice quivering; trembling/hand tremors; shakiness; increased respiration (sympathetic); urinary urgency (parasympathetic); increased pulse (sympathetic); pupil dilation (sympathetic); increased reflexes (sympathetic); abdominal pain (parasympathetic); sleep disturbance (parasympathetic); tingling in extremities (parasympathetic); cardiovascular excitation (sympathetic); increased perspiration; facial tension; anorexia (sympathetic); heart pounding (sympathetic); diarrhea (parasympathetic); urinary hesitancy (parasympathetic); fatigue (parasympathetic); dry mouth (sympathetic); weakness (sympathetic); decreased pulse (parasympathetic); facial flushing (sympathetic); superficial vasoconstriction (sympathetic); twitching (sympathetic); decreased blood pressure (parasympathetic); nausea (parasympathetic); urinary frequency (parasympathetic); faintness (parasympathetic); respiratory difficulties (sympathetic); increased blood pressure (sympathetic)

### Cognitive

Blocking of thought, confusion; preoccupation, forgetfulness, rumination, impaired attention, decreased perceptual field, fear of unspecified consequences, tendency to blame others, difficulty concentrating, diminished ability to problem solve and/or learn, awareness of physiologic symptoms

## Related Factors (r/t)

Exposure to toxins; unconscious conflict about essential values/goals of life; familial association/heredity; unmet needs; interpersonal transmission/contagion; situational/maturational crises; threat of death; threat to self-concept; stress; substance abuse; threat to or change in role status, health status, interaction patterns, role function, environment, and/or economic status

**NOC**

## Outcomes (Nursing Outcomes Classification)

### Suggested NOC Outcomes

Aggression Self-Control, Anxiety Level, Anxiety Self-Control, Coping, Impulse Self-Control

**Example NOC Outcome with Indicators**

**Anxiety Self-Control** as evidenced by the following indicators: Eliminates precursors of anxiety/Monitors physical manifestations of anxiety/Controls anxiety response (Rate each indicator of **Anxiety Self-Control:** 1 = never demonstrated, 2 = rarely demonstrated, 3 = sometimes demonstrated, 4 = often demonstrated, 5 = consistently demonstrated [see Section I].)

A

## Client Outcomes

**Client Will (Specify Time Frame):**

- Identify and verbalize symptoms of anxiety
- Identify, verbalize, and demonstrate techniques to control anxiety
- Verbalize absence of or decrease in subjective distress
- Have vital signs that reflect baseline or decreased sympathetic stimulation
- Have posture, facial expressions, gestures, and activity levels that reflect decreased distress
- Demonstrate improved concentration and accuracy of thoughts
- Identify and verbalize anxiety precipitants, conflicts, and threats
- Demonstrate return of basic problem-solving skills
- Demonstrate increased external focus
- Demonstrate some ability to reassure self

NIC

## Interventions (Nursing Interventions Classification)

### Suggested NIC Intervention

Anxiety Reduction

| Example NIC Activities—Anxiety Reduction |
|---|
| Use calm, reassuring approach; explain all procedures, including sensations likely to be experienced |

## Nursing Interventions and Rationales

- Assess the client's level of anxiety and physical reactions to anxiety (e.g., tachycardia, tachypnea, nonverbal expressions of anxiety). Use the Sheehan Patient-Rated Anxiety Scale (SPRAS). Validate observations by asking the client, "Are you feeling anxious now?" Consider the use of a "faces scale" to assess anxiety in critically ill clients. **EBN:** *Anxiety is known to intensify physical symptoms (Schreier & Davis, 2004).* **EBN:** *SPRAS was more effective in detecting asthmatics likely to be suffering from coexisting anxiety disorders (Davis et al, 2002).* **EBN:** *The Faces Anxiety Scale has minimal subject burden and elicits self-report from intensive care patients more often than do other simple scales (McKinley, 2003).* **EBN:** *In adolescents anxiety symptoms were correlated with physical complaints and depression (Puskar et al, 2003).* **EBN:** *Jong et al (2004) demonstrated in a study of heart failure and myocardial infarction clients that elevated heart rate and blood pressure did not accurately reflect the levels of anxiety reported.*
- If the situational response is rational, use empathy to encourage the client to interpret the anxiety symptoms as normal. **EBN:** *The way a nurse interacts with a client influences his/her quality of life. Enhancing self-esteem and providing information and psychological support promotes the client's well-being and his or her quality of life (Di Giulio, 2001).*
- If irrational thoughts or fears are present, offer the client accurate information and en-

courage him or her to talk about the meaning of the events contributing to the anxiety. **EBN:** *During the diagnosis and management of cancer, highlighting the importance of the meaning of events to an individual is an important factor in helping clients to identify what makes them anxious. Acknowledgment of this meaning may help to reduce anxiety (Stark & House, 2000).*

- Encourage the client to use positive self-talk such as, "Anxiety won't kill me," "I can do this one step at a time," "Right now I need to breathe and stretch," "I don't have to be perfect." **EBN:** *Cognitive therapies focus on changing behaviors and feelings by changing thoughts. Replacing negative self-statements with positive self-statements helps to decrease anxiety (Fishel, 1998).*
- Intervene when possible to remove sources of anxiety. *Anxiety is a normal response to actual or perceived danger; if the threat is removed, the response will stop.* **EBN:** *Anxiety has a negative effect on quality of life that persists over time (Scheirer & Williams, 2004).* **EBN:** *One study on children's posthospital adjustment suggests that mothers who know what behavior changes to expect in their children experienced less anxiety and participated more in their children's care during hospitalization (Melnyk & Feinstein, 2001).*
- Explain all activities, procedures, and issues that involve the client; use nonmedical terms and calm, slow speech. Do this in advance of procedures when possible, and validate the client's understanding. *With preadmission client education, clients experience less anxiety and emotional distress and have increased coping skills because they know what to expect (Review, 2000).*
- Ascertain client preferences about the desire to be distracted before and during noxious medical procedures. **EBN:** *Clients have individual preferences for the use of distraction during anxiety-provoking procedures (Kwekkeboom, 2003).*
- Explore coping skills previously used by client to relieve anxiety; reinforce these skills and explore other outlets. *Methods of coping with anxiety that have been successful in the past are likely to be helpful again.* **EBN:** *Listening to clients and helping them to sort through their fears and expectations encourages them to take charge of their lives (Fishel, 1998).*
- Provide backrubs/massage for the client to decrease anxiety. **EBN:** *Massage significantly decreased anxiety or perception of tension (Richards et al, 2000).*
- Use therapeutic touch and healing touch techniques. **EBN:** *Various techniques that involve intention to heal, laying on of hands, clearing the energy field surrounding the body, and transfer of healing energy from the environment through the healer to the subject can reduce anxiety (Fishel, 1998).* **EBN:** *Anxiety was significantly reduced in a therapeutic touch placebo condition. Healing touch may be one of the most useful nursing interventions available to reduce anxiety (Gagne & Toye, 1998).*
- Guided imagery can be used to decrease anxiety. **EBN:** *Anxiety was decreased with the use of guided imagery using audio tape intervention for post operative pain (Antall & Kresevic, 2004).*
- Provide clients with a means to listen to music of their choice or audiotapes. Provide a quiet place and encourage clients to listen for 20 minutes. **EBN:** *Immediately and 1 hour after listening to music for 20 minutes in a quiet environment, reductions in heart rate, respiratory rate, and myocardial oxygen demand were significantly greater in the experi-*

*mental group of clients with myocardial infarction (MI) than in the control group (White, 1999).* **EBN:** *Music therapy has the potential to reduce physiological signs of anxiety (heart rate and blood pressure) and the need for sedation among individuals undergoing colonoscopy (Smolen et al, 2002).* **EB:** *Researchers have documented that music listening reduces anxiety and pain (Lukas, 2004).* **EBN:** *In one study of chemotherapy patients by Williams & Schreirer (2004), patients who used audiotapes had lower anxiety than a control group.*

- Animal-assisted therapy (AAT) can be incorporated into the care of perioperative clients. **EBN:** *A study of perioperative clients has shown that interaction with animals reduces blood pressure and cholesterol, decreases anxiety, and improves a person's sense of well-being (Miller & Ingram, 2000).*
- Rule out withdrawal from alcohol, sedatives, or smoking as the cause of anxiety. **EB:** *One third of respondents in this study with an alcohol use disorder (abuse or dependence) were three times more likely to have an anxiety disorder (Burns & Teeson, 2002).*
- Identify and limit, discontinue, or be aware of the use of any stimulants such as caffeine, nicotine, theophylline, terbutaline sulfate, amphetamines, and cocaine. *Many substances cause or potentially cause anxiety symptoms.*

## Geriatric

- ▲ Monitor the client for depression. Use appropriate interventions and referrals. **EB:** *Anxiety often accompanies or masks depression in elderly adults. Patients who have depression and anxiety, are socially isolated or severely ill should be asked whether they've been thinking about ending their life or wanting to die (Bartels, 2002).* **EB:** *Anxiety and depression are associated with overall health status, emotional and cognitive functioning, and fatigue (Smith et al, 2003).*
- Provide a protective and safe environment. Use consistent caregivers and maintain the accustomed environmental structure. *Elderly clients tend to have more perceptual impairments and adapt to changes with more difficulty than younger clients, especially during illness (Halm & Alpen, 1993).*
- Observe for adverse changes if antianxiety drugs are taken. *Age renders clients more sensitive to both the clinical and toxic effects of many agents.*
- Provide a quiet environment with diversion. *Excessive noise increases anxiety; involvement in a quiet activity can be soothing to the elderly.*

## Multicultural

- Assess for the presence of culture-bound anxiety states. **EBN:** *The context in which anxiety is experienced, its meaning, and responses to it are culturally mediated. The following culture-bound syndromes are related to anxiety: Susto—Latin America; Nervios—Latin America; Dhat—Asia; Koro—Southeast Asia; Kayak angst—Eskimo; Taijin kyousho—Japan; Nervous breakdown or bad nerves—African Americans (Charron, 1998; Kavanagh, 1999; APA, 2000).*
- Assess for the influence of cultural beliefs, norms, and values on the client's perspective of a stressful situation. **EBN:** *What the client considers stressful may be based on cultural perceptions (Cochran, 1998; Doswell & Erlen, 1998; Leininger & McFarland, 2002).*
- *Identify how anxiety is manifested in the culturally diverse client.* **EBN:** *Anxiety is mani-*

*fested differently from culture to culture through cognitive to somatic symptoms (Charron, 1998).*

- Acknowledge that value conflicts from acculturation stresses may contribute to increased anxiety. **EBN:** *Challenges to traditional beliefs and values are anxiety provoking (Charron, 1998; Youn et al, 1999).*
- Acknowledge that socioeconomic factors may contribute to increased stress and anxiety. **EB:** *Job and marital instability, female-headed households, unstable finances, and housing issues create additional sources of stress (Lewis & Bernstein, 1996; Taylor, Jason, & Jahn, 2003).*
- For the diverse client experiencing preoperative anxiety, provide music of their choice. **EBN:** *Music intervention was found to have cross-cultural validity in the reduction of preoperative anxiety in Chinese male clients (Yung et al, 2002).*

## Home Care

- Above interventions may be adapted for home care use.
- Approach the client's anxiety in nonjudgmental fashion. *The inability of others to perceive the source of the client's anxiety does not make it any less distressing for the client.*
- Assist family to be supportive of the client in the face of anxiety symptoms. **EBN:** *Social support, self-esteem, and optimism were all positively related to positive health practices, and social support was positively related to self-esteem and optimism (McNicholas, 2002).*
- Adapt treatment needs to specific anxiety type. *Changes in usual approach may be needed to achieve same objective; for example, limiting physician visits and accompanying the client may be necessary if the client is agoraphobic.*
- Assess for influence of anxiety on medical regimen. *Anxiety may be a reaction to medical disorders, producing attentional fatigue, and may influence the ability to carry out the medical regimen.* **EBN:** *Preoperative anxiety was found to be a significant issue in women newly diagnosed with breast cancer. Higher anxiety drains attentional resources, and may result in attentional fatigue (Lehto & Cimprich, 1999). The ability to direct attention is necessary for self-care and independence, and was reduced for a several months after surgery in older women newly diagnosed with breast cancer (Cimprich & Ronis, 2001; Stark & Cimprich, 2003).*
- Assess for presence of depression. *Depression and anxiety co-occur frequently.*

▲ Consider referral for the prescription of antianxiety or antidepressant medications for clients who have panic disorder (PD) or other anxiety-related psychiatric disorders. **EBN:** *PD may be treated with drugs, psychosocial intervention, or both. In a recent study, the combination of imipramine and cognitive-behavioral therapy appeared to offer limited advantage in the short term but more substantial advantage by the end of maintenance (Barlow et al, 2000). In a study of older adults, anxiety was associated with increased disability and decreased well-being; although the use of health services was increased, appropriate care was often not received (de Beurs et al, 1999).*

▲ Assist the client/family to institute medication regimen appropriately. Instruct in side effects, importance of taking medications as ordered, and effects to report immediately to nurse or physician. *Antianxiety and antidepressant medications have side effects that may prompt the client to discontinue use, sometimes with additional uncomfortable effects. Some medications may be used to overdose. Antidepressant medications can take up to several weeks for full effect, and the client may discontinue use prematurely if there is little effect or if the medication is effective and the client considers it no longer necessary.*

- ▲ Assess for suicidal ideation. Implement emergency plan as indicated. *Suicidal ideation may occur in response to co-occurring depression or a sense of hopelessness over severe anxiety symptoms or once antidepressant medications have been started.* Refer to care plan for **Risk of Suicide**.
- ▲ Encourage use of appropriate community resources: family, friends, neighbors, self-help and support groups, volunteer agencies, churches, clubs and centers for recreation, and other persons with similar interests. *One of the most reassuring elements of care includes access to the family (Fishel, 1998). Vicarious experience provided through dyadic support is effective in helping clients undergoing cardiac surgery to cope with surgical anxiety and in improving self-efficacy expectations and self-reported activity after surgery (Parent & Fortin, 2000).*
- ▲ Refer for psychiatric home health care services for client reassurance and implementation of a therapeutic regimen. **EBN:** *Psychiatric home care nurses can address issues relating to the client's anxiety, including agoraphobia, with or without coexisting depression. Behavioral interventions in the home can assist the client to participate more effectively in the treatment plan (Patusky et al, 1996).*

## Client/Family Teaching

- Teach the client/family the symptoms of anxiety. **EBN:** *Information is empowering and reduces anxiety (Fishel, 1998).*
- Help client to define anxiety levels (from "easily tolerated" to "intolerable") and select appropriate interventions. **EBN:** *Mild anxiety enhances learning and adaptation, but moderate to severe anxiety may impede or immobilize progress (Peplau, 1963).*
- Teach the client techniques to self-manage anxiety. **EBN:** *Teaching patients anxiety reduction techniques can help them manage side effects with self care behaviors (Blanchard et al, 2001).*
- Teach progressive muscle relaxation techniques. **EBN:** *A significant reduction in anxiety level was obtained by using progressive muscle relaxation interventions (Weber, 1996).*
- Teach relaxation breathing for occasional use: client should breathe in through nose, fill slowly from abdomen upward while thinking "re," and then breathe out through mouth, from chest downward, and think "lax." **EBN:** *Anxiety management training effectively treats both specific and generalized anxiety (Fishel, 1998).*
- Teach the client to visualize or fantasize about the absence of anxiety or pain, successful experience of the situation, resolution of conflict, or outcome of procedure. **EBN:** *Use of guided imagery has been useful for reducing anxiety (Weber, 1996).*
- Teach relationship between a healthy physical and emotional lifestyle and a realistic mental attitude. *Health and well-being are influenced by how well-defined and well-met needs are in areas of safety, diet, exercise, sleep, work, pleasure, and social belonging.* **EBN:** *Exercise is an excellent means of decreasing anxiety (Fishel, 1998).* **EB:** *Aerobic exercise training has antidepressant and anxiolytic effects and protects against harmful consequences of stress (Salmon, 2001).*

A

- ▲ Teach use of appropriate community resources in emergency situations (e.g., suicidal thoughts), such as hotlines, emergency departments, law enforcement, and judicial systems. **EB:** *The method of suicide prevention found to be most effective is a systematic, direct-screening procedure that has a high potential for institutionalization (Shaffer & Craft, 1999).*
- ▲ Provide family members with information to help them to distinguish between a panic attack and serious physical illness symptoms. Instruct family members to consult a health care professional if they have questions. **EBN:** *Education on managing anxiety disorders must include family members because they are the ones usually called on to take the client for emergency care. Family members can be expert informants because of their familiarity with the client's history and symptoms (Fishel, 1998).*

## evolve WEBSITES FOR EDUCATION

See the EVOLVE website for World Wide Web resources for client education.

## REFERENCES


American Psychiatric Association: *Diagnostic and statistical manual of mental disorders,* ed 4-TR, Washington DC, 2000, The Association.

Antall GF, Kresevic D: The use of guided imagery to manage pain in an elderly orthopaedic population, *Orthop Nurs* 23(5):335-340, 2004.

Barlow DH Gorman JM, Shear MK et al: Cognitive-behavioral therapy, imipramine, or their combination for panic disorder: a randomized controlled trial, *JAMA* 283(19):2529-2536, 2000.

Bartels SJ: Patients with depression and anxiety might be contemplating suicide, *Geriatrics* 57:8, 2002.

Beck AT, Emery G: *Anxiety disorders and phobias: a cognitive perspective,* New York, 1985, Basic Books.

Blanchard CM, Courneya KS, Laing D: Effects of acute exercise on state anxiety in breast cancer survivors, *Oncol Nurs Forum* 28(10):1617-1621, 2001.

Burns L, Teeson M: Alcohol use disorders comorbid with anxiety, depression and drug use disorders: findings from the Australian National Survey of Mental Health and Well Being, *Drug Alcohol Depend* 68(3):299, 2002.

Charron HS: Anxiety disorders. In Varcarolis EM, editor: *Foundations of psychiatric mental health nursing,* ed 3, Philadelphia, 1998, WB Saunders.

Cimprich B, Ronis DL: Attention and symptom distress in women with and without breast cancer, *Nurs Res* 50(2):86, 2001.

Cochran M: Tears have no color, *Am J Nurs* 98(6):53, 1998.

Damrosch S: General strategies for motivating people to change their behavior, *Nurs Clin North Am* 26:833, 1991.

Davis TMA, Rocc CJM, MacDonald GF: Screening and assessing adult asthmatics for anxiety disorders, *Clin Nurs Res* 11(2):173, 2002.

De Beurs E et al: Consequences of anxiety in older persons: its effect on disability, well-being and use of health services, *Psychol Med* 29:583, 1999.

Di Giuli P: Cancer care: the unique contribution of nursing, *Int Nurs Perspect* 1(1):39, 2001.

Doswell W, Erlen J: Multicultural issues and ethical concerns in the delivery of revising care interventions, *Nurs Clin North Am* 33(2):353, 1998.

Fishel A: Nursing management of anxiety and panic, *Nurs Clin North Am* 33(1):135, 1998.

Gagne D, Toye FC: Nursing management of anxiety and panic, *Nurs Clin North Am* 33(1):135, 1998.

Halm MA, Alpen MA: The impact of technology on patients and families, *Nurs Clin North Am* 28:443, 1993.

Jong DE, Moser DK, An K et al: Anxiety is not manifested by elevated heart rate and blood pressure in acutely ill cardiac patients, *Eur J Cardiovasc Nurs* 3(3):248-53, 2004.

Kavanagh KH: The role of cultural diversity in mental health nursing. In Fontaine KL, Fletcher JS, editors: *Mental health nursing,* ed 4, Menlo Park, Calif, 1999, Addison-Wesley.

Kwekkeboom KL: Music versus distraction for procedural pain and anxiety in patients with cancer, *Oncol Nurs Forum* 30(3):433-440, 2003.

A

Lehto RH, Cimprich B: Anxiety and directed attention in women awaiting breast cancer surgery, *Oncol Nurs Forum* 26(4):767, 1999.
Leininger MM, McFarland MR: *Transcultural nursing: concepts, theories, research and practices,* ed 3, New York, 2002, McGraw-Hill.
Lewis JA, Bernstein J: *Women's health: a relational perspective across the life cycle,* Sudbury, Mass, 1996, Jones and Bartlett.
Lukas L: Orthopedic outpatients' perception of perioperative music listening as therapy, *J Theory Construction Testing* (8)1:7-12, 2004.
McKinley S: Development and testing of a Faces Scale for the assessment of anxiety in critically ill patients, *J Adv Nurs* 41(1):73, 2003.
McNicholas SL: Social support and positive health practices, *West J Nurs Res* 24(7):772, 2002.
Melnyk BM, Feinstein NF: Mediating functions of maternal anxiety and participation in care on young children's posthospital adjustment, *Res Nurs Health* 24:18, 2000.
Miller J, Ingram L: Perioperative nursing and animal-assisted therapy, *AORN J* 72(3):477, 2000.
Parent N, Fortin F: A randomized, controlled trial of vicarious experience through peer support for male first-time cardiac surgery patients: impact on anxiety, self-efficacy expectation, and self-reported activity, *Heart Lung* 29(6):389, 2000.
Patusky KL, Rodning C, Martinez-Kratz M: Clinical lessons in psychiatric home care: a case study approach, *J Home Health Case Manage* 9:18, 1996.
Peplau H: A working definition of anxiety. In Burd S, Marshall M, editors: *Some clinical approaches to psychiatric nursing,* New York, 1963, Macmillan.
Puskar KR, Sereika SM, Haller LL: Anxiety, somatic complaints, and depressive symptoms in rural adolescents, *J Child Adolesc Psychiatr Nurs* 16(3):102-111, 2003.
Review: A practical guide to improving patient outcomes, *Orthop Nurs* 19(suppl):22, 2000.
Richards KC, Gibson R, Overton-McCoy AL: Effects of massage in acute and critical care, *AACN Clin Issues* 11(1):77, 2000.
Salmon P: Effects of physical exercise on anxiety, depression, and sensitivity to stress: a unifying theory, *Clin Psychol Rev* 21(1):33, 2001.
Schreier AM, Williams SA: Anxiety and quality of life of women who receive radiation or chemotherapy for breast cancer, *Oncol Nurs Forum* 31(1):127-130, 2004.
Shaffer D, Craft L: Methods of adolescent suicide prevention, *J Clin Psychiatry* 60(suppl 2):70, 1999; discussion 60(suppl 2):75, 113, 1999.
Smith EM, Gomm SA, Dickens, CM: Assessing the independent contribution to quality of life from anxiety and depression in patients with advanced cancer, *Palliat Med* 17(6):509-13, 2003.
Smolen D, Topp R, Singer L: The effect of self-selected music during colonoscopy on anxiety, heart rate, and blood pressure, *Appl Nurs Res* 15(3):126, 2002.
Stark DP, House A: Anxiety in cancer patients, *Br J Cancer* 83(10):1261, 2000.
Stark MA, Cimprich B: Promoting attentional health: importance to women's lives, *Health Care Women Int* 24(2):93-102, 2003.
Taylor RR, Jason LA, Jahn SC: Chronic fatigue and sociodemographic characteristics as predictors of psychiatric disorders in a community-based sample, *Psychosom Med* 65(5):896-901, 2003.
Weber S: The effects of relaxation exercises on anxiety levels in psychiatric inpatients, *J Holist Nurs* 4(3):196, 1996.
White J: Effects of relaxing music on cardiac autonomic balance and anxiety after acute myocardial infarction, *Am J Crit Care* 8(4): 220, 1999.
Williams SA, Schreier AM: The effects of education in managing side effects in women receiving chemotherapy for management of breast cancer, *Oncol Nurs Forum* 31(1):E16-24, 2004.
Youn G, Knight BG, Jeong HS et al: Differences in familism values and caregiving outcomes among Korean, Korean American, and White American dementia caregivers, *Psychol Aging* 14(3):355-364, 1999.
Yung PMB, Chui-Kam S, French P et al: A controlled trial of music and pre-operative anxiety in Chinese men undergoing transurethral resection of the prostate, *J Adv Nurs* 39(4):352-359, 2002.

# Death Anxiety

*Teresa Howell*

## NANDA

### Definition

The apprehensions, worry, or fear related to death or dying

### Defining Characteristics

Worrying about impact of one's own death on significant others, powerless over issues related to dying, fear of loss of physical and/or mental abilities when dying, anticipated pain related to dying, deep sadness, fear of dying process, concerns of overworking caregiver as terminal illness incapacitates self, concern about meeting one's creator or feeling doubtful about existence of God or higher being, total loss of control over any aspect of one's own death, negative death images or unpleasant thoughts about any event related to death or dying, fear of delayed demise, fear of premature death because it prevents accomplishment of important life goals, worrying about being the cause of others' grief and suffering, fear of leaving family alone after death, fear of developing a terminal illness, denial of one's own mortality or impending death

### Related Factors (r/t)

To be developed—see Defining Characteristics

## NOC

### Outcomes (Nursing Outcomes Classification)

#### Suggested NOC Outcomes

Dignified Life Closure; Fear Self-Control; Health Beliefs: Perceived Threat

**Example NOC Outcome with Indicators**

**Dignified Life Closure** as evidenced by the following indicators: Expresses readiness for death/Resolves important issues and concerns/Shares feelings about dying/Discusses spiritual concerns (Rate each indicator of **Dignified Life Closure:** 1 = never demonstrated, 2 = rarely demonstrated, 3 = sometimes demonstrated, 4 = often demonstrated, 5 = consistently demonstrated [see Section I].)

### Client Outcomes

**Client Will (Specify Time Frame):**

- State concerns about impact of death on others
- Express feelings associated with dying
- Seek help in dealing with feelings

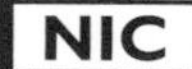

- Discuss concerns about God or higher being
- Discuss realistic goals
- Use prayer or other religious practice for comfort

NIC

## Interventions (Nursing Interventions Classification)

### Suggested NIC Interventions

Dying Care, Grief Work Facilitation, Spiritual Support

**Example NIC Activities—Dying Care**

Communicate willingness to discuss death; support client and family through stages of grief

## Nursing Interventions and Rationales

- Assess the psychosocial maturity of the individual. Erikson's scale of task accomplishment may be used. **EB:** *A study using the framework of Erikson indicates that the higher the ego integrity, the lower is the death anxiety (Fishman, 1992). As psychosocial maturity and age increase, death anxiety decreases. Findings have shown that psychosocial maturity is a better predictor of death anxiety than is age (Rasmussen & Brems, 1996).*
- Assist clients to identify with their culture and its values. **EB:** *The process of identification with one's culture is identified as a coping mechanism that may protect the individual from increased death anxiety (Tomer & Eliason, 1996).*
- Assess clients for pain and provide pain relief measures. **EBN:** *Barriers to optimal care of the dying, according to family members contacted by phone interview, include level of pain and management of pain (Tolle et al, 2000).*
- Assess client for fears related to death. **EBN:** *Acknowledging and responding to these fears is the core of end-of-life palliative care (Tarzian, 2000).*
- Assist clients with life planning: consider and redefine main life goals, focus on areas of strength and/or goals that will provide satisfaction, adopt realistic goals and recognize those that are impossible to achieve. **EB:** *Life planning processes affect self-esteem and self-concept. By changing unrealistic goals, the individual may be able to reduce the amount of future-related regret that the prospect of a not-too-distant death may produce (Tomer & Eliason, 1996).* **EB:** *Increased levels of death anxiety may block future thoughts (Martz & Livneh, 2003).*
- Assist clients with life review and reminiscence. **EB:** *Life reviewing can foster the integration of past conflicts. It can improve ego integrity and life satisfaction, lower depression, and reduce stress (Tomer & Eliason, 1996).*
- Provide music of a client's choosing. **EBN:** *Music therapy is a nonpharmacological nursing intervention that may be used to promote relaxation (Chlan, 2000).* **EB:** *Music may be beneficial in easing emotional, physical, and spiritual distress as death approaches (Hogan, 2003).*
- Provide social support for families receiving cardiopulmonary resuscitation (CPR) training to save the life of a family member at risk for sudden death. **EB:** *Findings sup-*

*port tailoring family CPR training so that instruction does not result in negative psychological states in clients. The findings also illustrate the efficacy of a simple intervention that combines CPR training with social support (Dracup et al, 1997).*

- Encourage clients to pray. **EBN:** *Participants in one study stated their belief that God listened to their prayers and answered them when they were seeking comfort. It was this reassurance that gave them the strength to face uncertainty and possible death (Hawley & Irurita, 1998).* **EBN:** *In one study, prayer, scripture reading, and clergy visits were found to comfort some hospice patients but sometimes specific religious tenets may be troubling and need to be resolved before the client can find peace (Forbes & Rosdahl, 2003).*

## Geriatric

- Carefully assess older adults for issues regarding death anxiety. **EB:** *Lower ego integrity, more physical problems, and more psychological problems are predictive of higher levels of death anxiety in the elderly (Fortner & Neimeyer, 1999).* **EBN:** *Elders differ in their readiness for death. Some still have goals that they want to reach. These goals may not always be realistic (Burgess, 1997).* **EB:** *Old age raises questions for many adults, such as whether we face a painful death, what happens after death, and if our lives had meaning (DePayola et al, 2003).*
- Provide back massage for clients who have anxiety regarding issues such as death. **EBN:** *Massage significantly decreased anxiety or perception of tension (Richards et al, 2000).*
- Refer to care plan for **Anticipatory Grieving.**

## Multicultural

- Refer to care plans for **Anxiety** and **Anticipatory Grieving.**

## Home Care

- Above interventions may be adapted for home care.
- Identify times and places when anxiety is greatest. Provide for psychological support at those times, using such strategies as personal contact, telephone contact, diversionary activities, or therapeutic self. *Anxiety may be related to earlier events associated with home setting or daily patterns that created pain and now serve as triggers.*
- Support religious beliefs; encourage client to participate in services and activities of choice. *Belief in a supreme being/higher power provides a feeling of ever-present help.*

▲ Refer to medical social services or mental health services, including support groups as appropriate (e.g., anticipatory grieving groups from hospice, visiting volunteers of hospice). *Referral to specialty groups may be a key part of the nursing plan.*

- Encourage the client to verbalize feelings to family/caregivers, counselors, and self. *Expression of feelings relieves fear burden and allows examination and validation of feelings.*
- Identify client's preferences for end of life care; provide assistance in honoring preferences as much as practicable. **EB:** *A review of issues with malignant mesothelioma found that many such clients expressed the preference of dying at home, but were often hospitalized in the days prior to death without returning home (Hawley & Monk, 2004).*
- Assist the client in making contact with death-related planning organizations, if ap-

propriate, such as the Cremation Society and funeral homes. *Planning and direct action (contracting for afterdeath care) often relieve anxiety and provide the client with a measure of control.*

- With client, create a memento book reflecting life achievements. Leave in the home for regular review by client. If family will be the recipient, a memento book serves as both an opportunity for life review and a means of proactively leaving something behind for survivors. *It gives client a sense of focus, decreasing feelings of powerlessness over death.* Refer to care plan for **Powerlessness.**
- With client/caregivers, establish realistic life goals for anticipated life span of self or others. Create manageable, tangible steps that client can refer to and use to measure activity. *Memento books and written life goals are tangible milestones related to life and death. They provide comfort, reassurance, hope, and direction for the client and more definition for client/caregiver expectations.*
- ▲ Refer for psychiatric home health care services for client reassurance and implementation of a therapeutic regimen. Psychiatric home care nurses can address issues relating to client's death anxiety, including family relationships. *Behavioral interventions in the home can assist client to participate more effectively in the treatment plan (Patusky et al, 1996).*

## Client/Family Teaching

- Promote more effective communication to family members engaged in the caregiving role. Encourage them to talk to their loved one about areas of concern. *One study investigated both the content and avoidance of communication between 84 spousal and filial caregivers and care receivers. The study findings indicate that both caregivers and care receivers avoid discussing issues of concern. Nurses working with families are well placed to promote more effective communication (Edwards & Forster, 1999).* **EBN:** *A study by Tarzian (2000) indicates that increasing the knowledge of and access to palliative care decreases suffering before death.*
- Allow family members to be physically close to their dying loved one, giving them permission, instruction, and opportunities to touch. Keep family members informed. **EBN:** *Tertiary care centers are criticized for not providing a peaceful death experience. A qualitative study was undertaken to ascertain suggestions of family members (N = 29) (Pierce, 1999). The suggestions mentioned came out of this study.* **EBN:** *One study relayed the importance of preparing clients and family members for what to expect during the dying process, including the possibility of the client developing air hunger (Tarzian, 2000).*
- To increase clients' knowledge about end-of-life issues, teach them and their family members about options for care, such as advance directives. **EB:** *A survey of 1000 clients suggests that greater public knowledge about end-of-life care is needed, and advance care planning must be preceded by education about options (Silveira et al, 2000).*

## evolve WEBSITES FOR EDUCATION

See the EVOLVE website for World Wide Web resources for client education.

## REFERENCES


Burgess AW: *Psychiatric nursing: promoting mental health,* Stamford, Conn, 1997, Appleton and Lange.

Chlan LL: Music therapy as a nursing intervention for patients supported by mechanical ventilation, *AACN Clin Issues* 11(1):128, 2000.

DePaola SJ, Griffen M, Yound JR et al: Death anxiety and attitudes toward the elderly among older adults: the role of gender and ethnicity, *Death Stud* 27(4):335-354, 2003.

Dracup K, Moser DK, Taylor SE et al: The psychological consequences of cardiopulmonary resuscitation training for family members of patients at risk for sudden death, *Am J Public Health* 87(9):1434-1439, 1997.

Edwards H, Forster E: Avoidance of issues in family care giving, *Contemp Nurse* 8(2):5, 1999.

Fishman S: Relationships among an older adult's life review, ego integrity, and death anxiety, *Int Psychogeriatr* 4(suppl 2):267, 1992.

Forbes MA, Rosdahl DR: The final journey of life, *J Hospice Palliative Nurs* 5(4):213-220, 2003.

Fortner BV, Neimeyer RA: Death anxiety in older adults: a quantitative review, *Death Stud* 23(5):387, 1999.

Hawley G, Irurita V: Seeking comfort through prayer, *Int J Nurs Pract* 4(1):9, 1998.

Hawley R, Monk A: Malignant mesothelioma: current practice and research directions, *Collegian* 11(2):22, 2004.

Hogan, BE: Soul music in the twilight years: music therapy and the dying process, *Top Geriatr Rehabil* 19(4), 275-281, 2003.

Martz E, Livneh H: Death anxiety as a predictor of future time orientation among individuals with spinal cord injuries, *Disabil Rehabil* 25(18):1024-1032, 2003.

Patusky KL, Rodning C, Martinez-Kratz M: Clinical lessons in psychiatric home care: a case study approach, *J Home Health Case Manage* 9:18, 1996.

Pierce SF: Improving end-of-life care: gathering suggestions from family members, *Nurs Forum* 34(2):5, 1999.

Rasmussen CA, Brems C: The relationship of death anxiety with age and psychosocial maturity, *J Psychol* 130(2):141, 1996.

Richards KC, Gibson R, Overton-McCoy AL: Effects of massage in acute and critical care, *AACN Clin Issues* 11(1):77, 2000.

Silveira MJ DiPiero A, Gerrity MS et al: Patients' knowledge of options at the end of life: ignorance in the face of death, *JAMA* 284(19):2483-2488, 2000.

Tarzian AJ: Caring for dying patients who have air hunger, *J Nurs Scholarship* 32(2):137, 2000.

Tolle SW, Tiblen VP, Rosenfeld AG et al: Family reports of barriers to optimal care of the dying, *Nurs Res* 49(6):310, 2000.

Tomer A, Eliason G: Toward a comprehensive model of death anxiety, *Death Stud* 20:343, 1996.


# Risk for Aspiration

evolve

*Betty J. Ackley*

**NANDA**

### Definition

At risk for entry of gastrointestinal secretions, oropharyngeal secretions, solids, or fluids into the tracheobronchial passages

### Risk Factors

Increased intragastric pressure; tube feedings; situations hindering elevation of upper body; reduced level of consciousness; presence of tracheostomy or endotracheal tube; medication administration; wired jaws; increased gastric residual; incomplete lower esophageal sphincter; impaired swallowing; gastrointestinal tubes; facial, oral, or neck surgery or trauma; depressed cough and gag reflexes; decreased gastrointestinal motility; delayed gastric emptying

# NOC

## Outcomes (Nursing Outcomes Classification)

### Suggested NOC Outcomes

Aspiration Prevention, Respiratory Status: Ventilation, Swallowing Status

**Example NOC Outcome with Indicators**

**Respiratory Status: Ventilation** as evidenced by the following indicators: Respiratory rate IER/Moves sputum out of airway/Adventitious breath sounds not present/SOB not present/Auscultated breath sounds IER/ Auscultated vocalization IER/Chest x-ray findings IER (Rate each indicator of **Respiratory Status: Ventilation:** 1 = severely compromised, 2 = substantially compromised, 3 = moderately compromised, 4 = mildly compromised, 5 = not compromised [see Section I].)

IER, In expected range; SOB, shortness of breath.

## Client Outcomes

### Client Will (Specify Time Frame):

- Swallow and digest oral, nasogastric, or gastric feeding without aspiration
- Maintain patent airway and clear lung sounds

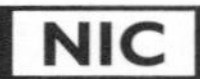

# NIC

## Interventions (Nursing Interventions Classification)

### Suggested NIC Intervention

Aspiration Precautions

**Example NIC Activities—Aspiration Precautions**

Monitor level of consciousness, cough reflex, gag reflex, and swallowing ability; check nasogastric or gastrostomy residual before feeding

## Nursing Interventions and Rationales

- Monitor respiratory rate, depth, and effort. Note any signs of aspiration such as dyspnea, cough, cyanosis, wheezing, or fever. *Signs of aspiration should be detected as soon as possible to prevent further aspiration and to initiate treatment that can be lifesaving. Because of laryngeal pooling and residue in clients with dysphagia, silent aspiration (i.e., not manifested by choking or coughing) may occur (Smith & Connolly, 2003; Smeltzer & Bare, 2004).*
- Auscultate lung sounds frequently and before and after feedings; note any new onset of crackles or wheezing. **EB:** *Bronchial auscultation of lung sounds was shown to be specific in identifying clients at risk for aspirating (Shaw et al, 2004).*
- Take vital signs frequently, noting onset of a temperature.

- Before initiating oral feeding, check client's gag reflex and ability to swallow by feeling the laryngeal prominence as the client attempts to swallow. *It is important to check client's ability to swallow before feeding. A client can aspirate even with an intact gag reflex (Smith & Connolly, 2003).*
- When feeding client, watch for signs of impaired swallowing or aspiration, including coughing, choking, spitting food, or excessive drooling. If client is having problems swallowing, see Nursing Interventions for **Impaired Swallowing**.
- Have suction machine available when feeding high-risk clients. If aspiration does occur, suction immediately. *A client with aspiration needs immediate suctioning and may need further lifesaving interventions such as intubation.*
- Keep head of bed elevated when feeding and for at least an hour afterward. *Maintaining a sitting position after meals can help decrease aspiration pneumonia in the elderly.* **EB:** *A study demonstrated that the number of clients developing a fever was significantly reduced when kept sitting upright after eating (Matsui et al, 2002).*

▲ Note presence of any nausea, vomiting, or diarrhea. Treat nausea promptly with antiemetics.

- Listen to bowel sounds frequently, noting if they are decreased, absent, or hyperactive. *Decreased or absent bowel sounds can indicate an ileus with possible vomiting and aspiration; increased high-pitched bowel sounds can indicate mechanical bowel obstruction with possible vomiting and aspiration (Kasper et al, 2005).*
- Note new onset of abdominal distention or increased rigidity of abdomen. *Abdominal distention or rigidity can be associated with paralytic or mechanical obstruction and an increased likelihood of vomiting and aspiration (Kasper et al, 2005).*

▲ If client has a tracheostomy, ask for referral to speech pathologist for swallowing studies before attempting to feed. After evaluation, decision should be made to have cuff either inflated or deflated when client eats. **EBN and EB:** *The presence of a tracheostomy tube increases the incidence of aspiration (Elpern et al, 1993). One study demonstrated that clients who had aspiration following a tracheostomy had aspiration before the tracheostomy, and if the client did not aspirate before the tracheostomy, they also did not aspirate after the tracheostomy procedure was done (Leder & Ross, 2000) For some clients, inflating the cuff may help decrease aspiration; for others, the inflated cuff will interfere with swallowing. This decision should be made following swallowing studies for the safety of the client's airway (Murray & Brzozowski, 1998).*

- If client shows symptoms of nausea and vomiting, position on side.
- If client needs to be fed, feed slowly and allow adequate time for chewing and swallowing. Position upright during and after feedings.

## Enteral Feedings

- Insert nasogastric feeding tube using the internal nares to distallower esophageal-sphincter distance. **EBN:** *A study demonstrated that this method was more accurate in predicting the correct distance than a traditional method, and another method based on research (Ellet et al, 2005).*

▲ Check to make sure initial nasogastric feeding tube placement was confirmed by x-ray, especially if a small-bore feeding tube is used. If unable to use x-ray for verification, check the pH of the aspirate. If pH reading is 4 or less, the tube is probably in the stomach. Also check bilirubin level of aspirate if possible. *X-ray verification of placement remains the gold standard for determining safe placement of feeding tubes (Metheny et al, 1998).* **EBN:** *Small-bore feeding tubes have been inadvertently placed in the respiratory tract, and clients did not demonstrate any signs of respiratory distress (Metheny et al, 1990a). Use of pH and bilirubin measurement has been found to be predictive of correct placement of feeding tubes, both gastric and intestinal. Bilirubin testing is done using urinary bilirubin test strip and a developed visual bilirubin scale (Metheny et al, 2000).*

- Keep nasogastric tube securely taped. Use pink tape to secure the tube. **EBN:** *Use of pink tape as opposed to clear tape or butterfly tape increases the length of time a tube stays taped (Burns et al, 1995).*
- Determine placement of feeding tube before each feeding or every 4 hours if client is on continuous feeding. Check pH of aspirate and note characteristic appearance of aspirate; do not rely on air insufflation method. **EBN:** *The auscultatory air insufflation method is often not reliable for differentiating between gastric or respiratory placement (Metheny et al, 1990b). Testing the pH generally predicts feeding tube position in the gastrointestinal tract, especially if combined with identification of appearance of aspirate (Metheny et al, 1994, 1998).*
- Check for gastric residual during continuous feedings or before feedings; if residual is greater than 400 mL, hold feedings following institutional protocol. *Monitoring gastric residual as evidence of intolerance to tube feedings has not been supported by research. The practice reduces the amount of calories given to the client If the client has an alteration in level of consciousness, or has gastrointestinal dysfunction, hold feedings for smaller amounts of gastric residual (Keithley & Swanson, 2004; Metheny, Schallom, & Edwards, 2004).* **EBN:** *A study of the effectiveness of either returning gastric residual volumes to the client, or discarding it resulted in inconclusive findings with complications when either action was taken, more research is needed in the area (Booker et al, 2000).*
- Test for the presence of glucose in tracheobronchial secretions or the presence of pepsin to detect aspiration of enteral feedings. Recognize that the glucose test may not be accurate if there is blood in the aspirate or if a low glucose feeding is being used (St. John, 2000). **EBN:** *Tracheobronchial secretions that test positive for glucose can indicate aspiration of enteral feedings (Metheny et al, 1998). The detection of pepsin in tracheal secretions is considered an indicator of aspiration of gastric contents, a flat position is strongly associated with the presence of pepsin in secretions (Metheny et al, 2002).*
- Do not use blue dye to tint enteral feedings. *The presence of blue and green skin and urine and serum discoloration has been associated with the death of two clients; the use of blue dye in feedings should be stopped (Maloney et al, 2002; Lucarelli et al, 2004). This technique is not reliable and use of a multiple-use bottle may result in contamination of feedings and spread bacteria (Fellows et al, 2000).*
- During enteral feedings, position client with head of bed elevated 30 to 40 degrees; maintain for 30 to 45 minutes after feeding. *Evidence confirms that a semirecumbant position can help reduce aspiration of tube feeding formula (Keithley & Swanson, 2004).* **EBN and EB:** *A study of mechanically ventilated clients receiving tube feedings demonstrated there was an increase of the presence of pepsin (from gastric contents) in pulmonary secretions if the client was in a flat position versus being positioned with head elevated*

*(Metheny et al, 2000). A study of mechanically ventilated clients receiving enteral feedings demonstrated a decreased incidence of nosocomial pneumonia if the client was positioned at a 45-degree semirecumbent position as opposed to a supine position (Drakulovic et al, 1999).*

- Use a closed versus an open enteral delivery system of tube feeding if possible. **EB:** *A study demonstrated that the closed delivery system did not result in contamination of the feeding, use of the open bags resulted in several tube feeding formulas becoming contaminated (Vanek, 2000).*
- Stop continual feeding temporarily when turning or moving client. *When turning or moving a client, it is difficult to keep the head elevated to prevent regurgitation and possible aspiration.*

## Geriatric

- Carefully check elderly client's gag reflex and ability to swallow before feeding. *Laryngeal nerve endings are reduced in the elderly, which diminishes the gag reflex (Miller, 2004).*
- Watch for signs of aspiration pneumonia in the elderly with cerebrovascular accidents, even if there are no apparent signs of difficulty swallowing or of aspiration. *Bedside evaluation for swallowing and aspiration can be inaccurate; silent aspiration can occur in this population (Smith & Connolly, 2003).*

▲ Use central nervous system depressants cautiously; elderly clients may have an increased incidence of aspiration with altered levels of consciousness. *Elderly clients have altered metabolism, distribution, and excretion of drugs. Some medications can interfere with the swallowing reflex (Miller, 2004).*

- Keep the elderly, mostly bedridden client sitting upright for 2 hours following meals. **EB:** *A study demonstrated that the number of clients developing a fever was significantly reduced when kept sitting upright after eating (Matsui et al, 2002).*
- Recommend to families that tube feedings not be used for clients with dementia, instead use increased feeding assistance, modified food consistency as needed, or environmental alterations. **EBN:** *Research has demonstrated that tube feedings in this population do not prevent malnutrition or aspiration, improve survival or reduce infections, instead there is an increased risk for aspiration pneumonia (Keithley & Swanson, 2004).*

## Home Care

- Above interventions may be adapted for home care use.
- For clients at high risk for aspiration, obtain complete information from the discharging institution regarding institutional management. *Continuity of care can prevent unnecessary stress for the client and family and can facilitate successful management in the home setting.*
- Assess the client and family for willingness and cognitive ability to learn and cope with swallowing, feeding, and related disorders. *Food and feeding habits may be strongly tied to family cultural values. Acknowledgment and/or adjustment to cultural values can facilitate compliance and successful family coping.*
- Assess caregiver understanding and reinforce teaching regarding positioning and assessment of the client for possible aspiration. *Caregiver is in the position to prevent and respond to aspiration difficulties.*

- Provide the client with emotional support in dealing with fears of aspiration. *Fear of choking can provoke extreme anxiety, which can interfere with the client's ability or willingness to adhere to the treatment plan.* Refer to care plan for **Anxiety.**
- Establish emergency and contingency plans for care of client. *Clinical safety of client between visits is a primary goal of home care nursing.*
- ▲ Have a speech and occupational therapist assess client's swallowing ability and other physiological factors and recommend strategies for working with client in the home (e.g., pureeing foods served to client; providing adaptive equipment for independence in eating). *Successful strategies allow the client to remain part of the family.*
- Obtain suction equipment for the home as necessary.
- Teach caregivers safe, effective use of suctioning devices. Inform client and family that only individuals instructed in suctioning should perform the procedure.
- ▲ Institute case management of frail elderly to support continued independent living. *Swallowing difficulties represent and can lead to increasing needs for assistance in using the health care system effectively. Case management combines nursing activities of client and family assessment, planning and coordination of care among all health care providers, delivery of direct nursing care, and monitoring of care and outcomes. These activities are able to address continuity of care, mutual goal setting, behavior management, and prevention of worsening health problems (Guttman, 1999).*

## Client/Family Teaching

- Teach the client and family signs of aspiration and precautions to prevent aspiration.
- Teach the client and family how to safely administer tube feeding.

## evolve WEBSITES FOR EDUCATION

See the EVOLVE website for World Wide Web resources for client education.

## REFERENCES


Booker KJ, Niedringhaus L, Eden B: Comparison of 2 methods of managing gastric residual volumes from feeding tubes, *Am J Crit Care* 9(5):318, 2000.

Burns SM, Martin M, Robbins V et al: Comparison of nasogastric tube securing methods and tube types in medical intensive care patients, *Am J Crit Care* 4:198, 1995.

Drakulovic MB, Torres A, Bauer TT et al: Supine body position as a risk factor for nosocomial pneumonia in mechanically ventilated patients: a randomised trial, *Lancet* 354(9193):1851, 1999.

Ellett ML, Beckstrand J, Flueckiger J et al: Predicting the insertion distance for placing gastric tubes, *Clin Nurs Res* 14(1):11, 2005.

Elpern EH, Jacobs ER, Bone RC: Incidence of aspiration in tracheally intubated adults, *Heart Lung* 16:527, 1993.

Fellows LS, Miller EH, Frederickson M et al: Evidence-based practice for enteral feedings: aspiration prevention strategies, bedside detection, and practice change, *Medsurg Nurs* 9(1):27, 2000.

Guttman R: Case management of the frail elderly in the community, *Clin Nurs Spec* 13(4):174, 1999.

Kasper DL, Braunwald E, Fauci AS et al: Harrison's principles of *internal medicine,* ed 16, New York, McGraw-Hill, 2005.

Keithley JK, Swanson B: Enteral nutrition: an update on practice recommendations, *Medsurg Nurs* 13(2):131, 2004.

Leder SB, Ross DA: Investigation of the causal relationship between tracheostomy and aspiration in the acute care setting, *Laryngoscope* 100(4):641, 2000.

Lucarelli MR, Shirk MB, Julian MW et al: Toxicity of Food Drug and Cosmetic Blue No. 1 dye in critically ill patients, *Chest* 125(2):793, 2004.

Maloney JP, Ryan TA, Brasel KJ et al: Food dye use in enteral feedings: a review and a call for a moratorium, *Nutr Clin Pract* 17(3):169, 2002.

Matsui T, Yamaya M, Ohrui T et al: Sitting position to prevent aspiration in bed-bound patients, *Gerontology* 48(3):194, 2002.
Metheny NA, Smith L, Stewart BJ: Development of a reliable and valid bedside test for bilirubin and its utility for improving prediction of feeding tube location, *Nurs Res* 49(6):302, 2000.
Metheny NA, St John RE, Clouse RE: Measurement of glucose in tracheobronchial secretions to detect aspiration of enteral feedings, *Heart Lung* 27(5):285, 1998.
Metheny N, Dettenmeier P, Hampton K et al: Detection of inadvertent respiratory placement of small-bore feeding tubes: a report of 10 cases, *Heart Lung* 19(6):631, 1990a.
Metheny N, McSweeney M, Wehrle MA et al: Effectiveness of the auscultatory method in predicting feeding tube location, *Nurs Res* 39(5):262, 1990b.
Metheny N, Reed L, Wiersema L et al: Effectiveness of pH measurements in predicting feeding tube placement: an update, *Nurs Res* 42(6):324, 1993.
Metheny N, Reed L, Berglund B et al: Visual characteristics of aspirates from feeding tubes as a method for predicting tube location, *Nurs Res* 43(5):282, 1994.
Metheny NA, Smith L, Wehrle MA et al: pH, color and feeding tubes, *RN* 1(1):25, 1998.
Metheny NA, Chang YH, Ye JS et al: Pepsin as a marker for pulmonary aspiration, *Am J Crit Care* 11(2):150, 2002.
Metheny NA, Schallom ME, Edwards SJ: Effect of gastrointestinal motility and feeding tube site on aspiration risk in critically ill patients: a review, *Heart Lung* 33(3):131, 2004.
Miller CA: *Nursing for wellness in older adults*, ed 4, Philadelphia, 2004, Lippincott.
Murray KA, Brzozowski LA: Swallowing in patients with tracheotomies, *AACN Clin Issues* 9(3):416, 1998.
Shaw JL, Sharpe S, Dyson SE et al: Bronchial auscultation: an effective adjunct to speech and language therapy bedside assessment when detecting dysphagia and aspiration? *Dysphagia* 19(4):211, 2004.
Smeltzer SC, Bare BG: *Brunner and Suddarths's textbok of medical-surgical nursing*, ed 10, Philadelphia, 2004, Lippincott.
Smith HA, Connolly MJ: Evaluation and treatment of dysphagia following stroke, *Topics Geriatr Rehab* 19(1):43, 2003.
St John RE: Ask the experts, *Crit Care Nurse* 20(4):100, 2000.
Vanek VW: Closed versus open enteral delivery systems: a quality improvement study, *Nutr Clin Pract* 15(5): 234, 2000.

## Risk for impaired parent/infant/child Attachment evolve

*Mary DeWys*

**NANDA**

### Definition

Disruption of the interactive process between parent/significant other and infant/child that fosters the development of a protective and nurturing reciprocal relationship

The terms *bonding* and *attachment* are used to describe the emotional connectedness that develops between the infant and his/her parent/primary caregiver over the first months and years of life. Bonding refers to the maternal process of emotional connectedness, whereas attachment is the infant process of emotionally connecting with the mother (Box III-3). The two unfolding processes describe the foundation of the mother-infant relationship that allows attachment to evolve (Ainsworth, 1978; Klaus, 1972)

### Risk Factors

Physical barriers; anxiety associated with the parent role; substance abuse; premature infant, ill infant/child who is unable to effectively initiate parental contact as a result of altered behavioral organization; lack of privacy; inability of parents to meet personal needs; separation

**BOX III-3 PARENT/INFANT/CHILD ATTACHMENT BEHAVIORS**

| Securely Attached | Avoidantly Attached | Ambivalently Attached |
|---|---|---|
| Mother (primary or caregiver) is warm, sensitively attuned, consistent. Quickly responds to baby's cries. | Mother is often emotionally unavailable or rejecting. Dislikes "neediness," may applaud independence. | Mother is unpredictable or chaotic. Often attentive but out of synch with baby. Most tune in to baby's fear. |
| Baby readily explores, using mother as secure base. Cries least of three groups, most compliant with mother, and most easily put down after being held. | By end of first year, baby seeks little physical contact with mother, randomly angry with her, unresponsive to being held, but often upset when put down. | Baby cries a lot, is clingy and demanding, often angry, upset by small separations, chronically anxious in relation to mother, limited in exploration. |
| Preschool: Easily makes friends. Popular. Flexible and resilient under stress. Spends more time with peers. Good self-esteem. | Preschool: Often angry, aggressive, defiant. May be isolated, disliked. Hangs around teachers. Withdraws when in pain. | Preschool: Fretful and easily overwhelmed by anxiety. Immature, overly dependent on teacher. May be victimized by bullies. |

From Karen R: *Becoming attached: first relationships and how they shape our capacity to love,* New York and Oxford, 1998, Oxford University Press, p 444.

***Parent***: maternal ambivalence toward pregnancy; unplanned/unwanted pregnancy; traumatic prenatal experience/birth trauma; unprepared for responsibility of parenting; poor parenting role models; history of abuse and neglect; substance abuse; insecure attachments within family of origin; social/emotional instability; homeless; maternal isolation, maternal depression; significant family stressors; prolonged separation from infant; hospitalization; teenage pregnancy; poverty; unsafe environment; low maternal education; use of corporal punishment; lack of empathy; lack of maternal sensitivity; unable to provide mutually satisfying interactions; lack of father's involvement/support; unstable/abusive relationship

***Infant/child:*** feeding difficulties; premature birth; prolonged hospitalization; colicky, episodes of prolonged, unexplained crying; genetic disposition-difficult temperament; unclear readable cues; disorganized behavior; inconsolable or difficult to console; frequent moves and placement homes; failed adoptions; inconsistent or inadequate day care, sudden maternal separation (illness, abandonment, death, prolonged hospitalization)

***Attachment behaviors***: eye contact; smiles; exchange of gentle touching/caressing; engages in positive reciprocal interactions; exchange of vocalizations/vocal play (coos, babbles pleasurably, responds, initiates and imitates infant); looks/reaches/touches parent for comfort when distressed; can be comforted with touch; comfortable with physical closeness, watches each other's face for sustained periods of time; relaxed in presence of each other; speaks positively of child (DeWys, 2005)

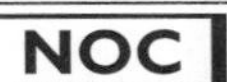

## Outcomes (Nursing Outcomes Classification)

### Suggested NOC Outcomes

Caregiver Adaptation to Patient Institutionalization; Child Development: 2 Months, 4 Months, 6 Months, 12 Months, 2 Years, 3 Years, 4 Years, Preschool; Coping; Parent-Infant Attachment; Family Physical Environment; Parenting Performance; Parenting: Psychosocial Safety; Safe Home Environment

#### Example NOC Outcomes with Indicators

Demonstrates appropriate **Child Development: 2 Months** as evidenced by the following indicators: Coos and vocalizes/Shows interest in visual stimuli/Shows interest in auditory stimuli/Smiles/Shows pleasure in interactions, especially with primary caregivers. **4 Months:** Looks at and becomes excited by mobile/Recognizes parents voices/Smiles, laughs and coos. **6 months:** Smiles, laughs, squeals, imitates noise/Shows beginning of stranger anxiety. **12 Months:** Plays social games/Imitates vocalizations/Pulls to stand (Rate each indicator of appropriate **Child Development:** 1 = never demonstrated, 2 = rarely demonstrated, 3 = sometimes demonstrated, 4 = often demonstrated, 5 = consistently demonstrated [see Section I].)

## Client Outcomes

### Parent(s) Will (Specify Time Frame):

- Display enjoyment with their infant/child
- Be able to provide a safe environment free of hazards
- Provide nurturing environment responding to infant/child's need for nutrition/feeding, sleeping, comfort, and social play
- Read and respond contingently to infant/child's behavior cues (approach/engagement, avoidance/disengagement)
- Be able to calm and relieve their infant/child's distress
- Engage in mutually satisfying interactions that provide an opportunity for attachment
- Engage in nurturing tactile/kinesthetic/vestibular communication (holding, cuddling, stroking, rocking, etc.)
- Demonstrate an awareness of developmentally appropriate activities that are interesting to the infant and growth fostering
- Not punish (inflict harm on) child for misbehavior
- Be knowledgeable of appropriate community resources and support services

NIC

## Interventions (Nursing Interventions Classification)

### Suggested NIC Interventions

Anticipatory Guidance, Attachment Process, Attachment Promotion, Coping Enhancement, Developmental Care, Developmental Enhancement: Child, Environmental

Management: Attachment Process, Family Integrity Promotion, Parent Education: Infant, Parenting Promotion, Role Enhancement

**Example NIC Activities—Anticipatory Guidance**

Instruct parent(s) about normal infant/child development and behavior, as appropriate; provide information on realistic expectations related to the infant/child's behavior; use case examples and/or model appropriate parenting behaviors to enhance the parent(s)' problem-solving skills, as appropriate

## Nursing Interventions and Rationales

- Establish a trusting relationship with the parents. *The effective model of "mothering mothers" is an important aspect of home visitation program utilizing nurses to provide nurturing, support and education with families (Olds, 1998). The quality of the nurse-client relationship was found to a key to success or failure (Sikma & Barnard, 1994; Barnard, 1998). There are instances when the parent is not able to focus on the child or is not emotionally available to the child, address the parent's developmental and psychological needs. Interventions must address both the infant's needs for stimulating responsive and secure environment and meet the parent's developmental and emotional challenges (Barnard, 1998).*
- Nurture parents so that they in turn can nurture their infant/child. *The therapeutic practice of nurses involves relationship-based caregiving, and when working with parents the nurse is nurturing the developing mother–infant relationship (Lawhon, 2003).*
- Allow parents to verbalize their childhood fears, "ghosts in the nursery." *Ghosts in the nursery are parents' early memories of fearful experiences occurring in their childhood surface surrounding the birth of a child. The painful legacy of parent's unanswered cries, chronic fear, pain, terror, abandonment in earliest life are communicated to the "listener" through powerful verbal and nonverbal behavior patterns with the child. Is anyone listening? "Hearing a mother's cries" is necessary in helping her "hear her child's cries," an important aspect toward therapeutic healing (Fraiberg et al, 1975).*
- Be an empathetic listener to parents' stories of childhood memories that may influence their struggle to attach with their child. **EBN:** *One study indicated that health care providers may recommend storytelling as the central mechanism of interactions in support groups that help participants to cope with daily anxieties of living (Dickerson et al, 2000).*
- Offer parent-to-parent support to parents of NICU hospitalized infants. **EBN:** *Findings from a study using one-to-one veteran parent support, in a nurse-managed program, may influence maternal and maternal-infant interaction outcomes (Roman et al, 1995).*
- Assist parents in learning to accurately read infant's physical states (sleep/wake) and behavior cues that communicate, approach/engagement and avoidance/disengagement, and respond in a contingent and sensitive way. When infants experience joyful and soothing responses to basic needs, infants experience satisfaction and emotional connectedness that evolves in building a secure relationship allowing for attachment bond between the two of them to form. *Provide nursing interventions that*

*recognizes and appraises positive parenting behaviors and provides knowledge of infant emotional states and strategies to manage crying promotes adaptive parent functioning (Elliot et al, 1996). When providing direct child interventions be sensitive in offering interventions that strengthen the parent-infant bond (Barnard, 1998).*

- Support parents' ability to respond and relieve their infant's/child's distress. **EB:** *The more the infant cries at 2 months of age, the less the mother responds to crying sets up negative feedback cycle that impairs infants attachment security at 18 months of age (Gunnar, 1996). Dr Karp identified five S's to effectively calm infants during the first three months of life or the "fourth trimester." The five S's include: swaddling/snug wrapping; side or stomach position (not for sleeping due to increase risk of sudden infant death syndrome (SIDS); Shushing, "Shhh" sounds louder than crying pitch, "white noise" (levels up to 80 dB); swinging/movement; and sucking, non-nutritive sucking (NNS). The suggested interventions stimulate the calming reflex an unreported "primitive" reflex that is an off switch when young babies fretfully cry (Karp, 2004).*
- Assist parents with recognizing how their infant/child learns through sensory motor experiences (sights/visual, sounds/auditory, touch/tactile, vestibular/movement and body awareness). *Guide parents in providing play activities at or slightly above the child's developmental level (Barnard, 1994).* **EBN:** *Encourage parents of premature infants to initially interact using mature sensory systems (tactile and vestibular) such as holding, rocking, stroking, touching etc., add one of the less mature sensory systems (auditory and visual) such as eye contact, "enface looking, vocalizing and avoid over stimulation.* **EBN:** *Over stimulated infants will look away, arch or fuss as an attempt to disengage (White-Traut, 1996).*
- Guide parents in adapting their behaviors and activities with infant/child cues and changing needs. *By assisting parents to be more responsive to infant/child's cues and their response to those cues are growth-fostering activities nurses can encourage (Barnard, 1994). Model calming interventions to provide parents with tools for positive interactions with their infant/child (Karl, 1999).*
- Identify factors related to depressive symptoms and offer appropriate interventions. *Postpartum disturbances in maternal mood have been associated with differences in maternal behavior toward infants and in the behavior of infants themselves (Miller, 1993). Interactions are altered when parent is unresponsive as with depressed, mentally ill, or have been abused as children (Rutter, 1990).* **EBN:** *Several studies reported mothers of hospitalized infants depressive symptoms decreased from hospital discharge over time except when infants remained hospitalized, technologically dependent or had chronic medical and developmental complications, maternal depressive symptoms did not decrease overtime (Miles et al, 1999).*
- Offer anticipatory developmental guidance including interactive play activities that are interesting to the child. *The unrealistic expectations of parents regarding infant/child abilities can negatively influence the parent-child relationship by expecting too much to soon. "Touchpoints" manual provides developmental guidance regarding what to expect and when, addresses parenting challenges and offers engaging play activities and parenting strategies (Brazelton, 1992).*
- Attend to both the parents and infant/child in an effort to strengthen high-quality parent-infant interactions. **EB:** *High-quality interactions parent-infant is important in*

*promoting child resiliency, and needs to be promoted in family-centered early interventions (LeTourneau, 1997). Identifying the infant/child's strengths and limitations can provide parents with more information regarding how they can encourage optimal growth and development (Barnard et al, 1993). Nurses are well prepared using the nursing process model as a framework for assessing infant, caregivers, and their environments and implementing interventions aimed at strengthening caregiver-infant affective process, adaptive behaviors and coping skills of all members of the relational field (Kearney, 1997).* **EB:** *Enabling and facilitation the interactive process of attunement and synchrony between infant and mother is the earliest years of life will enhance secure attachment that will provide a substantial buffer against life's slings and arrows (Svanberg, 1998).*

- Encourage parents of hospitalized infants to "personalize" their infant by bringing in baby clothes, pictures of themselves, toys, and tapes of their voices. *These actions help parents claim the infant as their own. Neonatal nurses are in a unique position to support families' competence and confidence in caring for their infant at their own pace and encouraging the developing mother-infant relationship (Lawhon, 2002).*
- Encourage physical closeness using skin-to-skin experiences for parents and infants as appropriate. The mothers studied perceived skin-to-skin contact with their very immature infants as a positive and helpful intervention. **EBN:** *Kangaroo care is an efficient method, although other interventions are effective including swaddling, pacifier, heartbeat sounds, sounds of mother's voice, rhythmic movement, and decreasing external stimuli (Ludington-Hoe et al, 2002). Skin-to-skin care has been found to increase a favorable perception of the infant by the caregiver, and result in parents who feel more competent in caring for their infant (Tessier et al, 1998).*
- Encourage parents and caregivers to massage their infants and children. *Infant massage/stroking offers enhances attachment by using proximal/physical stimulation of mature sensory systems (tactile/kinesthetic) that is an inexpensive tool that should be used as part of developmental care for premature infants (Beachy, 2003; Field, 2002).* **EB:** *One study demonstrated that massage therapy on infants and children with various medical conditions resulted in lower anxiety and stress hormones and improved clinical course. Having grandparent volunteers and parents provide the therapy enhances their own wellness and provides a cost-effective treatment for the infants/children (Field, 1995).*
- Assist parents in developing new caregiving practice competencies and/or revising and extending old ones. One model to consider for use with parents in guided participation, a process in which an experienced person helps another with less experience to become competent in practices that are personally and socially meaningful for everyday life. **EBN:** *Caregiving competencies foster a child's developments. Five domains of caregiving activities have been identified: (1) being with the infant, (2) knowing the infant as a person, (3) giving care to the infant, (4) communicating and engaging with others about needs (infant and parental), and (5) problem-solving/decision-making/learning (Pridham et al, 1998).*
- Plan ways for parents to interact with/assist with caregiving for their infant/child. **EBN:** *One nursing research study indicates that the ability to see an infant in the delivery room prior to transporting the infant to an intensive care unit may decrease parental stress, which can be a significant barrier to attachment (Shields-Poe & Pinelli, 1997).*

## Infant

- Provide lyrical, soothing music in the nursery and home as appropriate (with premature infants visual and auditory stimulation must be designed as appropriate with postconceptual age (PCA) and contingent with state and behavioral cues) premature infants). **EB:** *The results from one study suggest that soothing music may be a feasible intervention to help newborns demonstrate fewer high-arousal states and less state lability (Kaminski & Hall, 1996). Premature infants may find auditory and visual stimulation stressful (White-Traut, 1996).*
- Recognize and support infant/child's attention capabilities. *The ability to organize incoming sensory input and focus attention to animate and inanimate and interact is significant milestone to cognitive development.*
- Encourage opportunities for mutually satisfying interactions between infant and parent. *The process of attachment involves communication and patterns of interactions between parent and infant that are synchronous and rhythmic (Rosetti, 1990)*
- Encourage opportunities for physical closeness. *The infant "tunes in" to mothers heartbeat, respiration, body warmth, etc. Studies of bonding identifies that early physical contact enhances maternal qualities (Klaus et al, 1972).*
- Provide therapeutic touch for children with anxiety. **EBN:** *In one study the therapeutic touch (TT) intervention resulted in lower overall mean anxiety scores, whereas the mimic TT did not. These findings provide preliminary support for the use of TT in reducing the anxiety level of children with HIV infection (Ireland, 1998).*

## Multicultural

- Discuss cultural norms with families to provide care that is appropriate for enhancing attachment with the infant/child. **EBN:** *Misinterpretation of parenting behaviors can occur when the nurse and parent are from different cultures. It is inappropriate to pressure parents to relate to the infant/child in a way that is culturally unacceptable/abnormal for the family (Coffman, 1992; Guarnaccia, 1998). This limits family choice and sets up a tense environment rather than a trusting, supportive one.*
- Encourage a reciprocal attachment process. **EBN:** *Parents who develop a sensitivity to their infant's/child's communication patterns and behavioral cues will respond appropriately to the infant's/child's desire for increased interaction; the infant may then attempt to obtain the parent's attention. This encourages a process of mutual feedback that enhances the attachment process (Goulet et al, 1998).*
- Promote the attachment process by providing a treatment environment that is culturally based and women centered. **EBN:** *Pregnant and postpartum Asian/Pacific Islander women in substance abuse treatment identified provisions for the newborn, infant health care, parent education, and infant mother bonding as conducive to their treatment (Morelli et al, 2001).*
- Empower family members to draw on personal strengths in which multiple worldviews and values of individual members are recognized, incorporated, and negotiated. **EB:** *A respectful intervention process can reiterate a parallel process in the family in which multiple worldviews among different members are explored, accepted, appreciated, and negotiated for the benefit of the family (Lee & Mjelde-Mossey, 2004).*

A

- Encourage positive involvement and relationship development between children and non-custodial fathers to enhance health and development. **EB:** *Research with low-income African American fathers has shown that these fathers are strongly committed to their children, but there is a need for outside facilitation to overcome barriers that interfere with their positive involvement (Dubowitz et al, 2004).*

## Home Care

- Above interventions may be adapted for home care use.
- Assess quality of interaction between parent and infant/child. *Attachment provides the infant with a source of comfort when anxious and is a precursor to social interaction. Social interaction, beginning with parents, is important to child development.*
- ▲ Assess mother for depressive symptoms and initiate referral for mental health care as needed. Referral to psychiatric home health care, if available, can be helpful. **EBN:** *Depressive symptoms in low-income mothers have been shown to affect infant development negatively. Treatment in the home by masters prepared psychiatric nurses was helpful in reducing depressive symptoms (Beeber et al, 2004).*
- Use interaction coaching: teach mother about infant's behavioral cues and how to match infant's preferences; have mother position infant in direct line of sight; demonstrate responsive behaviors that can be modulated (e.g., facial, expression, voice, touch); encourage practice by trial and error; reinforce sensitive responsiveness as it occurs; give positive reinforcement for success. **EBN:** *Mothers with postpartum depressive symptoms who received interaction coaching demonstrated significantly greater maternal-infant responsiveness (Censullo, 1994; Horowitz et al, 2001).*

## evolve WEBSITES FOR EDUCATION

See the Evolve website for World Wide Web resources for client education.

## REFERENCES

Ainsworth M, Blehar M, Waters E et al: *Patterns of attachment: a psychological study of the strange situation*, Hillsdale, NJ, 1978, Lawrence Erlbaum.

Barnard KE, Morisset CE, Spieker SJL: Preventive interventions: enhancing parent-infant relationship. In Zeanah C, editor: *Handbook on infant mental health,* New York, 1993, The Guilford Press, pp. 386-401.

Barnard KE: *Caregiver/parent-child interaction feeding and teaching manual,* Seattle, 1994, University of Washington NCAST Publications.

Barnard KE, editor: Developing, implementing, and documenting interventions with parents and young children, *Zero to Three,* February and March, 1998, 23-29.

Barnard KE: Influencing parent-child interactions. In Guralnick MJ editor: *The effectiveness of early intervention,* Baltimore, 1997, Brooks Publishing, pp. 249-268.

Barnard KE: *Nursing systems toward effective parenting-preterm (NSTEP-P),* Seattle, 1987, University of Washington NCAST Publications.

Beachy JM: Premature infant massage in the NICU, *Neonatal Netw* 22(3):39-45, 2003.

Beeber LS, Holditch-Davis D, Belyea MJ et al: In-home intervention for depressive symptoms with low-income mothers of infants and toddlers in the United States, *Health Care Women Int* 25(6):561-580, 2004.

Brazelton TB, *Touchpoints,* New York, 1992, Addison-Wesley.

Caldwell BM, Bradley RH: *Infant-toddler home observation for measurement of the environment scale (HOME),* (Rev ed), Little Rock, 1984, University of Arkansas-Little Rock.

Coffman S: Parent and infant attachment: review of nursing research: 1981-1990, *Pediatr Nurs* 18(4):421-5, 1992.

Denehy J: Interventions related to parent-infant attachment, *Nurs Clin North Am* 27(2):425-443, 1992.

Dubowitz H, Lane W, Ross K et al: The involvement of low-income African American fathers in their children's lives, and the barriers they face, *Ambul Pediatr* 4(6):505-508, 2004.

Farel AM, Freeman VA, Keenan NL et al: Interaction between high-risk infants and their mothers: the NCAST as an assessment tool, *Res Nurs Health* 14(2):109-118, 1991.

Field T: Massage therapy for infants and children, *J Dev Behav Pediatr* 16(2):105-111, 1995.

Field T: Massage, *Med Clin North Am* 86(1):163-167, 2002.

Fraiberg S, Adelson E, Shapiro V: Ghosts in the nursery: a psychoanalytic approach to the problems of impaired infant-mother relationships, *J Am Acad Child Psychiatry* 14:387-421, 1975.

Goulet C et al: A concept analysis of parent-infant attachment, *J Adv Nurs* 28(5):1071-1081, 1998.

Guarnaccia P: Multicultural experiences of family caregiving: a study of African American, European American, and Hispanic American families, *New Dir Ment Health Serv* 77:45-61, 1998.

Gunnar MR, Brodersen L, Nachmias M et al: Stress reactivity and attachment security, *Dev Psychobiol* 29(3): 91-204, 1996.

Ireland M: Therapeutic touch with HIV-infected children: a pilot study, *J Assoc Nurses AIDS Care* 9(4):68-77, 1998.

Kaar-Moorse R, Wiley MS: *Ghosts from the nursery,* New York, 1997, Atlantic Monthly Press.

Kaminski J, Hall W: The effect of soothing music on neonatal behavioral states in the hospital newborn nursery, *Neonat Netw* 15(1):45-54, 1996.

Karen R: *Becoming attached, first relationships and how they shape our capacity to love*, New York and Oxford, 1998, Oxford University Press.

Karl D: The interactive newborn bath, *MCN Am J Matern Child Nurs* 24(6):280-286, 1999.

Karp H: The "fourth trimester: a framework and strategy for understanding and resolving colic, *Contemp Pediatr* 21(2):94-107, 2004.

Kearney JA: Emotional development in infancy: theoretical models and nursing implications, *J Child Adolesc Psychiatr Nurs* 10(4): 7-17, 1997.

Klaus MH, Jerauld R, Kreger NC et al: Maternal attachment. Importance of the first post-partum days, *New Engl J Med* 286(9)460-463, 1972.

LawhonG: Integrated nursing care: vital issues important in the humane care of the newborn, *Semin Neonatol* 7:441-446, 2002.

Le Tourneau N: Fostering resiliency in infants and young children through parent-infant interaction, *Infants Young Child* 9:36-45, 1997.

Lee MY, Mjelde-Mossey L: Cultural dissonance among generations: a solution-focused approach with East Asian elders and their families, *J Marital Fam Ther* 30(4):497-513, 2004.

Ludington-Hoe SM, Cong X, Hashemi F: Infant crying: nature, physiologic consequences, and select interventions, *Neonatal Netw* 21(2):29-36, 2002.

Rutter M: Commentary: Some focus and process considerations regarding effects of parental depression on children, *Dev Psychol* 26(1):60-67, 1990.

Mew AM, Holditch-Davis D, Belyea M et al: Correlates of depressive symptoms in mothers of preterm infants, *Neonatal Netw* 22(5):51-60, 2003.

Meyer EC, Carcia-Coll CT, Lester B et al: Family-based intervention improves maternal psychological well-being and feeding interaction of preterm infants, *Pediatrics* 98:241-246, 1994.

Miles MS, Carter MC: Assessing parental stress in intensive care unit, *MCN Am J Matern Child Nurs* 1983.

Miles MS, Holditch-Davis D, Burchinal P et al: Distress and growth outcomes in mothers of medically fragile infants, *Nurs Res* 48(3):129-140, 1999.

Miller AR, Barr RG, Eaton WO: Crying and motor behavior of six-week-old infants and postpartum maternal mood, *Pediatrics* 92(4):551-558, 1993.

Morelli PT, Fong R, Oliveria J: Culturally competent substance abuse treatment for Asian/Pacific Islander women, *J Hum Behav Soc Environ* 3(3/4):263, 2001.

NCAST*: Keys to caregiving: a video program.* Seattle, 1994, University of Washington NCAST Publications.

Olds D, Pettit LM, Robinson J et al: The potential for reducing antisocial behavior with a program of prenatal and early childhood home visitation, *J Community Psychol.* 26(1):65-83, 1998.

Pridham KF: Guided participation and development of care-giving competencies for families of low birth-weight infants, *J Adv Nurs* 28(5):948-958, 1998.

Robson AL: Low birth weight and parenting stress during early childhood, *J Pediatr Psychol* 22:297-311, 1997.

Roman LA, Lindsay JD, Boger RP et al: Parent-to-parent support initiated in the neonatal intensive care unit, *Res Nurs Health* 18: 385-394, 1995.

Rossetti LM: *Infant-toddler assessment*, Boston, 1990, Little-Brown and Company.
Shields-Poe D, Pinelli J: Variables associated with parental stress in neonatal intensive care units, *Neonat Netw* 16(1):29, 1997.
Sikma S, Barnard D: *Nurse-client relationship pilot study*, Poster presented at the NCAST National Institute, 1994, Seattle.
Sumner G, Spietz A: *Caregiver/parent-child interaction feeding and teaching manuals,* Seattle, 1994, University of Washington NCAST Publications.
Svanberg PG: Attachment, resilience and prevention, *J Ment Health*. 7(6):543-578, 1997.
Tessier R, Cristo M, Velez S et al: Kangaroo mother care and the bonding hypothesis, *Pediatrics* 102(2):e17, 1998.
van Ijzendoorn MH, Dijkstra J, Bus AG: Attachment, intelligence and language-a meta-analysis, *Soc Dev* 4:115-128, 1995.
White-Traut R: Environmental factors and alternative therapies in nursing, *AWHONN Voice* 4(9):1, 12-3, 1996.

# Autonomic dysreflexia

*Betty J. Ackley*

**NANDA**

## Definition

Life-threatening, uninhibited sympathetic response of the nervous system to a noxious stimulus after a spinal cord injury at T7 or above

## Defining Characteristics

Pallor (below the injury); paroxysmal hypertension (sudden, periodic elevated blood pressure where systolic pressure is >140 mm Hg and diastolic is > 90 mm Hg); red splotches on skin (above the injury); bradycardia or tachycardia (pulse rate of <60 or >100 beats/min); diaphoresis above the injury; headache (diffuse pain in different parts of the head, not confined to any nerve distribution area); blurred vision; chest pain; chilling; conjunctival congestion; Horner's syndrome (contraction of pupil on one side, partial ptosis of the eyelid, recession of eyeball into the head, occasional loss of sweating over the affected side of the face); metallic taste in mouth; nasal congestion; paresthesia; pilomotor reflex (gooseflesh formation when skin is cooled)

## Related Factors (r/t)

Bladder distention, bowel distention, skin irritation, lack of client and caregiver knowledge

**NOC**

## Outcomes (Nursing Outcomes Classification)

### Suggested NOC Outcomes

Neurological Status, Neurological Status: Autonomic, Vital Signs

**Example NOC Outcome with Indicators**

**Neurological Status: Autonomic** as evidenced by the following indicators: Systolic blood pressure WNL/Diastolic blood pressure WNL/Apical heart rate WNL/Perspiration response pattern/Goose bump response pattern/Pupil reactivity/Peripheral tissue perfusion (Rate each indicator of **Neurological Status: Autonomic:** 1 = severely compromised, 2 = substantially compromised, 3 = moderately compromised, 4 = mildly compromised, 5 = not compromised [see Section I].)

WNL, Within normal limits.

## Client Outcomes/Goals

**Client Will (Specify Time Frame):**

- Maintain normal vital signs
- Remain free of dysreflexia symptoms
- Explain symptoms, prevention, and treatment of dysreflexia

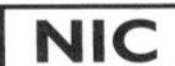

## Interventions (Nursing Interventions Classification)

### Suggested NIC Intervention

Dysreflexia Management

**Example NIC Activities—Dysreflexia Management**

Identify and minimize stimuli that may precipitate dysreflexia; monitor for signs and symptoms of autonomic dysreflexia

## Nursing Interventions and Rationales

- • Monitor the client for symptoms of dysreflexia. See Defining Characteristics. *Some clients are mostly asymptomatic (Dunn, 2004).*
- ▲ Observe with physician the cause of dysreflexia (e.g., distended bladder, impaction, pressure ulcer, urinary calculi, bladder infection, acute condition in the abdomen, penile pressure, ingrown toenail, or other source of noxious stimuli). *Noxious stimuli cause an uncontrolled sympathetic nervous system response (Walker, 2002; Dunn, 2004).*
- ▲ If symptoms of dysreflexia are present, place client in high Fowler's position, remove all support hoses or binders, and immediately determine the identity of the noxious stimuli causing the response. If blood pressure cannot be decreased within 1 minute, notify the physician STAT (Walker, 2002; Dunn, 2004). *These steps promote venous pooling, decrease venous return, and decrease blood pressure. The client should be rapidly evaluated by both the physician and nurse to find the possible cause (Kavchak-Keyes, 2000).*

- To determine the stimulus for dysreflexia:
  - First, assess bladder function. Check for distention, and if present catheterize using an anesthetic jelly as a lubricant. Do not use Valsalva maneuver or Crede's method to empty the bladder. Ensure existing catheter patency. Also note signs of urinary tract infection.
  - Second, assess bowel function. Numb the bowel area with a topical anesthetic as ordered, and once agent is effective (5 minutes), check for impaction.
  - Third, assess the skin looking for any points of pressure.

  *The stimulus for dysreflexia is most commonly bladder distention, then bowel impaction, then pressure on the skin (Travers, 1999; Essat, 2003).*

▲ Initiate antihypertensive therapy as soon as ordered. *A severely elevated blood pressure needs to be decreased for client safety (Walker, 2002; Dunn, 2004).*

▲ Be careful not to increase noxious sensory stimuli. If numbing agent is ordered, use it on anus and 1 inch of rectum before attempting to remove a fecal impaction. Also spray pressure ulcer with it. If necessary to replace an obstructed catheter, use an anesthetic jelly as ordered. *Increased noxious sensory stimuli can exacerbate the abnormal response and worsen the client's prognosis (Walker, 2002; Dunn, 2004).* **EB:** *In one study the use of topical lidocaine did not limit the development of autonomic dysreflexia during anorectal procedures in spinal cord injury clients (Cosman et al, 2002).*

- Monitor vital signs every 3 to 5 minutes during acute event; continue to monitor vital signs after event is resolved. *It is possible for the client to develop rebound hypotension after the acute event because of the use of antihypertensive medications, or symptoms of dysreflexia may reoccur(Kasper, Braunwald, & Fauci, 2005).*
- Watch for complications of dysreflexia, including signs of cerebral hemorrhage, seizures, MI, or intraocular hemorrhage. *Extremely high blood pressure can cause intracranial hemorrhage and death (Kasper, Braunwald, & Fauci, 2005).*
- Accurately and completely record any incidences of dysreflexia; especially note the precipitating stimuli. *It is imperative to determine both the causes of the condition and whether the condition is persistent, requiring the client to take medications routinely to prevent repeat incidences (Kavchak-Keyes, 2000).*
- Use the following interventions to prevent dysreflexia:
  - Ensure that drainage from Foley catheter is good and that bladder is not distended.
  - Ensure a regular pattern of defecation to prevent fecal impaction. *Bladder distention and bowel impaction are the most common causes of dysreflexia (Walker, 2002; Dunn, 2004).*
  - Frequently change position of client to relieve pressure and prevent the formation of pressure ulcers.
  - If ordered, apply an anesthetic agent to any wound below level of injury before performing wound care.

▲ Because episodes can reoccur, notify all health care team members of the possibility of a dysreflexia episode. *All health care personnel working with the client should be aware of the condition because symptoms could begin while the client is away from the nursing unit (Travers, 1999).*

## Home Care

- Above interventions may be adapted for home care use.
- Instruct the client with any known proclivity toward dysreflexia to wear a medical alert bracelet and carry a medical alert wallet card when not in a safe environment (i.e., not with someone who knows client has the condition and can respond appropriately). *Autonomic dysreflexia is life-threatening response (Kavchak-Keyes, 2000).*
- ▲ Establish an emergency plan: obtain physician orders for medications to be used in situations in which first aid does not work (e.g., nifedipine) (Wirtz et al, 1996). *Medication administered immediately can reverse early stage dysreflexia. Dysreflexia that is not recognized and treated can result in death (Kasper, Braunwald, & Fauci, 2005).*
- ▲ If orders have not been obtained or client does not have medications, use emergency medical services.
- If episode of dysreflexia is resolved, monitor blood pressure every 30 to 60 minutes for next 4 to 5 hours or admit to institution for observation. *After an episode of autonomic dysreflexia, it is not uncommon for a second episode or rebound to occur (Kasper, Braunwald, & Fauci, 2005).*
- ▲ Institute case management of frail elderly to support continued independent living. *Nervous system difficulties represent and can lead to increasing needs for assistance in using the health care system effectively. Case management combines nursing activities of client and family assessment, planning and coordination of care among all health care providers, delivery of direct nursing care, and monitoring of care and outcomes. These activities are able to address continuity of care, mutual goal setting, behavior management, and prevention of worsening health problems (Guttman, 1999).*

## Client/Family Teaching

- Teach recognition of the earliest symptoms of dysreflexia, the actions that should be taken when they occur, and the need to summon help immediately. Give client a written card that contains this information. *The client must know the symptoms and treatment well enough to instruct people in his or her environment how to relieve the symptoms (Kavchak-Keyes, 2000).*
- Teach steps to prevent dysreflexia episodes: care of bladder, bowel, and skin and prevention of other forms of noxious stimuli (i.e., not wearing clothing that is too tight). *Dysreflexia can occur anytime after discharge. Of clients with spinal cord lesions above C6, 85% experience dysreflexia (Kasper, Braunwald, & Fauci, 2005).*

## evolve WEBSITES FOR EDUCATION

See the EVOLVE website for World Wide Web resources for client education.

## REFERENCES

Cosman BC, Vu TT, Plowman BK: Topical lidocaine does not limit autonomic dysreflexia during anorectal procedures in spinal cord injury: a prospective, double-blind study, *Int J Colorectal Dis* 17(2):104, 2002.

Dunn KL: Identification and management of autonomic dysreflexia in the emergency department, *Top Emerg Med* 26(3):254, 2004.
Essat Z: Management of autonomic dysreflexia, *Nurs Stand* 17(32):42, 2003.
Guttman R: Case management of the frail elderly in the community, *Clin Nurs Spec* 13(4):174, 1999.
Kasper DL, Braunwald E, Fauci AS: *Harrison's principles of internal medicine,* ed 16, New York, 2005, McGraw-Hill.
Kavchak-Keyes MA: Autonomic hyperreflexia, *Rehabil Nurs* 25(1):31, 2000.
Travers PL: Autonomic dysreflexia: a clinical rehabilitation problem, *Rehabil Nurs* 24(1):19, 1999.
Walker JA: Autonomic dysreflexia, *Prof Nurse* 17(9):519-520, 2002.
Wirtz KM, LaFavor KM, Ang R: Managing chronic spinal cord injury: issues in critical care, *Crit Care Nurse* 16(4):24, 1996.

# Risk for Autonomic dysreflexia

*Betty J. Ackley*

**NANDA**

## Definition

At risk for life-threatening, uninhibited response of the sympathetic nervous system; post–spinal shock; in an individual with spinal cord injury or lesion at T6 or above (has been demonstrated in clients with injuries at T7 and T8)

## Defining Characteristics (Risk Factors)

An injury/lesion at T6 or above and at least one of the following noxious stimuli:

- Neurological stimuli: painful/irritating stimuli below the level of injury
- Urological stimuli: bladder distention, detrusor sphincter dyssynergia, bladder spasms, instrumentation or surgery, epididymitis, urethritis, urinary tract infection, calculi, cystitis, catheterization
- Gastrointestinal stimuli: bowel distention, fecal impaction, digital stimulation, suppositories, hemorrhoids, difficult passage of feces, constipation, enemas, gastrointestinal system pathology, gastric ulcers, esophageal reflux, gallstones
- Reproductive stimuli: menstruation, sexual intercourse, pregnancy, labor and delivery, ovarian cyst, ejaculation
- Regulatory stimuli: temperature fluctuations, extreme environmental temperatures
- Musculoskeletal-integumentary stimuli: cutaneous stimulations (e.g., pressure ulcer, ingrown toenail, dressings, burns, rash); heterotrophic bone; pressure over bony prominences or genitalia; spasm; fractures; range-of-motion exercises; wounds; sunburns
- Situational stimuli: positioning; drug reactions (e.g., decongestants, sympathomimetics, vasoconstrictors, narcotic withdrawal); constrictive clothing (e.g., straps, stockings, shoes); surgical procedures
- Cardiac/pulmonary problems: pulmonary emboli, deep vein thrombosis

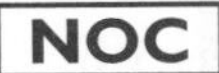

## Outcomes (Nursing Outcomes Classification)

### Suggested NOC Outcomes

Neurological Status, Neurological Status: Autonomic, Vital Signs

**Example NOC Outcome with Indicators**

**Neurological Status: Autonomic** as evidenced by the following indicators: Systolic blood pressure WNL/Diastolic blood pressure WNL/Apical heart rate WNL/Perspiration response pattern/Goose bumps response pattern/Pupil reactivity size/Peripheral tissue perfusion (Rate each indicator with regard to **Neurological Status: Autonomic:** 1 = severely compromised, 2 = substantially compromised, 3 = moderately compromised, 4 = mildly compromised, 5 = not compromised [see Section I].)

WNL, Within normal limits.

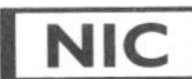

## Interventions (Nursing Interventions Classification)

### Suggested NIC Intervention

Dysreflexia Management

**Example NIC Activities—Dysreflexia Management**

Identify and minimize stimuli that may precipitate dysreflexia; monitor for signs and symptoms of autonomic dysreflexia

## Client Outcomes, Nursing Interventions and Rationales

Refer to care plan for **Autonomic dysreflexia.**

# Disturbed Body image

evolve

*Teresa Howell and Gail B. Ladwig*

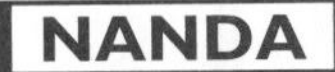

## Definition

Confusion in mental picture of one's physical self

## Defining Characteristics

Verbalization of feelings that reflect an altered view of one's body in appearance, structure, or function; verbalization of perceptions that reflect an altered view of one's body in

B

appearance, structure, or function; nonverbal response to actual or perceived change in body structure and/or function; behaviors of avoidance, monitoring, or acknowledgment of one's body

### Objective

Missing body part; trauma to nonfunctioning part; not touching body part; hiding or overexposing body part (intentional or unintentional); actual change in structure and/or function; change in social involvement; change in ability to estimate spatial relationship of body to environment; extension of body boundary to incorporate environmental objects; not looking at body part

### Subjective

Refusal to verify actual change, preoccupation with change or loss, personalization of part or loss by name, depersonalization of part or loss by impersonal pronouns, extension of body boundary to incorporate environmental objects

## Related Factors (r/t)

Psychosocial, biophysical, cognitive/perceptual, cultural, spiritual, or developmental changes; illness; trauma or injury; surgery; illness treatment

NOC

## Outcomes (Nursing Outcomes Classification)

### Suggested NOC Outcomes

Body Image; Child Development: 2 Years, 3 Years, 4 Years, Preschool, Middle Childhood, Adolescence; Distorted Thought Self-Control; Grief Resolution; Psychosocial Adjustment: Life Change; Self-Esteem

**NOC Outcome with Indicators**

**Body Image** as evidenced by the following indicators: Congruence between body reality, body ideal, and body presentation/Satisfaction with body appearance/Adjustment to changes in physical appearance (Rate each indicator of **Body Image:** 1 = never positive, 2 = rarely positive, 3 = sometimes positive, 4 = often positive, 5 = consistently positive [see Section I].)

## Client Outcomes

### Client Will (Specify Time Frame):

- State or demonstrate acceptance of change or loss and an ability to adjust to lifestyle change
- Call body part or loss by appropriate name
- Look at and touch changed or missing body part
- Care for changed or nonfunctioning part without inflicting trauma

- Return to previous social involvement
- Correctly estimate relationship of body to environment

B

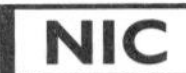

## Interventions (Nursing Interventions Classification)

### Suggested NIC Intervention

Body Image Enhancement

| Example NIC Activities—Body Image Enhancement |
|---|
| Determine client's body image expectations based on developmental stage; assist the client to identify activities that will enhance appearance |

## Nursing Interventions and Rationales

- Use a tool such as the Body Image Instrument (BII) to identify clients who have concerns about changes in body image. The five BII subscales—General Appearance, Body Competence, Others' Reaction to Appearance, Value of Appearance, and Body Parts—exhibited moderate to high internal reliability and concurrent validity (Kopel et al, 1998). **EBN:** *Using a body image scale can help nurses to identify possible body image disturbances and to plan individual nursing interventions (Souto & Garcia, 2002).*
- ▲ Assess for body dysmorphic disorder (BDD) and make appropriate referrals. *The severity of BDD varies. Some youth experience manageable distress about their appearance and are able to function well, although not up to their potential. Psychiatric treatment is often effective in decreasing BDD symptoms and the suffering they cause (Phillips, 2003).* **EB:** *In delusional and nondelusional clients with body dysmorphic disorder, fluoxetine hydrochloride was more effective than placebo (Rao, 2002).*
- Observe client's usual coping mechanisms during times of extreme stress and reinforce their use in the current crisis. **EBN:** *In this study of clients on hemodialysis, more psychosocial stressors were associated with greater use of problem solving, social support, and avoidance coping; avoidance coping was found to explain much of the relationship between psychosocial stressors and depression (Welch & Austin, 2001).*
- Explore opportunities to assist the client to develop a realistic perception of his or her body image. *Actual body size may not be consistent with the client's perceived body size. Inaccurate perception by the client can be unhealthy (Townsend, 2003).*
- Acknowledge denial, anger, or depression as normal feelings when adjusting to changes in body and lifestyle. **EB:** *The influence of emotion-focused coping (venting emotions and mental disengagement) on distress following disfiguring injury was associated with less body image disturbance (Fauerbach et al, 2002).*
- Identify clients at risk for body image disturbance (e.g., body builders, cancer survivors). **EB:** *Male body builders are at risk for body image disturbance and the associated psychological characteristics that have been commonly reported among eating disorder clients. These psychological characteristics also appear to predict steroid use in this group of males.*

*Steroid users reported an elevated drive to put on muscle mass in the form of bulk (Blouin & Goldfield, 1995).* **EBN:** *The female perception of body image contains passive assimilation of comments from others and acute observation of the media and the environment (Chang et al, 2004).*

- Clients should not be rushed into sharing their feelings. *Feelings associated with complicated and emotionally powerful issues involving an altered body image take time to work through and express (Johnson, 1994).*
- Do not ask clients to explore feelings unless they have indicated a need to do so. **EBN:** *Patients reported keeping their feelings to themselves as a frequently used coping strategy (Zacharia et al, 1994).*
- Explore strengths and resources with client. Discuss possible changes in weight and hair loss; select a wig before hair loss occurs. **EBN:** *Nurses play an important role in assisting the client to cope with alopecia and help clients move through a potentially devastating experience to a renewed sense of well-being (Bachelor, 2001).*
- Encourage the client to purchase clothes that are attractive and that deemphasize their disability. *Individuals with osteoporosis are not usually disabled but may perceive themselves as unattractive and experience social isolation as a result of ill-fitting clothes that accentuate the physical changes (Sedlak & Doheny, 2000).*
- Allow client and others gradual exposure to the body change. Begin by having the client touch the affected area; then use a mirror to look at it. Go to a hospital shop with a nurse or support person and discuss feelings associated with the reaction of others to the body change. *Part of the rehabilitation process is graded exposure—the client moves from a protected to an unprotected environment with the support of the nurse (MacGinley, 1993).*
- Encourage the client to discuss interpersonal and social conflicts that may arise. *Changes in physical appearance and function associated with disease processes (and sometimes treatment) need to be integrated into the interaction that occurs between clients and lay caregivers (Price, 2000).*
- Encourage the client to make own decisions, participate in plan of care, and accept both inadequacies and strengths. **EBN:** *It has been found that support given to women with breast cancer has a positive effect on their reactions to the illness and may even prolong their survival (Lindrop & Cannon, 2001).* **EB:** *The results of this study of clients with severe psoriasis indicate that the criterion for the management of psoriasis should be the clients' own perception of the consequences of the disease (Wahl et al, 2002).* **EBN:** *Data from one study suggest that satisfaction with body image is disturbed by surgery for breast cancer despite active participation in decisions regarding selection of treatment. These outcomes suggest that women need assistance in adjusting to alterations in body image from nurses (Newell, 1999).*
- Help client accept help from others; provide a list of appropriate community resources (e.g., Reach to Recovery, Ostomy Association). *Motivation, sharing of experiences, camaraderie with and support from peers, and knowledge of not being alone have been identified as advantages of group learning (Payne, 1993).*
- Help client describe self-ideal, identify self-criticisms, and be accepting of self. *The perception of self-image involves knowing the self and what is important and valued. Dis-*

*ability causes individuals to live as changed human beings regardless of whether they are willing to do so (Pohl & Winland-Brown, 1992).*

- Encourage the client to write a narrative description of their changes. **EB:** *One's experience of coping or adjustment to a disability is represented as narratives about himself or herself. Each person with traumatic brain injury (TBI) reconstructed certain self-narratives when coping with their changed self-images and daily lives (Nochi, 2000).*
- Avoid looks of distaste when caring for clients who have had disfiguring surgery or injuries. Provide privacy; care should be completed without unnecessary exposure. *Nurses must be aware of their nonverbal behavior; clients often become acutely aware of nurses' feelings as a result of the nurses' facial expressions, tone of voice, touch, or other behaviors (MacGinley, 1993).*
- Encourage the client to continue same personal care routine that was followed before the change in body image. It is preferable that this care be completed in the bathroom and not in bed. **EBN:** *This routine gives the client privacy and also prevents the client from settling into an "invalid" role. Research has shown that women who resume familiar routines and habits heal better and suffer less depression than those who settle into the role of client (Johnson, 1994).*

## Geriatric

- Focus on remaining abilities. Have client make a list of strengths. **EB:** *Results from unstructured interviews with women aged 61 to 92 years regarding their perceptions and feelings about their aging bodies suggest that women exhibit the internalization of ageist beauty norms, even as they assert that health is more important to them than physical attractiveness and comment on the "naturalness" of the aging process (Hurd, 2000).*

## Multicultural

- Assess for the influence of cultural beliefs, norms, and values on the client's body image. **EBN:** *The client's body image may be based on cultural perceptions, as well as influences from the larger social context. Use of pan-ethnic status such as Asian or Hispanic may obscure important ethnic group differences (Cochran, 1998; Doswell & Erlen, 1998; Leininger & McFarland, 2002; Yates, Edman, & Aruguete, 2004).*
- Validate the client's feelings with regard to the impact of health status on disturbances in body image. **EBN:** *Validation is a therapeutic communication technique that lets the client know that the nurse has heard and understands what was said and promotes the nurse-client relationship (Heineken, 1998).*
- Acknowledge that body image disturbances can affect all individuals regardless of culture, race, or ethnicity. **EBN:** *Body image disturbances are pervasive across western cultures and appear to increase in other cultures with acculturation to western ideals (Thomas & Ricciardelli, 2000; Hebl, King, & Lin J 2004).* **EB:** *Non-Caucasian girls were found to report higher internalization of the thin ideal than their Caucasian peers (Hermes & Keele, 2003).*
- Assess for the presence of conflicting cultural demands. **EBN:** *Poor peer socialization and family rigidity were found to be related to the preoccupation with body size and slimness in a young female Mexican-American population (Kuba & Harris, 2001).*

- Assess for the presence of depressive symptoms. **EBN:** *Recent studies have shown that body image attitudes were significantly related to depressive symptoms in a study of diverse postpartum women (Walker, Timmerman, King, & Sterling, 2002).*

## Home Care

- Above interventions may be adapted for home care use.
- Assess client's stage of grieving or acceptance of body change on return to home setting. Include the future role of sexuality in the psychological assessment of acceptance as appropriate. *Body change or loss of a body part raises multiple issues relating to self-concept, as well as continuing functional ability and dealing with responses of others.*
- Assess family/caregiver level of acceptance of client's body changes. *Negative feedback from family/caregiver can influence client's reactions and ability to adjust to body changes negatively.*
- Recognize that older women may continue their younger preoccupation with weight and recurrent dieting, despite being at normal weight. Assess source of low weight or weight loss with this in mind. **EB:** *Reports suggest that elderly women continue to be preoccupied with being thin. Increased awareness of eating habits and weight preoccupation in elderly women has been recommended (Fallaz et al, 1999).*
- Be accepting of body changes in all interactions with client and family/caregivers. *Acceptance promotes trust and assures client that others can be accepting of him or her.*
- Help client to see new or changing roles in family. Point out ways in which the community can help support client and family strengths.
- ▲ Refer to medical social services to address level of acceptance and possible financial impact of changes. *Social worker visits can support the client or caregivers with dedicated time and can work with the nurse to be supportive and adapt interventions to promote acceptance. The nurse or social worker can introduce or reinforce use of community resources.*
- Teach all aspects of care. Involve client and caregivers in self-care as soon as possible. Do this in stages if client still has difficulty looking at or touching changed body part. *The quicker the involvement in self-care, the greater are the chances for permanent acceptance and positive self-esteem.*
- Teach family and client complications of medical condition and when to contact physician.
- ▲ Refer to occupational therapy if necessary to evaluate home setting for safety and adaptive equipment and to assist client with return to normal activities. *The quicker the reinvolvement in activies of daily living (ADLs) and self-care, the greater are the chances for permanent acceptance and positive self-esteem.*
- ▲ If appropriate, provide home health aide support to help the client and family through ADL transition.
- ▲ Refer to physical therapy if necessary to build range-of-motion, flexibility, and strength; prevent contractures; assist with transfer or ambulation safety; or obtain use of a prosthetic device in the home setting.
- Assess for and promote good nutrition and sleep patterns. Adapt nutrition to specific physiological situations (e.g., client with ostomy). *Good nutrition and sleep patterns promote faster healing and better coping.*
- Assist family with obtaining needed supplies. *Cost of ostomy supplies and adaptive equipment can be an added stressor for the client. Community resources can assist.*

- • Be alert to the differential body image found in clients with schizophrenia that may contribute to the need for assisted living and avoidance of competitive situations. **EB:** *Five body image factors differentiated individuals with schizophrenia from those without: dullness in movement, powerlessness, unusually strong digestive function, lifelessness, and fragility (Koide, Iizuka, & Fujihara et al, 2002).* Refer to care plan for **Powerlessness.**
- ▲ Refer for psychiatric home health care services for client reassurance and implementation of a therapeutic regimen. Psychiatric home care nurses can address issues relating to client's distorted body image. *Behavioral interventions in the home can assist client to participate more effectively in treatment plan (Patusky et al, 1996).*

## Client/Family Teaching

- • Teach appropriate care of surgical site (e.g., mastectomy site, amputation site, ostomy site). *Patient teaching by enterostomal therapist (ET) nurses may alleviate problems associated with altered body image in relation to the presence of an ostomy (Tomaselli et al, 1991).*
- • Inform client of available community support groups; offer to make initial phone call. *Motivation, sharing of experiences, camaraderie with and support from peers, and knowledge of not being alone have been identified as advantages of group learning (Payne, 1993).*
- ▲ Refer the client to counseling for help adjusting to body change. *Counseling is important for a client who is trying to create a new body ideal or work through a grief process (Price, 1990).*
- • Provide printed material and didactic information for significant others. *Some significant others prefer to receive didactic material rather than vent their feelings as a way of showing support (Northouse & Peters-Golden, 1993).*
- • Encourage significant others to offer support. *Social support from significant others enhances both emotional and physical health (Badger, 1990).*
- • Direct social support as follows: instruct regarding practical care (bandaging); encourage appraisal support (listening); encourage self-esteem support (favorable comparisons between client's and others' appearance); and encourage sense of belonging (assist with socializing). The preceding are four categories of support recognized in the body-image care model. *Clients with an active social support network are likely to make better progress than those without support (Price, 1990).*
- ▲ Refer an interdisciplinary team to clients with ostomies who are having difficulty with personal acceptance, personal and social body image disruption, sexual concerns, reduced self-care skills, and the management of surgical complications. **EB:** *Many clinical studies have found clients with ostomies to be a group facing multiple adjustment demands. One of these demands is coping with a significant change in body image. At the Medical College of Wisconsin, a team approach has been initiated; the ET nurse, the psychologist, and the surgeon deal with body image concerns together. The multidisciplinary approach has been demonstrated to be successful in facilitating adaptation to an altered body image (Walsh et al, 1995).*

## evolve WEBSITES FOR EDUCATION

See the EVOLVE website for World Wide Web resources for client education.

## REFERENCES

B

Bachelor D: Hair and cancer chemotherapy: consequences and nursing care—a literature study, *Eur J Cancer Care* 10(3):147, 2001.
Badger V: Men with cardiovascular disease and their spouses: coping, health and marital adjustment, *Arch Psychiatr Nurs* 4:319, 1990.
Blouin AG, Goldfield GS: Body image and steroid use in male bodybuilders, *Int J Eat Disord* 18(2):159, 1995.
Cochran M: Tears have no color, *Am J Nurs* 98(6):53, 1998.
Doswell W, Erlen J: Multicultural issues and ethical concerns in the delivery of revising care interventions, *Nurs Clin North Am* 33(2):353, 1998.
Fallaz AF, Bernstein M, Van Nes MC et al: Weight loss preoccupation in aging women: a review, *J Nutr Health Aging* 3:177-181, 1999.
Fauerbach JA, Heinberg LJ, Lawrence JW et al: Coping with body image changes following a disfiguring burn injury, *Health Psychology* 21(2):115-121, 2002.
Harris M, Eberly M, Cumella EJ: Helping teenagers with eating disorders, *Nursing* 34(10):24-25, 2004.
Hebl MR, King EB, Lin J: The swimsuit becomes us all: ethnicity, gender, and vulnerability to self-objectification, *Pers Soc Psychol Bull* 30(10):1322-1331, 2004.
Heineken J: Patient silence is not necessarily client satisfaction: communication in home care nursing, *Home Healthc Nurse* 16(2): 115-120, 1998.
Hermes SF, Keel PK: The influence of puberty and ethnicity on awareness and internalization of the thin ideal, *Int J Eat Disord* 33(4):465-467, 2003.
Hurd LC: Older women's body image and embodied experience: an exploration, *J Women Aging* 12(3-4):77-97, 2000.
Johnson J: Caring for the woman who's had a mastectomy, *Am J Nurs* 94:24-31, 1994.
Koide R, Iizuka S, Fujihara K et al: Body image, symptoms and insight in chronic schizophrenia, *Psychiatry Clin Neurosci* 56(1): 9-15, 2002.
Kopel SJ, Eiser C, Cool P et al: Brief report: assessment of body image in survivors of childhood cancer, *J Pediatr Psychol* 23(2): 141-147, 1998.
Kuba SA, Harris DJ: Eating disturbances in women of color: an exploratory study of contextual factors in the development of disordered eating in Mexican American women, *Health Care Women Int* 22(3):281-298, 2001.
Leininger MM, McFarland MR: *Transcultural nursing: concepts, theories, research and practices,* ed 3, New York, 2002, McGraw-Hill.
Lindop E, Cannon S: Evaluating the self-assessed support needs of women with breast cancer, *J Adv Nurs* 34(6):760-771, 2001.
MacGinley K: Nursing care of the patient with altered body image, *Br J Nurs* 2:1098-1102, 1993.
Newell RJ: Altered body image: a fear-avoidance model of psycho-social difficulties following disfigurement, *J Adv Nurs* 30(5): 1230-1238, 1999.
Nochi M: Reconstructing self-narratives in coping with traumatic brain injury, *Soc Sci Med* 51(12):1795-1804, 2000.
Northouse L, Peters-Golden H: Cancer and the family: strategies to assist spouses, *Semin Oncol Nurs* 9:74-82, 1993.
Patusky KL, Rodning C, Martinez-Kratz M: Clinical lessons in psychiatric home care: a case study approach, *J Home Health Case Manage* 9:18, 1996.
Payne J: The contribution of group learning to the rehabilitation of spinal cord injured adults, *Rehabil Nurs* 18:375-379, 1993.
Phillips K: Child and Adolescent Action Center, *Nami E-News,* 2003. Available at http://www.nami.org/youth/dysmorphic.html, accessed on March 12, 2003.
Pohl C, Winland-Brown J: The meaning of disability in a caring environment, *J Nurs Adm* 22(6):29-35, 1992.
Price B: A model for body-image care, *J Adv Nurs* 15(5):585-593, 1990.
Price B: Altered body image: managing social encounters, *Int J Palliat Nurs* 6(4):179-185, 2000.
Rao S: Fluoxetine was safe and effective for body dysmorphic disorder, *Evid Based Ment Health* 5(4):119, 2002.
Sedlak CA, Doheny MO: Fashion tips for women with osteoporosis, *Orthop Nurs* 19(5):31-35, 2000.
Souto CMR, Garcia TR: Construction and validation of a body image rating scale: a preliminary study *Int J Nurs Terminol Classif* 13(4):117-126, 2002.
Thomas K, Ricciardelli I: Gender traits and self-concept as indicators of problem eating and body dissatisfaction among children, *Sex Roles* 43(7/8):441, 2000.
Tomaselli N, Jenks J, Morin K: Body image in patients with stomas: a critical review of the literature, *J ET Nurs* 18:95-9, 1991.
Townsend MC: *Psychiatric mental health nursing: concepts of care,* Saddle River, NJ, 2003, FA Davis.
Wahl AK, Gjengedal E, Hanestad BR: The bodily suffering of living with severe psoriasis: in-depth interviews with 22 hospitalized patients with psoriasis, *Q Health Res* 12(2):250-261, 2002.

Walker L, Timmerman GM, Kim M et al: Relationships between body image and depressive symptoms during postpartum in ethnically diverse, low income women, *Women Health* 36(3):101-121, 2002.
Walsh BA et al: Multidisciplinary management of altered body image in the patient with an ostomy, *J Wound Ostomy Continence Nurs* 22(5):227-236, 1995.
Welch JL, Austin JK: Stressors, coping and depression in haemodialysis patients, *J Adv Nurs* 33(2):200-207, 2001.
Yates A, Edman J, Aruguete M: Ethnic differences in BMI and body/self-dissatisfaction among Whites, Asian subgroups, Pacific Islanders, and African-Americans, *J Adolesc Health* 34(4):300-307, 2004.
Yu-Jen C, Yiing-Mei L, Shuh-Jen S et al: Unbearable weight: young adult women's experiences of being overweight, *J Nurs Res* 12(2):153-160, 2004.
Zacharias DR, Gilig CA, Foxall MJ: Quality of life and coping in patients with gynecologic cancer and their spouses, *Oncol Nurs Forum* 21:1699-1706, 1994.

# Risk for imbalanced Body temperature

*Betty J. Ackley*

**NANDA**

## Definition

At risk for failure to maintain body temperature within a normal range

## Risk Factors

Altered metabolic rate, extremes of age or weight, exposure to cool/cold or hot/warm environments, dehydration, inactivity or vigorous activity, medications that cause vasoconstriction or vasodilatation, sedation, clothing inappropriate for environmental temperature, illness or trauma that affects body temperature regulation

## Related Factors (r/t)

See Risk Factors

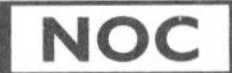

## Outcomes (Nursing Outcomes Classification)

### Suggested NOC Outcomes

Thermoregulation, Thermoregulation: Newborn

**Example NOC Outcome with Indicators**

**Thermoregulation** as evidenced by the following indicators: Body temperature WNL/Skin temperature IER/Skin color changes not present/Hydration adequate/Reported thermal comfort (Rate each indicator of **Thermoregulation:** 1 = severely compromised, 2 = substantially compromised, 3 = moderately compromised, 4 = mildly compromised, 5 = not compromised [see Section I].)

IER, In expected range; WNL, within normal limits.

## Client Outcomes

B

### Client Will (Specify Time Frame):

- Maintain temperature within normal range.
- Explain measures needed to maintain normal temperature
- Identify symptoms of hypothermia or hyperthermia

NIC

## Interventions (Nursing Interventions Classification)

### Suggested NIC Interventions

Temperature Regulation, Temperature Regulation: Intraoperative, Vital Signs Monitoring

**Example NIC Activities—Temperature Regulation**

Institute a continuous core temperature monitoring device as appropriate; promote adequate fluid and nutritional intake

## Nursing Interventions and Rationales

- Monitor temperature q1 to 4 hours or use continuous temperature monitoring as appropriate. *Normal adult temperature is usually identified at 98.6° F (37° C), but in actuality the normal temperature fluctuates throughout the day. In the early morning, it may be as low as 96.4° F (35.8° C) and in the late afternoon or evening as high as 99.1° F (37.3° C) (Bickley & Szilagyj, 2002). Disease, injury, or pharmacological agents may impair regulation of body temperature (Kasper et al, 2005).*
- If client is awake, take the temperature orally in the adult, instead of by use of a tympanic thermometer or an axillary temperature. **EBN:** *Oral temperatures provide a more accurate temperature than tympanic thermometers (Fisk & Arcona, 2001; Giuliano et al, 2000; Lee et al, 1999). Axillary temperatures are often inaccurate (Fulbrook, 1997). The oral temperature is usually accurate even in the intubated client (Fallis, 2002). The SolarTherm and DataTherm devices correlated strongly with core body temperatures obtained from a pulmonary artery catheter (Smith, 2004).*
- Take vital signs q1 to 4 hours, noting changes associated with hypothermia: first, increased blood pressure, pulse, and respirations; then, decreased values as hypothermia progresses (Edwards, 1999).
- Monitor the client for signs of hypothermia (e.g., shivering, cool skin, piloerection, pallor, slow capillary refill, cyanotic nailbeds, decreased mentation, dysrhythmias) (Edwards, 1999).
- Note changes in vital signs associated with hyperthermia: rapid, bounding pulse; increased respiratory rate; and decreased blood pressure with orthostatic hypotension present (Worfolk, 2000). *Consistent monitoring promotes prevention and early intervention in clients with altered cardiopulmonary status associated with hypothermia or hyperthermia.*

- Monitor the client for signs of hyperthermia (e.g., headache, nausea and vomiting, weakness, absence of sweating, delirium, and coma) (Worfolk, 2000). *Monitoring for defining characteristics of hypothermia and hyperthermia allows for prevention and/or early intervention.*
- Maintain a consistent room temperature (72° F; 22.2° C). *A consistent temperature limits environmental effects on thermoregulation.*
- Promote adequate nutrition and hydration. *These measures help maintain a normal body temperature.*
- Adjust clothing to facilitate passive warming or cooling as appropriate. *This will help maintain a normal body temperature.*
- See Nursing Interventions and Rationales for **Hypothermia** or **Hyperthermia** as appropriate.

## Geriatric

- Do not allow geriatric clients to become chilled. Keep covered when giving a bath or doing a procedure. Offer socks to wear when in bed and a head covering if desired. *Older adults have a decreased ability to adapt to temperature extremes and need protection from extreme environmental temperatures. Older adults have a higher threshold of central temperature for sweating, diminished or absent sweating, impaired warmth or cold perception, impaired shiver response, diminished thermogenesis, abnormal peripheral blood flow response to warmth or cold, and compromised cardiovascular reserve (Ballester & Harchelroad, 1999; Florez-Duquet & McDonald, 1998).*

▲ Assess medication profile for potential risk of drug-related altered body temperature. *Anesthetics, barbiturates, salicylates, nonsteroidal anti-inflammatory drugs (NSAIDs), diuretics, antihistamines, anticholinergics, beta-blockers, and thyroid hormones have been linked to altered body temperatures (Carroll, 2002; Haskell et al, 1997).*

▲ Ensure that elderly clients receive sufficient fluids during hot days and stay out of the sun. *The elderly may have trouble walking independently to obtain fluids, have decreased thirst sensation, and have chronic illnesses that predispose to heat stroke (Carroll, 2002).*

## Pediatric

- Recognize that pediatric clients have a decreased ability to adapt to temperature extremes. Take the following actions to maintain body temperature in the infant or young child:
  - Keep the head covered.
  - Use blankets to keep the client warm.
  - Keep client covered during procedures, transport, and diagnostic testing.
  - Maintain a consistent room temperature of 72° F (22.2° C).

  *These measures can help prevent hypothermia in the child, which is a very possible occurrence, especially in the pediatric trauma client (Bernardo & Henker, 1999). The combination of a relatively larger body surface area, smaller body fluid volume, less well-developed temperature control mechanisms, and smaller amount of protective body fat*

B

*limits the infant and child's ability to maintain normal temperatures (Hockenberry, 2005).*

- Recognize that the infant and small child are vulnerable to develop heat stroke in hot weather and ensure they receive sufficient fluids and are protected from hot environments. *Infants and young children are at risk for heat stroke for many reasons including a decreased thermoregulatory ability in the young body and the inability to obtain their own fluids (Carroll, 2002).*

### Home Care

- Above interventions may be adapted for home care use.

#### Prevention of Hypothermia in Cold Weather

- Avoid prolonged exposure outside. Wear a hat and gloves. Wool or fleece clothing can help to maintain body heat.
- Keep room temperature at 68° to 72° F (20° to 22.2° C).
- Ensure adequate source of heat; refer to social services if client is low income and heat could be turned off.
- Help elderly client determine a warm environment they can go to for safety in cold weather if his or her home environment is no longer warm.

#### Prevention of Hyperthermia in Hot Weather

- Encourage the client to wear lightweight loose-fitting cotton clothing. Help the elderly remove their usual sweaters.
- Ensure that client drinks adequate amounts of fluids (2000 mL/day), avoiding caffeine and alcohol. *Adequate fluids are needed during hot weather to replace fluids lost from sweating. Fluids containing caffeine and alcohol can serve as diuretics and decrease fluid volume in the body.*
- Help client obtain a fan to increase evaporation, or an air conditioner as needed, using social services if needed. *Air moving across the skin enhances evaporative cooling if the temperature is below 95° F (35° C)(Carroll, 2002).*
- Take the temperature of the elderly in hot weather. *The elderly may not be able to tell that they are hot because of decreased sensation (Worfolk, 2000).*
- Help elderly client determine a cool environment they can go to for safety in hot weather.

### Client/Family Teaching

- Teach the client and family the signs of hypothermia and hyperthermia and the appropriate actions they should take if either condition develops. *Adequate teaching improves compliance and promotes safety.*
- Teach the client and family proper method for taking temperature. *Optimal placement of the appropriate device is essential for accurate monitoring.*
- Teach to avoid alcohol and medications that depress cerebral function. *When the client is sedated or under the influence of alcohol, mentation is depressed, resulting in decreased activities to maintain an adequate body temperature. In addition, traumatic injuries are associated with alcohol and illicit drug use (Ruffolo, 2002).*

B

## evolve WEBSITES FOR EDUCATION

See the EVOLVE website for World Wide Web resources for client education.

## REFERENCES


Ballester JM, Harchelroad FP: Hypothermia: an easy-to-miss, dangerous disorder in winter weather, *Geriatrics* 54(2):51, 1999.

Bernardo LM, Henker R: Thermoregulation in pediatric trauma: an overview, *Int J Trauma Nurs* 5(3):101, 1999.

Bickley LS, Szilagyj PJ: *Bate's guide to physical examination and history taking*, ed 8, Philadelphia, 2002, JB Lippincott.

Carroll P: The heat is on: protecting your patients from nature's silent killer, *Home Healthcare Nurse* 20(6): 376, 2002.

Edwards SL: Hypothermia, *Prof Nurse* 14(4):253, 1999.

Elliott F: You'd better watch out, *Occup Health Safe* 73(11):76, 2004.

Fallis WM: Monitoring urinary bladder temperature in the intensive care unit: state of the science, *Am J Crit Care* 11(1):38, 2002.

Fisk J, Arcona S: Comparing tympanic membrane and pulmonary artery catheter temperatures, *Dimens Crit Care Nurs* 20(2):44, 2001.

Florez-Duquet M, McDonald RB: Cold-induced thermoregulation and biological aging, *Physiol Rev* 78(2):339, 1998.

Fulbrook P: Core body temperature measurement: a comparison of axilla, tympanic membrane and pulmonary artery blood temperature, *Intensive Crit Care Nurs* 13(5):266, 1997.

Giuliano KK, Giuliano AJ, Scott SS et al: Temperature measurement in critically ill adults: a comparison of tympanic and oral methods, *Am J Crit Care* 9(4):254, 2000.

Haskell RM, Boruta B, Rotondo MF et al: Hypothermia, *AACN Clin Issues* 8(3):368, 1997.

Hockenberry MJ: *Wong's essentials of pediatric nursing*, ed 7, St Louis, 2005, Mosby.

Kasper DL, Braunwald E, Fauci AS, et al: *Harrison's principles of internal medicine*, ed 16, New York, 2005, McGraw-Hill.

Lee VK, McKenzie NE, Cathcart M: Ear and oral temperatures under usual practice conditions, *Res Nurs Pract* 1(1), 1999.

Ruffolo D: Hypothermia in trauma: the cold hard facts, *RN* 65(2):46, 2002.

Smith LS: Temperature measurement in critical care adults: a comparison of thermometry and measurement routes, *Biol Res Nurs* 6(2):117, 2004.

Worfolk JB: Heat waves: their impact on the health of elders, *Geriatr Nurs* 21(2):70, 2000.


# Bowel incontinence evolve

*Mikel Gray*

**NANDA**

## Definition

Change in normal bowel elimination habits characterized by involuntary passage of stool

## Defining Characteristics

Constant dribbling of soft stool, fecal odor; inability to delay defecation; rectal urgency; self-report of inability to feel rectal fullness or presence of stool in bowel; fecal staining of underclothing; recognition of rectal fullness but reported inability to expel formed stool; inattention to urge to defecate; inability to recognize urge to defecate; irritation of perianal skin

## Related Factors (r/t)

Change in stool consistency (diarrhea, constipation, fecal impaction); abnormal motility (metabolic disorders, inflammatory bowel disease, infectious disease, drug induced motil-

B

ity disorders, food intolerance); defects in rectal vault function (low rectal compliance from ischemia, fibrosis, radiation, infectious proctitis, Hirschprung's disease, local or infiltrating neoplasm, severe rectocele); sphincter dysfunction (obstetric- or traumatic-induced incompetence, fistula or abscess, prolapse, third-degree hemorrhoids, high-tone pelvic floor muscle dysfunction); neurological disorders impacting gastrointestinal motility, rectal vault function and sphincter function (cerebrovascular accident, spinal injury, traumatic brain injury, central nervous system tumor, advanced stage dementia, encephalopathy, profound mental retardation, multiple sclerosis, myelodysplasia and related neural tube defects, gastroparesis of diabetes mellitus, heavy metal poisoning, chronic alcoholism, infectious or autoimmune neurological disorders, myasthenia gravis)

NOC

## Outcomes (Nursing Outcomes Classification)

### Suggested NOC Outcomes

Bowel Continence; Bowel Elimination

**Example NOC Outcome with Indicators**

**Bowel Continence** as evidenced by the following indicators: Maintains predictable pattern of evacuation of stool/Maintains control of passage of stool/Evacuates stool at least every 3 days (Rate each indicator of **Bowel Continence:** 1 = never demonstrated, 2 = rarely demonstrated, 3 = sometimes demonstrated, 4 = often demonstrated, 5 = consistently demonstrated [see Section I].)

## Client Outcomes

**Client Will (Specify Time Frame):**

- Have regular, complete evacuation of fecal contents from the rectal vault (pattern may vary from every day to every 3 to 5 days) (Roig et al, 1993)
- Have regulation of stool consistency (soft, formed stools)
- Reduce or eliminate frequency of incontinent episodes
- Demonstrate intact skin in the perianal/perineal area
- Demonstrate the ability to isolate, contract and relax pelvic muscles (when incontinence related to sphincter incompetence or high-tone pelvic floor dysfunction)
- Increase pelvic muscle strength (when incontinence related to sphincter incompetence)

NIC

## Interventions (Nursing Interventions Classification)

### Suggested NIC Interventions

Bowel Incontinence Care, Bowel Incontinence Care: Encopresis, Bowel Training

**Example NIC Interventions—Bowel Incontinence Care**

Determine physical or psychological cause of fecal incontinence; instruct client family to record fecal output, as appropriate

B

## Nursing Interventions and Rationales

- In a reasonably private setting, directly question any client at risk about the presence of fecal incontinence. If the client reports altered bowel elimination patterns, problems with bowel control or "uncontrollable diarrhea," complete a focused nursing history including previous and present bowel elimination routines, dietary history, frequency and volume of uncontrolled stool loss, aggravating and alleviating factors. *Unless questioned directly, clients are unlikely to report the presence of fecal incontinence (Schultz et al, 1997). The nursing history determines the patterns of stool elimination, to characterize involuntary stool loss, and the likely etiology of the incontinence (Norton & Chelvanaygam, 2000).*
- Complete a focused physical assessment including inspection of perineal skin, pelvic muscle strength assessment, digital examination of the rectum for presence of impaction and anal sphincter strength, and evaluation of functional status (mobility, dexterity, visual acuity). *A focused physical examination assists in determining the severity of fecal leakage, and its likely etiology. A functional assessment provides information concerning the impact of functional status on stool elimination patterns and incontinence (Gray & Burns, 1996).*
- Complete an assessment of cognitive function. *Dementia, acute confusion, and mental retardation are risk factors for fecal incontinence (O'Donnell et al, 1992; Norton & Chelvanaygam, 2000).*
- Document patterns of stool elimination and incontinent episodes through a bowel record, including frequency of bowel movements, stool consistency, frequency and severity of incontinent episodes, precipitating factors, and dietary and fluid intake. *This document, used to confirm the verbal history, assists in determining the likely etiology of stool incontinence and serves as a baseline to evaluate treatment efficacy (Norton & Chelvanaygam, 2000).*
- Assess stool consistency and its influence on risk for stool loss. *Several classification systems for stool have been promulgated (Bliss et al, 2001). They assist the nurse and client to differentiate between normal soft, formed stool, hardened stools associated with constipation, and liquid stools associated with diarrhea.* **EBN:** *A study of stool consistency found good reliability when evaluated by professional nurses, student nurses, and clients. Word-only descriptors yielded equivocal consistency when assessed by subjects as did tools that combined words with illustrations of various stool consistencies (Bliss et al, 2001).*
- Identify conditions contributing to or causing fecal incontinence. *Fecal incontinence is frequently multifactorial. Accurate assessment of the probable etiology of fecal incontinence is necessary to select a treatment plan likely to control or eliminate the condition (Norton & Chelvanaygam, 2000).*

B

- Improve access to toileting:
  - Identify usual toileting patterns among persons in the acute care or long-term care facility and plan opportunities for toileting accordingly.
  - Provide assistance with toileting for clients with limited access or impaired functional status (mobility, dexterity, access).
  - Institute a prompted toileting program for persons with impaired cognitive status (retardation, dementia).
  - Provide adequate privacy for toileting.
  - Respond promptly to requests for assistance with toileting.

  *Acute or transient fecal incontinence frequently occurs in the acute care or long-term care facility because of inadequate access to toileting facilities, insufficient assistance with toileting, or inadequate privacy when attempting to toilet (Bliss et al, 2000; Gray and Burns, 1996).*
- Counsel clients with fecal incontinence associated with liquid stools (diarrhea) about methods to normalize stool consistency via dietary fiber or fiber supplements. *A liquid stool is associated with an increased likelihood of fecal incontinence (Bliss et al, 2000).* **EBN:** *Daily supplementation of dietary fiber using a product containing psyllium improved stool consistency and reduced frequency of incontinent stools (Bliss et al, 2001).*
- For the client with intermittent episodes of fecal incontinence related to acute changes in stool consistency, begin a bowel re-education program consisting of:
  - Cleansing the bowel of impacted stool if indicated
  - Normalizing stool consistency by adequate intake of fluids (30 mL/kg of body weight/day) and dietary or supplemental fiber
  - Establishing a regular routine of fecal elimination based on established patterns of bowel elimination (patterns established prior to onset of incontinence)

  *Bowel reeducation is designed to reestablish normal defecation patterns and to normalize stool consistency in order to reduce or eliminate the risk of recurring fecal incontinence associated with changes in stool consistency (Doughty, 1996).*
- Begin a prompted defecation program for the adult with dementia, mental retardation, or related learning disabilities. *Prompted urine and fecal elimination programs have been shown to reduce or eliminate incontinence in the long-term care facility and in community settings (Doughty, 1996; Smith et al, 1994).*
- Begin a scheduled, stimulation defecation program for persons with neurological conditions causing fecal incontinence including the following steps:
  - Cleanse the bowel of impacted fecal material before beginning the program.
  - Implement strategies to normalize stool consistency including adequate intake of fluid and fiber and avoidance of foods associated with diarrhea.
  - Determine a regular schedule for bowel elimination (typically every day or every other day) based on prior patterns of bowel elimination whenever feasible.
  - Provide a stimulus before assisting the client to a position on the toilet; digital stimulation, a stimulating suppository, "mini-enema," or pulsed evacuation enema may be used for stimulation.

  *The scheduled, stimulated program relies on consistency of stool, and a mechanical or chemical stimulus to produce a bolus contraction of the rectum with evacuation of fecal material*

B

*(Doughty, 1996; Dunn & Galka; 1994; King et al, 1994, Munchiando & Kendall, 1993).*

- ▲ Begin a reeducation or pelvic floor muscle exercise program for the person with sphincter incompetence or high-tone pelvic floor muscle dysfunction of the pelvic muscles, or refer persons with fecal incontinence related to sphincter dysfunction to a nurse specialist or other therapist with clinical expertise in these techniques of care. *A systematic review found insufficient evidence to conclude that bowel reeducation or pelvic floor muscle exercise programs are effective for the management of fecal incontinence in adults, but the existing evidence does provide adequate support to consider implementing this intervention in selected patients, particularly given the potential for benefit in the absence of harmful side effects (Norton et al, 2003).*
- • Begin a pelvic muscle biofeedback program among clients with urgency to defecate and fecal incontinence related to recurrent diarrhea. *Pelvic muscle reeducation, including biofeedback, can reduce uncontrolled loss of stool among persons who experience urgency and diarrhea as provocative factors for fecal incontinence (Chiarioni et al, 1993).*
- • Thoroughly cleanse and dry the perianal and perineal skin daily using a cleanser capable of removing irritants, including urine, stool, and materials. Select a product with a slightly acidic pH designed to preserve its acid mantle. Select a product that is designed to remove irritants from the skin with minimal physical force. Avoid vigorous scrubbing with water, soap, and a washcloth. Consider selection of a product with a moisturizer. *Traditional soaps tend to be alkaline, interfering with the natural acid mantle of the integument and increasing its susceptibility to irritant dermatitis and secondary infection. Brisk scrubbing may exacerbate skin erosion and further increase the risk of irritation and infection (Gray, Ratliff, & Donovan, 2002; Gray, 2004).*
- • Cleanse the perineal and perianal skin following each episode of fecal incontinence. *Frequent cleaning with soap and water may compromise perianal skin integrity and enhance the irritation produced by fecal leakage (Gray et al, 2002; Gray, 2004).*
- • Apply a moisture barrier containing dimethicone or zinc oxide to patients with severe urinary incontinence or those with double urinary and fecal incontinence. *Clients with very severe incontinence and those with double fecal and urinary incontinence (particularly when the stool is liquified) typically require a product with vigorous moisture barrier qualities. Petrolatum based products containing dimethicone or zinc oxide are preferred (Gray, Ratliff, & Donovan, 2002; Gray, 2004).*
- • When cleansing a client with a moisture barrier containing zinc oxide, avoid vigorous scrubbing or use of a traditional washcloth to remove the paste. Instead, cleanse fecal materials away from the skin, leaving a clean layer of zinc oxide paste when cleansing after a single episode or gently removing the paste with mineral oil. *Pastes containing zinc oxide are difficult to remove, and it is not necessary to completely remove the product every time the perineal skin is cleansed. When deep cleansing and inspection of the underlying skin are indicated, mineral oil can be used to remove the paste without the need for brisk scrubbing.*
- ▲ Consult the physician concerning use of a moisture barrier with active healing ingredients when perineal dermatitis exists. Apply and teach care providers to use

B

the product sparingly when applying to affected areas. **EBN:** *Xenaderm contains active ingredients (Balsam Peru, trypsin, and castor oil) that have been shown more effective than placebo for the management of partial thickness wounds in patients with urinary or fecal incontinence (Gray & Jones, 2004). An thin layer of an antifungal powders may be layered beneath the ointment, but application of excessive may paradoxically retain moisture and diminish its effectiveness (Evans & Gray, 2003; Gray, Ratliff, & Donovan, 2002).*

- • Assist the client to select and apply a containment device for occasional episodes of fecal incontinence. *A fecal containment device will prevent soiling of clothing and reduce odors in the client with uncontrolled stool loss (Brazelli et al, 2003).*
- • Teach the caregiver of the client with frequent episodes of fecal incontinence and limited mobility to regularly monitor the sacrum and perineal area for pressure ulcerations. *Limited mobility, particularly when combined with fecal incontinence, increases the risk of pressure ulceration. Routine cleansing, pressure reduction techniques, and management of fecal and urinary incontinence reduce this risk (Johanson et al, 1997; Schnelle et al, 1997).*
- ▲ Teach the client with more frequent stool loss to apply an anal continence plug in consultation with the physician. *The anal continence plug is a device that can reduce or eliminate persistent liquid or solid stool incontinence in selected clients (Doherty, 2004).*
- • Apply a fecal pouch to the client with frequent stool loss, particularly when fecal incontinence produces altered perianal skin integrity. *Fecal pouches contain stool loss, reduce odor, and protect the perianal skin from chemical irritation related to contact with stool (Fiers & Thayer, 2000; Waldrop & Doughty, 2000).*
- ▲ For the patient with acute fecal incontinence and liquid stools, consult with a nurse practitioner or physician concerning placement of a specialized bowel management system. *The Zassi Bowel management system was specially designed for the management of fecal output in patients who are bedridden or immobile for a prolonged period. Initial clinical experience supports the use of this specially designed product is more effective in containing fecal outpour than large bore urinary catheters or similar "home built" systems (Echols et al, 2004).*

## Geriatric

- • Evaluate all elderly clients for established or acute fecal incontinence when the elderly client enters the acute or long-term care facility and intervene as indicated. *The rate of fecal incontinence in the acute care facility is as high as 3% and as high as 50% of residents in long-term care facilities (Egan et al, 1983).*
- • Evaluate cognitive status in the elderly person with a NEECHAM confusion scale (Neelan et al, 1992) for acute cognitive changes, a Folstein Mini-Mental Status Examination (Folstein et al, 1975), or other tool as indicated. *Acute or established dementias increase the risk of fecal incontinence among the elderly.*

## Home Care

- • Above interventions may be adapted for home care use.

B

- Assess and teach a bowel management program to support continence. Address timing, diet, fluids, and actions taken independently to deal with bowel incontinence. *Identifying factors that change level of incontinence may guide interventions. If client has been taking over-the-counter medications or home remedies, it is important to consider their influence.*
- Instruct caregiver to provide clothing that is nonrestrictive, can be manipulated easily for toileting, and can be changed with ease. *Avoidance of complicated maneuvers increases the chance of success in toileting programs and decreases the client's risk for embarrassing incontinent episodes.*
- Assist the family in arranging care in a way that allows the client to participate in family or favorite activities without embarrassment. *Careful planning can both help client retain dignity and maintain integrity of family patterns.*
- ▲ If the client is limited to bed (or bed and chair), provide a commode or bedpan that can be easily accessed. If necessary, refer the client to physical therapy services to learn side transfers and to build strength for transfers.
- ▲ If the client is frequently incontinent, refer for home health aide services to assist with hygiene and skin care.
- Teach the client and family to perform a bowel reeducation program, scheduled, stimulated program, or other strategies to manage fecal incontinence.
- Teach the client and family about common dietary sources for fiber, as well as supplemental fiber or bulking agents as indicated.
- ▲ Refer the family to support services to assist with in-home management of fecal incontinence as indicated.
- Teach nursing colleagues and nonprofessional care providers the importance of providing toileting opportunities and adequate privacy for the client in an acute or long-term care facility.

NOTE: Refer to nursing diagnoses **Diarrhea** and **Constipation** for detailed management of these related conditions.

## evolve WEBSITES FOR EDUCATION

See the EVOLVE website for World Wide Web resources for client education.

## REFERENCES

Bliss DZ, Larson SJ, Burr JK et al: Reliability of a stool consistency classification system, *J Wound Ostomy Cont Nurs* 28(6):305-313, 2001.

Bliss DZ, Johnson S, Savik K et al: Fecal incontinence in hospitalized patients who are acutely ill, *Nurs Res* 49(2):101-108, 2000.

Bliss DZ, Jung HJ, Savik K et al: Supplementation with dietary fiber improves fecal incontinence, *Nurs Res* 50(4):203-213, 2001.

Brazzelli M, Shirran E, Vale L: Absorbent products for containing urinary and/or fecal incontinence in adults, *Cochrane Database Syst Rev* 3:CD001406, 1999.

Chiarioni G, Scattolini C, Bonfante F et al: Liquid stool incontinence with severe urgency: anorectal function and effective biofeedback treatment, *Gut* 34(11):1576-1580, 1993.

Doughty DB: A physiologic approach to bowel training, *J Wound Ostomy Cont Nurs* 23:46, 1996.

Doherty W: Managing faecal incontinence or leakage: the Peristeen Anal Plug, *Br J Nurs* 13(21):1293-1297, 2004.

Dunn KL, Galka ML: A comparison of the effectiveness of Therevac SB and bisacodyl suppositories in SCI patients' bowel programs, *Rehabil Nurs* 19:334-338, 1994.
Echols J, Freidman B, Mullins RF et al: *Initial experience with a new system for the control of fecal output for the protection of patients in a large burn center* (Abstract.) John A. Boswick Burn and Wound Care Symposium, February 2004.
Egan M, Plymad K, Thomas T: Incontinence in patients in two district general hospitals, *Nurs Times* 79:22, 1983.
Fiers S, Thayer D: Management of intractable incontinence. In: Doughty DB, editor: *Urinary and fecal incontinence: nursing management,* ed 2, St Louis, 2000, Mosby.
Folstein MF, Folstein EF, McHugh P: Mini Mental State: a practical method of grading the cognitive status of the patient for the clinician, *J Psychiatric Rev* 12:189, 1975.
Gray M, Jones DP: The effect of different formulations of equivalent active ingredients on the performance of two topical wound treatment products, *Ostomy Wound Manage* 50(3):34-44, 2004.
Gray M: Preventing and managing perineal dermatitis: a shared goal for wound and continence care, *J Wound Ostomy Cont Nurs* 31(1 Suppl):S2-S9, 2004.
Gray M, Ratliff C, Donovan A: Perineal skin care for the incontinent patient, *Adv Skin Wound Care* 15(4):170-175, 2002.
Gray ML, Burns SM: Continence management, *Crit Care Nurs Clin North Am* 8:29, 1996.
Grogan TA, Kramer DJ: The rectal trumpet: use of a nasopharyngeal airway to contain fecal incontinence in critically ill patients, *J Wound Ostomy Cont Nurs* 29(4):193, 2002.
Johanson JF, Irizarry F, Doughty A: Risk factors for fecal incontinence in a nursing home population, *J Clin Gastroenterol* 24:156, 1997.
King JC, Currie DM, Wright E: Bowel training in spina bifida: importance of education, patient compliance, age, and anal reflexes, *Arch Phys Med Rehabil* 75:243, 1994.
Munchiando JF, Kendall K: Comparison of the effectiveness of two bowel programs for CVA patients, *Rehabil Nurs* 18:168, 1993.
Neelan VJ et al: Use of the NEECHAM confusion scale to assess acute confusional states of hospitalized older patients. In Funk SG et al, editors: *Key aspects of elder care: managing falls, incontinence and cognitive impairment,* New York, 1992, Springer.
Norton C, Chelvanayagam S: A nursing assessment tool for adult with fecal incontinence, *J Wound Ostomy Cont Nurs* 27:279, 2000.
Norton C, Hosker G, Brazzelli M: Biofeedback and/or sphincter exercises for the treatment of faecal incontinence in adults, *Cochrane Database Syst Rev* 2:CD002111, 2000.
O'Donnell BF, Drachman DA, Barnes HJ et al: Incontinence and troublesome behaviors predict institutionalization in dementia, *J Geriatr Psychiatry Neurol* 5(1):45-52, 1992.
Roig Vila JV, Garcia Garcia A, Flors Alandi C et al: The defecation habits in a normal working population, *Rev Esp Enferm Dig* 84(4):224-230, 1993.
Schnelle JF, Adamson GM, Cruise PA et al: Skin disorders and moisture in incontinent nursing home residents: intervention implications, *J Am Geriatr Soc* 45(10):1182-1188, 1997.
Schultz A, Dickey G, Skoner M: Self-report of incontinence in acute care, *Urol Nurs* 17(1):23-28, 1997.
Smith LJ, Franchetti B, McCoull K et al: A behavioural approach to retraining bowel function after long-standing constipation and faecal impaction in people with learning disabilities, *Dev Med Child Neurol* 36(1):41-49, 1994.
Waldrop J, Doughty DB: Pathophysiology of bowel dysfunction and fecal incontinence. In Doughty DB, editor: *Urinary and fecal incontinence: nursing management,* ed 2, St Louis, 2000, Mosby.

# Effective Breastfeeding

*Arlene Farren*

**NANDA**

## Definition

Mother-infant dyad/family exhibits adequate proficiency and satisfaction with the breastfeeding process

• = Independent; ▲ = Collaborative; EBN = Evidence-Based Nursing; EB = Evidence-Based

B

## Defining Characteristics

Effective mother/infant communication patterns, regular and sustained suckling/swallowing at the breast, appropriate infant weight pattern for age, infant content after feeding, mother able to position infant at breast to promote a successful latch-on response, signs and/or symptoms of oxytocin release, adequate infant elimination patterns for age, eagerness of infant to nurse, maternal verbalization of satisfaction with the breastfeeding process

## Related Factors (r/t)

Infant gestational age >34 weeks, support source, normal infant oral structure, maternal confidence, basic breastfeeding knowledge, normal breast structure

**NOC**

## Outcomes (Nursing Outcomes Classification)

### Suggested NOC Outcomes

Breastfeeding Establishment: Infant, Maternal; Breastfeeding Maintenance

**Example NOC Outcome with Indicators**

**Breastfeeding Establishment: Infant** as evidenced by the following indicators: Proper alignment and latch-on/Proper areolar grasp/Proper areolar compression/Correct suck and tongue placement/Swallowing a minimum of 5 to 10 minutes per breast/Minimum eight feedings per day/Urinations per day appropriate for age/Weight gain appropriate for age (Rate each indicator of **Breastfeeding Establishment: Infant:** 1 = not adequate, 2 = slightly adequate, 3 = moderately adequate, 4 = substantially adequate, 5 = totally adequate [see Section I].)

## Client Outcomes

**Client Will (Specify Time Frame):**

- Maintain effective breastfeeding
- Maintain normal growth patterns (infant)
- Verbalize satisfaction with breastfeeding process (mother)

**NIC**

## Interventions (Nursing Interventions Classification)

### Suggested NIC Interventions

Breastfeeding Assistance, Lactation Counseling

**Example NIC Activities—Breastfeeding Assistance**

Discuss with parents an estimate of effort and length of time they would like to put toward breastfeeding; provide early mother/infant contact opportunity to breastfeed within 2 hours after birth

## Nursing Interventions and Rationales

B

- Encourage and facilitate early skin-to-skin contact (SSC) (position includes contact of the naked baby with the mother's bare chest within 2 hours after birth). *Early SSC is thought to assist with maternal milk production, aid in establishing breastfeeding, and have a positive effect on duration of breast feeding (Anderson et al, 2004; Spatz, 2004).* **EBN:** *While clinical benefits of SSC have been supported in the literature (Anderson et al, 2004), researchers agree that methodological limitations in previous studies make firm conclusions regarding SSC and the duration of breastfeeding impossible, therefore, further research is needed (Anderson, Moore, Hepworth et al, 2004; Carfoot, Williamson, & Dickson, 2003).*
- Encourage rooming-in and breastfeeding on demand. *Rooming-in and breastfeeding on demand are positively associated with breastfeeding success (Maternity Center Association, 2004; Palda et al, 2004; Renfew et al, 2001; U.S. Department of Health and Human Services, 2000).* **EBN:** *Demand feedings have been associated with continuation of breastfeeding 4 to 6 weeks postpartum in comparison to restricted feeding intervals (Renfew et al, 2001).* **EB:** *A U.S. national survey and a Canadian team reporting a systematic review, conclude that there is good evidence to recommend rooming-in as an effective intervention to promote breastfeeding (Maternity Center Association, 2004; Palda et al, 2004).*
- Monitor the breastfeeding process. *The nurse's presence and involvement allows for early detection of areas in need of clarification and fosters breastfeeding success in primiparous and multiparous women (Association of Women's Health Obstetric and Neonatal Nurses, 2000; Gill, 2001; Hong et al, 2003).* **EBN:** *Nurses provide assistance with technique and informational needs while observing mothers. Breastfeeding mothers expect nurses to observe and provide feedback during breastfeeding (Gill, 2001).* **EB:** *Breastfeeding support consistent with the Baby Friendly Hospital Initiative is recommended and findings from a systematic review indicate there is a beneficial effect on any breastfeeding and exclusive breastfeeding when extra professional support is provided (Maternity Center Association, 2004; Sikorski et al, 2005).*
- Identify opportunities to enhance knowledge and experience regarding breastfeeding. Support and teaching must be individualized to the client's level of understanding. *Exposure to a variety of sources of information is an important predictor of breastfeeding duration (Dennis, 2002; deOlivera et al, 2001; Lauver et al, 2002; Palda et al, 2004; Tiedje et al, 2002).* **EBN:** *Initial and continued breastfeeding was positively influenced by the use of written instructions and individual follow-up by nurses (Hoyer & Horvat, 2000).* **EB:** *Findings from a systematic review indicate there is a beneficial effect on any breastfeeding and exclusive breastfeeding when extra professional support is provided (Sikorski et al, 2005).*
- Give encouragement/positive feedback related to breastfeeding mother-infant interactions. *These activities foster maternal satisfaction with care and promote maternal confidence which can predict breastfeeding outcomes (Blyth et al, 2002; Gill, 2001).* **EBN:** *High breastfeeding self-efficacy (maternal confidence) was associated with breastfeeding initiation, continuing to breastfeed at 4 months, and exclusive breastfeeding (Blyth et al, 2002).*
- Monitor for signs and symptoms of nipple pain and/or trauma. *These factors have been identified as impacting the continuation of breastfeeding in the first weeks of motherhood. Early detection and treatment of problems are important for successful breastfeeding (Associa-*

B

*tion of Women's Health Obstetric and Neonatal Nurses, 2000; Smith and Tully, 2001; Riordan et al, 2001).* **EBN:** *Women with breast/nipple comfort continued to breastfeed longer in comparison with women with less breast or nipple comfort (Riordan et al, 2001).*

- Discuss prevention and treatment of common breastfeeding problems. *Permits the nurse to identify the need for information and clarification. Common problems that can lead to early termination of breastfeeding are mainly preventable or can be overcome with assistance and support (Association of Women's Health Obstetric and Neonatal Nurses, 2000; Registered Nurses Association of Ontario, 2003; Tiedje et al, 2002).* **EBN:** *Evidence-based practice guidelines support the need to evaluate breastfeeding women's knowledge regarding the prevention and management of common problems (e.g., sore nipples, breast engorgement) associated with breastfeeding (Association of Women's Health Obstetric and Neonatal Nurses, 2000; Registered Nurses Association of Ontario, 2003).*
- Monitor infant responses to breastfeeding. *Ongoing evaluation of the adequacy of infant intake such as weight, number of excretions (urine and stool) per 24 hours, and assessment of the presence of jaundice is important to support ongoing effective breastfeeding and for early detection of problems (Association of Women's Health Obstetric and Neonatal Nurses, 2000; Registered Nurses Association of Ontario, 2003).* **EBN:** *Evidence-based practice guidelines include monitoring infant responses as described above (Association of Women's Health Obstetric and Neonatal Nurses, 2000; Registered Nurses Association of Ontario, 2003).*
- Identify current support person network and opportunities for continued breastfeeding support. *Support from family, professionals, and peer support have been found to improve outcomes such as postpartal complications (psychosocial), duration of breastfeeding, and satisfaction with breastfeeding (Adams et al, 2001; Association of Women's Health Obstetric and Neonatal Nurses, 2000; Dennis et al, 2002; McKeever et al, 2002; Pugh et al, 2001).* **EBN:** *In a randomized controlled trial, mothers receiving support through a peer support program were continuing to breastfeed longer and reported greater satisfaction with their breastfeeding experience than their counterparts receiving conventional care (Dennis et al, 2002).*
- Avoid supplemental bottle feedings and do not provide samples of formula on discharge. *Supplemental/formula/bottle feedings can interfere with the infant's desire to breastfeed, increases the risk of allergies, and conveys the subtle message that the mother's breast milk is not adequate. These practices are associated with poor breastfeeding success (Dennis, 2002; DiGirolamo et al, 2001; Donnelly, Snowden, Renfrew et al, 2001).* **EBN:** *Supplemental feedings were identified as one of two strong risk factors for early breastfeeding termination (DiGirolamo et al, 2001).* **EB:** *Use of commercial discharge packages have been shown to decrease breastfeeding rates (Donnelly, Snowden, Renfrew et al, 2001; Palda, Guise, Wathen et al, 2004).*

▲ Provide follow-up contact; as available provide home visits and/or peer counseling. *Outreach of this type is associated with management of client problems and better outcomes including breastfeeding duration (Adams et al, 2001; Association of Women's Health Obstetric and Neonatal Nurses, 2000; McKeever et al, 2002; McNaughton, 2004; Palda et al, 2004; Pugh et al, 2002).* **EBN:** *Breastfeeding women receiving nurse and peer counselor support had longer duration of breastfeeding and infants had fewer sick visits and reported use of fewer medications than those receiving usual care (Pugh et al, 2002).*

B

### Multulticultural

- Assess for the influence of cultural beliefs, norms, and values on current breastfeeding practices. *The client's knowledge of breastfeeding may be based on cultural perceptions, as well as influences from the larger social context (Cricco-Lizza, 2004; Gill et al, 2004; Kong & Lee, 2004; Leininger & McFarland, 2002).* **EBN:** *A study of African-American women revealed formula-feeding experiences were the norm and infant-feeding beliefs reflected responses to life experiences (Cricco-Lizza, 2004).*
- Assess mothers' timing preference to begin breastfeeding. *Women from different cultures may have different beliefs about the best time to begin breastfeeding (Purnell & Paulanka, 2003).* **EBN:** *Although usual hospital practice is to begin breastfeeding immediately, some cultures (e.g., Arab heritage) do not regard colostrum as appropriate for newborns and may prefer to wait until milk is present at about 3 days of age (Purnell & Paulanka, 2003).*
- Validate the client's concerns about the amount of milk taken. **EBN:** *Some cultures may add semisolid food within the first month of life as a result of concerns that the infant is not getting enough to eat and the perception that "big is healthy" (Higgins, 2000).*

### Home Care

- Above interventions may be adapted for home care use.

## Client/Family Teaching

- Include the father and other family members in education about breastfeeding. *Allaying the misconceptions and the social embarrassment associated with breastfeeding can encourage fathers to be more supportive (DDHS, 2000; Shepherd et al, 2000; Wolfberg et al, 2004).* **EB:** *Researchers conducting a randomized controlled trial with a 2-hour intervention class on infant care and breastfeeding promotion found that the fathers in the intervention group were influential advocates for breastfeeding (Wolfberg et al, 2004).*
- Teach the client the importance of maternal nutrition. **EB:** *Generally, no special diet is required; however, 500 calories above the non-pregnant recommendations (or adjusting caloric intake to need) is thought to assist in sustaining breastfeeding and consuming a healthy diet using foods from a variety of sources is recommended (Breslin & Lucas, 2003; US Department of Health and Human Services & US Department of Agriculture, 2005).*
- Reinforce the infant's subtle hunger cues (e.g., quiet-alert state, rooting, sucking, hand-to-mouth activity) and encourage the client to nurse whenever signs are apparent. *Parents need to know infant characteristics and the early feeding readiness cues of infants so that they can respond appropriately (Association of Women's Health Obstetric and Neonatal Nurses, 2000; Karl, 2004; Milligan et al, 2000).* **EBN:** *Evidence-based practice guidelines support the teaching/reinforcement of these skills as important to effective breastfeeding (Association of Women's Health Obstetric and Neonatal Nurses, 2000).*
- Review guidelines for frequency (every 2 to 3 hours, or 8 to 12 feedings per 24 hours) and duration (until suckling and swallowing slow down and satiety is reached) of feeding times. *In the first few days, frequent and regular stimulation of the breasts is important to establish an adequate milk supply; after breastfeeding is established, feeding lasts until*

B

*the breasts are drained (Association of Women's Health Obstetric and Neonatal Nurses, 2000; Neifert, 2004).* **EBN:** *Evidence-based guidelines recommend assessment of infant satisfaction/satiety including infant cues and patterns of weight (Association of Women's Health Obstetric and Neonatal Nurses, 2000).*

- Provide anticipatory guidance about common infant behaviors. *Being able to anticipate and manage behaviors and problems promote parental confidence (Association of Women's Health Obstetric and Neonatal Nurses, 2000; Milligan et al, 2000).* **EBN:** *Lack of knowledge about infant growth spurts, temperament, sleep/wake cycles, and introduction of other foods can create parental anxiety and lead to premature termination of breastfeeding (Milligan et al, 2000).*
- Provide information about additional breastfeeding resources. **EBN:** *Evidence-based clinical practice guidelines suggest that breastfeeding books, materials, websites, and breastfeeding support groups, which provide current and accurate information, can enhance maternal success and satisfaction with the breastfeeding process (Association of Women's Health Obstetric and Neonatal Nurses, 2000).*

## evolve WEBSITES FOR EDUCATION

See the EVOLVE website for World Wide Web resources for client education.

## REFERENCES


Adams C, Berger R, Conning P et al: Breastfeeding trends at a community breastfeeding center: an evaluative survey, *J Gynecol Neonat Nurs* 30(4):392-400, 2001.

Anderson GC, Moore E, Hepworth J et al: Early skin-to-skin contact for mothers and their healthy newborn infants, *Cochrane Database Syst Rev* (2):CD003519, 2003.

Association of Women's Health Obstetric and Neonatal Nurses: *Evidence-based clinical practice guideline: breastfeeding support: prenatal care through the first year (practice guideline),* Washington, DC, 2000, The Association.

Blyth R, Creedy DK, Dennis CL et al: Effect of maternal confidence on breastfeeding duration: an application of breastfeeding self-efficacy theory, *Birth* 29(4):278-84, 2002.

Breslin ET, Lucas VA: *Women's health nursing: toward evidence-based practice,* St. Louis, 2003, WB Saunders.

Carfoot S, Williamson PR, Dickson R: A systematic review of randomized controlled trials evaluating the effect of mother/baby skin-to-skin care on successful breastfeeding, *Midwifery* 19(2):148-55, 2003.

Corry MP; Maternity Center Association: Recommendations from Listening to Mothers: the first national US survey of women's childbearing experiences, *Birth* 31(1):61-5, 2004.

Cricco-Lizza R: Infant-feeding beliefs and experiences of black women enrolled in WIC in the New York metropolitan area, *Qual Health Res* 14(9):1197-210, 2004.

de Oliveira MI, Camacho LA, Tedstone AE: Extending breastfeeding duration through primary care: a systematic review of prenatal and postnatal interventions, *J Hum Lact* 17(4):326-43, 2001.

Dennis CL: Breastfeeding initiation and duration: a 1990-2000 literature review, *J Obstet Gynecol Neonatal Nurs*, 31(1):12-32, 2002a.

Dennis CL: Breastfeeding peer support: maternal and volunteer perceptions from a randomized controlled trial, *Birth* 29(3):169-76, 2002b.

Dennis CL, Hodnett E, Gallop R: The effect of peer support on breast-feeding duration among primiparous women: a randomized controlled trial, *CMAJ* 166(1):21-8, 2002.

DiGirolamo AM, Grummer-Strawn LM, Fein S: Maternity care practices: implications for breastfeeding, *Birth* 28(2):94-100, 2001.

Dochterman JM, Bulecheck GM: *Nursing interventions classification (NIC),* ed 4, St. Louis, 2004, Mosby.

B

Donnelly A et al: The influence of discharge packs on breastfeeding. In Neilson J et al, editors: *Pregnancy and childbirth module of the Cochrane Database of Systematic Reviews.* Available in the Cochrane Library [database on disk and CD ROM]. The Cochrane Collaboration, Issue 1. Oxford, UK: Updata Software (updated quarterly), 2001.

Gill SL: The little things: perceptions of breastfeeding support, *J Obstet Gynecol Neonat Nurs* 30(4):401-9, 2001.

Gill SL, Reifsnider E, Mann AR et al: Assessing infant breastfeeding belief among low-income Mexican Americans, *J Perinat Educ* 13:29, 2004.

Higgins B: Puerto Rican cultural beliefs: influence on infant feeding practices in western New York, *J Transcult Nurs* 11(1):19-30, 2000.

Hong TM, Callister LC, Schwartz R: First time mothers' views of breastfeeding support from nurses, *MCN Am J Matern Child Nurs* 28(1):10-5, 2003.

Johnson M, Maas M, Moorehead S: *Nursing outcomes classification (NOC)*, ed 3, St Louis, 2004, Mosby.

Karl DJ: Using principles of newborn behavioral state organization to facilitate breastfeeding, *MCN Am J Matern Child Nurs* 29(5): 292-8, 2004.

Kong SK, Lee DT: Factors influencing decision to breastfeed, *J Adv Nurs* 46(4):369-79, 2004.

Lauver DR, Ward SE, Heidrich SM et al: Patient-centered interventions, *Res Nurs Health* 25(4):246-55, 2002.

Leininger MM, McFarland MR: *Transcultural nursing: concepts, theories, research and practices,* ed 3, New York, 2002, McGraw-Hill.

McKeever P, Stevens B, Miller KL et al: Home versus hospital breastfeeding support for newborns: a randomized controlled trial, *Birth* 29(4):258-65, 2002.

McNaughton DB: Nurse home visits to maternal-child clients, *Public Health Nurs* 21(3):207-19, 2004.

Milligan RA, Pugh LC, Bronner YL et al: Breastfeeding duration among low income women, *J Midwif Womens Health* 45(3):246-52, 2000.

Neifert MR: Breastmilk transfer: positioning, latch-on, and screening for problems in milk transfer, *Clin Obstet Gynecol* 47(3):656-75, 2004.

Palda VA, Guise JM, Wathen CN et al: Interventions to promote breast-feeding: applying the evidence in clinical practice, *CMAJ* 170(6):976-8, 2004.

Pugh LC, Milligan RA, Frick KD et al: Breastfeeding duration, costs, and benefits of a support program for low-income breastfeeding women, *Birth* 29(2):95-100, 2002.

Purnell LD, Paulanka BJ: *Transcultural health care: a culturally competent approach,* ed 2, Philadelphia, 2003, FA Davis.

Registered Nurses Association of Ontario (RNAO): *Breastfeeding best practice guidelines for nurses*, Toronto, 2003, The Association.

Renfrew M et al: Feeding schedules in hospitals for newborn infants. In Neilson J et al, editors: *Pregnancy and childbirth module of the Cochrane Database of Systematic Reviews.* Available in The Cochrane Library [data-base on disk and CD ROM]. The Cochrane Collaboration, Issue 1. Oxford, UK: Updata Software (updated quarterly), 2001.

Riordan J, Bibb D, Miller M et al: Predicting breastfeeding duration using the LATCH breastfeeding assessment tool, *J Hum Lact* 17(1):20-3, 2001.

Shepherd CK, Power KG, Carter H: Examining the correspondence of breastfeeding and bottle-feeding couples' infant feeding attitudes, *J Adv Nurs* 31(3):651-60, 2000.

Sikorski J, Renfrew M J, Pindoria S et al: Support for breastfeeding mothers, *Cochrane Database Syst Rev,* (1):CD001141, 2002.

Smith JW, Tully MR: Midwifery management of breastfeeding: using the evidence, *J Midwif Womens Health* 46(6):423-38, 2001.

Spatz DL: Ten steps for promoting and protecting breastfeeding for vulnerable infants, *J Perinat Neonatal Nurs* 18(4):385-96, 2004.

Tiedje LB, Schiffman R, Omar M et al: An ecological approach to breastfeeding, *MCN Am J Matern Child Nurs* 27(3):154-61, 2002.

US Department of Health and Human Services: *HHS blueprint for action on breastfeeding*, Washington, DC, 2000, US Department of Health and Human Services, Office on Women's Health.

US Department of Health and Human Services and US Department of Agriculture: *Dietary guidelines for Americans 2005*, Washington, DC, 2005, The Departments.

Wolfberg AJ, Michels KB, Shields W et al: Dads as breastfeeding advocates: results from a randomized controlled trial of an educational intervention, *Am J Obstet Gynecol* 191(3):708-12, 2004.

# Ineffective Breastfeeding

evolve

B

*Arlene Farren*

NANDA

## Definition

Dissatisfaction or difficulty a mother, infant, or child experiences with the breastfeeding process

## Defining Characteristics

Unsatisfactory breastfeeding process; nonsustained suckling at the breast; resisting latching on; unresponsive to comfort measures; persistence of sore nipples beyond first week of breastfeeding; observable signs of inadequate infant intake; insufficient emptying of each breast per feeding; infant inability to latch on to maternal breast correctly; infant arching and crying at the breast; infant exhibiting fussiness and crying within the first hour after breastfeeding; actual or perceived inadequate milk supply; no observable signs of oxytocin release; insufficient opportunity for suckling at the breast

## Related Factors (r/t)

Nonsupportive partner/family; previous breast surgery; infant receiving supplemental feedings with artificial nipple; prematurity; previous history of breastfeeding failure; poor infant sucking reflex; maternal breast anomaly; maternal anxiety or ambivalence; interruption in breastfeeding; infant anomaly; knowledge deficit

NOC

## Outcomes (Nursing Outcomes Classification)

### Suggested NOC Outcomes

Breastfeeding Establishment: Infant, Maternal; Breastfeeding Maintenance; Breastfeeding Weaning; Knowledge: Breastfeeding

### Example NOC Outcome with Indicators

**Breastfeeding Establishment: Infant** as evidenced by the following indicators: Proper alignment and latch-on/Proper areolar grasp/Proper areolar compression/Correct suck and tongue placement/Swallowing a minimum of 5 to 10 minutes per breast/Minimum eight feedings per day/Urinations per day appropriate for age/Weight gain appropriate for age (Rate each indicator of **Breastfeeding Establishment: Infant**: 1=not adequate, 2 = slightly adequate, 3 = moderately adequate, 4 = substantially adequate, 5 = totally adequate [see Section I].)

## Client Outcomes

B

### Client Will (Specify Time Frame):

- Achieve effective breastfeeding (dyad)
- Verbalize/demonstrate techniques to manage breastfeeding problems (mother)
- Manifest signs of adequate intake at the breast (infant)
- Manifest positive self-esteem in relation to the infant feeding process (mother)
- Explain alternative method of infant feeding if unable to continue exclusive breastfeeding (mother)

NIC

## Interventions (Nursing Interventions Classification)

### Suggested NIC Interventions

Breastfeeding Assistance; Lactation Counseling

**Example NIC Activities—Breastfeeding Assistance**

Discuss with parents an estimate of effort and length of time they would like to put toward breastfeeding; provide early mother/infant contact opportunity to breastfeed within 2 hours after birth

## Nursing Interventions and Rationales

- Identify women with risk factors for lower breastfeeding initiation and continuation rates (age <20 years, low socioeconomic status) as well as factors contributing to ineffective breastfeeding as early as possible in the perinatal experience. *Early identification of potential problems make individualized, targeted interventions that are culturally sensitive possible (Association of Women's Health Obstetric and Neonatal Nurses, 2000a; Mozingo et al, 2000; Schwartz et al, 2002).* **EBN:** *A prospective cohort study of more than 900 revealed younger and less educated women, those with nipple/breast pain, mastitis, and bottle use were among those more likely to discontinue breastfeeding early. The researchers concluded that these women need additional assistance and counseling (Schwartz et al, 2002).*
- Use valid and reliable tools to measure breastfeeding performance and to predict early discontinuance of breastfeeding whenever possible/feasible. *Using instruments to measure clinically relevant constructs in a consistent manner permits identification of women/infants at risk and provides for systematic clinical outcome measurement (Dick et al, 2002; Hall et al, 2002).* **EBN:** *Researchers estimated internal consistency reliability and predictive validity of the Breastfeeding Attrition Prediction Tool (BAPT) in a sample of postpartal women and concluded that the BAPT (modified version) showed promise for clinical use (Dick et al, 2002).* **EB:** *Breastfeeding Assessment Score (BAS) has been used to identify infants at risk for early cessation of breastfeeding and may predict exclusive breastfeeding failure (Gianni, Veni, Ferraris et al, 2004).*
- Encourage and facilitate early SSC (position includes contact of the naked baby with the mother's bare chest within 2 hours after birth). *Early SSC is thought to assist with*

*maternal milk production, aid in establishing breastfeeding, and have a positive effect on duration of breast feeding (Anderson, Moore, Hepworth et al, 2003; Spatz, 2003).* **EBN:** *While clinical benefits of SSC have been supported in the literature (Anderson, Moore, Hepworth et al, 2003), researchers agree that methodological limitations in previous studies make firm conclusions regarding SSC and the duration of breastfeeding impossible, therefore, further research is needed (Anderson, Moore, Hepworth et al, 2003; Carfoot, Williamson, & Dickson, 2003).*

- Encourage rooming-in and feeding on demand. *These approaches have been positively associated with breastfeeding success (US Department of Health and Human Services, 2000; Renfrew et al, 2001).* **EB:** *A US national survey and a Canadian team reporting a systematic review conclude that there is good evidence to recommend rooming-in as an effective intervention to promote breastfeeding (Maternity Center Association, 2004; Palda, Guise, Wathen et al, 2004).*
- Evaluate the breast and nipple structures and provide appropriate measures as needed. *Normal nipple and breast structure and early detection and treatment of abnormalities with continuing support are important for successful breastfeeding. Nipple trauma is associated with latch-on problems and increased risk for mastitis (Association of Women's Health Obstetric and Neonatal Nurses, 2000b; Foxman et al, 2002; Smith & Tully, 2001).* **EBN:** *Sore/cracked nipples were found to be strongly associated with mastitis (Foxman et al, 2002). Breast/nipple comfort has been linked to continuation of breastfeeding (Riordan et al, 2001).*
- Observe a full breastfeeding session (every 8 hours in the early postpartum and once per visit on follow-up). *The nurse's presence and involvement allows for identification of those areas of the breastfeeding process for which assistance and support are needed and promotes maternal confidence (Association of Women's Health Obstetric and Neonatal Nurses, 2000a; Gill, 2001; Hong et al, 2003; Raisler, 2000).* **EBN:** *Women identified nurses' activities such as assessment, teaching, and assistance as being sources of emotional, informational, and tangible support (Hong et al, 2003).*
- Provide evidence-based teaching and breastfeeding assistance appropriate to the client's individualized needs (see Client/Family Teaching). *Accurate, consistent information and providing practical assistance with breastfeeding techniques that are based on evidence and in response to individualized client needs are associated with successful breastfeeding, longer duration breastfeeding, promotion of maternal confidence, and client satisfaction (Association of Women's Health Obstetric and Neonatal Nurses, 2000b; Gill, 2001; Hailes & Wellard, 2000; Lauver et al, 2002; Mozingo et al, 2000; Raisler, 2000).* **EBN:** *In a qualitative study, mothers described factors contributing to early termination of breastfeeding (e.g., incomplete and inconsistent information about breastfeeding). Mothers experiencing confusion, frustration, and dissatisfaction discontinued breastfeeding (Hailes & Wellard, 2000; Mozingo et al, 2000).*
- Promote comfort and relaxation to reduce pain and anxiety. *Discomfort and increased tension are factors associated with reduced let-down reflex and premature discontinuance of breastfeeding. Anxiety and fear are associated with decreased milk production (Association of Women's Health Obstetric and Neonatal Nurses, 2000a; Mezzacappa & Katkin, 2002; Tait, 2000).* **EBN:** *Evidence-based practice guidelines include employing comfort measures for breastfeeding mothers such as providing analgesia approximately 30 minutes before feeding (Association of Women's Health Obstetric and Neonatal Nurses, 2000a).*

B

- Provide time for clients to express expectations and concerns and give emotional support. *Discussing concerns and differences between expectations and experiences provide an opportunity for mothers to ventilate and may contribute to positive coping strategies and increase breastfeeding duration (Porteous et al, 2000; Vari et al, 2000).* **EBN:** *In an intervention study examining a social support intervention, women receiving the intervention (professionally mediated peer support) were more satisfied, were exclusively breastfeeding, and breastfeeding duration was longer than those receiving the usual care (Vari et al, 2000).*
- Avoid supplemental feedings. *Supplementation with formula feedings has been associated with higher risk of discontinuance of breastfeeding (DiGirolamo et al, 2001; Hall et al, 2002).* **EBN:** *Supplementing breast milk with formula was one of eight factors that significantly predicted breastfeeding cessation within 7 to 10 days of age in a large sample of mothers who intended to breastfeed their infants (Hall et al, 2002).* **EB:** *Researchers conducting a large-scale study of first-week feeding patterns found that supplementary bottle feeds were clearly associated with discontinued breastfeeding at 6 weeks (Casiday, Wright, Panter-Brick et al, 2004).*
- Monitor infant behavioral cues and responses to breastfeeding. *Infant behaviors contribute to oxytocin release and let down, contribute to effective feeding, indicate effective breastfeeding, manifest satiety, and indicate adequacy of the feeding while contributing to positive maternal-infant attachment (Association of Women's Health Obstetric and Neonatal Nurses, 2000a, 2000b; Matthiesen et al, 2001; White et al, 2002).* **EBN:** *In a small sample, researchers analyzed videotaped behaviors from birth to 2 hours and measured maternal oxytocin levels. The findings suggest that infants use their hands and mouths to stimulate maternal oxytocin release thereby influencing milk ejection (Matthiesen et al, 2001).*
- Collect data and monitor signs of adequate infant intake/nutrition. *Signs such as number of feedings in 24 hours, weight loss/gain pattern, and elimination patterns indicate that the infant is getting sufficient infant nutrition for normal patterns of growth and development and permit early identification and treatment of problems (Association of Women's Health Obstetric and Neonatal Nurses, 2000a).* **EBN:** *Evidence-based practice guidelines include assessment and monitoring of the above noted signs of adequate infant intake (Association of Women's Health Obstetric and Neonatal Nurses, 2000a; Spatz, 2004).*
- Provide necessary equipment/instruction/assistance for milk expression as needed. *While infant suckling is optimal, expressing human milk is done to stimulate the breasts, when the infant is unable to suckle, or when mother and baby are separated (such as mother returning to work). Expression of human milk is done either by hand or pump (Association of Women's Health Obstetric and Neonatal Nurses, 2000a; Jones et al, 2001; Phillips & Merewood, 2003).* **EBN:** *In a randomized control trial, researchers found that a combination of breast massage and simultaneous (both breasts at the same time) pumping increased the volume of milk produced and also increased maternal satisfaction (Jones et al, 2001). Breast massage using the Oketani method (first reported in Japan) was associated with improved quality of milk and growth and development patterns (Foda, Kawashima, Takaaki et al, 2004).*
- Provide anticipatory guidance in relation to home management of breastfeeding. *Mothers who are prepared for the needs of home management and possible problems (such as fatigue) can institute self-care measures, will feel more confident, and be less likely to dis-*

*continue breastfeeding (Blyth et al, 2002; Ertem et al, 2001; Schwartz et al 2002).* **EBN:** *Maternal confidence (breastfeeding self-efficacy) is a significant predictor of breastfeeding duration. The researchers identified implications for practice such as the use of self-efficacy enhancing strategies (Blyth et al, 2002).*

- Assist the client to identify and utilize support network. *Support from family, significant others, professionals, and peer support has been found to improve outcomes such as postpartal complications (psychosocial), duration of breastfeeding, and satisfaction with breastfeeding (Adams et al, 2001; Association of Women's Health Obstetric and Neonatal Nurses, 2000a; Dennis et al, 2002; McKeever et al, 2002).* **EBN:** *In a randomized controlled trial, mothers receiving support through a peer support program were continuing to breast-feed longer and reported greater satisfaction with their breastfeeding experience than their counterparts receiving conventional care (Dennis et al, 2002).*
- Do not provide samples of formula on discharge. *Supplemental/formula/bottle feeding are associated with poor breastfeeding success and can interfere with the infant's desire to breastfeed and increase the risk of allergies, and these practices convey subtle messages that the mother's breast milk is not adequate (Dennis, 2002; DiGirolamo et al, 2001; Donnelly et al, 2000).* **EBN:** *Supplemental feeding was identified as one of two strong risk factors for early breastfeeding termination (DiGirolamo et al, 2001).*
- Initiate breastfeeding follow-up after hospital discharge. *Follow-up provides the opportunity for review of information, feedback about proper technique, and identification of and assistance with problems, and promotes maternal confidence and satisfaction (Escobar et al, 2001; Hogan, 2001; Pugh et al, 2002).* **EBN:** *Breastfeeding women receiving nurse and peer counselor support had longer duration of breastfeeding and infants had fewer sick visits and reported use of fewer medications than those receiving usual care (Pugh et al, 2002).*

▲ Provide referrals and resources. *Lactation consultants, nurse and peer support programs, community organizations, and written and electronic sources of information contribute to successful breastfeeding and have been supported through outcomes such as knowledge, maternal confidence, duration of breastfeeding, and client satisfaction (Ahluwalia et al, 2000; Association of Women's Health Obstetric and Neonatal Nurses, 2000a).* **EBN:** *Evidenced-based guidelines and systematic reviews support the use of professionals with special skills in breastfeeding and other support programs to promote continued breastfeeding (Association of Women's Health Obstetric and Neonatal Nurses, 2000a).*

- If unsuccessful in achieving effective breastfeeding, help client accept and learn an alternate method of infant feeding. *Once the decision has been made to provide an alternate method of infant feeding, the mother needs support and education (Mozingo et al, 2000).* **EBN:** *In a qualitative study of women's experiences with short-term breastfeeding, researchers uncovered women's concerns about breastfeeding failure and their feelings of relief versus guilt and shame for which women may need assistance and support (Mozingo et al, 2000).*

## Multicultural

- Assess for the influence of cultural beliefs, norms, and values on breastfeeding attitudes. *The client's knowledge of breastfeeding may be based on cultural perceptions, as well as influences from the larger social context (Cricco-Lizza, 2004; Gill, Reifsnider, Mann et al,*

*2004; Kong & Lee, 2004; Leininger & McFarland, 2002).* **EBN:** *A study of African-American women revealed formula-feeding experiences were the norm and infant-feeding beliefs reflected responses to life experiences (Cricco-Lizza, 2004).*

- Assess whether the client's concerns about the amount of milk taken during breastfeeding is contributing to dissatisfaction with the breastfeeding process. **EBN:** *Some cultures may add semisolid food within the first month of life as a result of concerns that the infant is not getting enough to eat and the perception that "big is healthy" (Higgins, 2000).*
- Assess the influence of family support on the decision to continue or discontinue breastfeeding. **EBN:** *Women are the keepers and transmitters of culture in families. Female family members can play a dominant role in how infants are fed (Cesario, 2001).* **EB:** *In one Italian study, a description of mother characteristic that may indicate the need for more support included mothers that smoke and have had their first newborn (Bertini, Perugi, Dani et al, 2003). Recent research has found that the mother's partner and family are most influential in the choice of infant feeding method and, thus, should be included in breastfeeding promotion programs for ethnically diverse women (Rose et al, 2004).*
- Assess for the influence of mother's weight on attempts to initiate and sustain breastfeeding. **EB:** *Prepregnant overweight and obesity have been associated with failure to initiate and to sustain breastfeeding among Caucasian and Hispanic women (Kugyelka, Rasmussen, & Frongillo, 2004).*
- Validate the client's feelings regarding the difficulty or dissatisfaction with breastfeeding. **EBN:** *Evidence-based practice guidelines recommend exploring concerns or ambivalence about breastfeeding to identify misconceptions and other barriers to successful breastfeeding (Association of Women's Health, Obstetric, and Neonatal Nurses, 2000a).*

## Home Care

- Above interventions may be adapted for home care use.
- Investigate availability/refer to public health department, hospital home follow-up breastfeeding program, or other post-discharge support. *Some hospitals and public health departments have follow-up breastfeeding programs, particularly for high-risk mothers (e.g., older mothers, past history substance use, risk of physical abuse). Instructions and support initiated during hospitalization are continued, and identification of client problems are addressed by professional nurses (McNaughton, 2004).* **EBN:** *Primiparous breastfeeding mothers receiving peer support by telephone (48 hours after discharge and as frequently after as deemed necessary by the mother) were more likely to still be breastfeeding at 12 weeks postpartum (Ennis, Hodnett, Gallop et al, 2002).*
- Monitor for specific difficulties contributing to bonding difficulties between mother and infant. Refer to care plan for **Risk for impaired parent/infant/child Attachment.**

## Client/Family Teaching

- Review maternal and infant benefits of breastfeeding. **EBN:** *Information about benefits of breastfeeding can assist women/families to make informed decisions about breastfeeding*

*(Association of Women's Health Obstetric and Neonatal Nurses, 2000a,b; U.S. Department of Health and Human Services, 2000).*

- Instruct the client on maternal breastfeeding behaviors/techniques (preparation for, positioning, initiation of/promoting latch-on, burping, completion of session, and frequency of feeding). *Difficulties in these practices contribute to ineffective breastfeeding. Teaching behaviors/techniques of importance to breastfeeding will provide the woman with the necessary information and skills to initiate and continue breastfeeding and instill maternal confidence (Association of Women's Health Obstetric and Neonatal Nurses, 2000a,b; Ertem et al, 2001; Foda, Kawashima, Nakamura et al, 2004; Khoury, Mitra, Hinton et al, 2002; US Department of Health and Human Services, 2000).* **EBN:** *Researchers found preliminary support for a teaching intervention in the form of a breastfeeding promotion video addressing barriers to breastfeeding for low-income women (Khoury, Mitra, Hinton et al, 2002).*
- Teach the client self-care measures for the breastfeeding woman (e.g., breast care, management of breast/nipple discomfort, nutrition/fluid, rest/activity). *Nipple trauma, pain, mastitis, and fatigue are some of the problems a breastfeeding woman may experience. Developing knowledge and skill facilitates prevention and self-care management of these potential problems, fosters maternal confidence, and improves breastfeeding duration (Association of Women's Health Obstetric and Neonatal Nurses, 2000a; Foda, Kawashima, Nakamura et al, 2004; Foxman et al, 2002; Ruchala, 2000; Smith and Tully, 2001; Tait, 2000).* **EBN:** *In a sample of low-risk early postpartum women, the researcher found mothers perceived that receiving teaching regarding their own care (in contrast to newborn care) was the priority (Ruchala, 2000).*
- Provide information regarding infant cues and behaviors related to breastfeeding and appropriate maternal responses (e.g., cues that infant is ready to feed, behaviors during feeding that contribute to effective breastfeeding, measures of infant feeding adequacy). *Mothers who correctly interpret the infant's behaviors and responses and are able to provide comfort measures are more likely to continue to breastfeed, experience maternal confidence and satisfying maternal-infant interaction (Association of Women's Health Obstetric and Neonatal Nurses, 2000a,b; Bryan, 2000; Schwartz et al, 2002; Smith & Tully, 2001; White et al, 2002).* **EBN:** *In a research utilization project, researchers asserted that nurses are vital to helping parents understand infant states, cues, and behaviors and by providing that information postnatally, will foster a mutually satisfying interaction between parent and infant (White et al, 2002).*
- Provide education to father/family/significant others as needed. *Informed support people have a desire to learn, may be needed to assist mothers with breastfeeding management issues (e.g., fatigue and sleep pattern disturbances), and may have an impact on breastfeeding duration (Association of Women's Health Obstetric and Neonatal Nurses, 2000a; Gay, Lee, & Lee, 2004; Moore, 2000; Pollock et al, 2002; Quillin & Glenn, 2004; Wolfberg, Michels, Shields et al, 2004).* **EBN:** *In a descriptive study, men at perinatal settings indicated a preference for their babies to be breastfed and wanted to be included in decisions concerning breastfeeding (Pollock et al, 2002).* **EB:** *In a small, randomized controlled trial, an educational intervention demonstrated the critical role of dads in encouraging a women to breastfeed her newborn (Wolfberg, Michels, Shields, et al, 2004).*

## evolve WEBSITES FOR EDUCATION

B

See the EVOLVE website for World Wide Web resources for client education.

## REFERENCES


Adams C, Berger R, Conning P et al: Breastfeeding trends at a community breastfeeding center: an evaluative survey, *J Gynecol Neonat Nurs* 30(4):392-400, 2001.

Ahluwalia IB, Tessaro I, Grummer-Strawn LM et al: Georgia's breastfeeding promotion program for low-income women, *Pediatrics* 105(6):E85, 2000.

Anderson GC, Moore E, Hepworth J et al: Early skin-to-skin contact for mothers and their healthy newborn infants, *Cochrane Database Sys Rev* (2), 2003.

Association of Women's Health Obstetric and Neonatal Nurses: *Evidence-based clinical practice guideline: breastfeeding support: prenatal care through the first year (practice guideline),* Washington, DC, 2000a, The Association.

Association of Women's Health Obstetric and Neonatal Nurses: *Evidence-based clinical practice guideline: breast-feeding support: prenatal care through the first year (monograph),* Washington, DC, 2000b, The Association.

Bertini G, Perugi S, Dani C et al: Maternal education and the incidence and duration of breast feeding: a prospective study, *J Pediatr Gastroenterol Nutr* 37(4):447-452, 2003.

Blyth R, Creedy DK, Dennis CL et al: Effect of maternal confidence on breastfeeding duration: an application of breastfeeding self-efficacy theory, *Birth* 29(4):278-284, 2002.

Carfoot S, Williamson PR, Dickson R: A systematic review of randomized controlled trials evaluating the effect of mother/baby skin-to-skin care on successful breastfeeding, *Midwifery* 19(2):148-155, 2003.

Casiday RE, Wright CM, Panter-Brick C et al: Do early infant feeding patterns relate to breast-feeding continuation and weight gain? Data from a longitudinal cohort study, *Eur J Clin Nutr* 58(9):1290-1296, 2004.

Cesario S: Care of the Native American woman: strategies for practice, education, and research, *J Obstet Gynecol Neonatal Nurs* 30(1):13-19, 2001.

Corry MP; Maternity Center Association: Recommendations from Listening to Mothers: the first national U.S. survey of women's childbearing experiences, *Birth* 31(1):61-65, 2004.

Cricco-Lizza R: Infant-feeding beliefs and experiences of black women enrolled in WIC in the New York metropolitan area, *Qual Health Res* 14(9):1197-1210, 2004.

Dennis CL, Hodnett E, Gallop R: The effect of peer support on breast-feeding duration among primiparous women: a randomized controlled trial, *CMAJ* 166(1):21-28, 2002.

Dick MJ, Evans ML, Arthurs JB et al: Predicting early breastfeeding attrition, *J Hum Lact* 18(1):21-28, 2002.

DiGirolamo AM, Grummer-Strawn LM, Fein S: Maternity care practices: implications for breastfeeding, *Birth* 28(2):94-100, 2001.

Dochterman JM, Bulecheck GM: *Nursing interventions classification (NIC),* ed 4, St. Louis, 2003, Mosby.

Donnelly A et al: The influence of discharge packs on breastfeeding. In Neilson J et al, editors: *Pregnancy and childbirth module of the Cochrane Database of Systematic Reviews.* Available in the Cochrane Library [database on disk and CD ROM], *The Cochrane Collaboration,* Issue 1, Oxford, UK: Updata Software (updated quarterly), 2001.

Ertem IO, Votto N, Leventhal JM: The timing and predictors of the early termination of breastfeeding, *Pediatrics* 107(3):543-548, 2001.

Escobar GJ, Braveman PA, Ackerson L et al: A randomized comparison of home visits and hospital-based group follow-up visits after early postpartum discharge, *Pediatrics* 108(3):719-727, 2001.

Foda MI, Kawashima T, Nakamura S et al: Composition of milk obtained from unmassaged versus massaged breasts of lactating mothers, *J Pediatr Gastroentrol Nutr* 38(5):484-487, 2004.

Foxman B, D'Arcy H, Gillespie B et al: Lactation mastitis: occurrence and medical management among 946 breastfeeding women in the United States, *Am J Epidemiol* 155(2):103-114, 2002.

Gay CL, Lee KA, Lee SY: Sleep patterns and fatigue in new mothers and fathers, *Biol Res Nurs* 5(4):311-8, 2004.

Gianni ML, Vegni C, Ferraris G et al: 96 usefulness of an early breastfeeding assessment score to predict exclusive breastfeeding failure, *Pediatr Res* 56:480, 2004.

Gill SL: The little things: perceptions of breastfeeding support, *J Obstet Gynecol Neonatal Nurs* 30(4):401-9, 2001.

Hailes JF, Wellard SJ: Support for breastfeeding in the first postpartum month: perceptions of breastfeeding women, *Breastfeed Rev* 8(3):5-9, 2000.

Hall RT et al: A breast-feeding assessment score to evaluate the risk for cessation of breast-feeding by 7 to 10 days of age, *J Pediatr* 141(5):659-664, 2002.
Higgins B: Puerto Rican cultural beliefs: influence on infant feeding practices in western New York, *J Transcult Nurs* 11(1):19-30, 2000.
Hogan SE: Overcoming barriers to breastfeeding: suggested breastfeeding promotion programs for communities in eastern Nova Scotia, *Can J Public Health* 92(2):105-108, 2001.
Hong TM, Callister LC, Schwartz R: First time mothers' views of breastfeeding support from nurses, *MCN Am J Matern Child Nurs* 28(1):10-15, 2003.
Johnson M, Maas M, Moorehead S: *Nursing outcomes classification (NOC)*, ed 2, St Louis, 2000, Mosby.
Jones E, Dimmock PW, Spencer SA: A randomized controlled trial to compare methods of milk expression after preterm delivery, *Arch Dis Child Fetal Neonatal Ed* 85(2):F91-95, 2001.
Khoury AJ, Mitra AK, Hinton A et al: An innovative video succeeds in addressing barriers to breastfeeding among low-income women, *J Hum Lact* 18(2):125-131, 2002.
Kugyelka JG, Rasmussen KM, Frongillo EA: Maternal obesity is negatively associated with breastfeeding success among Hispanic but not Black women, *J Nutr* 134(7):1746-1753, 2004.
Lauver DR, Ward SE, Heidrich SM et al: Patient-centered interventions, *Res Nurs Health* 25(4):246-255, 2002.
Leininger MM, McFarland MR: *Transcultural nursing: concepts, theories, research and practices,* ed 3, New York, 2002, McGraw-Hill.
Matthiesen AS et al: Postpartum maternal oxytocin release by newborns: effects of infant hand massage and sucking, *Birth* 28(1): 13-19, 2001.
McKeever P, Stevens B, Miller KL et al: Home versus hospital breastfeeding support for newborns: a randomized controlled trial, *Birth* 29(4):258-265, 2002.
Meier PP, Brown LP, Hurst NM et al: Nipple shields for preterm infants: effect on milk transfer and duration of breastfeeding, *J Hum Lact* 16(2):106-114, quiz 129-131, 2000.
Mezzacappa ES, Katkin ES: Breast-feeding is associated with reduced perceived stress and negative mood in mothers, *Health Psychol* 21(2):187-193, 2002.
Moore ML: Perinatal nursing research: a 25-year review—1976-2000, *MCN Am J Matern Child Nurs* 25(6):305-310, 2000.
Mozingo JN, Davis MW, Droppleman PG et al: "It wasn't working." Women's experiences with short-term breastfeeding, *MCN Am J Matern Child Nurs* 25(3):120-126, 2000.
Palda VA, Guise JM, Wathen CN et al: Interventions to promote breast-feeding: applying the evidence in clinical practice, *CMAJ* 170(6):976-978, 2004.
Philipp B: Encouraging patients to use a breast pump, *Contemp Ob Gyn* 1:88-100, 2003.
Pollock CA, Bustamante-Forest R, Giarratano G: Men of diverse cultures: knowledge and attitudes about breastfeeding, *J Obstet Gynecol Neonatal Nurs* 31(6):673-679, 2002.
Porteous R, Kaufman K, Rush J: The effect of individualized professional support on duration of breastfeeding: a randomized controlled trial, *J Hum Lact* 16(4):303-308, 2000.
Pridham K, Lin CY, Brown R: Mothers' evaluation of their caregiving for premature and full-term infants through the first year: contributing factors, *Res Nurs Health* 24(3):157-169, 2001.
Pugh LC, Milligan RA, Frick KD et al: Breastfeeding duration, costs, and benefits of a support program for low-income breastfeeding women, *Birth* 29(2):95-100, 2002.
Quillin SI, Glenn LL: Interaction between feeding method and co-sleeping on maternal-newborn sleep, *J Obstet Gyneol Neonat Nurs* 33(5):580-588, 2004.
Raisler J: Against the odds: breastfeeding experiences of low income mothers, *J Midwifery Womens Health* 45(3):253-263, 2000.
Riordan J, Bibb D, Miller M et al: Predicting breastfeeding duration using the LATCH breastfeeding assessment tool, *J Hum Lact* 17(1):20-23, 2001.
Rose VA, Warrington VO, Linder R et al: Factors influencing infant feeding method in an urban community, *J Natl Med Assoc* 96(3):325-331, 2004.
Ruchala PL: Teaching new mothers: priorities of nurses and postpartum women, *J Obstet Gynecol Neonat Nurs* 29(3):265-273, 2000.
Schwartz K, D'Arcy HJ, Gillespie B et al: Factors associated with weaning in the first 3 months postpartum, *J Fam Pract* 51(5): 439-444, 2002.
Smith JW, Tully MR: Midwifery management of breastfeeding: using the evidence, *J Midwif Womens Health* 46(6):423-438, 2001.
Spatz DL: Ten steps for promoting and protecting breastfeeding for vulnerable infants, *J Perinat Neonatal Nurs* 18(4):385-396, 2004.

Tait P: Nipple pain in breastfeeding women: causes, treatment, and prevention strategies, *J Midwifery Womens Health* 45(3):212-215, 2000.

U.S. Department of Health and Human Services: *HHS blueprint for action on breastfeeding*, Washington, DC, 2000, US Department of Health and Human Services, Office on Women's Health.

Vari PM, Camburn J, Henly SJ: Professionally mediated peer support and early breastfeeding success, *J Perinat Educ* 9:22, 2000.

White C, Simon M, Bryan A: Using evidence to educate birthing center nursing staff: about infant states, cues, and behaviors, *MCN Am J Matern Child Nurs* 27(5):294-298, 2002.

Wolfberg AJ, Michels KB, Shields W et al: Dads as breastfeeding advocates: results from a randomized controlled trial of an educational intervention, *Am J Obstet Gynecol* 191(3):708-712, 2004.



# Interrupted Breastfeeding

*Arlene Farren*

## NANDA

### Definition

Break in the continuity of the breastfeeding process as a result of inability or inadvisability to putting the infant to the breast for feeding

### Defining Characteristics

Infant does not receive nourishment at the breast for some or all feedings; maternal desire to maintain and provide (or eventually provide) her breast milk for her infant's nutritional needs; lack of knowledge regarding expression and storage of breast milk; separation of mother and infant

### Related Factors (r/t)

Contraindications to breastfeeding; maternal employment; maternal or infant illness; need to abruptly wean infant; prematurity

## NOC

### Outcomes (Nursing Outcomes Classification)

#### Suggested NOC Outcomes

Breastfeeding Establishment: Infant, Maternal; Breastfeeding Maintenance; Knowledge: Breastfeeding; Parent-Infant Attachment

**Example NOC Outcome with Indicators**

**Breastfeeding Establishment: Infant** as evidenced by the following indicators: Proper alignment and latch on/Proper areolar grasp/Proper areolar compression/Correct suck and tongue placement/Swallowing a minimum of 5 to 10 minutes per breast/Minimum eight feedings per day/Urinations per day appropriate for age/Weight gain appropriate for age (Rate each indicator of **Breastfeeding Establishment: Infant:** 1 = not adequate, 2 = slightly adequate, 3 = moderately adequate, 4 = substantially adequate, 5 = totally adequate [see Section I].)

## Client Outcomes

### Client Will (Specify Time Frame):

#### Infant

- Receive mother's breast milk if not contraindicated by maternal conditions (e.g., certain drugs, infections) or infant conditions (e.g., true breast milk jaundice)

#### Maternal

- Maintain lactation
- Achieve effective breastfeeding or satisfaction with the breastfeeding experience
- Demonstrate effective methods of breast milk collection and storage

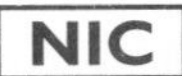

## Interventions (Nursing Interventions Classification)

### Suggested NIC Interventions

Bottle Feeding; Breastfeeding Assistance; Emotional Support; Kangaroo Care; Lactation Counseling

**Example NIC Activities—Lactation Counseling**

Instruct parents on how to differentiate between perceived and actual insufficient milk supply; encourage employers to provide opportunities for and private facilities for lactating mothers to pump and store breast milk during work times

## Nursing Interventions and Rationales

- Discuss mother's desire/intention to begin or resume breastfeeding. *Mothers' commitment/attitude about breastfeeding are associated with breastfeeding success (Kloeblen-Tarver et al, 2002; Mozingo et al, 2000; Pinelli et al, 2001).* **EBN:** *Researchers examining the efficacy of an intervention to improve duration of breastfeeding in very-low-birth-weight infants suggested that high motivation to breast feed may have accounted for the lack of demonstrated differences in breastfeeding duration of parents who did and did not receive the intervention (Pinelli et al, 2001).*
- Provide anticipatory guidance to the mother/family regarding potential duration of the interruption when possible/feasible. *When conditions (e.g., certain maternal drugs/substances; setting/maternal or infant illness) require a temporary interruption of breastfeeding, having an approximate duration of the interruption will assist the mother/family to plan and will provide reassurance of the temporary nature of the interruption (Davis et al, 2000; Ito, 2000; Nystorm & Axelsson, 2002; Ward et al, 2001; U.S. Department of Health and Human Services, 2000).* **EBN:** *Mothers who experienced separation from their infants due to the infant needing to go to the neonatal intensive care unit (NICU) shared that they desired someone to speak with them and provide explanations about what was happening with their baby (Nystrom & Axelsson, 2002). Using a case study methodology describing in detail the experiences of two mothers of premature infants, nurse researchers suggest that*

*women with a history of breast augmentation be monitored for the possible complication of lactation insufficiency (Hill, Wilhelm, Aldag et al, 2004).*

- Reassure mother/family that early measures to sustain lactation and promote parent-infant attachment can make it possible to resume breastfeeding when the condition/situation requiring interruption is resolved. *Early breast stimulation assists in establishing lactation, and efforts to maintain lactation during interrupted breastfeeding can assist in the resumption of breastfeeding (Association of Women's Health Obstetric and Neonatal Nurses, 2000a; Hill, 2000; Jones et al, 2001; Jones & Spencer, 2001).* **EBN:** *Researchers found that delays in suckling and milk expression may cause maternal prolactin levels to decrease suggesting the chance for difficulty in resuming lactation unless early measures are taken (Jones et al, 2001).*
- Reassure the mother/family that the infant will benefit from any amount of breast milk provided. *The benefits of breast milk include protection (immunity, reduced risk of allergies, and so on). Breast milk is the preferable nutrition source (Association of Women's Health Obstetric and Neonatal Nurses, 2000a,b; U.S. Department of Health and Human Services, 2000; World Health Organization, 2001).* **EBN:** *Evidence-based clinical practice guidelines recommend teaching women/families about the benefits of breast milk and providing professional support during transition times (return to work and other interruptions) (Association of Women's Health Obstetric and Neonatal Nurses, 2000a).* **EB:** *Reviews of the literature have agreed with professional standards recommending exclusive breastfeeding and have identified studies supporting the beneficial effects in relation to growth and development, protection from asthma, allergies, and so on; however, findings from studies over time have been inconsistent and questions remain regarding nutritional enhancement for very-low-birth-weight babies (Fulhan, Collier, & Duggan, 2003; O'Connor, Merko, & Brennan, 2004).*
- Provide time for mother/family to express their expectations and concerns and give emotional support. Emotional responses regarding events leading to the interruption that may arise include feelings of grief/loss, guilt, anxiety, and failure. *Discussing concerns and differences between expectations and experiences provide an opportunity for the client to ventilate and may contribute to positive coping strategies (Mozingo et al, 2000; Nystrom & Axelsson, 2002; Porteous et al, 2000; Rojjanasrirat, 2004; Schaefer, 2004).* **EBN:** *In a qualitative study, mothers who were separated from their newborns revealed emotional strain and anxiety regardless of the presence of serious illness (Nystrom & Axelsson, 2002). In one case study describing breastfeeding problems, nurses provided psychosocial support and three consecutive skin-to-skin breastfeedings with positive outcomes (Burkhammer, Anderson, & Chiu, 2004).*

▲ Collaborate with the mother/family/health care providers/employers (as needed) to develop a plan for expression of breast milk/infant feeding/kangaroo care/SSC. *Clients' participation will assure the success of the plan, promote maternal confidence and self-esteem, and/or facilitate maternal role performance (Burkhammer, Anderson, & Chiu, 2004; Charpak et al, 2001; Griffin et al, 2000; Libbus & Bullock, 2002; Matthiesen et al, 2001; Stevens & Janke, 2003).* **EBN:** *In a qualitative arm of a larger study, responses to open-ended questions provided by 50 women were content analyzed. Four themes emerged related to support, attitudes, having a strategic plan, and psychological distress and the researcher suggests clinical implications for nurse advocacy, collaborating with women to* *develop a plan for pumping and maintaining lactation, and providing support (Rojjanasrirat, 2004).*



- Monitor for signs indicating infants' ability to and interest in breastfeeding. *The infant must be able to demonstrate the ability to breastfeed and demonstrate responsiveness for the mother to begin/resume breastfeeding. The interplay between mother and baby is an important factor in maternal confidence and breastfeeding success (Mennella, 2001; Pridham et al, 2001; Thomas, 2000).* **EBN:** *Researchers found that an infant's contentedness and ability to be soothed (aspects of responsiveness) contribute to mothers' evaluation of self in relation to confidence and competence (Pridham et al, 2001).*
- Provide evidence-based teaching and practical assistance with milk expression, storage, temporary feeding techniques, and breastfeeding techniques appropriate to the client's individualized needs (see Client/Family Teaching). *Accurate, consistent information and providing practical assistance based on evidence and in response to individualized needs are associated with maternal confidence, client satisfaction, and successful breastfeeding (Association of Women's Health Obstetric and Neonatal Nurses, 2000b; Jones et al, 2001; Lauver et al, 2002; Meier et al, 2000; Nyqvist, 2002; Philipp & Merewood, 2003).* **EBN:** *In a prospective study of a small number of mothers delivering preterm twins, the researcher elicited mothers' need for special support and nurses practical assistance, encouragement, and emotional support (Nyqvist, 2002). In an expert review of one teaching video, the content and medium were evaluated as meeting the needs of breastfeeding mothers of babies being cared for in the NICU (Hayes, 2003).*
- Observe mother performing psychomotor skill (expression, storage, alternative feeding, kangaroo care, and/or breastfeeding) and assist as needed. *The nurse's presence and involvement allow for identification of those areas for which assistance, clarification, and/or support are needed and promotes maternal confidence (Association of Women's Health Obstetric and Neonatal Nurses, 2000a; Gill, 2001; Hong, Callister, & Schwartz, 2003; US Department of Health and Human Services, 2000).* **EBN:** *Evidence-based guidelines include observation and practical assistance with psychomotor skills for all women/families (Association of Women's Health Obstetric and Neonatal Nurses, 2000a; U.S. Department of Health and Human Services, 2000).*
- ▲ Provide and/or assist with arrangements and/or necessary equipment. *Pumping and other equipment recommendations should be based on each mother's/infant's situation and needs (Association of Women's Health Obstetric and Neonatal Nurses, 2000a; Meier et al, 2000; Rojjanasrirat, 2004; Schaefer, 2004).* **EBN:** *Nurse researchers have found that working women and those with chronic illness have specific needs including assistance with arrangement of space and time for milk expression (hand or pump) and anticipatory guidance for planning for pumping schedules, using alternative feeding positions/approaches to promote successful breastfeeding (Ortiz, McGilligan, & Kelly, 2004; Rojjanasrirat, 2004; Schaefer, 2004).*
- ▲ Use supplementation only as medically indicated. *If human milk can be provided and fed to the infant, it is preferable (Association of Women's Health Obstetric and Neonatal Nurses, 2000a; Fenton et al, 2000; Fulhan, Collier, & Duggan, 2003; O'Connor, Merko, & Brennan, 2004).* **EBN:** *Researchers found that mothers of very-low-birth-weight infants who used commercial breast milk–enhancing powder products with expressed breast milk were able to achieve lactation durations closer to their stated goals (Fenton et al, 2000).* **EB:**

B

*Literature reviews suggest that while human breast milk is beneficial, the needs of infants with nutritional vulnerabilities, especially those of very-low-birth-weight, may require micronutrient fortification after hospital discharge to promote catch-up growth, accretion of lean body mass, and improved bone mineralization (Fulhan, Collier, & Duggan, 2003; O'Connor, Merko, & Brennan, 2004).*

- Provide anticipatory guidance for common problems associated with interrupted breastfeeding (e.g., incomplete emptying of milk glands, diminishing milk supply, infant difficulty with resuming breastfeeding, or infant refusal of alternative feeding method). *Mothers who know what to expect will feel more confident and be more likely to cope with any difficulties that may arise (Blyth et al, 2002; Libbus & Bullock, 2002; Modrcin-Talbott, Harrison, Groer et al, 2003; Thoyre, 2000).* **EBN:** *Researchers found that the most common reason for discontinuation of breastfeeding was insufficient milk supply (Blyth et al, 2002).*
- Initiate follow-up and make appropriate referrals. *Follow-up provides the opportunity for review of information, feedback about techniques, identification of and assistance with problems, and promotes maternal confidence and satisfaction (Association of Women's Health Obstetric and Neonatal Nurses, 2000a; Pugh et al, 2002).* **EBN:** *Breastfeeding women receiving nurse and peer counselor support had longer duration of breastfeeding, and infants had fewer sick visits and reported use of fewer medications than those receiving usual care (Pugh et al, 2002).*
- Assist the client to accept and learn an alternative method of infant feeding if effective breastfeeding is not achieved. *If it is clear that breastfeeding cannot be achieved after the interruption and an alternative feeding method must be instituted, the mother needs support and education (Mozingo et al, 2000).* **EBN:** *In a qualitative study of women's experiences with short-term breastfeeding, researchers uncovered women's concerns about breastfeeding failure and their feelings of relief versus guilt and shame for which women may need assistance and support (Mozingo et al, 2000).*

## Multicultural

- Assess for the influence of cultural beliefs, norms, and values on current decision to stop breastfeeding. **EBN:** *The client's decision to halt breastfeeding may be based on cultural perceptions, as well as influences from the larger social context (Cricco-Lizza, 2004; Leininger & McFarland, 2002; deOliveira, 2003; Newton, 2004). A study of Thai nurses suggests that beliefs about breastfeeding and postpartum practices of the nurse care provider may also have implications for clients' breastfeeding experiences (Kaewsarn, Moyle, & Creedy, 2003).*
- Assess the influence of family support on the decision to continue or discontinue breastfeeding. **EBN:** *Women are the keepers and transmitters of culture in families. Female family members can play a dominant role in how infants are fed (Cesario, 2001). Recent research has found that the mother's partner and family are most influential in the choice of infant feeding method and thus should be included in breastfeeding promotion programs for ethnically diverse women (Rose et al, 2004).*
- Assess whether the client's concerns about the amount of milk taken during breastfeeding is contributing to decision to stop breastfeeding. **EBN:** *Some cultures may add*

*semisolid food within the first month of life as a result of concerns that the infant is not getting enough to eat and the perception that "big is healthy" (Higgins, 2000).*

- Teach culturally appropriate techniques for maintaining lactation. **EBN:** *The Oketani method of breast massage is used by Japanese and other Asian women. Researchers have found that Oketani breast massage improved quality of human milk by increasing total solids, lipids, casein concentration and gross energy (Foda, Kawashima, Nakamura et al, 2004).*
- Validate the client's feelings with regard to the difficulty of or her dissatisfaction with breastfeeding. **EBN:** *Scandinanvian researchers examined psychosocial factors related to length of breastfeeding and found that the first 5 weeks was a vulnerable period and found factors associated with continuing to breast-feed. They concluded that interventions should be aimed at improving self-efficacy and resources available to those at risk (Kronborg & Vaeth, 2004).*

### Home Care

- Above interventions may be adapted for home care use.

## Client/Family Teaching

- Teach mother effective methods to express breast milk. *There are a variety of methods of expression and these involve psychomotor skills requiring instruction; breast stimulation is essential to continuing lactation (Association of Women's Health Obstetric and Neonatal Nurses, 2000a; Fewtrell et al, 2001; Foda, Kawashima, Nakamura et al, 2004; Jones et al, 2001; Matthiesen et al, 2001; Phillip & Merewood, 2003).* **EBN:** *In a sample of women who delivered preterm infants, researchers testing the use of electric and manual pumps found that those using the electric pump had shorter expression times but produced no more milk than those using the manual pump (Fewtrell et al, 2001).*
- Teach mother/parents about kangaroo care. *Indirect stimulation of lactation through close contact with the infant can occur and kangaroo care has been associated with positive neonatal out comes (Charpak et al, 2001; Daley & Kennedy, 2000; Mellien, 2001).* **EBN:** *In a small study of very-low-birth-weight preterm infants, the infants maintained a stable temperature in their mothers' arms with no indication of increased metabolic activity (Mellien, 2001). Although clinical benefits of SSC have been supported in the literature (Anderson, Moore, Hepworth et al, 2003), researchers agree that methodological limitations in previous studies make firm conclusions regarding SSC and the duration of breastfeeding impossible and suggest that further research is needed (Anderson, Moore, Hepworth et al, 2004; Carfoot, Williamson, & Dickson, 2003).*
- Instruct mother on safe breast milk handling techniques. *Storage and handling practices can optimize the nutritional value and provide protection against contaminants (Association of Women's Health Obstetric and Neonatal Nurses, 2000a; Phillipp & Merewood, 2003; Tully, 2000).* **EBN:** *Evidence-based guidelines address the importance of expression, storage, and provision of stored human milk in cases of mother-infant separation particularly as it relates to women returning to work (Association of Women's Health Obstetric and Neonatal Nurses, 2000a,b).*
- Provide education to father/family/significant others as needed. *Informed support people have a desire to learn, may be needed to assist mothers who are separated from their infants,*

*and may have an impact on breastfeeding duration (Association of Women's Health Obstetric and Neonatal Nurses, 2000a; Guttman & Zimmerman, 2000; Hill, 2000; Moore, 2000; Pollock et al, 2002; Wolfberg, Michels, Shields et al, 2004).* **EB:** *Researchers conducting a randomized controlled trial with a 2-hour intervention class on infant care and breastfeeding promotion found that the fathers in the intervention group were influential advocates for breastfeeding (Wolfberg, Michels, Shields et al, 2004).*

## evolve WEBSITES FOR EDUCATION

See the EVOLVE website for World Wide Web resources for client education.

## REFERENCES


Anderson GC, Moore E, Hepworth J et al: Early skin-to-skin contact for mothers and their healthy newborn infants, *Cochrane Database Sys Rev* (2), 2003.

Association of Women's Health Obstetric and Neonatal Nurses: *Evidence-based clinical practice guideline: breastfeeding support: prenatal care through the first year (practice guideline),* Washington, DC, 2000a, The Association.

Association of Women's Health Obstetric and Neonatal Nurses: *Evidence-based clinical practice guideline: breast-feeding support: prenatal care through the first year (monograph),* Washington, DC, 2000b, The Association.

Blyth R, Creedy DK, Dennis CL et al: Effect of maternal confidence on breastfeeding duration: an application of breastfeeding self-efficacy theory, *Birth* 29(4):278-284, 2002.

Burkhammer MD, Anderson GC, Chiu SH: Grief, anxiety, stillbirth, and perinatal problems: healing with kangaroo care, *J Obstet Gynecol Neonat Nurs* 33(6):774-782, 2004.

Carfoot S, Williamson PR, Dickson R: A systematic review of randomized controlled trials evaluating the effect of mother/baby skin-to-skin care on successful breastfeeding, *Midwifery* 19(2):148-155, 2003.

Cesario S: Care of the Native American woman: strategies for practice, education, and research, *J Obstet Gynecol Neonatal Nurs* 30(1):13-19, 2001.

Charpak N, Ruiz-Pelaez JG, Figueroa de CZ et al: A randomized, controlled trial of kangaroo mother care: results of follow-up at 1 year of corrected age, *Pediatrics* 108(5):1072-1079, 2001.

Daley HK, Kennedy CM: Meta analysis: effects of interventions on premature infants feeding, *J Perinat Neonat Nurs* 14(3):62-77, 2000.

Davis LJ, Okuboye S, Ferguson SL: Healthy people 2010. Examining a decade of maternal and infant health, *AWHONN Lifelines* 4(3):26-33, 2000.

Brady S de O: Protecting breastfeeding: Brazil's story, *Pract Midwife* 6(10):14-16, 2003.

Dochterman JM, Bulecheck GM: *Nursing interventions classification (NIC),* ed 4, St. Louis, 2003, Mosby.

Fenton TR, Tough SC, Belik J: Breast milk supplementation for preterm infants: parental preferences and postdischarge lactation duration, *Am J Perinatol* 17(6):329-333, 2000.

Fewtrell MS, Lucas P, Collier S et al: Randomized trial comparing the efficacy of a novel manual breast pump with a standard electric breast pump in mothers who delivered preterm infants, *Pediatrics* 107(6):1291-1297, 2001.

Foda MI, Kawashima T, Nakamura S et al: Composition of milk obtained from unmassaged versus massaged breasts of lactating mothers, *J Pediatr Gastroentrol Nutr* 38(5):484-487, 2004.

Fulhan J, Collier S, Duggan C: Update on pediatric nutrition: breastfeeding, infant nutrition, and growth, *Curr Opin Pediatr* 15(3): 323-332, 2003.

Gill SL: The little things: perceptions of breastfeeding support, *J Obstet Gynecol Neonatal Nurs* 30(4):401-409, 2001.

Griffin TL, Meier PP, Bradford LP et al: Mothers' performing creamatocrit measures in the NICU: accuracy, reactions, and cost, *J Obstet Gynecol Neonat Nurs* 29(3):249-257, 2000.

Guttman N, Zimmerman DR: Low-income mothers' views on breastfeeding, *Soc Sci Med* 50(10):1457-1473, 2000.

Hattori R, Hattori H: Breastfeeding twins: guidelines for success, *Birth* 26(1):37-42, 1999.

Hayes B: A premie needs his mother: first steps to breastfeeding your premature baby, *Birth* 30(1):69, 2003.

Higgins B: Puerto Rican cultural beliefs: influence on infant feeding practices in western New York, *J Transcult Nurs* 11(1):19-30, 2000.

Hill PD: Update on breastfeeding: Healthy People 2010 objectives, *MCN Am J Matern Child Nurs* 25:248, 2000.

Hill PD, Wilhelm PA, Aldag JC et al: Breast augmentation and lactation outcomes: a case report, *MCN Am J Matern Child Nurs* 29:238, 2004.

Hong TM, Callister LC, Schwartz R: First-time mothers' views of breastfeeding support from nurses, *MCN Am J Matern Child Nurs* 28:10, 2003.

International Lactation Consultant Association: *Evidence-based guidelines for breastfeeding management during the first fourteen days,* Raleigh, NC, 1999, The Association.

Ito S: Drug therapy: drug therapy for breast-feeding women, *N Engl J Med* 343:118, 2000.

Johnson M, Maas M, Moorehead S: *Nursing outcomes classification (NOC)*, ed 2, St Louis, 2000, Mosby.

Jones E, Dimmock PW, Spencer SA: A randomized controlled trial to compare methods of milk expression after preterm delivery, *Arch Dis Child Fetal Neonatal Ed* 85(2):F91-95, 2001.

Jones E, Spencer SA: Promoting successful breastfeeding for mothers of preterm infants, *Prof Care Mother Child* 10:145, 2001.

Kaewsarn P, Moyle W, Creedy D: Thai nurses' beliefs about breastfeeding and postpartum practices, *J Clin Nurs* 12:467, 2003.

Kloeblen-Tarver AS, Thompson NJ, Miner KR: Intent to breast-feed: the impact of attitudes, norms, parity, and experience, *Am J Health Behav* 26:182, 2002.

Kronborg H & Vaeth M: The influence of psychosocial factors on the duration of breastfeeding, *Scand J Public Health* 32:210, 2004.

Lauver DR, Ward SE, Heidrich SM et al: Patient-centered interventions, *Res Nurs Health* 25(4):246-255, 2002.

Leininger MM, McFarland MR: *Transcultural nursing: concepts, theories, research and practices,* ed 3, New York, 2002, McGraw-Hill.

Libbus MK, Bullock LFC: Breastfeeding and employment: an assessment of employers' attitudes, *J Hum Lact* 18:247, 2002.

Matthiesen AS et al: Postpartum maternal oxytocin release by newborns: effects of infant hand massage and sucking, *Birth* 28(1): 13-19, 2001.

Meier PP, Brown LP, Hurst NM et al: Nipple shields for preterm infants: effect on milk transfer and duration of breastfeeding, *J Hum Lact* 16(2):106-14, quiz 129-131, 2000.

Mellien AC: Incubators versus mothers' arms: body temperature conservation in very-low-birth-weight premature infants, *J Gynecol Neonat Nurs* 30:157, 2001.

Mennella JA: Regulation of milk intake after exposure to alcohol in mothers' milk, *Alcoholism* 25:590, 2001.

Modrcin-Talbott MA, Harrison LL, Groer MW et al: The biobehavioral effects of gentle human touch on preterm infants, *Nurs Sci Q* 16:60, 2003.

Mozingo JN, Davis MW, Droppleman PG et al: "It wasn't working." Women's experiences with short-term breastfeeding, *MCN Am J Matern Child Nurs* 25(3):120-126, 2000.

Newton ER: The epidemiology of breastfeeding, *Clin Obstet and Gynecol* 47:613, 2004.

Nyqvist KH: Breast-feeding in preterm twins: development of feeding behavior and milk intake during hospital stay and related caregiving practices, *J Pediatr Nurs* 17:246, 2002.

Nystrom K, Axelsson K: Mothers' experience of being separated from their newborns, *J Gynecol Neonat Nurs* 31: 275, 2002.

O'Connor DL, Merko S, Brennan J: Human milk feeding of very low birth weight infants during initial hospitalization and after discharge, *Nutri Today* 39:102, 2004.

Ortiz J, McGilligan K, Kelly P: Duration of breast milk expression among working mothers enrolled in an employer-sponsored lactation program, *Pediatric Nurs* 30:111, 2004.

Philipp B: Encouraging patients to use a breast pump, *Contemp Ob Gyn* 1:88-100, 2003.

Pinelli J, Atkinson SA, Saigal S: Randomized trial of breastfeeding support in very low-birth-weight infants, *Arch Pediatr Adolesc Med* 155:548, 2001.

Pollock CA, Bustamante-Forest R, Giarratano G: Men of diverse cultures: knowledge and attitudes about breastfeeding, *J Obstet Gynecol Neonatal Nurs* 31(6):673-679, 2002.

Porteous R, Kaufman K, Rush J: The effect of individualized professional support on duration of breastfeeding: a randomized controlled trial, *J Hum Lact* 16(4):303-308, 2000.

Pridham K, Lin CY, Brown R: Mothers' evaluation of their caregiving for premature and full-term infants through the first year: contributing factors, *Res Nurs Health* 24(3):157-169, 2001.

Pugh LC, Milligan RA, Frick KD et al: Breastfeeding duration, costs, and benefits of a support program for low-income breastfeeding women, *Birth* 29(2):95-100, 2002.

Rojjanasrirat W: Working women's breastfeeding experiences, *MCN Am J Matern Child Nurs* 29:222, 2004.

Schaefer KM: Breastfeeding in chronic illness: the voices of women with fibromyalgia, *MCN Am J Matern Child Nurs* 29:248, 2004.

B

Stevens KV, Janke J: Breastfeeding experiences of active duty military women, *Milit Med* 168:380, 2003.
Thomas KA: Differential effects of breast-and formula-feeding on preterm infants sleep-wake patterns, *J Gynecol Neonat Nurs* 29: 145, 2000.
Thoyre SM: Mothers' ideas about their role in feeding their high-risk infants, *J Gynecol Neonat Nurs* 29:613, 2000.
Tully MR: Recommendations for handling of mothers' own milk, *J Hum Lact* 16:149, 2000.
US Department of Health and Human Services: *HHS blueprint for action on breastfeeding,* Washington, DC, 2000, US Department of Health and Human Services, Office on Women's Health.
Vari PM, Camburn J, Henly SJ: Professionally mediated peer support and early breastfeeding success, *J Perinat Educ* 9:22, 2000.
Ward RM et al: The transfer of drugs and other chemicals into human milk, *Pediatrics* 108:776, 2001.
Wolfberg AJ, Michels KB, Shields W et al: Dads as breastfeeding advocates: results from a randomized controlled trial of an educational intervention, *Am J Obstet Gynecol* 191(3):708-712 2004.
World Health Organization: *Report of the expert consultation on the optimal duration of exclusive breastfeeding,* Geneva, Switzerland, 2001, WHO.

# Ineffective Breathing pattern

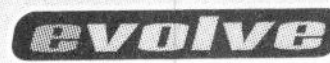

*Betty J. Ackley*

**NANDA**

## Definition

Inspiration and/or expiration that does not provide adequate ventilation

## Defining Characteristics

Decreased inspiratory/expiratory pressure; decreased minute ventilation; use of accessory muscles to breathe; nasal flaring; dyspnea; altered chest excursion; shortness of breath; assumption of a three-point position; pursed-lip breathing; prolonged expiration phases; increased anteroposterior diameter; respiratory rate/min: infants = <25 or >60, ages 1-4 = <20 or >30, ages 5-14 = <14 or >25, adults over 14 = <11 or >24; depth of breathing: adult tidal volume = 500 mL at rest, infant tidal volume = 6-8 mL/Kg; timing ratio; decreased vital capacity

## Related Factors (r/t)

Hyperventilation, hypoventilation syndrome, bony deformity, pain, chest wall deformity, anxiety, decreased energy/fatigue, neuromuscular dysfunction, musculoskeletal impairment, perception/cognitive impairment, obesity, spinal cord injury, body position, neurological immaturity, respiratory muscle fatigue

**NOC**

## Outcomes (Nursing Outcomes Classification)

### Suggested NOC Outcomes

Respiratory Status: Airway Patency, Ventilation; Vital Signs

B

**Example NOC Outcome with Indicators**

**Respiratory Status: Ventilation** as evidenced by the following indicators: Respiratory rate IER/Respiratory rhythm IER/Depth of inspiration/Chest expansion symmetrical/Ease of breathing/Accessory muscle use not present/Chest retraction not present/Auscultated breath sounds IER/Tidal volume IER/Vital capacity IER (Rate each indicator of **Respiratory Status: Ventilation:** 1 = severely compromised, 2 = substantially compromised, 3 = moderately compromised, 4 = mildly compromised, 5 = not compromised [see Section I].)

IER, In expected range.

## Client Outcomes

### Client Will (Specify Time Frame):

- Demonstrate a breathing pattern that supports blood gas results within the client's normal parameters
- Report ability to breathe comfortably
- Demonstrate ability to perform pursed-lip breathing and controlled breathing and use relaxation techniques effectively
- Identify and avoid specific factors that exacerbate episodes of ineffective breathing patterns

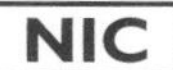

## Interventions (Nursing Interventions Classification)

### Suggested NIC Interventions

Airway Management, Respiratory Monitoring

**Example NIC Activities—Airway Management**

Encourage slow, deep breathing; turning; and coughing; monitor respiratory and oxygenation status as appropriate

## Nursing Interventions and Rationales

- Monitor respiratory rate, depth, and ease of respiration. Normal respiratory rate is 12 to 16 breaths/min in the adult. *When the respiratory rate exceeds 24 breaths/min, significant respiratory or cardiovascular disease is evident.* See Defining Characteristics for guidelines for children.
- Note pattern of respiration. If client is dyspneic, note what seems to cause the dyspnea, the way in which the client deals with the condition, and how the dyspnea resolves or gets worse. Note amount of anxiety associated with the dyspnea. *A normal respiratory pattern is regular in a healthy adult. To assess dyspnea, it is important to consider all of its dimensions, including antecedents, mediators, reactions, and outcomes.* **EBN:** *A qualitative study demonstrated that experienced nurses working with COPD clients fre-*

*quently used the degree of anxiety as an indicator of an acute exacerbation of COPD (Bailey, Colella, & Mossey, 2004).*

- Attempt to determine if client's dyspnea is physiological or psychological in cause. *Psychological dyspnea includes dyspnea caused by anxiety or fear and can be associated with a panic attack (Meuret, Wilhelm, & Roth, 2004).*

## Psychological Dyspnea—Hyperventilation

- Assess cause of hyperventilation by asking client about current emotions and psychological state. **EB:** *A study demonstrated that clients with idiopathic hyperventilation were more anxious and had a higher depression score than control subjects (Jack et al, 2004).*
- Ask the client to breathe with you to slow down respiratory rate. Maintain eye contact and give reassurance. *By making the client aware of respirations and giving support, the client may gain control of the breathing rate.*
- ▲ If pain is the cause of hyperventilation, provide medication routinely as ordered to prevent severe pain. Use distraction techniques to help client deal with pain. See interventions for **Acute Pain.** *An increased respiratory rate is one sign of pain. Providing pain relief will cause the respiratory rate to return to normal.*
- If client has chronic problems with hyperventilation, numbness and tingling in extremities, dizziness, and other signs of panic attacks, refer for counseling. *Cognitive behavioral therapy can be helpful for panic attacks, as can also respiratory feedback utilizing measurement of $CO_2$ levels using a capnometry device to give the client feedback on rate and depth of breathing (Meuret, Wilhelm, & Roth, 2004).*

## Physiological Dyspnea

- Ensure that client in acute dyspneic state has received medications, oxygen, and any other treatment needed. *Pharmacological treatment of dyspnea exists but may not suffice to relieve dyspnea (Bruera et al, 2000; Janssens, 2000).*
- Determine severity of dyspnea using a rating scale such as the modified Borg scale, rating dyspnea 0 (best) to 10 (worst) in severity. An alternative scale is the Visual Analogue Scale (VAS) with dyspnea rated as 0 (best) to 100 (worst). **EBN and EB:** *In a study in an emergency room, the modified Borg scale correlated well with clinical measurements of respiratory function and was found helpful by both clients and nurses (Kendrick et al, 2000). Another study comparing the Borg and the VAS scales found that they measured symptoms reproducibly during steady-state exercise and can detect the effect of a drug intervention (Grant et al, 1999).*
- Note abdominal breathing, use of accessory muscles, nasal flaring, retractions, irritability, confusion, or lethargy. *These symptoms signal increasing respiratory difficulty and increasing hypoxia.*
- Observe color of tongue, oral mucosa, and skin. *Cyanosis of the tongue and oral mucosa is central cyanosis and generally represents a medical emergency. Peripheral cyanosis of nail beds or lips may or may not be serious (Kasper et al, 2005).*
- Auscultate breath sounds, noting decreased or absent sounds, crackles, or wheezes. *These abnormal lung sounds can indicate a respiratory pathology associated with an altered breathing pattern.*
- ▲ Monitor client's oxygen saturation and blood gases. *An oxygen saturation of less than*

*90% (normal: 95% to 100%) or a partial pressure of oxygen of less than 80 (normal: 80 to 100) indicates significant oxygenation problems (Berry & Pinard, 2002; Grap, 2002).*

- ▲ Monitor for presence of pain and provide pain medication for comfort as needed. *Pain causes the client to hypoventilate and take shallow breaths that predispose the client to atelectasis.*
- • Using touch on the shoulder, coach the client to slow respiratory rate, demonstrating slower respirations; making eye contact with the client; and communicating in a calm, supportive fashion. *The nurse's presence, reassurance, and help in controlling the client's breathing can be very beneficial in decreasing anxiety (Truesdell, 2000).* **EBN:** *Anxiety can exacerbate dyspnea, causing the client to enter into a dyspneic panic state (Gift et al, 1992). A study demonstrated that anxiety is an important indicator of severity of client's disease with COPD (Bailey, 2004).*
- • Support the client in using pursed-lip and controlled breathing techniques. *Pursed-lip breathing results in increased use of intercostal muscles, decreased respiratory rate, increased tidal volume, and improved oxygen saturation levels (Collins et al, 2001; Dechman & Wilson, 2004).* **EB:** *A study demonstrated that pursed-lip breathing was effective in decreasing breathlessness (Bianchi et al, 2004).*
- • Position the client in an upright or semi-Fowler's position. *An upright position facilitates lung expansion.* See Nursing Interventions and Rationales for **Impaired Gas exchange** for further information on positioning.
- ▲ Administer oxygen as ordered. *Oxygen therapy helps decrease dyspnea through reduction in the central drive mediated via peripheral chemoreceptors in the carotid body (Meek, 1999).*
- • Increase client's activity to walking three times per day as tolerated. Assist the client to use oxygen during activity as needed. See Nursing Interventions and Rationales for **Activity intolerance**. *Supervised exercise has been shown to decrease dyspnea and increase tolerance to activity (Kasper et al, 2005).* **EBN:** *A group of COPD clients who participated in a systematic movement program used less emotion-focused coping than did nonexercisers (Gift & Austin, 1992).*
- • Schedule rest periods before and after activity. *Respiratory clients with dyspnea are easily exhausted and need additional rest.*
- ▲ Evaluate the client's nutritional status. Refer to a dietitian if needed. Use nutritional supplements to increase nutritional level if need indicated. *Improved nutrition may help increase inspiratory muscle function and decrease dyspnea (Meek, 1999).*
- • Provide small, frequent feedings. *Small feedings are given to avoid compromising ventilatory effort and to conserve energy. Clients with dyspnea often do not eat sufficient amounts of food because their priority is breathing.*
- • Offer a fan to move the air in the environment. *The movement of cool air on the face may help relieve dyspnea in pulmonary clients (Meek, 1999).*
- • Encourage the client to take deep breaths at prescribed intervals and do controlled coughing.
- • Help the client with chronic respiratory disease to evaluate dyspnea experience to determine if similar to previous incidences of dyspnea and to recognize that he or she made it through those incidences. Encourage the client to be self-reliant if possible, use problem solving skills, and maximize use of social support. *The focus of attention on sensations of breathlessness has an impact on judgment used to determine the intensity of*

*the sensation (Meek, 2000).* **EBN:** *One study demonstrated that the most frequently used coping styles for clients with COPD were being optimistic and self-reliant, using problem-solving skills, and receiving social support (Baker & Scholz, 2002).*

- See **Ineffective Airway clearance** if client has a problem with increased respiratory secretions.
- ▲ Refer COPD client for pulmonary rehabilitation. **EB:** *Pulmonary rehabilitation has been shown to relieve dyspnea and fatigue, and enhance clients' sense of control over client's disease. Rehabilitation is an important component of the management of COPD (Lacasse et al, 2002). Pulmonary rehabilitation was effective in reducing the utilization of health care resources (California Pulmonary Rehabilitation Collaborative Group, 2004).*

### Geriatric

- Encourage ambulation as tolerated. *Immobility is harmful to the elderly because it decreases ventilation and increases stasis of secretions (Fletcher, 2005).*
- Encourage elderly clients to sit upright or stand and to avoid lying down for prolonged periods during the day. *Thoracic aging results in decreased lung expansion; an erect position fosters maximal lung expansion (Fletcher, 2005).*

### Home Care

- Above interventions may be adapted for home care use.
- Assist the client and family with identifying other factors that precipitate or exacerbate episodes of ineffective breathing patterns (i.e., stress, allergens, stairs, activities that have high energy requirements). *Awareness of precipitating factors helps clients avoid them and decreases risk of ineffective breathing episodes.*
- Assess client knowledge of and compliance with medication regimen. *Client/family may need repetition of instructions received at hospital discharge, and may require reiteration as fear of a recent crisis decreases. Fear interferes with the ability to assimilate new information.*
- Teach the client and family the importance of maintaining regimen and having PRN drugs easily accessible at all times. *Appropriate and timely use of medications can decrease the risk of exacerbating ineffective breathing.* **EBN:** *Parents/family have been found to have inadequate knowledge about recognition of asthma attacks, triggers, and management (Navaie-Waliser et al, 2004).*
- Provide the client with emotional support in dealing with symptoms of respiratory difficulty. Provide family with support for care of a client with chronic or terminal illness. *Breathing difficulty can provoke extreme anxiety, which can interfere with the client's ability or willingness to adhere to the treatment plan.* Refer to care plan for **Anxiety.** *Witnessing breathing difficulties and facing concerns of dealing with chronic or terminal illness can create fear in caregiver. Fear inhibits effective coping.* **EBN:** *Social support helped asthma sufferers fight the sense of powerlessness caused by their illness (Makinen, Suominen, & Lauri, 2000). Parents of a child with cystic fibrosis particularly benefit from nursing support. Parents deal with devastation upon receiving the diagnosis, a sense of fear and isolation, an overwhelming sense of guilt and powerlessness, vigilance, and returning to normalcy (Carpenter & Narsavage, 2004).* Refer to care plan for **Powerlessness.**

- When respiratory procedures (e.g., apneic monitoring for an infant) are being implemented, explain equipment and procedures to family members, and provide needed emotional support. *Family members assuming responsibility for respiratory monitoring often find this stressful. They may not have been able to assimilate fully any instructions provided by hospital staff (McNeal, 2000).*
- When electrically based equipment for respiratory support is being implemented, evaluate home environment for electrical safety, proper grounding, etc. Ensure that notification is sent to the local utility company, the emergency medical team, police and fire departments. *Notification is important to provide for priority service (McNeal, 2000).*
- Refer to GOLD and ACP-ASIM/ACCP guidelines for management of home care and indications of hospital admission criteria (Chojnowski, 2003).
- Support clients' efforts at self-care. Ensure they have all the information they need to participate in care. **EBN:** *Self-care study participants showed competence at managing care of their own asthma (Makinen et al, 2000).* **EB:** *In another study of asthma clients, less self-efficacy, more depressive symptoms, expectation to be cured of asthma, having difficult access to care, and being Hispanic or African American predicted lower scores on quality-of-life questionnaires (Mancuso, Rincon, McCulloch, et al, 2001).*
- Identify an emergency plan including when to call the physician or 911. *Having a ready emergency plan reassures the client and promotes client safety.*

▲ Refer the client to an outpatient pulmonary rehabilitation program or a home-based training program for COPD. **EB:** *Outpatient rehabilitation programs can achieve worthwhile benefits including decreased perception of dyspnea, increased walking distance, and less fatigue (Guell et al, 2000; Lacasse et al, 2002). A simple home-based program of exercise training can help COPD clients achieve improvement in exercise tolerance, dyspnea, and quality of life (Hernandez et al, 2000).*

▲ Refer to occupational therapy for evaluation and teaching of energy conservation techniques.

▲ Refer to home health aide services as needed to support energy conservation. *Energy conservation decreases the risk of exacerbating ineffective breathing.*

▲ Institute case management of frail elderly to support continued independent living. *Respiratory difficulties represent and can lead to increasing needs for assistance in using the health care system effectively. Case management combines nursing activities of client and family assessment, planning and coordination of care among all health care providers, delivery of direct nursing care, and monitoring of care and outcomes. These activities are able to address continuity of care, mutual goal setting, behavior management, and prevention of worsening health problems (Guttman, 1999).*

## Client/Family Teaching

- Teach pursed-lip and controlled breathing techniques. *Pursed-lip breathing results in increased use of intercostal muscles, decreased respiratory rate, increased tidal volume, and improved oxygen saturation levels (Collins et al, 2001; Dechman & Wilson, 2004).* **EB:** *A study demonstrated that pursed-lip breathing was effective in decreasing breathlessness (Bianchi et al, 2004).*
- Using a prerecorded tape, teach client progressive muscle relaxation techniques. **EBN:** *Relaxation therapy can help reduce dyspnea and anxiety (Gift et al, 1992).*

B

- Teach about dosage, actions, and side effects of medications. *Inhaled steroids and bronchodilators can have undesirable side effects, especially when taken in inappropriate doses.*
- Teach the client to identify and avoid specific factors that exacerbate ineffective breathing patterns, such as exposure to other sources of air pollution, especially smoking.

## evolve WEBSITES FOR EDUCATION

See the EVOLVE website for World Wide Web resources for client education.

## REFERENCES


Baker CF, Scholz JA: Coping with symptoms of dyspnea in chronic obstructive pulmonary disease, *Rehabil Nurs* 27(2):67, 2002.

Bailey PH: The dyspnea-anxiety-dypnea cycle—COPD patients stories of breathlessness: "It's scary when you can't breathe," *Qual Health Res* 14(6):760, 2004.

Bailey PH, Colella T, Mossey S: COPD-intuition or template: nurses' stories of acute exacerbations of chronic obstructive pulmonary disease, *J Clin Nurs* 13(6):756, 2004.

Berry BE, Pinard AE: Assessing tissue oxygenation, *Crit Care Nurse* 22(3):22, 2002.

Bianchi R, Gigliotti F, Romagnoli I et al: Chest wall kinematics and breathlessness during pursed-lip breathing in patients with COPD, *Chest* 125(2):459, 2004.

Bruera E, Schmitz B, Pither J et al: The frequency and correlates of dyspnea in patients with advanced cancer, *J Pain Symptom Manage* 19(5):357, 2000.

California Pulmonary Rehabilitation Collaborative Group: Effects of pulmonary rehabilitation on dyspnea, quality of life and healthcare costs in California, *J Cardiopulm Rehabil* 24(1):52, 2004.

Carpenter DR, Narsavage GL: One breath at a time: Living with cystic fibrosis, *J Pediatr Nurs* 19(1):25, 2004.

Chojnowski D: "GOLD" standards for acute exacerbation in COPD, *Nurs Practitioner* 28(5):26, 2003.

Collins EG, Langbein WE, Fehr L et al: Breathing pattern retraining and exercise in person with chronic obstructive pulmonary disease. *AACN Clin Issues* 12(2):202, 2001.

Dechman G, Wilson CR: Evidence underlying breathing retraining in people with stablechronic obstructive pulmonary disease, *Physical Therapy* 84(12):1189, 2004.

Dyspnea. Mechanisms, assessment, and management: a consensus statement. American Thoracic Society, *Am J Respir Crit Care Med* 159(1):321, 1999.

Fletcher K: Immobility: geriatric self-learning module, *Medsurg Nursing* 14(1):35, 2005.

Gift A, Austin D: The effects of a program of systematic movement on COPD patients, *Rehabil Nurs* 17(1):6, 1992.

Gift A, Moore T, Soeken K: Relaxation to reduce dyspnea and anxiety in COPD patients, *Nurs Res* 41(4):242, 1992.

Guell R, Casan P, Belda J et al: Long-term effects of outpatient rehabilitation of COPD: a randomized trial, *Chest* 117(4):976, 2000.

Grant S, Aitchison T, Henderson E et al: A comparison of the reproducibility and the sensitivity to change of visual analogue scales, Borg scales, and Likert scales in normal subjects during submaximal exercise, *Chest* 116(5):1208, 1999.

Grap MJ: Protocols for practice: applying research at the bedside: pulse oximetry, *Crit Care Nurse* 22(3):69, 2002.

Guttman R: Case management of the frail elderly in the community, *Clin Nurs Spec* 13(4):174, 1999.

Hernandez MT, Rubio TM, Ruiz FO et al: Results of a home-based training program for patients with COPD, *Chest* 188(1):106, 2000.

Jack S, Rossiter HB, Pearson MG et al: Ventilatory responses to inhaled carbon dioxide, hypoxia, and exercise in idiopathic hyperventilation, *Am J Respir Crit Care Med* 170(2):118, 2004.

Janssens JP, Muralt BD, Titelion V: Management of dyspnea in severe chronic obstructive pulmonary disease, *J Pain Symptom Manage* 19(5):378, 2000.

Kasper DL et al: *Harrison's principles of internal medicine,* ed 16, New York, 2005, McGraw-Hill.

Kendrick KR, Baxi SC, Smith RM: Usefulness of the modified 1-10 Borg scale in assessing the degree of dyspnea in patients with COPD and asthma, *J Emerg Nurs* 26(3):216, 2000.

Lacasse Y, Brosseau L, Milne S et al: Pulmonary rehabilitation for chronic obstructive pulmonary disease, *Cochrane Database Syst Rev* (3):CD003793, 2002.
Makinen S, Suominen T, Lauri S: Self-care in adults with asthma: how they cope, *J Clin Nurs* 9:557, 2000.
Mancuso CA, Rincon M, McCulloch CE et al: Self-efficacy, depressive symptoms, and patients' expectations predict outcomes in asthma, *Med Care* 39(12):1326, 2001.
McNeal GJ: *AACN guide to acute care procedures in the home,* Philadelphia, 2000, Lippincott.
Meek PM: Influence of attention and judgment on perception of breathlessness in healthy individuals and patients with chronic obstructive pulmonary disease, *Nurs Res* 49(1):11, 2000.
Meuret AE, Wilhelm FH, Roth WT: Respiratory feedback for treating panic disorder, *J Clin Psychol* 60(2):197, 2004.
Navaie-Waliser M, Misener M, Mersman C et al: Evaluating the needs of children with asthma in home care: The vital role of nurses as caregivers and educators, *Public Health Nurs* 21(4):306, 2004.
Truesdell S: Helping patients with COPD manage episodes of acute shortness of breath, *Medsurg Nurs* 9(4):178, 2000.

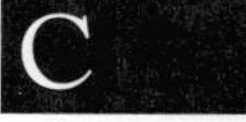

# Decreased Cardiac output

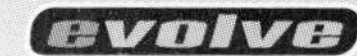

*Terri Ellis and Betty Ackley*

**NANDA**

## Definition

Inadequate blood pumped by the heart to meet metabolic demands of the body

## Defining Characteristics

**Altered heart rate/rhythm:** Dysrhythmias (tachycardia, bradycardia); palpitations; electrocardiographic changes
**Altered preload:** Jugular vein distention; fatigue; edema; murmurs; increased/decreased central venous pressure (CVP); increased/decreased pulmonary artery wedge pressure (PAWP); weight gain
**Altered afterload:** Cold/clammy skin; shortness of breath/dyspnea; oliguria; prolonged capillary refill; decreased peripheral pulses; variations in blood pressure readings; increased/decreased systemic vascular resistance (SVR); increased/decreased pulmonary vascular resistance (PVR); skin color changes
**Altered contractility:** Crackles; cough; orthopnea/paroxysmal nocturnal dyspnea; cardiac output less than 4 L/min; cardiac index less than 2.5 L/min; decreased ejection fraction; stroke volume index (SVI); left ventricular stroke work index (LVSWI); S3 or S4 sounds
**Behavioral/emotional:** Anxiety; restlessness

## Related Factors (r/t)

Altered heart rate/rhythm; altered stroke volume: altered preload, altered afterload, altered contractility

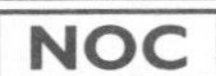

## Outcomes (Nursing Outcomes Classification)

C

### Suggested NOC Outcomes

Cardiac Pump Effectiveness; Circulation Status; Tissue Perfusion: Abdominal Organs, Peripheral; Vital Signs

**Example NOC Outcome with Indicators**

**Cardiac Pump Effectiveness** as evidenced by the following indicators: Blood pressure/Heart rate/ Cardiac index/Ejection fraction/Activity tolerance/Peripheral pulses strong/NVD not present/ Dysrhythmias not present/Abnormal heart sounds not present/Angina not present/Peripheral edema not present/ Pulmonary edema not present (Rate each indicator of **Cardiac Pump Effectiveness:** 1 = severely compromised, 2 = substantially compromised, 3 = moderately compromised, 4 = mildly compromised, 5 = not compromised [see Section I].)

## Client Outcomes

### Client Will (Specify Time Frame):

- Demonstrate adequate cardiac output as evidenced by blood pressure and pulse rate and rhythm within normal parameters for client; strong peripheral pulses; and an ability to tolerate activity without symptoms of dyspnea, syncope, or chest pain
- Remain free of side effects from the medications used to achieve adequate cardiac output
- Explain actions and precautions to take for cardiac disease

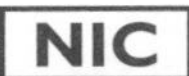

## Interventions (Nursing Interventions Classification)

### Suggested NIC Interventions

Cardiac Care; Cardiac Care: Acute

**Example NIC Activities—Cardiac Care**

Evaluate chest pain (e.g., intensity, location, radiation, duration, and precipitating and alleviating factors); document cardiac dysrhythmias

## Nursing Interventions and Rationales

- Monitor for symptoms of heart failure and decreased cardiac output; listen to heart sounds, lung sounds; note symptoms, including dyspnea, orthopnea, paroxysmal nocturnal dyspnea, Cheyne-Stokes respirations, fatigue, weakness, third and fourth heart sounds, crackles in lungs, increased venous pressure greater than 16 cm $H_2O$, and positive hepatojugular reflex. *These are major criteria for diagnosis of heart failure—the Framingham Criteria (Kasper et al, 2005).*

- Recognize the importance of cardiac index estimated by thermodilution in the intensive care unit (ICU) patient. **EBN:** *The cardiac index reflects with good precision the cardiac output of ICU patients and provides immediate results; in addition, the measurements are easy to repeat (Oliva & Cruz 2003).*
- Be aware of the utilization of impedance cardiography in noninvasive hemodynamic monitoring of heart failure. **EB:** *Impedance cardiography has demonstrated diagnostic and prognostic value in emergent and chronic heart failure. It has been shown to aid in the diagnosis of cardiac versus noncardiac heart failure patients (Yancy & Abraham, 2003); results of cardiac output and index measured by noninvasive bioimpedance and invasive thermodilution method were significantly correlated, supporting the efficacy of bioimpendance for measuring cardiac output/index (Albert et al, 2004). In the critically ill client, a study demonstrated that bioimpedance cardiac output is not accurate enough to replace the thermodilution method (Engoren et al, 2005).*
- Recognize the effect of sleep disordered breathing in heart failure. **EBN:** *Sleep disordered breathing, including obstructive sleep apnea and Cheyne-Stokes with central sleep apnea, are common organic sleep disorders in patients with chronic heart failure and are a poor prognostic sign associated with higher mortality (Brostrom, 2004).*
- Observe for chest pain or discomfort; note location, radiation, severity, quality, duration, associated manifestations such as nausea, indigestion, and diaphoresis, also note precipitating and relieving factors. *Chest pain/discomfort is generally indicative of an inadequate blood supply to the heart, which can compromise cardiac output. Clients with heart failure can continue to have chest pain with angina or can reinfarct.*
- If chest pain is present, have client lie down, monitor cardiac rhythm, give oxygen, check vital signs, run a monitor strip, medicate for pain, and notify the physician. *Prompt assessment of the client with acute coronary symptoms is critical because the incidence of ventricular fibrillation is 15 times greater during the first hour after symptoms of an acute myocardial infarction (Newberry, 2003).*
- Monitor intake and output. If client is acutely ill, measure hourly urine output and note decreases in output. *Decreased cardiac output results in decreased perfusion of the kidneys, with a resulting decrease in urine output.*
- Note results of electrocardiography and chest radiography. *Heart failure is strongly suggested by the presence of cardiomegaly or pulmonary vascular congestion on the chest radiograph. The probability of heart failure is increased by anterior Q waves or left bundle branch block on the electrocardiogram (Dosh, 2004).*
- Note results of diagnostic imaging studies such as echocardiogram, radionuclide imaging, or dobutamine stress echocardiography. *The echocardiogram is of critical importance determining the cause and severity of heart failure (Kasper et al, 2005). The ejection fraction (EF) is often quoted as a measure of left ventricular function, with an EF < 40% indicating clinical heart failure (Williams & Kearney, 2002).*
- Watch laboratory data closely, especially arterial blood gases, electrolytes including potassium, and B-type natriuretic peptide (BNP assay). *Client may be receiving cardiac glycosides and the potential for toxicity is greater with hypokalemia; hypokalemia is common in heart clients because of diuretic use (Kasper et al, 2005).* **EB:** *Rapid measurement of BNP is useful in establishing or eliminating the diagnosis of heart failure in the client with dyspnea (Kasper et al, 2005; Maisel et al, 2002).*

C

- Monitor laboratory work such as complete blood count (CBC), sodium level, and serum creatinine. *Routine blood work can provide insight into the etiology of heart failure and extent of decompensation. A low serum sodium level often is observed with advanced heart failure and can be a poor prognostic sign (Kasper et al, 2005). Serum creatinine levels will elevate in clients with severe heart failure because of decreased perfusion to the kidneys.*
- ▲ Administer oxygen as needed per physician's order. *Supplemental oxygen increases oxygen availability to the myocardium.*
- Place client in semi-Fowler's position or position of comfort. *Elevating the head of the bed may decrease the work of breathing, and also decrease venous return and preload.*
- ▲ Check blood pressure, pulse, and condition before administering cardiac medications such as angiotensin-converting enzyme (ACE) inhibitors, digoxin, calcium channel blockers, and beta-blockers such as Carvedilol. Notify physician if heart rate or blood pressure is low before holding medications. *It is important that the nurse evaluate how well the client is tolerating current medications before administering cardiac medications; do not hold medications without physician input. The physician may decide to have medications administered even though the blood pressure or pulse rate has lowered.*
- During acute events, ensure client remains on short-term bed rest or maintains activity level that does not compromise cardiac output. *In severe heart failure, restriction of activity reduces the workload of the heart (Kasper et al, 2005).*
- Gradually increase activity when client's condition is stabilized by encouraging slower paced activities or shorter periods of activity with frequent rest periods following exercise prescription; observe for symptoms of intolerance. Take blood pressure and pulse before and after activity and note changes. *Activity of the cardiac client should be closely monitored.* See **Activity intolerance.**
- Serve small sodium-restricted, low-cholesterol meals. *Sodium-restricted diets help decrease fluid volume excess. Low-cholesterol diets help decrease atherosclerosis, which causes coronary artery disease. Clients with cardiac disease tolerate smaller meals better because they require less cardiac output to digest.*
- Serve only small amounts of coffee or caffeine-containing beverages if requested (no more than four cups per 24 hours) if no resulting dysrhythmia. **EBN and EB:** *A review of studies on caffeine and cardiac arrhythmias concluded that moderate caffeine consumption does not increase the frequency or severity of cardiac arrhythmias (Hogan et al, 2002; Myers & Harris, 1990; Schneider, 1987).*
- Monitor bowel function. Provide stool softeners as ordered. Caution client not to strain when defecating. *Decreased activity can cause constipation. Straining when defecating that results in the Valsalva maneuver can lead to dysrhythmia, decreased cardiac function, and sometimes death.*
- Have clients use a commode or urinal for toileting and avoid use of a bedpan. *Getting out of bed to use a commode or urinal does not stress the heart any more than staying in bed to toilet. In addition, getting the client out of bed minimizes complications of immobility and is often preferred by the client (Winslow, 1992).*
- Provide a restful environment by minimizing controllable stressors and unnecessary

disturbances. Schedule rest periods after meals and activities. *Rest helps lower arterial pressure and reduce the workload of the myocardium by diminishing the requirements for cardiac output (Kasper et al, 2005).*

- Weigh client at same time daily (after voiding). *An accurate daily weight is needed to guide the administration of diuretics (Kasper et al, 2005). Daily weight is also a good indicator of fluid balance. Increased weight and severity of symptoms can signal decreased cardiac function with retention of fluids.*
- Apply graduated compression stockings as ordered. Ensure proper fit by measuring accurately. Remove the stocking at least twice a day, in the morning with the bath and in the evening, to assess the condition of the extremity, then reapply. **EBN and EB:** *A meta-analysis of 11 studies demonstrated that the use of graduated compression stockings reduced the incidence of deep vein thrombosis in a high-risk surgical population and that implementation of additional antithrombotic measures along with stocking use decreased the incidence even further (Joanna Briggs Institute, 2001). Graduated compression stockings, alone or used in conjunction with other prevention modalities, help prevent deep vein thrombosis in hospitalized patients (Amarigiri & Lees, 2005).*
- Assess for presence of anxiety. Consider using music to decrease anxiety and improve cardiac function. See Nursing Interventions and Rationales for **Anxiety** to facilitate reduction of anxiety in clients and family. **EBN:** *Music has been shown to reduce heart rate, blood pressure, anxiety, and cardiac complications (Guzzetta, 1994). Watch for signs of depression: flat affect, poor sleeping, loss of appetite, listlessness.*

▲ Refer for treatment if present. *Depression is very common in heart failure clients and can result in increased mortality (Thomas et al, 2003).*

▲ Closely monitor fluid intake, including intravenous lines. Maintain fluid restriction if ordered. *In clients with decreased cardiac output, poorly functioning ventricles may not tolerate increased fluid volumes.*

▲ Observe for symptoms of cardiogenic shock, including impaired mentation, hypotension with blood pressure lower than 90 mm Hg, decreased peripheral pulses, cold clammy skin, signs of pulmonary congestion and decreased organ function. If present, notify physician immediately. *Cardiogenic shock is a state of circulatory failure from loss from cardiac function associated with inadequate organ perfusion with a high mortality rate (Clark & Kruse, 2003).* **EBN:** *In a study the defining characteristics of decreased cardiac output were best indicated by decreased peripheral pulses and decreased peripheral perfusion (Oliva & Cruz, 2003).*

- If shock is present, monitor hemodynamic parameters for an increase in pulmonary wedge pressure, an increase in systemic vascular resistance, or a decrease in cardiac output and index. *Hemodynamic parameters give a good indication of cardiac function (Sole et al, 2001).*
- Titrate inotropic and vasoactive medications within defined parameters to maintain contractility, preload, and afterload per physician's order. *By following parameters, the nurse ensures maintenance of a delicate balance of medications that stimulate the heart to increase contractility, while maintaining adequate perfusion of the body.*

▲ Refer to heart failure program or cardiac rehabilitation program for education, evaluation, and guided support to increase activity and rebuild life. **EB:** *Exercise can help*

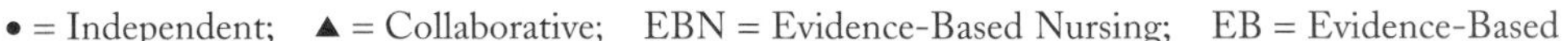

*many clients with heart failure. Whereas rest was commonly recommended a few years ago, it has become clear that inactivity can worsen the skeletal muscle myopathy in these clients. A carefully monitored exercise program can improve both exercise capacity and quality of life in mild to moderate heart failure clients (Rees et al, 2004). Exercise-based cardiac rehabilitation is effective in reducing the number of cardiac deaths, also decreasing cholesterol levels, systolic blood pressure and reduced self-reported smoking (Taylor et al, 2004; Jolliffe 2001).*

## Geriatric

- • Observe for atypical pain; the elderly often have jaw pain instead of chest pain or may have silent myocardioal infarctions (MIs) with symptoms of dyspnea or fatigue. *Symptoms, when present in older patients with an acute MI, may be extremely vague, and, as with myocardial ischemia, the diagnosis may be easily missed. Atypical symptoms of MI include dyspnea, neurologic symptoms, or gastrointestinal (GI) symptoms (Aronow, 2003).*
- ▲ If client has heart disease causing activity intolerance, refer for cardiac rehabilitation. **EB:** *Elderly clients with coronary artery disease in exercise regimens after hospitalization have exercise trainability comparable to that of younger clients participating in similar experiences (Shepard, 1990).*
- • Consider the use of graphic feedback with the elderly in exercise adherence. **EBN:** *The graphic format may be especially helpful because graphs provide a clear picture of the patient's exercise goals and recent progress. Graphic feedback serves as a visual reminder of exercise goals, and visualization of recent exercise participation may help motivate a continuation of exercise (Duncan, 2003).*
- ▲ Observe for syncope, dizziness, palpitations, or feelings of weakness associated with an irregular heart rhythm. *Dysrhythmias are common in the elderly.*
- ▲ Observe for side effects from cardiac medications. *The elderly have difficulty with metabolism and excretion of medications due to decreased function of the liver and kidneys; therefore toxic side effects are more common.*

## Home Care

- • Some of the above interventions may be adapted for home care use.
- ▲ Begin discharge planning as soon as possible with case manager or social worker to assess home support systems and the need for community or home health services. Consider referral for advanced practice nurse (APN) follow-up. Support services may be needed to assist with home care, meal preparations, housekeeping, personal care, transportation to doctor visits, or emotional support. *Clients often need help on discharge.* **EBN:** *In a randomized control trial, the assignment of an APN to assist with transition to the home for elders with heart failure resulted in greater length of time between hospitalizations, fewer total hospitalizations, and decreased health care costs. The intervention included specialized training in the needs of older adults during acute heart failure, use of quality care management, and implementation of an evidence-based protocol (Naylor, Brooten, Campbell et al, 2004). A study of transitional care using nonspecialist nurses found an improvement in the quality of life and a reduction in the number of emergency department visits with congestive heart failure (CHF) clients (Clark & Nadash, 2004).*

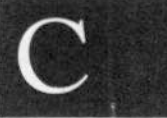


- Adopt a clinical pathway to address focused interventions with CHF, coronary artery bypass graft (CABG). *National Practice Guidelines for Cardiac Home Care are available to direct intervention for the client post-CABG who is recovering at home (Frantz & Walters, 2001a).* **EBN:** *Study of the outcome of a CHF clinical pathway revealed a 45% reduction in rehospitalization (Hoskins et al, 2001). Home health nurses reported that use of an evidence-based clinical pathway had a beneficial influence, including increased client knowledge of medications and diet (Young, McShane, O'Connor et al, 2004).*
- ▲ Assess or refer to case manager or social worker to evaluate client ability to pay for prescriptions. *The cost of drugs may be a factor in filling prescriptions and adhering to a treatment plan.*
- Continue to monitor client closely for exacerbation of heart failure when discharged home. Transition to home can create increased stress and physiological instability related to diagnosis. **EBN:** *Home visits and phone contacts that emphasize patient education and recognition of early symptoms of exacerbation can decrease rehospitalization (Gorski & Johnson, 2003).*
- Monitor women for differential symptoms of MI and institute emergency treatment measures as indicated. **EBN:** *Continuing research is exploring differences in MI symptoms between men and women. A qualitative study of 40 women following MI noted prodromal symptoms (0 to 11 per woman) a few weeks to 2 years prior. Most frequent were unusual fatigue, discomfort in the shoulder blade area, and chest sensations. Most common acute symptoms were chest sensations, shortness of breath, feeling hot and flushed, and unusual fatigue. Severe pain during the acute phase was experienced by only 11 women (McSweeney & Crane, 2000). African-American and Caucasian women have different physical recovery trajectories from acute MI (prolonged) but similar psychosocial recovery trajectories (Ranking, 2002).*
- Instruct women in the differential symptoms of MI in women, and the need to take symptoms seriously and seek help as indicated. **EBN:** *In one study, women delayed seeking help a median of 6.25 hours. Help-seeking behavior was influenced by beliefs about women's susceptibility to MI and differential symptom awareness. Symptoms presenting in this study were rarely consistent with those described in the health promotion literature (Holliday, Lowe, & Outram, 2000).*
- Assess client for understanding of and compliance with medical regimen, including medications, activity level, and diet. Client/family may need repetition of instructions received at hospital discharge, and may require reiteration as fear of a recent crisis decreases. *Fear interferes with the ability to assimilate new information.*
- ▲ Assess and monitor for signs of depression (particularly in adults age 65 years or older) or social isolation. Refer for mental health treatment as indicated. **EBN:** *Mood disturbance, social isolation, low socioeconomic status, and nonwhite ethnicity predicted lower functional status of clients with left ventricular dysfunction after 1 year (Clarke et al, 2000).* **EB:** *Depression has been noted as prevalent after acute MI in clients over age 65. Depressed older adults post-MI had greater comorbidity than those who were nondepressed and almost four times the risk of dying within 4 months of hospital discharge. Inability to follow recommendations to reduce cardiac risk may have been the cause (Romanelli et al, 2002). Depression and social isolation were suggested as a significant predictor of mortality with cli-*

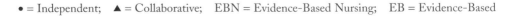

C

*ents in CHF (Murberg & Bru, 2001; Murberg & Furze, 2004). Depression has been shown to be an independent risk factor for heart failure in elderly women but not in elderly men (Williams et al, 2002).*

- Assess for signs/symptoms of cognitive impairment. **EBN:** *Cognitive function may decline in late-stage CHF (Quaglietti, Lovett, Hawthorne, et al, 2004).*
- Assess for fatigue and weakness frequently. Assess home environment for safety, as well as resources/obstacles to energy conservation. Instruct client and family members on need for behavioral pacing, energy conservation. **EBN:** *Fatigue and weakness limit activity level and quality of life. Assistive devices and other techniques of work simplification can help the client participate in and respond to the healthcare regimen more effectively (Quaglietti et al, 2004).*
- Instruct family and client about the disease process, complications of disease process, information on medications, need for weighing daily, and when it is appropriate to call doctor. *Early recognition of symptoms facilitates early problem solving and prompt treatment. Decreased cardiac output can be life threatening.* **EBN:** *Clients with heart failure need intensive education about these topics to help prevent readmission to the hospital (Moser, 2000). Home instruction (covering physical sensations and their management) regarding CABG recovery was found to be an effective intervention to prepare clients for home recovery. In one study, women experienced positive effects on physical functioning; men experienced positive effects on psychological distress, vigor, and fatigue (Moore & Dolansky, 2001). In another study, women reported more shortness of breath and depression, less activity, vigor, and overall health than men following CABG (Kereszíes, Merritt, Holm, et al, 2003).*
- Help family adapt daily living patterns to establish life changes that will maintain improved cardiac functioning in the client. Take the client's perspective into consideration, and use a holistic approach in assessing and responding to client planning for the future. *Transition to the home setting can cause risk factors such as inappropriate diet to reemerge.* **EBN:** *A study of women recovering from MI revealed that these women lived with a feeling of insecurity, based on a new inability to trust their bodies. Caring for women post-MI, researchers concluded, must approach health as being more than the absence of illness (Johansson et al, 2003).*
- Assist client to recognize and exercise power in using self-care management to adjust to health change. **EBN:** *Women post-MI reported that not participating in their health process increased their suffering and left them feeling powerless (Johansson et al, 2003).* Refer to care plan for **Powerlessness.** *A study of end-stage heart failure patients found that perceived powerlessness predicted mental health status (Scott, 2000).*
- Support client self-efficacy to increase physical activity by creating a supportive environment, offering encouragement, providing anticipatory guidance, and supplying a realistic assessment of the client's abilities. *Increasing self-efficacy takes time, but can lead to increased physical activity, decreased symptomatology, and improved quality of life for the client (Borsody et al, 1999).*

▲ Explore barriers to medical regimen adherence. Review medications and treatment regularly for needed modifications. Take complaints of side effects seriously and serve as client advocate to address changes as indicated. *The presence of uncomfortable side effects frequently motivates clients to deviate from the medication regimen. A discussion of treatment regimen with coronary heart disease noted that physicians do not always adhere to guideline recommendations; adherence to guidelines and long-term strategies would prompt use of the most effective agents with the lowest incidence of side effects (Erhardt, 1999).*

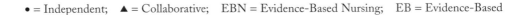

- ▲ Refer for cardiac rehabilitation, strengthening exercises if client is not involved in outpatient cardiac rehabilitation. Refer to agency cardiac care program if available. *Cardiac rehabilitation safely increases aerobic capacity, muscular strength, and endurance in older clients (Ades, 1999). Specialized cardiac care programs have addressed the needs to CABG clients discharged from the hospital early (Frantz & Walters, 2001b) and are especially indicated for women in order to modify risk factors (Rankin, 2002).*
- ▲ Refer to medical social services as necessary for counseling about the impact of severe or chronic cardiac disease. *Social workers can assist the client and family with acceptance of life changes.*
- ▲ Institute case management of frail elderly to support continued independent living. *Difficulties with cardiac output represent and can lead to increasing needs for assistance in using the health care system effectively. Case management combines nursing activities of client and family assessment, planning and coordination of care among all health care providers, delivery of direct nursing care, and monitoring of care and outcomes. These activities are able to address continuity of care, mutual goal setting, behavior management, and prevention of worsening health problems (Guttman, 1999).*
- ▲ As client condition warrants, refer to hospice. *The multidisciplinary hospice team can reduce hospital readmission, increase functional capacity, and improve quality of life in end-stage heart failure (Coviello et al, 2002).*
- ▲ Provide specific written materials and self-care plan for client/caregivers to use for reference. Consult dietitian or assist client in understanding the need for a sodium-restricted diet. Provide alternatives for salt such as spices, herbs, lemon juice, or vinegar. *Although the initial elimination of salt from the diet is very difficult for a person used to its taste, the taste of salt can be unlearned. The above can enhance the taste appeal of food while the preference for salt is changing (Cataldo, DeBruyne, & Whitney, 2003).*
- • Identify emergency plan, including use of cardiopulmonary resuscitation (CPR). Encourage family members to become certified in cardiopulmonary resuscitation. **EBN:** *CPR training significantly increased perceived control in spouses of recovering cardiac clients (Moser & Dracup, 2000).*

## Client/Family Teaching

- • Teach symptoms of heart failure and appropriate actions to take if client becomes symptomatic.
- • Teach importance of smoking cessation and avoidance of alcohol intake. *Smoking is a well-established risk factor for coronary artery disease. Help patients who smoke stop by informing them of potential consequences and by helping them find an effective cessation method. Excessive intake of alcohol can produce alcoholic cardiomyopathy or worsen heart*

C

*failure (Caboral & Mitchell, 2003).* **EB:** *Smoking cessation advice and counsel given by nurses can be effective, and should be available to clients to help stop smoking (Rice & Stead, 2000).*

- Teach stress reduction (e.g., imagery, controlled breathing, muscle relaxation techniques).
- Explain necessary restrictions, including consumption of a sodium-restricted diet, guidelines on fluid intake, and the avoidance of Valsalva maneuver. Teach the importance of pacing activities, work simplification techniques, and the need to rest between activities to prevent becoming overly fatigued. *Sodium retention leading to fluid overload is a common cause of hospital readmission (Bennett et al, 2000).*

▲ Assist the client in understanding the need for and how to incorporate lifestyle changes. Refer to cardiac rehabilitation for assistance with coping and adjustment. *Psychoeducational programs including information on stress management and health education have been shown to reduce long-term mortality and recurrence of MI in heart patients (Benson, 2000).*

▲ Teach the client actions, side effects, and importance of consistently taking cardiovascular medications. *Medications can prolong the lives of heart failure clients but often are not taken, resulting in hospital readmissions (Agency for Health Care Policy and Research, 1994).* **EBN:** *A research study demonstrated that heart failure clients were not knowledgeable of the medications, but also the need for weight monitoring and recognizing the definition for heart failure (Artinian et al, 2002).*

- Provide client/family with advance directive information to consider. Allow client to give advance directions about medical care or designate who should make medical decisions if he or she should lose decision-making capacity.
- Instruct the client on importance of getting a pneumonia shot (usually one per lifetime) and yearly influenza shots as prescribed by physician. *Clients with decreased cardiac output are considered higher risk for complications or death if they do not get immunization injections.*
- Instruct client/family on the need to weigh daily and keep a weight log. Ask if client has a scale at home; if not, assist in getting one. Instruct on establishing baseline weight on own scale when gets home. *Daily weighing is an essential aspect of self-management. A scale is necessary (Campbell, 1998). Scales vary; the client needs to establish a baseline weight on his or her home scale.*
- Provide specific written materials and self-care plan for client/caregivers to use for reference.

▲ Consult dietitian or assist client in understanding the need for a sodium-restricted diet. Provide alternatives for salt such as spices, herbs, lemon juice, or vinegar. *Although the initial elimination of salt from the diet is very difficult, the taste of salt can be unlearned. The spices and seasonings above can enhance the taste appeal of food while the preference for salt is changing (Cataldo, DeBruyne, & Whitney, 2003). Taste sensation is often diminished as a function of age, producing a greater desire for salty foods (Forman & Rich, 2003).*

- Instruct family regarding cardiopulmonary resuscitation.

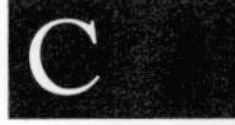

## evolve WEBSITES FOR EDUCATION

See the EVOLVE website for World Wide Web resources for client education.

## REFERENCES


Ades PA: Cardiac rehabilitation in older coronary patients, *J Am Geriatr Soc* 47:98, 1999.

Agency for Health Care Policy and Research (AHCPR): *Guidelines for patients with heart failure,* AHCPR Publication No 942, Rockville, Md, 1994, US Department of Health and Human Services.

Albert NM, Hail MD, Li J et al: Equivalence of the bioimpedance and thermodilution methods in measuring cardiac output in hospitalized patients with advanced, decompensated chronic heart failure, *Am J Crit Care* 13(6):469, 2004.

Amarigiri SV, Lees TA: Elastic compression stockings for prevention of deep vein thrombosis, *Cochrane Database Syst Rev* (3): CD001484, 2005.

Aronow W: Silent MI. Prevalence and prognosis in older patients diagnosed by routine electrocardiograms, *Geriatrics* 58(1):24-26, 36-38, 40, 2003.

Artinian NT, Magnan M, Christian W et al: What do patients know about their heart failure? *Appl Nurs Res* 15(4):200, 2002.

Bennett SJ, Cordes DK, Westmoreland G et al: Self-care strategies for symptom management in patients with chronic heart failure, *Nurs Res* 49(3):139, 2000.

Benson G: Review: psychoeducational programmes reduce long-term mortality and recurrence of myocardial infarction in cardiac patients, *Evidence-Based Nurs* 49(3):80, 2000.

Borsody JM, Courtney M, Taylor K et al: Using self-efficacy to increase physical activity in patients with heart failure, *Home Healthc Nurse* 17:113, 1999.

Brostrom A, Stromberg A, Dahlstrom U et al: Sleep difficulties, daytime sleepiness, and health-related quality of life in patients with chronic heart failure, *J Cardiovasc Nurs* 19(4):234, 2004.

Caboral M, Mitchell J: New guidelines for heart failure focus on prevention, *Nurse Pract* 28(1):13, 16, 22-23, 2003.

Campbell RL, Banner R, Konick-McMahan J et al: Discharge planning and home follow-up of the elderly patient with heart failure, *Geriatr Nurs* 33(3):497, 1998.

Cataldo CB, DeBruyne LK, Whtney EN: *Nutrition and diet therapy*, ed 6, Belmont, 2003, Thomson Wadsworth.

Clark A, Nadash P: The effectiveness of a nurse-led transitional care model for patients with congestive heart failure, *Home Healthc Nurs* 22(3):160, 2004.

Clarke SP, Frasure-Smith N, Lesperance F et al: Psychosocial factors as predictors of functional status at 1 year in patients with left ventricular dysfunction, *Res Nurs Health* 23:290, 2000.

Coviello JS, Hricz L, Masulli PS: Client challenge: accomplishing quality of life in end-stage heart failure: a hospice multidisciplinary approach, *Home Healthc Nurs* 20:195, 2002.

Dosh S: Diagnosis of heart failure in adults, *Am Fam Physician* 70(11):2145, 2004.

Duncan K, Pozehl B: Effects of an exercise adherence intervention on outcomes in patients with heart failure, *Cardiac Rehab* 28(4):117, 2003.

Engoren M, Barbee D: Comparison of cardiac output determined by bioimpedance, thermodilution, and the Fick method, *Am J Crit Care* 14(1):40, 2005.

Erhardt ER: The essence of effective treatment and compliance is simplicity, *Am J Hypertens* 12(10 Pt 2):105SS, 1999.

Forman D, Rich M: Heart failure in the elderly, *Congest Heart Fail* 9(6):311, 2003.

Frantz AK, Walters JI: Recovery from coronary artery bypass grafting at home: is your practice current? *Home Healthc Nurs* 19:417, 2001a.

Frantz AK, Walters JI: Cardiac home care programs impact patients after coronary artery bypass grafting, *Home Healthc Nurs* 19: 495, 2001b.

Gorski LA, Johnson K: A disease management program for heart failure: collaboration between a home care agency and a care management organization, *Home Healthc Nurs* 21(11):734, 2003.

Guttman R: Case management of the frail elderly in the community, *Clin Nurs Spec* 13(4):174, 1999.

Guzzetta CE: Soothing the ischemic heart, *Am J Nurs* 94:24, 1994.

Hogan E, Hornick B, Bouchoux A: Communicating the message: clarifying the controversies about caffeine, *Nutr Today* 37(1):28, 2002.

Holliday JE, Lowe JM, Outram S: Women's experience of myocardial infarction, *Intl J Nurs Pract* 6:307, 2000.

Hoskins LM, Clark HM, Schroeder MA et al: A clinical pathway for congestive heart failure, *Home Healthc Nurs* 19:207, 2001.

Joanna Briggs Institute: Best practice: graduated compression stockings for the prevention of post-operative venous thromboembolism, *Evidenced Based Practice Information Sheets for Health Professions* 5:2, 2001.

Johansson A, Dahlberg K, Ekebergh M: Living with experiences following a myocardial infarction, *Euro J Cardiovasc Nurs* 2:229, 2003.

Jolliffe JA, Rees K, Taylor RS et al: Exercise-based rehabilitation for coronary heart disease, *Cochrane Database Syst Rev* (1): CD001800, 2001.

Kasper DL et al: *Harrison's principles of internal medicine,* 16th ed, New York, 2005, McGraw-Hill.

Keresztes PA, Merritt SL, Holm K et al: The coronary artery bypass experience: gender differences, *Heart Lung* 32:308, 2003.

Maisel AS, Krishnaswamy P, Nowak RM et al: Rapid measurement of B-type natriuretic peptide in the emergency diagnosis of heart failure, *N Engl J Med* 347(3):11, 2002.

McSweeney JC, Crane PB: Challenging the rules: women's prodromal and acute symptoms of myocardial infarction, *Res Nurs Health* 23:135, 2000.

Moore SM, Dolansky MA: Randomized trial of a home recovery intervention following coronary artery bypass surgery, *Res Nurs Health* 24:93, 2001.

Moser DK: Heart failure management: optimal health care delivery programs, *Annu Rev Nurs* Res 18:91, 2000.

Moser DK, Dracup K: Impact of cardiopulmonary resuscitation training on perceived control in spouses of recovering cardiac patients, *Res Nurs Health* 23:270, 2000.

Murberg TA, Bru E: Social relationships and mortality in patients with congestive heart failure, *J Psychosom Res* 51:521, 2001.

Murberg TA, Furze G: Depressive symptoms and mortality in patients with congestive heart failure: a six-year follow-up study, *Med Sci Monit* 10(12):CR643, 2004.

Myers MG, Harris L: High dose caffeine and ventricular arrhythmias, *Can J Cardiol* 6(3):95, 1990.

Naylor MD, Brooten DA, Campbell RL et al: Transitional care of older adults hospitalized with heart failure: arandomized, controlled trial, *J Am Geriatr Soc* 52:675, 2004.

Newberry L: *Sheehy's emergency nursing,* ed 5, St Louis, 2003, Mosby.

Oliva PC, Cruz DD: Decreased cardiac output: validation with postoperative heart surgery patients, *Dimens Crit Care Nurs* 22(1): 39, 2003.

Peckenpaugh NJ, Poleman C: *Nutrition essentials and diet therapy,* ed 8, Philadelphia, 1999, WB Saunders.

Quaglietti S, Lovett S, Hawthorne C et al: Management of the patient with congestive heart failure in the home care and palliative care setting, *Ann Long Term Care* 12(1):33, 2004.

Rankin SH: Women recovering from acute myocardial infarction: psychosocial and physical functioning outcomes for 12 months after acute myocardial infarction, *Heart Lung* 31(6):399, 2002.

Rees K, Taylor RS, Singh S et al: Exercise based rehabilitation for heart failure, *Cochrane Database Syst Rev* (3):CD003331, 2004.

Rice VH, Stead LF: Nursing interventions for smoking cessation, *Cochrane Database Syst Rev* (2):CD001188, 2000.

Romanelli J, Fauerbach JA, Bush DE et al: The significance of depression in older patients after myocardial infarction, *J Am Geriatr Soc* 50:817, 2002.

Schneider JR: Effects of caffeine ingestion on heart rate, blood pressure, myocardial oxygen consumption, and cardiac rhythm in acute myocardial infarction patients, *Heart Lung* 16:167, 1987.

Scott LD: Caregiving and care receiving among a technologically dependent heart failure population, *Adv Nurs Sci* 23(2):82, 2000.

Sole ML, Lamborn ML, Hartshorn JC: *Introduction to critical care nursing,* ed 3, Philadelphia, 2001, WB Saunders.

Taylor RS, Brown A, Ebrahim S et al: Exercise-based rehabilitation for patients with coronary heart disease: systematic review and meta-analysis of randomized controlled trials, *Am J Med* 116(10):682, 2004.

Thomas SA, Friedmann E, Khatta M et al: Depression in patients with heart failure: physiologic effects, incidence, and relation to mortality, *AACN Clin Issues* 14(1):3, 2003.

Williams H, Kearney M: Chronic heart failure, *Pharma J* 269:325, 2002

Williams SA, Kasl SV, Heiat A et al: Depression and risk of heart failure among the elderly: a prospective community-based study, *Psychosom Med* 64(1):6, 2002.

Winslow EH: Panning bedpans, *Am J Nurs* 92:16G, 1992.


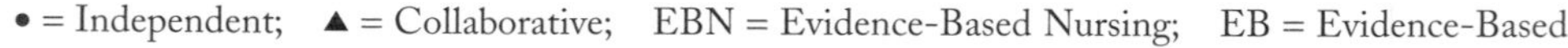

Yancy C, Abraham W: Noninvasive hemodynamic monitoring in heart failure: utilization of impedance cardiography, *Congest Heart Fail* 9(5):241, 2003

Young W, McShane J, O'Connor T et al: Registered nurses' experiences with an evidence-based home care pathway for myocardial infarction clients, *Can J Cardiovasc Nurs* 14(3):24, 2004.

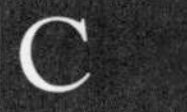

# Caregiver role strain

evolve

*Barbara Given and Paula Sherwood*

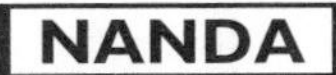

## Definition

Difficulty in performing family caregiver role

## Defining Characteristics

### Caregiving Activities

Difficulty performing/completing required tasks, preoccupation with care routine, apprehension about the future regarding care receiver's health and the caregiver's ability to provide care, apprehension about care receiver's care if caregiver becomes ill or dies, dysfunctional change in caregiving activities, apprehension about possible institutionalization of care receiver

### Caregiver Health Status—Physical

GI upset (e.g., mild stomach cramps, vomiting, diarrhea, recurrent gastric ulcer episodes); weight change; rash; hypertension; cardiovascular disease; diabetes; fatigue; headaches

### Caregiver Health Status—Emotional

Impaired individual coping, feeling depressed, disturbed sleep, anger, stress, somatization, increased nervousness, increased emotional lability, irritability, impatience, lack of time to meet personal needs, frustration

### Caregiver Health Status—Socioeconomic

Withdrawal from social life, changes in leisure activities, low work productivity, refuses career advancement

### Caregiver–Care Receiver Relationship

Grief/uncertainty regarding changed relationship with care receiver; difficulty watching care receiver go through the illness

### Family Processes

Family conflict, concerns about family members

## Related Factors (r/t)

### Care Receiver Health Status

Illness severity, illness chronicity, increasing care needs/dependency, unpredictability of illness course, instability of care receiver's health, problem behaviors, psychological or cognitive problems, addiction or codependency

### Caregiving Activities

Amount of activities, complexity of activities, 24-hour care responsibilities, ongoing changes in activities, discharge of family members to home with significant care needs, years of caregiving, unpredictability of care situation

### Caregiver Health Status

Physical problems, psychological or cognitive problems, addiction or codependency, marginal coping patterns, unrealistic expectations of self, inability to fulfill one's own or others' expectations

### Socioeconomic Factors

Isolation from others; competing role commitments; alienation from family, friends, and coworkers; insufficient recreation

### Caregiver–Care Receiver Relationship

History of poor relationship, presence of abuse or violence, unrealistic expectations of caregiver by care receiver, mental status of elder inhibiting conversation

### Family Processes

History of marginal family coping; history of family dysfunction

### Resources

Inadequate physical environment for providing care (e.g., housing, temperature, safety); inadequate equipment for providing care; inadequate transportation; inadequate community resources (e.g., respite services, recreational resources); insufficient finances; lack of support; caregiver is not developmentally ready for caregiver role; inexperience with caregiving; insufficient time; lack of knowledge about or difficulty assessing community resources; lack of caregiver privacy; emotional strength; physical energy; assistance and support (formal and informal)

**NOC**

## Outcomes (Nursing Outcomes Classification)

### Suggested NOC Outcomes

Caregiver Emotional Health; Caregiver Lifestyle Disruption; Caregiver Performance: Direct Care, Indirect Care; Caregiver Physical Health; Caregiver Stressors; Caregiver Well-Being; Role Performance; Caregiver Self-Esteem; Caregiver Mastery; Caregiver Competence; Caregiver Role Adjustment

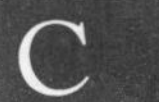

**Example NOC Outcome with Indicators**

**Caregiver Emotional Health** with plans for a positive future as evidenced by the following indicators: Satisfaction with life/Sense of control/Self-esteem/Free of anger/Free of guilt/Free of depression/Perceived social connectedness/Perceived spiritual well-being (Rate each indicator of 1 = severely compromised, 2 = substantially compromised, 3 = moderately compromised, 4 = mildly compromised, 5 = not compromised [see Section I].)

## Client Outcomes

- Caregiver will feel supported.
- Caregiver will report low or no feelings of burden or distress.
- Caregiver will maintain physical and psychological/emotional health.
- Caregiver will identify resources available to help in giving care.
- Caregiver will verbalize mastery of the care situation.
- Care receiver will obtain appropriate care.

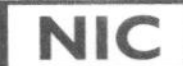

## Interventions (Nursing Interventions Classification)

### Suggested NIC Intervention

Caregiver Support

**Example NIC Activities—Caregiver Support**

Determine caregiver's acceptance of care role; accept expressions of negative emotion

## Nursing Interventions and Rationales

- Use an evaluation tool to determine caregiver burden and role strain. Various instruments have been developed, including the Burden Interview, the Caregiver Strain Index, the Caregiver Burden Inventory, Caregiver Reaction Assessment, Screen for Caregiver Burden, and the Subjective and Objective Burden Scale (Deeken et al, 2003; Given et al, 1992; Vitaliano et al, 1991). **EBN and EB:** *Research has validated the effectiveness of a number of evaluation tools for caregiver stress, including the Caregiver Reaction Assessment (Given et al, 1992), Burden Interview (Zarit et al, 1980), the Caregiver Strain Index (Robinson, 1983), and the Caregiver Burden Inventory (Novak & Guest, 1989). Caregiver assessment tools should be multidimensional and evaluate the impact of providing care on multiple aspects of the caregiver's life, such as burden, depression, and distress.*
- Use an evaluation tool to determine potential caregiver resources such as mastery, social support, optimism, and positive aspects of care.
- Screen for caregiver role strain at the onset of the care situation, at regular intervals throughout the care situation, and with changes in care recipient status and care transitions. *Care situations that last for several months or years can cause wear and tear that exhaust caregivers' coping mechanisms and available resources. In addition, changes in the*

*care recipient's health status necessitate new skills and monitoring from the caregiver and affect the caregiver's ability to continue to provide care.*

- Watch for signs of depression and deteriorating health in the caregiver, especially if the marital relationship is poor, the care recipient has cognitive or neuropsychiatric symptoms, there is little social support available, the caregiver becomes enmeshed in the care situation, the caregiver is elderly, female, or has poor preexisting physical or emotional health. Intervene to provide support and to help the caregiver obtain counseling to cope. If signs are present, refer to the care plan for **Hopelessness.** *Caregiving may weaken the immune system and predispose the caregiver to illness in some situations (Mills et al, 2004; Redwine et al, 2004). The incidence of depression in family caregivers is estimated to be 40% to 50% (Schulz & Martire, 2004; Knop, Bergman-Evans, & McCabe, 1998).* **EBN:** *Intervening early to help the caregiver can result in improved care for the stroke client and, it is hoped, improved health for the caregiver (Bakas & Burgener, 2002; Teel, Duncan, & Lai, 2001). Psychiatric nurses can play an important role in the assessment and treatment of caregiver depression (Buckwalter, 1999).*
- Watch for caregivers who become enmeshed in the care situation (e.g., becoming overinvolved or unable to disentangle themselves from the caregiver role). **EB:** *Role training (assisting caregivers to understand and define their role) may prevent caregivers from becoming enmeshed, which can in turn prevent burden and depression (Hepburn et al, 2002).*
- Monitor the quality of care by the caregiver for adequacy and need for improvement.
- Arrange for intervals of respite care for the caregiver; encourage use if available. *Respite care is beneficial to caregivers, if they can be convinced to use it (Hayes, 1999).*
- Help the caregiver to identify support systems and be assertive in using them. *Caregivers sometimes feel abandoned (Given et al, 1992) and need assistance to activate their support systems (Kleffel, 1998).*
- Encourage the caregiver to grieve over changes in the care receiver's condition. Give the caregiver permission to share angry feelings in a safe environment. Refer to nursing interventions for **Grieving.** *Caregivers grieve the loss of function of their loved one, especially when dementia is involved (Narayan et al, 2001; Liken & Collins, 1993).*
- Identify with the caregiver the factors that can and cannot be controlled.
- Help the caregiver find personal time to meet his or her own needs, learn stress management techniques, schedule regular health screenings, and schedule regular respite time. *Self-care is important for the caregiver. Maintaining personal wellness can increase stamina, energy, and self-esteem and enhance the quality of care given (Ruppert, 1996).*
- Encourage the caregiver to schedule and keep routine health care appointments (i.e., annual physicals and screening tests). **EB:** *Caregivers who report being strained are at risk for lower perceptions of their own health status, increased risky behaviors such as smoking, and higher use of prescription drugs (Beach, Schulz, & Yee et al, 2000; Burton, Newsom, Schulz et al, 1997).*
- Support the caregiver in setting boundaries and determining the legitimate caregiving role. **EBN:** *Women in caregiving roles can develop "fraying connections", lose a sense of self when their own needs are not met (Wuest, 1998), and are more prone to depression.*

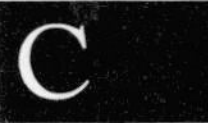


- Encourage the caregiver to use humor to cope when appropriate, including cartoons, stories, and jokes. **EBN:** *Humor is a healthy distancing technique, helping the caregiver feel liberated from oppressive stimuli. It can help relieve pain, loss, grief, or unpleasantness (Buffum & Brod, 1998).*
- Encourage the caregiver to talk about feelings, concerns, uncertainties, and fears. Acknowledge the frustration associated with caregiver responsibilities. *Professionals need to listen to caregiving spouses and note expressions of positive and negative responses to caregiving (Narayan et al, 2001).*
- Observe for any evidence of caregiver or care receiver violence or abuse; if evidence is present, speak with the caregiver and care receiver separately. *Caregiver violence is possible, especially if the care receiver was violent to the caregiver in the past (Brandle & Raymond, 1997)*

▲ Involve the family in care transitions; use a multidisciplinary team to provide medical and social serves for instruction and planning. **EBN:** *Caregivers who reported involvement in discharge planning reported better acceptance of the caregiving role and better health (Bull, Hansen, & Gross, 2000). Use of an interdisciplinary team to provide discharge planning was seen by elders as a "proper discharge" (Bull & Roberts, 2001).*

- Give the caregiver permission to arrange custodial care in an extended care facility if necessary; support both caregiver and care receiver during this difficult transition.
- Help the caregiver deal with elements of placing the care receiver in a long term care facility, planning for stress, and seeking solace in support from others. *Placing a loved one in an extended care facility can relieve the burden of care but does not relieve the stress resulting from financial concerns, guilt, loss of control, or lack of support (Schulz et al, 2004).*
- Encourage regular communication with the care recipient and with the health care team.
- Help caregiver assess his/or her socioeconomic status (services reimbursed by insurance, available support through community and religious organizations). **EB and EBN:** *Low incomes and limited financial resources can cause strain for the caregiver, particularly if there are substantial out-of-pocket costs involved in providing care (Nijboer et al, 2001; Hayman et al, 2001).*
- Help the caregiver identify competing occupational demands and potential ways to modify the work role in order to provide care (enact the Family Leave Act, change from full to part time, work from home, take a leave of absence or early retirement). **EB:** *Employed caregivers report missed days, interruptions at work, leaves of absence, and reduced productivity because of the need to be involved with cancer care (Cameron, Franche, Cheung et al, 2002). Older caregivers may take early retirement when care demands increase (Grunfield, 2004).*
- Validate the family's feelings regarding the impact of caregiving on family and personal lifestyle. **EBN:** *Validation is a therapeutic communication technique that lets the individual know that the nurse has heard and understood what was said (Heineken, 1998).*

## Geriatric

- Monitor the caregiver for psychological distress and signs of depression, especially if caring for a mentally impaired elder or if there was an unsatisfactory marital relation-

C

ship before caregiving. **EBN:** *A difficult marriage before caregiving predisposes the caregiver to depression (Knop, Bergman-Evans, & McCabe, 1998).*

- Assess the health of caregivers at intervals, especially if they have their own chronic illness in addition to caregiving role. **EB:** *If caregiving is associated with self-reported physical or emotional strain, the older caregiver has an increased risk of mortality (Schulz & Beach, 1999).*
- Recognize that it is hard for the elderly to accept a change in caregivers or in the environment. *Help the caregiver identify ways to equitably distribute workload among family or significant others, to ask for help and accept social support.*
- Assess social support and encourage the use of secondary caregivers with elderly caregivers. *Older caregivers often become enmeshed in the care situation (often because they provide care by themselves) and isolate themselves from social and family support to become completely focused on providing care for their spouse.*
- Provide skills training related to direct care, performing complex monitoring tasks, supervision interpreting patient symptoms, assisting with decision-making, providing emotional support and comfort, and coordinating care. **EBN:** *Each task demands different skills and knowledge, organizational capacities, role demands, and social and psychological strengths from family members (Schumacher et al, 2000).*
- Teach symptom management techniques (assessment, potential causes, aggravating factors, potential alleviating factors, reassessment), particularly for fatigue, constipation, anorexia and pain. **EB and EBN:** *Certain patient symptoms such as fatigue, constipation, anorexia, pain, and depression have been associated with caregiver strain (Kurtz et al, 2004; Newton et al, 2002; Yurk et al, 2002; Miaskowski et al, 1997).*

## Multicultural

- Assess for the influence of cultural beliefs, norms, values, and expectations on the family's experience of caregiving. **EBN:** *How the family views caregiving may be based on cultural perceptions (Leininger & McFarland, 2002; Cochran, 1998; Doswell and Erlen, 1998; Guarnaccia, 1998).* **EB:** *Caregiving can be complicated by the distrust that many African Americans hold toward the health care system, which has resulted from years of exclusion, racism, and discrimination. It is important to hear from African-American families to gain an understanding of what services are needed (Turner et al, 2004).*
- Assess for conflicts between the caregiver's cultural obligations to provide care and competing factors like employment, time management and arrangements, their own health, competing role demands, and low rewards. **EBN:** *Conflicts between cultural expectations and competing factors can increase caregiver stress (Jones, 1996). Interventions to develop and maintain work environments support not only the older employee's work performance, but participation in the role of elder caregiver as well (Beitman et al, 2004).*
- Assess and identify the effect of the caregiver's own health on role overload. **EB:** *Feelings of role overload were correlated among caregivers who have health problems of their own is associated with greater depressive symptomatology (Leblanc, Driscoll, & Pearlin, 2004).*
- Negotiate with the client regarding the aspects of caregiving that can be modified

while still honoring cultural beliefs. **EBN:** *Give and take with the client will lead to culturally congruent care (Leininger & McFarland, 2002).*

▲ Refer the family to social services or other supportive services to assist with the impact of caregiving. **EBN:** *African-American caregivers of dementia clients evidence less desire than others to institutionalize their family members and are more likely to report unmet service needs (Hinrichsen & Ramirez, 1992). African-American and Caucasian families of dementia clients report restricted social activity (Haley et al, 1995).*

▲ Assist the family/caregiver in identifying barriers that would prevent the use of social services or other supportive services that could help reduce the impact of caregiving. **EBN:** *Expectations of discrimination, lack of knowledge about services, expectations embedded in familism, lack of sense of prevention, lack of health insurance, preference for traditional remedies, and neglect or abuse were barriers identified by researchers studying the low utilization of skilled home care nursing services among elderly Hispanic individuals (Crist, 2002). Language may present another barrier to the access of supportive services (McGrath, Vun, & McLeod, 2001). Nearly one half of Asian-American caregivers reported service barriers. Some barriers were related to personal issues that caregivers often felt "too proud to accept it" or "didn't want outsiders coming in." Other frequently reported barriers were related to service providers, including "service is not available," "bureaucracy too complex," or "can't find qualified providers." More than one half of caregivers reported that services provided did not meet care receivers' needs (Li, 2004).*

▲ Encourage the family to use support groups or other service programs. **EBN:** *Studies indicate that minority families of clients with dementia use few support programs even though these programs could have a positive impact on caregiver well-being (Cox, 1999).*

• Encourage caregiver use of spirituality or religion as a source of support for the caregiver. **EBN:** *Studies indicate that African-American and other diverse caregivers cited religion and spirituality as their greatest source of support (Leblanc, Driscoll, & Pearlin, 2004; Roff et al, 2004; Poindexter & Linsk, 1998).*

• Validate the family's feelings regarding the impact of caregiving on family and personal lifestyle. **EBN:** *Validation is a therapeutic communication technique that lets the individual know that the nurse has heard and understood what was said (Heineken, 1998).*

## Home Care

• Identify client and caregiver factors that necessitated the use of formal home care services, and that may affect provision of care or that need to be addressed before the client can be safely discharged from home care. **EBN:** *A study noted that limitations of the client in the ability to perform the activities of daily living (ADLs) predicted referral to home care, while diagnosis and presence of physical impairment did not. Elders living alone or with fewer household members were more likely to use home care. On the part of the caregiver, factors included lack of mobility outside of the home, need to rearrange work schedules, and need for provision of bowel or bladder care (Houde, 1998). Problem solving should address each of these elements as possible prior to discharge from home care.*

C

- Assess the level of caregiver strain; use of a measurement tool may be helpful. **EB:** *The Modified Caregiver Strain Index is a useful and easily used measure of caregiver strain (Thornton & Travis, 2003).*
- Assess caregiver levels of optimism or pessimism. **EBN:** *In a study of caregivers for patients with Parkinson's disease, the Life Orientation Test was used to measure optimism and pessimism. Pessimism early in the caregiving situation was a warning sign of poor current and future caregiver health (Lyons et al, 2004).*
- Assess the client and caregiver at every visit for quality of care provided, functional disability of care recipient, caregiver coping, and signs of caregiver stress. Document all observations objectively. **EB:** *A study of caregiver burden found that caregivers are most burdened by client behavior, with client physical and cognitive impairments and amount of care provision contributing. Coping processes and caregiver receipt of social support may moderate the relationship between caregiving demands and caregiving outcomes. The researchers concluded that caregivers need interventions that will reduce client behavior problems and increase caregivers' skills in handling behavioral difficulties (Pinquart & Sorensen, 2003).*
- Assess the client and caregiver at every visit for quality of relationship, and for the quality of caring that exists. **EBN:** *A phenomenological study of caregivers for clients with multiple sclerosis (MS) found that caring equated with worrying about the partner, about their relationship with the partner, about their future, their own health, institutional care, and lack of support (Cheung & Hocking, 2004). A study of caregivers for clients post-stroke found that caregivers in lower functioning families reported worse mental health. Clients with a combination of high memory/behavior changes and low motor function were particularly stressful to care for. Family conflict appeared to increase problems (Clark et al, 2004).* **EB:** *Negative relationships were found to exist when there was a poor person-environment fit between the amount of care a spouse provided, and the client's need for independence (Martire et al, 2002). A study found that negative interactions for older adults were stable over a 6-year period, suggesting that interpersonal conflicts were chronic stressors for older adults (Krause & Rook, 2003). The latter finding suggests that nurses should be realistic in their assessment of potential change in older adults' relationships; established patterns may be resistant to change.*
- Assess family caregiving skill. The identification of caregiver difficulty with any of a core set of processes highlights areas for intervention. **EBN:** *The ability to engage effectively and smoothly in nine processes has been identified as constituting family caregiving skill: monitoring client behavior, interpreting changes accurately, making decisions, taking action, making adjustment to care, accessing resources, providing hands-on care, working together with the ill person, and negotiating the health care system (Schumacher et al, 2000).*
- Assess perceived level of power experienced by the caregiver in ability to complete daily activities. *Decreased perceived power level can lead to caregiver overload, possibly because of a burden of financial management the caregiver must assume when ill prepared.*
- Assess preexisting strengths and weaknesses the caregiver brings to the situation, as well as current responses, depression, and fatigue levels. **EBN:** *Low individual and family hardiness was found to foster depression and fatigue in caregivers; coping strategies did not mediate the relationship (Clark, 2002). The type of empathy shown by caregivers can influence outcomes. Caregivers with high cognitive empathy (i.e., ability to under-*

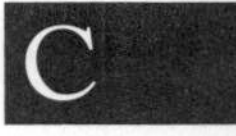

*stand another's feelings while maintaining emotional distance) viewed caregiving as less stressful, were less depressed, and reported higher life satisfaction than those with low cognitive empathy. Emotional empathy (i.e., vicarious emotional response to the perceived feelings of others) was associated with lower life satisfaction, presumably because caregivers were unable to detach themselves from the clients' feelings (Lee, Brennan, & Daly, 2001).*

- Identify and support strengths of the caregiver and efforts to gain control of unpredictable situations. **EB:** *The use of external services may be helpful to gain control of the situation, and was often implemented when caregivers showed signs of depressive symptomatology. However, when clients had memory and behavior problems, fewer services were called in. As caregivers experienced difficulty performing IADLs, more depressive symptoms and greater service use were seen (Bookwala et al, 2004). The nurse will need to monitor service need and use over time.*
- Help the caregiver to stay connected with the client who may be behaving differently than usual, to make life as routine as possible, to help the client set goals and sustain hope, and to allow the client space to experience progress. *Identifying and acknowledging positive caregiver responses to the client's illness will help the caregiver to maintain a positive relationship with the client.* **EBN:** *Family members of persons with severe mental illness have found it helpful to work at staying connected to the person with mental illness, finding a role that they can feel comfortable with, and helping the relative move forward (Rose, 1998).*
- Recognize that caregiver disabilities may not prevent them from providing care; assess each situation individually. *Caregivers with mental illness need not be considered incapable of the caregiving role.* **EBN:** *Adult children with mental illness have been shown to provide their mothers help with a range of daily living tasks, thus decreasing maternal subjective burden (Greenberg, 1995).*
- Form a trusting and supportive relationship with the caregiver. Allow the caregiver to verbalize frustrations. *Providing attention to the caregiver can decrease caregiver stress and reduce the risk of caregiver violence.*
- Assist the caregiver in identifying sources of concern and areas of stress in dealing with the client's illness. **EBN:** *A study identified the need for support of heart transplantation clients' spouses (Bohachick et al, 2001). Prior to transplantation, spouses experienced high levels of distress because of an inability to participate in social activities, as their time was spent in caregiving and maintaining the home. Anxiety, depression, worry, vocational disruption, and sexual adjustment difficulties occurred. Improvements in all of these areas were found by 1 year after transplantation, in part due to relief of fears that the client might die before a donor could be found. After transplantation, spouses were more relaxed and able to resume social activities.*
- Instruct the caregiver in the care needs of the client, disease processes, medications, and what to expect; use a variety of instructional techniques (e.g., explanations, demonstrations, visual aids) until the caregiver is able to express a degree of comfort with care delivery. *Knowledge and confidence are separate concepts. Self-assurance in caregiving will improve performance of the role in client maintenance that caregivers assume (Scott, 2000).*
- Assist the caregiver and client in arranging care so that it is compatible with other household patterns. **EBN:** *Caregivers of elders have been identified as using home envi-*

C

*ronmental modification strategies for specific purposes: organizing the home, supplementing the elder's function, structuring the elder's day, protecting the elder, working around limitations or deficits in the home environment, enriching the home environment, and transitioning to a new home setting (Messecar et al, 2002).*

- • Explore the state of the relationship between the client and the caregiver before the onset of chronic illness or dementia; identify the strengths and weaknesses of each party. Formulate a plan to assist the couple in dealing with likely worsening of dementia. *Chronic illness, especially dementia, can represent a gradual and devastating loss of the marital relationship as it existed formerly. An understanding of the prior relationship is needed before the couple can be helped to anticipate continuing care needs or deterioration (Zarit, 2001). In a study of cancer clients and spousal caregivers, past relationships characterized by mutual concern and responsiveness (communal) led to caregiver depression, as loss of intimacy and affection predicted restriction of caregiver's routine activity. When past relationships were less communal, activity restriction was predicted by the severity of client symptoms and led to resentment of the care recipient and the caregiving role (Williamson, Shaffer, & Schultz, 1998).*
- • Explore with the spouse the process of understanding the client's behavior that the spouse has been undergoing; assist with reframing that understanding to be as realistic and positive as possible. Consider use of the Progressively Lowered Stress Threshold psychoeducational nursing intervention to help the spouse understand and handle the behavior changes associated with Alzheimer's disease. **EBN:** *In a qualitative study, wives of clients with Alzheimer's disease described a process of recognizing changes, drawing inferences about their observations, rewriting identities for themselves and their husbands as they took on the husbands' roles and responsibilities, and constructing a new daily life. Reframing interventions can help caregivers consider positive aspects of caring along with grief and frustration (Perry, 2002). Nurses can help caregivers normalize events, making these events more manageable and less threatening (Ayres, 2000a, 2000b). The Progressively Lowered Stress Threshold psychoeducational nursing intervention has been shown to have a positive effect in decreasing the frequency of disruptive behavior and improving the response of the caregiver to the behaviors of the Alzheimer's client (Gerdner, Buckwalter, & Reed, 2002).*
- ▲ Refer the client to home health aide services for assistance with ADLs and light housekeeping. Allow the caregiver to gain confidence in the respite provider. *Home health aide services can provide physical relief and respite for the caregiver.* **EB:** *The greatest caregiver burden was reported to occur as physical demands increased, especially during the last 3 months of the client's life (Brazil, Bedard, Willison, et al, 2003).*
- ▲ Identify appropriate individual and group interventions for the caregiver; assess for appropriateness of referrals given the caregiver's needs and mobility. **EBN:** *Individual interventions (family-focused individual therapy, cognitive behavioral therapy, cognitive stimulation training, professional and peer counseling, stress management and problem solving) and group interventions (professional versus self-help support groups, stress management, respite care, multimedia training groups, caregiver training in behavior management and social skills) have been identified as effective in reducing caregiver stress (Yin, Zhou, & Bashford, 2002).*
- ▲ Refer to a caregivers support group if available or recommend an online support

• = Independent; ▲ = Collaborative; EBN = Evidence-Based Nursing; EB = Evidence-Based

group—see suggested websites listed on the Evolve website. **EBN:** *Sharing concerns with others can mitigate loneliness. Increased caregiver loneliness has been associated with depression, relational deprivation, and poorer quality of the current caregiver–client relationship (Beeson et al, 2000). Because members read and send messages 24 hours per day every day of the week, online support groups offer the advantage of immediate communication with others offering support. When nurses assist with online support groups, the groups can help caregivers learn, give them a sense of community, and encourage a sense of empowerment (White & Dorman, 2000).*

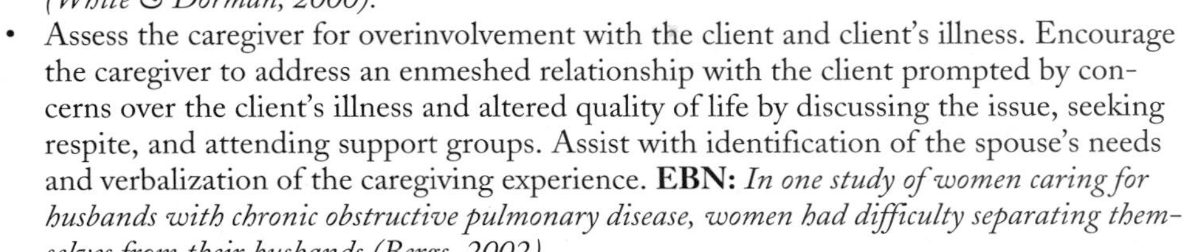

- • Assess the caregiver for overinvolvement with the client and client's illness. Encourage the caregiver to address an enmeshed relationship with the client prompted by concerns over the client's illness and altered quality of life by discussing the issue, seeking respite, and attending support groups. Assist with identification of the spouse's needs and verbalization of the caregiving experience. **EBN:** *In one study of women caring for husbands with chronic obstructive pulmonary disease, women had difficulty separating themselves from their husbands (Bergs, 2002).*
- ▲ Refer to case managers as necessary for community resource assistance, financial planning, and supportive counseling for both client and caregiver. **EBN:** *Individualized counseling in problem solving by nurses was shown to be effective in reducing the number of admissions to nursing homes (Roberts et al, 1999).*
- ▲ Refer for homemaker or psychiatric home health care services for respite, client reassurance, and implementation of a therapeutic regimen. *Taking responsibility for a person needing extensive care results in high caregiver stress. Respite decreases caregiver stress. The presence of caring individuals is reassuring to both the client and caregivers, especially during periods of client anxiety or agitation. Counseling may be necessary to address unresolved family relationship issues that threaten to impede the delivery of care.* **EB:** *Home care services for frail elderly clients with dementia were shown to decrease caregiver stress (Tibaldi, Aimonino, Ponzetto, et al, 2004). Home care services provided to children with intellectual disabilities was shown to improve significantly the mental health of caregivers (Shu, Lung, & Huang, 2002).*
- • As indicated by client status, assist the caregiver in examining the option of adult day care and maintaining realistic expectations of adult day care. **EB:** *Studies have not shown a major impact of day care on the anxiety or depression of older adults, or on caregiver burden. However, a study did find subjective reports of reduced loneliness, anxiety, and depression among clients, and decreased perceived burden on caregivers (Baumgarten, Lebel, Laprise, et al, 2002).*
- ▲ As indicated by deterioration of the client's condition, assist the caregiver in examining options for institutional placement. **EBN:** *Caregiver overload leads to decreased physical health and increased anxiety over time. The caregiver may require instruction in the client's need for formal supports as condition deteriorates (Winslow, 1997). Caregiver burden has been shown to decrease following institutional placement (Winslow et al, 1999).*
- • Assess the caregiver's emotional response to placement of the client and provide support, cognitive interventions, and problem solving as needed. *A variety of difficulties may impede the caregiver's acceptance of the need for the client's placement, including financial concerns, inability to accept the client's level of need for increased supervision, guilt, or unresolved relationship issues. It is important to identify the relevant concerns and options, as well*

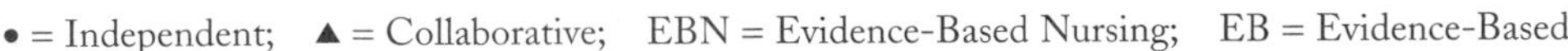

• = Independent; ▲ = Collaborative; EBN = Evidence-Based Nursing; EB = Evidence-Based

C

as to address psychological issues. **EBN:** *Placement of a family member involves a struggle to make a decision, find reassurance, and remain connected to the client (Butcher et al, 2001).*

- Be aware that physical demands on the caregiver tend to increase during the last 3 months of a care recipient's life, and more assistance with ADLs foretells greater risk of caregiver burden. Both emotional and instrumental support of the caregiver may increase toward recipient's end of life. **EB:** *Families of terminally ill clients are especially vulnerable to caregiver role strain because the timing of the impending death is unpredictable, caregiver effort and resources are disproportionately spent early in the caregiving process, and increased physical care demands are associated with caregiver burden (Brazil, Bedard, Willison, et al, 2003).*

## Caregiver/Family Teaching

- Assess the caregiver's need for information such as information on symptom management, disease progression, specific skills, available support.
- Teach the caregiver warning signs for burnout, depression, and anxiety. Help them identify a resource in case they begin to feel overwhelmed.
- Teach the caregiver methods for managing disruptive behavioral symptoms if present. Refer to the care plan for **Chronic Confusion.** *Multicomponent interventions can be particularly effective in caregivers of persons with neurologic sequelae (Gitlin et al, 2003).*
- Teach the caregiver how to provide the physical care needed.
- Provide information and problem-solving techniques for symptom management in the care receiver.
- Provide ongoing support and evaluation of care skills as the care situation and care demands change.
- Provide information regarding the care recipient's diagnosis, treatment regimen, and expected course of illness.

▲ Refer to counseling or support groups to assist in adjusting to the caregiver role.

## evolve WEBSITES FOR EDUCATION

See the EVOLVE website for World Wide Web resources for caregiver education.

## REFERENCES

Ayres L: Narratives of family caregiving: four story types, *Res Nurs Health* 23(5):359-371, 2000a.

Ayres L: Narratives of family caregiving: the process of making meaning, *Res Nurs Health* 23(6):424-434, 2000b.

Bakas T, Burgener S: Predictors of emotional distress, general health, and caregiving outcomes in family caregivers of stroke survivors, *Top Stroke Rehabil* 9(1):34-45, 2002.

Baumgarten M, Lebel P, Laprise H et al: Adult day care for the frail elderly: outcomes, satisfaction, and cost, *J Aging Health* 14(2): 237-259, 2002.

Beach S, Schulz R, Yee J et al: Negative and positive health effects of caring for a disabled spouse: longitudinal findings from the caregiver health effects study, *Psychol Aging* 15(2):259-271, 2000.

Beeson R, Horton-Deutsch S, Farran C et al: Loneliness and depression in caregivers of persons with Alzheimer's disease or related disorders, *Issues Ment Health Nurs* 21(8):779-806, 2000.

Beitman CL, Johnson JL, Clark AL et al: Caregiver role strain of older workers, *Work* 22(2):99-106, 2004.

Bergs D: "The hidden client"—women caring for husbands with COPD: their experience of quality of life, *J Clin Nurs* 11(5):613-21, 2002.

Bohachick P, Reeder S, Taylor MV et al: Psychosocial impact of heart transplantation on spouses, *Clin Nurs Res* 10(1):6-25, 2001.

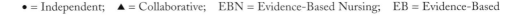

Boland D, Sims S: Family caregiving at home as a solitary journey, *Image J Nurs Sch* 28(1):55-58, 1996.
Bookwala J, Zdaniuk B, Burton L et al: Concurrent and long-term predictors of older adults' use of community-based long-term care services: the Caregiver Health Effects Study, *J Aging Health* 16(1):88-115, 2004.
Brandl B, Raymond J: Unrecognized elder abuse victims. Older abused women, *J Case Manag* 6(2):62-68, 1997.
Brazil K, Bedard M, Willison K et al: Caregiving and its impact on families of the terminally ill, *Aging Ment Health* 7(5):376-382, 2003.
Buckwalter KC, Gerdner L, Kohout F et al: A nursing intervention to decrease depression in family caregivers of person with dementia, *Arch Psychiatr Nurs* 13(2):80-88, 1999.
Buffum MD, Brod M: Humor and well-being in spouse caregivers of patients with Alzheimer's disease, *Appl Nurs Res* 11(1):12-18, 1998.
Bull MJ, Hansen HE, Gross CR: Differences in family caregiver outcomes by their level of involvement in discharge planning, *Appl Nurs Res* 13(2):76-82, 2000.
Bull MJ, Roberts J: Components of a proper hospital discharge for elders, *J Adv Nurs* 35(4):571-581, 2001.
Burton L, Newsom J, Schulz R et al: Preventive health behaviors among spousal caregivers, *Prev Med* 26(2):162-169, 1997.
Butcher HK, Holkup PA, Park M et al: Thematic analysis of the experience of making a decision to place a family member with Alzheimer's disease in a special care unit, *Res Nurs Health* 24(6):470-480, 2001.
Cameron J, Franche RL, Cheung AM et al: Lifestyle interference and emotional distress in family caregivers of advanced cancer patients, *Cancer* 94(2):521-527, 2002.
Cheung J, Hocking P: Caring as worrying: the experience of spousal carers, *J Adv Nurs* 47(5):475-482, 2004.
Clark MC: A causal functional explanation of maintaining a dependent elder in the community, *Res Nurs Health* 20(6):515-526, 1997.
Clark PC, Dunbar SB, Shields CG et al: Influence of stroke survivor characteristics and family conflict surrounding recovery on caregivers' mental and physical health, *Nurs Res* 53(6):406-413, 2004.
Clark PC: Effects of individual and family hardiness on caregiver depression and fatigue, *Res Nurs Health* 25(1):37-48, 2002.
Cochran M: Tears have no color, *Am J Nurs* 98(6):53, 1998.
Coon D, Rubert M, Solano N et al: Well-being, appraisal, and coping in Latina and Caucasian female dementia caregivers: findings from the REACH study, *Aging Ment Health* 8(4):330-345, 2004.
Cox C: Race and caregiving: patterns of service use by African-American and white caregivers of persons with Alzheimer's disease, *J Gerontol Soc Work* 32(2):5-19, 1999.
Crist JD: Mexican American elders' use of skilled home care nursing services, *Public Health Nurs* 19(5):366-376, 2002.
Deeken J, Taylor K, Mangan P et al: Care for the caregivers: a review of self-report instruments developed to measure the burden, needs, and quality of life of informal caregivers, *J Pain Symptom Manage* 26(4):922-953, 2003.
Doswell W, Erlen J: Multicultural issues and ethical concerns in the delivery of nursing care interventions, *Nurs Clin North Am* 33(2):353-361, 1998.
Gerdner LA, Buckwalter KC, Reed D: Impact of a psychoeducational intervention on caregiver response to behavior problems, *Nurs Res* 51(6):363-374, 2002.
Gitlin L, Belle SH, Burgio LD et al: Effect of multicomponent interventions on caregiver burden and depression: the REACH multisite initiative at 6-month follow-up, *Psychol Aging* 18(3):361-374, 2003.
Given CW, Given B, Stommel M et al: The caregiver reaction assessment (CRA) for caregivers to persons with chronic physical and mental impairments, *Res Nurs Health* 15(4):271-383, 1992.
Grunfeld E et al: Family caregiver burden: results of a longitudinal study of breast cancer patients and their principal caregivers, *CMAJ* 170(12):1795-1801, 2004.
Guarnaccia P: Multicultural experiences of family caregiving: a study of African American, European American, and Hispanic American families, *New Dir Ment Health Serv* (77):45-61, 1998.
Hayes JM: Respite for caregivers. A community-based model in a rural setting, *J Gerontol Nurs* 25(1):22-26, 1999.
Hayman J, Langa KM, Kabeto MU et al: Estimating the cost of informal caregiving for elderly patients with cancer, *J Clin Oncol* 19(13):3219-3225, 2001.
Heineken J: Patient silence is not necessarily client satisfaction: communication in home care nursing, *Home Healthc Nurse* 16(2): 115-120, 1998.
Hepburn K, Tornatore J, Center B et al: Dementia family caregiver training: affecting beliefs about caregiving and caregiver outcomes, *J Am Geriatr Soc* 49(4):450-457, 2001.
Houde SC: Predictors of elders' and family caregivers' use of formal home services, *Res Nurs Health* 21(6):533-543, 1998.
Jones PS: Asian American women caring for elderly parents, *J Fam Nurs* 2(1):56, 1996.
Kleffel D: Lives on hold: evaluation of a caregivers' support program, *Home Healthc Nurse* 16(7):465-472, 1998.

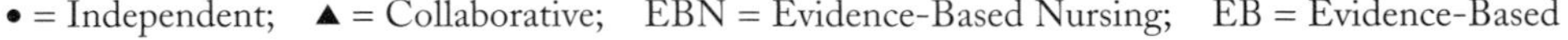

Knop DS, Bergman-Evans B, McCabe BW: In sickness and in health: an exploration of the perceived quality of the marital relationship, coping, and depression in caregivers of spouses with Alzheimer's disease, *J Psychosoc Nurs Ment Health Serv* 36(1):16-21, 1998.

Krause N, Rook K: Negative interaction in late life: issues in the stability and generalizability of conflict across relationships, *J Gerontol B Psychol Sci Soc Sci* 58(2):P88-99, 2003.

Kurtz M, Kurtz JC, Given CW et al: Depression and physical health among family caregivers of geriatric patients with cancer—a longitudinal view, *Med Sci Monit* 10(8):CR447-456, 2004.

Lampley-Dallas V, Mold J, Flori D: Perceived needs of African-American caregivers of elders with dementia, *J Natl Med Assoc* 93(2):47-57, 2001.

Leblanc AJ, Driscoll AK, Pearlin LI: Religiosity and the expansion of caregiver stress, *Aging Ment Health* 8(5):410-421, 2004.

Lee H, Cameron, M: Respite care for people with dementia and their carers, *Cochrane Database Syst Rev* (2):CD004396, 2004.

Li H: Barriers to and unmet needs for supportive services: experiences of Asian-American caregivers, *J Cross Cult Gerontol,* 19(3): 241-260, 2004.

Leininger MM, McFarland MR: *Transcultural nursing: concepts, theories, research and practices,* ed 3, New York, 2002, McGraw-Hill.

Liken MA, Collins CE: Grieving: facilitating the process for dementia caregivers, *J Psychosoc Nurs Ment Health Serv* 31(1):21-26, 1993.

Lyons KS, Stewart BJ, Archbold PG et al: Pessimism and optimism as early warning signs for compromised health for caregivers of patients with Parkinson's disease, *Nurs Res* 53(6):354-362, 2004.

Martire LM, Stephens MA, Druley JA et al: Negative reactions to received spousal care: predictors and consequences of miscarried support, *Health Psychol* 21(2):167-276, 2002.

McGrath P, Vun M, McLeod L: Needs and experiences on non-English speaking hospice patients and families in an English speaking country, *Am J Hosp Palliat Care* 18(5):305-312, 2001.

Messecar DC, Archbold PG, Stewart BJ et al: Home environmental modification strategies used by caregivers of elders, *Res Nurs Health* 25(5):357-370, 2002.

Miaskowski C, Kragness L, Dibble S et al: Differences in mood states, health status, and caregiver strain between family caregivers of oncology outpatients with and without cancer-related pain, *J Pain Symptom Manag* 13(3):138-147, 1997.

Mills P, Adler KA, Dimsdale JE et al: Vulnerable caregivers of Alzheimer disease patients have a deficit in beta 2-adrenergic receptor sensitivity and density, *Am J Geriatr Psychiatry* 12(3):281-286, 2004.

Narayan S, Lewis M, Tornatore J et al: Subjective responses to caregiving for a spouse with dementia, *J Gerontol Nurs* 27(3):19-28, 2001.

Newton M, Bell D, Lambert S et al: Concerns of hospice patient caregivers. *ABNF J,* 13(6):140-244, 2002.

Nijboer C, Tempelaar R, Triemstra M et al: The role of social and psychologic resources in caregiving of cancer patients, *Cancer* 91(5):1029-1039, 2001.

Northouse L, Mood D, Templin T et al: Couples' patterns of adjustment to colon cancer, *Soc Sci Med* 50(2):271-284, 2000.

Novak M, Guest C: Application of a multidimensional caregiver burden inventory, *Gerontologist* 29(6):798-803, 1989.

Perry J: Wives giving care to husbands with Alzheimer's disease: a process of interpretive caring, *Res Nurs Health* 25(4):307-316, 2002.

Pinquart M, Sorensen S: Associations of stressors and uplifts of caregiving with caregiver burden and depressed mood: a meta-analysis, *J Gerontol B Psychol Sci Soc Sci* 58(2):P112-128, 2003.

Poindexter CC, Linsk NL: Sources of support in a sample of HIV-affected older minority caregivers, *Fam Soc* 79(5):491, 1998.

Redwine L, Mills P, Sada M et al: Differential immune cell chemotaxis responses to acute psychological stress in Alzheimer caregivers compared to non-caregiver controls, *Psychosom Med* 66(5):770-775, 2004.

Roberts J, Browne G, Milne C et al: Problem-solving counseling for caregivers of the cognitively impaired: effective for whom? *Nurs Res* 48(3):162-272, 1999.

Robinson B: Validation of a Caregiver Strain Index, *J Gerontol* 38(3):344-348, 1983.

Roff LL, Burgio LD, Gitlin L et al: Positive aspects of Alzheimer's caregiving: the role of race, *J Gerontol B Psychol Sci Soc Sci* 59(4):P185-190, 2004.

Rose LE: Gaining control: family members relate to persons with severe mental illness, *Res Nurs Health* 21(4):363-373, 1998.

Ruppert RA: Caring for the lay caregiver, *Am J Nurs* 96(3):40-5, 1996.

Schulz R, Beach SR: Caregiving as a risk factor for mortality: the Caregiver Health Effects Study, *JAMA* 282(23):2215-2219, 1999.

Schulz R, Belle S, Czaja S et al: Long-term care placement of dementia patients and caregiver health and well-being, *JAMA* 292(8):961-967, 2004.

Schulz R, Martire L: Family caregiving of persons with dementia: prevalence, health effects, and support strategies, *Am J Geriatr Psychiatry* 12(3):240-249, 2004.

Schumacher KL, Stewart BJ, Archbold PG et al: Family caregiving skill: development of the concept, *Res Nurs Health* 23(3): 191-203, 2000.
Scott LD: Caregiving and care receiving among a technologically dependent heart failure population, *Adv Nurs Sci* 23(2):82-97, 2000.
Shu BC, Lung FW, Huang C: Mental heath of primary caregivers with children with intellectual disability who receive a home care programme, *J Intellec Disabil Res* 46(Pt 3):257-263, 2002.
Silveira JM, Winstead-Fry P: The needs of patients with cancer and their caregivers in rural areas, *Oncol Nurs Forum* 24(1):71-76, 1997.
Smith M, Gerdner LA, Hall GR et al: History, development, and future of the progressively lowered stress threshold: a conceptual model for dementia care, *J Am Geriatr Soc* 52(10):1755-1760, 2004.
Strang V: Caregiver respite: coming back after being away, *Perspectives* 24(4):10-20, 2000.
Teel CS, Duncan P, Lai SM: Caregiving experiences after stroke, *Nurs Res* 50(1):53, 2001.
Thornton M, Travis SS: Analysis of the reliability of the Modified Caregiver Strain Index, *Gerontol B Psychol Sci Soc Sci* 58(2): S127-132, 2003.
Tribaldi V, Aimonino N, Ponzetto M et al: A randomized controlled trial of a home hospital intervention for frail elderly demented patients: behavioral disturbances and caregiver's stress, *Arch Gerontol Geriatr* (Suppl 9):431-436, 2004.
Turner WL, Wallace BR, Anderson JR et al: The last mile of the way: understanding caregiving in African American families at the end-of-life, *J Marital Fam Ther* 30(4):427-438, 2004.
Vitaliano P, Russo J, Young H et al: The screen for caregiver burden, *The Gerontologist* 31(1):76-83, 1991.
White MH, Dorman SM: Online support for caregivers: analysis of an internet Alzheimer mailgroup, *Comput Nurs* 18(4):168-176, 2000.
Williamson GM, Shaffer DR, Schulz R: Activity restriction and prior relationship history as contributors to mental health outcomes among middle-aged and older spousal caregivers, *Health Psychol* 17(2):152-62, 1998.
Winslow BW: Effects of formal supports on stress outcomes in family caregivers of Alzheimer's patients, *Res Nurs Health* 20(1): 527-537, 1997.
Wuest J: Setting boundaries: a strategy for precarious ordering of women's caring demands, *Res Nurs Health* 21(1):39-49, 1998.
Yin T, Zhou Q, Bashford C: Burden on family members: caring for frail elderly: a meta-analysis of interventions, *Nurs Res* 51(3): 199-208, 2002.
Yurk R, Morgan D, Franey S et al: Understanding the continuum of palliative care for patients and their caregivers, *J Pain Symptom Manage* 24(5):459-470, 2002.
Zarit J: A tribute to adaptability: mental illness and dementia in intimate late-life relationships, *Generations* 25(2):70, 2001.
Zarit SH et al: Relatives of the impaired elderly: correlates of feelings of burden, *Gerontologist* 20(6):649, 1980.
Zhan L: Caring for family members with Alzheimer's disease: perspectives from Chinese American caregivers, *J Gerontol Nurs* 30(8):19-29, 2004.

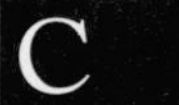


# Risk for Caregiver role strain

*Betty J. Ackley*

**NANDA**

## Definition

Caregiver is vulnerable for felt difficulty in performing the family caregiver role

## Risk Factors

Caregiver not developmentally ready for caregiver role (e.g., a young adult needing to provide care for a middle-aged person); inadequate physical environment for providing care (e.g., housing, transportation, community services, equipment); unpredict-

C

able illness course or instability in care receiver's health; psychological or cognitive problems in care receiver; presence of situational stressors that normally affect families (e.g., significant loss, disaster, or crisis; economic vulnerability; major life events); presence of abuse or violence; premature birth/congenital defect; past history of poor relationship between caregiver and care receiver; marginal family adaptation or dysfunction prior to the caregiving situation; marginal caregiver's coping patterns; lack of respite and recreation for caregiver; inexperience with caregiving; caregiver is female; addiction or codependency; care receiver exhibits deviant, bizarre behavior; Caregiver's competing role commitments; caregiver health impairment; illness severity of care receiver; caregiver is spouse; developmental delay or retardation of care receiver or caregiver; complexity/amount of caregiving tasks; discharge of family member with significant home care needs; duration of caregiving required; family/caregiver isolation

NOC

## Outcomes (Nursing Outcomes Classification)

### Suggested NOC Outcomes

Caregiver Emotional Health, Caregiver Lifestyle Disruption, Caregiver Performance: Direct Care, Caregiver Performance: Indirect Care, Caregiver Physical Health, Caregiver Stressors, Caregiver Well-Being, Role Performance

**Example NOC Outcome with Indicators**

**Caregiver Emotional Health** with plans for a positive future as evidenced by the following indicators: Satisfaction with life/Sense of control/Self-esteem/Free of anger/Free of guilt/Free of depression/Perceived social connectedness/Perceived spiritual well-being (Rate each indicator of **Caregiver Emotional Health:** 1 = severely compromised, 2 = substantially compromised, 3 = moderately compromised, 4 = mildly compromised, 5 = not compromised [see Section I].)

## Client Outcomes

### Client/Caretaker Will (Specify Time Frame):

- Maintain physical and psychological health
- Identify resources available to help in giving care
- Obtain appropriate care

NIC

## Interventions (Nursing Interventions Classification)

### Suggested NIC Interventions

Caregiver Support, Family Support, Home Maintenance Assistance, Normalization Promotion, Respite Care, Support Group

**Example NIC Activities—Caregiver Support**

Determine caregiver's acceptance of role; accept expressions of negative emotion

C

## Nursing Interventions and Rationales and Client/Family Teaching

Refer to the care plan for **Caregiver role strain.**

# Impaired Comfort[1]

evolve

*Scott C. Lamont*

**NANDA**

## Definition

State in which an individual experiences an uncomfortable sensation in response to a noxious stimulus (Carpenito, 2000); unpleasant sensation of being physically ill at ease that may be localized or generalized but is not described in terms of tissue damage (Lamont, 2002)

## Defining Characteristics

Verbalization of discomfort (e.g., aches, pruritus, photophobia); observed behaviors indicative of discomfort; shifting and/or restlessness; tenseness; shivering and covering up or removing of covers; avoidance of particular stimuli; malaise; aching; stiffness; distention; hunger and thirst; reduced mobility; itching; reddened, irritated skin (pruritus)

## Related Factors (r/t)

Reaction to chemical irritants, including allergies; dry skin; illness and/or immobility; unmet physical needs (food, fluid, bathing, and so on); fever; disease processes; pregnancy; immobility; musculoskeletal disorders; inflammation; intestinal gas, colic; medication side effects; contagious diseases (chickenpox, meningitis, and so on)

**NOC**

## Outcomes (Nursing Outcomes Classification)

### Suggested NOC Outcomes

Comfort Level, Symptom Control

[1]Impaired Comfort is not a NANDA-I–approved nursing diagnosis.

### Example NOC Outcome with Indicators

**Comfort Level** as evidenced by the following indicators: Physical well-being/Symptom control (Rate each indicator of **Comfort Level:** 1 = not at all satisfied, 2 = somewhat satisfied, 3 = moderately satisfied, 4 = very satisfied, 5 = completely satisfied [see Section I].)

## Client Outcomes

### Client Will (Specify Time Frame):

- State he or she is comfortable
- State that his or her uncomfortable sensations (aches, itching, and so on) are relieved or diminished to an acceptable level
- Explain methods to decrease own discomfort
- Display improved physical mobility
- Appear less restless and more at ease

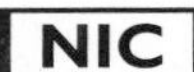

## Interventions (Nursing Interventions Classification)

### Suggested NIC Interventions

Acupressure, Bathing, Cutaneous Stimulation, Distraction, Environmental Management: Comfort, Exercise Promotion, Exercise Promotion: Stretching, Heat/Cold Application, Medication Administration, Music Therapy, Nausea Management, Positioning, Progressive Muscle Relaxation, Pruritus Management, Simple Guided Imagery, Simple Massage, Simple Relaxation Therapy, Skin Care: Topical Treatments, Touch

### Example NIC Activities—Pruritus Management

Apply medicated creams and lotions as appropriate; instruct client to limit bathing to once or twice a week as appropriate

## Nursing Interventions and Rationales

- Assess client needs holistically. *Physical discomfort often coexists with and is exacerbated by emotional and spiritual discomfort; therefore addressing nonphysical needs can improve the client's perception of physical comfort. The nurse's therapeutic approach and demeanor can have a profound impact on perception of comfort.* **EBN:** *One small, quantitative study found that female breast cancer clients undergoing radiation therapy rated their overall comfort as being greater than the sum of the hypothesized components of comfort, which lent support to the theory of the holistic nature of comfort (Kolcaba & Steiner, 2000). A grounded theory study of clients' perceptions of nurses' comfort work found that, although physical care provided was important, empathy and interpersonal skills were the dominant issue for clients (Walker, 2002).*

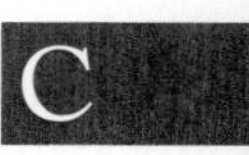


- ▲ Consult with the physician for medication to reduce discomforting symptoms such as aching. *Medications can reduce many discomforting sensations.*
- • Provide distraction techniques such as music, television, or games. *These activities help to temporarily distract the client from discomforting sensations.* **EB and EBN:** *Music therapy was found to reduce reported discomfort and anxiety compared to a control condition of no music in a study of individuals undergoing flexible sigmoidoscopy (Chlan et al, 2000). A 3-month clinical effectiveness study of single-session music therapy with terminally ill clients found significant improvements in reported pain control, physical comfort, and relaxation (Krout, 2001).*
- • Encourage early mobilization and provide routine position changes to decrease physical discomforts associated with bed rest. **EBN:** *A study of the comfort and complications associated with a 6-hour bed rest versus a 4-hour bed rest after cardiac catheterization found no significant differences and concluded that shorter periods may be acceptable (Wang et al, 2001). A study of 420 individuals following nonemergency cardiac catheterization found consistently lower scores for back discomfort with no increase in bleeding in the intervention group, who were turned every hour (Chair et al, 2003). A review comparing the Chair et al study to others found its results to be consistent with other studies which have found that backrest elevation, side lying, and early ambulation all improved comfort (Benson, 2004).*
- • Position the client to maximize comfort. **EBN:** *A qualitative study reported that some clients found positioning by nurses, such as leg elevation following injury, to be helpful (Hawley, 2000).*
- • Provide simple massage. *Massage may be helpful by reducing discomfort and anxiety, and promoting relaxation and sleep.* **EBN:** *A review of 22 articles on the effects of massage in acute care settings noted that the majority of studies found a significant decrease in anxiety or perception of tension, and some studies found decreased discomfort (Richards, Gibson, & Overton-McCoy, 2000). A quasi-experimental study of subjects in a rehabilitation facility found that subjects provided with 3 days of massage had improved physiological measures and reported a positive response to the massage (Holland & Pokorny, 2001).*
- • Provide gentle, soothing touch, which may be well-suited for clients who cannot tolerate more stimulating interventions such as simple massage. **EBN:** *A study of 1-to 3-week-old neonates in a level III neonatal intensive care unit (NICU) found that infants receiving gentle human touch showed evidence of being soothed compared with a control group but that the intervention must be carefully monitored in this client group because episodes of physiological instability were experienced by some subjects (Harrison et al, 2000).*
- • Skin-to-skin contact (SSC) and selection of most effective method improves the comfort of newborns during routine blood draws. **EB:** *A small, randomized clinical trial of healthy, full-term infants showed a decrease in pain reactions in the group receiving SSC with their mothers during heel lancing (Gray, Watt, & Blass, 2000). Another randomized study found that infants who had blood obtained by venipuncture on the dorsal side of the hand instead of heel lancing demonstrated less discomfort, and required fewer skin punctures (Larsson et al, 1998).*
- • Inform the client of options for control of discomfort such as self-hypnosis and

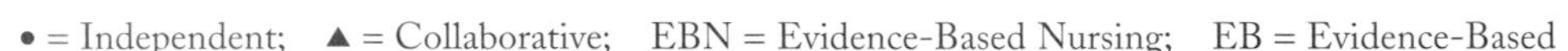

C

guided imagery, and provide these interventions if appropriate. **EBN:** *A study found that female breast cancer clients treated with guided imagery while undergoing radiation therapy had significant improvements in comfort (using one of two scales) compared with the control group (Kolcaba & Steiner, 2000).*

- Individualize the timing and type of bathing for each client; bathing may be distressing or comforting. **EB and EBN:** *Clients in labor may find discomfort and anxiety reduced if allowed to bathe for approximately 60 minutes early in labor (Benfield et al, 2001). This study and a second study found no maternal or neonatal ill effects associated with early labor bathing (Benfield et al, 2001; Ohlsson et al, 2001). Conversely, an experiment comparing a modified type of bed bathing using a no-rinse cleanser with standard tub bathing for elderly clients with dementia found that agitated behaviors were significantly lower for the bed-bathing group and that the effect was greater for men than for women. These clients may therefore experience less discomfort if not subjected to tub baths (Dunn, Thiru-Chelvam, & Beck, 2002).*
- Limit potentially uncomfortable interventions. Implement only when clearly needed and include the impetus for or timing of discontinuation in the plan of care. **EBN:** *A descriptive study of clients who had urinary catheters placed found that for 15 of 51 observed individuals there was no plan of care associated with their urinary catheterization, and for only 8 was there a plan for the discontinuation of catheter use (Brennan & Evans, 2001).*
- Tailor uncomfortable interventions to individual client needs or responses to therapy. Be aware of current research on alternatives to uncomfortable therapies that may benefit specific client groups or subgroups. **EB and EBN:** *A descriptive study of two specific groups of individuals experiencing leg ulcers found that reduced compression bandaging resulted in little or no discomfort without compromising wound healing (Arthur & Lewis, 2000). An experimental study of pressure bandaging to reduce bleeding after coronary angiography found that although the incidence of femoral bleeding was higher and the time of its onset was earlier in the nonbandage group, the overall incidence was low, the extent of bruising was the same for both groups, and the incidence of severe physical discomfort was higher in the bandage group. Based on these findings, the authors did not recommend the routine application of pressure bandaging after angiography (Botti et al, 1998).*
- Utilize careful, safe technique when transferring patients in and out of beds or chairs. **EBN:** *A descriptive study of orthopedic nurses and their clients found that clients felt safer and more comfortable during transfers when the nurses used safe technique as measured by work technique score (Kjellberg, Lagerstrom, & Hagberg, 2004).*
- Offer acupressure with either finger technique or with antinausea wrist bands for clients experiencing or at risk for nausea. **EBN:** *A randomized trial involving 150 postoperative patients resulted in significant decreases in the incidence of nausea and vomiting in the intervention groups (Ming et al, 2002).*
- Lower fevers with medication rather than sponging alone or in combination with medication unless there is a clear need to rapidly lower the client's temperature. **EBN:** *Medications such as acetaminophen reduce fever more quickly than sponging alone, and some studies found that children perceived sponging as discomforting (Joanna Briggs Institute, 2001).*

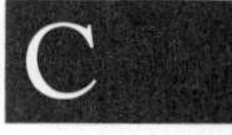


### Geriatric

- Comforting touch is helpful for elders because they respond to touch more than to verbal comforting. **EBN:** *A study of outcomes of comfort touch with elderly institutionalized women found that perceptions of self-esteem, well-being, health status, and other measures improved significantly in the experimental group (Butts, 2001).*
- Frail elderly clients should be protected from cold discomfort and can be offered warmed blankets to decrease discomfort. *Frail elders are at risk for cold discomfort and hypothermia, even in warm environments and may not be able to meet their own needs by means such as adding a layer of clothing (Worfolk, 1997). A pre- and postdesign study of 49 clients found that they reported a significantly lower level of discomfort one hour after the application of a warm blanket (Robinson & Benton, 2002).*

### Multicultural

- Assess for the influence of cultural beliefs, norms, and values on the client's perceptions of skin and/or hair status and practices. **EBN:** *What the client considers normal and abnormal skin and hair condition may be based on cultural perceptions (Leininger & McFarland, 2002; Cochran, 1998; Doswell & Erlen, 1998).*
- Identify and clarify cultural language used to describe skin and hair. **EBN:** *Clients may interchange words meaning discomfort and pain, may refer to minor discomforts as pain, or may not discuss nonpainful discomforts at all (Lamont, 2002). Specific words and nonverbal expression are related to health beliefs, practices, and values (Leininger & McFarland, 2002).*
- Assess skin for ashy appearance. **EBN:** *Black skin and the skin of other people of color will appear ashy as a result of the flaking off of the top layer of the epidermis (Smith & Burns, 1999; Jackson, 1998).*
- Encourage the use of lanolin-based lotions for African-American clients with dry skin. **EBN:** *Vaseline may clog the pores and cause cellulitis or other skin problem (Jackson, 1998).*
- Offer hair oil and lanolin-based lotion for dry scalp and skin. **EBN:** *Black skin seems to produce less oil than lighter-colored skin; therefore African Americans may use more lubricants as a normal part of skin hygiene (Smith & Burns, 1999).*
- Use soap sparingly if the skin is dry. **EBN:** *Black skin tends to be dry, and soap will exacerbate this condition (Jackson, 1998).*

### Home Care

- Assist the client and family in identifying and providing comfort measures that are effective and safe for the condition and situation.
- Encourage mobilization as frequently as is appropriate for the client.
- Keep the temperature of the home moderate to warm for frail clients.

## Client/Family Teaching

- Teach techniques to use when the client is uncomfortable, including relaxation techniques, guided imagery, hypnosis, and music therapy. *Interventions such as progressive muscle relaxation training, guided imagery, hypnosis, and music therapy can effectively decrease the perception of uncomfortable sensations.*

- Instruct the client and family on prescribed medications and therapies that improve comfort.
- ▲ Teach the client to follow up with the physician or other practitioner if discomfort persists.



## Pruritus

- Perform a complete assessment to determine the cause of pruritus (e.g., dry skin, contact with irritating substance, medication side effect, insect bite, infection, healing burns, underlying systemic disease). **EB and EBN:** *The cause of pruritus helps direct treatment (Bueller & Bernhard, 1998). Pruritus may be caused by serious illnesses such as renal failure, liver failure, malignancy, or diabetes (Bueller & Bernhard, 1998; Eaglestein, McKay, & Pariser, 1994), as well as by dry skin and various skin conditions. Treatment should be individualized (Bueller & Bernhard, 1998).*
- Assess for sleep disturbances. **EB:** *One study found that a majority of clients reported difficulty falling asleep and that itching was more frequent at night (Yosipovitch et al, 2002).*
- Implement soaks with cool or cold washcloths or offer cool baths if appropriate. **EB:** *Some clients report that bathing with cool or cold water can depress the itching sensation (Yosipovitch et al, 2002). Bathing with salts may improve skin barrier protection and have an emollient effect. Baking soda, colloidal oatmeal (with and without oil), and bath oils may also be comforting. A study with an experimental irritant design demonstrated reduced transepidermal water loss and improved skin water capacitance with the use of sea water and water containing sodium choloride (NaCl) and potassium choloride (KCl) (Yoshizawa et al, 2001). A study comparing postburn itching in individuals showering with either a 5% colloidal oatmeal and liquid paraffin combination or a plain liquid paraffin bath oil found the colloidal oatmeal and oil combination significantly more effective (Matheson, Clayton, & Muller, 2001).*
- Keep the client's fingernails short; have the client wear mitts if necessary. *Scratching with fingernails can excoriate the area and increase skin damage and risk of cellulitis.*
- Leave pruritic area open to the air if possible. *Covering the area with a nonventilated dressing can increase itching sensation and warmth in the area.*
- Use nonallergenic mild soap and use it sparingly. **EB:** *Many soaps can be irritating to the skin and increase the itching sensation (Bueller & Bernhard, 1998).*
- Keep skin well-lubricated. After bathing, while the skin is still moist, apply nonallergenic moisturizers such as Medilan that are alcohol free and available in cream or ointment form. Apply moisturizers daily. **EB:** *These agents lubricate the skin surface and make the skin feel smoother and less dry (Hardy, 1996). Medilan is a hypoallergenic lanolin that has soothing and hydrating properties. It can be helpful for the treatment of eczema and other dry skin conditions (Stone, 2000). Creams and ointments are more effective than lotions because they contain more oil and less water (Bueller & Bernhard, 1998). Apply emollients within 3 to 5 minutes of exiting bath to trap absorbed water; pat rather than rub dry after application (Koblenzer, 1999). Daily application of moisturizers can have the persistent clinical effect of relieving dry skin (Tabata et al, 2000).*
- Provide simple massage for select client groups, such as those recovering from burns. **EBN:** *Two studies of the effects of massage on burn wounds demonstrated reduced pruri-*

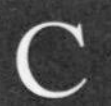

*tus: one involved the remodeling phase of wound healing (Field et al, 2000), and the other involved hypertrophic scars (Patino et al, 1999).*

- Behavior modification may reduce self-injury due to scratching and improve quality of life. *Incorporating a behavioral model for care using a habit reversal technique into nursing care plans for clients with atopic eczema has been advocated (Buchanan, 2001).*
- ▲ Advocate for altering or substituting medications if pruritus is potentially a side effect of the current regimen.

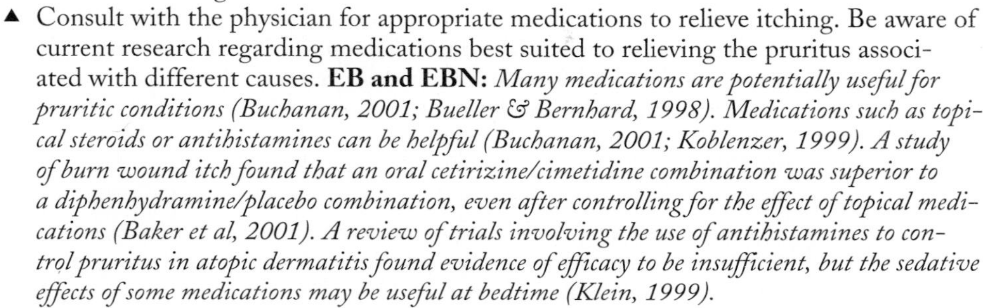

- ▲ Consult with the physician for appropriate medications to relieve itching. Be aware of current research regarding medications best suited to relieving the pruritus associated with different causes. **EB and EBN:** *Many medications are potentially useful for pruritic conditions (Buchanan, 2001; Bueller & Bernhard, 1998). Medications such as topical steroids or antihistamines can be helpful (Buchanan, 2001; Koblenzer, 1999). A study of burn wound itch found that an oral cetirizine/cimetidine combination was superior to a diphenhydramine/placebo combination, even after controlling for the effect of topical medications (Baker et al, 2001). A review of trials involving the use of antihistamines to control pruritus in atopic dermatitis found evidence of efficacy to be insufficient, but the sedative effects of some medications may be useful at bedtime (Klein, 1999).*

## Geriatric

- Limit the number of complete baths to no more than one every other day. Consider the use of no-rinse skin cleansers as a bathing alternative for select clients. *Excessive bathing, especially in hot water, depletes aging skin of moisture and increases dryness. Use a tepid water temperature (e.g., 90° to 105° F [32° C]) for bathing, and limit immersion to less than 20 minutes (Bueller & Bernhard, 1998).* **EBN:** *One study showed no clinical difference in outcome between use of a regular skin detergent for bathing and use of a no-rinse cleanser in a long-term care setting, but the no-rinse cleanser is more than double the cost. Selected clients with pruritus may benefit from the no-rinse preparations, but further research is required (Dawson et al, 2001).*
- Use a superfatted soap such as Dove, Tone, Basis, or Caress. *Superfatted soaps help retain moisture in dry skin of elderly clients (Hardy, 1996). Dove is reported to be the mildest soap available (Bueller & Bernhard, 1998).*
- Increase fluid intake within cardiac or renal limits to a minimum of 1500 mL/day. *Dry skin is caused by loss of fluid through the skin; increasing fluid intake rehydrates the skin. Adequate hydration helps decrease itching (Koblenzer, 1999).*
- Use a humidifier or place a container of water on a heat source to increase humidity in the environment, especially during winter. *Increasing moisture in the air helps to keep moisture in the skin (Bueller & Bernhard, 1998; Hardy, 1996). During times of cold weather and low humidity, dermatitis of the hands is common (Uter, Gefeller, & Schwanitz, 1998).*

## Home Care

- Assist the client and family in identifying and avoiding irritants that exacerbate pruritus (e.g., wool, cleansers, allergens). *Avoidance of irritants decreases discomfort of pruritus (Koblenzer, 1999).*

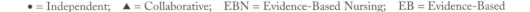

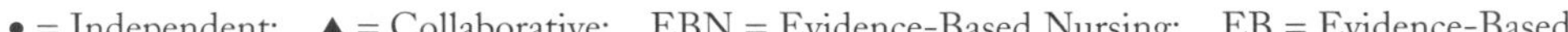

C

- Teach the family to use mild, nonscented, and non–bleach-containing laundry products. *Chemical irritants increase the discomfort of pruritus.*
- Keep the temperature of the home moderate to cool. Use a humidifier. *Overheated home environments increase sweating, which adds salts to the skin and increases irritation. Raising the moisture in the air helps to keep moisture in the skin (Hardy, 1996).* **EB:** *Cool ambient temperature has been reported to reduce pruritus in some clients (Yosipovitch et al, 2002).*
- Support the use of the client's preferred body lotion, as long as it has not been found to exacerbate pruritus. Have the client apply lotion after bathing before blotting skin dry. *Clients are more likely to continue past practices. Applying lotion while the skin is still wet increases the moisturizing action of the lotion.*

## Client/Family Teaching

- Teach techniques to use when the client is uncomfortable, including relaxation techniques, guided imagery, hypnosis, and music therapy. *Interventions such as progressive muscle relaxation, guided imagery, hypnosis, and music therapy can effectively decrease the itching sensation.*
- Teach the client with pruritus and the family to substitute rubbing, massage, pressure, or vibration for scratching when itching is severe and irrepressible. *Scratching may be self-injurious and may not relieve the pruritus (Buchanan, 2001).*
- Teach the client and the family correct application or administration of prescribed medications or therapies. *Some clients may benefit from education regarding the link between stress and pruritus caused by certain conditions (Koblenzer, 1999).*

▲ Instruct the client to see the primary care practitioner if itching persists and no cause is found. *Itching can be a symptom of other conditions (Koblenzer, 1999; Eaglestein, McKay, & Pariser, 1994).*

## evolve WEBSITES FOR EDUCATION

See the EVOLVE website for World Wide Web resources for client education.

## REFERENCES

Arthur J, Lewis P: When is reduced-compression bandaging safe and effective? *J Wound Care* 9(10):469-471, 2000.

Baker RA, Zeller RA, Klein RL et al: Burn wound itch control using H1 and H2 antagonists, *J Burn Care Rehabil* 22(4):263-268, 2001.

Benfield RD, Herman J, Katz VL et al: Hydrotherapy in labor, *Res Nurs Health* 24(1):57-67, 2001.

Benson G: Changing patients' position in bed after non-emergency coronary angiography reduced back pain, *Evid Based Nurs* 7(1):19, 2004.

Botti M, Williamson B, Steen K et al: The effect of pressure bandaging on complications and comfort in patients undergoing coronary angiography: a multicenter randomized trial, *Heart Lung* 27(6):360-373, 1998.

Brennan ML, Evans A: Why catheterize? Audit findings on the use of urinary catheters, *Br J Nurs* 10(9):580-590, 2001.

Buchanan PI: Behavior modification: a nursing approach for young children with atopic eczema, *Dermatol Nurs* 13(1):15-8, 21-23, 2001.

Bueller HA, Bernhard JD: Review of pruritus therapy, *Dermatol Nurs* 10(2):101-17, 1998.

Butts JB: Outcomes of comfort touch in institutionalized elderly female residents, *Geriatr Nurs* 22(4):180-14, 2001.

Carpenito JL: *Nursing diagnosis: application to clinical practice,* ed 8, Philadelphia, 2000, JB Lippincott.

Chair SY, Taylor-Piliae RE, Lam G et al: Effect of positioning on back pain after coronary angiography, *J Adv Nurs* 42(5):470-478, 2003.

Chlan L, Evans D, Greenleaf M et al: Effects of a single music therapy intervention on anxiety, discomfort, satisfaction, and compliance with screening guidelines in outpatients undergoing flexible sigmoidoscopy, *Gastroenterol Nurs* 23(4):148-156, 2000.

Cochran M: Tears have no color, *Am J Nurs* 98(6):53, 1998.

Dawson M, Pilgrim A, Moonsawmy C et al: An evaluation of two bathing products in a chronic care setting, *Geriatr Nurs* 22(2): 91, 2001.

Doswell W, Erlen J: Multicultural issues and ethical concerns in the delivery of nursing care interventions, *Nurs Clin North Am* 33(2):353-361, 1998.

Dunn JC, Thiru-Chelvam B, Beck CH: Bathing. Pleasure or pain? *J Gerontol Nurs* 28(11):6-13, 2002.

Eaglestein WH, McKay M, Pariser DM: The problems that plague aging skin, *Patient Care* 28:89, 1994.

Field T, Peck M, Scd, Hernandez-Reif M et al: Postburn itching, pain, and psychological symptoms are reduced with massage therapy, *J Burn Care Rehabil* 21(3):189-193, 2000.

Gray L, Watt L, Blass EM: Skin-to-skin contact is analgesic in healthy newborns, *Pediatrics* 105(1):e14, 2000.

Hardy MA: What can you do about your patient's dry skin? *J Gerontol Nurs* 22(5):10-18, 1996.

Harrison LL et al: Physiologic and behavioral effects of gentle human touch on preterm infants, *Res Nurs Health* 23(6):435-446, 2000.

Hawley MP: Nurse comforting strategies: perceptions of emergency department patients, *Clin Nurs Res* 9(4):441-459, 2000.

Holland B, Pokorny ME: Slow stroke back massage: its effect on patients in a rehabilitation setting, *Rehabil Nurs* 26(5):182-186, 2001.

Jackson F: The ABC's of black hair and skin care, *ABNF J* 9(5):100-104, 1998.

The Joanna Briggs Institute For Evidence Based Nursing And Midwifery (JBIEBNM): Management of the child with fever, *Best Practice* 5(5), Australia, 2001, Blackwell Science-Asia.

Kjellberg K, Lagerstrom M, Hagberg M: Patient safety and comfort during transfers in relation to nurses' work technique, *J Adv Nurs* 47(3):251-259, 2004.

Klein PA: An evidence-based review of the efficacy of antihistamines in relieving pruritus in atopic dermatitis, *Arch Dermatol* 135(12):1522-1525, 1999.

Koblenzer CS: Itching and the atopic skin, *J Allergy Clin Immunol* 104(3 Pt 2):S109-113, 1999.

Kolcaba K, Steiner R: Empirical evidence for the nature of holistic comfort, *J Holist Nurs* 18(1):46-62, 2000.

Krout RE: The effects of single-session music therapy interventions on the observed and self-reported levels of pain control, physical comfort, and relaxation of hospice patients, *Am J Hosp Palliat Care* 18(6):383-390, 2001.

Lamont SC: "Discomfort" as a potential nursing diagnosis: a concept analysis and review of the literature. Paper presented at the NNN 2002 Conference, April 10-13, 2002, Chicago.

Larsson BA, Tannfeldt G, Lagercrantz H et al: Alleviation of the pain of venepuncture in neonates, *Acta Paediatr.* 87(7):774-9, 1998.

Leininger MM, McFarland MR: *Transcultural nursing: concepts, theories, research and practices,* ed 3, New York, 2002, McGraw-Hill.

Matheson JD, Clayton J, Muller MJ: The reduction of itch during burn wound healing, *J Burn Care Rehabil* 22(1):76-81, 2001.

Ming JL, Kuo BI, Lin JG et al: The efficacy of acupressure to prevent nausea and vomiting in post-operative patients, *J Adv Nurs* 39(4):343-351, 2002.

Ohlsson G, Buchhave P, Leandersson U et al: Warm tub bathing during labor: maternal and neonatal effects, *Acta Obstet Gynecol Scand* 80(4):311-34, 2001.

Patino O, Novick C, Merlo A et al: Massage in hypertrophic scars, *J Burn Care Rehabil* 20(3):268-71, 1999.

Robinson S, Benton G: Warmed blankets: an intervention to promote comfort for elderly hospitalized patients, *Geriatr Nurs* 23(6):320-323, 2002.

Richards KC, Gibson R, Overton-McCoy AL: Effects of massage in acute and critical care, *AACN Clin Issues* 11(1):77-96, 2000.

Smith W, Burns C: Managing the hair and skin of African-American pediatric patients, *J Pediatr Health Care* 13(2):72-78, 1999.

Stone L: Product focus: Medilan: a hypoallergenic lanolin for emollient therapy, *Br J Nurs* 9(1)54-57, 2000.

Tabata N, O'Goshi K, Zhen YX et al: Biophysical assessment of persistent effects of moisturizers after their daily applications: evaluation of corneotherapy, *Dermatology* 200(4):308-313, 2000.

Uter W, Gefeller O, Schwanitz HJ: An epidemiological study of the influence of season (cold and dry air) on the occurrence of irritant skin changes of the hands, *Br J Dermatol* 138(2):266-272, 1998.
Walker AC: Safety and comfort work of nurses glimpsed through patient narratives, *Int J Nurs Pract* 8(1):42-48, 2002.
Wang S, Redeker NS, Moreyra AE et al: Comparison of comfort and local complications after cardiac catheterization, *Clin Nurs Res* 10(1):29-39, 2001.
Worfolk JB: Keep frail elders warm! *Geriatr Nurs* 18(1):7-11, 1997.
Yoshizawa, Y, Tanojo H, Kim SJ et al: Sea water or its components alter experimental irritant dermatitis in man, *Skin Res Technol* 7(1):36-39, 2001.
Yosipovitch G, Goon AT, Wee J et al: Itch characteristics in Chinese patients with atopic dermatitis using a new questionnaire for the assessment of pruritus, *Int J Dermatol* 41(4):212-216, 2002.

## Readiness for enhanced Communication

*Gail B. Ladwig*

**NANDA**

### Definition

Pattern of exchanging information and ideas with others that is sufficient for meeting one's needs and life's goals and can be strengthened

### Defining Characteristics

Expresses willingness to enhance communication; able to speak or write a language; forms words, phrases, and language; expresses thoughts and feelings; uses and interprets nonverbal cues appropriately; expresses satisfaction with ability to share information and ideas with others

### Related Factors (r/t)

To be developed

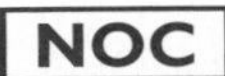

### Outcomes (Nursing Outcomes Classification)

#### Suggested NOC Outcomes

Communication; Communication: Expressive, Receptive

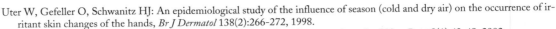

**Example NOC Outcome with Indicators**

**Communication** as evidenced by the following indicators: Use of spoken language/Use of written language/Acknowledgment of messages received/Exchanges messages accurately with others (Rate each indicator of **Communication:** 1 = severely compromised, 2 = substantially compromised, 3 = moderately compromised, 4 = mildly compromised, 5 = not compromised [see Section I].)

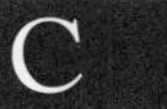

## Client Outcomes

**Client Will (Specify Time Frame):**

- Express willingness to enhance communication
- Demonstrate ability to speak or write a language
- Form words, phrases, and language
- Express thoughts and feelings
- Use and interpret nonverbal cues appropriately
- Express satisfaction with ability to share information and ideas with others

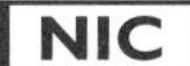

## Interventions (Nursing Interventions Classification)

### Suggested NIC Interventions

Active Listening; Communication Enhancement: Hearing Deficit; Communication Enhancement: Speech Deficit

| Example NIC Activities—Communication Enhancement: Hearing Deficit |
|---|
| Listen attentively; validate understanding of messages by asking client to repeat what was said |

## Nursing Interventions and Rationales

- Establish a good nurse-client relationship: provide appropriate education for the client, demonstrate caring by being present to the client. **EB:** *A good nurse-client relationship is essential to meet the clinical, psychological, and social needs of the client to optimize treatment in clients with renal disease. In this context, the importance of effective client education to increase client compliance played a vital role (Jenkins et al, 2002).* **EBN:** *Studies have demonstrated the importance of presence and caring communication (Sundin, Jansson, & Norberg, 2002).*
- Carefully assess the client's readiness to communicate. **EBN:** *Best practice with regard to communication in palliative care was achieved by using a sensitive assessment of how each client chooses to cope with his or her situation rather than a uniform approach to care (Dean, 2002).*
- Assess the client's literacy level. **EB:** *Health literacy is increasingly recognized as a critical factor affecting communication across the continuum of cancer care. According to the National Adult Literacy Survey, considered the most accurate portrait of literacy in our society, about one in five American adults may lack the necessary literacy skills to function adequately in our society (Davis et al, 2002).*
- Listen attentively and provide a comfortable environment for communicating; use these practical guidelines to assist in communication:
  - Slow down and listen to the client's story.
  - Use "living room" language.
  - Use pictures and stories to illustrate important points.

- Repeat instructions; limit the amount of information given.
- Have the client "teach back" to confirm understanding.
- Avoid asking, "Do you understand?"
- Be respectful, caring, and sensitive.

**EB:** *Practical communication aids can help bridge the cancer communication gap (Davis et al, 2002).* **EBN:** *A descriptive qualitative study of the nurse-client relationship identified helping influences that included consistency, pacing, listening, positive initial impressions, and attention to comfort and control (Forchuk et al, 2000).*

▲ Provide communication with specialty nurses who have knowledge about the client's situation. **EBN:** *Evidence suggests that clients supported by a nurse specialist are well informed and have a high degree of satisfaction (Greenhill, Betts, & Pickard, 2002).*

▲ Refer couples in maladjusted relationships to psychosocial intervention and social support to strengthen communication; consider nurse specialists. **EB:** *One study examined the relationship between coping and distress in couples faced with prostate cancer. Findings suggest that the relationship between coping and distress depends on the quality of dyadic functioning. Being part of a strong dyad may serve as a buffering factor; this implies the need for psychosocial intervention for couples in maladjusted relationships (Banthia et al, 2003).* **EBN:** *Social support intervention may be most useful when delivered by clinical nurse specialists who have additional education, training in communication, and teaching and consulting skills (Daugherty et al, 2002).*

• Consider using music to enhance communication between client and family of a client who is dying and having difficulty expressing feelings and emotions. **EB:** *Music therapy is described as a way to ease communication and sharing between dying patients and their loved ones (Krout, 2003).*

## Pediatric

▲ All individuals involved in the care and everyday life of children with learning difficulties need to have a collaborate approach to communication. **EBN:** *Collaboration has the potential to enable health professionals to adopt methods of communication that are familiar to the child, such as those used in the school setting. The advantage of such collaboration will enable health professionals to learn some of the methods used in the education of children with learning difficulties, which could be transferred to the health care setting (Kerzman & Smith, 2004).*

## Geriatric

▲ Assess for hearing and vision impairments and make appropriate referrals for hearing aids. **EB:** *One study recommended that clinicians assess each client's vision and conversational performance along with hearing thresholds before considering directions for rehabilitation. During face-to-face interaction, many people with adequate vision can compensate for a high-frequency hearing loss through lip reading, which precludes the need for hearing aids; many people with poor vision cannot compensate for a high-frequency hearing loss through lip reading and may require hearing aids (Erber, 2002).*

• Use touch if culturally acceptable when communicating with older clients and their families. *Touch can be useful for improving comfort and communication among terminally ill older adults and their loved ones (Bush, 2001).* **EBN:** *Provision of comfort touch to 45 institutionalized elderly women significantly improved perceptions of self-esteem, well-being and social processes, health status, life satisfaction and self-actualization, faith or belief, and self-responsibility (Butts, 2001).*

C

- Caregivers may sing when delivering care and instructions. **EBN:** *During caregiver singing, the client communicated with an increased understanding of the situation, both verbally and behaviorally (Gtell, Brown, & Ekman, 2002).*
- ▲ Use reminiscence therapy as a way to promote self-esteem and self-healing, to elevate mood and to relieve stress and aid in communication. **EBN:** *This study showed a significant difference in mood status and self-health perception in elderly clients who used reminiscence therapy in long-term care facilities. It is a way to promote healthy aging (Wang et al, 2004) This study suggests reminiscence therapy is an appropriate intervention for communication and to relieve stress in elders (Stokes & Gordon, 2003).*

## Multicultural

- Nurses should become more sensitive to the meaning of a culture's nonverbal communication modes such as eye contact, facial expression, touching, and body language. Nurses should realize that their good intentions and their usual nonverbal communication style may sometimes be interpreted as offensive and insulting by a specific cultural group. **EBN:** *To give a client a positive signal during a therapy session, a nurse may display the American sign of thumbs up. In Iran, however, thumbs extended upward are considered a vulgar gesture (Campinha-Bacote, 1998).*
- Assess for the influence of cultural beliefs, norms, and values on the client's communication process. **EBN:** *What the client considers normal and abnormal communication may be based on cultural perceptions (Leininger & McFarland, 2002; Johnson, 1999; Cochran, 1998; Doswell & Erlen, 1998). An affirmative answer does not necessarily mean "yes"; a client may be showing respect to the caregiver or avoiding the embarrassment of saying "no" (Galanti, 1997).*
- Assess personal space needs, acceptable communication styles, acceptable body language, interpretation of eye contact, perception of touch, and use of paraverbal modes when communicating with the client. **EBN:** *Nurses need to consider multiple factors when interpreting verbal and nonverbal messages (Purnell, 2000). Native Americans may consider avoiding direct eye contact to be a sign of respect and asking questions to be rude and intrusive (Seiderman et al, 1996). Empirical findings suggest that Chinese Americans and European Americans differ in the ways that they describe emotional experience, with Chinese Americans using more somatic and social words than Americans (Tsai, Simeonova, & Watanabe, 2004).*
- Assess for how language barriers contribute to health disparities among ethnic and racial minorities. **EBN:** *Studies indicate that language barriers are associated with longer visit time per clinic visit, less frequent clinic visits, less understanding of physician's explanation, more laboratory tests, more emergency department visits, less follow-up care, and less satisfaction with health services (Yeo, 2004).*
- Take extreme care when using touch. **EBN:** *Touch is largely culturally defined (Leninger & McFarland, 2002). Touch is believed by some cultures to be a source of illness. Touching a baby's head requires parental permission in some Southeast Asian cultures. Many*

C

*Latinos believe that excessive admiration of a child without touching will result in physical illness of the child (*mal de ojo*—"evil eye"). In some Islamic and Latino cultures, physical touch between a nurse and client is acceptable only if the individuals are of the same sex (Kelley, 1998). Some Asian cultures believe that touching the head is a sign of disrespect (Galanti, 1997).*

- Modify and tailor the communication approach in keeping with the client's particular culture. **EBN:** *Modification of communication will convey respect to the client and may increase patient's satisfaction with care (Purnell, 2000; Taylor & Lurie, 2004). Culturally tailored communication interventions were positively viewed by African-American women (Kreuter et al, 2004).*
- Use an interpreter if the client speaks a different language. **EB:** *An experienced interpreter will allow for accurate translation and is cost effective (Jacobs, Shepard, Suaya, & Stone, 2004).*
- Use therapeutic communication techniques that emphasize acceptance, offer the self, validate the client's concerns, and convey respect. **EBN:** *Validation is a therapeutic communication technique that lets the client know that the nurse has heard and understood what was said, and it promotes the nurse-client relationship (Heineken, 1998). Studies show that, even when language is not a barrier, some ethnic clients may be reluctant to discuss their beliefs and practices because of fear of criticism or ridicule (Evans & Cunningham, 1996).*
- Use reminiscence therapy as a language intervention. **EBN:** *Reminiscence therapy is well-suited as a language intervention for older adults from culturally and linguistically diverse backgrounds (Harris, 1997).*
- Use of the Office of Minority Health (OMH) of the US Department of Health and Human Services (DHHS) standards on culturally and linguistically appropriate services (CLAS) in health care should be used as needed. **EB:** *The recommended standards cover three broad areas of competence requirements for health care for racial or ethnic minorities: (1) culturally competent care, (2) language access services, and (3) organizational support for cultural competence.*

## Home Care

- The interventions described previously may be used in home care.
- Refer to the care plan **Impaired verbal Communication.**

## evolve WEBSITES

See the EVOLVE website for World Wide Web resources for client education.

## REFERENCES

Banthia R, Malcarne VL, Varni JW et al: The effects of dyadic strength and coping styles on psychological distress in couples faced with prostate cancer, *J Behav Med* 26(1):31-52, 2003.

Bush E: The use of human touch to improve the well-being of older adults: a holistic nursing intervention, *J Holist Nurs* 19(3): 256-270, 2001.

Butts JB: Outcomes of comfort touch in institutionalized elderly female residents, *Geriatr Nurs* 22(4):180-184, 2001.

Campinha-Bacote J: *A model of practice to address cultural competence in rehabilitation nursing*, Continuing Education, Association of Rehabilitation Nurses, 1998. Available at http://www.rehabnurse.org/ce/010201/010201_a.htm, accessed on February 12, 2003.

Cochran M: Tears have no color, *Am J Nurs* 98(6):53, 1998.

Daugherty J, Saarmann L, Riegel B et al: Can we talk? Developing a social support nursing intervention for couples, *Clin Nurse Spec* 16(4):211-218, 2002.

Davis TC, Williams MV, Marin E et al: Health literacy and cancer communication, *CA Cancer J Clin* 52(3):130-149, 2002.

Dean A: Talking to dying clients of their hopes and needs, *Nurs Times* 98(43):34-35, 2002.

Doswell WM, Erlen JA: Multicultural issues and ethical concerns in the delivery of nursing care interventions, *Nurs Clin North Am* 33(2):353-361, 1998.

Erber NP: Hearing, vision, communication, and older people, *Semin Hearing* 23(1):35-42, 2002.

Evans CA, Cunningham BA: Caring for the ethnic elder, *Geriatr Nurs* 17(3):105-110, 1996.

Forchuk C, Westwell J, Martin M et al: The developing nurse-client relationship: nurses' perspectives, *J Am Psychiatr Nurses Assoc* 6(1):3-10, 2000.

Galanti G: *Caring for patients from different cultures: case studies from American hospitals,* ed 2, Philadelphia, 1997, University of Pennsylvania Press.

Greenhill L, Betts T, Pickard N: The epilepsy nurse specialist—expendable handmaiden or essential colleague? *Seizure* 11(suppl A):615-620, 2002.

Gotell E, Brown S, Ekman SL: Caregiver singing and background music in dementia car, *West J Nurs Res* 24(2):195-216, 2002.

Heineken J: Patient silence is not necessarily client satisfaction: communication in home care nursing, *Home Healthc Nurse* 16(2):115-121, 1998.

Jacobs EA, Shepard DS, Suaya JA et al: Overcoming language barriers in health care: costs and benefits of interpreter services, *Am Pub Health* 94(5):866-869, 2004.

Jenkins K, Bennett L, Lancaster L et al: Improving the nurse-patient relationship: a multi-faceted approach, *EDTNA ERCA J* 28(3):145-150, 2002.

Johnson M: Focus. Communication in healthcare: a review of some key issues, *NT Res* 4(1):18, 1999.

Kelley J: Cultural and ethnic considerations. In Frisch NC, Frisch LE, editors: *Psychiatric mental health nursing,* Albany, NY, 1998, Delmar.

Kerzman B, Smith P: Lessons from special education: enhancing communication between health professionals and children with learning difficulties, *Nurse Educ Pract* 4(4): 230-25, 2004.

Kreuter MW, Skinner CS, Steger-May K et al: Responses to behaviorally vs culturally tailored cancer communication among African American women, *Am J Health Behav* 28(3):195-207, 2004.

Krout RE: Music therapy with imminently dying hospice patients and their families: facilitating release near the time of death, *Am J Hosp Palliat Care* 20(2):129-134, 2003.

Leininger MM, McFarland MR: *Transcultural nursing: concepts, theories, research and practices,* ed 3, New York, 2002, McGraw-Hill.

Maltby HJ: Interpreters: a double-edged sword in nursing practice, *J Transcult Nurs* 10(3):248-254, 1999.

Purnell L: A description of the Purnell Model for Cultural Competence, *J Transcult Nurs* 11(1):40-46, 2000.

Seideman RY, Jacobson S, Primeaux M et al: Assessing American Indian families, *MCN Am J Matern Child Nurs* 21(6):274-279, 1996.

Shaw-Taylor Y: Culturally and linguistically appropriate health care for racial or ethnic minorities: analysis of the U.S. Office of Minority Health's recommended standards, *Health Policy* 62(2):211-221, 2002.

Stokes SA, Gordon SE: Common stressors experienced by the well elderly. Clinical implications, *J Gerontol Nurs* 29(5):38-46, 2003.

Sundin K, Jansson L, Norberg A: Understanding between care providers and patients with stroke and aphasia: a phenomenological hermeneutic inquiry, *Nurs Inq* 9(2):93-103, 2002.

Taylor SL, Lurie N: The role of culturally competent communication in reducing ethnic and racial healthcare disparities, *Am J Managed Care* 10(Spec No):SP1-4, 2004.

Tsai JL, Simeonova DI, Watanabe JT: Somatic and social: Chinese Americans talk about emotion, *Pers Soc Psychol Bull* 30(9): 1226-1238, 2004.

Wang JJ: The comparative effectiveness among institutionalized and non-institutionalized elderly people in Taiwan of reminiscence therapy as a psychological measure, *J Nurs Res* 12(3):237-245, 2004.

Yeo S: Language barriers and access to care, *Annu Rev Nurs Res* 22:59-73, 2004.

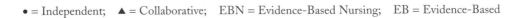

# Impaired verbal Communication

evolve

*Gail B. Ladwig*

C

**NANDA**

## Definition

Decreased, delayed, or absent ability to receive, process, transmit, and use a system of symbols

## Defining Characteristics

Willful refusal to speak; disorientation in the three spheres of time, space, and person; inability to speak dominant language; does not or cannot speak; speaks or verbalizes with difficulty; inappropriate verbalizations; difficulty forming words or sentences (e.g., aphonia, dyslalia, dysarthria); difficulty expressing thoughts verbally (e.g., aphasia, dysphasia, apraxia, dyslexia); stuttering; slurring; dyspnea; absence of eye contact or difficulty in selectively attending; difficulty in comprehending and maintaining usual communication pattern; partial or total visual deficit; inability to use or difficulty in using facial or body expressions

## Related Factors (r/t)

Decrease in circulation to brain; cultural differences; psychological barriers (e.g., psychosis, lack of stimuli); physical barrier (e.g., tracheostomy, intubation); anatomical defect (e.g., cleft palate; alteration of neuromuscular visual system, auditory system, phonatory apparatus); brain tumor; differences related to developmental age; side effects of medication; environmental barriers; absence of significant others; altered perceptions; lack of information; stress; alteration of self-esteem or self-concept; physiological conditions; alteration of central nervous system; weakening of musculoskeletal system; emotional conditions

**NOC**

## Outcomes (Nursing Outcomes Classification)

### Suggested NOC Outcomes

Communication; Communication: Expressive, Receptive

**Example NOC Outcome with Indicators**

**Communication** as evidenced by the following indicators: Use of spoken language/Use of written language/Acknowledgment of messages received/Exchanges messages accurately with others (Rate each indicator of **Communication:** 1 = Severely compromised, 2 = substantially compromised, 3 = moderately compromised, 4 = mildly compromised, 5 = not compromised [see Section I].)

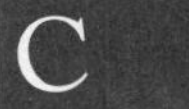

## Client Outcomes

**Client Will (Specify Time Frame):**

- Use effective communication techniques
- Use alternative methods of communication effectively
- Demonstrate congruency of verbal and nonverbal behavior
- Demonstrate understanding even if not able to speak
- Express desire for social interactions

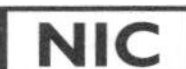

## Interventions (Nursing Interventions Classification)

### Suggested NIC Interventions

Active Listening; Communication Enhancement: Hearing Deficit; Communication Enhancement: Speech Deficit

**Example NIC Activities—Communication Enhancement: Hearing Deficit**

Listen attentively; validate understanding of messages by asking client to repeat what was said

## Nursing Interventions and Rationales

▲ When the client is having difficulty communicating, assess and refer for consultation for hearing problems. Suspect hearing loss when:
  - Client frequently complains that people mumble, speech is not clear, or they hear only parts of conversations when people are talking.
  - Client often asks people to repeat what they said.
  - Client's friends or relatives tell them that they don't seem to hear very well.
  - Client does not laugh at jokes because they miss too much of the story.
  - Client needs to ask others about the details of a meeting that they just attended.
  - Others say that the client plays the television or radio too loudly.
  - Client cannot hear the doorbell or the telephone.
  - Client finds that looking at people when they talk to them makes it somewhat easier to understand, especially when they're in a noisy place or where there are competing conversations.

  *People with hearing disorders do not hear sounds clearly. Such disorders may range from hearing speech sounds faintly or in a distorted way to profound deafness (American Speech-Language-Hearing Association, 2004).*

• Involve a familiar person when attempting to communicate with a person who has difficulty with communication **EB:** *Conversation partners of individuals with aphasia, including health care professionals, families, and others, play a role that is as important for communication for individuals with aphasia (Roth, 2004).*

▲ Identify the language spoken; obtain a language dictionary or interpreter if possible

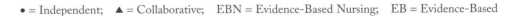

• = Independent; ▲ = Collaborative; EBN = Evidence-Based Nursing; EB = Evidence-Based

C

and accepted by the client. **EB:** *Language barriers can negatively affect health outcomes, patient satisfaction, efficient use of resources and quality of care. Professional interpreters are not only better able to communicate medical terms but also to help reduce the ever-present risk of breaching patient privacy and confidentiality. Study after study shows that optimal communication enhances patient satisfaction, improves outcomes and provides greater patient safety (Greenbaum & Flores, 2004).*

- Listen carefully. Validate verbal and nonverbal expressions particularly when dealing with pain. **EBN:** *In a study of caring behavior involving 200 nurse practitioners, listening was identified as one of the top ten caring behaviors (Brunton & Beaman, 2000).* **EBN:** *Nonverbal indicators of pain observed by nurses in this study of clients with intellectual disabilities (moaning during manipulation, crying during manipulation, painful facial expression during manipulation, swelling, screaming during manipulation, not using (affected) body part, and moving the body in a specific way of behaving) (Zwakhalen et al, 2004).*
- Spend time communicating with the client. **EBN:** *In a qualitative study, psychological well-being was found to be enhanced by humanistic and personal interaction with the nurse (Richardson, 2002).*
- Use simple communication; speak in a well-modulated voice, smile, and show concern for the client. **EBN:** *This research revealed that affective questions and tentative speech, together with continuers, facilitated active participation by patients (Kettunen, 2003).*
- Maintain eye contact at the client's level. **EBN:** *Good communication involves many familiar concepts, including good eye contact (Summers, 2002).*
- When working with the hearing impaired, remove masks and reduce background noise whenever possible. **EB:** *One study of hearing-impaired children receiving dental care indicated that removing masks while talking, reducing background noise, and learning to use simple signs may improve communication with these children (Champion and Holt, 2000).*
- Use touch as appropriate. **EBN:** *Physical touch is integral to nursing practice (Gleeson & Timmins, 2004).* **EBN:** *Physical touch in caring has physical, emotional, social, and spiritual significance and needs to be treated in a holistic way. It is possible to enrich the meanings and methods of physical touch in nursing so that its application may produce positive impacts on clients' well-being and comfort (Chang, 2001).*
- Use presence. Spend time with the client, allow time for responses, and make the call light readily available. **EBN:** *Attentive presence makes explicit that the other is cherished; it is a universal lived experience that is important to health and quality of life(Carroll, 2002).* **EBN:** *This study of perioperative clients indicated time with the nurse was experienced by them as having a positive effect on the healing process and recovery (Rudolfsson, et al, 2003).*
- Explain all health care procedures. *The nurse cannot assume that a person will not understand, even if that person is nonverbal. A person's receptive language skills may be better than his or her expressive language skills (Hahn, 1999).*
- Obtain communication equipment such as electronic devices, letter boards, picture boards, and magic slates. **EBN:** *A study demonstrated that communication technology enables humanness (Dickerson et al, 2002).*
- Consider electronic voice output communication aids for intubated clients. **EBN:** *This study showed that use of VOCAs is possible with selected critically ill adults and may con-*

*tribute to greater ease of communication during respiratory tract intubation particularly with family members. (Happ et al, 2004).*

- Establish an alternative method of communication such as writing or pointing to letters, word phrases, picture cards, or simple drawings of basic needs. **EB:** *Alternative methods of communication are necessary when the client is unable to use verbal communication. A booklet of drawings (visual language) representing the most common needs was used with a group of 34 clients affected by severe dysarthria or motor aphasia causing severe language disorders. Most of these clients used this booklet to express their basic needs (Marquez-Rebollo & Tornel-Costa, 1997).*
- Consider use of an intelligent keyboard to facilitate communication for clients unable to express themselves verbally **EBN:** *A new 'intelligent' keyboard, which was developed as an aid for people with a handicap, was evaluated by ventilated patients in this center and compared with the letter board. Patients and nurses considered the keyboard to be significantly better than the traditional letter board (van den Boogaard & van Grunsven, 2004).*
- Consultation with a speech therapist may be helpful. Supplement the work of the speech therapist with appropriate exercises. **EB:** *Consultation and collaboration with a specialist may be necessary to provide the best approach to improving communication. The main conclusion of one review is that speech and language therapy for people with aphasia after a stroke has not been shown to be either clearly effective or clearly ineffective in a randomized controlled trial (Greener, Enderby, & Whurr, 2000).*
- Encourage the family to bring in familiar pictures or calendars.
- Establish an understanding of the client's symbolic speech, especially with schizophrenic clients. Ask the client to clarify particular statements. *Clarification is a necessary communication skill. Psychoeducation covers the practical problems of living with schizophrenia. Families learn when to ignore problem behaviors and when to intervene (Huddleston, 1992).*
- If a comprehension deficit is present, keep the environment quiet when communicating and get the client's attention before attempting to communicate (e.g., touch the client's shoulder, call the client's name). **EB:** *Conditions that are tolerable for normally hearing adults in casual conversation can be difficult for adults and children in learning situations, and intolerable for persons with deficits of hearing, language, attention, or processing. Sound-field amplification can improve the speech audibility index for all listeners in a noisy room (Boothroyd, 2004).*
- Do not raise your voice or shout at the client. *A loud voice can be frightening and decrease communication.*

## Pediatric

- Observe behavioral communication cues in infants **EBN:** *Infant pain is encoded into observable manifestations through which an infant communicates behavioral and physiological changes such as altered vital signs, characteristic cries, and facial expressions (Byers & Thornley, 2004).*
- Identify and define variations of communication that may be used by children with significant disabilities. Teach at least two new forms of socially acceptable communication alternatives to teach as repairs when communication breaks down. Example:

C

Teach use of one-word requests or teach the child to point, reinforce appropriate responses. **EB:** *Young children with significant disability often have limited communicative repertoires. The means they have available to communicate with others might include natural gesturing, vocalizing, and occasionally challenging behavior. These forms frequently are unconventional, ambiguous, and idiosyncratic and are therefore difficult for partners to understand. As a result of these compromised repertoires, communication breakdowns are the rule rather than the exception and the children's capacity to repair these breakdowns becomes critical (Halle, Brady, & Drasgow, 2004).*

- • Teach children with severe disabilities functional communication skills related to requesting and rejecting. **EB:** *In this study it was demonstrated that children with severe disabilities can be taught new forms of communicative rejecting to replace prelinguistic behaviors associated with escape or avoidance (Sigafoos et al, 2004).*
- ▲ Refer children with primary speech and language delay/disorder for speech and language therapy interventions. **EBN:** *This review shows that overall there is a positive effect of speech and language therapy interventions for children with expressive phonological and expressive vocabulary difficulties (Law, Garrett, & Nye, 2003).*

## Geriatric

- • Carefully assess all clients for hearing difficulty using an audiometer. **EB:** *The prevalence of hearing impairment in hospitalized elderly clients was found to be very high during screening with an audiometer (Lim & Yap, 2000).* **EB:** *One study demonstrated that decreases in speech understanding in noise and declines in central auditory processing are common in the growing population of older women (Garstecki & Erler, 2001).*
- • Avoid use of "elderspeak." **EBN:** *Care providers unknowingly may communicate messages of dependence, incompetence, and control to older adults by using elderspeak, a speech style similar to baby talk that fails to communicate appropriate respect. Therapeutic communication is a critical tool for nurses who provide health care to the growing population of older adults (Williams, Kember, & Hummert, 2004).*
- • Initiate communication with the client with dementia. **EBN:** *In a qualitative study, participants were more often responders than initiators in social interactions (Fitzgerald, 2001).*
- • Encourage the client to wear hearing aids. **EB:** *In this 5-year longitudinal study of adults mean age 68, 24% had a moderate-to-severe hearing loss, and 28% had a mild hearing loss. Severity is associated with reduced quality of life in older adults. Identifying individuals with hearing loss and supplying appropriate hearing aids or other listening devices and teaching coping strategies may have a positive effect on quality of life for older people (Dalton et al, 2003).* **EB:** *Clients with dementia in this study were screened for hearing impairment and fitted with hearing aids. Disability from hearing impairment was reduced (Allen et al, 2003).*
- • When communicating with a client, face toward his or her unaffected side or better ear. *Correct positioning increases the client's awareness of the interaction and enhances the client's ability to interact.*
- • Provide sufficient light and remove distractions such as glare and background noise. *Background noise further impairs the elderly client's hearing.*
- • Use low voice tones and recognize that perception of the sounds f, s, th, ch, sh, b, t, p,

k, and d is impaired with age-related hearing loss. *Presbycusis decreases the ability to hear high-pitched sounds and the consonant sounds listed earlier. Perception of consonants is important to understanding language.*

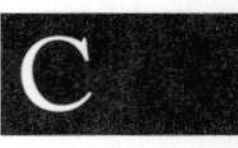



- Facilitate communication and reminiscing with remembering boxes that contain objects, photographs, and writings that have meaning for the client. **EB:** *These communication tools helped staff learn more about clients and enhanced interactions with staff and client's families (Hagens et al, 2003).*
- Use touch as culturally appropriate. **EBN:** *A number of studies suggest that the appropriate use of touch by nurses can be useful for improving comfort and communication in terminally ill older adults and their loved ones (Bush, 2001).*

## Multicultural

- Nurses should become more sensitive to the meaning of a culture's nonverbal communication modes, such as eye contact, facial expression, touching, and body language. Nurses should realize that their good intentions and their usual nonverbal communication style may sometimes be interpreted as offensive and insulting by a specific cultural group. **EBN:** *To give a client a positive signal during a therapy session, a nurse may display the American sign of thumbs up. In Iran, however, thumbs extended upward are considered a vulgar gesture (Campinha-Bacote, 1998).*
- Assess for the influence of cultural beliefs, norms, and values on the client's communication process. **EBN:** *What the client considers normal and abnormal communication may be based on cultural perceptions (Leininger & McFarland, 2002; Johnson, 1999; Cochran, 1998; Doswell & Erlen, 1998). An affirmative answer does not necessarily mean "yes"; a client may be showing respect to the caregiver or avoiding the embarrassment of saying "no" (Galanti, 1997).*
- Assess personal space needs, acceptable communication styles, acceptable body language, interpretation of eye contact, perception of touch, and use of paraverbal modes when communicating with the client. **EBN:** *Nurses need to consider multiple factors when interpreting verbal and nonverbal messages (Purnell, 2000). Native Americans may consider avoiding direct eye contact to be a sign of respect and asking questions to be rude and intrusive (Seiderman et al, 1996). Empirical findings suggest that Chinese Americans and European Americans differ in the ways that they describe emotional experience, with Chinese Americans using more somatic and social words than Americans (Tsai, Simeonova, & Watanabe, 2004).*
- Assess for how language barriers contribute to health disparities among ethnic and racial minorities. **EBN:** *Studies indicate that language barriers are associated with longer visit time per clinic visit, less frequent clinic visits, less understanding of physician's explanation, more laboratory tests, more emergency department visits, less follow-up, and less satisfaction with health services (Yeo, 2004).*
- Take extreme care when using touch. **EBN:** *Touch is largely culturally defined (Leininger & McFarland, 2002). Touch is believed by some cultures to be a source of illness. Touching a baby's head requires parental permission in some Southeast Asian cultures. Many Latinos believe that excessive admiration of a child without touching will result in physical illness of the child (*mal de ojo*—"evil eye"). In some Islamic and Latino cultures, physical touch between a nurse and client is acceptable only if the individuals are of the same sex (Kelley,*

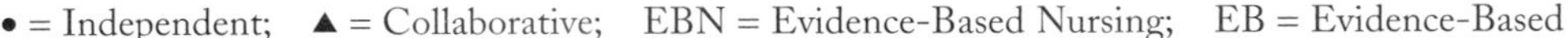

C

*1998). Some Asian cultures believe that touching the head is a sign of disrespect (Galanti, 1997).*

- Modify and tailor the communication approach in keeping with the client's particular culture. **EBN:** *Modification of communication will convey respect to the client and may increase patient's satisfaction with care (Purnell, 2000; Taylor & Lurie, 2004). Culturally tailored communication interventions were positively viewed by African-American women (Kreuter et al, 2004).*
- Use an interpreter if the client speaks a different language. **EB:** *An experienced interpreter will allow for accurate translation and is cost effective (Jacobs et al, 2004).*
- Use therapeutic communication techniques that emphasize acceptance, offer the self, validate the client's concerns, and convey respect. **EBN:** *Validation is a therapeutic communication technique that lets the client know that the nurse has heard and understood what was said, and it promotes the nurse-client relationship (Heineken, 1998). Studies show that, even when language is not a barrier, some ethnic clients may be reluctant to discuss their beliefs and practices because of fear of criticism or ridicule (Evans & Cunningham, 1996).*
- Use reminiscence therapy as a language intervention. **EBN:** *Reminiscence therapy is well-suited as a language intervention for older adults from culturally and linguistically diverse backgrounds (Harris, 1997).*
- Use of the Office of Minority Health (OMH) of the US Department of Health and Human Services (DHHS) standards on culturally and linguistically appropriate services (CLAS) in health care should be used as needed. **EB:** *The recommended standards cover three broad areas of competence requirements for health care for racial or ethnic minorities: (1) culturally competent care, (2) language access services, and (3) organizational support for cultural competence.*

## Home Care

- • The interventions described previously may be adapted for home care use.
- ▲ Begin discharge planning as soon as possible with the case manager or social worker to assess the need for home support systems, assistive devices, and community or home health services.
- ▲ Continue with speech therapy services per the physician's order. Support the speech therapy plan of care. *With appropriate support, clients can continue to make significant progress toward resuming normal or improved communication function.*
- ▲ Assess the cause of communication difficulty and the psychological response to communication difficulty. Refer for mental health assessment as indicated. **EB:** *Seemingly willful refusal to speak may indicate a psychiatric disorder or a medication reaction (e.g., severe dystonia). Major depression has been diagnosed in an average of 20% of post-stroke clients (Tateno, Kimura, & Robinson, 2002). Impaired communication as a result of stroke may increase depressed mood.*
- ▲ Use an understanding of the client's specific physiological changes to implement actions that will assist client communication, provide support, and decrease stress. *Inability to express oneself and be understood by others is frustrating and stressful. Acknowledging the experience for the client can be helpful. The specific pathophysiological cause can*

*indicate appropriate expectations of the client; for example, an expressive aphasic condition will interfere with coherent speech but does not mean that the client does not understand what is said to him or her. It is inappropriate to assume that the client has lost global communication functions.*



- ▲ Assess the family for possible role changes resulting from communication impairment of a family member. *An impairment that prevents a family member from fulfilling the usual role can change the family constellation.*
- ▲ When possible, encourage the family to include the client in family activities using enhanced communication techniques with sensitivity. *Involving the client in family activities promotes earlier return to normal life patterns, but doing so in an awkward or embarrassing way can diminish interest.*
- ▲ Refer to medical social services as necessary for help in obtaining funds for communication devices and counseling for dealing with the long-term effect of the communication changes in the family.
- ▲ Institute case management of the frail elderly to support continued independent living. *Difficulties with communication can lead to increasing needs for assistance in using the health care system effectively. Case management combines the nursing activities of client and family assessment, planning and coordination of care among all health care providers, delivery of direct nursing care, and monitoring of care and outcomes. These activities can address continuity of care, mutual goal setting, behavior management, and prevention of worsening health problems (Guttman, 1999).*
- ▲ Refer for psychiatric home health care services for client reassurance and implementation of a therapeutic regimen. **EBN:** *Psychiatric home care nurses can address issues relating to the client's ability to adjust to communication difficulties. Behavioral interventions in the home can assist the client in participating more effectively in the treatment plan (Patusky, Rodning, & Martinez-Kratz, 1996).*

## Client/Family Teaching

- • Teach the client and family techniques to increase communication. *Alternative methods of communication are necessary when the client is unable to use verbal communication.*
- • Encourage significant others to use touch, such as holding the client's hand or stroking the arm. **EBN:** *Touch can be useful for improving comfort and communication among terminally ill older adults and their loved ones (Bush, 2001).*
- • Teach the client how to use communication devices.
- ▲ Refer the client to a speech-language pathologist or audiologist. *The purpose of audiological assessment is to quantify and qualify hearing in terms of the degree of hearing loss, the type of hearing loss and the configuration of the hearing loss. Once a particular hearing loss has been identified, a treatment and management plan is put into place (American Speech Language-Hearing Association, 2004).*
- ▲ Refer to a specialist for possible surgical intervention when clients have surgical defects caused by cancer of the maxillary sinus and alveolar ridge. **EB:** *Obturators have been developed for surgical defects caused by cancer of the maxillary sinus and alveolar ridge. In a study of 32 consecutively treated maxillectomy clients with the obturator inserted, mean speech intelligibility was 94%, speaking rate was 164 words/min, and nasality was rated as*

*1.6. Clients' mean self-perceived communication effectiveness was 75% of what it was before the diagnosis of cancer (Sullivan et al, 2002).*

C

evolve **WEBSITES FOR EDUCATION**

See the EVOLVE Website for World Wide Web resources for client education.

## REFERENCES

American Speech-Language-Hearing Association: *How do I know if I have a hearing loss*? Available at www.asha.org/public/hearing/disorders/how_know.htm, accessed on August 9, 2004.

American Speech-Language-Hearing Association: *Hearing assessment.* Available at www.asha.org/public/hearing/testing/assess.htm, accessed on August 9, 2004.

Allen NH, Burns A, Newton V et al: The effects of improving hearing in dementia, *Age Ageing,* 32(2):189-193, 2003.

Boothroyd A: Room acoustics and speech perception, *Seminars in Hearing* 25(2):155-166, 2004.

Brunton B, Beaman M: Nurse practitioners' perceptions of their caring behaviors, *J Am Acad Nurse Pract* 11:451, 2000.

Bush E: The use of human touch to improve the well-being of older adults: a holistic nursing intervention, *J Holist Nurs* 19(3):256, 2001.

Byers JF, Thornley K: Cueing into infant pain, *MCN Am J Matern Child Nurs* 29(2):84-91, 2004.

Campinha-Bacote J: *A model of practice to address cultural competence in rehabilitation nursing,* Continuing Education, Association of Rehabilitation Nurses, 1998. Available at www.rehabnurse.org/ce/010201/010201_a.htm, accessed on February 12, 2003.

Carroll KA: Attentive presence: a lived experience of human becoming. Loyola University of Chicago doctoral dissertation (136 p). UMI Order #AAI3056410, 2002.

Champion J, Holt R: Dental care for children and young people who have a hearing impairment, *Br Dent J* 189(3):155, 2000.

Chang SO: The conceptual structure of physical touch in caring, *J Adv Nurs* 33(6):820, 2001.

Cochran M: Tears have no color, *Am J Nurs* 98(6):53, 1998.

Dalton DS, Cruickshanks KJ, Klein BE et al: The impact of hearing loss on quality of life in older adults, *Gerontologist* 43(5):661-668, 2003.

Dickerson SS et al: The meaning of communication: experiences with augmentative communication devices, *Rehabil Nurs* 27(6):215, 2002.

Doswell W, Erlen J: Multicultural issues and ethical concerns in the delivery of nursing care interventions, *Nurs Clin North Am* 33(2):353, 1998.

Evans CA, Cunningham BA: Caring for the ethnic elder, *Geriatr Nurs* 17(3):105, 1996.

Fitzgerald DC: *Descriptive study of the social interactions of older adults diagnosed with dementia*, doctoral dissertation, Washington, DC, The Catholic University of America, 2001.

Galanti G: *Caring for patients from different cultures: case studies from American hospitals,* ed 2, Philadelphia, 1997, University of Pennsylvania Press.

Garstecki D, Erler SF: Personal and social conditions potentially influencing women's hearing loss management, *Am J Audiol* 10(2):78, 2001.

Gleeson M, Timmins F: Touch: a fundamental aspect of communication with older people experiencing dementia, *Nurs Older People* 16(2):18-21, 2004.

Greenbaum M, Flores G: Lost in translation. Professional interpreters needed to help hospitals treat immigrant patients, *Mod Healthc* 34(18):21, 2004.

Greener J, Enderby P, Whurr R: Speech and language therapy for aphasia following stroke, *Cochrane Database Syst Rev* (2):CD000425, 2000.

Guttman R: Case management of the frail elderly in the community, *Clin Nurs Spec* 13(4):174, 1999.

Hahn J: Cueing in to patient language, *Reflections* 25(1):8, 1999.

Hagens C, Beaman A, Ryan EB: Reminiscing, poetry writing, and remembering boxes: personhood-centered communication with cognitively impaired older adults, *Activ Adapt Aging*; 27(3/4):97-112, 2003.

Halle J, Brady NC, Drasgow E: Enhancing socially adaptive communicative repairs of beginning communicators with disabilities, *Am J Speech Lang Pathol* 13(1):43-54, 2004.

Happ MB, Roesch TK, Garrett K: Electronic voice-output communication aids for temporarily nonspeaking patients in a medical intensive care unit: a feasibility study, *Heart Lung* 33(2):92-101, 2004.

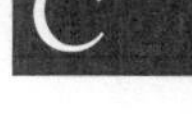

Huddleston J: Family and group psychoeducational approaches in the management of schizophrenia, *Clin Nurs Spec* 6:118, 1992.
Jacobs EA, Shepard DS, Suaya JA et al: Overcoming language barriers in health care: costs and benefits of interpreter services, *Am J Public Health* 94(5):866-869, 2004.
Johnson M: Focus. Communication in healthcare: a review of some key issues, *NT Res* 4(1):18, 1999.
Kelley J: Cultural and ethnic considerations. In Frisch NC, Frisch LE, editors: *Psychiatric mental health nursing,* Albany, NY, 1998, Delmar.
Kettunen T, Poskiparta M, Karhila P: Speech practices that facilitate patient participation in health counseling—a way to empowerment? *Health Educ J* 62(4):326-340, 2003.
Kreuter MW, Skinner CS, Steger-May K et al: Responses to behaviorally vs. culturally tailored cancer communication among African American women, *Am J Health Behav* 28(3):195-207, 2004.
Law J, Garrett Z, Nye C: Speech and language therapy interventions for children with primary speech and language delay or disorder, *Cochrane Database Syst Rev* (3):CD004110, 2003.
Leininger MM, McFarland MR: *Transcultural nursing: concepts, theories, research and practices,* ed 3, New York, McGraw-Hill, 2002.
Lim JK, Yap KB: Screening for hearing impairment in hospitalized elderly, *Ann Acad Med Singap* 29(2):237, 2000.
Marquez-Rebollo MC, Tornel-Costa MC: Design of a non-verbal method of communication using cartoons, *Rev Neurol* 25(148): 2045, 1997.
Patusky KL, Rodning C, Martinez-Kratz M: Clinical lessons in psychiatric home care: a case study approach, *J Home Health Case Manag* 9:18, 1996.
Purnell L: A description of the Purnell model for cultural competence, *J Transcult Nurs* 11(1):40, 2000.
Richardson J: Health promotion in palliative care: the patients' perception of therapeutic interaction with the palliative nurse in the primary care setting, *J Adv Nurs* 40(4):432, 2002.
Roth EJ: Grand rounds. A set of observational measures for rating support and participation in conversation between adults with aphasia and their conversation partners, *Top Stroke Rehabil* 11(1):67-83, 2004.
Rudolfsson G, Hallberg LRM, Ringsberg KC et al: The nurse has time for me: the perioperative dialogue from the perspective of patients, *J Adv Perioperative Care* 1(3):77-84, 2003.
Seiderman RY et al: Assessing American Indian families, *MCN Am J Matern Child Nurs* 21(6):274, 1996.
Sigafoos J, Drasgow E, Reichle J et al: Tutorial: teaching communicative rejecting to children with severe disabilities, *Am J Speech Lang Pathol* 13(1):31-42, 2004.
Stokes SA, Gordon SE: Common stressors experienced by the well elderly. Clinical implications, *J Gerontol Nurs* 29(5):38-46, 2003.
Sullivan M, Gaebler C, Beukelman D et al: Impact of palatal prosthodontic intervention on communication performance of patients' maxillectomy defects: a multilevel outcome study, *Head Neck* 24(6):530, 2002.
Summers LC: Mutual timing: an essential component of provider/patient communication, *J Am Acad Nurse Pract* 14(1):19, 2002.
Tateno A, Kimura M, Robinson RG: Phenomenological characteristics of poststroke depression. Early- versus late-onset, *Am J Geriatr Psychiatry* 10:575, 2002.
Taylor SL, Lurie N: The role of culturally competent communication in reducing ethnic and racial healthcare disparities, *Am J Manag Care* 10:SP1-4, 2004.
Tsai JL, Simeonova DI, Watanabe JT: Somatic and social: Chinese Americans talk about emotion, *Pers Soc Psychol Bull* 30(9): 1226-1238, 2004.
van den Boogaard M, van Grunsven A: A new communication aid for mechanically ventilated patients, *Connect: The World of Critical Care Nursing* 3(1):20-23, 2004.
Williams K, Kemper S, Hummert L: Enhancing communication with older adults: overcoming elderspeak, *J Gerontol Nurs* 30(10): 17-25, 2004.
Yeo S: Language barriers and access to care, *Ann Rev Nurs Res* 22:59-73, 2004.
Zwakhalen SMG, van Dongen KAJ, Hamers JPH et al: Pain assessment in intellectually disabled people: non-verbal indicators, *J Adv Nurs* 45(3):236-245, 2004.

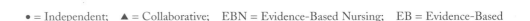

# Decisional Conflict (specify)

*Gail B. Ladwig*

C

**NANDA**

## Definition

Uncertainty about course of action to be taken when choice among competing actions involves risk, loss, or challenge to personal life values

## Defining Characteristics

Verbalization of uncertainty about choices; verbalization of undesired consequences of alternative actions being considered; vacillation between alternative choices; delayed decision making; verbalization of feelings of distress while attempting to make a decision; self-focusing; physical signs of distress or tension (e.g., increased heart rate, increased muscle tension, restlessness); questioning of personal values and beliefs while attempting to make a decision

## Related Factors (r/t)

Support system deficit, perceived threat to value system, lack of experience or interference with decision making, multiple or divergent sources of information, lack of relevant information, unclear personal values/beliefs

**NOC**

## Outcomes (Nursing Outcomes Classification)

### Suggested NOC Outcomes

Decision Making, Information Processing, Participation in Health Care Decisions

**Example NOC Outcome with Indicators**

**Decision Making** as evidenced by the following indicators: Identifies relevant information/Identifies alternatives/Identifies potential consequences of each alternative/Identifies resources necessary to support each alternative (Rate each indicator of **Decision Making:** 1 = severely compromised, 2 = substantially compromised, 3 = moderately compromised, 4 = mildly compromised, 5 = not compromised [see Section I].)

## Client Outcomes

**Client Will (Specify Time Frame):**

- State the advantages and disadvantages of choices
- Share fears and concerns regarding choices and responses of others
- Make an informed choice

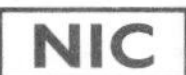

## Interventions (Nursing Interventions Classification)

### Suggested NIC Intervention

Decision-Making Support

C

**Example NIC Activities—Decision-Making Support**

Inform client of alternative views or solutions; facilitate client's articulation of goals for care

## Nursing Interventions and Rationales

- Observe for factors causing or contributing to conflict (e.g., value conflicts, fear of outcome, poor problem-solving skills). **EB:** *This trial demonstrates that, among patients facing a real treatment decision, interventions to inform patients about hypertension and to clarify patients' values concerning outcomes of treatment are effective in reducing decisional conflict and increasing patient knowledge (Montgomery, Fahey, & Peters, 2003).*
- Work with and allow the client to make decisions in a way that is comfortable for the client, such as deferring (allowing others to decide), delaying (choosing an alternative that meets basic requirements), or deliberating (looking at all alternatives). **EB:** *This study of intervention efforts designed to promote repeat HIV test acceptance among low-income, African-American women should focus on changing perceptions of barriers, and enhancing supportive factors to enhance decision making (Bonney, Crosby, & Odenat, 2004).* **EB:** *This study indicates that clients can be more involved in treatment decisions, and risks and benefits of treatment options can be explained in more detail, without adversely affecting patient-based outcomes (Edwards et al, 2004).*
- Give the client time and permission to express feelings associated with decision making. **EB:** *For decisions that are high risk and have more than one choice informed consent and shared decision making are both applicable. The physician should take time to explore the patient's values, concerns, and emotional and social needs; educate the patient and the family about the problem; and outline the available choices (Whitney, McGuire, & McCullough, 2004).*
- Demonstrate reassurance with unconditional respect for and acceptance of the client's values, spiritual beliefs, and cultural norms. **EB:** *This study indicates that trust in the client's physician is important in shared decision making. Supporting client's autonomy is important (Kraetschmer et al, 2004).*

▲ Use decision aids or computer based decision aid to assist clients in making decisions. **EBN:** *Trials indicate that decision aids improve knowledge and realistic expectations, enhance active participation in decision making, lower decisional conflict, decrease the proportion of people remaining undecided, and improve agreement between values and choice (O'Connor, 2003).* **EB:** *In this randomized controlled trial an interactive computer program was more effective than standard genetic counseling for increasing knowledge of breast cancer and genetic testing among women at low risk of carrying a BRCA1 or BRCA2 mutation. These results suggest that this computer program has the potential to stand alone as*

C

*an educational intervention for low-risk women but should be used as a supplement to genetic counseling for those at high risk (Green et al, 2004).*

- ▲ Initiate health teaching and referrals when needed. *Advanced practice nurses as case managers can make a positive contribution toward individualizing care for the elderly (Mick & Ackerman, 2002).*
- ▲ Facilitate communication between the client and family members regarding the final decision; offer support to the person actually making the decision. **EB:** *Formulation of an advance proxy plan is important to ensure that the client's previous wishes or best interests are considered when decisions about treatment strategies are made (Volicer, 2001).*
- ▲ Provide detailed information on benefits and risks using functional terms and probabilities tailored to clinical risk, plus steps for considering the issues and means for making a decision, including values clarification and decision aides, when clients are faced with difficult treatment choices. **EB:** *Informed choices require information that is relevant, valid and accessible (Oxman, 2004).*

### Geriatric

- • Carefully assess clients with dimension regarding ability to make decisions. In evaluating reasoning it may be helpful to take person through the reasoning process. First learn about the social and situational context for the health care decision and then by asking about the consequences of treatment alternatives for those contexts. Check if information is excluded because it was not remembered or because it was not important to individual. **EB:** *Most adults with mild dementia can participate in medical decision making as defined by legal standards. In dementia, assessments of reasoning about treatment options should focus on whether a person can describe salient reasons for a specific choice, whereas assessments of appreciation of the meaning of diagnostic and treatment information should focus on whether a person can describe the implications of various choices for future states (Moye et al, 2004).*
- • If end-of-life discussions are being avoided, describe the possible consequences. **EBN:** *Participants in one study thought that a "do not resuscitate" decision should be discussed with clients and also with relatives if appropriate. However, there was ambivalence about whether individuals would like to be involved personally in such a decision because of the anxiety this would produce (Phillips & Woodward, 1999).*
- ▲ Discuss the purpose of a living will and advance directives. **EBN:** *Elderly clients and their significant others need to know how to legally make end-of-life decisions (Note: Laws differ in each state.) Research has demonstrated that the presence of an advance directive can be very helpful in decreasing family stress when end-of-life decisions need to be made (Tilden et al, 2001).*
- • Discuss choices or changes to be made (e.g., moving in with children, into a nursing home, or into an adult foster care home). *Caregivers need to provide support when the client and family are facing difficult decisions (Hurley & Volicer, 2002).*
- • Teach family members how to be supportive of the final decision or how to refrain from being destructive if they are unable to be supportive. *It is important to support the decisions that the client makes.*

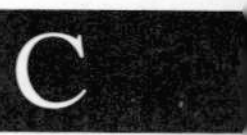


## Multicultural

- Assess for the influence of cultural beliefs, norms, and values on the client's decision-making conflict. **EBN:** *Cultural influences may interfere with the client's decision-making process (Wong & Anderson, 2003; Wright, Leininger, & McFarland, 2002; Doswell & Erlen, 1998; Cochran, 1998; Cohen & Caroselli, 1997). Individuals of Chinese and Korean descent, as well as individuals of the Muslim religion, may accept the health provider's decision regarding medical needs rather than assert their own wishes (Valle, 2001; Moazam, 2000). African-American women may use fatalistic and destiny beliefs to guide their health decisions (Green et al, 2004).*
- Identify who will be involved in the decision-making process. **EBN:** *In a group of frail elderly clients, ethnic variations were found with regard to the family member identified as the decision maker (Hornug et al, 1998). Contrary to expectations, Latinas will often make decisions related to prenatal care and services (Browner, Preloran, & Cox, 1999). Korean American clients and other Asian clients may consider some decisions to be a family affair (D'Avanzo et al, 2001; Blackhall et al, 1999). Elders may play a key role in decision making in some Asian populations (Davis, 2001). Some Native-American societies are matriarchal in structure, and the matriarch's approval and support may be required for compliance with a treatment plan (Cesario, 2001). Other studies have shown that the role of family and physicians recommendations were highly valued in the decision-making process by Hispanic women (Ellington et al, 2003).*
- Use cross-cultural decision aids whenever possible to enhance an informed decision making process. **EBN:** *Consumer-based cross-cultural decision aids inform clients of potential risks and benefits so that they can make value- and evidence-integrated decisions (Lawrence et al, 2000). In one study, Latinas' assessment of risk and uncertainty with procedures was associated with decisions to refuse certain procedures (Browner, Preloran, & Cox, 1999). Another study found that African-American women underwent immediate breast reconstruction at significantly lower rates compared with Caucasian, Hispanic, and Asian women. The decision pathways found that African-American women were less likely to be offered referrals for reconstruction, were less likely to accept offered referrals, were less likely to be offered reconstruction, and were less likely to elect reconstruction if it was offered (Tseng et al, 2004).*
- Validate the client's feelings regarding the decisional conflict. **EBN:** *Validation is a therapeutic communication technique that lets the client know that the nurse has heard and understood what was said, and it promotes the nurse-client relationship (Heineken, 1998).*

## Home Care

NOTE: Before addressing decisional conflict, nurses should be aware of their existing biases and preconceptions, and avoid superimposing them on the client's decision-making process. For example, clients making end-of-life decisions must process multiple issues regarding their choices; nurses' discomfort with end-of-life issues could interfere with clients' ability to reflect on choices.

- The interventions described previously may be adapted for home care use.

C

- ▲ Before providing any home care, assess the client plan for advance directives (living will and power of attorney). If a plan exists, place a copy in the client file. If no plan exists, offer information on advance directives according to agency policy. Refer for assistance in completing advance directives as necessary. Do not witness a living will. *This is a legal requirement of the Consolidated Omnibus Budget Reconciliation Act (COBRA).*
- • Determine the relevance of the decisional conflict to the plan of care.
- • Assess the client and family for consensus (or lack thereof) regarding the issue in conflict. When the conflict involves end-of-life decisions, work to shift the client's and family's expectations from curative to palliative. **EBN:** *A study of the means by which providers worked with clients and families at the end of life revealed that the focus was on changing expectations from unrealistic (curative) to realistic (palliative). Helping the client and family accurately understand the client's condition involved the following: laying the groundwork (teaching, planting the seeds); shifting the picture (working together, arranging family meetings, creating new expectations, changing the scope of choice, changing the value of treatment options, changing indicators); and accepting the new picture (involving others, redirecting hope, repeating and reiterating information) (Norton & Bowers, 2001).*
- ▲ If a decision is relevant to the plan of care, the primary nurse or medical social services may evaluate the need for a family conference and call such a conference. If a consensus cannot be reached, continue efforts to resolve the conflict. Clients, unless medically incompetent (by legal guidelines) or under authorized power of attorney, may make their own decisions. *Guided family conferences allow all persons affected by the decision to be heard and the value system of the client to be validated. The nurse or social worker serves as the facilitator and client advocate.*
- • Assist the client and family in initiating problem solving and in identifying options, pros and cons, and consequences of choices. *Situations involving illness may create tunnel vision or a sense of being overwhelmed. Assistance is needed to help the client and family perceive that options do exist and to help them evaluate these options.* Refer to the care plan for **Anxiety** as indicated.
- ▲ If the decision is not relevant to the plan of care, refer to community support services appropriate to the type of decision and client need.

## Client/Family Teaching

- ▲ Instruct the client and family members to provide advance directives in the following areas:
  - Person to contact in an emergency
  - Preference (if any) to die at home or in the hospital
  - Desire to sign a living will
  - Desire to donate an organ
  - Funeral arrangements (i.e., burial, cremation)

  **EB:** *A large discrepancy exists between the wishes of dying patients and their actual end-of-life care. However, retrospective clinical experience suggests that early advance care planning can markedly reduce this discrepancy (Schwartz et al, 2002).*

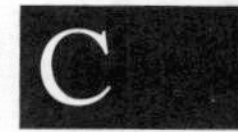


- ▲ Inform the family of treatment options; encourage and defend self-determination. **EBN:** *The Patient Self-Determination Act, effective since December 1991, has changed the importance of introducing life support options to clients (Beland & Froman, 1995).*
- • Identify reasons for family decisions regarding care. Explore ways in which family decisions can be respected. **EBN:** *A high proportion of elders and their caregivers report substantial unmet transitional care needs, with the need for information and increased access to services consistently among the top priorities. Differences in expectations between and among clients, families, and health care providers, and the need for increased client and family involvement in decision making are common themes in discharge planning studies (Naylor, 2002).*
- • Recognize and allow the client to discuss the selection of complementary therapies available, such as spiritual support, relaxation, imagery, exercise, lifestyle changes, diet (e.g., macrobiotic, vegetarian), and nutritional supplementation. **EBN:** *A study of cancer clients found that the clients unanimously believed that complementary therapies helped to improve their quality of life by helping them to cope more effectively with stress, decreasing the discomforts of treatment and illness, and giving them a sense of control (Sparber et al, 2000).* **EB:** *One study demonstrated that the use of complementary/alternative medicine for cancer care is widespread. There is clearly an expressed need for complementary/alternative medical treatments by clients and a willingness to pay for them (Lewith, Broomfield, & Prescott, 2002).*
- ▲ Provide the Physician Orders for Life-Sustaining Treatment (POLST) form for clients and families faced with end-of-life choice across the health care continuum. **EBN:** *This study demonstrated that the POLST form assures end-of-life choices can be implemented in all settings, from the home through the health care continuum. An informed consent process was evidenced in 16 of 21 cases, and the POLST form was congruent with residents' existing advance directives for health care. The findings support the continued use, development, and evaluation of this promising tool for improving end-of-life care (Meyers et al, 2004).*

## evolve WEBSITES FOR EDUCATION

See the EVOLVE Website for World Wide Web resources for client education.

## REFERENCES


Beland K, Froman R: Preliminary validation of a measure of life support preferences, *Image J Nurs Sch* 27:307, 1995.

Blackhall LJ, Frank G, Murphy ST et al: Ethnicity and attitudes towards life sustaining technology, *Soc Sci Med* 48(12):1779-1789, 1999.

Bonney EA, Crosby R, Odenat L: Repeat HIV testing among low-income minority women: a descriptive analysis of factors influencing decisional balance, *Ethn Dis* 14(3):330-335, 2004.

Browner CH, Preloran HM, Cox SJ: Ethnicity, bioethics, and prenatal diagnosis: the amniocentesis decisions of Mexican-origin women and their partners, *Am J Public Health* 89(11):1658-1666, 1999.

Cesario S: Care of the Native American woman: strategies for practice, education, and research, *J Obstet Gynecol Neonatal Nurs* 30(1):13-19, 2001.

C

Cochran M: Tears have no color, *Am J Nurs* 98(6):53, 1998.
D'Avanzo CE et al: Developing culturally informed strategies for substance-related interventions. In Naegle MA, D'Avanzo CE, editors: *Addictions and substance abuse: strategies for advanced practice nursing,* St Louis, 2001, Mosby.
Davis RE: The convergence of health and family in the Vietnamese culture, *J Fam Nurs* 6:136-156, 2000.
Doswell W, Erlen J: Multicultural issues and ethical concerns in the delivery of nursing care interventions, *Nurs Clin North Am* 33(2):353-361, 1998.
Edwards A, Elwyn G, Hood K et al: Patient-based outcome results from a cluster randomized trial of shared decision making skill development and use of risk communication aids in general practice, *Fam Pract* 21(4):347-354, 2004.
Ellington L, Wahab S, Sahami S et al: Decision-making issues for randomized clinical trial participation among Hispanics, *Cancer Control 10*(5 Suppl):84-86, 2003.
Green BL, Lewis RK, Wang MQ et al: Powerlessness, destiny, and control: the influence on health behaviors of African Americans, *J Community Health* 29(1):15-27, 2004.
Green MJ, Peterson SK, Baker MW et al: Effect of a computer-based decision aid on knowledge, perceptions, and intentions about genetic testing for breast cancer susceptibility: a randomized controlled trial, *JAMA* 292(4):442-452, 2004.
Heineken J: Patient silence is not necessarily client satisfaction: communication in home care nursing, *Home Healthc Nurse* 16(2): 115-120, 1998.
Hornung CA, Eleazer GP, Strothers HS 3rd et al: Ethnicity and decision makers in a group of frail elderly, *J Am Geriatr Soc* 46(3): 280-286, 1998.
Hurley AC, Volicer L: Alzheimer disease: "It's okay, Mama, if you want to go, it's okay," *JAMA* 288(18):2324-2331, 2002.
Kraetschmer N, Sharpe N, Urowitz S et al: How does trust affect patient preferences for participation in decision-making? *Health Expect* 7(4):317-326, 2004.
Lawrence VA et al: A cross-cultural consumer based decision aid for screening mammography, *Prev Med* 30(3): 200-208, 2000.
Leininger MM, McFarland MR: *Transcultural nursing: concepts, theories, research and practices,* ed 3, New York, 2002, McGraw-Hill.
Lewith GT, Broomfield J, Prescott P: Complementary cancer care in Southampton: a survey of staff and patients, *Complement Ther Med* 10(2):100-106, 2002.
Mick DJ, Ackerman MH: New perspectives on advanced practice nursing case management for aging patients, *Crit Care Nurs Clin North Am* 14(3):281-291, 2002.
Moazam F: Families, patients, and physicians in medical decision making, *Hastings Cent Rep* 30(6):28-37, 2000.
Montgomery AA, Fahey T, Peters TJ: A factorial randomised controlled trial of decision analysis and an information video plus leaflet for newly diagnosed hypertensive patients, *Br J Gen Pract* 53(491):446-453, 2003.
Moye J, Karel MJ, Azar AR et al: Capacity to consent to treatment: empirical comparison of three instruments in older adults with and without dementia, *Gerontologist* 44(2):166-175, 2004.
Naylor MD: Transitional care of older adults, *Annu Rev Nurs Res* 20:127-147, 2002.
Norton SA, Bowers BJ: Working toward consensus: providers' strategies to shift patients from curative to palliative treatment choices, *Res Nurs Health* 24:258-269, 2001.
O'Connor AM, Stacey D, Entwistle V et al: Decision aids for people facing health treatment or screening decisions, *Cochrane Database Syst Rev* (2):CD001431, 2003.
Oxman AD: You cannot make informed choices without information, *J Rehabil Med* (43 Suppl):5-7, 2004.
Phillips K, Woodward V: The decision to resuscitate: older people's views, *J Clin Nurs* 8(6):753-761, 1999.
Schwartz CE, Wheeler HB, Hammes B et al: Early intervention in planning end-of-life care with ambulatory geriatric patients: results of a pilot trial, *Arch Intern Med* 162(14):1611-1618, 2002.
Sparber A, Bauer L, Curt G et al: Use of complementary medicine by adult patients participating in cancer clinical trials, *Oncol Nurs Forum* 27(4):623-630, 2000.
Tilden VP, Tolle SW, Nelson CA et al: Family decision making to withdraw life-sustaining treatments from hospitalized patients, *Nurs Res* 50(2):105-115, 2001.
Tseng JF, Kronowitz SJ, Sun CC et al: The effect of ethnicity on immediate reconstruction rates after mastectomy for breast cancer, *Cancer 101*(7):1514-1523, 2004.
Valle R: Cultural assessment in bioethical advocacy—toward cultural competency and bioethical practice, *Bioethics Forum* 17(1): 15-26, 2001.
Volicer L: Management of severe Alzheimer's disease and end-of-life issues, *Clin Geriatr Med* 17(2):377-391, 2001.
Whitney SN, McGuire AL, McCullough LB: A typology of shared decision making, informed consent, and simple consent, *Ann Intern Med* 140(1):54-59, 2004.

Wong FW, Anderson SM: Team approach in cross-cultural ethical decision making: a case study, *Prog Transplant* 13(1):38-41, 2003.

Wright F, Cohen S, Caroselli C: Diverse decisions. How culture affects ethical decision-making, *Crit Care Nurs Clin North Am* 9(1):63-74, 1997.

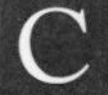


## Parental role Conflict

evolve

*Gail B. Ladwig*

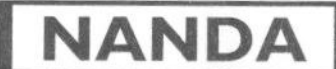


### Definition

Parent's experience of role confusion and conflict in response to crisis

### Defining Characteristics

Expresses concerns about changes in parental role, family functioning, family communication, family health; expresses concerns/feelings of inadequacy with regard to providing for child's physical and emotional needs during hospitalization or at home; reluctant to participate in usual caregiving activities, even with encouragement and support; demonstrates disruption in caretaking routines; expresses concern about perceived loss of control regarding decisions relating to child; verbalizes or demonstrates feelings of guilt, anger, fear, anxiety, and frustration concerning effect of child's illness on family processes

### Related Factors (r/t)

Change in marital status; home care of child with special needs (e.g., apnea monitoring, postural drainage, hyperalimentation); interruptions of family life as a result of home care regimens (e.g., treatments, caregivers, lack of respite); specialized care center policies; separation from child as a result of chronic illness; intimidation by invasive or restrictive modalities (e.g., isolation, intubation)

NOC

### Outcomes (Nursing Outcomes Classification)

#### Suggested NOC Outcomes

Caregiver Adaptation to Patient Institutionalization, Caregiver Home Care Readiness, Caregiver Lifestyle Disruption, Coping, Parenting Performance, Family Coping

#### Example NOC Outcome with Indicators

**Family Coping** as evidenced by the following indicators: Demonstrates role flexibility/Manages family problems/Uses family-centered stress reduction activities (Rate each indicator of **Family Coping:** 1 = never demonstrated, 2 = rarely demonstrated, 3 = sometimes demonstrated, 4 = often demonstrated, 5 = consistently demonstrated [see Section I].)

## Client Outcomes

**Client Will (Specify Time Frame):**

- Express feelings and perceptions regarding impacts of illness, disability, and/or hospitalization on parental role
- Participate in hospital and home care as much as able to given the availability of resources and support systems
- Exhibit assertiveness and responsibility in active family decision making regarding care of the child
- Describe and select available resources to support parental management of the child's and family's needs

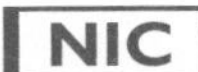

## Interventions (Nursing Interventions Classification)

### Suggested NIC Interventions

Abuse Protection Support: Child, Caregiver Support, Counseling, Crisis Intervention, Decision-Making Support, Environmental Management: Attachment Process, Family Process Maintenance, Family Therapy, Role Enhancement

**Example NIC Activities—Role Enhancement**

Teach new behaviors needed by parent to fulfill a role; serve as role model for learning new behaviors

## Nursing Interventions and Rationales

- Assess and support parents' previous coping behaviors. **EB:** *Chronic illness in children affects the psychological health of the parents. Active coping strategies are associated with fewer distress indices and thus if inculcated may improve the ability to bear the burden of the illness without becoming themselves affected by psychiatric illnesses (Rao, 2004).*
- Explore parent/family sources of stress, usual methods of coping, and perceptions of illness/condition. Capitalize on the strengths identified. **EB:** *This study demonstrated that caregivers of children with disabilities experience stress that should be addressed by therapists to maximize compliance with home programs. As caregiver and family problems increased, noncompliance with home programs increased (Rone-Adams, Stern, & Walker, 2004).*
- Evaluate the family's perceived strength of its social support system. Encourage the family to use social support to increase its resiliency and to moderate stress. **EBN:** *Perceived social support is a factor influencing resiliency and ability to cope with stress (Tak & McCubbin, 2002).* **EBN:** *This study demonstrates that parental support had the strongest direct effect on mothers' quality of life (Sgarbossa & Ford-Gilboe, 2004).*
- Determine the older-than-average mother's support systems and self-expectations for motherhood. **EB:** *Increasing numbers of women have delayed childbearing until after they reach their thirties. The researchers who studied early maternal role attainment in women over 30 failed to reflect on the challenges of raising a child to adulthood. The importance of these challenges was identified in this study (Dobrzykowski & Stern, 2003).*

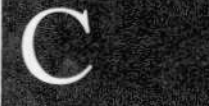

- Consider the use of family theory as a framework to help guide interventions (e.g., family stress theory, role theory, social exchange theory). **EBN:** *This study demonstrated that use of a family assessment tool is an effective way of appraising families and addressing suffering. Formative evaluations demonstrated improvements in team members' perceptions of their knowledge, family centeredness, and ability to assess and intervene with families (Hogan & Logan, 2004).*
- Sustain parental involvement in shared decision making with regard to care by using the following steps:
  - Incorporate parents' information concerning the child's typical routines, behaviors, fears, likes, and dislikes.
  - Provide clear and direct firsthand information concerning the child's condition and progress.
  - Normalize the home/hospital environment as much as possible.
  - Collaborate in care by providing choices when possible.

  **EB:** *For decisions that are high risk and have more than one choice informed consent and shared decision making are both applicable. The physician should take time to explore the patient's values, concerns, and emotional and social needs; educate the patient and the family about the problem; and outline the available choices (Whitney, McGuire, & McCullough, 2004).*
- Seek and support parental participation in care. **EBN:** *The importance of family centred caregiving over 6 years was documented through the Colorado Consortium of Intensive Care Nurseries. Results of surveys described the significance of more open hours for parents and siblings to be with their baby, less punitive and restrictive language, and a move toward viewing parents as participants in their baby's care, rather than as visitors (Brown et al, 2004).*
- Provide support for each parent's primary coping strategies. **EBN:** *Mothers may require additional support in their role in caring for chronically ill children. Mothers exhibit greater efforts than fathers in coping patterns, including strategies to acquire social support outside the family, increase self-worth, and decrease psychological tensions (Brazil & Krueger, 2002).*
- Offer respite care to assist parents in maintaining sufficient energy and personal resources to continue caregiving responsibilities. **EBN:** *A retrospective pilot study was conducted to describe perceived stressors and coping strategies of the primary caregiver of a child with a tracheostomy and gastrostomy. Data revealed that caregivers believed there was disruption of social interactions within and outside the family because of the child's condition. Data indicate a need for developing home care plans that include respite services (Montagnino & Mauricio, 2004).*
- Be available to discuss concerns and be a good listener. **EBN:** *In this study of pediatric oncology, clients supportive care that focuses on informational and emotional support appears to be most important from diagnosis to treatment (Kerr et al, 2004).*
- Encourage the parent to meet his or her own needs for rest, nutrition, and hygiene. Provide facilities so that the parent may stay with the sick child (e.g., cot, reclining chair). *A parent is unable to meet the child's needs when his or her basic self-needs are unmet.*
- Provide family-centered care: Demonstrate safe places where the parent may touch or

C

stroke the child. Encourage the parent to talk or sing to the child. Adjust equipment so that the parent is able to hold the child, and provide a comfortable chair, preferably a rocking chair. Provide opportunities and offer praise for successful care giving. **EBN:** *This study illustrated that the family-centered care model could be successfully implemented in the clinical pediatric unit in a large hospital setting. The children are happier. The families openly and continuously communicate with the nurses, being confident in caring for the children and satisfied with nursing care (Attharos et al, 2004).*

- Refer parents to available telephone counseling services. **EB:** *This study demonstrated that phone interviews are a reliable method of interviewing for use in assessing patients for post-traumatic stress disorder and major depressive disorder (Aziz & Kenford, 2004).*
- Support young grandmothers of teen mothers in areas of mother-daughter conflict such as childrearing decisions, time with friends, household chores, and teens' choices/priorities with appropriate community referrals. **EBN:** *This study indicates that community- and home-based multigenerational parent support interventions for young grandmothers of teen mothers may address some of these grandmothers' concerns (Sadler & Clemmons, 2004).*

## Multicultural

- Acknowledge racial/ethnic differences at the onset of care. **EBN:** *Acknowledgment of race/ethnicity issues will enhance communication, establish rapport, and promote treatment outcomes (D'Avanzo et al, 2001; Ludwick & Siva, 2000).*
- Assess for the influence of cultural beliefs, norms, and values on the client's perceptions of the parental role. **EBN:** *What the client considers a normal or abnormal parental role may be based on cultural perceptions (Leininger & McFarland, 2002; Cochran, 1998; Doswell & Erlen, 1998). Some Mexican-American families may engage in an intergenerational family ritual called La Cuarentena, which lasts for 40 days after birth and involves prescriptions for maternal food, clothing, and paternal role (Niska, Snyder, & Lia-Hoagberg, 1998).*
- Acknowledge that value conflicts arising from acculturation stresses may contribute to increased anxiety and significant conflict with the parental role. **EBN:** *Challenges to traditional beliefs and values are anxiety provoking (Charron, 1998). Less acculturated parents may experience conflict with their more acculturated children as the children demand greater independence and freedom (True, 1995).*
- Promote the female parenting role by providing a treatment environment that is culturally based and woman centered. **EBN:** *Pregnant and postpartum Asian and Pacific Islander women in substance abuse treatment identified provisions for the newborn, infant health care, parent education, and infant-mother bonding as conducive to their treatment (Morelli, Fong, & Oliveria, 2001). African-American mothers of medically fragile infants reported the sights and sounds of the hospital environment as an additional stress (Miles et al, 2002).*
- Validate the client's feelings with regard to parental role confusion and conflict. **EBN:** *Validation is a therapeutic communication technique that lets the client know that the nurse has heard and understood what was said, and it promotes the nurse-client relationship (Heineken, 1998).*

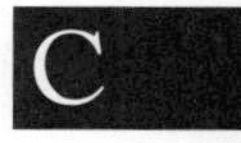

### Home Care

- • The interventions described previously may be adapted for home care use.
- • Assess family adjustment prenatally and postpartum; assist new parents to renegotiate behavior around issues such as amount of time spent together, sexual relationship, resolution of disagreements, and provision of sufficient time for leisure/recreational activities. Encourage the father to take an active role in infant care. **EBN:** *Declining satisfaction in family function indicates a need for supportive nursing intervention. Most decline has been shown to occur during the first 4 months postpartum, with little change thereafter. Less decline was evident when fathers were involved in infant care and household tasks. Prenatal satisfaction with family functioning influenced mothers' sense of competence at 4 and 8 months postpartum (Knauth, 2000).*
- ▲ Assess interference with family functioning. Refer for family counseling as indicated. *Parental role conflict can influence all areas of family life, creating additional stress and family dysfunction. Family therapy or counseling provides an opportunity to address stressors and improve family functioning.*

## Client/Family Teaching

- • Furnish clear explanations about condition, disease or disability, associated treatments, and prognosis. Describe circumstances involving emotional and physical reactions of the child and types of family member reactions that might be anticipated in response to the condition or crisis. Provide ample time for skill practice. *Providing information to families decreases confusion and anxiety, increases understanding, and allows a feeling of competence and control. Providing information about the disease and treatment process helps build parents' feelings of confidence (Baker, 1994).*
- • For parents of children with chronic disabilities, tailor educational opportunities based on the experiential phase of the parents (protection, survival, or development of the parent as a central person) as parents develop an identity as the central caregivers for their child. *As parents of physically and/or cognitively disabled children gain knowledge and become more involved in caregiving activities, their caregiver identity emerges (Perkins, 1993).*
- ▲ Refer parents of children with behavioral problems to parenting programs. **EB:** *This study showed that parenting programs significantly reduced child behavior problems and improved mental health. At immediate and 6-month follow-ups parents reported gains in confidence and feeling less stressed. Some also reported beneficial changes in their own and their children's behavior and improved relationships with their children (Stewart-Brown, 2004).*
- ▲ Involve parents in formal and/or informal social support situations, such as internet support groups. **EBN:** *This exploratory study describes factors related to use of Internet parent support groups (IPSGs) by primary caregivers of children with special health care needs (CSHCN). The majority of participants not only obtained what they sought, but found more than expected in terms of insight and people to trust. The strongest outcome factor related to satisfaction was improved caregiver-CSHCN relationship, and nearly 90% of the sample suggested participating in an IPSG as soon as possible (Baum, 2004).*

C

- ▲ Teach the client about available community resources (e.g., therapists, ministers, counselors, self-help groups). **EBN:** *Families need assistance in coping with health changes. The nurse is often perceived as the individual who can help them obtain necessary social support (Tak & McCubbin, 2002; Northouse et al, 2002).*
- ▲ Encourage parents with human immunodeficiency virus/acquired immune deficiency syndrome (HIV/AIDS) to implement custody plans for their children. **EB:** *This study of parents living with HIV/AIDS in New Your City indicates that an increasing number of children are likely to lose one or both of their parents to HIV disease. However, many parents have not formalized custody plans for their children, which can endanger the child's future. Interventions are needed to help affected families develop viable custody plans (Lightfoot & Rotheram-Borus, 2004).*

## evolve WEBSITES FOR EDUCATION

See the EVOLVE website for World Wide Web resources for client education.

## REFERENCES


Attharos T, Khampalikit S, Phuphaibul R et al: Development of a family-centered care model for children with cancer in a pediatric cancer unit, *Thai J Nurs Res* 8(1):52-63, 2004.

Aziz MA, Kenford S: Comparability of telephone and face-to-face interviews in assessing patients with posttraumatic stress disorder, *J Psychiatr Pract* 10(5):307-313, 2004.

Baker NA: Avoid collisions with challenging families, *MCN Am J Matern Child Nurs* 19:97-101, 1994.

Baum LS: Internet parent support groups for primary caregivers of a child with special health care needs, *Pediatr Nurs* 30(5):381-388, 401, 389-90, 2004.

Brazil K, Krueger P: Patterns of family adaptation to childhood asthma, *J Pediatr Nurs* 17(3):167-1673, 2002.

Browne JV, Sanchz E, Langlois A et al: From visitation policies to family participation guidelines in the NICU: the experience of the Colorado Consortium of Intensive Care Nurseries, *J Neonat Paediatr Child Health Nurs* 7(2):16-23, 2004.

Charron HS: Anxiety disorders. In Varcarolis EM, editor: *Foundations of psychiatric mental health nursing,* ed 3, Philadelphia, 1998, WB Saunders.

Cochran, M: Tears have no color, *Am J Nurs* 98(6):53, 1998.

D'Avanzo CE et al: Developing culturally informed strategies for substance-related interventions. In Naegle MA, D'Avanzo CE, editors: *Addictions and substance abuse: strategies for advanced practice nursing,* St Louis, 2001, Mosby.

Dobrzykowski TM, Noerager Stern P: Out of sync: a generation of first-time mothers over 30, *Health Care Women Int* 24(3):242-253, 2003.

Doswell W, Erlen J: Multicultural issues and ethical concerns in the delivery of nursing care interventions, *Nurs Clin North Am* 33(2):353-61, 1998.

Heineken J: Patient silence is not necessarily client satisfaction: communication in home care nursing, *Home Healthc Nurse* 16(2):115-20, 1998.

Hogan DL, Logan J: The Ottawa Model of Research Use: a guide to clinical innovation in the NICU, *Clin Nurse Spec* 18(5):255-261, 2004.

Kerr LMJ, Harrison MB, Medves J et al: Supportive care needs of parents of children with cancer: transition from diagnosis to treatment, *Oncol Nurs Forum* 31(6):E116-126, 2004.

Knauth DG: Predictors of parental sense of competence for the couple during the transition to parenthood, *Res Nurs Health* 23:496-509, 2000.

Leininger MM, McFarland MR: *Transcultural nursing: concepts, theories, research and practices,* ed 3, New York, McGraw-Hill, 2002.

Ludwick R, Silva M: Nursing around the world: cultural values and ethical conflicts, *Online J Issues Nurs,* August 14, 2000. Available at www.nursingworld.org/ojin/ethcol/ethics_4.htm, accessed on June 19, 2003.

Lightfoot M, Rotheram-Borus MJ: Predictors of child custody plans for children whose parents are living with AIDS in New York City, *Social Work* 49(3):461-469, 2004.

Miles MS, Burchinal P, Holditch-Davis D et al: Perceptions of stress, worry, and support in black and white mothers of hospitalized, medically fragile infants, *J Pediatr Nurs* 17(2):82-88, 2002.
Montagnino BA, Mauricio RV: The child with a tracheostomy and gastrostomy: parental stress and coping in the home—a pilot study, *Pediatr Nurs* 30(5):373-380, 401, 389-390, 2004.
Morelli PT, Fong R, Oliveria J: Culturally competent substance abuse treatment for Asian/Pacific Islander women, *J Hum Behav Soc Environ* 3(3/4):263, 2001.
Niska K, Snyder M, Lia-Hoagberg B: Family ritual facilitates adaptation to parenthood, *Public Health Nurs* 15(5):329-337, 1998.
Northouse LL, Mood D, Kershaw T et al: Quality of life of women with recurrent breast cancer and their family members, *J Clin Oncol* 20(19):4050-4064, 2002.
Perkins MT: Parent-nurse collaboration: using the caregiver identity emergence phases to assist parents of hospitalized children with disabilities, *J Pediatr Nurs* 8:2-9, 1993.
Rao P, Pradhan PV, Shah H: Psychopathology and coping in parents of chronically ill children, *Indian J Pediatr* 71(8):695-699, 2004
Ray LD, Ritchie JA: Caring for chronically ill children at home: factors that influence parents' coping, *J Pediatr Nurs* 8:217-25, 1993.
Rone-Adams SA, Stern DF, Walker V: Stress and compliance with a home exercise program among caregivers of children with disabilities, *Pediatr Phys Ther* 16(3):140-148, 2004.
Sadler LS, Clemmens DA: Ambivalent grandmothers raising teen daughters and their babies, *J Fam Nurs* 10(2):211-231, 2004.
Stewart-Brown S, Patterson J, Mockford C et al: Impact of a general practice based group parenting programme: quantitative and qualitative results from a controlled trial at 12 months, *Arch Dis Child* 89(6):519-525, 2004.
Sgarbossa D, Ford-Gilboe M: Mother's friendship quality, parental support, quality of life, and family health work in families led by adolescent mothers with preschool children, *J Fam Nurs* 10(2):232-261, 2004.
Tak YR, McCubbin M: Family stress, perceived social support and coping following the diagnosis of a child's congenital heart disease, *J Adv Nurs* 39(2):190-198, 2002.
True RH: Mental health issues of Asian/Pacific island women. In Adams DL, editor: *Health issues for women of color: a cultural diversity perspective,* Thousand Oaks, Calif, 1995, Sage.
Whitney SN, McGuire AL, McCullough LB: A typology of shared decision making, informed consent, and simple consent, *Ann Intern Med* 140(1):54-59, 2004.

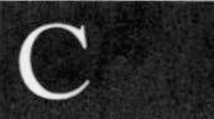

## Acute Confusion

evolve

*Kimberly Hickey*

**NANDA**

### Definition

Abrupt onset of a cluster of global, transient changes and disturbances in attention, cognition, psychomotor activity level, level of consciousness, and/or sleep-wake cycle

### Defining Characteristics

Lack of motivation to initiate and/or follow through with goal-directed or purposeful behavior; fluctuation in psychomotor activity; misperceptions; fluctuation in cognition; increased agitation or restlessness; fluctuation in level of consciousness; fluctuation in sleep-wake cycle, hallucinations

### Related Factors (r/t)

Over 60 years of age; alcohol abuse; delirium; dementia; drug abuse

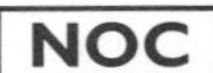

## (Nursing Outcomes Classification)

C

### Suggested NOC Outcomes

Cognitive Orientation; Distorted Thought Self-Control; Information Processing; Memory; Neurological Status: Consciousness; Sleep

**Example NOC Outcome with Indicators**

**Cognitive Orientation** as evidenced by the following indicators: Communicates clearly and appropriately for age and ability/Demonstrates control over selected events and situations/Attentiveness/Orientation (Rate each indicator of **Cognitive Orientation:** 1 = severely compromised, 2 = substantially compromised, 3 = moderately compromised, 4 = mildly compromised, 5 = not compromised [see Section I].)

## Client Outcomes

**Client Will (Specify Time Frame):**

- Demonstrate restoration of cognitive status to baseline
- Obtain adequate amount of sleep
- Demonstrate appropriate motor behavior
- Maintain functional capacity
- Optimize hydration and nutrition

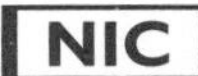

## Interventions (Nursing Interventions Classification)

### Suggested NIC Interventions

Delirium Management; Delusion Management

**Example NIC Activities—Delirium Management**

Orient to time, place, and person; present information in small, concrete portions

## Nursing Interventions and Rationales

- Assess the client's behavior and cognition systematically and continually throughout the day and night, as appropriate. **EB:** *Rapid onset and fluctuating course are hallmarks of delirium (Murphy, 2000). The Confusion Assessment Method is sensitive, specific, reliable, and easy to use (Inouye et al, 1990). Other tools to consider include the Delirium Rating Scale (DRS) and the Neelon/Champagne (NEECHAM) Confusion Scale. Selection depends on the population and reason for assessment (Rapp et al, 2000; Schuurmans et al, 2003).* **EBN:** *Nurses play a vital role in assessing acute confusion because they provide 24-hour care and see the client in a variety of circumstances (Inouye, 2000; Marr, 1992).* **EB:** *Delirium always involves an acute change in mental status; therefore, knowledge of the client's baseline mental status is key in assessing delirium (Flacker & Marcantonio, 1998).* **EBN**: *It is necessary to pay attention to behavioral changes because recent research has shown that there may*

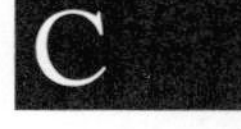

*be a prodromal phase of delirium in which sudden disorientation and urgent calls for attention may precede the onset of delirium (Duppils & Wikblad, 2004).*

- Perform an accurate mental status examination that includes the following:
  - Overall appearance, manner, and attitude
  - Behavior characteristics and level of psychomotor behavior
  - Mood and affect (presence of suicidal or homicidal ideation as observed by others and reported by the client)
  - Insight and judgment
  - Cognition as evidenced by level of consciousness, orientation (to time, place, and person), thought process, and content (perceptual disturbances such as illusions and hallucinations, paranoia, delusions, abstract thinking)
  - Attention

  *Missing a diagnosis of delirium can lead to serious negative consequences. Delirium in adults should be considered a medical emergency (Rosen, 1994). Early intervention in the case of delirium may decrease the severity and length of the delirious episode (Milisen et al, 2001).* **EB:** *Abnormal attention is an important diagnostic feature of delirium (Flacker & Marcantonio, 1998). Delirium is a state of mind, whereas agitation is a behavioral manifestation. Some clients may be delirious without agitation and may actually exhibit withdrawn behavior. This is a hypoactive form of delirium. Some clients present with a mixed hypoactive and hyperactive type of delirium (O'Keefe & Lavan, 1999).*

▲ Assess and report possible physiological alterations (e.g., sepsis, hypoglycemia, hypoxia, hypotension, infection, changes in temperature, fluid and electrolyte imbalance, use of medications with known cognitive and psychotropic side effects). **EBN:** *Such alterations may be contributing to confusion and must be corrected (Matthiesen et al, 1994).* **EB:** *Early attention to these risk factors may prevent delirium (Inouye et al, 2000). Medications are considered the most common cause of delirium in the ICU (Harvey, 1996).*

▲ Treat the underlying causes of delirium in collaboration with the health care team:
  - Establish/maintain normal fluid and electrolyte balance; establish/maintain normal nutrition, normal body temperature, normal oxygenation (if the client experiences low oxygen saturation, deliver supplemental oxygen), normal blood glucose levels, normal blood pressure.
  - Communicate client status, cognition, and behavioral manifestations to all necessary providers.
  - Monitor for any trends occurring in these manifestations.

  **EBN:** *Recognize that the client's fluctuating cognition and behavior are the hallmark of delirium and are not to be construed as client preference for certain caregivers (Inouye et al, 1990).* **EB:** *Careful monitoring is needed to identify the potential etiologic factors for delirium (Foreman, 2004).*

▲ Laboratory results should be closely monitored and physiological support given as appropriate. **EB:** *Dehydration is a significant risk factor for delirium and should be addressed aggressively (Inouye, 2000).* **EBN:** *Once acute confusion has been identified, it is vital to recognize and treat the associated underlying causes (Rapp & Iowa Veterans Affairs Nursing Research Consortium, 1997).*

- Establish or maintain elimination patterns. **EBN and EB:** *Disruption in elimination may be a cause of confusion (Rapp & Iowa Veterans Affairs Nursing Research Consortium,*

C

*1997). Urinary retention or a urinary tract infection, as well as constipation, may lead to delirium. These conditions may also present as a symptom of acute confusion and/or as a consequence of delirium and so attention to elimination patterns is essential. Prompt response to requests for assistance with elimination in addition to timed voids may assist in maintaining regular elimination, orientation, and patient safety (Rosen, 1994).*

- • Plan care that allows for an appropriate sleep-wake cycle. **EBN:** *Disruptions in usual sleep and activity patterns should be minimized because those clients with nocturnal exacerbations experience more complications from delirium (Inouye, 2000).*
- • Conduct a medication review. **EBN and EB:** *Medication use is one of the most important modifiable factors that can cause or worsen delirium, especially the use of anticholinergics, antipsychotics, and hypnosedatives (Flacker & Marcantonio, 1998; Han et al, 2001; Agostini, Leo-Summers, & Inouye, 2002).*
- • Modulate sensory exposure and establish a calm environment. **EBN:** *Extraneous lights and noise can give rise to agitation, especially if misperceived. Sensory overload or sensory deprivation can result in increased confusion (Rosen, 1994).* **EB**: *Clients with a hyperactive form of delirium often have increased irritability and startle responses and may be acutely sensitive to light and sound (Casey et al, 1996).*
- • Manipulate the environment to make it as familiar to the client as possible. Use a large clock and calendar. Encourage visits by family and friends. Place familiar objects in sight. **EBN:** *An environment that is familiar provides orienting clues, maintains an appropriate balance of sensory stimulation, and secures safety (Rosen, 1994).*
- • Identify yourself by name at each contact even if you have met the client before; call the client by his or her preferred name. *People with short-term memory deficits or dementia are at high risk for the development of delirium.*
- • Use appropriate communication techniques for clients at risk for confusion including communicating clearly and providing simple explanations as needed (Inouye, 2000; Foreman, 2004).
- • Use orientation techniques. If the client becomes distressed or argumentative about what is real, however, do not argue with the client. Rather, explore the emotion behind the client's non–reality-based statements (Rosen, 1994).
- • Offer reassurance to the client and use therapeutic communication at frequent intervals. **EBN:** *Client reassurance and communication are nursing skills that promote trust and orientation and reduce anxiety (Harvey, 1996).*
- • Provide supportive nursing care including meeting of basic needs such as feeding, toileting, and hydration. **EBN:** *Delirious clients are unable to care for themselves due to their confusion. Their care and safety needs must be anticipated by the nurse (Foreman et al, 1999).*
- ▲ Identify, evaluate, and treat pain quickly (see care plans for **Acute Pain** or **Chronic Pain**). **EB and EBN:** *Untreated pain is a potential cause of delirium (Inouye, 2000; Milisen et al, 2001).*
- ▲ Anticipate pain-producing conditions and treat pain with around-the-clock medications. *Clients experiencing delirium often will not report their pain nor be able to request medications prescribed on a prn basis.*
- ▲ Facilitate appropriate sensory input by having clients use aids (e.g., glasses, hearing

aids) as needed. *Sensory impairment contributes to misinterpretation of the environment and significantly contributes to delirium (Inouye, 2000).*

▲ Recognize that delirium is frequently treated with an antipsychotic medication. Watch for side effects of the medications. **EB:** *Be aware of paradoxical effects and side effects such as extrapyramidal symptoms, agitation, sedation, and arrhythmias, because these may exacerbate the delirium (Schwartz & Masand, 2002). In some situations, highly sensitive response to any of the antipsychotic medication may be cause to believe that a dementia underlies the delirium.*

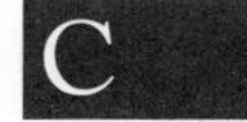

## Geriatric

- Mobilize the client as soon as possible; provide active and passive range of motion. **EBN and EB:** *Older clients who had a low level of physical activity before injury are at particular risk for acute confusion (Inouye, 2000; Matthiesen et al, 1994).*

▲ Provide sufficient medication to relieve pain. **EBN and EB:** *Older clients may give inaccurate pain histories, underreport symptoms, not want to bother the nurse, or exhibit restlessness, agitation, or increased confusion (Matthiesen et al, 1994).*

- Explain hospital routines and procedures slowly and in simple terms; repeat information as necessary. **EBN:** *Anxiety and sensory impairment decrease the older client's ability to integrate new information (Matthiesen et al, 1994).*
- Provide continuity of care when possible (e.g., provide the same caregivers, avoid room changes) (Foreman, 2004). **EBN:** *Continuity of care helps decrease the disorienting effects of hospitalization (Matthiesen et al, 1994).*
- If clients know that they are not thinking clearly, acknowledge the concern. *Fear is frequently experienced by people with delirium.* **EBN and EB:** *Confusion is very frightening, and the memory of the delirium can be equally frightening (Breitbart, Gibson, & Tremblay, 2002; Matthiesen et al, 1994).*
- Do not use the intercom to answer a call light. **EBN:** *The intercom may be frightening to an older confused client (Matthiesen et al, 1994).*
- Keep the client's sleep-wake cycle as normal as possible (e.g., avoid letting the client take daytime naps, avoid waking the client at night, give sedatives but not diuretics at bedtime, provide pain relief and back rubs). **EBN and EB:** *Acute confusion is accompanied by disruption of the sleep-wake cycle (Inouye, 2000; Matthiesen et al, 1994).*
- Maintain normal sleep-wake patterns (treat with bright light for 2 hours in the early evening). **EBN:** *Light treatment facilitates normal sleep-wake patterns (Rapp & Iowa Veterans Affairs Nursing Research Consortium, 1997).*

## Home Care

- Some of the interventions described previously may be adapted for home care use.
- Assess and monitor for acute changes in cognition and behavior. *An acute change in cognition and behavior is the classic presentation of delirium. It should be considered a medical emergency.*
- Delirium is reversible but can become chronic if untreated. The client may be discharged from the hospital to home care in a state of undiagnosed delirium. **EBN:** *Staff should receive training in the assessment of acute confusion; assessment may be complicated*

C

*by the presence of periods of lucidity (Mentes et al, 1999).* **EB:** *In a study of delirium among clients in a convalescent hospital following an acute care hospital stay for a variety of precipitating factors, 22% presented with delirium, and 93% of these had developed the delirium prior to convalescent home admission. Multiple precipitating factors were frequently present (Pi-Figueras et al, 2004).*

- Use brief self-report measures to improve identification and clinical management of at-risk cases. **EB:** *A brief test battery has been developed to identify subclinical cognitive problems, using six items (repetition of three words, back-spelling of the word "sport," problem searching in a complex picture, recall of the three words, three progressive colored matrices, clock drawing test). Abnormal findings suggest the need for deeper neuropsychological assessment; the tool cannot be used to diagnose dementia (Cucinotta et al, 2004).*
- Assess for treatable causes of changes in cognition and behavior. *The mnemonic DEMENTIA can be used to remember potential causes of acute or chronic confusion (Smith, 2002):*

  **D:** Drugs and alcohol—including over-the-counter drugs
  **E:** Eyes and ears—disorientation due to visual/auditory distortion
  **M:** Medical disorders—e.g., diabetes, hypothyroidism
  **E:** Emotional and psychological disturbances—e.g., mood or paranoid disorders
  **N:** Neurological disorders—e.g., multiinfarct dementia
  **T:** Tumors and trauma
  **I:** Infections—e.g., urinary tract or upper respiratory tract
  **A:** Arteriosclerosis—leading to heart failure, insufficient blood supply to heart and brain, confusion
- Assess fluid intake, dementia status, and occurrence of a fall within the past 30 days in evaluating confusion. **EBN:** *Confusion may be explained by inadequate fluid intake, dementia, or a fall. In the last case, it is unclear if falls are a precipitating event or indicative of frailty (Mentes et al, 1999).*
- Avoid preconceptions about the source of acute confusion; assess each occurrence on the basis of available evidence. *Delirium may not be readily recognized, in part because of its varying presentations and in part because preconceptions interfere with accurate assessment. For example, although delirium may occur in advanced cancer clients prior to death, it also may arise in response to reversible causes that should be identified and treated, depending on the goals of care (Lawlor, 2001).*

▲ Institute case management of frail elderly clients to support continued independent living. *Difficulties with acute confusion lead to increasing needs for assistance in using the health care system effectively. Case management combines the nursing activities of client and family assessment, planning and coordination of care among all health care providers, delivery of direct nursing care, and monitoring of care and outcomes. These activities are able to address continuity of care, mutual goal setting, behavior management, and prevention of worsening health problems (Guttman, 1999).*

## Client/Family Teaching

▲ Teach the family to recognize signs of early confusion and seek medical help. **EBN:** *Early intervention prevents long-term complications (Rapp & Iowa Veterans Affairs Nursing Research Consortium, 1997).*

- Counsel the client and family regarding the symptoms of delirium, its management, and its sequelae. **EB:** *Families experience a high degree of distress when observing a loved one in delirium. Families should be told that symptoms of delirium may persist for months following a delirious episode so that appropriate plans can be made for continuing care (Marcantonio et al, 2003; Breitbart, Gibson, & Tremblay, 2002).*

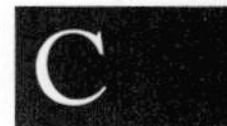


## REFERENCES


Agostini JV, Leo-Summers LS, Inouye SK: Cognitive and other adverse effects of diphenhydramine use in hospitalized older patients, *Arch Intern Med* 161(17):2091-2097, 2001.

Breitbart W, Gibson C, Tremblay A: The delirium experience: delirium recall and delirium related distress in hospitalized patients with cancer, their spouses/caregivers, and their nurses, *Psychosomatics* 43(3):183-194, 2002.

Casey DA, DeFazio JV Jr, Vansickle K et al: Delirium: quick recognition, careful evaluation, and appropriate treatment, *Postgrad Med* 100(1):121-124, 1996.

Cucinotta D, Reggiani A, Galleiti L et al: Preventive Comprehensive Assessment (PCA): a new screening method for subclinical cognitive problems, *Arch Gerontol Geriatr* (Suppl 9):97, 2004.

Duppils GS, Wikblad K: Delirium: behavioural changes before and during prodromal phase, *J Clin Nurs* 13(5):609-616, 2004.

Flacker JM, Marcantonio ER: Delirium in the elderly: optimal management, *Drugs Aging* 13(2):119, 1998.

Foreman MD, Mion LC, Tryostad L et al: Standard of practice protocol: acute confusion/delirium, NICHE Faculty, *Geriatr Nurs* 20(3):147-152, 1999.

Guttman R: Case management of the frail elderly in the community, *Clin Nurs Spec* 13(4):174, 1999.

Han L, McCusker J, Cole M et al: Use of medications with anticholinergic effect predicts clinical severity of delirium symptoms in older medical inpatients, *Arch Intern Med* 161(8):1099-1105, 2001.

Harvey M: Managing agitation in critically ill patients, *Am J Crit Care* 5:7, 1996.

Inaba-Roland K, Maricle R: Assessing delirium in the acute care setting, *Heart Lung* 21:49, 1992.

Inouye SK: Prevention of delirium in hospitalized older patients: risk factors and targeted intervention strategies, *Ann Med* 32(4): 257, 2000.

Inouye SK, Bogardus ST Jr, Baker DI et al: The Hospital Elder Life Program: a model of care to prevent cognitive and functional decline in older hospitalized patients. Hospital Elder Life Program, *J Am Geriatr Soc* 48(12):1697-1706, 2000.

Inouye SK, van Dyck CH, Alessi CA et al: Clarifying confusion: the confusion assessment method: a new method for detection of delirium, *Ann Intern Med* 113(12):941-948, 1990.

Lawlor PG: Assessment of delirium in patients with advanced cancer, *Home Health Care Consult* 8(9):10, 2001.

Marcantonio ER, Simon SE, Bergmann MA et al: Delirium symptoms in post-acute care: prevalent, persistent, and associated with poor recovery, *J Am Geriatr Soc* 51(1):4-9, 2003.

Marr J: Acute confusion, *Nurs Times* 88:16, 1992.

Matthiesen V, Sivertsen L, Foreman MD et al: Acute confusion: nursing interventions in older patients, *Orthop Nurs* 13:25, 1994.

Mentes J, Culp K, Maas M et al: Acute confusion indicators: risk factors and prevalence using MDS data, *Res Nurs Health* 22(2):95-105, 1999.

Milisen K, Foreman MD, Abraham IL et al: A nurse-led interdisciplinary intervention program for delirium in elderly hip fracture patients, *J Am Geriatr Soc* 49(5):523-532, 2001.

Murphy BA: Delirium, *Emerg Med Clin North Am* 18:243, 2000.

Pi-Figueras M, Aguilera A, Arellano M et al: Prevalence of delirium in a geriatric convalescent hospital unit: patient's clinical characteristics and risk precipitating factor analysis, *Arch Gerontol Geriatr* (Suppl 9):333, 2004.

O'Keefe ST, Lavan JN: Clinical significance of delirium subtypes in older people, *Age Ageing* 28(2):115, 1999.

Rapp C, Iowa Veterans Affairs Nursing Research Consortium: *Acute confusion/delirium,* Iowa City, 1997, The Consortium.

Rapp CG, Wakefield B, Kundrat M et al: Acute confusion assessment instruments: clinical versus research usability, *Appl Nurs Res* 13(1):37-45, 2000.

Rosen SL: Managing delirious older adults in the hospital, *MedSurg Nurs* 3(3):181, 1994.

Schuurmans MJ, Deschamps PI, Markham SW et al: The measurement of delirium: review of scales, *Res Theory Nurs Pract* 17(3): 207-224, 2003.

Schwartz TL, Masand PS: The role of atypical antipsychotics in the treatment of delirium, *Psychosomatics* 43:171, 2002.

Smith GB: Case management guideline: Alzheimer disease and other dementias, *Lippincotts Case Manag* 7(2):77-84, 2002.

# Chronic Confusion

evolve

*Kimberly Hickey*

C

## NANDA

### Definition

Irreversible, long-standing, and/or progressive deterioration of intellect and personality characterized by decreased ability to interpret environmental stimuli; decreased capacity for intellectual thought processes; and manifested by disturbances of memory, orientation, and behavior

### Defining Characteristics

Altered interpretation/response to stimuli; clinical evidence of organic impairment; progressive/long-standing cognitive impairment; altered personality; impaired memory (short- and long-term); impaired socialization; no change in level of consciousness

### Related Factors (r/t)

Multiinfarct dementia; Korsakoff's psychosis; head injury; Alzheimer's disease; cerebral vascular accident

## NOC

### Outcomes (Nursing Outcomes Classification)

#### Suggested NOC Outcomes

Cognition; Cognitive Orientation; Distorted Thought Self-Control

**Example NOC Outcome with Indicators**

**Cognition** as evidenced by the following indicators: Communicates clearly and appropriately for age and ability/Demonstrates control over selected events and situations/Attentiveness/Orientation (Rate each indicator of **Cognition:** 1 = severely compromised, 2 = substantially compromised, 3 = moderately compromised, 4 = mildly compromised, 5 = not compromised [see Section I].)

### Client Outcomes

**Client Will (Specify Time Frame):**

- Remain content and free from harm
- Function at maximal cognitive level
- Participate in activities of daily living at the maximum of functional ability
- Have minimal episodes of agitation since agitation occurs in up to 70% of patients with dementia

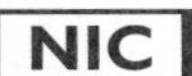

## Interventions (Nursing Interventions Classification)

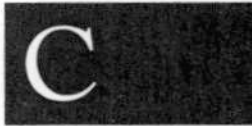

### Suggested NIC Interventions

Dementia Management; Environmental Management; Reality Orientation; Surveillance: Safety

**Example NIC Activities—Dementia Management**

Use distraction rather than confrontation to manage behavior; give one simple direction at a time

## Nursing Interventions and Rationales

- Determine the client's cognitive level using a screening tool such as the Mini-Mental State Exam (MMSE). The Mini-Cog is also a useful screening tool to be used in a busy setting. **EB:** *Use of a standard evaluation tool such as the MMSE can help determine the client's abilities and assist in planning appropriate nursing interventions (Agostinelli et al, 1994; Bodner et al, 2004; Borsen et al, 2003; Schuurmans et al, 2003).*
- Gather information about the client's predementia functioning, including social situation, physical condition, and psychological functioning. **EBN and EB:** *Knowing the client's background can assist the nurse in identifying agenda behavior and using validation therapy, and will provide guidance for reminiscence. This information may also be useful to the nurse in understanding behavior if the client becomes delusional and hallucinates (Fine and Rouse-Bane, 1995; Cohen-Mansfield, Golander, & Arnheim, 2000).*
- Assess the client for signs of depression: insomnia, poor appetite, flat affect, and withdrawn behavior. **EBN:** *Up to 50% of clients with dementia have depressive symptoms (Cleeland, 1997).*
- Place an identification bracelet on client. **EB:** *Clients with dementia wander and can become lost; identification bracelets increase their safety (Painter, 1996).*
- Avoid as much as possible exposing the client to unfamiliar situations and people. Maintain continuity of caregivers. Maintain routines of care by observing established eating, bathing, and sleeping schedules. Send a familiar person with the client when the client goes for diagnostic testing or into unfamiliar environments. **EBN:** *Situational anxiety associated with environmental, interpersonal, or structural change can escalate into agitated behavior (Gerdner and Buckwalter, 1994).*
- Keep the environment quiet. Avoid or minimize sights and sounds that have a high potential for misinterpretation, such as buzzers, alarms, and overhead paging systems. **EB and EBN:** *Sensory overload can result in agitated behavior in a client with dementia. Misinterpretation of the environment can also contribute to agitation (Doody et al, 2001).*
- Begin each interaction with the client by identifying yourself and calling the client by name. Approach the client with a caring, loving, and accepting attitude, and speak calmly and slowly. **EBN:** *Dementia clients can sense feelings of compassion; a calm, slow manner projects a feeling of comfort to the client (Stolley, 1994).*

C

- Give one simple direction at a time and repeat it as necessary. Use verbal and physical prompts, and model the desired action if needed and possible. **EBN:** *People with dementia need time to assimilate and interpret your directions; if you rephrase your question, you give them something new to process, which increases their confusion (Stolley, 1994).*
- Break down self-care tasks into simple steps (e.g., instead of saying, "Take a shower," say to the client, "Please follow me. Sit down on the bed. Take off your shoes. Now take off your socks."). **EBN:** *Dementia clients are unable to follow complex commands; breaking down an activity into simple steps makes the activity more feasible (Agostinelli et al, 1994).*
- Keep questions simple; yes or no questions are often preferable. Use positive statements and actions and avoid negative communication. *Negative feedback leads to increased confusion and agitation. It is more effective to go along with the client and then redirect as necessary.*
- If eating in the dining room increases agitation, let the client leave and eat in a quieter environment with a smaller number of people. **EB and EBN:** *The noise and confusion in a large dining room can be overwhelming for a dementia client and result in agitated behavior. It is preferable to have dementia clients eat in small groups (Sloane, 1998).*
- Provide finger food if the client has difficulty using eating utensils or is unable to sit to eat. **EB:** *Feeding oneself is a complex task and may prove challenging for someone with significant dementia (Finley, 1997).*
- Provide boundaries by placing red or yellow tape on the floor or by using a stop sign. *Boundaries help the client identify safe areas; older clients can more easily see red and yellow.*
- Assess the cause of wandering rather than or before attempting to control the wandering. **EBN:** *Wandering indicates a problem and need for intervention; therefore, the reason for the wandering behavior must be determined (Algase, 1999).*
- Write the client's name in large block letters in the room and on the client's clothing and possessions.
- Use symbols rather than words to identify areas such as the bathroom or kitchen. Utilize environmental cues such as clocks and a sign with mealtimes to decrease common mealtime questions and thus decrease agitation around mealtimes. **EBN:** *The results of a study in which a large clock and a sign with large lettering that identified mealtimes were hung in the dining area suggest a simple, inexpensive environmental intervention can reduce repetitive questions commonly exhibited by individuals with dementia (Nolan & Mathews, 2004).*
- Limit visitors to two and provide them with guidelines on what are appropriate topics to discuss with the client and how to best communicate with the client. (See how to converse with a memory-impaired person in the Client/Family Teaching section.)
- Set up scheduled quiet periods in a recliner or room. Use afghans and environmental cues to define rest periods. **EBN:** *Quiet times allow the client's anxiety and building tension levels to decrease (Hall et al, 1995). Fatigue has been associated with the onset of increased confusion and agitation (Stolley, 1994).*
- Provide quiet activities such as listening to music of the client's preference or introduce other cues that promote relaxation in the afternoon or early evening. **EB and EBN:**

*An increase in confusion and agitation may occur in the late afternoon and early evening and is referred to as "sundowning syndrome." Quiet activities can provide a calming environment (Doody et al, 2001).*

- Provide simple activities for the client, such as folding washcloths and sorting or stacking activities. Avoid misleading and frightening stimuli, which may include the television, mirrors, and pictures of people or animals. **EBN:** *Repetitive activities give clients a positive outlet for behavior (Burgener et al, 1998). They see, hear, and perceive a different world; they may not recognize themselves in the mirror and be afraid of the stranger they see so close to them.*
- If the client becomes increasingly confused and agitated, perform the following steps:
  - Assess the client for physiological causes, including acute hypoxia, pain, medication effects, malnutrition, infections such as urinary tract infection, fatigue, electrolyte disturbances, and constipation. *An acute change in behavior is a medical emergency and should be evaluated.* **EBN and EB:** *Many physiological factors can result in increased agitation of clients with dementia (Gerdner &Buckwalter, 1994; Alexopoulos et al, 1998).*
  - Assess for psychological causes, including changes in the environment, caregiver, and routine; demands to perform beyond capacity; or multiple competing stimuli, including discomfort. **EB and EBN:** *It is important for the nurse to recognize precipitating events and subsequent behavior to prevent further incidents of agitation (Bair et al, 1999).*
  - Avoid confrontations with the client; allow the client to dissipate energy by performing repetitive tasks or by pacing.
  - If the client is delusional or hallucinating, do not confront him or her with reality.
- Use validation therapy to verbally reflect back the emotions that the client appears to be feeling. Use statements such as, "It must be frightening to see a fire at the end of your bed," "I can see you are afraid," "I will stay with you," or "Can you tell me more about what is going on right now?" **EB and EBN:** *Orienting the client to reality can increase agitation; validation therapy conveys empathy and understanding and can help determine the internal stimulus that is creating the change in behavior (Feil, 1993). Staff training in validation therapy resulted in a decrease in the doses of psychotherapeutic medications used and in incidences of behavior problems in one study (Fine & Rouse-Bane, 1995).*
- Reality orientation (RO) techniques may be used if individualized. For some people with dementia, RO may enhance a sense of understanding of one's environment and hence their self-esteem, but in others, it may negatively effect self-esteem. **EB:** *The use of reality orientation has met with mixed responses and therefore must be used only as appropriate for the client and the situation (Spector et al, 2004).*
- Decrease stimuli in the environment (e.g., turn off the television, take the client to a quiet place). Institute activities associated with pleasant emotions, such as playing soft music the client likes, looking through a photo album, providing favorite food, or using simulated presence therapy. **EBN:** *Decreasing stimuli can decrease agitation. Reassuring activities can help bring pleasant emotions to help soothe the client; these include*

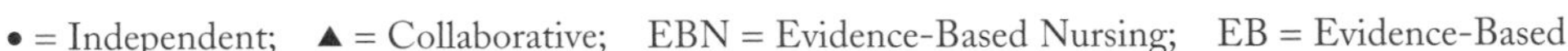

C

*simulated presence therapy in which the client listens to a tape of a conversation with a loved one (Woods & Ashley, 1995).*

- Avoid using restraints if at all possible. **EB:** *Restraints are not benign interventions and should be used sparingly and judiciously and only when alternatives to manage the behaviors have been tried and have proven unsuccessful. Side effects of restraints include falls, increased confusion, deconditioning, and incontinence (Tinetti, Liu, & Ginter, 1992).*
- When bathing a patient with dementia, minimize the patient's discomfort by using the Bag Bath (if available). Bathtime is an opportunity to emphasize person-centered nursing. **EBN and EB:** *Bathing is known to be stressful for patients with dementia as evidenced by the frequently seen agitation that occurs during this activity. The Bag Bath decreases discomfort during bathing, and the person-centered approach maintains self-esteem and a sense of control for the patient (Somboontanont et al, 2004).*
- Use PRN or low-dose regular dosing of psychotropic or antianxiety drugs only as a last resort. They are effective in managing symptoms of psychosis and aggressive behavior. Start with the lowest possible dose. **EB:** *Psychotropic drugs such as haloperidol (Haldol) and risperidone (Risperdal) may decrease client function and have side effects that need to be monitored (Katz et al, 1999).*

▲ Avoid the use of anticholinergic medications such as Benadryl. *Anticholinergic medications have a high side-effect profile that includes disorientation, urinary retention, and excessive drowsiness (Han et al, 2001). The anticholinergic side effects outweigh the antihistaminic effects.*

- For predictable difficult times, such as during bathing and grooming, try the following:
  - Massage the client's hands lovingly or use therapeutic touch to relax the client. **EBN:** *Hand massage and therapeutic touch have been shown to induce relaxation that may allow care activities to take place without difficulty (Snyder, Egan, & Burns, 1995).*
  - Avoid questioning the client or highlighting situations in which the client is unable to remember, since this can result in frustration and contribute to agitation.
  - Approach the client in a patient-centered framework as this offers a sense of control and promotes self-esteem.
  - Use positive behavioral reinforcement for each small step of bathing, such as praising the client for walking toward the shower, sitting in the shower chair, and removing items of clothing. **EBN:** *Positive behavioral reinforcement for desired behavior is effective for clients with dementia (Boehm et al, 1995). Consider a towel bath if shower or tub bathing is too stressful for the client (Hall & Buckwalter, 1999).*
- Treat the client with the utmost respect and give individualized care. **EBN:** *Treating confused clients with respect and individualizing care can decrease aggression and increase nursing staff satisfaction (Maxfield, Lewis, & Cannon, 1996).*
- For care of early dementia clients with primarily symptoms of memory loss, see the care plan for **Impaired Memory.**
- For care of clients with self-care deficits, see the appropriate care plan **(Feeding Self-care deficit; Dressing Self-care deficit;** and **Toileting Self-care deficit).**

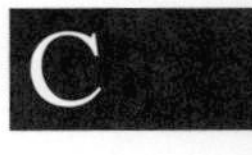


## Geriatric

NOTE: Most of the aforementioned interventions apply to the geriatric client.

- Use reminiscence and life review therapeutic interventions; ask questions about the client's work, child raising, or time spent in military service. Ask questions such as, "What was really important to you as you look back?" **EBN:** *Reminiscence and life review can help an older person reframe and accept life events.*
- Assess and treat pain. *Many older people with dementia also have at least one, and many times several, chronic condition that has associated discomfort or pain. While some older people with dementia are able to respond to pain assessment questions, there are increasing numbers of people who cannot. It is essential to assess for the presence of painful conditions and to treat it. Likewise it is important to anticipate when the pain may be worse and proactively treat it. The response to pain will need to be monitored by assessing how best the client demonstrates pain or discomfort. Agitation may be one manner in which pain is demonstrated (Buffem et al, 2001; Fuchs-Lacelle & Hadjistavropoulos, 2004; Kaasalainen & Crook, 2004). Memories and reminiscence have been used successfully with elderly persons to evoke pleasure and achieve therapeutic goals (Woods & Ashley, 1995). Reminiscence can activate past sources of self-esteem and aid coping (Nugent, 1995).*

## Multicultural

- Assess for the influence of cultural beliefs, norms, and values on the family's or caregiver's understanding of chronic confusion or dementia. **EBN:** *What the family considers normal and abnormal health behavior may be based on cultural perceptions (Leininger & McFarland 2002; Cochran, 1998; Doswell & Erlen, 1998; Guarnaccia, 1998). Research indicates that Caucasian older adults are significantly more knowledgeable about Alzheimer's disease (AD) than African-American, Asian, and Latino older adults (Ayalon & Arean, 2004). Another study showed African Americans showed less awareness of facts about AD, reported fewer sources of information, and indicated less perceived threat of the disorder (Roberts et al, 2003).*
- Inform the client's family or caregiver of the meaning of and reasons for common behavior observed in clients with dementia. **EBN:** *An understanding of dementia behavior will enable the client's family or caregiver to provide the client with a safe environment. Black and Latino community-dwelling patients with moderate to severe dementia have a higher prevalence of dementia-related behaviors than whites (Sink et al, 2004).*
- Assist the family or caregiver in identifying barriers that would prevent the use of social services or other supportive services that could help reduce the impact of caregiving. **EBN:** *Expectations of discrimination, lack of knowledge about services, expectations embedded in familism, lack of sense of prevention, lack of health insurance, preference for traditional remedies, and neglect or abuse were barriers identified by researchers studying the low utilization of skilled home care nursing services by elderly Hispanic clients (Crist, 2002). Language may present another barrier to the access of supportive services (McGrath, Vun, & McLeod, 2001). The lack of health insurance, and financial resources for a substantial proportion of Mexican-American people means many do not receive medical care, so their Alzheimer's disease remains undiagnosed and untreated (Briones et al, 2002).*

- Assess the client for the presence of an instrumental activity of daily living (IADL) disability and chronic health conditions. **EBN:** *African-American clients with cognitive impairments had higher IADL disability, poorer self-rated health, higher cognitive errors, and more chronic health conditions (Chumbler et al, 2001).*
- ▲ Refer the family to social services or other supportive services to assist in meeting the demands of caregiving for the client with dementia. **EBN:** *African-American caregivers of dementia clients may evidence less desire than others to institutionalize their family members and are more likely to report unmet service needs (Hinrichsen & Ramirez, 1992). Families of dementia clients may report restricted social activity (Haleyet al, 1995). Korean families reported waiting waited 3-4 years before seeking help for their family member with dementia. Help was sought when memory decline was accompanied by other problems (Watari & Gatz, 2004).*
- ▲ Encourage the family to make use of support groups or other service programs. **EBN:** *Studies indicate that some minority families of clients with dementia may use few support programs even though these programs could have a positive impact on caregiver well-being (Cox, 1999).*
- Validate the family members' feelings with regard to the impact of the client's behavior on family lifestyle. **EBN:** *Validation lets family members know that the nurse has heard and understood what was said, and it promotes the relationship between the nurse and family members (Heineken, 1998).*
- *Black and Latino community-dwelling patients with moderate to severe dementia have a higher prevalence of dementia-related behaviors than Caucasian patients. Therefore, as the aging minority population grows, it will be especially important to target caregiver education, in-home support, and resources to minority communities (Sink et al, 2004).*

## Home Care

NOTE: Keeping the client as independent as possible is important. Because community-based care is usually less structured than institutional care, however, in the home setting the goal of maintaining safety for the client takes on primary importance.

- The interventions described previously may be adapted for home care use.
- Assess and monitor the client for acute changes in cognition and behavior. *An acute change in cognition and behavior is the classic presentation of delirium. Delirium is reversible, should be considered a medical emergency, and can occur in conjunction with dementia. Delirium can become chronic if untreated, and clients may be discharged from hospitals to home care in states of undiagnosed delirium.*
- Use brief self-report measures to improve identification and clinical management of at-risk cases. **EB:** *A brief test battery has been developed to identify subclinical cognitive problems, using six items (repetition of three words, back-spelling of the word "sport," problem searching in a complex picture, recall of the three words, three progressive colored matrices, clock drawing test). Abnormal findings suggest the need for deeper neuropsychological assessment; the tool cannot be used to diagnose dementia (Cucinotta et al, 2004).*
- Assess for treatable causes of changes in cognition and behavior. *The mnemonic DEMENTIA can be used to remember potential causes (Smith, 2002):*
  **D:** Drugs and alcohol—including over-the-counter drugs
  **E:** Eyes and ears—disorientation due to visual/auditory distortion

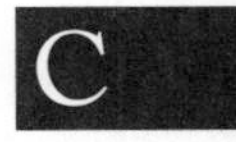


**M:** Medical disorders—e.g., diabetes, hypothyroidism
**E:** Emotional and psychological disturbances—e.g., mood or paranoid disorders
**N:** Neurological disorders—e.g., multiinfarct dementia
**T:** Tumors and trauma
**I:** Infections—e.g., urinary tract or upper respiratory tract
**A:** Arteriosclerosis—leading to heart failure, insufficient blood supply to heart and brain, and confusion

- ▲ Before providing any home care, assess the client plan for advance directives (living will and power of attorney). If a plan exists, place a copy in the client file. If no plan exists, offer information on advance directives according to agency policy. Refer for assistance in completing advance directives as necessary. Do not witness a living will. *This is a legal requirement of the Consolidated Omnibus Budget Reconciliation Act (COBRA). The ability of the client to plan advance directives legally depends on the stage of dementia, the degree of certainty of the client's wishes for end-of-life care, and the degree of distress experienced by the client with dementia. Successful completion of advance directives by clients with mild to moderate dementia has been reported (Rempusheski & Hurley, 2000).*
- • Assess the client's memory and executive function deficits before assuming the inability to make any medical decisions. **EB:** *A review of existing research on the decision-making competence of cognitively impaired older adults concluded that many persons with dementia are capable of decision making and that, at least in the early stages of dementia, interventions may improve decisional abilities (Kim, Karlawish, & Caine, 2002).*
- ▲ Assess the home for safety features and client needs for assistive devices. Explore with the client and family areas of concern. Refer to an occupational therapist for adaptive measures. Problem solve personal and environmental solutions for client protection. *Assistance from an occupational therapist offers sustained benefits in modifying the home environment for optimal adaptation (Gitlin, 2001). A variety of personal items (e.g., shoes, clothing) or environmental aspects (e.g., ready access to stove, loose rugs, flimsy outer door lock) may threaten client safety. Adaptations may include shoes or clothing with Velcro fasteners, stove knob locks, nonskid rugs or removal of rugs, and alarmed doors.*
- • Elements of reality orientation therapy may be applied in the home, incorporating person-centered respect, reminiscence, validation, and sensory-motor stimulation. **EB:** *In one study, participants with dementia were led in ecological exercises (e.g., a game around using money); personal, spatial, and social orientation; verbal and visual memory; verbal fluency; categorization; and auditory and visual attention. Improvement in cognition, language, memory, and affective function were noted (Savorani et al, 2004).*
- ▲ Evaluate the client's use or history of use of alcohol or drugs; continued use should be halted if the client can be persuaded. Instruct the client and family regarding the influence of substance use on cognition and behavior. Assess for the potential for withdrawal; refer to a physician for withdrawal protocol as indicated. *Continued substance use serves as a barrier to achieving effective outcomes in addressing dementia (Smith, 2002).*
- • Provide support to the family of the client with a chronic and disabling condition; be prepared to offer support and information to family members who live at a distance as well. **EB:** *A study compared primary caregivers of clients having dementia with relatives living more than an hour distant. Both groups sought similar information about the cli-*

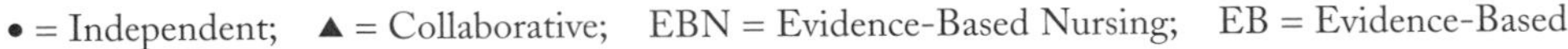

C

*ent's disorder and reported similar subjective distress, but the distant relatives were more often dissatisfied with the information received and were less likely to seek out reading materials or lay societies (Thompsell & Lovestone, 2002).*

- Use familiar aspects of the environment (smells, music, foods, pictures) to cue the client, capitalizing on habit to remind the client of activities in which the client can participate (e.g., cooperating with medication administration). **EBN:** *While clients with dementia are probably unable to learn new activities because of deteriorated explicit memory, preserved implicit memory or habit may be useful in maximizing functional ability (Son, Therrien, & Whall, 2002).*
- Instruct the caregiver to provide a balanced activity schedule that neither stresses the client nor deprives him or her of stimulation; avoid sustained low- or high-stimulation activity. **EBN:** *In one study, imbalances in the pacing of sensory stimulation and sensory calming (i.e., sustained low- and high-stimulation activity) contributed to agitation and functional decline (Kovach & Wells, 2002).*
- ▲ If the client will require extensive supervision on an ongoing basis, evaluate the client for day care programs. Refer the family to medical social services to assist with this process if necessary. Day care programs provide safe, structured care for the client and respite for the family. *Respite care for caregivers is an essential part of successful long-term care for a confused client.* **EB:** *Studies have not shown a major impact of day care on the anxiety or depression of older adults, or on caregiver burden. However, a study did find subjective reports of reduced loneliness, anxiety, and depression among clients, and decreased perceived burden on caregivers (Baumgarten et al, 2002).*
- Encourage the family to include the client in family activities when possible. Reinforce the use of therapeutic communication guidelines (see Client/Family Teaching) and sensitivity to the number of people present. *These steps help the client maintain dignity and lead to familial socialization of the client.*
- Assess family caregivers for caregiver stress, loneliness, and depression. *Caring for a loved one with a dementing process is highly stressful. Respite care is a necessary component of the overall care plan.*
- Refer to the care plan for **Caregiver role strain. EBN:** *Caregiver loneliness has been associated with depression, relational deprivation, and poorer quality of the current caregiver-client relationship (Beeson et al, 2000).*
- Explore the state of the relationship that existed between the client and caregiver before the onset of dementia, including the strengths and weaknesses of each party. Formulate a plan to assist married couples in dealing with the likely worsening of dementia. *Dementia represents a gradual and devastating loss of the marital relationship as it existed formerly. An understanding of the prior relationship is needed before the couple can be helped to anticipate continuing deterioration (Zarit, 2001).*
- Explore with the spouse the process he or she is undergoing to understand the client's behavior; assist with reframing that understanding to be as realistic and positive as possible. **EBN:** *In a qualitative study, wives of clients with Alzheimer's disease described a process of recognizing changes, drawing inferences about their observations, rewriting identities for themselves and their husbands as they took on their husbands' roles and responsibilities, and constructing a new daily life. Reframing interventions can assist caregivers in considering positive aspects of caring along with grief and frustration (Perry, 2002).*

- ▲ Refer the client to medical social services as necessary to evaluate financial resources and initiate benefits or access to providers. *Limited resources serve as barriers to effective outcomes in addressing dementia (Smith, 2002).*
- ▲ Institute case management for frail elderly clients to support continued independent living. *Difficulties with chronic confusion lead to increasing needs for assistance in using the health care system effectively. Case management combines the nursing activities of client and family assessment, planning and coordination of care among all health care providers, delivery of direct nursing care, and monitoring of care and outcomes. These activities are able to promote continuity across multiple sites of care, mutual goal setting, behavior management, and prevention of worsening health problems (Guttman, 1999; Tichawa, 2002).*
- ▲ Refer for homemaker or psychiatric home health care services for respite, client reassurance, and implementation of a therapeutic regimen. *Having responsibility for a person who is chronically confused results in high caregiver stress. Respite decreases caregiver stress. The presence of caring individuals is reassuring to both the client and caregivers, especially during periods of client anxiety. The client who shows chronic confusion, especially if it is accompanied by depression, can benefit from the interventions described previously, modified for the home setting (Di Gioacchino et al, 2004; Fabris et al, 2004).*

## Client/Family Teaching

- • In the early stages of confusion (e.g., initial period following stroke), provide the caregiver with information on illness processes, needed care, and likely trajectory of progress. **EBN:** *In one study, family caregivers of stroke survivors felt abandoned by staff. Caregivers wanted information to ensure that they felt competent, confident, and able to provide care safely; they wanted to understand likely future demands (Brereton & Nolan, 2002; Kuhn & Fulton, 2004).*
- • Recommend that the family develop a memory aid wallet or booklet for the client, which contains pictures and text that chronicle the client's life. **EB:** *Using memory aids such as wallets or booklets helps dementia clients make more factual statements and stay on topic, and decreases the number of confused, erroneous, and repetitive statements (Bourgeois, 1992).*
- • Teach the family how to converse with a memory-impaired person. Guidelines include the following:
  - ■ Ask the client to have a conversation with you.
  - ■ Guide the conversation to specific, nonthreatening topics and redirect the conversation back on topic when the client begins to ramble.
  - ■ Reassure and help out when the client gets stuck or cannot find the right words.
  - ■ Smile and act interested in what the client is saying even if unsure what it means.
  - ■ Thank the client for talking.
  - ■ Avoid quizzing the client or asking a lot of specific questions.
  - ■ Avoid correcting or contradicting something that was stated even if it is wrong.

  **EB:** *These guidelines can help families interact more effectively with clients and decrease frustration levels (Bourgeois, 1992).*
- • Teach the family how to set up the environment and use the care techniques/interventions listed so that cognitive and functional impairments that interact with the client's progressively lowered stress threshold (PLST) will be addressed. Identify

C

stressors and initiate compensatory modifications of the environment. **EBN:** *Alzheimer's clients are unable to deal with stress and have decreased tolerance to stimuli; decreasing stress can decrease confusion and changes in behavior. PLST instruction of caregivers has had a positive influence on response to problem behaviors. A typical PLST care plan includes a structured routine with regular rest periods. Teach the family compensatory modifications of the environment; for example, reduce the temperature on the hot water heater to prevent scalding; replace the toilet seat with one of contrasting color to aid visualization; remove mirrors to reduce misinterpretation of environmental stimuli (Gerdner, Buckwalter, & Reed, 2002).*

- • Instruct the family and care providers that faith, humor, patience, and contact with friends and family have been identified as positive approaches in keeping a client with dementia engaged in their care. **EBN:** *This has been found to work in keeping a client with dementia from displaying passive behaviors (Colling, 2004).*
- • Discuss with the family what to expect as the dementia progresses.
- ▲ Counsel the family about resources available regarding end-of-life decisions and legal concerns.
- ▲ Inform the family that as dementia progresses, hospice care may be available in the home in the terminal stages to help the caregiver. **EBN:** *Hospice services in the late stages of dementia can help support the family with nursing services and visitation by the primary care provider, home health aides, social services personnel, volunteer visitors, and a spiritual counselor if desired as the client is dying (Boyd & Vernon, 1998).*

NOTE: The nursing diagnoses **Impaired Environmental interpretation syndrome** and **Chronic Confusion** are very similar in definition and interventions. **Impaired Environmental interpretation** must be interpreted as a syndrome when other nursing diagnoses would also apply. **Chronic Confusion** may be interpreted as the human response to a situation or situations that require a level of cognition of which the individual is no longer capable. Further research is under way to make this distinction clear to the practicing nurse.

## evolve WEBSITES FOR EDUCATION

See the EVOLVE website for World Wide Web resources for client education.

## REFERENCES


Agostinelli B, Demers K, Garrigan D et al: Targeted interventions: use of the Mini-Mental State Exam, *J Gerontol Nurs* 20(8): 15-23, 1994.

Alexopoulos GS, Silver JM, Kahn DA et al, editors: *Treatment of agitation in older persons with dementia.* Postgraduate medicine special report. Expert consesus guideline series, Minneapolis, 1998, McGraw-Hill Healthcare Information Programs.

Algase D: Wandering: a dementia-compromised behavior, *J Gerontol Nurs* 25(9):10, 1999.

Ayalon L, Arean PA: Knowledge of Alzheimer's disease in four ethnic groups of older adults, *Int J Geriatr Psychiatr* 19(1):51-7, 2004.

C

Bair B, Toth W, Johnson MA et al: Interventions for disruptive behaviors, *J Gerontol Nurs* 25(1):13-21, 1999.

Baumgarten M, Lebel P, Laprise H et al: Adult day care for the frail elderly: outcomes, satisfaction, and cost, *J Aging Health* 14(2): 237, 2002.

Beeson R, Horton-Deutsch S, Farran C et al: Loneliness and depression in caregivers of persons with Alzheimer's disease or related disorders, *Issues Ment Health Nurs* 21:779, 2000.

Bodner T, Delazer M, Kemmler G et al: Clock drawing, clock reading, clock setting, and judgment of clock faces in elderly people with dementia and depression, *J Am Geriatr Soc* 52(7):1146-1150, 2004.

Boehm S, Whall AL, Cosgrove KL et al: Behavioral analysis and nursing interventions for reducing disruptive behaviors of patients with dementia, *Appl Nurs Res* 8(3):118-122, 1995.

Borson S, Scanlan JM, Chen P et al: The Mini-Cog as a screen for dementia: validation in a population-based sample, *J Am Geriatr Soc* 51(10):1451-1454, 2003.

Bourgeois MS: *Conversing with memory impaired individuals using memory aids: a memory aid workbook,* Gaylord, Mich, 1992, Northern Speech Services.

Boyd CO, Vernon GM: Primary care of the older adult with end-stage Alzheimer's disease, *Nurse Pract* 23(4):63, 1998.

Brereton L, Nolan M: Seeking: a key activity for new family carers of stroke survivors, *J Clin Nurs* 11:22, 2002.

Briones DF, Ramirez AL, Guerrero M et al: Determining cultural and psychosocial factors in Alzheimer disease among Hispanic populations, *Alzheimer Dis Assoc Disord* 16(Suppl 2):S86-88, 2002.

Buckwalter K, Gerdner L, Kohout F et al: A nursing intervention to decrease depression in family caregivers of AD patients, *Arch Psychiatr Nurs* 13(2):80-88, 1999.

Buffum MD, Miaskowski C, Sands L et al: A pilot study of the relationship between discomfort and agitation in patients with dementia, *Geriatr Nurs* 22(2):80-85, 2001.

Burgener SC, Bakas T, Murray C et al: Effective caregiving approaches for patients with Alzheimer's disease, *Geriatr Nurs* 19(3): 121-126, 1998.

Chumbler NR, Hartmann DJ, Cody M et al: Differences by race in the health status of rural cognitively impaired Arkansans, *Clin Gerontol* 24(1/2):103-121, 2001.

Cleeland EA: Depression in people with dementia, *Home Healthc Nurse* 15:781, 1997.

Cochran M: Tears have no color, *Am J Nurs* 98(6):53, 1998.

Cohen-Mansfield J, Golander H, Arnheim G: Self-identity in older persons suffering from dementia: preliminary results, *Soc Sci Med* 51(3):381, 2000.

Colling KB: Caregiver interventions for passive behaviors in dementia: links to the NDB model, *Aging Ment Health* 8(2):117-125, 2004.

Cox C: Race and caregiving: patterns of service use by African-American and white caregivers of persons with Alzheimer's, *J Gerontol Soc Work* 32(2):5, 1999.

Crist JD: Mexican American elders' use of skilled home care nursing services, *Public Health Nurs* 19(5):366, 2002.

Cucinotta D, Reggiani A, Galleiti L et al: Preventive Comprehensive Assessment (PCA): a new screening method for subclinical cognitive problems, *Arch Gerontol Geriatr* (Suppl 9):97, 2004.

Di Gioacchino CF, Ronzoni S, Mariano A et al: Home care prevents cognitive and functional decline in frail elderly, *Arch Gerontol Geriatr* (Suppl 9):121, 2004.

Doody RS, Stevens JC, Beck C et al: Practice parameter: management of dementia (an evidence-based review). Report of the Quality Standards Subcommittee of the American Academy of Neurology, *Neurology* 56(9):1154-1166, 2001.

Doswell W, Erlen J: Multicultural issues and ethical concerns in the delivery of nursing care interventions, *Nurs Clin North Am* 33(2):353, 1998.

Espino DV, Jules-Bradley AC, Johnston CL et al: Diagnostic approach to the confused elderly patient, *Am Fam Physician* 57(6): 1358, 1998.

Fabris F, Molaschi M, Aimonino N et al: Home care for demented subjects: new models of care and home care allowance, *Arch Gerontol Geriatr* (Suppl 9):155, 2004.

Feil N: *The validation breakthrough: simple techniques for communicating with people with Alzheimer's-type dementia,* Baltimore, 1993, Health Professions.

Fine J, Rouse-Bane S: Using validation techniques to improve communication with cognitively impaired older adults, *J Gerontol Nurs* 21(6):39, 1995.

Finley B: Nutritional needs of the person with Alzheimer's disease: practical approaches to quality care, *J Am Diet Assoc* 97(Suppl 10):S177, 1997.

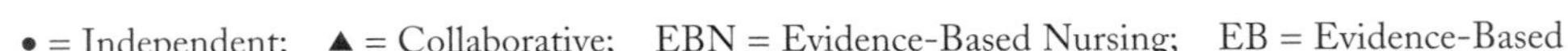

Fuchs-Lacelle S, Hadjistavropoulos T: Development and preliminary validation of the Pain Assessment Checklist for Seniors with Limited Ability to Communicate (PACSLAC), *Pain Manag Nurs* 5(1):37-49, 2004.

Gerdner LA, Buckwalter KC: A nursing challenge: assessment and management of agitation in Alzheimer's patients, *J Gerontol Nurs* 20(4):11, 1994.

Gerdner LA, Buckwalter KC, Reed D: Impact of a psychoeducational intervention on caregiver response to behavior problems, *Nurs Res* 51(6):363, 2002.

Gitlin LN: Effectiveness of home environmental interventions for individuals with dementia and family caregivers, *Home Health Care Consult* 8(9):22, 2001.

Guarnaccia P: Multicultural experiences of family caregiving: a study of African American, European American, and Hispanic American families, *New Dir Ment Health Serv* 77:45, 1998.

Guttman R: Case management of the frail elderly in the community, *Clin Nurs Spec* 13(4):174, 1999.

Haley WE, West CA, Wadley VG et al: Psychological, social, and health impact of caregiving: a comparison of black and white dementia family caregivers and noncaregivers, *Psychol Aging* 10(4):540, 1995.

Hall GR, Buckwalter KC, Stolley JM et al: Standardized care plan: managing Alzheimer's patients at home, *J Gerontol Nurs* 21(1): 37, 1995.

Hall GR, Buckwalter KC: *Bathing persons with dementia,* Iowa City, Ia, 1999, University of Iowa Gerontological Nursing Interventions Research Center.

Heineken J: Patient silence is not necessarily client satisfaction: communication in home care nursing, *Home Health Nurse* 16(2): 115, 1998.

Hinrichsen GA, Ramirez M: Black and white dementia caregivers: a comparison of their adaptation, *Gerontologist* 32(3):375, 1992.

Kaasalainen S, Crook J: An exploration of seniors' ability to report pain, *Clin Nurs Res* 13(3):199-215, 2004.

Katz IR, Jeste DV, Mintzer JE et al: Comparison of risperidone and placebo for psychosis and behavioral disturbances with dementia: a randomized, double-blind trial. Risperidone Study Group, *J Clin Psychiatry* 60(2):107-115, 1999.

Kim SY, Karlawish JH, Caine ED: Current state of research on decision-making competence of cognitively impaired elderly persons, *Am J Geriatr Psychiatry* 10:151, 2002.

Kovach CR, Wells T: Pacing of activity as a predictor of agitation for persons with dementia in acute care, *J Gerontol Nurs* 22:28, 2002.

Kuhn D, Fulton BR: Efficacy of an educational program for relatives of persons in the early stages of Alzheimer's disease, *J Gerontol Soc Work* 42(3/4):109-130, 2004.

Leininger MM, McFarland MR: *Transcultural nursing: concepts, theories, research and practices*, ed 3, New York, 2002, McGraw-Hill.

Maxfield MC, Lewis RE, Cannon S: Training staff to prevent aggressive behavior of cognitively impaired elderly patients during bathing and grooming, *J Gerontol Nurs* 22(1):37, 1996.

McGrath P, Vun M, McLeod L: Needs and experiences of non-English-speaking hospice patients and families in an English-speaking country, *Am J Hosp Palliat Care* 18(5):305, 2001.

Nolan BAD, Mathews RM: Facilitating resident information seeking regarding meals in a special care unit: an environmental design intervention, *J Gerontol Nurs* 30(10):12-16, 55-56, 2004.

Nurses Drug Alert: Delirium with single dose of diphenhydramine, *Nurses Drug Alert* 19(1):4, 1995.

Painter J: Home environment considerations for people with Alzheimer's disease, *Occup Ther Health Care* 10(3):45, 1996.

Perry J: Wives giving care to husbands with Alzheimer's disease: a process of interpretive caring, *Res Nurs Health* 25:307, 2002.

Rempusheski VF, Hurley AC: Advance directives and dementia, *J Gerontol Nurs* 26(10):27, 2000.

Roberts JS, Connell CM, Cisewski D et al: Differences between African Americans and whites in their perceptions of Alzheimer disease, *Alzheimer Dis Assoc Disord* 17(1):19-26, 2003.

Savorani G, Chattat R, Capelli E et al: Immediate effectiveness of the "new identity" reality orientation therapy (ROT) for people with dementia in a geriatric day hospital, *Arch Gerontol Geriatr* (Suppl 9):359, 2004.

Schuurmans MJ, Deschamps PI, Markham SW et al: The measurement of delirium: review of scales, *Res Theory Nurs Pract* 17(3): 207-224, 2003.

Sink KM, Covinsky KE, Newcomer R et al: Ethnic differences in the prevalence and pattern of dementia-related behaviors, *J Am Geriatr Soc* 52(8):1277-1283, 2004.

Sloane PD: Advances in the treatment of Alzheimer's disease, *Am Fam Physician* 58(7):1577, 1998.

Smith GB: Case management guideline: Alzheimer disease and other dementias, *Lippincotts Case Manag* 7:77, 2002.

Snyder M, Egan EC, Burns KR: Interventions for decreasing agitation behaviors in persons with dementia, *J Gerontol Nurs* 21(7): 34, 1995.
Somboontanont W, Sloane PD, Floyd FJ et al: Assaultive behavior in Alzheimer's disease: identifying immediate antecedents during bathing, *J Gerontol Nurs* 30(9):22-29, 55-56, 2004.
Son G, Therrien B, Whall A: Implicit memory and familiarity among elders with dementia, *J Nurs Sch* 34:263, 2002.
Spector A, Orrell M, Davies S et al: Reality orientation for dementia, *Cochrane Database Syst Rev* (3):CD001119, 2000.
Stolley JM: When your patient has Alzheimer's disease, *Am J Nurs* 94(8):34, 1994.
Thompsell A, Lovestone S: Out of sight out of mind? Support and information given to distant and near relatives of those with dementia, *Int J Geriatr Psychiatry* 17:804, 2002.
Tichawa U: Creating a continuum of care for elderly individuals, *J Gerontol Nurs* 28:46, 2002.
Tinetti ME, Liu WL, Ginter SF: Mechanical restraint use and fall-related injuries among residents of skilled nursing facilities, *Ann Intern Med* 116:369, 1992.
Watari KF, Gatz M: Pathways to care for Alzheimer's disease among Korean Americans, *Cultur Divers Ethnic Minor Psychol* 1(1): 23-28, 2004.
Woods P, Ashley J: Simulated presence therapy: using selected memories to manage problem behaviors in Alzheimer's disease patients, *Geriatr Nurs* 16(1):9-14, 1995.
Zarit J: A tribute to adaptability: mental illness and dementia in intimate late-life relationships, *Generations* 25(2):70, 2001.

# Constipation

evolve

*Betty J. Ackley*

**NANDA**

## Definition

Decrease in normal frequency of defecation, accompanied by difficult or incomplete passage of stool and/or passage of excessively hard, dry stool

## Defining Characteristics

Change in bowel pattern; bright red blood with stool; presence of soft, pastelike stool in rectum; distended abdomen; dark, black, or tarry stool; increased abdominal pressure; percussed abdominal dullness; pain with defecation; decreased volume of stool; straining with defecation; decreased frequency of stool; dry, hard, formed stool; palpable rectal mass; feeling of rectal fullness or pressure; abdominal pain; inability to pass

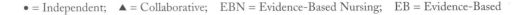

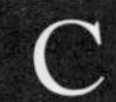

stool; anorexia; headache; change in abdominal growling (borborygmi); indigestion; atypical presentation in older adults (e.g., change in mental status, urinary incontinence, unexplained falls, elevated body temperature); severe flatus; generalized fatigue; hypoactive or hyperactive bowel sounds; palpable abdominal mass; abdominal tenderness with or without palpable muscle resistance; nausea and/or vomiting; oozing of liquid stool

## Related Factors (r/t)

### Functional

Recent environmental changes; habitual denial or ignoring of urge to defecate; insufficient physical activity; irregular defecation habits; inadequate toileting (e.g., timeliness, positioning for defecation, privacy); abdominal muscle weakness

### Psychological

Depression, emotional stress, mental confusion

### Pharmacological

Antilipemic agents; overdose of laxatives; calcium carbonate; aluminum-containing antacids; nonsteroidal antiinflammatory drugs (NSAIDs); opiates; anticholinergics; diuretics; iron salts; phenothiazines; sedatives; sympathomimetics; bismuth salts; antidepressants; calcium channel blockers

### Mechanical

Rectal abscess or ulcer; pregnancy; rectal anal fissure; tumor; megacolon (Hirschsprung's disease); electrolyte imbalance; rectal prolapse; prostate enlargement; neurological impairment; rectal anal stricture; rectocele; postsurgical obstruction; hemorrhoids; obesity

### Physiological

Poor eating habits, decreased motility of gastrointestinal tract, inadequate dentition or oral hygiene, insufficient fiber intake, insufficient fluid intake, change in usual foods and eating patterns, dehydration

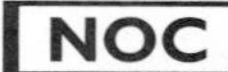

## Outcomes (Nursing Outcomes Classification)

### Suggested NOC Outcomes

Bowel Elimination, Hydration

**Example NOC Outcome with Indicators**

**Bowel Elimination** as evidenced by the following indicators: Elimination pattern in expected range/Stool soft and formed/Passage of stool without aids/Ease of stool passage (Rate each indicator of **Bowel Elimination:** 1 = severely compromised, 2 = substantially compromised, 3 = moderately compromised, 4 = mildly compromised, 5 = not compromised [see Section I].)

## Client Outcomes

**Client Will (Specify Time Frame):**

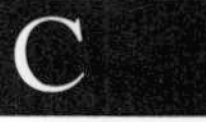

- Maintain passage of soft, formed stool every 1 to 3 days without straining
- State relief from discomfort of constipation
- Identify measures that prevent or treat constipation

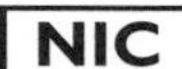

## Interventions (Nursing Interventions Classification)

### Suggested NIC Intervention

Constipation/Impaction Management

| Example NIC Activities—Constipation/Impaction Management |
| --- |
| Identify factors (e.g., medications, bed rest, and diet) that may cause or contribute to constipation/impaction |

## Nursing Interventions and Rationales

- • Assess usual pattern of defecation, including time of day, amount and frequency of stool, consistency of stool; history of bowel habits or laxative use; diet, including fluid intake; exercise patterns; personal remedies for constipation; obstetrical/ gynecological history; surgeries; alterations in perianal sensation; present bowel regimen. *There often are multiple reasons for constipation; the first step is assessment of the usual patterns of bowel elimination.*
- • Have the client or family keep a diary of bowel habits using a Management of Constipation Assessment Inventory, including information such as time of day; usual stimulus; consistency, amount, and frequency of stool; fluid consumption; and use of any aids to defecation. **EBN:** *A diary of bowel habits is valuable in treatment of constipation; the use of a diary has proven to be more accurate than client recall in determining the presence of constipation (Karam & Nies, 1994; Hinrichs et al, 2001).*
- ▲ Review the client's current medications. **EB:** *Many medications are associated with chronic constipation including opiates, antidepressants, antispasmodics, diuretics, anticonvulsants, and antacids containing aluminum (Talley et al, 2003).*
- ▲ If the client is receiving opioids, request an order for stool softeners from the primary care practitioner and institute a bowel regimen before the onset of constipation. *The use of opioids is commonly associated with constipation because of decreased peristalsis, and prevention is the best route of action.*
- • If new onset of constipation, determine if the client has recently stopped smoking. **EB:** *Constipation happens in one in six people who stop smoking and in some people can be very severe (Hajek, Gillison, & McRobbie, 2003).*
- • Palpate for abdominal distention, percuss for dullness, and auscultate bowel sounds. *In clients with constipation the abdomen is often distended, with abdominal rigidity and tenderness and a palpable colon. Bowel sounds will be present (Hinrichs et al, 2001).*
- ▲ Check for impaction; if present, perform digital removal per physician's order. *If im-*

C

*paction is present, manual removal is necessary before a bowel routine can be instituted (Hinrichs et al, 2001).*

▲ If the client is uncomfortable or in pain due to constipation or has acute or chronic constipation that does not respond to increased fiber, fluid, activity, and appropriate toileting, refer the client to the primary care practitioner for an evaluation of bowel function and health status. *There can be multiple causes of constipation, such as hypothyroidism, depression, somatization, bowel obstruction, and Hirschsprung's disease (Arce, Ermocilla, & Costa, 2002).*

- Provide privacy for defecation. Help the client to the bathroom and close the door if possible. *Toileting is recommended 5 to 15 minutes after meals, especially after breakfast when the gastrocolic reflex is strongest (Hinrichs et al, 2001). Bowel elimination is a very private act, and a lack of privacy can contribute to constipation (Weeks, Hubbartt, & Michaels, 2000).*
- Ask the client to keep a food log of the foods eaten during the last 24 hours. If needed, instruct the client in the need to eat five to nine fruits and vegetables per day, and at least three servings of whole-grain foods. *If the client eats a healthy diet with sufficient fruits and vegetables and sufficient servings of whole-grains foods, the soluble and insoluble fiber that is present in the foods will naturally prevent constipation.*
- Encourage fiber intake of 25 to 30 g/day for adults. Emphasize foods such as fresh fruits, beans, vegetables, and bran cereals. Add fiber to diet gradually with increased intake of fluids. **EBN:** *A daily intake of 25 to 30 g of fiber can increase the frequency of stools in clients with constipation (Ouellet et al, 1996; Cheskin et al, 1995; Gibson et al, 1995). Fiber helps prevent constipation by giving stool bulk. Add fiber to the diet gradually, because a sudden increase can cause bloating, gas, and diarrhea (Doughty, 1996).* **EB:** *Dietary supplements of fiber in the form of bran or wheat fiber are helpful for women experiencing constipation during pregnancy (Jewell & Young, 2001). Increasing fiber is helpful for some clients with constipation, but also can make other cases of constipation worse (Muller-Lissner et al, 2005).*
- Use a mixture of 1 cup of bran cereal, 1 cup applesauce, and 1 cup of prune juice; begin administration in small amounts and gradually increase amount. Keep refrigerated. Always check with the primary care practitioner before initiating this intervention. It is important that the client also ingest sufficient fluids. **EBN:** *This bran mixture has been shown to be effective even with short-term use in elderly clients recovering from acute conditions. NOTE: Giving fiber without sufficient fluid has resulted in worsening of constipation (Muller-Lissner et al, 2005). A study involving institutionalized elderly men with chronic constipation demonstrated that, with use of a bran mixture, clients were able to discontinue use of oral laxatives (Howard, West, & Ossip-Klein, 2000). A number of bran mixtures have been shown to effectively decrease constipation (Gibson et al, 1995; Beverley & Travis, 1992), including a mixture known as "power pudding" (Neal, 1995).*

▲ If client would prefer to increase fiber intake using a pill, recommend that client use a tablet that contains methylcellulose. **EB:** *A study demonstrated that 75% of clients using caplets containing methylcellulose had very good or excellent results in resolution of constipation (Smith, Hellebusch, & Mandel, 2003).*

- Encourage a fluid intake of 1.5 to 2 L/day (6 to 8 glasses of liquids per day). If oral in-

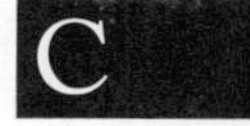

take is low, gradually increase fluid intake. *Fluid intake must be within the cardiac and renal reserve. Increasing fluid intake to 1.5 to 2 L/day while maintaining a fiber intake of 25 g can significantly increase the frequency of stools in clients with constipation (Weeks, Hubbartt, & Michaels, 2000; Anti, 1998).* **EB:** *Increasing fluid intake is not helpful for constipation alone or else the client is dehydrated (Muller-Lissner, 2005).*

- • Encourage the client to be out of bed as soon as possible and to perform the activities of daily living himself or herself as able. Encourage exercise such as turning and changing positions in bed, lifting the hips off the bed, performing range-of-motion exercises, alternately lifting each knee to the chest, doing wheelchair lifts, doing waist twists, stretching the arms away from the body, and pulling in the abdomen while taking deep breaths. *Activity, even minimal, increases peristalsis, which is necessary to prevent constipation (Weeks, Hubbartt, & Michaels, 2000).* **EB and EBN:** *Increases in activity do not appear to relieve chronic constipation (Annels & Koch, 2003; Lembo & Carilleri, 2003).*
- • Initiate a regular schedule for defecation, using the client's normal evacuation time whenever possible. Offer hot coffee, hot lemon water, or prune juice before breakfast, or while the client sits on the toilet if necessary. An optimal time for many individuals is 30 minutes after breakfast because of the gastrocolic reflex. *Establishing a schedule gives the client a sense of control, but more importantly it promotes evacuation before drying of stool and constipation occur. Ingestion of hot liquids can stimulate peristalsis and result in defecation (Weeks, Hubbartt, & Michaels, 2000).*
- • Help the client onto a bedside commode or toilet with the client's hips flexed and feet flat.
- • Have the client deep breathe through the mouth to encourage relaxation of the pelvic floor muscle and use the abdominal muscles to help evacuation.
- ▲ Provide laxatives, suppositories, and enemas only as needed if other more natural interventions are not effective, and as ordered only; establish a client goal of eliminating their use. *Use of stimulant laxatives should be avoided because they result in laxative dependence and loss of normal bowel function (Merli & Graham, 2003).*
- • Avoid the use of both soapsuds and tap water enemas if possible, or use a low concentration of Castile soap only. If enemas are ordered, measure the amount of fluid given and the amount expelled. *Enema fluid can be retained, and this retained fluid can be harmful for the client prone to fluid overload.* **EBN:** *Soap sud enemas can damage the colonic mucosa (Schmelzer & Wright, 1993). The use of a soapsuds enema was shown to increase stool output compared with a tap water enema in preoperative liver transplant clients; the amount of mucosal irritation was unknown. Several clients retained large amounts of fluid (Schmelzer et al, 2000).*
- ▲ For the stable neurological client, consider use of a bowel routine of a Therevac enema instead of suppositories every other day. For persistent constipation, refer to a physician for evaluation. **EBN:** *Use of the Therevac SB minienema was found to reduce the time needed for bowel care by as much as 1 hour or more compared with the use of suppositories (Dunn & Galka, 1994).*

## Geriatric

- • Explain the importance of adequate fiber intake, fluid intake, activity, and established toileting routines to ensure soft, formed stool. *Fiber intake, fluid intake, and activity*

C

*are often decreased in elderly clients. Increasing fiber and fluids can effectively prevent constipation in the elderly (Hinrichs et al, 2001).* **EB:** *Increasing activity has been shown to be helpful for the elderly with constipation (Muller-Lissner, 2005).* **EBN:** *A study involving institutionalized elderly men with chronic constipation demonstrated that, with use of a bran mixture, clients were able to discontinue use of oral laxatives (Howard, West, & Ossip-Klein, 2000).*

- • Determine the client's perception of normal bowel elimination; promote adherence to a regular schedule. *Misconceptions regarding the frequency of bowel movements can lead to anxiety and overuse of laxatives.*
- • Explain Valsalva maneuver and the reason it should be avoided. *Valsalva maneuver can cause bradycardia and even death in cardiac clients.*
- • Respond quickly to the client's call for help with toileting.
- • Avoid regular use of enemas in the elderly. *Enemas can cause fluid and electrolyte imbalances and damage to the colonic mucosa (Schmelzer & Wright, 1993).*
- ▲ Use opioids cautiously. If they are ordered, use stool softeners and bran mixtures to prevent constipation. *Use of opioids can cause constipation (Kurz & Sessler, 2003).*
- • Position the client on the toilet or commode and place a small footstool under the feet. *Placing a small footstool under the feet increases intraabdominal pressure and makes defecation easier for an elderly client with weak abdominal muscles.*

## Home Care

- • The interventions described previously may be adapted for home care use.
- • Take complaints seriously and evaluate claims of constipation in a matter-of-fact manner. *Continued constipation can lead to bowel obstruction, a medical emergency. Use of a matter-of-fact manner will limit positive reinforcement of the behavior if actual constipation does not exist.* Refer to the care plan for **Perceived Constipation.**
- • Assess the self-care management activities the client is already using. **EBN:** *Many older adults seek solutions to constipation, with laxative use a frequent remedy that creates its own problems (Annells & Koch, 2002).*
- • The following treatment recommendations have been offered (Annells & Koch, 2002):
  - ■ Acknowledge the client's life-long experience of bowel function; respect beliefs, attitudes, and preferences, and avoid patronizing responses.
  - ■ Make available comprehensive, useful written information about constipation and possible solutions.
  - ■ Make available empathetic and accessible professional care to provide treatment and advice; a multidisciplinary approach (including physician, nurse, and pharmacist) should be used.
  - ■ Institute a bowel management program.
  - ■ Consider affordability when suggesting solutions to constipation; discuss cost-saving strategies.
  - ■ Discuss a range of solutions to constipation and allow the client to choose the preferred options.
  - ■ Have orders in place for a suppository and enema as the need may occur.

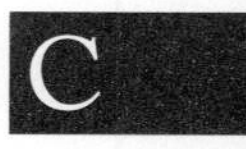

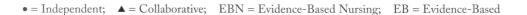

*As part of a bowel management program, suppositories or enemas may become necessary (Annels & Koch, 2002).*

- Although the use of a bedside commode may be necessitated by the client's condition, allow the client to use the toilet in the bathroom when possible and provide assistance. *Bowel elimination is a very private act, and a lack of privacy can contribute to constipation (Weeks, Hubbartt, & Michaels, 2000).*
- In older clients, routinely advise consumption of fluids, fruits, and vegetables as part of the diet, and ambulation if the client is able. Introduce a bowel management program at the first sign of constipation. *Constipation is a major problem for terminally ill or hospice clients, who may need very high doses of opioids for pain management (Miller & Miller, 2002).*
- ▲ Refer for consideration of the use of polyethylene glycol 3350 (PEG-3350) for constipation. **EBN:** *In a study of PEG-3350 use for idiopathic constipation, researchers concluded that it appeared to be safe and efficacious when dietary and lifestyle changes were ineffective. Clients reported increased perceived bowel control, with reduced complaints of straining, stool hardness, bloating, and gas (Stoltz et al, 2001).* **EB:** *There is good evidence to support the use of PEG for chronic constipation (Ramkumar & Rao, 2005).*
- Advise the client against attempting to remove impacted feces on his or her own. *Older or confused clients in particular may attempt to remove feces and cause rectal damage.*
- Instruct the client and family in appropriate expectations for having bowel movements. *The client and family may have unrealistic expectations regarding the frequency and type of bowel movements. Failure to so instruct may result in the client's and family's acting on expectations and resorting to laxatives inappropriately.*
- When using a bowel program, establish a pattern that is very regular and allows the client to be part of the family unit. *Regularity of the program promotes psychological and/or physiological readiness to evacuate stool. Families of home care clients often cannot proceed with normal daily activities until bowel programs are complete.*

## Client/Family Teaching

- Instruct the client on normal bowel function and the need for adequate fluid and fiber intake, activity, and a defined toileting pattern in a bowel program.
- Encourage the client to heed defecation warning signs and develop a regular schedule of defecation by using a stimulus such as a warm drink or prune juice. *Most cases of constipation are mechanical and result from habitual neglect of impulses that signal the appropriate time for defecation. The reflex that causes the urge to defecate diminishes after a few minutes and may remain quiet for several hours; as a result, the stool becomes hardened and more difficult to expel (American Academy of Family Physicians, 2005; Folden, 2002).*
- Encourage the client to avoid long-term use of laxatives and enemas and to gradually withdraw from their use if they are used regularly. *Use of stimulant laxatives should be avoided, long-term use can result in dependence on laxative for defecation (American Academy of Family Physicians, 2005).*
- If not contraindicated, teach the client how to do bent-leg sit-ups to increase abdominal tone; also encourage the client to contract the abdominal muscles frequently

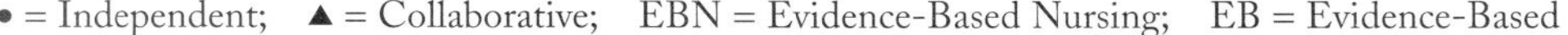

throughout the day. Help the client develop a daily exercise program to increase peristalsis.

C

## evolve WEBSITES FOR EDUCATION

See the EVOLVE website for World Wide Web resources for client education.

## REFERENCES


American Academy of Family Physicians: Information from your family doctor: constipation, *Am Fam Physician* 71(3):539-540, 2005.

Annells M, Koch T: Older people seeking solutions to constipation: the laxative mire, *J Clin Nurs* 11:603, 2002.

Anti M: Water supplementation enhances the effect of high-fiber diet on stool frequency and laxative consumption in adult patients with functional constipation, *Hepatogastroenterology* 45(21):727, 1998.

Arce DA, Ermocilla CA, Costa H: Evaluation of constipation, *Am Fam Physician* 65:11, 2002.

Beverley L, Travis I: Constipation: proposed natural laxative mixtures, *J Gerontol Nurs* 18(10):5, 1992.

Cheskin LJ, Kamal N, Crowell MD et al: Mechanisms of constipation in older persons and effects of fiber compared with placebo, *J Am Geriatr Soc* 43(6):666-669, 1995.

Doughty D: A physiologic approach to bowel training, *J Wound Ostomy Continence Nurs* 23(1):46, 1996.

Dunn KL, Galka ML: A comparison of the effectiveness of Therevac SB and bisacodyl suppositories in SCI patients' bowel programs, *Rehabil Nurs* 19:334, 1994.

Gibson CJ, Opalka PC, Moore CA et al: Effectiveness of bran supplement on the bowel management of elderly rehabilitation patients, *J Gerontol Nurs* 21(10):21, 1995.

Hajek P, Gillison F, McRobbie H: Stopping smoking can cause constipation, *Addiction* 98(11):1563, 2003.

Hinrichs M, Huseboe J, Tang JH et al: Research-based protocol. Management of constipation, *J Gerontol Nurs* 27(2):17, 2001.

Howard LV, West D, Ossip-Klein DJ: Chronic constipation management for institutionalized older adults, *Geriatr Nurs* 21(2):78, 2000.

Jewell DJ, Young G: Interventions for treating constipation in pregnancy, *Cochrane Database Syst Rev,* (2):CD001142, 2001.

Karam SE, Nies DM: Student/staff collaboration: a pilot bowel management program, *J Gerontol Nurs* 20:3, 1994.

Kurz A, Sessler DI: Opiod-induced bowel dysfunction: pathophysiology and potential new therapies, *Drugs* 63:7, 2003.

Lembo A, Camilleri M: Current concepts in chronic constipation, *New Engl J Med* 349:14, 2003.

Merli GJ, Graham MG: Three steps to better management of constipation, *Patient Care,* 37:6, 2003.

Miller KE, Miller M: Managing common gastrointestinal symptoms at the end of life, *J Hosp Palliat Nurs* 4:1, 2002.

Muller-Lissner SA, Kamm MA, Scarpignato C et al: Myths and misconceptions about constipation, *AM J Gastroenterol* 100(1): 232-242, 2005.

Neal LJ: "Power pudding": natural laxative therapy for the elderly who are homebound, *Home Healthcare Nurse* 13(3):66, 1995.

Ouellet LL, Turner TR, Pond S et al: Dietary fiber and laxation in postop orthopedic patients, *Clin Nurs Res* 5:4, 1996.

Ramkumar D, Rao SS: Efficacy and safety of traditional medical therapies for chonic constipation: systematic review, *Am J Gastroenterol* 100(4):936-971, 2005.

Schmelzer M, Case P, Chappell SM et al: Colonic cleansing, fluid absorption, and discomfort following tap water and soapsuds enemas, *Appl Nurs Res* 13(2):83, 2000.

Schmelzer M, Wright K: Working smart, *Am J Nurs* 93:55, 1993.

Smith C, Hellebusch SJ, Mandel KG: Patient and physician evaluation of a new bulk fiber laxative tablet, *Gastroenterol Nurs* 26(1): 31, 2003.

Stolz R, Weiss LM, Merkin DH et al: An efficacy and consumer preference study of polyethylene glycol 3350 for the treatment of constipation in regular laxative users, *Home Healthc Consult* 8(2):21, 2001.

Talley NJ, Jones M, Nuyts G et al: Risk factors for chronic constipation based on a general practice sample, *Am J Gastroenterol* 98(5):1107, 2003.

Weeks SK, Hubbartt E, Michaels TK: Keys to bowel success, *Rehabil Nurs* 25(2):66, 2000.

Wong PN, Kadakia S: How to deal with chronic constipation, *Postgrad Med* 106(6):199, 1999.

# Perceived Constipation

*Betty J. Ackley*

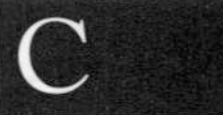

## NANDA

### Definition

Self-diagnosis of constipation and abuse of laxatives, enemas, and suppositories to ensure a daily bowel movement

### Defining Characteristics

Expectation of a daily bowel movement that results in overuse of laxatives, enemas, and suppositories; expectation of a passage of stool at same time every day

### Related Factors (r/t)

Cultural or family health beliefs, faulty appraisals, impaired thought processes

## NOC

### Outcomes (Nursing Outcomes Classification)

#### Suggested NOC Outcomes

Bowel Elimination, Health Beliefs, Health Beliefs: Perceived Threat

#### Example NOC Outcome with Indicators

**Bowel Elimination** as evidenced by the following indicators: Elimination pattern/Stool soft and formed/Passage of stool without aids/Ease of stool passage (Rate each indicator of **Bowel Elimination:** 1 = severely compromised, 2 = substantially compromised, 3 = moderately compromised, 4 = mildly compromised, 5 = not compromised [see Section I].)

### Client Outcomes

#### Client Will (Specify Time Frame):

- Regularly defecate soft, formed stool without using any aids
- Explain the need to decrease or eliminate the use of stimulant laxatives, suppositories, and enemas
- Identify alternatives to stimulant laxatives, enemas, and suppositories for ensuring defecation
- Explain that defecation does not have to occur every day

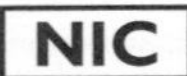

## Interventions (Nursing Interventions Classification)

### Suggested NIC Interventions

Bowel Management; Medication Management

| Example NIC Activities—Bowel Management |
|---|
| Note preexistent bowel problems, bowel routine, and use of laxatives |

## Nursing Interventions and Rationales

- Have the client keep a diary of bowel habits using a Management of Constipation Assessment Inventory, including information such as time of day; usual stimulus; consistency, amount, and frequency of stool; fluid consumption; and use of any aids to defecation. **EBN:** *A diary of bowel habits is valuable in the treatment of constipation; the use of a diary has proven to be more accurate than client recall in determining the presence of constipation (Hinrichs et al, 2001; Karam & Nies, 1994).*
- Determine the client's perception of an appropriate defecation pattern. *The client may need to be taught that one bowel movement every 1 to 3 days is normal (American Academy of Family Physicians, 2005).*
- Monitor the use of laxatives, suppositories, or enemas and suggest replacing them with increased fiber intake along with increased fluids to 2 L/day. *Long-term use of laxatives may result in a cathartic colon, with the inability to have a bowel movement without use of laxatives (Hinrichs et al, 2001). An increase in fiber intake to 25 to 30 g/day along with an increase in fluid intake can help clients with chronic constipation (Wong & Kadakia, 1999).*
- Ask the client to keep a food log of the foods eaten for the last 24 hours or recall the usual foods eaten. If necessary, teach the client the need to eat at least five and preferably nine servings of fruits and vegetables per day, and at least three servings of whole-grain foods (American Academy of Family Physicians, 2005). *If the client eats a healthy diet with sufficient fruits and vegetables and servings of whole-grains foods, the soluble and insoluble fiber that is present in the foods will naturally prevent constipation.*
- Use a mixture of 1 cup of bran cereal, 1 cup applesauce, and 1 cup prune juice; begin administration in small amounts and gradually increase amount. Keep refrigerated. Always check with the primary care practitioner before initiating this intervention. It is important that the client also ingest sufficient fluids. **EBN:** *This bran mixture has been shown to be effective even with short-term use in elderly clients recovering from acute conditions. Note: Giving fiber without sufficient fluid has resulted in worsening of constipation (Muller-Lissner et al, 2005). A study involving institutionalized elderly men with chronic constipation demonstrated that, with use of a bran mixture, clients were able to discontinue use of oral laxatives (Howard, West, & Ossip-Klein, 2000). A number of bran mixtures have been shown to effectively decrease constipation (Gibson et al, 1995; Beverley & Travis, 1992), including a mixture known as "power pudding" (Neal, 1995).*

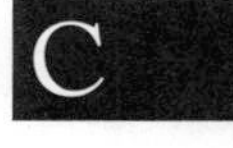

- If client would prefer to increase fiber intake using a pill, recommend that client use a tablet that contains methylcellulose. **EB:** *A study demonstrated that 75% of clients using caplets containing methylcellulose had very good or excellent results in resolution of constipation (Smith, Hellebusch, & Mandel, 2003).*
- Encourage the client to respond promptly to the defecation reflex. *The reflex that causes the urge to defecate diminishes after a few minutes and may remain quiet for several hours; as a result, the stool becomes hardened and more difficult to expel (Folden, 2002).*
- ▲ If the client is uncomfortable or in pain due to constipation or has chronic constipation that does not respond to increased fiber and fluid intake, activity, and appropriate toileting, refer the client to a gastroenterologist for an evaluation of bowel function and health status. *The multiple causes of constipation include hypothyroidism, depression, somatization, bowel obstruction, and Hirschsprung's disease (Arce, Ermocilla, & Costa, 2002).*
- ▲ Obtain a dietary referral for analysis of the client's diet and input on how to improve the diet to ensure adequate fiber intake and nutrition.
- ▲ Assess for signs of depression, a sedentary lifestyle, a history of sexual abuse, and obesity. Refer for counseling as appropriate. *All of these factors can contribute to constipation (Wong & Kadakia, 1999).*
- Encourage the client to increase activity, walking for at least 30 minutes at least 5 days a week as tolerated. *Increased activity increases bowel motility, which decreases constipation (Hinrichs et al, 2001). Not being active predisposes to constipation (American Academy of Family Physicians, 2005).*
- ▲ Observe for the presence of an eating disorder, the use of laxatives to control or decrease weight; refer for counseling if needed.

## Home Care

- The interventions described previously may be adapted for home care use.
- Take complaints seriously and evaluate claims of constipation in a matter-of-fact manner. *Continued constipation can lead to bowel obstruction, a medical emergency. Presence of a pattern of perceived constipation does not mean actual constipation cannot occur. However, use of a matter-of-fact manner will limit positive reinforcement of the behavior.*
- Obtain family and client histories of bowel or other patterned behavior problems. *History may reveal a psychological cause for the constipation (e.g., withholding).*
- Observe family cultural patterns related to eating and bowel habits. *Cultural patterns may control bowel habits.*
- Encourage a mindset and program of self-care management. Elicit from the client the self-talk he or she uses to describe body perceptions; correct fatalistic interpretations.
- Instruct the client in a healthy lifestyle that supports normal bowel function (e.g., activity, fluid intake, diet) and encourage progressive inclusion of these elements into daily activities. *A study of cognitive patterns in individuals with somatization syndrome showed that body perceptions were assumed to be a sign of catastrophic occurrence (e.g., "physical complaints are always signs of disease") and concepts of health were very restrictive. Somatizing individuals were acutely aware of bodily sensations that would normally be considered automatic and would seek help immediately to obtain medications or other solutions. They did not participate in other types of health-seeking behavior (Rief, Hiller, & Margraf, 1998).*

- Discuss the client's self image. Help the client to reframe the self-concept as capable. *Somatizing individuals tend to see themselves as weak and therefore avoid exercise (Rief, Hiller, & Margraf, 1998). Developing the ability to see themselves as capable of self-care management may take time, as will making lifestyle changes.*
- Instruct the client and family in appropriate expectations for having bowel movements.
- Offer instruction and reassurance regarding explanations for variation from the previous pattern of bowel movements. *The client may have unrealistic expectations regarding the frequency or type of bowel movements and may assume that constipation exists when there is a reasonable explanation for deviation from the past pattern. The client may resort to the use of laxatives inappropriately.*
- Contract with the client and/or a responsible family member regarding the use of laxatives. Have the client maintain a bowel pattern diary. Observe for diarrhea or frequent evacuation. *Intermittent care does not allow for 24-hour supervision. Contracting allows guided control of care by the client in partnership with the nurse, and the diary promotes more accurate reporting.*
- ▲ Teach the family to carry out the bowel program per the physician's orders.
- ▲ Refer for home health aide services to assist with personal care, including the bowel program, if appropriate.
- Identify a contingency plan for bowel care if the client is dependent on outside persons for such care.

## Client/Family Teaching

- Explain normal bowel function and the necessary ingredients for a regular bowel regimen (e.g., fluid, fiber, activity, and regular schedule for defecation).
- Work with the client and family to develop a diet that fits the client's lifestyle and includes increased fiber.
- Teach the client that it is not necessary to have daily bowel movements and that the passage of anywhere from three stools each day to three stools each week is considered normal.
- Explain to the client the harmful effects of the continual use of defecation aids such as laxatives and enemas.
- Encourage the client to gradually decrease the use of the usual laxatives and or enemas, and recognize it may take months for the process to do it gradually (American Academy of Family Physicians, 2005).
- Determine a method of increasing the client's fluid intake and fit this practice into the client's lifestyle.
- Explain what Valsalva maneuver is and why it should be avoided.
- Work with the client and family to design a bowel training routine that is based on previous patterns (before laxative or enema abuse) and incorporates the consumption of warm fluids, increased fiber, and increased fluids; privacy; and a predictable routine.

## Additional Nursing Interventions and Rationales, Client/Family Teaching

See care plan for **Constipation.**

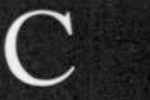

## evolve WEBSITES FOR EDUCATION

See the EVOLVE website for World Wide Web resources for client education.

## REFERENCES


American Academy of Family Physicians: Information from your family doctor: constipation, *Am Fam Physician* 71(3):539-540, 2005.

Anti M, Pignataro G, Armuzzi A et al: Water supplementation enhances the effect of high-fiber diet on stool frequency and laxative consumption in adult patients with functional constipation, *Hepatogastroenterology* 45(21):727, 1998.

Arce DA, Ermocilla CA, Costa H: Evaluation of constipation, *Am Fam Physician* 65:11, 2002.

Beverley L, Travis I: Constipation: proposed natural laxative mixtures, *J Gerontol Nurs* 18(10):5, 1992.

Folden SL: Practice guidelines for the management of constipation in adults, *Rehabil Nurs* 27(5):169, 2002.

Gibson CJ, Opalka PC, Moore CA et al: Effectiveness of bran supplement on the bowel management of elderly rehabilitation patients, *J Gerontol Nurs* 21(10):21, 1995.

Hinrichs M, Huseboe J, Tang JH et al: Research-based protocol. Management of constipation, *J Gerontol Nurs* 27(2):17, 2001.

Howard LV, West D, Ossip-Klein DJ: Chronic constipation management for institutionalized older adults, *Geriatr Nurs* 21(2):78, 2000.

Karam SE, Nies DM: Student/staff collaboration: a pilot bowel management program, *J Gerontol Nurs* 20(3):32, 1994.

Muller-Lissner SA, Kamm MA, Scarpignato C et al: Myths and misconceptions about constipation, *Am J Gastroenterol* 100(1):232-242, 2005.

Neal LJ: "Power pudding": natural laxative therapy for the elderly who are homebound, *Home Healthc Nurse* 13(3):66, 1995.

Rief W, Hiller W, Margraf J: Cognitive aspects of hypochondriasis and somatization syndrome, *J Abnorm Psychol* 107:587, 1998.

Wong PW, Kadakia S: How to deal with chronic constipation: a stepwise method of establishing and treating the source of the problem, *Postgrad Med* 106(6):199, 1999.


# Risk for Constipation

*Betty J. Ackley*

**NANDA**

## Definition

At risk for a decrease in normal frequency of defecation accompanied by difficult or incomplete passage of stool and/or passage of excessively hard, dry stool

## Related Factors (r/t)

### Functional

Habitual denial/ignoring urge to defecate; recent environmental changes; inadequate toileting (e.g., timeliness, positioning for defecation, privacy); irregular defecation habits; insufficient physical activity; abdominal muscle weakness

### Psychological

Depression; emotional stress; mental confusion

C

### Physiological

Insufficient fiber intake, dehydration, inadequate dentition or oral hygiene, poor eating habits, insufficient fluid intake, change in usual foods and eating patterns, decreased motility of gastrointestinal tract

### Pharmacological

Anticonvulsants, phenothiazines, nonsteroidal antiinflammatory agents, sedatives, aluminum-containing antacids, laxative overuse, iron salts, anticholinergics, antidepressants, antilipemic agents, calcium channel blockers, calcium carbonate, diuretics, sympathomimetics, opiates, bismuth salts

### Mechanical

Rectal abscess or ulcer; pregnancy; rectal anal structure; postsurgical obstruction; rectal and anal fissures; megacolon (Hirschsprung's disease); electrolyte imbalance; tumors; prostate enlargement; rectocele; rectal prolapse; neurological impairment; hemorrhoids; obesity

**NOC**

## Outcomes (Nursing Outcomes Classification)

### Suggested NOC Outcome

Bowel Elimination

**Example NOC Outcome with Indicators**

**Bowel Elimination** as evidenced by the following indicators: Elimination pattern/Stool soft and formed/ Passage of stool without aids/Ease of stool passage (Rate each indicator of **Bowel Elimination:** 1 = severely compromised, 2 = substantially compromised, 3 = moderately compromised, 4 = mildly compromised, 5 = not compromised [see Section I].)

## Client Outcomes

**Client Will (Specify Time Frame):**

- Maintain passage of soft, formed stool every 1 to 3 days without straining
- Identify measures that prevent constipation
- Explain rationale for not using laxatives and enemas

**NIC**

## Interventions (Nursing Interventions Classification)

### Suggested NIC Intervention

Constipation/Impaction Management

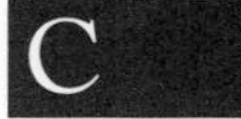


**Example NIC Activities—Constipation/Impaction Management**

Identify factors (e.g., medications, bed rest, and diet) that may cause or contribute to constipation/impaction

## Nursing Interventions and Rationales, Client/Family Teaching

See care plan for **Constipation.**

# Ineffective Coping

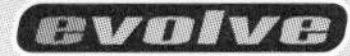


*Ann Keeley*

**NANDA**

## Definition

Inability to form a valid appraisal of internal or external stressors, inadequate choices of practiced responses, and/or inability to access or use available resources

## Defining Characteristics

Lack of goal-directed behavior or resolution of problem, including inability to attend, difficulty with organized information, sleep disturbance, abuse of chemical agents, decreased use of social support, use of forms of coping that impede adaptive behavior, poor concentration, fatigue, inadequate problem solving, verbalized inability to cope or ask for help, inability to meet basic needs, destructive behavior toward self or others, inability to meet role expectations, high illness rate, change in usual communication patterns, risk taking

## Related Factors (r/t)

Gender differences in coping strategies, inadequate level of confidence in ability to cope, uncertainty, inadequate social support created by characteristics of relationships, inadequate level of perception of control, inadequate resource availability, high degree of threat, situational crises, maturational crises, disturbance in pattern of tension release, inadequate opportunity to prepare for stressor, inability to conserve adaptive energies, disturbance in pattern of appraisal of threat

**NOC**

## Outcomes (Nursing Outcomes Classification)

### Suggested NOC Outcomes

Coping; Decision Making; Impulse Self-Control; Information Processing

C

**Example NOC Outcome with Indicators**

**Coping** as evidenced by the following indicator: Identifies effective and ineffective coping patterns; modifies lifestyle as needed (Rate the indicator of **Coping:** 1 = never demonstrated, 2 = rarely demonstrated, 3 = sometimes demonstrated, 4 = often demonstrated, 5 = consistently demonstrated [see Section I].)

## Client Outcomes

**Client Will (Specify Time Frame):**

- Verbalize ability to cope and ask for help when needed
- Demonstrate ability to solve problems related to current needs
- Remain free of destructive behavior toward self or others
- Communicate needs and negotiate with others to meet needs
- Discuss how recent or ongoing life stressors have overwhelmed normal coping strategies
- Demonstrate new effective coping strategies
- Have illness and accident rates not excessive for age and developmental level

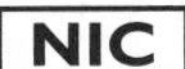

## Interventions (Nursing Interventions Classification)

### Suggested NIC Interventions

Coping Enhancement; Decision-Making Support

**Example NIC Activities—Coping Enhancement**

Assist the client in developing an objective appraisal of the event; explore with the client previous methods of dealing with problems

## Nursing Interventions and Rationales

- Observe for causes of ineffective coping such as poor self-concept, grief, lack of problem-solving skills, lack of support, or recent change in life situation. **EBN:** *Psychological manifestations of ineffective coping can be understood only after a thorough inquiry into the client's framework for appraisal (Dudley-Brown, 2002).*
- Observe for strengths such as the ability to relate the facts and to recognize the source of stressors. **EBN:** *Successful adaptation requires a coordination of efforts to fit the nursing interventions to the client's perception of the threat, personal values and beliefs, and recognition of personal strengths (Norris & Spelic, 2002).*
- Assess the risk of the client's harming self or others and intervene appropriately. See the care plan for **Risk for Suicide. EBN:** *The value an individual attaches to a stressor will affect the level and type of emotional reaction (Norris & Spelic, 2002). Hopelessness associated with depression is an indicator of a higher risk of suicidal behavior (Szanto, 2003).*

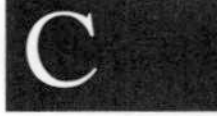

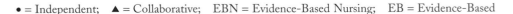

- Help the client set realistic goals and identify personal skills and knowledge. **EB:** *Providing validation of actual stressors and available coping resources and/or strategies aids in a positive adaptation to stress (Pakenham, 2001).* **EBN:** *Efforts to educate regarding possible and/or potential effects of a specific diagnosis and the resources available to assist with coping are a positive factor in successful adaptation (Wassem, Beckham, & Dudley, 2001).*
- Use empathetic communication and encourage the client and family to verbalize fears, express emotions, and set goals. **EBN:** *A nurse's holistic presence with clients is considered to be vital (Cote & Pepler, 2002). "The interview process itself can be therapeutic" (Overcash, 2004). "Health professionals could alleviate some psychological distress by spending time listening to patients and channeling their fears and worries into meaningful discussions about fatigue" (Potter, 2004). Connectedness to others helps with coping (Lin & Bauer, 2003).*
- Encourage the client to make choices and participate in the planning of care and scheduled activities. **EB:** *Active involvement in coping plans increases the possibility of a positive adjustment (Pakenham, 2001). Involving young males in the planning of a clinic increased its likelihood of success (Raine et al, 2003).* **EBN:** *The inclusion of consumer consultants in preparing discharge planning programs would increase client satisfaction (Cleary, Horsfall, & Hunt, 2003). Collaborative 'triadic' decision-making processes result in greater effectiveness of care (Dalton, 2003).*
- Provide mental and physical activities within the client's ability (e.g., reading, television, radio, crafts, outings, movies, dinners out, social gatherings, exercise, sports, games). **EBN:** *Activities that decrease stress and/or increase self-efficacy provide a positive approach to perceived stressors (Fisher & Laschinger, 2001). Nurses working with individuals with nonhealing ulcers helped them find ways to normalized their experience and positively impacted the individuals' adjustment (Hopkins, 2004).*
- If the client is physically able, encourage moderate aerobic exercise. **EBN:** *Exercise is effective in alleviating anxiety (Blanchard, Courneya, & Laing, 2001).* **EB:** *Exercise was found to improve quality of life in female cardiac patients (Tyni-Lenn et al, 2002).*
- Provide information regarding care before care is given. *When providing information take into account the client's individual coping style (Nikoletti et al, 2003). Before psychiatric clients can make decisions regarding treatment, they must have appropriate information (Linhorst et al, 2002).* **EBN:** *In women with post–breast cancer lymphedema information is necessary for informed choice with highest potential for a good outcome (Radina, 2004).*
- Discuss changes with the client before making them. **EBN:** *Nurses are pivotal in communicating to clients the information needed to ensure the best outcome. They are identified by clients as necessary in coordinating all aspects of their care (Hodgkinson & Lester, 2002).* **EBN:** *The nurse's ongoing interaction with individuals with non-healing ulcers involved honest assessment and communication (Hopkins, 2004).*
- Discuss the client's and family's power to change a situation or the need to accept a situation. **EBN:** *An honest assessment of a particular situation as shared by the nurse is important to the family's sense of what is expected of them in adapting to a health care change (Weiss & Chen, 2002).*
- Use active listening and acceptance to help the client express emotions such as sadness, guilt, and anger (within appropriate limits). **EBN:** *Nurses need to provide an opportunity for clients to address all aspects of the impact of a health status change on their lives*

C

*(Richer & Ezer, 2002). "The interview process itself can be therapeutic" (Overcash, 2004). "Health professionals could alleviate some psychological distress by spending time listening to patients and channeling their fears and worries into meaningful discussions about fatigue" (Potter, 2004). Connectedness to others helps with coping (Lin & Bauer, 2003).*

- • Encourage the client to describe previous stressors and the coping mechanisms used. **EBN:** *Recounting previous experiences that were perceived by the client as having been dealt with successfully strengthens effective coping and helps eliminate ineffective coping mechanisms (Northouse et al, 2002).* **EBN:** *Evaluation of pessimism and optimism in family members of Parkinson's patients can help identify those who are at greater risk for negative health consequences (Lyons, 2004).*
- • Be supportive of coping behaviors; allow the client time to relax. **EBN:** *Sharing of innermost cares and concerns requires that nurses provide opportunities for clients to feel safe enough to share (Richer & Ezer, 2002).* **EBN:** *The relationship the nurse has with her patient as a positive effect on the coping of individuals with nonhealing ulcers (Hopkins, 2004).*
- • Help the client to define what meaning his or her symptoms might have for the client. **EBN:** *Exploring the meaning of health status change and the adjustments required for a successful adaptation within the client's life experience fosters positive growth (Norris & Spelic, 2002; Richer & Ezer, 2002). "The most positive strategies used by the participants involved having opportunities to talk about their experience and receiving explanations about what was happening to them" (Potter, 2004).*
- • Encourage the use of cognitive behavioral relaxation (e.g., music therapy, guided imagery). **EBN:** *Relaxation training has been demonstrated to improve overall coping ability (Tyni-Lenne et al, 2002).*
- • Use distraction techniques during procedures that cause the client to be fearful. *Distraction has been demonstrated to be effective in coping with pain of older people (Blomquist & Edberg, 2002). "Virtual reality, as an emotion-focused distraction intervention, decreases the symptom distress associated with chemotherapy treatments" (Schneider et al, 2004).*
- ▲ Refer for counseling as needed. **EBN:** *Nurses are perceived as the bridge between the client and all other resources needed to manage an adaptive response to a health care change (Hodgkinson & Lester, 2002).*

### Geriatric

- • Engage the client in reminiscence. *Reminiscence activates positive memories and evokes well-being (Puentes, 2002).* **EBN:** *Life review as an intervention had a significant effect of lowering depression in individuals with cerebral vascular accident (Davis, 2004).*
- ▲ Assess and report possible physiological alterations (e.g., sepsis, hypoglycemia, hypotension, infection, changes in temperature, fluid and electrolyte imbalances, and use of medications with known cognitive and psychotropic side effects).
- • Determine if the individual is displaying a change in personality as a manifestation of difficulty with coping. *An older individual's responses to age-related stress will depend on the balance of personality strengths and weaknesses.* **EBN:** *Negative life events will vary in the degree to which they affect the symptoms observed in the elderly (Kraaij, 2001).*
- • Increase and mobilize the support available to the elderly client. Encourage interaction

with family and friends. **EBN:** *Relationships are pivotal in supporting coping in older adults (Cutcliffe & Grant, 2001).*

- Actively listen to complaints and concerns. **EBN:** *The quality of care provided to elderly chronic pain patients living at home could be improved by active listening (Blonquist, 2002).*

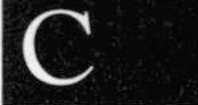


## Multicultural

- Assess for the influence of cultural beliefs, norms, and values on the client's perceptions of effective coping. *"Healthcare providers must recognize, respect, and integrate clients' cultural beliefs and practices into health prescriptions" (Purnell, 2005).* **EBN:** *The client's coping behavior may be based on cultural perceptions of normal and abnormal coping behavior (Sterling & Peterson, 2003; Leininger & McFarland, 2002; D'Avanzo et al, 2001; Doswell & Erlen, 1998). Culture influences perceptions of stressors and perceptions of potential coping behaviors as well as resources (Cuellar, 2002).* **EBN:** *Chinese women may be less likely to seek mental health services for postnatal depression (Chan, 2002). Gender and age mediate a woman's response to signs and symptoms of cardiac disease (Lefler, 2004). For Mexican-American adolescents, positive reinterpretation, focusing and venting emotions, instrumental social support, active coping, religious, restraint, emotional support, acceptance and planning were all forms of coping were all associated with positive psychological and physical health (Vaughn & Roesch, 2003).*
- Assess the influence of fatalism on the client's coping behavior. **EBN:** *Fatalistic perspectives, which involve the belief that one cannot control one's own fate, may influence health behaviors in some Asian-American, African-American, and Latino populations (Chen, 2001).* **EBN:** *A study of patients with non–small cell lung cancer in Taiwan yielded that one response was to accept the outcome as fate (Kuo, 2002).*
- Assess the influence of cultural conflicts that may affect coping abilities. **EBN:** *It may be necessary to help the client to identify and find coping strategies that do not conflict with cultural expectations (Shibusawa & Mui, 2001).*
- Assess for intergenerational family problems that can overwhelm coping abilities. **EBN:** *Family assessment is integral to nursing care of clients (Northouse et al, 2002).*
- Encourage spirituality as a source of support for coping. **EBN:** *Many African Americans and Latinos identify spirituality, religiousness, prayer, and church-based approaches as coping resources (Abrums, 2004; Coon et al, 2004; Weaver & Flannelly, 2004; Samuel-Hodge et al, 2000). A sense of faith is an important component of psychosocial well-being in individuals with advanced cancer (Lin, 2003). Spirituality has a positive effect on coping (Kelly, 2004).*
- Negotiate with the client with regard to the aspects of coping behavior that will need to be modified. **EBN:** *As a part of the assessment of coping behaviors, alternate methods may be introduced and offered to the client as a possible choice in new coping strategies (Wassem, Beckham, & Dudley, 2001).*
- Identify which family members the client can count on for support. **EBN:** *In a variety of different cultures family members are relied on to cope with stress (Aziz & Rowland, 2002; Donnelly, 2002; Gleeson-Kreig, Bernal, & Woolley, 2002; White et al, 2002).*
- Support the inner resources that clients use for coping. **EBN:** *African-American women in one study used inner resources to develop self-help strategies to cope with reactions following involuntary pregnancy loss (Van & Meleis, 2003).*
- Use an empowerment framework to redefine coping strategies. **EBN:** *Use of an em-*

C

*powerment framework will allow individuals to redefine behaviors as coping strategies to confront their environment and connect to natural supports in the community (Dancy et al, 2001).* **EB:** *Empowerment strategies are important for people with sever mental illness (Linhort, 2002).*

## Home Care

- The interventions described previously may be adapted for home care use.
- Observe the family for coping behavior patterns. Obtain family and client history as possible. **EBN:** *Family assessment is necessary to guide interventions (Weiss & Chen, 2002; Northouse et al, 2002).* **EBN:** *The assessment of caregivers coping and information styles is an important part of nursing care of women with advanced cancer (Nikiletti, 2003).*
- ▲ Assess for suicidal tendencies. Refer for mental health care immediately if indicated.
- Identify an emergency plan should the client become suicidal. *Ineffective coping can occur in a crisis situation and can lead to suicidal ideation if the client sees no hope for a solution. A suicidal client is not safe in the home environment unless supported by professional help.* Refer to the care plan for **Risk for Suicide**.
- ▲ Assess for affective symptoms after CVA in the elderly, particularly emotional lability and depression. Refer for evaluation and treatment as indicated. **EB:** *In a study of elderly with first ever stroke, in the immediate post–acute phase, 48.5% of clients showed evidence of emotional lability, 57.6% showed evidence of depression, while showing normal global cognitive level. Prevalence of emotional lability was shown in previous studies to decrease over the first 6 months post-stroke. Apathy (15.2%) and anhedonia (6.1%) were significantly and negatively associated with the Barthel Index measure of functional ability (Piamarta, Iurlaro, Isella, et al, 2004).*
- Encourage the client to use self-care management to increase the experience of personal control. Identify with the client all available supports and sense of attachment to others. Refer to the care plan for **Powerlessness. EBN:** *In a study of heart transplantation clients, personal control was positively associated with optimism, well-being, and satisfaction with life, and was negatively associated with anger and depression. Perceived social support helpfulness and attachment were positively associated with better psychological and functional outcomes (Bohachick et al, 2002).* **EBN:** *Patients experiencing cancer related fatigue report feeling loss of control which can lead to helplessness (Potter, 2004).*
- ▲ Refer to medical social services for evaluation and counseling, which will promote adequate coping as part of the medical plan of care. If no primary medical diagnosis has been made, request medical social services to assist with community support contacts. *If the client is involved with the mental health system, actively participate in mental health team planning. Based on knowledge of the home and family, home care nurses can often advocate for clients. These nurses are frequently requested to monitor medication use and therefore need to know the plan of care.*
- ▲ Refer the client and family to support groups. **EBN:** *Support groups provide an essential resource to clients and their families when adapting to health status change (Fung & Chien, 2002). Support groups have appositive effect on individuals receiving chemotherapy (Ekman, 2004).* **EBN:** *An HIV self-care symptom management program implemented with African-American mothers produced positive outcomes in mental and physical health measures (Miles, 2003).*

- ▲ If monitoring medication use, contract with the client or solicit assistance from a responsible caregiver. *Prepouring of medications may be helpful with some clients. Caregivers in the home benefit from interventions that promote self-efficacy and provide a nurse for support (Dibartolo, 2002).*
- ▲ Institute case management for frail elderly clients to support continued independent living. *Difficulties in coping with changes in health care needs can lead to increasing needs for assistance in using the health care system effectively. Case management combines the nursing activities of client and family assessment, planning and coordination of care among all health care providers, delivery of direct nursing care, and monitoring of care and outcomes. These activities are able to address continuity of care, mutual goal setting, behavior management, and prevention of worsening health problems (Guttman, 1999).*
- ▲ If the client is homebound, refer for psychiatric home health care services for client reassurance and implementation of a therapeutic regimen. **EBN:** *Psychiatric home care nurses can address issues relating to the client's ability to adjust to changes in health status. Behavioral interventions in the home can help the client to participate more effectively in the treatment plan (Patusky, Rodning, & Martinez-Kratz, 1996).* **EB:** *Elderly stroke patients receiving home care were shown to have lower depression scores, and lower rates of admission to nursing homes (Ricauda et al, 2004).*

NOTE: All of the previously mentioned interventions may be applied in the home setting. Home care may offer psychiatric nursing or the services of a licensed clinical social worker under special programs. Traditionally, insurance does not reimburse for counseling that is not related to a medical plan of care unless it falls under one of the programs just described. Public health agencies generally do not have the clinical support needed to offer psychiatric nursing services to clients. Clients are usually treated in the ambulatory mental health system.

## Client/Family Teaching

- Teach the client to problem solve. Have the client define the problem and cause, and list the advantages and disadvantages of the options. **EBN:** *Interventions that support hardiness and self-efficacy facilitate positive adaptation to stressors (Dibartolo, 2002; Wassem, Beckham, & Dudley, 2001; Fisher and Laschinger, 2001). Cognitive behavioral therapy is a useful intervention when working on issues of hope (Collins, 2003).*
- Provide the seriously ill client and his or her family with needed information regarding the condition and treatment. **EB:** *Clients and families benefit from a sense of trust in health care providers that is based on honest communication regarding their condition and options (Fallowfield, Jenkins, & Beveridge, 2002).*
- Teach relaxation techniques. **EBN:** *Relaxation training has been demonstrated to improve self-efficacy in family caregivers of clients with Alzheimer's disease (Fisher & Laschinger, 2001).* **EB:** *Quality of life is enhanced in women with coronary syndrome X when they incorporated exercise and relaxation therapy into their coping behaviors (Tyni-Lenne, 2002).*
- Work closely with the client to develop appropriate educational tools that address individualized needs. **EBN:** *Educational level may affect the client's level of concern and ability to process information (Miles et al, 2002). Caregiver and patient coping patterns may vary (Kershaw, et al 2004).*

C

▲ Teach the client about available community resources (e.g., therapists, ministers, counselors, self-help groups). **EBN:** *Families need assistance in coping with health changes. The nurse is often perceived as the individual who can help them obtain necessary social support (Northouse et al, 2002; Tak & McCubbin, 2002). The degree of economic impact of the illness on a family will affect their ability to seek out and accept help from community resources (Mantagnino & Mauricio, 2004).*

## evolve WEBSITES FOR EDUCATION

See the EVOLVE website for World Wide Web resources for client education.

## REFERENCES


Abrums M: Faith and feminism: how African American women from a storefront church resist oppression in healthcare, *ANS Adv Nurs Sci* 27(3):187-201, 2004.

Antoni MH: Stress management effects on psychological, endocrinological, and immune functioning in men with HIV infection: empirical support for a psychoneuroimmunoligical model, *Stress* 6(3):173-188, 2003.

Aziz N, Rowland JH: Cancer survivorship research among ethnic minority and medically underserved groups, *Oncol Nurs Forum* 29(5):789-801, 2002.

Blanchard CM, Courneya KS, Laing D: Effects of acute exercise on state anxiety in breast cancer survivors, *Oncol Nurs Forum* 28(10):1617-1621, 2001.

Blomquist, K, Edberg AK: Living with persistent pain: experiences of older people receiving home care, *J Adv Nurs* 40(3):297-306, 2002.

Bohachick P, Taylor MV, Sereika S et al: Social support, personal control, and psychological recovery following heart transplant, *Clin Nurs Res* 11:34-51, 2002.

Chan SW, Levy V, Chung TK et al: A qualitative study of a group of Hong Kong Chinese women diagnosed with postnatal depression, *J Adv Nurs* 39(6):571-579, 2002.

Chen YC: Chinese values, health and nursing, *J Adv Nurs* 36(2):270-273, 2001.

Cleary M, Horsfall J, Hunt GE: Consumer feedback on nursing care and discharge planning, *J Adv Nurs* 42(3):269-277, 2003.

Coon DW, Rubert M, Solano N et al: Well-being, appraisal, and coping in Latina and Caucasian female dementia caregivers: findings from the REACH study, *Aging Ment Health* 8(4):330-345, 2004.

Cote JK, Pepler C: A randomized trial of a cognitive coping intervention for acutely ill HIV-positive men, *Nurs Res* 51(4):237-244, 2002.

Cuellar NG: A comparison of African American and Caucasian American female caregivers of rural, post-stroke, bedbound older adults, *J Gerontol Nurs* 28(1):36-45, 2002.

Cutcliffe JR, Grant G: What are the principles and processes of inspiring hope in cognitively impaired older adults within a continuing care environment? *J Psychiatr Ment Health Nurs* 8(5):427-46, 2001.

Dancy BL, McCreary L, Daye M et al: Empowerment: a view of two African American communities, *J Natl Black Nurses Assoc* 12(2):49-52, 2001.

Davis MC: Life review therapy as an intervention to manage depression and enhance life satisfaction in individuals with right hemisphere cerebral vascular accidents, *Issues Ment Health Nurs* 25(5):503-515, 2004.

D'Avanzo CE et al: Developing culturally informed strategies for substance-related interventions. In Naegle MA, D'Avanzo CE, editors: *Addictions and substance abuse: strategies for advanced practice nursing,* St Louis, 2001, Mosby.

Dalton JM: Development and testing of the theory of collaborative decision-making in nursing practice for triads, *J Adv Nurs* 41(1):22-33, 2003.

Dibartolo M: Exploring self-efficacy and hardiness in spousal caregivers of individuals with dementia, *J Gerontol Nurs* 28(4):24-33, 2002.

Dombeck MT: Chaos and self-organization as a consequence of spiritual disequilibrium. 1996, *Clin Nurse Spec* 16(1):42-47, 2002.

Donnelly TT: Contextual analysis of coping: implications for immigrants' mental health care, *Issues Ment Health Nurs* 23:715-732, 2002.

Doswell W, Erlen J: Multicultural issues and ethical concerns in the delivery of nursing care interventions, *Nurs Clin North Am* 33(2):353-361, 1998.

Dudley-Brown S: Prevention of psychological distress in persons with inflammatory bowel disease, *Issues Ment Health Nurs* 23: 403-422, 2002.
Ekman I, Bergbom I, Ekman T et al: Maintaining normality and support are central issues when receiving chemotherapy for ovarian cancer, *Cancer Nurs* 27(3):177-182, 2004.
Fallowfield LJ, Jenkins VA, Beveridge HA: Truth may hurt but deceit hurts more: communication in palliative care, *Palliat Med* 16(4):297-303, 2002.
Fisher PA, Laschinger HS: A relaxation training program to increase self-efficacy for anxiety control in Alzheimer family caregivers, *Holist Nurs Pract* 15(2):47-58, 2001.
Fung WY, Chien WT: The effectiveness of a mutual support group for family caregivers of a relative with dementia, *Arch Psychiatr Nurs* 26(3):134-144, 2002.
Gleeson-Kreig J, Bernal H, Woolley S: The role of social support in the self-management of diabetes mellitus among a Hispanic population, *Public Health Nurs* 19(3):215-222, 2002.
Hodgkinson R, Lester H: Stresses and coping strategies of mothers living with a child with cystic fibrosis: implications for nursing professionals, *J Adv Nurs* 39(4):377-383, 2002.
Howell D, Fitch MI, Deane KA: Women's experiences with recurrent ovarian cancer, *Cancer Nurs* 26:10-17, 2003.
Kershaw T, Northouse L, Kritpracha C: Coping strategies and quality of life in women with advanced breast cancer and their family caregivers, *Psychol Health* 19(2):139-155, 2004.
Kraaij V, de Wilde EJ: Negative life events and depressive symptoms in the elderly: a life span perspective, *Aging Ment Health* 5(1): 84-91, 2001.
Kelly J: Spirituality as a coping mechanism, *Dimen Crit Care Nurs* 23(4):162-168, 2004.
Kuo TT, Ma FC: Symptoms distresses and coping strategies in patients with non-small cell lung cancer, *Cancer Nurs* 25(4): 309-317, 2002.
Lefler L , Bondy KN: Women's delay in seeking treatment with myocardial infarction: a meta-synthesis, *J Cardiovasc Nurs* 19(4): 251-268, 2004.
Leininger MM, McFarland MR: *Transcultural nursing: concepts, theories, research and practices,* ed 3, New York, 2002, McGraw-Hill.
Linhorst DM, Hamilton G, Young E et al: Opportunities and barriers to empowering people with severe mental illness through participation in treatment planning, *Soc Work* 47(4):425-434, 2002.
Lyons KS, Stewart BJ, Archbold PG et al: Pessimism and optimism as early warning signs for compromised health for caregivers of patients with Parkinson's disease, *Nurs Res* 53(6):354-362, 2004.
Miles MS, Burchinal P, Holditch-Davis D et al: Perceptions of stress, worry, and support in black and white mothers of hospitalized, medically fragile infants, *J Pediatr Nurs* 17(2):82-88, 2002.
Miles MS, Holditch-Davis D, Eron A et al: An HIV self-care symptom management intervention for African American mothers, *Nurs Res* 52(6):350-360, 2003.
Montagnino BA, Mauricio RV: The child with a tracheostomy and gastrostomy: parental stress and coping in the home—a pilot study, *Pediatr Nurs* 30(5):373-401, 2004.
Nikoletti S, Kristjanson LJ, Tataryn D et al: Information needs and coping styles of primary family caregivers of women following breast cancer surgery, *Oncol Nurs Forum* 30(6):987-996, 2003.
Norris J, Spelic SS: Supporting adaptation to body image disruption, *Rehabil Nurs* 27(1):8-12, 38, 2002.
Northouse L, Walker J, Schafenacker A et al: A family-based program of care for women with recurrent breast cancer and their family members, *Oncol Nurs Forum* 29(10):1411-1419, 2002.
Overcash JA: Using narrative research to understand the quality of life of older women with breast cancer, *Oncol Nurs Forum* 31(6): 1153-1159, 2004.
Pakenham KI: Application of a stress and coping model to caregiving in multiple sclerosis, *Psychol Health Med* 6(1):13-27, 2001.
Patusky KL, Rodning C, Martinez-Kratz M: Clinical lessons in psychiatric home care: a case study approach, *J Home Health Case Manag* 9:18, 1996.
Piamarta F, Iurlaro S, Isella V et al: Unconventional affective symptoms and executive functions after stroke in the elderly, *Arch Gerontol Geriatr* Suppl(9):315-323, 2004.
Puentes WJ: Simple reminiscence: a stress-adaptation model of the phenomenon, *Issues Ment Health Nurs* 23(5):497-511, 2002.
Purnell LD, Paulanka BJ: *Guide to culturally competent health care,* Philadelphia, 2005, FA Davis Company.
Radina ME, Armer JM, Culbertson SC et al: Post-breast cancer lymphedema: understanding women's knowledge of their condition, *Oncol Nurs Forum* 31(1):97-104, 2004.

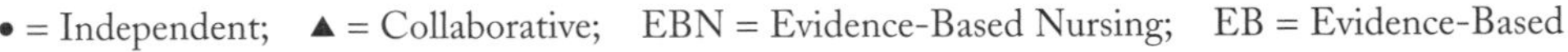

Raine T, Marcell AV, Rocca CH et al: The other half of the equation: serving young men in a young women's reproductive health clinic, *Perspect Sex Reprod Health* 35(5):208-214, 2003.
Ricauda NA, Bo M, Molaschi M et al: Home hospitalization service for acute uncomplicated first ischemic stroke in elderly patients: a randomized trial: *J Am Geriatr Soc* 52:278-283, 2004.
Richer MC, Ezer H: Living in it, living with it, and moving on: dimensions of meaning during chemotherapy, *Oncol Nurs Forum* 29(1):113-119, 2002.
Samuel-Hodge CD: Influences on day-to-day self-management of type 2 diabetes among African-American women: spirituality, the multi-caregiver role, and other social context factors, *Diabetes Care* 23(7),928-33, 2000.
Schneider SM, Prince-Paul M, Allen JJ et al: Virtual reality as a distraction intervention for women receiving chemotherapy, *Oncol Nurs Forum* 31(1):81-88, 2004.
Shibusawa T, Mui AC: Stress, coping and depression among Japanese American elders, *J Gerontol Soc Work* 36(1/2):63, 2001.
Sterling YM, Peterson JW: Characteristics of African American women caregivers of children with asthma, *MCN Am J Matern Child Nurs* 28(1):32-38, 2003.
Tak YR, McCubbin M: Family stress, perceived social support and coping following the diagnosis of a child's congenital heart disease, *J Adv Nurs* 39(2):190-198, 2002.
Tyni-Lenne R, Stryjan S, Eriksson B et al: Beneficial therapeutic effects of physical training and relaxation therapy in women with coronary syndrome X, *Physiother Res Int* 7(1):35-43, 2002.
Van P, Meleis AI: Coping with grief after involuntary pregnancy loss: perspectives of African American women, *J Obstet Gynecol Neonatal Nurs* 32(1):28-39, 2003.
Vaughn AA, Roesch SC: Psychological and physical health correlates of coping in minority adolescents, *J Health Psychol* 8(6): 671-683, 2003.
Wassem R, Beckham N, Dudley W: Test of a nursing intervention to promote adjustment to fibromyalgia, *Orthop Nurs* 20(3): 33-45, 2001.
Weaver AJ, Flannelly KJ: The role of religion/spirituality for cancer patients and their caregivers, *South Med J* 97(12):1210-1214, 2004.
Weiss SJ, Chen JL: Factors influencing maternal mental health and family functioning during the low birth-weight infant's first year of life, *J Pediatr Nurs* 17(2):114-125, 2002.
Wengstrom Y, Haggmark C, Forsberg C: Coping with radiation therapy: effects of a nursing intervention on coping ability for women with breast cancer, *Int J Nurs Pract* 7(1):8-15, 2001.
White N, Bichter J, Koeckeritz J et al: A cross-cultural comparison of family resiliency in hemodialysis clients, *J Transcult Nurs* 13(3):218-217, 2002.

# Readiness for enhanced Coping

*Gail B. Ladwig*

**NANDA**

## Definition

Pattern of cognitive and behavioral efforts to manage demands that is sufficient for well-being and can be strengthened

## Defining Characteristics

Defines stressors as manageable, seeks social support, uses a broad range of problem-oriented and emotion-oriented strategies, uses spiritual resources, acknowledges power, seeks knowledge of new strategies, is aware of possible environmental changes

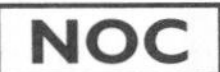

## Outcomes (Nursing Outcomes Classification)

### Suggested NOC Outcomes

Coping, Personal Well-Being, Social Interaction Skills, Quality of life

**Example NOC Outcome with Indicators**

**Coping** as evidenced by the following indicator: Identifies effective coping patterns/Uses effective coping strategies (Rate the indicator of **Coping:** 1 = never demonstrated, 2 = rarely demonstrated, 3 = sometimes demonstrated, 4 = often demonstrated, 5 = consistently demonstrated [see Section I].)

## Client Outcomes

**Client Will (Specify Time Frame):**

- Verbalize ability to cope and ask for help when needed
- Demonstrate ability to solve problems related to current needs
- Communicate needs and negotiate with others to meet needs
- State that stressors are manageable
- Demonstrate new effective coping strategies
- Seek social support for problems associated with coping
- Seek spiritual support of personal choice

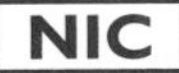

## Interventions (Nursing Interventions Classification)

### Suggested NIC Interventions

Coping Enhancement, Decision-Making Support

**Example NIC Activities—Coping Enhancement**

Assist client in developing an objective appraisal of the event; Explore with client previous methods of dealing with problems

## Nursing Interventions and Rationales

- Observe for strengths such as the ability to relate the facts and to recognize the source of stressors. **EBN:** *Successful adaptation requires a coordination of efforts to fit the nursing interventions to the client's perception of the threat, personal values and beliefs, and recognition of personal strengths (Norris & Spelic, 2002).*
- Use empathetic communication and encourage the client and family to verbalize fears, express emotions, and set goals. Be present for clients. **EBN:** *A nurse's holistic presence with clients is considered to be vital (Cote & Pepler, 2002).*
- Help the client set realistic goals and identify personal skills and knowledge. **EBN and**

C

**EB:** *Providing validation of actual stressors and available coping resources and/or strategies aids in a positive adaptation to stress (Pakenham, 2001). Efforts to educate the client regarding possible and/or potential effects of a specific diagnosis and the resources available to assist with coping are a positive factor in successful adaptation (Wassem, Beckham, & Dudley, 2001).*

- • Encourage expression of positive thoughts and emotions. **EB:** *Positive emotions initiate upward spirals toward enhanced emotional well-being (Fredrickson & Joiner, 2002).* **EBN:** *This study shows that clients believe that coping is important to their well-being (Edgar, 2004).*
- • Encourage the use of cognitive behavioral relaxation (e.g., music therapy, guided imagery). **EBN:** *Relaxation training has been demonstrated to improve overall coping ability (Tyni-Lenne et al, 2002).*
- ▲ Refer for cognitive behavioral therapy. **EBN:** *A cognitive behavioral nursing program was effective in increasing adjustment to fibromyalgia. Treatment subjects had improved post-treatment adjustment and symptom severity compared to control subjects (Wassem, Beckham, & Dudley, 2001).*
- • Encourage the client to use spiritual coping mechanisms such as faith and prayer. **EBN:** *Addressing spiritual needs is acknowledged to be an essential component of holistic nursing care (Narayanasamy, 2002).*
- • Help the client with depression to maintain social support networks or assist in building new ones. **EBN:** *Lay support is vital in restoring the depressed client's health and assisting the client in getting well and resuming his or her place in the public domain. An important task for the nurse is therefore to support the client in maintaining the client's existing social network or in building a new one (Skärsäter et al, 2003).*
- ▲ Consider a workplace stress management program to enhance coping skills. **EB:** *A work site program that focuses on stress, anxiety, and coping measurement along with small group educational intervention can significantly reduce illness and health care use (Rahe et al, 2002).*
- ▲ Refer the client with breast cancer to a psychosocial group intervention for coping skills training, stress management, relaxation exercises, and psychosocial support. **EB:** *In women with primary breast carcinoma, a psychosocial group intervention reduced psychological distress and enhanced coping (Schulz, 2001).*
- • Refer to the care plans for **Readiness for enhanced Communication** and **Readiness for enhanced Spiritual well-being**.

## Pediatric

- • Encourage exercise for children and adolescents to promote positive self-esteem, to enhance coping, and to prevent behavioral and psychological problems. **EBN:** *The results of this review indicate that exercise has positive short-term effects on self-esteem in children and young people. Since there are no known negative effects of exercise and many positive effects on physical health, exercise may be an important measure in improving children's self-esteem (Ekland et al, 2004).*

## Geriatric

- • Consider the use of telephone support for caregivers of family members with dementia. **EBN:** *Results from this study suggest family caregivers can be helped through a variety of*

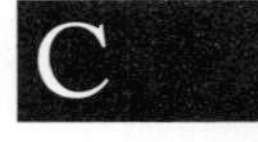


*social support mechanisms including telephone support. Participants reported assistance in sharing thoughts and feelings, expressing feelings of being overwhelmed, discussing physical and psychosocial problems, forgetting the situation, seeking reassurance, and asking for information (Chang et al, 2004).*

- ▲ Refer the client with Alzheimer's disease who is terminally ill to hospice. **EBN:** *Home care and hospice nurses can provide invaluable care in helping families cope with this disease and end-of-life issues (Head, 2003).*
- ▲ Refer the widowed older client to self-help support groups. **EBN:** *Bereaved older clients who attended face-to-face support groups for 20 weeks reported increased hope, improved skills in developing social relationships, enhanced coping, new role identities, and less loneliness (Stewart et al, 2001).*

## Multicultural

- Assess for the influence of cultural beliefs, norms, and values on the client's perceptions of effective coping. **EBN:** *The client's coping behavior may be based on cultural perceptions of normal and abnormal coping behavior (Leininger & McFarland, 2002; D'Avanzo et al, 2001; Cochran, 1998; Doswell & Erlen, 1998). Culture influences perceptions of stressors and perception of potential coping behaviors as well as resources (Cuellar, 2002).*
- Encourage spirituality as a source of support for coping. **EBN:** *Many African Americans and Latinos identify spirituality, religiousness, prayer, and church-based approaches as coping resources (Abrums, 2004; Coon et al, 2004; Weaver & Flannelly, 2004; Samuel-Hodge et al, 2000).*
- Identify which family members the client can count on for support. **EBN:** *In a variety of different cultures family members are relied on to cope with stress (Aziz & Rowland, 2002; Donnelly, 2002; Gleeson-Kreig, Bernal, & Woolley, 2002; White et al, 2002).*
- Support the inner resources that clients use for coping. **EBN:** *African-American women in one study used inner resources to develop self-help strategies to cope with reactions following involuntary pregnancy loss (Van & Meleis, 2003).*
- Use an empowerment framework to redefine coping strategies. **EBN:** *Use of an empowerment framework will allow individuals to redefine behaviors as coping strategies to confront their environment and connect to natural supports in the community (Dancy et al, 2001; Washington & Moxley, 2003).*

## Home Care

- The interventions described previously may be adapted for home care use.
- Observe the family for coping behavior patterns. Obtain family and client history as possible. **EBN:** *Family assessment is necessary to guide interventions (Weiss & Chen, 2002; Northouse et al, 2002).*
- Encourage the client to use self-care management to increase the experience of personal control. Identify with the client all available supports and sense of attachment to others. **EBN:** *In a study of heart transplantation clients, personal control was positively associated with optimism, well-being, and satisfaction with life, and was negatively associated with anger and depression. Perceived social support helpfulness and attachment were positively associated with better psychological and functional outcomes (Bohachick et al, 2002).*

▲ Refer the client and family to support groups. **EBN:** *Support groups provide an essential resource to clients and their families when adapting to health status change (Fung & Chien, 2002).*

C

## Client/Family Teaching

- Teach relaxation techniques. **EBN:** *Relaxation training has been demonstrated to improve self-efficacy in family caregivers of clients with Alzheimer's disease (Fisher & Laschinger, 2001).*

▲ Teach the client about available community resources (e.g., therapists, ministers, counselors, self-help groups). **EBN:** *Families need assistance in coping with health changes. The nurse is often perceived as the individual who can help them obtain necessary social support (Tak & McCubbin, 2002; Northouse et al, 2002).*

## evolve WEBSITES FOR EDUCATION

See the EVOLVE website for World Wide Web resources for client education.

## REFERENCES


Abrums M: Faith and feminism: how African American women from a storefront church resist oppression in healthcare, *Adv Nurs Science* 27(3):187-201, 2004.

Aziz N, Rowland JH: Cancer survivorship research among ethnic minority and medically underserved groups, *Oncol Nurs Forum* 29(5):789, 2002.

Bohachick P, Taylor MV, Sereika S et al: Social support, personal control, and psychological recovery following heart transplant, *Clin Nurs Res* 11(1):34-51, 2002.

Chang BL, Nitta S, Carter PA et al: Technology innovations. Perceived helpfulness of telephone calls: providing support for caregivers of family members with dementia, *J Gerontol Nurs* 30(9):14-21, 2004.

Cochran, M: Tears have no color, *Am J Nurs* 98(6):53, 1998.

Coon DW, Rubert M, Solano N et al: Well-being, appraisal, and coping in Latina and Caucasian female dementia caregivers: findings from the REACH study, *Aging Ment Health* 8(4):330-345, 2004.

Cote JK, Pepler C: A randomized trial of a cognitive coping intervention for acutely ill HIV-positive men, *Nurs Res* 51(4):237, 2002.

Cuellar NG: A comparison of African American and Caucasian American female caregivers of rural, post-stroke, bedbound older adults, *J Gerontol Nurs* 28(1):36, 2002.

Dancy BL, McCreary L, Daye M et al: Empowerment: a view of two African American communities, *J Natl Black Nurses Assoc* 12(2):49-52, 2001.

D'Avanzo CE et al: Developing culturally informed strategies for substance-related interventions. In Naegle MA, D'Avanzo CE, editors: *Addictions and substance abuse: strategies for advanced practice nursing,* St Louis, 2001, Mosby.

Donnelly TT: Contextual analysis of coping: implications for immigrants' mental health care, *Issues Ment Health Nurs* 23:715, 2002.

Doswell W, Erlen J: Multicultural issues and ethical concerns in the delivery of nursing care interventions, *Nurs Clin North Am* 33(2):353, 1998.

Watt S, Edgar L: Nucare, a coping skills training intervention for oncology patients and families: participants' motivations and expectations, *Can Oncol Nurs J* 14(2):84-95, 2004.

Ekeland E, Heian F, Hagen KB et al: Exercise to improve self-esteem in children and young people, *Cochrane Database Syst Rev* (1):CD003683, 2004.

Gleeson-Kreig J, Bernal H, Woolley S: The role of social support in the self-management of diabetes mellitus among a Hispanic population, *Public Health Nurs* 19(3):215, 2002.

Fisher PA, Laschinger HS: A relaxation training program to increase self-efficacy for anxiety control in Alzheimer family caregivers, *Holist Nurs Pract* 15(2):47, 2001.

Fredrickson BL, Joiner T: Positive emotions trigger upward spirals toward emotional well-being, *Psychol Sci* 13(2):172, 2002.

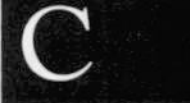



Fung WY, Chien WT: The effectiveness of a mutual support group for family caregivers of a relative with dementia, *Arch Psychiatr Nurs* 26(3):134, 2002.
Gleeson-Kreig J, Bernal H, Woolley S: The role of social support in the self-management of diabetes mellitus among a Hispanic population, *Public Health Nurs* 19(3):215, 2002.
Head G: Palliative care for persons with dementia, *Home Healthc Nurse* 21(1):53, 2003.
Leininger MM, McFarland MR: *Transcultural nursing: concepts, theories, research and practices,* ed 3, New York, 2002, McGraw-Hill.
Narayanasamy A: Spiritual coping mechanisms in chronically ill patients, *Br J Nurs* 11(22):1461, 2002.
Norris J, Spelic SS: Supporting adaptation to body image disruption, *Rehabil Nurs* 27(1):8, 2002.
Northouse LL, Mood D, Kershaw T et al: Quality of life of women with recurrent breast cancer and their family members, *J Clin Oncol* 20(19):4050-4064, 2002.
Pakenham KI: Application of a stress and coping model to caregiving in multiple sclerosis, *Psychol Health Med* 6(1):13, 2001.
Rahe RH, Taylor CB, Tolles RL et al: A novel stress and coping workplace program reduces illness and healthcare utilization, *Psychosom Med* 64(2):278-286, 2002.
Samuel-Hodge CD, Headen SW, Skelly AH et al: Influences on day-to-day self-management of type 2 diabetes among African-American women: spirituality, the multi-caregiver role, and other social context factors, *Diabetes Care* 23(7):928-933, 2000.
Schulz K: A psychosocial group intervention reduced psychological distress and enhanced coping in primary breast cancer, *Evid Based Ment Health* 4(1):15, 2001.
Skarsater I, Dencker K, Haggstrom L et al: A salutogenetic perspective on how men cope with major depression in daily life, with the help of professional and lay support, *Int J Nurs Stud* 40(2):153, 2003.
Stewart M, Craig D, MacPherson K et al: Promoting positive affect and diminishing loneliness of widowed seniors through a support intervention, *Public Health Nurs* 18(1):54, 2001.
Tak YR, McCubbin M: Family stress, perceived social support and coping following the diagnosis of a child's congenital heart disease, *J Adv Nurs* 39(2):190, 2002.
Tyni-Lenne R, Stryjan S, Eriksson B et al: Beneficial therapeutic effects of physical training and relaxation therapy in women with coronary syndrome X, *Physiother Res Int* 7(1):35-43, 2002.
Van P, Meleis AI: Coping with grief after involuntary pregnancy loss: perspectives of African American women, *J Obstet Gynecol Neonatal Nurs* 32(1):28, 2003.
Washington OG, Moxley DP: Promising group practices to empower low-income minority women coping with chemical dependency, *Am J Orthopsychiatry* 73(1):109-16, 2003.
Wassem R, Beckham N, Dudley W: Test of a nursing intervention to promote adjustment to fibromyalgia, *Orthop Nurs* 20(3):33-45, 2001.
Weaver AJ, Flannelly KJ: The role of religion/spirituality for cancer patients and their caregivers, *South Med J* 97(12):1210-1214, 2004.
Weiss SJ, Chen JL: Factors influencing maternal mental health and family functioning during the low birth-weight infant's first year of life, *J Pediatr Nurs* 17(2):114, 2002.
White N, Bichter J, Koeckeritz J et al: A cross-cultural comparison of family resiliency in hemodialysis clients, *J Transcult Nurs* 13(3):218-227, 2002.


# Ineffective community Coping

*Margaret Lunney*

**NANDA**

## Definition

Pattern of community activities (for adaptation and problem solving) that is unsatisfactory for meeting the demands or needs of the community

• = Independent; ▲ = Collaborative; EBN = Evidence-Based Nursing; EB = Evidence-Based

C

## Defining Characteristics

Expressed community powerlessness; failure of community to meet its own expectations; deficits of community participation; deficits in communication methods; excessive community conflicts; expressed vulnerability; high illness rates; stressors perceived as excessive; increased social problems (e.g., homicides, vandalism, arson, terrorism, robbery, infanticide, abuse, divorce, unemployment, poverty, militancy, mental illness)

## Related Factors (r/t)

Natural or manmade disasters; ineffective or nonexistent community systems (e.g., lack of emergency medical, transportation, or disaster planning systems); deficits in community social support services and resources; inadequate resources for problem solving

**NOC**

## Outcomes (Nursing Outcomes Classification)

### Suggested NOC Outcomes

Community Competence, Community Health Status, Community Violence Level

**Example NOC Outcome with Indicators**

**Community Competence** as evidenced by the following indicators: Participation rates in community activities/Common and competing interests among groups are considered when solving community problems/Representation of all segments of the community in problem solving/Effective use of conflict management strategies (Rate each indicator of **Community Competence:** 1 = poor, 2 = fair, 3 = good, 4 = very good, 5 = excellent [see Section I].)

## Community Outcomes

**A Broad Range of Community Members Will (Specify Time Frame):**

- Participate in community actions to improve power resources
- Develop improved communication among community members
- Participate in problem solving
- Demonstrate cohesiveness in problem solving
- Develop new strategies for problem solving
- Express power to deal with change and manage problems

**NIC**

## Interventions (Nursing Interventions Classification)

### Suggested NIC Interventions

Community Health Development; Program Development

NIC Interventions developed for use with individuals can be adapted for use with communities: Coping Enhancement, Culture Brokerage, Mutual Goal Setting, Support System Enhancement

**Example NIC Activities—Community Health Development**

Enhance community support networks; identify and mentor potential community leaders; unify community members behind a common mission; ensure that community members maintain control over decision making

C

## Nursing Interventions and Rationales

NOTE: The diagnosis of **Ineffective Coping** does not apply and should not be used when stress is being imposed by external sources or circumstance. If the community is a victim of circumstances, using the nursing diagnosis **Ineffective Coping** is equivalent to blaming the victim. See the care plans for **Ineffective community Therapeutic regimen management** and **Readiness for enhanced community Coping.**

- Establish a collaborative partnership with the community (see the care plan for **Ineffective community Therapeutic regimen management** for references). **EB:** *In a study conducted by Mt. Sinai researchers and clinicians with community leaders of east and central Harlem, the collaborative partnerships of researchers, clinicians and community leaders were key assets to accomplish community health goals (Horowitz et al, 2004).*
- Assist the community with team building. **EB:** *After completing a survey of 105 counties in Kansas, the researcher concluded that "encouraging a teambuilding approach during coalition development, emphasizing key exercises for coalition cohesion" (p. 25) and so forth may have helped to address some of the limitations reported by communities (Curtis, 2002). A nurse-community health advocate team successfully contributed to the health of urban immigrants (Elmurray, Park, & Buseh, 2003).*
- Participate with community members in the identification of stressors and assessment of distress; for example, observe and participate in community meetings and task forces. **EBN:** *From nurses' stories related to community health nursing (N = 25), it was suggested that attendance at community meetings helps nurses to gain a community and population perspective (Diekemper, Smithbattle, & Drake, 1999).*
- Identify community strengths with community members. **EBN:** *In an ethnographic study of health, environment, culture and poverty, it was found that community members can describe their strengths and goals for future health-related activities (Bent, 2003).*
- Identify the health services and information resources that are currently available in the community. **EBN:** *Helping a community to cope requires an understanding of the contextual nature of coping, including social, cultural, political, economic, and historical conditions (Donnelly, 2002).*
- Work with community members to increase awareness of ineffective coping behaviors (e.g., conflicts that prevent community members from working together, anger and hate that paralyze the community). **EBN:** *Problem solving is essential for effective coping. Community members in partnership with providers can modify behaviors that interfere with problem solving (Anderson & McFarlane, 2003; Chinn, 2001).*
- Provide support to the community and help community members to identify and mobilize additional supports. **EBN:** *In a 13-month three-group randomized clinical trial involving 125 women diagnosed with early-stage breast cancer, women in the two groups that received regular social support reported more positive outcomes, such as less mood distur-*

C

*bance and less loneliness, in the three phases of data collection (Samarel, Tulman, & Fawcett, 2002). Often people need help in mobilizing supports that are available (Pender, Murdaugh, & Parsons, 2002).*

- Use focus group methods to evaluate and strengthen interventions. **EBN:** *Focus group methodology strengthened population interventions in a Medicaid managed care population in Nebraska (Kaiser, Barry, & Kaiser, 2002).*
- Use mentoring strategies for community members. **EBN:** *In a focus group study of 43 African-American teens and adults on the community problem of teenage pregnancy, the participants selected mentoring as a strategy to teach, counsel, and provide information (Tabi, 2002).*
- Advocate for the community in multiple arenas (e.g., television, newspapers, and governmental agencies). **EBN:** *Advocacy is a specific form of caring that enhances power resources for community coping (Chinn, 2001).* **EB:** *In a study of the conduct of community health assessment of 105 counties in Kansas, it was identified that increased state level support would have helped those communities who did not complete health assessments (Curtis, 2002).*
- Work with community groups to improve the economic status and reduce unemployment. **EB:** *Analysis of population and labor force data from 1992 to 2002 indicated a strong significant correlation of penetrating trauma/crime indices and economic conditions, including unemployment (Cinat et al, 2004).*
- Write grant proposals to help community members obtain funds for programs that reduce stress or improve coping. (See Coley and Scheinberg, 2000, for program proposal-writing methods.) **EBN:** *The programs that are necessary may be expensive, and often funds may not be available without the assistance of public or privately funded grants (Anderson & McFarland, 2003).*
- Work with members of the community to identify and develop coping strategies that promote a sense of power (e.g., obtaining sources for funding, collaborating with other communities). **EBN:** *In a study of 39 blind subjects, those experiencing power as defined by Barrett's theory of power (power is being aware of what one is choosing to do, feeling free to do it, and doing it intentionally) reported better emotional and general health than individuals lacking power (Leksell et al, 2001). A first step in power enhancement is for the community to identify and develop its own coping strategies (Chinn, 2001).*
- Obtain police support for community partnerships aimed at healthy coping. **EB:** *Police programs have led to innovative programs that contribute to community health (Frommer & Papouchado, 2000).*
- Support positive attitudes and feelings as a basis for change. **EBN:** *In a qualitative study using key informants from a South-African community characterized by violence, community members described positive and negative experiences from living with violence. Positive experiences included feelings of solidarity, bravery, and increased appreciation (Madela & Poggenpoel, 1993).*
- Protect children from exposure to community conflicts. **EB:** *In numerous studies of children exposed to community conflict, it was found that permanent negative effects result from exposure to community conflicts, including using coping strategies such as distrust, detachment, distraction, and minimization (Shiavone, 2000), participation in acts of violence*

*(Feigelman & Howard, 2000), engaging in HIV sexual risk behaviors (Voisin, 2003), and psychological distress (Rosenthal & Wilson, 2003).*

### Multicultural

C

- Acknowledge the stressors unique to racial/ethnic communities. **EBN:** *Targeted alcohol and tobacco marketing, high levels of unemployment, lack of health insurance, and racism are stressors unique to culturally diverse communities (D'Avanzo et al, 2001).*
- Work with members of the community to prioritize and target health goals specific to the community. **EB:** *Such prioritization and targeting will increase feelings of control over and sense of ownership of programs (Anderson & McFarlane, 2003; Chinn, 2001; National Institutes of Health, 1998).*
- Approach community leaders and members of color with respect, warmth, and professional courtesy. **EBN:** *Instances of disrespect and lack of caring have special significance for individuals of color (D'Avanzo et al, 2001).*
- Establish and sustain partnerships with key individuals within communities when developing and implementing programs. **EBN:** *Local leaders are excellent sources of information and their participation will enhance the credibility of programs (National Institutes of Health, 1998).*
- Use community church settings as a forum for advocacy, teaching, and program implementation. **EBN:** *Evaluation of a faith-based program supplied to 125 people from 18 congregations showed an increase in health promotion knowledge, rise in consumer satisfaction, and improvement in health (Kotecki, 2002). A literature review of church-based health promotion programs showed that they are successful in helping people to adopt health-promoting behaviors (Peterson, Atwood, & Yates, 2002). Church-based programs are especially effective in communities of color.*
- Ask political leaders to become part of the partnership process. **EB:** *The Carnegie Commission on Preventing Deadly Conflict established the importance of political leaders' working to prevent community conflicts and violence (Hamburg, George, & Ballentine, 1999).*

### Community Teaching

- Teach strategies for stress management.
- Explain the relationship between enhancing power resources and coping.

## evolve WEBSITES FOR EDUCATION

See the EVOLVE website for World Wide Web resources for client education.

## REFERENCES

Anderson ET, McFarlane J: *Community as partner: theory and practice in nursing,* ed 4, Philadelphia, 2003, Lippincott Williams & Wilkins.

Bent KN: "The people know what they want": an empowerment process of sustainable, ecological community health, *Adv Nurs Science* 26(3):215-226, 2003.

Chinn PL: *Peace and power: building communities for the future,* ed 5, Boston, 2001, Jones & Bartlett.

Cinat ME, Wilson SE, Lush S et al: Significant correlation of trauma epidemiology with economic conditions of a community, *Arch Surg* 139(12):1350-1355, 2004.

Coley SM, Scheinberg CA: *Proposal writing,* ed 2, Thousand Oaks, Calif, 2000, Sage.
Curtis DC: Evaluation of community health assessment in Kansas, *J Public Health Manag Pract* 8(4):20-25, 2002.
D'Avanzo CE et al: Developing culturally informed strategies for substance-related interventions. In Naegle MA, D'Avanzo CE, editors: *Addictions and substance abuse: strategies for advanced practice nursing,* St Louis, 2001, Mosby.
Diekemper M, Smithbattle L, Drake MA: Bringing the population into focus: a natural development in community health nursing practice, part I, *Public Health Nurs* 16(1):3, 1999.
Donnelly TT: Contextual analysis of coping: implications for immigrants' mental health care, *Issues Ment Health Nurs* 23(7):715, 2002.
Drevdahl D: Meanings of community in a community health center, *Public Health Nurs* 16(6):417, 1999.
Frommer P, Papouchado K: Police as contributors to healthy communities: Aiken, South Carolina, *Public Health Rep* 115(2-3): 249, 2000.
Hamburg DA, George A, Ballentine K: Preventing deadly conflict: the critical role of leadership, *Arch Gen Psychiatry* 56(11):971, 1999.
Horowitz CR, Arniella A, James S et al: Using community-based participatory research to reduce health disparities in East and Central Harlem, *Mt. Sinai J Med* 71(6):368-374, 2004.
Kaiser MM, Barry TL, Kaiser KL: Using focus groups to evaluate and strengthen public health nursing population-focused interventions, *J Transcult Nurs* 13(4):303, 2002.
Kotecki CN: Developing a health promotion program for faith-based communities, *Holist Nurs Pract* 16(3):61, 2002.
Leksell JK, Johansson I, Wibell LB et al: Power and self-perceived health in blind diabetic and nondiabetic individuals, *J Adv Nurs* 34(4):511-519, 2001.
Madela EN, Poggenpoel M: The experience of a community characterized by violence: implications for nursing, *J Adv Nurs* 18(5): 691, 1993.
McElmurry BJ, Park CG, Buseh AG: The nurse-community health advocate team for urban immigrant primary health care, *J Nurs Schol* 35(3):275-281, 2003.
Miller LS, Wasserman GA, Neugebauer R et al: Witnessed community violence and anti-social behavior in high risk, urban boys, *J Clin Child Psychol* 28(1):2-11, 1999.
National Institutes of Health: *Salud para su corazon: bringing heart health to Latinos—a guide for building community programs,* DHHS Pub No 98-3796, Washington, DC, 1998, US Government Printing Office.
Pender NJ, Murdaugh CL, Parsons MA: *Health promotion in nursing practice,* ed 4, Upper Saddle River, NJ, 2002, Prentice Hall.
Peterson J, Atwood JR, Yates B: Key elements for church-based health promotion programs: outcome-based literature review, *Public Health Nurs* 19(6):401, 2002.
Rosenthal BS, Wilson WC: The association of ecological variables and psychological distress with exposure to community violence among adolescents, *Adolescence* 38(151):459-479, 2003.
Samarel N, Tulman L, Fawcett J: Effects of two types of social support and education on adaptation to early-stage breast cancer, *Res Nurs Health* 25(6):459, 2002.
Tabi MM: Community perspective on a model to reduce teenage pregnancy, *J Adv Nurs* 40(3):275, 2002.
Wright RJ, Mitchell H, Visness CM et al: Community violence and asthma morbidity: the inner city Asthma study, *Am J Public Health* 94(4):625-632, 2004.

# Readiness for enhanced community Coping

*Margaret Lunney*

**NANDA**

## Definition

Pattern of community activities for adaptation and problem solving that is satisfactory for meeting the demands or needs of the community but that can be improved for management of current and future problems/stressors

## Defining Characteristics

One or more of the following characteristics that indicate effective coping: positive communication between community/aggregates and larger community, availability of programs for recreation and relaxation, sufficiency of resources for managing stressors, agreement that community is responsible for stress management, active planning by community for predicted stressors, active problem solving by community when faced with issues, positive communication among community members

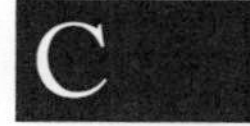

## Related Factors (r/t)

Community has sense of power to manage stressors, social supports available, resources available for problem solving

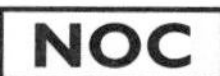

## Outcomes (Nursing Outcomes Classification)

### Suggested NOC Outcomes

Community Competence; Community Health Status

**Example NOC Outcome with Indicators**

**Community Health Status** as evidenced by the following indicators: Prevalence of health promotion programs/Health status of infants, children, adolescents, adults, elders/Attendance at programs for healthy states (Rate each indicator of **Community Health Status:** 1 = poor, 2 = fair, 3 = good, 4 = very good, 5 = excellent [see Section I].)

## Community Outcomes

**Community Will (Specify Time Frame):**

- Develop enhanced coping strategies
- Maintain effective coping strategies for management of stress

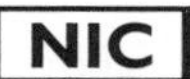

## Interventions (Nursing Interventions Classification)

### Suggested NIC Interventions

Environmental Management: Community, Health Policy Monitoring

NIC Interventions developed for use with individuals can be adapted for use with communities: Coping Enhancement, Culture Brokerage, Mutual Goal Setting, Support System Enhancement

**Example NIC Activities—Coping Enhancement**

Explore with community members previous methods of dealing with life problems; assist the community to solve problems in a constructive manner

## Nursing Interventions and Rationales

C

NOTE: Interventions depend on the specific aspects of community coping that can be enhanced (e.g., planning for stress management, communication, development of community power, community perceptions of stress, community coping strategies). Nursing interventions are conducted in collaboration with key members of the community, community/public health nurses, and members of other disciplines (Anderson & McFarlane, 2003; Chinn, 2001).

- Describe the roles of community/public health nurses in working with healthy communities. **EBN:** *Nurses at general and specialists levels (bachelor's and master's degrees) have significant roles in helping communities to achieve optimum health, including coping with stress (Logan, 2004; Stanhope & Lancaster, 2004).*
- Help the community to obtain funds for additional programs. (See Coley and Scheinberg, 2000, for proposal-writing methods.) **EBN:** *Healthy communities may need additional funding sources to strengthen community resources (Anderson & McFarlane, 2003).*
- Encourage positive attitudes toward the community through the media and other sources. **EB:** *Negative attitudes or stigmas create additional stress and deficits in social support (Anderson & McFarlane, 2003; Stanhope & Lancaster, 2004).*
- Help community members to collaborate with one another for power enhancement and coping skills. **EBN:** *Community members may not have sufficient skills to collaborate for enhanced coping. Health care providers can promote effective collaboration skills can be promoted (Chinn, 2001).*
- Encourage critical thinking. **EBN:** *Critical thinking supports problem-solving ability (Scheffer & Rubenfeld, 2000).*
- Demonstrate optimum use of the power resources. **EBN:** *Optimum use of power resources and working for community empowerment supports coping (Bent, 2003).*
- Reduce poverty whenever possible. **EB:** *Public health studies in most countries of the world show that poverty is an important predictor of health status in all categories (Wagstaff et al, 2004). Socioeconomic inequalities are most likely relevant to the health of people in all age groups.*

▲ Collaborate with community members to improve educational levels within the community. **EBN:** *In a study of 18 randomly selected communities and 900 elders living in those communities, higher educational levels were associated with less stress pertaining to health, and fewer helpers were needed by the educated elderly (Preston & Bucher, 1996). Higher educational levels are associated with lower levels of emotional and physical distress (Ross & Van Willigen, 1997).*

### Multicultural

- Acknowledge the stresses unique to racial/ethnic communities. **EBN:** *Targeted alcohol and tobacco marketing, high levels of unemployment, lack of health insurance, and racism are stressors unique to culturally diverse communities (D'Avanzo et al, 2001).*

▲ Identify what health services and information are currently available in the commu-

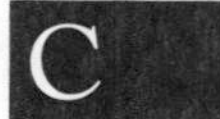

nity. **EB:** *This will assist with focusing efforts and promote wise use of valuable resources (National Institutes of Health, 1998).*

- Work with members of the community to prioritize and target health goals specific to the community. **EB:** *This will increase feelings of control over and sense of ownership of programs (National Institutes of Health, 1998).*
- Approach community leaders and members of color with respect, warmth, and professional courtesy. **EBN:** *Instances of disrespect and lack of caring have special significance for individuals of color (D'Avanzo et al, 2001).*
- Establish and sustain partnerships with key individuals within communities when developing and implementing programs. **EB:** *Local leaders are excellent sources of information and their participation will enhance the credibility of programs (National Institutes of Health, 1998).*
- Use community church settings as a forum for advocacy, teaching, and program implementation. **EBN:** *Evaluation of a faith-based program supplied to 125 people from 18 congregations showed an increase in health promotion knowledge, rise in consumer satisfaction, and improvement in health (Kotecki, 2002). Literature reviews of church-based health promotion programs showed that they are successful in helping people to adopt health-promoting behaviors (DeHaven et al, 2004; Peterson, Atwood, & Yates, 2002). Church-based programs are especially effective in communities of color.*

### Community Teaching

- Review coping skills, power for coping, and the use of power resources.

## evolve WEBSITES FOR EDUCATION

See the EVOLVE website for World Wide Web resources for client education.

## REFERENCES


Anderson ET, McFarlane J: *Community as partner: theory and practice in nursing,* ed 4, Philadelphia, 2003, Lippincott Williams & Wilkins.

Chinn PL: *Peace and power: building communities for the future,* ed 5, Boston, 2001, Jones & Bartlett.

Coley SM, Scheinberg CA: *Proposal writing,* ed 2, Thousand Oaks, Calif, 2000, Sage.

D'Avanzo CE et al: Developing culturally informed strategies for substance-related interventions. In Naegle MA, D'Avanzo CE, editors: *Addictions and substance abuse: strategies for advanced practice nursing,* St Louis, 2001, Mosby.

DeHaven M, Hunter I, Wilder L et al: Health programs in faith-based organizations: are they effective? *Am J Public Health* 94(6): 1030-1036, 2004.

Kotecki CN: Developing a health promotion program for faith-based communities, *Holist Nurs Pract* 16(3):61, 2002.

Logan L: The practice of certified community health CNSs, *Clin Nurse Spec* 19(1):43-48, 2005.

National Institutes of Health: *Salud para su corazón: bringing heart health to Latinos—a guide for building community programs,* DHHS Pub No 98-3796, Washington, DC, 1998, US Government Printing Office.

Peterson J, Atwood JR, Yates B: Key elements for church-based health promotion programs: outcome-based literature review, *Public Health Nurs* 19(6):401, 2002.

Preston DB, Bucher JA: The effects of community differences on health status, health stress, and helping networks in a sample of 900 elderly, *Public Health Nurs* 13:72, 1996.

Ross CE, Van Willigen M: Education and subjective quality of life, *J Health Soc Behav* 38:275, 1997.

Scheffer BK, Rubenfeld MG: A consensus statement on critical thinking, *J Nurs Educ* 15:350, 2000.
Stanhope M, Lancaster J: Community and public health nursing, ed 6, St. Louis, 2004, Mosby.
Wagstaff A, Bustreo F, Bryce J et al: Child health: reaching the poor, *Am J Public Health* 94(5):726-36, 2004.

# Defensive Coping

*Ann Keeley*

## NANDA

### Definition

Repeated projection of falsely positive self-evaluation based on self-protective pattern that defends against underlying perceived threats to positive self-regard

### Defining Characteristics

Grandiosity, rationalization of failures, hypersensitivity to slight/criticism, denial of obvious problems/weaknesses, projection of blame/responsibility, lack of follow-through or participation in treatment or therapy, superior attitude toward others, hostile laughter or ridicule of others, difficulty in perception of reality/reality testing, difficulty establishing/maintaining relationships

### Related Factors (r/t)

To be developed

## NOC

### Outcomes (Nursing Outcomes Classification)

#### Suggested NOC Outcomes

Coping, Decision Making, Impulse Self-Control, Information Processing

**Example NOC Outcome with Indicators**

**Coping** as evidenced by the following indicators: Identifies effective and ineffective coping patterns/Modifies lifestyle as needed (Rate each indicator of **Coping:** 1 = never demonstrated, 2 = rarely demonstrated, 3 = sometimes demonstrated, 4 = often demonstrated, 5 = consistently demonstrated [see Section I].)

### Client Outcomes

#### Client Will (Specify Time Frame):

- Acknowledge need for change in coping style
- Accept responsibility for own behavior
- Establish realistic goals with validation from caregivers
- Solicit caregiver validation in decision making

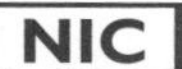

## Interventions (Nursing Interventions Classification)

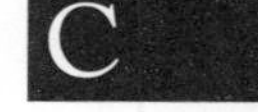

### Suggested NIC Intervention

Self-Awareness Enhancement

**Example NIC Activities—Self-Awareness Enhancement**

Encourage client to recognize and discuss thoughts and feelings; assist client in identifying behaviors that are self-destructive

## Nursing Interventions and Rationales

- Assess for the presence of denial as a coping mechanism. **EB:** *A thorough assessment for behaviors indicating the presence of denial is necessary in order to address issues of non-adherence in persons with HIV (Power et al, 2003).*
- Do not confront denial if its consequences are not a significant threat to health. **EBN:** *A period of denial may be necessary for the client to develop a construct within which the given information has meaning and can be appraised as not being a threat to survival (Norris & Spelic, 2002). Denial may be protective (Stephenson, 2004).*
- Determine whether the client has a positive or negative overall appraisal of a given event. **EB:** *Adolescent cannabis abusers present with a variety of challenges in outpatient treatment. Accurate assessment is necessary for successful outcome (Tims et al, 2002).*
- Develop a trusting, therapeutic relationship with the client and family. *The interview process itself can be therapeutic (Overcash, 2004).*
- Ask appropriate questions using an assessment tool such as Fast Alcohol Screening Test (FAST) to assess whether denial is being used in association with alcoholism. For each question, the client is asked to circle the appropriate response: Less than monthly, Monthly, Weekly, Daily, or Almost Daily.
  1. **Men:** How often do you have EIGHT or more drinks on one occasion?
     **Women:** How often do you have SIX or more drinks on one occasion?
  2. How often during the last year have you been unable to remember what happened the night before because you had been drinking?
  3. How often during the last year have you failed to do what was normally expected of you because of drinking?
  4. In the last year has a relative or friend, or a doctor or other health worker been concerned about your drinking or suggested you cut down?

  **EB:** *The four-item FAST alcohol questionnaire had good sensitivity and specificity across a range of settings when the Alcohol Use Disorders Identification Test (AUDIT) alcohol assessment score was used as the gold standard. The FAST questionnaire is quick to administer, since more than 50% of clients are categorized using just one question (Hodgson et al, 2002). Include drug use in addition to drinking in the questionnaire (Hinkin et al, 2001). T-ACE and TWEAK are modified to be used with women.* **EBN:** *Alcoholism rates are increasing in women, and women may have distinct assessment risk factors (Becker & Walton-Moss, 2001). Brief addiction screening tools are available (Gorski, 2002).*

- Determine the client's perception of the problem and then provide reality-based examples of the true situation (e.g., witnesses to an accident, blood alcohol levels, problems caused by alcohol). **EBN:** *Psychological manifestations of defensive coping can be understood only after a thorough inquiry into the client's framework for appraisal (Dudley-Brown, 2002).*
- Help the client identify patterns of response in life that may be maladaptive. A clear, honest recounting of life incidents and their consequences in a trusting relationship may provide the motivation necessary to seek a change in behavior (Faltz & Skinner, 2002).
- ▲ Promote the client's feelings of self-worth by using group or individual therapy, role playing, one-to-one interactions, and role modeling. **EBN:** *A variety of methods may be used to assist clients in their attempts to assimilate the implications of a health status change (Whittemore et al, 2002).*
- Support strengths and normal observations with "I note that" or "I want you to notice." Tell clients when they do something well. **EBN:** *Nurses effectively support adaptation to a change in health status by actively listening to the client at all stages and encouraging reflection and self-understanding throughout the process (Whittemore et al, 2002).*
- Teach the client to use positive thinking by blocking negative thoughts with the word "Stop!" and inserting positive thoughts (e.g., "I'm a good [person, friend, student]"). *Interventions that encourage the cognitive reframing of a change in health status within a more positive framework support adaptation to a change in health status (Dudley-Brown, 2002).*
- Provide feedback regarding others' perceptions of the client's behavior through group or milieu therapy or one-to-one interactions. **EBN:** *Group therapy is an effective component of treatment in women with a dual diagnosis (Moser, Sowell, & Phillips, 2001).*
- Encourage the client to use "I" statements and to accept responsibility for and consequences of actions. **EB:** *Interventions that support self-efficacy and a building of the sense of self as an individual who can control his or her own response facilitate the client's meeting of his or her goals (Brun & Rapp, 2001).*
- Refer to the care plans for **Ineffective Denial** and **Dysfunctional Family processes: alcoholism.**

## Geriatric

- Assess the client for anger and identify previous outlets for anger. *Nurses can help individuals to cope effectively with a change in health status by teaching them alternative methods of coping (Reynaud & Meeker, 2002).*
- Explore new outlets for anger, including physical activities within the client's capabilities (e.g., hitting a pillow, woodworking, sanding, scrubbing floors). **EB:** *Stress, along with the client's method of coping with it, is a risk factor for substance abuse behavior. Instruction in effective stress-reducing strategies may lower the risk (Brady & Sonne, 1999).*
- Use the CAGE tool with this population and include drug use along with drinking.

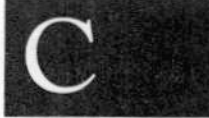

An affirmative answer to two or more of the following questions is considered a basis for suspicion of alcohol abuse:

**C:** Have you ever felt you ought to **Cut down** on drinking?
**A:** Have people **Annoyed** you by criticizing your drinking?
**G:** Have you ever felt bad or **Guilty** about your drinking?
**E:** Have you ever had a drink the first thing in the morning to steady your nerves or get rid of a hangover **(Eye opener)?**

**EBN:** *Alcoholism and drug abuse are present in the geriatric population, and the CAGE tool is effective in identifying individuals at risk (Hinkin et al, 2001). Individuals with these problems are more likely to be found in health care settings that are not substance abuse specific (Weisner, 2001).*

- Assess the client for dementia or depression. *A thorough assessment must be conducted to determine if the aberrant behavior has an organic origin (Green, 2002). Clients may not readily admit to psychological or substance abuse symptoms (Boyd & Stanley, 2002).*
- If a traumatic event has occurred, support positive religious coping behaviors. **EBN:** *Religious coping behaviors, when positive, can facilitate a more constructive health outcome (Bell Meisenhelder, 2002). Women with cancer who are involved in religious activities and groups report a more positive adaptation (Ferrell, 2003).*

## Multicultural

- Assess for the influence of cultural beliefs, norms, and values on the client's feelings of defensiveness. **EBN:** *The "denial" perceived by the nurse may be an expected behavior within the culture of the client (Lindenberg et al, 2002).*
- Acknowledge racial/ethnic differences at the onset of care. **EBN:** *Acknowledgment of race/ethnicity issues will enhance communication, establish rapport, and promote treatment outcomes (D'Avanzo et al, 2001). African-American parents who denied experiences of racism reported higher rates of behavior problems in their children, in contrast to African-American parents who actively coped with racism and reported lower levels of behavior problems in their children (Caughy, O'Campo, & Muntaner, 2004).*
- Use therapeutic communication techniques that emphasize acceptance, offer the self, validate the client's concerns, and convey respect. **EBN:** *Open communication by the nurse will facilitate the use of health care resources by immigrant populations. Care needs to be taken to incorporate the concept of health and healing prevalent in the client's culture (Chen & Rankin, 2002; White et al, 2002; Donnelly, 2002). The therapeutic use of* dichos *(Spanish language proverbs and sayings) decreased defensiveness in a repopulation of Hispanic/Latino psychiatric inpatients (Aviera, 1996).*
- Give a rationale when assessing ethnically diverse clients for alcohol use/misuse or other sensitive behaviors. **EBN:** *Depending on the culture, aspects of responsibility may have different values than in the Western health care system (Shin, 2002; Rungreangkulkij et al, 2002; White et al, 2002). African Americans and other people of color may expect Caucasian caregivers to hold negative and preconceived ideas about people of color. Giving a rationale for questions asked will help reduce this perception (D'Avanzo et al, 2001).*

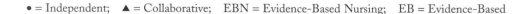

C

## Home Care

- The interventions described previously may be adapted for home care use.
- Include in the initial assessment client and family histories of mental health problems. **EBN:** *A thorough understanding of the family history of mental health problems, the attempts made to seek help, and the cultural context of the behavior will facilitate a successful intervention by the nurse (Aziz & Rowland, 2002; Donnelly, 2002; Rungreangkulkij et al, 2002; Shin, 2002).*
- Observe family dynamics for dysfunctional and supportive communication. **EBN:** *An understanding of the family structure, patterns of communication, health care history, and cultural influences will facilitate effective interventions on the part of the nurse. In the context of some family patterns of communication, defensive coping may be a learned behavior (Hellemann, Lee, & Kury, 2002).*
- ▲ Refer to a mental health professional for possible psychodrama therapy, especially if the client experiences difficulty in coping with a traumatic event. **EB:** *Psychodrama has been shown to help people begin to reframe their feelings of victimization as feelings of survival and begin to see the future as hopeful (Carbonell & Parteleno-Barehmi, 1999).*
- ▲ In the absence of primary medical diagnoses, refer to medical social services for assistance in contacting appropriate community services. **EBN:** *The nurse is often perceived as the "constant" in a client's relationship with the health care system and as such can help bridge the gap between the client and available resources (Northouse et al, 2002; Tak & McCubbin, 2002).*
- ▲ If medical diagnoses coexist with defensive coping, confirm and validate the client's mental health plan and progress. **EBN:** *The nurse is often perceived as the"constant" in a client's relationship with the health care system and as such can help bridge the gap between the client and available resources (Northouse et al, 2002; Tak & McCubbin, 2002).*
- ▲ Refer to a therapist for debriefing if a traumatic or critical event has occurred. *Critical incident debriefing has decreased the number of psychological problems caused by traumatic events (Johal & Bennett, 1999).* **EB:** *A review of psychological debriefing, however, has concluded that there is little evidence for its use. Early intervention recommendations are to assess the need for sustained treatment, to provide psychological first aid, and to supply education about trauma and information about treatment resources. Recommendations for secondary prevention of posttraumatic stress disorder include education, anxiety management, cognitive restructuring, exposure, and relapse prevention (Litzet al, 2002).*
- ▲ Refer for psychiatric home health care services for client reassurance and implementation of a therapeutic regimen. **EBN:** *Psychiatric home care nurses can address issues relating to the client's ability to adjust to changes in health status. Behavioral interventions and reality orientation in the home can help the client to participate more effectively in the treatment plan (Patusky, Rodning, & Martinez-Kratz, 1996).*

## Client/Family Teaching

- ▲ Teach the client the actions and side effects of medications and the importance of taking them as prescribed, even when the client is feeling good. **EBN:** *Education about the desired effects and potential side effects increases the knowledge and effective decision-making ability of the client (Moser, Sowell, & Phillips, 2001).*

▲ Work with the client's support group to identify harmful behaviors and to seek help for the client if he or she is unable to control behavior. **EBN:** *When possible, the client's family system should be a component of the treatment (Cook, 2001). Families need assistance in identifying resources and therapeutic responses as they adapt to the individual client's behaviors (Faltz & Skinner, 2002).*

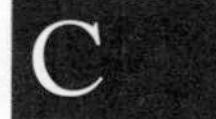

- Support family efforts using religious coping behaviors. **EBN:** *Interventions to enhance positive religious coping facilitate recovery (Bell Meisenhelder, 2002; Newlin, Knafi, & Meldus, 2002).*

## evolve WEBSITES FOR EDUCATION

See the EVOLVE website for World Wide Web resources for client education.

## REFERENCES


Aviera A: "Dichos" therapy group: a therapeutic use of Spanish language proverbs with hospitalized Spanish-speaking psychiatric patients, *Cult Divers Ment Health* 2(2):73-87, 1996.

Aziz N, Rowland JH: Cancer survivorship research among ethnic minority and medically underserved groups, *Oncol Nurs Forum* 29(5):789, 2002.

Becker K, Walton-Moss B: Detecting and addressing alcohol abuse in women, *Nurse Pract* 26(10):13, 2001.

Bell Meisenhelder J: Terrorism, posttraumatic stress, and religious coping, *Issues Ment Health Nurs* 23(8):771, 2002.

Boyd MA, Stanley M: Mental health assessment of the elderly. In Boyd MA, editor: *Psychiatric nursing in contemporary practice,* ed 2, Philadelphia, 2002, Lippincott.

Brady KT, Sonne SC: The role of stress in alcohol use, alcoholism treatment, and relapse, *Alcohol Res Health* 23(4):263, 1999.

Brun C, Rapp RC: Strengths-based case management: individual's perspectives on strengths and the case manager relationship, *Soc Work* 46(3):278, 2001.

Carbonell DM, Parteleno-Barehmi C: Psychodrama groups for girls coping with trauma, *Int J Group Psychother* 49(3):285-306, 1999.

Caughy MO, O'Campo PJ, Muntaner C: Experiences of racism among African American parents and the mental health of their preschool-aged children, *Am J Public Health* 94(12):2118-2124, 2004.

Chen J-L, Rankin SH: Using the resiliency model to deliver culturally sensitive care to Chinese families, *J Pediatr Nurs* 17(3):157, 2002.

Cook LS: Adolescent addiction and delinquency in the family system, *Issues Ment Health Nurs* 22:151, 2001.

D'Avanzo CE et al: Developing culturally informed strategies for substance-related interventions. In Naegle MA, D'Avanzo CE, editors: *Addictions and substance abuse: strategies for advanced practice nursing,* St Louis, 2001, Mosby.

Donnelly TT: Contextual analysis of coping: implications for immigrants' mental health care, *Issues Ment Health Nurs* 23:715, 2002.

Dudley-Brown S: Prevention of psychological distress in persons with inflammatory bowel disease, *Issues Ment Health Nurs* 23:403, 2002.

Faltz BG, Skinner MK: Substance abuse disorders. In Boyd MA, editor: *Psychiatric nursing in contemporary practice,* ed 2, Philadelphia, 2002, Lippincott.

Ferrell BR, Smith SL, Juarez G et al: Meaning of illness and spirituality in ovarian cancer survivors, *Oncol Nurs Forum* 30(2):249, 2003.

Gorski T: *Women at risk: brief addiction screening tools,* 2002. Available at www.tgorski.com/clin_mod/atp/women_at_risk-brief_sceening_tools.htm, accessed on March 30, 2005.

Green GC: Guidelines for assessing and diagnosing acute psychosis: a primer, *J Emerg Nurs* 28:S1, 2002.

Hellemann MV, Lee KA, Kury FS: Strengths and vulnerabilities of women of Mexican descent in relation to depressive symptoms, *Nurs Res* 51(3):175, 2002.

Hinkin CH, Castellon SA, Dickson-Fuhrman E et al: Screening for drug and alcohol abuse among older adults using a modified version of the CAGE, *Am J Addict* 10:319, 2001.

Hodgson R, Alwyn T, John B et al: The FAST Alcohol Screening Test, *Alcohol Alcohol* 37(1):61-66, 2002.

Lefler L, Bondy KN: Women's delay in seeking treatment with myocardial infarction: a meta-synthesis, *J Cardiovasc Nurs* 19(4): 251, 2004.

Lindenberg CS, Solorzano RM, Bear D et al: Reducing substance use and risky sexual behavior among young, low-income, Mexican-American women: comparison of two interventions, *Appl Nurs Res* 16(2):137-148, 2002.
Litz BT, Gray M, Bryant LA et al: Early intervention for trauma: current status and future direction, *Clin Psychol Sci Pract* 9:112, 2002.
Moser KM, Sowell RL, Phillips KD: Issues of women dually diagnosed with HIV infection and substance use problems in the Carolinas, *Issues Ment Health Nurs* 22:23, 2001.
Newlin K, Knafi K, Meldus GD: African-American spirituality: a concept analysis, *ANS Adv Nurs Sci* 25(2):57, 2002.
Norris J, Spelic SS: Supporting adaptation to body image disruption, *Rehabil Nurs* 27(1):8, 2002.
Northouse L, Walker J, Schafenacker A et al: A family-based program of care for women with recurrent breast cancer and their family members, *Oncol Nurs Forum* 29(10):1411-1419, 2002.
Overcash JA: Using narrative reseach to undrstand the quality of life of older women with breast cancer, *Oncol Nurs Forum* 31(6): 1153, 2004.
Power R, Koopman C, Volk J et al: Social support, substance use, and denial in relationship to antiretroviral treatment adherence among HIV-infected persons, *Aids Patient Care* 17(5):245, 2003.
Purnell LD, Paulanka BJ: *Guide to culturally competent health care,* Philadelphia, 2004, FA Davis.
Reynaud SN, Meeker BJ: Coping styles of older adults with ostomies, *J Gerontol Nurs* 28(5):30, 2002.
Rungreangkulkij S, Chafetz L, Chesla C et al: Psychological morbidity of Thai families of a person with schizophrenia, *Int J Nurs Stud* 39(1):35-50, 2002.
Shin JK: Help-seeking behaviors by Korean immigrants for depression, *Issues Ment Health Nurs* 23:461, 2002.
Stephenson PS: Understanding denial, *Oncol Nurs Forum* 31(5):985, 2004.
Tak YR, McCubbin M: Family stress, perceived social support and coping following the diagnosis of a child's congenital heart disease, *J Adv Nurs* 39(2):190, 2002.
Tims FM, Dennis ML, Hamilton N et al: Characteristics and problems of 600 adolescent cannabis abusers in outpatient treatment, *Addiction,* 97(Suppl 1):46, 2002.
Weisner C: The provision of services for alcohol problems: a community perspective for understanding access, *J Behav Health Serv Res* 28(2):130, 2001.
White N, Bichter J, Koeckeritz J et al: A cross-cultural comparison of family resiliency in hemodialysis clients, *J Transcult Nurs* 13(3): 218, 2002.
Whittemore R, Chase SK, Mandle CL et al: Lifestyle change in type 2 diabetes, *Nurs Res* 51(1):18, 2002.

# Compromised family Coping

evolve

*Gail B. Ladwig*

**NANDA**

## Definition

Situation in which usually supportive primary person (family member or close friend) provides insufficient, ineffective, or compromised support, comfort, assistance, or encouragement that may be needed by client to manage or master adaptive tasks related to health challenge

## Defining Characteristics

### Objective

Significant person attempts assistive or supportive behaviors with less than satisfactory results; significant person displays protective behavior disproportionate (too little or too much) to client's abilities or need for autonomy; significant person withdraws or enters into limited or temporary personal communication with client at time of need

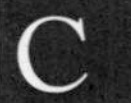

### Subjective

Client expresses or confirms a concern or complaint about significant other's response to his or her health problem; significant person describes or confirms an inadequate understanding or knowledge base, which interferes with effective assistance or supportive behaviors; significant person describes preoccupation with personal reaction (e.g., fear, anticipatory grief, guilt, or anxiety) to client's illness, disability, or other situational or developmental crisis

## Related Factors (r/t)

Temporary preoccupation of a significant person who tries to manage emotional conflicts and personal suffering and is unable to perceive or act effectively with regard to client's needs; temporary family disorganization and role changes; prolonged disease or disability progression that exhausts supportive capacity of significant people; other situational or developmental crises or problems significant person may be facing; inadequate or incorrect information or understanding by primary person; little support provided by client, in turn, for primary person

**NOC**

## Outcomes (Nursing Outcomes Classification)

### Suggested NOC Outcomes

Caregiver Emotional Health, Caregiver-Patient Relationship, Family Coping, Family Participation in Professional Care, Family Support during Treatment

**Example NOC Outcome with Indicators**

**Family Coping** as evidenced by the following indicators: Confronts family problems/Manages family problems/Seeks family assistance when appropriate (Rate each indicator of **Family Coping:** 1 = never demonstrated, 2 = rarely demonstrated, 3 = sometimes demonstrated, 4 = often demonstrated, 5 = consistently demonstrated [see Section I].)

## Client Outcomes

### Family/Significant Person Will (Specify Time Frame):

- Verbalize internal resources to help deal with the situation
- Verbalize knowledge and understanding of illness, disability, or disease
- Provide support and assistance as needed
- Identify need for and seek outside support

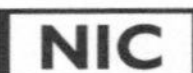

## Interventions (Nursing Interventions Classification)

C

### Suggested NIC Interventions

Caregiver Support, Coping Enhancement, Family Involvement Promotion, Family Mobilization, Family Support, Mutual Goal Setting, Normalization Promotion, Sibling Support

**Example NIC Activities—Family Support**

Appraise family's emotional reaction to client's condition; promote trusting relationship with family

## Nursing Interventions and Rationales

- Assess the strengths and deficiencies of the family system. **EBN:** *Assessments allow for anticipatory care and guidance to help members acquire and maintain supports and coping strategies (Thomas, 2000).* **EB:** *Chronic illness in children affects the psychological health of the parents. Active coping strategies are associated with fewer distress indices and thus if inculcated may improve the ability to bear the burden of the illness without becoming themselves affected by psychiatric illnesses (Rao, 2004).*
- Assess how family members interact with each other; observe verbal and nonverbal communication and individual and group responses to stress. **EBN:** *Understanding how families cope with stress is important. Family cohesion, presence of a partner, emotional support, and a mother's satisfaction with her family all contributed to her better mental health in a research study focusing on mothers of low-birth-weight infants (Weiss & Chen, 2002).*
- Establish rapport with families by providing accurate communication **EBN:** *This qualitative exploratory study of families in psychiatric settings indicated that family care can be improved by focusing on building rapport and communicating problems and concerns between families and health professionals (Rose, Mallinson, & Walton-Moss, 2004).*
- Consider the use of family theory as a framework to help guide interventions (e.g., family stress theory, role theory, social exchange theory). **EBN:** *This study demonstrated that use of a family assessment tool is an effective way of appraising families and addressing suffering. Formative evaluations demonstrated improvements in team members' perceptions of their knowledge, family centeredness, and ability to assess and intervene with families (Hogan & Logan, 2004.)*
- Help family members recognize the need for help and teach them how to ask for it. **EBN:** *Recognizing the need for help and knowing how to ask for it enables family members to maintain control (Szabo & Strang, 1999).*
- Encourage expression of positive thoughts and emotions. **EB:** *Positive emotions initiate upward spirals toward enhanced emotional well-being (Fredrickson & Joiner, 2002).* **EBN:** *This study shows that clients believe that coping is important to their well-being (Edgar, 2004).*
- Encourage family members to verbalize feelings. Spend time with them, sit down and make eye contact, and offer coffee and other nourishment. **EBN:** *The expression of*

*feelings helps family caregivers to regain and maintain control (Szabo & Strang, 1999). Acceptance of nourishment indicates a beginning acceptance of the situation.*

- Provide opportunities for families to discuss spirituality. **EB:** *This research provided by survivors of haematological malignancies gives insight into factors impacting their need to talk about spiritual issues (McGrath & Clarke, 2003).*
- Mothers may require additional support in their role of caring for chronically ill children. **EBN:** *Mothers exhibit greater efforts than fathers in coping patterns, including strategies to acquire social support outside the family, increase self-worth, and decrease psychological tensions (Brazil & Krueger, 2002).*
- Provide privacy during family visits. If possible, maintain flexible visiting hours to accommodate more frequent family visits. If possible, arrange staff assignments so the same staff members have contact with the family. Familiarize other staff members with the situation in the absence of the usual staff member. *Providing privacy, maintaining flexible hours, and arranging consistent staff assignments will reduce stress, enhance communication, and facilitate the building of trust.*
- Determine whether the family is suffering from additional stressors (e.g., child care issues, financial problems). **EBN:** *One study found that in mothers of low-birth-weight infants, the presence of other life stressors and the family's use of internally focused coping strategies contributed to worse mental health outcomes for the mother (Weiss & Chen, 2002).*

▲ Refer the family with ill family members to appropriate resources for assistance as indicated (e.g., counseling, psychotherapy, financial or spiritual support). **EBN:** *The findings of this study demonstrate the importance of supporting family functioning in the families of people with heart disease is an important challenge for family nursing. The most important predictors of family health were family structural factors. It was found that the better the family structure and relationships, the better the family health (stedt-Kurki et al, 2003).*

## Pediatric

- Assess the adolescent's perception of support from family and friends during crisis. **EBN:** *Some teens find parents and friends burdensome during a time of grief, whereas others find their support critical for coping with crises. Recognition of individual perception can assist families in negotiating times of crisis (Rask, Kaunonen, & Paunonen-Ilmonen, 2002).*
- Provide educational interventions and psychosocial interventions such as coping skills training in treatment for families and their adolescents who have type 1 diabetes. **EB:** *Education interventions increase diabetes knowledge but are not consistently helpful in improving metabolic outcomes. Psychosocial interventions such as coping skills training and behavioral family systems therapy have demonstrated improvements in metabolic control, self-efficacy, diabetes stress, quality of life, and parent-adolescent conflict. Family interventions are emerging as a positive way to improve interpersonal relations and assist the adolescent in transitioning from family-management toward self-management of their diabetes (Urban, Berry, & Grey, 2004).*
- Encourage the use of family rituals such as connection, spiritual, love, recreation, celebration, and evolving especially in single parent families. **EBN:** *Data from this study indicated that these rituals were found to be used by single-parent families as a way to facilitate family cohesion and instill family values (Moriarty & Wagner, 2004).*

C

- Encourage laughing, playing, singing, talking, and praying with seriously injured children. **EBN:** *This interpretive study examined the experiences of 16 pediatric burn intensive care unit nurses for the purpose of uncovering and articulating practices that help critically burned children to heal holistically. These everyday practices were identified as maintaining or reestablishing harmony of the children's mind, body, and spirit (Zengerle-Levy, 2004).*
- ▲ Link trained volunteers with "vulnerable" first-time parents. Provide social support and information related to age appropriate expectations of infants. **EBN:** *This descriptive comparative design demonstrated participant's satisfaction with the program and improvement in family functioning. The program could be appropriate for all parents (Kelleher & Johnson, 2004).*

## Geriatric

- Perform a holistic assessment of all needs of informal spousal caregivers. **EBN:** *The role of informal spousal caregivers has increased as the population ages. This research highlighted the interconnectedness of factors in the experiences of caregivers, reinforcing the need for holistic assessment beyond a focus on the "continence issue" alone (Cassells & Watt, 2003).*
- Help caregivers establish one's priorities and concentrate on them, believe in themesleves and their ability to handle the situation, taking life 1 day at a time, looking for positive things in each situation, and relying on their own individual expertise and experience. **EBN:** *The most helpful coping strategies identified in this major international research project on caregivers' work and coping in four countries (Kuuppelomäki et al, 2004).*
- ▲ Refer caregivers of Alzheimer's clients to a monthly psychoeducational support group. **EB:** *Nonpharmacologic interventions can be used for the management of Alzheimer's clients. This support group intervention has been well accepted by patients, families, and physicians in this study (Guerriero Austrom et al, 2004).*
- ▲ Consider the use of telephone support for caregivers of family members with dementia. **EBN:** *Results from this study suggest family caregivers can be helped through a variety of social support mechanisms including telephone support. Participants reported assistance in sharing thoughts and feelings, expressing feelings of being overwhelmed, discussing physical and psychosocial problems, forgetting the situation, seeking reassurance, and asking for information (Chang et al, 2004).*
- Assist in finding transportation to enable family members to visit. *If a family member is homebound and unable to visit, encourage alternative contact (e.g., telephone, cards and letters, e-mail) to provide ongoing scheduled progress reports. Reducing loneliness and isolation has many positive psychosocial and physical health benefits (Bulechek & McCloskey, 1992).*

## Multicultural

- Acknowledge racial/ethnic differences at the onset of care. **EBN:** *Acknowledgment of race/ethnicity issues will enhance communication, establish rapport, and promote treatment outcomes (D'Avanzo et al, 2001; Ludwick & Silva, 2000; Vontress & Epp, 1997).*
- Approach families of color with respect, warmth, and professional courtesy. **EB:** *Instances of disrespect and lack of caring have special significance for families of color*

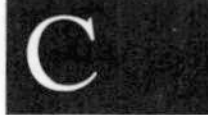

*(D'Avanzo et al, 2001; Vontress & Epp, 1997). Latina mothers of developmentally disabled adults reported their relationship with the educational and service delivery systems to be characterized by poor communication, low effort in providing services, negative attitudes of professionals toward the client-children, and negative treatment of parents by professionals (Shapiro et al, 2004).*

- Assess for the influence of cultural beliefs, norms, and values on the family's perceptions of coping. **EBN:** *What the family considers normal and abnormal coping behavior may be based on cultural perceptions (Leininger & McFarland, 2002; Cochran, 1998; Doswell & Erlen, 1998).*
- Give a rationale when assessing families with regard to sensitive issues. **EBN:** *African Americans and other people of color may expect Caucasian caregivers to hold negative and preconceived ideas about them. Giving a rationale for questions asked will help reduce this perception (D'Avanzo et al, 2001; Vontress & Epp, 1997). Topics such as smoking in the household, financial difficulties, and emotional support available to the parent were more likely to be asked of parents of African-American and Hispanic children than of parents of Caucasian children (Kogan et al, 2004).*
- Use a family-centered approach when working with Latino, Asian, African-American, and Native-American clients. **EBN:** *Latinos may perceive the family as a source of support, solver of problems, and source of pride. Asian Americans may regard the family as the primary decision maker and influence on individual family members (D'Avanzo et al, 2001; Guarnaccia, 1998). Elders may play a key role in decision making for some Asian populations (Davis, 2000). Native-American families have extended structures and exert powerful influences over functioning (Seiderman et al, 1996). Use of a family-based intervention among American-Indian families resulted in higher levels of child prosocial behavior and lowered drug use (Boyd-Ball, 2003). Among Mexican Americans with type 2 diabetes, higher levels of perceived family support and greater self-efficacy were associated with higher reported levels of diet and exercise self-care (Wen, Shepherd, & Parchman 2004).*
- Facilitate modeling and role playing for family regarding healthy ways to communicate and interact. **EBN:** *It is helpful for families and the client to practice communication skills in a safe environment before trying them in a real-life situation (Rivera-Andino & Lopez, 2000).*
- Validate the family's feelings regarding the impact of the client's illness on the family's lifestyle. **EBN:** *Validation lets family members know that the nurse has heard and understood what was said, and it promotes the relationship between nurse and family members (Heineken, 1998).*
- Work to provide caregivers who understand the importance of cultural beliefs and values the family may hold. **EBN:** *There are differences in some cultures regarding health beliefs, practices, and values (Camphinha-Bacote & Narayan, 2000).*

## Home Care

- The interventions described previously may be adapted for home care use.
- Assess the reason behind the breakdown of family coping. *Knowledge of the reasons behind compromised coping will assist in identification of appropriate interventions. Are family members physically able to aid client? Is there a lack of resources? Do past relationship*

C

*issues interfere with motivation? Are family members feeling stressed dealing with client's care needs?* Refer to the care plan for **Caregiver role strain.**

- • During the time of compromised coping, increase visits to ensure the safety of the client, support of the family, and assistance with coping strategies. Provide reassurance regarding expectations for prognosis as appropriate. *Increased time for expressions of support, active listening, and empathy can nurture the client and family and move them toward more effective coping.* **EBN:** *A study identified the need for support of the spouses of heart transplantation clients (Bohachick et al, 2001).*
- ▲ Assess the needs of the caregiver in the home. Intervene to meet needs as appropriate to total case management and explore all available resources that may be used to provide adequate home care (e.g., parish nursing as an effective adjunct, home health aide services to relieve caregiver's fatigue). Encourage caregivers not to neglect their own physical, mental, and spiritual health and give more specific information about the client's needs and ways to meet them. *Meeting the needs of caregivers supports their ability to meet the needs of the client. Assess the client and caregiver separately and in interaction. Do not assume that the client and his or her spouse experience similar patterns of distress or psychological adjustment.* **EBN:** *In one study, the highest level of distress in heart transplantation clients related to effects on their ability to work, while spouses felt higher levels of psychological distress (Bohachick et al, 2001).*
- ▲ Refer the family to medical social services for evaluation and supportive counseling. Dedicating time for nurturing the caregivers and reassuring the client allows them to express feelings and feel hope.
- ▲ Serve as an advocate, mentor, and role model for caregiving. Write down or contract for the care needed by the client. *Therapeutic use of self by the nurse and concrete task definition and assignment reinforce positive coping strategies and allow caregivers to feel less guilty when tasks are delegated to multiple caregivers.*
- ▲ When a terminal illness is the precipitating factor for ineffective coping, offer hospice services and support groups as possible resources. *Nonjudgmental support from helpers with no agenda allows verbalization of feelings. The hospice paradigm addresses the physical, emotional, and spiritual needs of the dying and their loved ones.*
- • With a cancer client, encourage family discussion of stressors (including the meaning of the illness, fear of recurrence, the client's employment status) and resources (family social support). **EBN:** *Stressors and resources have been shown to play an important role in determining family quality of life among cancer survivors (Mellon & Northouse, 2001).*
- • Encourage the client and family to discuss changes in daily functioning and routines created by the client's illness. Validate discomfort resulting from changes. *Individuals who live together for a long period tend to become entrained to each others' patterns: meals are expected at certain times, a spouse becomes accustomed to the client's sleep habits. Changes in these patterns may result in a vague discomfort that may be relieved when its source is known.*
- • Support positive individual and family coping efforts. *Positive feedback reinforces desired behaviors and supports the family unit.*
- ▲ If compromised family coping interferes with the ability to support the client's treat-

ment plan, refer for psychiatric home health care services for family counseling and implementation of a therapeutic regimen. **EBN:** *Psychiatric home care nurses can address issues relating to family members' ability to adjust to changes in the client's health status. Behavioral interventions in the home can help the family to participate more effectively in the treatment plan (Patusky, Rodning, & Martinez-Kratz, 1996).*

## Client/Family Teaching

- • Provide truthful information and support for the family and significant people regarding the client's specific illness or condition. **EBN:** *The results of this study indicate that attention needs to be given to methods of providing information and support to couples coping with prostate cancer. Both patients and partners need to be included in discussions about the effect of the illness and treatments so that both can feel more prepared to manage them (Harden et al, 2002).*
- ▲ Refer women with recurrent breast cancer and their family caregivers to a FOCUS Program (family involvement, optimistic attitude, coping effectiveness, uncertainty reduction, and symptom management), a family-based program of care. **EBN:** *Patients with recurrent breast cancer and their family members reported high satisfaction with the FOCUS Program. This study indicates that a need exists for family-based programs of care that enable both patients and their family members to manage the multiple demands associated with recurrent breast cancer (Northouse et al, 2002).*
- • Promote individual and family relaxation and stress-reduction strategies. *The immune system weakens in response to stress; relaxation elicits the opposite, healthful response (Bulechek & McCloskey, 1992).*
- ▲ Provide a parent support and education group to provide opportunities for parents to access support, learn new parenting skills, and, ultimately, optimize their relationships with their children in families of children in residential care. **EB:** *Working with the families of children in residential care is critical to the success of the placement. In this study a parent support and education group was designed and implemented. The responses of both parents and staff to this program were favorable. It served as a springboard to enhance family involvement in other program areas (Modlin, 2003).*

## evolve WEBSITES FOR EDUCATION

See the EVOLVE website for World Wide Web resources for client education.

## REFERENCES


Bohachick P, Reeder S, Taylor MV et al: Psychosocial impact of heart transplantation on spouses, *Clin Nurs Res* 10:6, 2001.

Boyd-Ball, AJ: A culturally responsive, family intervention model, *Alcohol Clin Exp Res* 27(8):1356-1360, 2003.

Brazil K, Krueger P: Patterns of family adaptation to childhood asthma, *J Pediatr Nurs* 17(3):167, 2002.

Bulechek G, McCloskey J: *Advanced nursing interventions,* Philadelphia, 1992, WB Saunders.

Camphinha-Bacote J, Narayan M: Culturally competent health care at home, *Home Care Provid* 5(6):213, 2000.

Cassells C, Watt E: The impact of incontinence on older spousal caregivers, *J Adv Nurs* 42(6):607-616, 2003.

Chang BL, Nitta S, Carter PA et al: Technology innovations. Perceived helpfulness of telephone calls: providing support for caregivers of family members with dementia, *J Gerontol Nurs* 30(9):14-21, 2004.

Cochran M: Tears have no color, *Am J Nurs* 98(6):53, 1998.

D'Avanzo CE et al: Developing culturally informed strategies for substance-related interventions. In Naegle MA, D'Avanzo CE, editors: *Addictions and substance abuse: strategies for advanced practice nursing,* St Louis, 2001, Mosby.
Davis RE: The convergence of health and family in the Vietnamese culture, *J Fam Nurs* 6(2):136, 2000.
Doswell W, Erlen J: Multicultural issues and ethical concerns in the delivery of nursing care interventions, *Nurs Clin North Am* 33(2):353, 1998.
Watts S, Edgar L: Nucare, a coping skills training intervention for oncology patients and families: participants' motivations and expectations, *Can Oncol Nurs J* 14(2):84-95, 2004.
Fredrickson BL, Joiner T: Positive emotions trigger upward spirals toward emotional well-being, *Psychol Sci* 13(2):172, 2002.
Gordon PA, Perrone KM: When spouses become caregivers: counseling implications for younger couples, *J Rehab* 70(2):27-32, 2004.
Guarnaccia P: Multicultural experiences of family caregiving: a study of African American, European American, and Hispanic American families, *New Dir Ment Health Serv* 77:45, 1998.
Guerriero Austrom M, Damush TM, Hartwell CW et al: Development and implementation of nonpharmacologic protocols for the management of patients with Alzheimer's disease and their families in a multiracial primary care setting, *Gerontologist* 44(4):548-553, 2004.
Harden J, Schafenacker A, Northouse L et al: Couples' experiences with prostate cancer: focus group research, *Oncol Nurs Forum* 29(4):701-709, 2002.
Heineken, J: Patient silence is not necessarily client satisfaction: communication in home care nursing, *Home Healthc Nurse* 16(2): 115, 1998.
Hogan DL, Logan J: The Ottawa Model of Research Use: a guide to clinical innovation in the NICU, *Clin Nurse Spec* 18(5): 255-261, 2004.
Kelleher L, Johnson M: An evaluation of a volunteer-support program for families at risk, *Pub Health Nurs* 21(4):297-305, 2004.
Kogan MD, Schuster MA, Yu SM et al: Routine assessment of family and community health risks: parent views and what they receive, *Pediatrics* 113(6 Suppl):1934-1943, 2004.
Kuuppelomäki M, Sasaki A, Yamada K et al: Coping strategies of family carers for older relatives in Finland, *J Clin Nurs* 13(6): 697-706, 2004.
Leininger MM, McFarland MR: *Transcultural nursing: concepts, theories, research and practices,* ed 3, New York, 2002, McGraw-Hill.
Ludwick R, Silva M: Nursing around the world: cultural values and ethical conflicts, *Online J Issues Nurs,* 2000. Available at www.nursingworld.org/ojin/ethcol/ethics_4.htm, accessed on January 10, 2003.
Mellon S, Northouse LL: Family survivorship and quality of life following a cancer diagnosis, *Res Nurs Health* 24:446, 2001.
McGrath P, Clarke H: Creating the space for spiritual talk: insights from survivors of haematological malignancies, *Aust Health Rev* 26(3):116-132, 2003.
Modlin H.: The development of a parent support group as a means of initiating family involvement in a residential program, *Child Youth Serv Rev* 25(1/2):169-189, 2003.
Moriarty PH, Wagner LD: Family rituals that provide meaning for single-parent families, *J Fam Nurs* 10(2):190-210, 2004.
Northouse LL, Walker J, Schafenacker A et al: A family-based program of care for women with recurrent breast cancer and their family members, *Oncol Nurs Forum* 29(10):1411-1419, 2002.
Patusky KL, Rodning C, Martinez-Kratz M: Clinical lessons in psychiatric home care: a case study approach, *J Home Health Case Manag* 9:18, 1996.
Rao P, Pradhan PV, Shah H: Psychopathology and coping in parents of chronically ill children, *Indian J Pediatr* 71(8):695-699, 2004.
Rask K, Kaunonen MM, Paunonen-Ilmonen M: Adolescent coping with grief after the death of a loved one, *Int J Nurs Pract* 8(3): 137, 2002.
Rivera-Andino J, Lopez L: When culture complicates care, *RN* 63(7):47, 2000.
Seideman RY, Jacobson S, Primeaux M et al: Assessing American Indian families, *MCN Am J Matern Child Nurs* 21(6):274-279, 1996.
Rose LE, Mallinson RK, Walton-Moss B: Barriers to family care in psychiatric settings, *J Nurs Scholarsh* 36(1):39-47, 2004.
Shapiro J, Monzo LD, Rueda R et al: Alienated advocacy: perspectives of Latina mothers of young adults with developmental disabilities on service systems, *Ment Retard* 42(1):37-54, 2004.
stedt-Kurki P, Lehti K, Tarkka M et al: Determinants of perceived health in families of patients with heart disease, *J Adv Nurs* 48(2):115-123, 2004.

Szabo V, Strang V: Experiencing control in caregiving, *Image J Nurs Sch* 31(1):71, 1999.
Thomas DJ, King MA: Parish nursing assessment—what should you know? *Home Healthcare Nurs Manag* 4(5):11-13, 2000.
Urban AD, Berry D, Grey M: Optimizing outcomes in adolescents with type 1 diabetes and their families, *J Clin Outcomes Manag* 11(5):299-306, 2004
Vontress CE, Epp LR: Historical hostility in the African American client: implications for counseling, *J Multicult Counseling Dev*, 25:170, 1997.
Weiss S, Chen J: Factors influencing maternal mental health and family functioning during the low birthweight infant's first year of life, *J Pediatr Nurs* 17(2):114, 2002.
Wen LK, Shepherd MD, Parchman ML: Family support, diet, and exercise among older Mexican Americans with type 2 diabetes, *Diabetes Educ* 30(6):980-993, 2004.
Zengerle-Levy K: Practices that facilitate critically burned children's holistic healing, *Qual Health Res* 14(9):1255-1275, 2004.

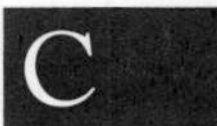

# Disabled family Coping

*Gail B. Ladwig*

**NANDA**

## Definition

Behavior of significant person (family member or other primary person) that disables his/her capacity and the client's capacity to effectively address tasks essential to either person's adaptation to the health challenge

## Defining Characteristics

Intolerance; agitation, depression, aggression, hostility; taking on of illness signs of client; rejection; psychosomaticism; neglectful relationships with other family members; neglectful care of client with regard to basic human needs and/or illness treatment; distortion of reality regarding client's health problem, including extreme denial about its existence or severity; impaired restructuring of meaningful life for self; impaired individualization, prolonged overconcern for client; desertion; decisions and actions that are detrimental to economic or social well-being; carrying on usual routines, disregarding client's needs; abandonment; client's development of helpless, inactive dependence; disregarding needs

## Related Factors (r/t)

Significant person with chronically unexpressed feelings of guilt, anxiety, hostility, despair, etc.; arbitrary handling of family's resistance to treatment, which tends to solidify defensiveness by dealing inadequately with underlying anxiety; dissonant or discrepant coping styles for dealing with adaptive tasks by significant person and client or among significant people; highly ambivalent family relationships

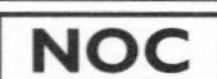

## Outcomes (Nursing Outcomes Classification)

C

### Suggested NOC Outcomes

Caregiver-Patient Relationship; Caregiver Performance: Direct Care, Indirect Care; Caregiver Well-Being; Family Coping; Caregiver Emotional Health; Caregiver Stressors; Coping

**Example NOC Outcome with Indicators**

**Coping** as evidenced by the following indicators: Identifies effective coping patterns/Verbalizes sense of control/Seeks information concerning illness and treatment/Uses available social support/Identifies multiple coping strategies (Rate each indicator of **Coping:** 1 = never demonstrated, 2 = rarely demonstrated, 3 = sometimes demonstrated, 4 = often demonstrated, 5 = consistently demonstrated [see Section I].)

## Client Outcomes

**Family/Significant Person Will (Specify Time Frame):**

- Express realistic understanding and expectations of the client
- Participate positively in the client's care within the limits of his or her abilities
- Identify responses that are harmful
- Acknowledge and accept the need for assistance with circumstances
- Express feelings openly, honestly, and appropriately

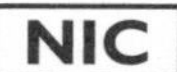

## Interventions (Nursing Interventions Classification)

### Suggested NIC Interventions

Family Support, Family Therapy, Anxiety Reduction, Coping Enhancement, Counseling, Crisis Intervention, Family Integrity Promotion, Family Involvement Promotion, Family Mobilization, Mutual Goal Setting, Normalization Promotion

**Example NIC Activities—Family Therapy**

Determine the client's usual roles within the family system; monitor for adverse therapeutic responses

## Nursing Interventions and Rationales

- Assess the strengths and deficiencies of the family system. **EBN:** *Assessments allow for anticipatory care and guidance to help members acquire and maintain supports and coping strategies (Thomas, 2000).* **EB:** *Chronic illness in children affects the psychological health of the parents. Active coping strategies are associated with fewer distress indices and thus if in-*

C

*culcated may improve the ability to bear the burden of the illness without becoming themselves affected by psychiatric illnesses (Rao, 2004).*

- • Identify current behaviors of family members, such as withdrawal (e.g., not visiting, briefly visiting, ignoring client when visiting), anger and hostility toward the client and others, or expression of guilt. *Many of these behaviors are defense mechanisms used by the ego to protect itself until it can fully accept the implications of the illness.* **EBN:** *Family cohesion, presence of a partner, emotional support, and a mother's satisfaction with her family all contributed to her better mental health in a research study focusing on mothers of low-birth-weight infants (Weiss & Chen, 2002).*
- • Note other stressors in the family (e.g., financial, job related). *This information allows the nurse to develop an appropriate plan of care.* **EBN:** *One study found that, in mothers of low-birth-weight infants, the presence of other life stressors and the family's use of internally focused coping strategies contributed to worse mental health outcomes for the mother (Weiss & Chen, 2002).*
- ▲ Evaluate the family's perceived strength of its social support system. Encourage the family to use social support to increase its resiliency and to moderate stress. *Perceived social support is a factor influencing resiliency and ability to cope with stress (Tak & McCubbin, 2002).*
- • Consider the use of family theory as a framework to help guide interventions (e.g., family stress theory, role theory, social exchange theory). **EBN:** *This study demonstrated that use of a family assessment tool is an effective way of appraising families and addressing suffering. Formative evaluations demonstrated improvements in team members' perceptions of their knowledge, family centeredness, and ability to assess and intervene with families (Hogan & Logan, 2004).*
- • Encourage family members to verbalize feelings by discussing ways to solve problems associated with the client's condition. *Many families find it difficult to maintain open and empathetic communication during times of acute stress. Interventions that help mobilize family strengths, such as problem-solving communication, may effectively promote the adaptation of families of critically injured clients (Leske & Jiricka, 1998).*
- • Encourage expression of positive thoughts and emotions. **EB:** *Positive emotions initiate upward spirals toward enhanced emotional well-being (Fredrickson & Joiner, 2002).* **EBN:** *This study shows that clients believe that coping is important to their well-being (Edgar, 2004).*
- • Mothers may require additional support in their role of caring for chronically ill children. *Mothers exhibit greater efforts than fathers in coping patterns, including strategies to acquire social support outside the family, increase self-worth, and decrease psychological tensions (Brazil & Krueger, 2002).*
- ▲ Encourage family members to participate in appropriate support programs (e.g., chronic obstructive pulmonary disease [COPD] support groups, Arthritis I Can Cope groups, Alzheimer's support groups). *Support group participation develops coping skills, enhances communication skills, and facilitates exchange of useful information (Northouse & Peters-Golden, 1993).*
- ▲ Observe for any symptoms of elder or child abuse or neglect. *Abuse can take several forms, such as physical assaults that may or may not result in injury, verbal attacks, isolation,*

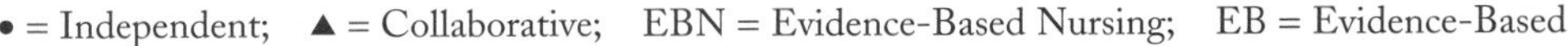
• = Independent; ▲ = Collaborative; EBN = Evidence-Based Nursing; EB = Evidence-Based

*and social and emotional neglect. Prompt reporting of abuse according to local and state law is necessary. In most states, the law mandates reporting abuse.*



## Pediatric

- Assess the adolescent's perception of support from family and friends during crisis. *Some teens find parents or friends burdensome during time of grief, while others find their support critical for coping with crises. Recognition of individual perception can assist families in negotiating times of crisis (Rask, Kaunonen, & Paunonen-Ilmonen, 2002).*
- Encourage the use of family rituals such as connection, spiritual, love, recreation, celebration, and evolving especially in single parent families. **EBN:** *Data from this study indicated that these rituals were found to be used by single-parent families as a way to facilitate family cohesion and instill family values (Moriarty & Wagner, 2004).*
- Encourage laughing, playing, singing, talking, and praying with seriously injured children. **EBN:** *This interpretive study examined the experiences of 16 pediatric burn intensive care unit nurses for the purpose of uncovering and articulating practices that help critically burned children to heal holistically. These everyday practices were identified as maintaining or reestablishing harmony of the children's mind, body, and spirit (Zengerle-Levy et al, 2004).*
- ▲ Link trained volunteers with "vulnerable" first-time parents. Provide social support and information related to age appropriate expectations of infants. **EBN:** *This descriptive comparative design demonstrated participant's satisfaction with the program and improvement in family functioning. The program could be appropriate for all parents (Kelleher & Johnson, 2004).*

## Geriatric

- Perform a holistic assessment of all needs of informal spousal caregivers. **EBN:** *The role of informal spousal caregivers has increased as the population ages. This research highlighted the interconnectedness of factors in the experiences of caregivers, reinforcing the need for holistic assessment beyond a focus on the "continence issue" alone (Cassells & Watt, 2003).*
- Help caregivers establish priorities and concentrate on them, believe in themselves and their ability to handle the situation, taking life 1 day at a time, looking for positive things in each situation, and relying on their own individual expertise and experience. **EBN:** *The most helpful coping strategies identified in this major international research project on caregivers' work and coping in four countries (Kuuppelomäki et al, 2004).*
- ▲ Refer caregivers of Alzheimer's clients to a monthly psychoeducational support group. **EB:** *Nonpharmacological interventions can be used for the management of Alzheimer's clients. This support group intervention has been well accepted by patients, families, and physicians in this study (Guerriero Austrom et al, 2004).*
- ▲ Consider the use of telephone support for caregivers of family members with dementia. **EBN:** *Results from this study suggest family caregivers can be helped through a variety of social support mechanisms including telephone support. Participants reported assistance in sharing thoughts and feelings, expressing feelings of being overwhelmed, discussing physical and psychosocial problems, forgetting the situation, seeking reassurance, and asking for information (Chang et al, 2004).*

- ▲ Refer the family to appropriate senior community resources (e.g., senior centers, Medicare assistance, meal programs, parish nursing services, charitable organizations). *Many federal, state, and local community-based resources for seniors are underused.*
- ▲ If actual or potential abuse or neglect is an issue, report it to the appropriate agency. *All who provide care to an elder must be aware of the potential signs of abuse and the remedies available (Birke, 2004).*
- ▲ Encourage the family member to participate in appropriate support groups (e.g., COPD support groups, Arthritis I Can Cope groups, Alzheimer's support groups). *Support groups provide people with a setting in which they can discuss their illness-related problems with others who have the same problems.*
- • Work with the family to manage common challenges related to normal aging. Having knowledge of the normal developmental challenges of aging can reduce the stress such challenges place on families.

C

## Multicultural

- • Work to provide caregivers who understand the importance of cultural beliefs and values the family may hold. **EBN:** *Cultures can differ with regard to health beliefs, practices, and values (Camphinha-Bacote & Narayan, 2000; Guarnaccia, 1998).*
- • Acknowledge racial/ethnic differences at the onset of care. **EBN:** *Acknowledgment of race/ethnicity issues will enhance communication, establish rapport, and promote treatment outcomes (D'Avanzo et al, 2001; Ludwick & Silva, 2000; Vontress & Epp, 1997).*
- • Approach families of color with respect, warmth, and professional courtesy. **EBN:** *Instances of disrespect and lack of caring have special significance for families of color (D'Avanzo et al, 2001; Vontress & Epp, 1997). Latina mothers of developmentally disabled adults reported their relationship with the educational and service delivery systems to be characterized by poor communication, low effort in providing services, negative attitudes of professionals toward the client-children, and negative treatment of parents by professionals (Shapiro et al, 2004).*
- • Assess for the influence of cultural beliefs, norms, and values on the family's perceptions of coping. **EB:** *What the family considers normal and abnormal coping behavior may be based on cultural perceptions (Leininger & McFarland, 2002; Cochran, 1998; Doswell & Erlen, 1998). Give a rationale when assessing families with regard to sensitive issues.* **EBN:** *African Americans and other people of color may expect Caucasian caregivers to hold negative and preconceived ideas about people of color. Giving a rationale for questions asked will help reduce this perception (D'Avanzo et al, 2001; Vontress & Epp, 1997).*
- • Use a family-centered approach when working with Latino, Asian-American, African-American, and Native-American clients. **EBN:** *Latinos may perceive the family as a source of support, solver of problems, and source of pride. Asian Americans may regard the family as the primary decision maker and influence on individual family members (D'Avanzo et al, 2001). Native-American families may have extended structures and exert powerful influences over functioning (Seideman et al, 1996). Use of a family based intervention among Native-American families resulted in higher levels of child prosocial behavior and lowered drug use (Boyd-Ball, 2003). Among Mexican Americans with type 2 diabetes, higher levels of perceived family support and greater self-efficacy were associated*

*with higher reported levels of diet and exercise self-care (Wen, Shepherd, & Parchman 2004).*

- Facilitate modeling and role playing for the family regarding healthy ways to communicate and interact. **EBN:** *It is helpful for family members and the client to practice communication skills in a safe environment before trying them in a real-life situation (Rivera-Andino & Lopez, 2000).*
- Validate the feelings of family members or significant caregivers regarding the impact of the client's illness on family lifestyle. **EBN:** *Validation is a therapeutic communication technique that lets the individual know that the nurse has heard and understood what was said and promotes the relationship between the nurse and that individual (Heineken, 1998).*

## Home Care

NOTE: This diagnosis presents the complex and difficult problem of securing an appropriate response by the family to a client's illness and caregiving needs. The same problem in the home setting creates an unusually high risk for abuse of the client. The nurse is cautioned that the margin of time for planning and effectively supporting the family unit to avoid abuse may be minimal or even negligible. Suspected or actual abuse should be reported to adult protective services.

- The interventions described previously may be adapted for home care use.
- If the client has been in an institution, establish empathetic contact with the client and family before discharge. *Contact with the family in a nonthreatening manner helps establish a trusting relationship, easing the transition to home.*
- Assess the family member's ability and willingness to assist in client care. Determine if the family member is an appropriate source of support for the client. *Knowledge of the reasons behind disabled coping will assist in identification of appropriate interventions. Is the family member's response consistent with the previous relationship with the client or have illness or other factors influenced the relationship? Is there a history of psychiatric disorder that is being exacerbated? Is there a lack of resources that places additional stress on the caregiver? Is the family member feeling stressed in dealing with the client's care needs?* Refer to the care plan for **Caregiver role strain.** *Alter expectations of the family member's assistance to the client, depending on assessment findings.*
- Assess the family member's understanding of the client's illness and behavior. Instruct in appropriate expectations of the client and correct any misconceptions. *The family member may be proceeding from false assumptions about the client's illness or behavior. For example, in the absence of comprehension of dementia, the family member may assume that the client's illness-related behaviors are signs of stubbornness, laziness, or willful acting out.*
- During the time of compromised coping, increase visits to assess the safety of the client and family, provide assistance with coping strategies, identify dysfunctional coping mechanisms, and intervene as necessary. *Increased opportunity for interaction and appropriate intervention will enhance the safety and health status of the client and family. Frequent assessment of the client's health status promotes early detection and treatment of problems. Changes in the client's health status (especially any deterioration in status) can pre-*

*cipitate more problems with the family or caregiver and place the client at greater risk.*

- • Identify any changes in skills needed for client care and support caregiving efforts. Assess the needs of the caregiver in the home. Intervene to meet needs as appropriate to total case management and explore all available resources that may be used to provide adequate home care (e.g., add home health aide services; coordinate services with mental health agencies; encourage caregivers not to neglect their own physical, mental, and spiritual health; and give more specific information about the client's needs and ways to meet them). *Support from the nurse through teaching and positive feedback helps caregivers to have a realistic perception of what can be expected of the client and shows them they are valued for the efforts made; meeting the needs of caregivers supports their ability to meet the needs of the client; home health aides may be used as role models for caregiving and can observe the status of the client and family. Caution the home health aide to document objectively.*
- ▲ Serve as an advocate, mentor, and role model for appropriate behavior. Write down or contract for the care needed by the client. *Therapeutic use of self by the nurse and concrete task definition and assignment reinforce positive coping strategies.*
- ▲ When a terminal illness is the precipitating factor for ineffective coping, offer hospice services and support groups as possible resources. *Nonjudgmental support from helpers with no agenda allows verbalization of feelings. The hospice paradigm addresses the physical, emotional, and spiritual needs of the dying and their loved ones.*
- • Support positive individual and family coping efforts. *Positive feedback reinforces desired behaviors and supports the family unit.*
- ▲ If disabled family coping interferes with the family member's ability to support the client's treatment plan, refer for psychiatric home health care services for family and client counseling and implementation of a therapeutic regimen. **EBN:** *Psychiatric home care nurses can address issues relating to the family member's and client's ability to adjust to changes in health status. Behavioral interventions in the home can help the family member and client to participate more effectively in the treatment plan (Patusky, Rodning, & Martinez-Kratz, 1996).*

## Client/Family Teaching

- • Encourage family members to ask for a break in caregiving and to spend time away from the client. *Caregivers who were able to maintain control recognized when they were losing control and needed a break from caregiving (Szabo & Strang, 1999).*
- • Provide truthful information and support for the family and significant people regarding the client's specific illness or condition. **EBN:** *The results of this study indicate that attention needs to be given to methods of providing information and support to couples coping with prostate cancer. Both patients and partners need to be included in discussions about the effect of the illness and treatments so that both can feel more prepared to manage them (Harden et al, 2002).*
- • Involve the client and family in the planning of care as often as possible; mutual goal setting is often an effective strategy. *Family members of any trauma client admitted to the level I trauma center are invited by the trauma staff to attend weekly multidisciplinary meetings. In this way family concerns can become a positive care factor, and the tasks of nurses, doctors, and social workers are made easier (Boettcher & Schiller, 1990).*

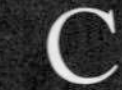

- Discuss with the family appropriate ways to demonstrate feelings. *Learning basic components of therapeutic communication helps family members to express feelings appropriately.*
- Help the family identify the health care needs of the client and family; teach the skills necessary to address health care needs. *Once needs are identified, skill mastery by the family will optimize health status. Skill mastery is an empowering and positive coping mechanism.*
- Promote individual and family relaxation and stress-reduction strategies. *The immune system weakens in response to stress; relaxation elicits the opposite, healthful response (Bulechek & McCloskey, 1992).*

## evolve WEBSITES FOR EDUCATION

See the EVOLVE website for World Wide Web resources for client education.

## REFERENCES


Boettcher M, Schiller W: The use of a multidisciplinary group meeting for families of critically ill trauma patients, *Intensive Care Nurs* 6(3):129, 1990.

Boyd-Ball, AJ: A culturally responsive, family intervention model, *Alcohol Clin Exp Res* 27(8):1356-1360, 2003.

Brazil K, Krueger P: Patterns of family adaptation to childhood asthma. *J Pediatr Nurs* 17(3):167, 2002.

Bulechek G, McCloskey J: *Advanced nursing interventions,* Philadelphia, 1992, WB Saunders.

Birke MG: Elder law, Medicare, and legal issues in older patients, *Semin Oncol* 31(2): 282-292, 2004.

Cassells C, Watt E: The impact of incontinence on older spousal caregivers, *J Adv Nurs* 42(6):607-616, 2003.

Camphinha-Bacote J, Narayan M: Culturally competent health care at home, *Home Care Provid* 5(6):213, 2000.

Chang BL, Nitta S, Carter PA et al: Technology innovations. Perceived helpfulness of telephone calls: providing support for caregivers of family members with dementia, *J Gerontol Nurs* 30(9):14-21, 2004.

Cochran M: Tears have no color, *Am J Nurs* 98(6):53, 1998.

D'Avanzo CE et al: Developing culturally informed strategies for substance-related interventions. In Naegle MA, D'Avanzo CE, editors: *Addictions and substance abuse: strategies for advanced practice nursing,* St Louis, 2001, Mosby.

Doswell W, Erlen J: Multicultural issues and ethical concerns in the delivery of nursing care interventions, *Nurs Clin North Am* 33(2):353, 1998.

Watts S, Edgar L: Nucare, a coping skills training intervention for oncology patients and families: participants' motivations and expectations, *Can Oncol Nurs J* 14(2):84-95, 2004.

Fredrickson BL, Joiner T: Positive emotions trigger upward spirals toward emotional well-being, *Psychol Sci* 13(2):172, 2002.

Guarnaccia P: Multicultural experiences of family caregiving: a study of African American, European American, and Hispanic American families, *New Dir Ment Health Serv* 77:45, 1998.

Guerriero Austrom M, Damush TM, Hartwell CW et al: Development and implementation of nonpharmacologic protocols for the management of patients with Alzheimer's disease and their families in a multiracial primary care setting, *Gerontologist* 44(4):548-553, 2004.

Harden J, Schafenacker A, Northouse L et al: Couples' experiences with prostate cancer: focus group research, *Oncol Nurs Forum* 29(4):701-79, 2002.

Heineken J: Patient silence is not necessarily client satisfaction: communication in home care nursing, *Home Healthc Nurse* 16(2): 115, 1998.

Hogan DL, Logan J: The Ottawa Model of Research Use: a guide to clinical innovation in the NICU, *Clin Nurse Spec* 18(5):255-261, 2004.

Kelleher L, Johnson M: An evaluation of a volunteer-support program for families at risk, *Pub Health Nurs* 21(4):297-305, 2004.

Kuuppelomäki M, Sasaki A, Yamada K et al: Coping strategies of family carers for older relatives in Finland, *J Clin Nurs* 13(6): 697-706, 2004.

Leininger MM, McFarland MR: *Transcultural nursing: concepts, theories, research and practices,* ed 3, New York, 2002, McGraw-Hill.

Leske J, Jiricka M: Impact of family demands and family strengths and capabilities on family well-being and adaptation after critical injury, *Am J Crit Care* 7(5):383, 1998.

Ludwick R, Silva M: Nursing around the world: cultural values and ethical conflicts, *Online J Issues Nurs,* August 14, 2000. Available at www.nursingworld.org/ojin/ethcol/ethics_4.htm, accessed on June 19, 2003.
Northouse L, Peters-Golden H: Cancer and the family: strategies to assist spouses, *Semin Oncol Nurs* 9:74, 1993.
Moriarty PH, Wagner LD: Family rituals that provide meaning for single-parent families, *J Fam Nurs* 10(2):190-210, 2004.
Patusky KL, Rodning C, Martinez-Kratz M: Clinical lessons in psychiatric home care: a case study approach, *J Home Health Case Manag* 9:18, 1996.
Rao P, Pradhan PV, Shah H: Psychopathology and coping in parents of chronically ill children, *Indian J Pediatr* 71(8):695-699, 2004.
Rask K, Kaunonen M, Paunonen-Ilmonen M: Adolescent coping with grief after the death of a loved one, *Int J Nurs Pract* 8(3): 137, 2002.
Rivera-Andino J, Lopez L: When culture complicates care, *RN* 63(7):47, 2000.
Seideman RY et al: Assessing American Indian families, *MCN Am J Matern Child Nurs* 21(6):274, 1996.
Shapiro J, Monzo LD, Rueda R et al: Alienated advocacy: perspectives of Latina mothers of young adults with developmental disabilities on service systems, *Ment Retard* 42(1):37-54, 2004.
Ludwick R, Silva M: Nursing around the world: cultural values and ethical conflicts, *Online J Issues Nurs,* August 14, 2000.
Szabo V, Strang V: Experiencing control in caregiving, *Image J Nurs Sch* 31(1):71, 1999.
Tak YR, McCubbin M: Family stress, perceived social support and coping following the diagnosis of a child's congenital heart disease, *J Adv Nurs* 39(2):190, 2002.
Thomas DJ, King MA: Parish nursing assessment—what should you know? *Home Healthcare Nurs Manag* 4(5):11-13, 2000.
Vontress CE, Epp LR: Historical hostility in the African American client: implications for counseling, *J Multicul Counseling Dev* 25:170, 1997.
Weiss S, Chen J: Factors influencing maternal mental health and family functioning during the low birthweight infant's first year of life, *J Pediatr Nurs* 17(2):114, 2002.
Zengerle-Levy K: Practices that facilitate critically burned children's holistic healing, *Qual Health Res* 14(9):1255-1275, 2004.

# Readiness for enhanced family Coping

*Gail B. Ladwig*

**NANDA**

## Definition

Effective management of adaptive tasks by family member involved with client's health challenge, who now exhibits desire and readiness for enhanced health and growth with regard to self and in relation to client

## Defining Characteristics

Individual expresses interest in making contact on a one-to-one basis or through mutual aid group with another person who has experienced a similar situation; attempts to describe growth impact of the crisis on his or her own values, priorities, goals, or relationships; moves in the direction of health promotion and health-enriching lifestyle that supports and monitors maturational processes; audits and negotiates treatment programs and generally chooses experiences that optimize wellness

## Related Factors (r/t)

Needs sufficiently gratified and adaptive tasks effectively addressed to enable goals of self-actualization to surface

**NOC**

## Outcomes (Nursing Outcomes Classification)



### Suggested NOC Outcomes

Caregiver Emotional Health; Caregiver-Patient Relationship; Caregiver Well-Being; Family Coping; Health-Seeking Behavior; Participation in Health Care Decisions

**Example NOC Outcome with Indicators**

**Coping** as evidenced by the following indicators: Identifies effective coping patterns/Verbalizes sense of control/Seeks information concerning illness and treatment/Uses available social support/Identifies multiple coping strategies (Rate each indicator of **Coping:** 1 = never demonstrated, 2 = rarely demonstrated, 3 = sometimes demonstrated, 4 = often demonstrated, 5 = consistently demonstrated [see Section I].)

## Client Outcomes

**Family Will (Specify Time Frame):**

- State a plan for growth
- Perform tasks needed for change
- State positive effects of changes made

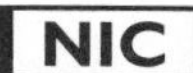

## Interventions (Nursing Interventions Classification)

### Suggested NIC Interventions

Anticipatory Guidance, Family Integrity Promotion, Family Involvement Promotion, Family Mobilization, Family Support, Mutual Goal Setting

**Example NIC Activities—Family Support**

Facilitate communication of concerns and feelings between client and family or among family members; identify and respect family's coping mechanisms

## Nursing Interventions and Rationales

- Assess how family members interact with each other; observe verbal and nonverbal communication and individual and group responses to stress. **EBN:** *Understanding how families cope with stress is important. Family cohesion, presence of a partner, emotional support, and a mother's satisfaction with her family all contributed to her better mental health in a research study focusing on mothers of low-birth-weight infants (Weiss & Chen, 2002).*
- Evaluate the family's perceived strength of its social support system. Encourage the family to use social support to increase its resiliency and to moderate stress. *Perceived*

*social support is a factor influencing resiliency and ability to cope with stress (Tak & McCubbin, 2002).*

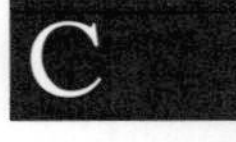

- Consider the use of family theory as a framework to help guide interventions (e.g., family stress theory, role theory, social exchange theory). **EBN:** *This study demonstrated that use of a family assessment tool is an effective way of appraising families and addressing suffering. Formative evaluations demonstrated improvements in team members' perceptions of their knowledge, family centeredness, and ability to assess and intervene with families (Hogan & Logan, 2004).*
- Establish rapport with families by providing accurate communication. **EBN:** *This qualitative exploratory study of families in psychiatric settings indicated that family care can be improved by focusing on building rapport and communicating problems and concerns between families and health professionals (Rose, Mallinson, & Walton-Moss, 2004).*
- Provide opportunities for families to discuss spirituality. **EB:** *This research provided by survivors of haematological malignancies gives insight into factors impacting their need to talk about spiritual issues (McGrath & Clarke, 2003).*
- When a client is having surgery, give the family a 5- to 10-minute progress report about halfway through the surgical procedure. **EBN:** *Family members who were given progress reports during an intraoperative waiting period experienced lower anxiety scores and had significantly lower mean arterial pressures and heart rates than those who did not receive the reports (Leske, 1995).*
- Allow the family to be present during invasive procedures and resuscitation efforts. **EBN:** *Recent research suggests family member presence during life-saving efforts may help families cope with the devastating outcomes of unsuccessful resuscitation (York, 2004).*
- Encourage setting aside leisure time free of obligatory tasks for family members to enjoy each other's company; because everyone is busy, family members may need to set up a schedule for leisure time. *Help family members communicate with each other using techniques they are comfortable with, such as role playing, letter writing, or tape recording messages. These techniques give the family an opportunity to communicate in an effective yet nonthreatening manner.*

▲ Identify support groups that discuss problems and concerns similar to those of the family (e.g., Al-Anon, Arthritis I Can Cope). *Such groups allow family members to discuss issues and concerns with others who share the same lived experience.*

## Pediatric

- Encourage the use of family rituals such as connection, spiritual, love, recreation, celebration, and evolving especially in single-parent families. **EBN:** *Data from this study indicated that these rituals were found to be used by single-parent families as a way to facilitate family cohesion and instill family values (Moriarty & Wagner, 2004).*
- Encourage laughing, playing, singing, talking, and praying with seriously injured children. **EBN:** *This interpretive study examined the experiences of 16 pediatric burn intensive care unit nurses for the purpose of uncovering and articulating practices that help critically burned children to heal holistically. These everyday practices were identified as maintaining or reestablishing harmony of the children's mind, body, and spirit (Zengerle-Levy et al, 2004).*
- Provide educational interventions and psychosocial interventions such as coping skills

C

training in treatment for families and their adolescents who have type 1 diabetes. **EB:** *Education interventions increase diabetes knowledge but are not consistently helpful in improving metabolic outcomes. Psychosocial interventions such as coping skills training and behavioral family systems therapy have demonstrated improvements in metabolic control, self-efficacy, diabetes stress, quality of life, and parent-adolescent conflict. Family interventions are emerging as a positive way to improve interpersonal relations and assist the adolescent in transitioning from family-management toward self-management of their diabetes (Urban, Berry, & Grey, 2004).*

▲ Link trained volunteers with "vulnerable" first-time parents. Provide social support and information related to age appropriate expectations of infants. **EBN:** *This descriptive comparative design demonstrated participant's satisfaction with the program and improvement in family functioning. The program could be appropriate for all parents (Kelleher & Johnson, 2004).*

## Geriatric

- Perform a holistic assessment of all needs of informal spousal caregivers. **EBN:** *The role of informal spousal caregivers has increased as the population ages. This research highlighted the interconnectedness of factors in the experiences of caregivers, reinforcing the need for holistic assessment beyond a focus on the "continence issue" alone (Cassells & Watt, 2003).*
- Help caregivers establish one's priorities and concentrate on them, believe in themesleves and their ability to handle the situation, taking life 1 day at a time, looking for positive things in each situation, and relying on their own individual expertise and experience. **EBN:** *The most helpful coping strategies identified in this major international research project on caregivers' work and coping in four countries (Kuuppelomäki et al, 2004).*

▲ Consider the use of telephone support for caregivers of family members with dementia. **EBN:** *Results from this study suggest family caregivers can be helped through a variety of social support mechanisms including telephone support. Participants reported assistance in sharing thoughts and feelings, expressing feelings of being overwhelmed, discussing physical and psychosocial problems, forgetting the situation, seeking reassurance, and asking for information (Chang et al, 2004).*

▲ Refer caregivers of Alzheimer's clients to a monthly psychoeducational support group. **EB:** *Nonpharmacologic interventions can be used for the management of Alzheimer's clients. This support group intervention has been well accepted by patients, families, and physicians in this study (Guerriero Austrom et al, 2004).*

- Encourage family members to reminisce with the older family member.
- Start and maintain a log of anecdotal stories about the older family member.
- Encourage children in the family to spend time with and share activities with the older family member. *These activities allow for knowledge of and respect for one another; they support the normal developmental tasks of aging.*

▲ Refer the family to parenting classes and classes for coping with the needs of older parents. *Such groups allow family members to discuss the challenges of aging parents with others who share the same experience.*

C

## Multicultural

- Acknowledge racial/ethnic differences at the onset of care. *Acknowledgment of race/ethnicity issues will enhance communication, establish rapport, and promote treatment outcomes (D'Avanzo et al, 2001).*
- Approach families of color with respect, warmth, and professional courtesy. **EB:** *Instances of disrespect and lack of caring have special significance for families of color (D'Avanzo et al, 2001). Latina mothers of developmentally disabled adults reported their relationship with the educational and service delivery systems to be characterized by poor communication, low effort in providing services, negative attitudes of professionals toward the client-children, and negative treatment of parents by professionals (Shapiro et al, 2004).*
- Assess for the influence of cultural beliefs, norms, and values on the family's perceptions of coping. *What the family considers normal and abnormal coping behavior may be based on cultural perceptions (Leininger, 2002).*
- Use a family-centered approach when working with Latino, Asian-American, African-American, and Native-American clients. *Latinos may perceive the family as a source of support, solver of problems, and source of pride. Asian Americans may regard the family as the primary decision maker and influence on individual family members (D'Avanzo et al, 2001). Native-American families may have extended structures and exert powerful influences over functioning (Seideman et al, 1996). Use of a family based intervention among Native-American families resulted in higher levels of child pro-social behavior and lowered drug use (Boyd-Ball, 2003). Among Mexican Americans with type 2 diabetes, higher levels of perceived family support and greater self-efficacy were associated with higher reported levels of diet and exercise self-care (Wen, Shepherd, & Parchman 2004).*
- Facilitate modeling and role playing for family with regard to healthy ways to communicate and interact. *It is helpful for family members and the client to practice communication skills in a safe environment before trying them in a real-life situation (Rivera-Andino & Lopez, 2000).*
- Validate family members' feelings regarding the impact of the client's illness on family lifestyle. *Validation lets the individual know that the nurse has heard and understood what was said, and it promotes the relationship between the nurse and the individual (Stuart & Laraia, 2001; Giger & Davidhizar, 1995).*

## Home Care

- The nursing interventions described previously for **Readiness for enhanced Family coping** should be used in the home environment with adaptations as necessary.
- Provide a videophone network for peer support for frail elderly people living at home. **EB:** *A videophone network appears to be helpful for elderly people in their peer support relationships. It supports and improves the functional independence of frail elderly people at home (Ezumi et al, 2003).*
- Encourage families to assist women caring for husbands with COPD to provide respite care so the women may have recreation time. **EBN:** *Women caregivers of husbands with COPD were dissatisfied with their lack of recreation, as well as support from friends, families, and health care providers (Bergs, 2002).*

C

## Client/Family Teaching

- Provide truthful information and support for the family and significant people regarding the client's specific illness or condition. **EBN:** *The results of this study indicate that attention needs to be given to methods of providing information and support to couples coping with prostate cancer. Both patients and partners need to be included in discussions about the effect of the illness and treatments so that both can feel more prepared to manage them (Harden et al, 2002).*
- Promote individual and family relaxation and stress-reduction strategies. *The immune system weakens in response to stress; relaxation elicits the opposite, healthful response (Bulechek & McCloskey, 1992).*
- ▲ Refer women with recurrent breast cancer and their family caregivers to a FOCUS Program (family involvement, optimistic attitude, coping effectiveness, uncertainty reduction, and symptom management), a family-based program of care. **EBN:** *Patients with recurrent breast cancer and their family members reported high satisfaction with the FOCUS Program. This study indicates that a need exists for family-based programs of care that enable both patients and their family members to manage the multiple demands associated with recurrent breast cancer (Northouse et al, 2002).*

## evolve WEBSITES FOR EDUCATION

See the EVOLVE website for World Wide Web resources for client education.

## REFERENCES


Boyd-Ball, AJ: A culturally responsive, family intervention model, *Alcohol Clin Exp Res* 27(8):1356-1360, 2003.

Bulechek G, McCloskey J: *Advanced nursing interventions,* Philadelphia, 1992, WB Saunders.

Cassells C, Watt E: The impact of incontinence on older spousal caregivers, *J Adv Nurs* 42(6):607-616, 2003.

Chang BL, Nitta S, Carter PA et al: Technology innovations. Perceived helpfulness of telephone calls: providing support for caregivers of family members with dementia, *J Gerontol Nurs* 30(9):14-21, 2004.

D'Avanzo CE et al: Developing culturally informed strategies for substance-related interventions. In Naegle MA, D'Avanzo CE, editors: *Addictions and substance abuse: strategies for advanced practice nursing,* St Louis, 2001, Mosby.

Giger JN, Davidhizar RE: *Transcultural nursing,* ed 2, St Louis, 1995, Mosby.

Guerriero Austrom M, Damush TM, Hartwell CW et al: Development and implementation of nonpharmacologic protocols for the management of patients with Alzheimer's disease and their families in a multiracial primary care setting, *Gerontologist* 44(4):548-553, 2004.

Harden J, Schafenacker A, Northouse L et al: Couples' experiences with prostate cancer: focus group research, *Oncol Nurs Forum* 29(4):701-709, 2002.

Kelleher L, Johnson M: An evaluation of a volunteer-support program for families at risk, *Pub Health Nurs* 21(4):297-305, 2004.

Kuuppelomäki M, Sasaki A, Yamada K et al: Coping strategies of family carers for older relatives in Finland, *J Clin Nurs* 13(6): 697-706, 2004.

Leininger MM: *Transcultural nursing: theories, research and practices,* ed 2, Hilliard, Ohio, 1996, McGraw-Hill.

Leske JS: Effects of intraoperative progress reports on anxiety levels of surgical patients' family members, *Appl Nurs Res* 8(4):169, 1995.

Moriarty PH, Wagner LD: Family rituals that provide meaning for single-parent families, *J Fam Nurs* 10(2):190-210, 2004.

Northouse LL, Walker J, Schafenacker et al: A family-based program of care for women with recurrent breast cancer and their family members, *Oncol Nurs Forum* 29(10):1411-1419, 2002.

Rose LE, Mallinson RK, Walton-Moss B: Barriers to family care in psychiatric settings, *J Nurs Scholarsh* 36(1):39-47, 2004.

Rivera-Andino J, Lopez L: When culture complicates care, *RN* 63(7):47, 2000.

Seideman RY, Jacobson S, Primeaux M et al: Assessing American Indian families, *MCN Am J Matern Child Nurs* 21(6):274-279, 1996.

Shapiro J, Monzo LD, Rueda R et al: Alienated advocacy: perspectives of Latina mothers of young adults with developmental disabilities on service systems, *Ment Retard* 42(1):37-54, 2004.
Stuart GW, Laraia MT: Therapeutic nurse-patient relationship. In Stuart GW, Laraia MT, editors: *Principles and practice of psychiatric nursing,* St Louis, 2001, Mosby.
Tak YR, McCubbin M: Family stress, perceived social support and coping following the diagnosis of a child's congenital heart disease, *J Adv Nurs* 39(2):190, 2002.
Urban AD, Berry D, Grey M: Optimizing outcomes in adolescents with type 1 diabetes and their families, *J Clin Outcomes Manag* 11(5):299-306, 2004.
Weiss S, Chen J: Factors influencing maternal mental health and family functioning during the low birthweight infant's first year of life, *J Pediatr Nurs* 17(2):114, 2002.
Wen LK, Shepherd MD, Parchman ML: Family support, diet, and exercise among older Mexican Americans with type 2 diabetes, *Diabetes Educ* 30(6):980-993, 2004.
York NL: Implementing a family presence protocol option, *Dimens Crit Care Nurs* 23(2):84-88, 2004.

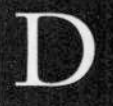

# Risk for sudden infant Death syndrome

*Betty J. Ackley*

## NANDA

### Definition

Presence of risk factors for sudden death of an infant under 1 year of age

### Risk Factors

**Modifiable:** Infants placed to sleep in the prone or side-lying position; prenatal and/or postnatal infant smoke exposure; infant overheating/overwrapping; soft underlayment/loose articles in the sleep environment; delayed or nonattendance of prenatal care

**Potentially Modifiable:** Low birth weight; prematurity; young maternal age

**Nonmodifiable:** Male gender; ethnicity (e.g., African-American, Native-American race of mother); seasonality of sudden infant death syndrome (SIDS) deaths (higher in winter and fall months); SIDS mortality peaks between infant age of 2 to 4 months

### Related Factors (r/t)

See Risk Factors

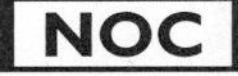

### Outcomes (Nursing Outcomes Classification)

#### Suggested NOC Outcomes

Knowledge: Child Physical Safety, Parenting Performance, Safe Home Environment

### Example NOC Outcome with Indicators

**Knowledge: Child Physical Safety** as evidenced by the following indicators: Description of methods to prevent SIDS/Description of first aid techniques (Rate each indicator of **Knowledge: Child Physical Safety:** 1 = none, 2 = limited, 3 = moderate, 4 = substantial, 5 = extensive [see Section I].)

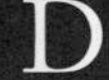

## Client Outcomes

### Client Will (Specify Time Frame):

- Explain appropriate measures to prevent SIDS
- Demonstrate correct techniques for positioning the infant, protecting the infant from harm

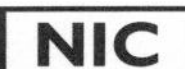

## Interventions (Nursing Interventions Classification)

### Suggested NIC Interventions

Infant Care, Teaching: Infant Safety

### Example NIC Activities—Teaching: Infant Safety

Place infant on back to sleep and keep loose bedding, pillows, and toys out of crib; avoid holding infant while smoking or drinking

## Nursing Interventions and Rationales

- Position infant on back to sleep, do not position in the prone position. **EB:** *Research has demonstrated that the prone position for sleeping infants is a risk factor for SIDS (Li et al, 2003; Malloy & Freeman, 2004). Population studies have demonstrated a striking trend in decreased incidence of SIDS since parents have been taught to* not *place infants in the prone position (Ponsonby et al, 2002).*
- Avoid use of loose bedding such as blankets and sheets for sleeping. If blankets are used, they should be tucked in around the crib mattress so the infant's face is less likely to become covered by bedding. "One strategy is to make up the bedding so that the infant's feet are able to reach the foot of the crib with the blankets tucked in around the crib mattress and reaching only the level of the infant's chest" (American Academy of Pediatrics, 2000, p. 653). **EB:** *Epidemiological studies have identified soft surfaces as a significant risk factor for SIDS, especially when these items are placed under the sleeping infant (Mitchell et al, 1998; Ponsonby et al, 1998).*
- Avoid overheating the infant by lightly clothing the child for sleep, and avoiding over-bundling. The infant should not feel hot to touch. **EB:** *Overheating the infant has been associated with increased risk of SIDS (Gilbert et al, 1992; Ponsonby et al, 1992).*

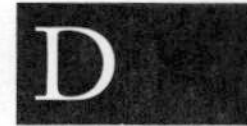


- Provide the infant a certain amount of time in prone position or "tummy time" while the infant is awake and observed. *A period on the tummy is recommended for developmental reasons and to help prevent flat spots on the back of the head (American Academy of Pediatrics, 2000).*
- Use electronic respiratory or cardiac monitors to detect cardiorespiratory arrest only if ordered. **EB:** *There is no evidence that infants prone to SIDS can be identified by monitoring of respiratory or cardiac function in the hospital (Malloy & Hoffman, 1996; Committee on Fetus & Newborn, 2003).*

### Home Care

- Most of the interventions above are relevant.
- Evaluate home for potential safety hazards such as inappropriate cribs, cradles, or strollers.
- Determine where and how the child sleeps and provide instructions on safe sleeping positions and environments as needed.

### Multicultural

- Discuss cultural norms with families in order to provide care that is appropriate for promoting safety for the infant in sleeping arrangements and care. **EBN:** *Misinterpretation of parenting behaviors can occur when the nurse and parent are from different cultures (Guarnaccia, 1998).*
- Encourage American-Indian mothers to avoid drinking and to avoid wrapping infants in excessive blankets or clothing. **EB:** *In one study an association was shown between binge drinking during pregnancy and having two or more layers of clothing on the infant in the American-Indian population (Iyasu et al, 2002).*
- Encourage African-American mothers to find alternatives to bed sharing and to avoid placing pillows, soft toys, and soft bedding in the sleep environment. **EB:** *Studies have demonstrated a higher incidence of SIDS in African-American infants. In one study the infants in death were commonly found in the supine position, but they were more likely to be sharing a bed with another person (Unger et al, 2003). Another study indicated that the greatest impact for SIDS reduction in the African-American population was the need to change behaviors regarding sleep locations by reducing placing infants for sleep on adult beds, sofas, or cots (Rasinski et al, 2003; Hauck et al, 2003).*

## Client/Family Teaching

- Teach families to position the infant on their back to sleep, do not position in the prone position. **EB:** *Research has demonstrated that the prone position for sleeping infants is a risk factor for SIDS (Li et al, 2003; Malloy & Freeman, 2004). Population studies have demonstrated a striking trend in decreased incidence of SIDS since parents have been taught to* not *place infants in the prone position (Ponsonby et al, 2002).*
- Teach the parents to place the infant supine to sleep with the head rotated to one side for a week, and then to the other side for a week. Parents should also change the orientation of the crib at intervals so the infant turns the head in alternate directions. *This is necessary to prevent the infant from developing a flat area on the back of the head (American Academy of Pediatrics, 2000; Persing et al, 2003).*

D

- Recommend the following infant care practices to parents:
  - Infants should not be put to sleep on soft surfaces such as waterbeds, sofas, or soft mattresses.
  - Avoid placing soft materials in the infant's sleeping environment such as pillows, quilts, and comforters. Do not use sheepskins under a sleeping infant.
  - Avoid placing soft objects such as stuffed toys and other gas-trapping objects in an infant's sleeping environment.
  - Avoid the use of loose bedding, such as blankets and sheets. If blankets are to be used, they should be tucked in around the crib mattress so the infant's face is less likely to become covered by bedding. "One strategy is to make up the bedding so that the infant's feet are able to reach the foot of the crib (feet to foot), with the blankets tucked in around the crib mattress and reaching only the level of the infant's chest. Another strategy is to use sleep clothing with no other covering over the infant" (American Academy of Pediatrics, 2000, p 653).

  **EB:** *Epidemiological studies have identified soft surfaces as a significant risk factor for SIDS, especially when these items are placed under the sleeping infant (Brook et al, 1997; Mitchell et al, 1998; Ponsonby et al, 1998).*
- Teach parents the need to obtain a crib that conforms to the safety standards of the Consumer Product Safety Commission. *Although many cradles and bassinets also may provide safe sleeping enclosures, safety standards have not been established for these items (American Academy of Pediatrics, 2000).*
- Teach parents not to place the infant in an adult bed to sleep, or a sofa or chair. Infants should sleep in a crib. *Sleep surfaces designed for adults have the risk of entrapment between the mattress and the structure of the bed (e.g., the headboard, footboard, side rails, and frame), the wall, or adjacent furniture, as well as between railings in the headboard or footboard (American Academy of Pediatrics, 2000).* **EB:** *In one study of SIDS deaths, over half of the infants were sleeping in the same bed as an adult, which suggests that some of the deaths were due to unintentional suffocation from the adult or from compressible bedding (Person et al, 2002). Another student demonstrated that the risk of suffocation increased by two times when infants were placed to sleep in an adult bed rather than in a crib (Scheers, 2003).*
- Teach parents not to sleep with an infant, especially if alcohol or medications/illicit drugs are used by the parents. **EB:** *A study demonstrated that parents who were under the influence of alcohol or illicit drugs or were smoking were more likely to have a SIDS result (James et al, 2003). Another study demonstrated that mother's who consumed three or more alcoholic drinks in the past 24 hours increased the risk of SIDS when bedsharing with an infant (Carpenter et al, 2004).*
- Recommend an alternative to sleeping with an infant; parents might consider placing the infant's crib near their bed to allow for more convenient breastfeeding and parent contact. *The safety of mother-infant sleeping is debated in the research literature, because results of studies vary (Mesich, 2005).*
- Teach parents to avoid overheating the infant by lightly clothing the child for sleep and avoiding overbundling. The infant should not feel hot to touch. The bedroom

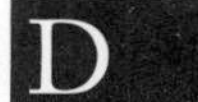

temperature should be comfortable to an adult wearing light bedclothing. **EB:** *Overheating the infant has been associated with an increased risk of SIDS (Gilbert et al, 1992; Ponsonby et al, 1992).*

- Question parents regarding following recommendations for the prevention of SIDS at each well-baby visit or visit with health care practitioner for illness. Strongly encourage compliance with precautions to prevent SIDS. **EB:** *A survey of mothers in Britain demonstrated that while the majority of the moms knew the precautions, 25% of the moms were not following the recommended practice (Roberts & Upton, 2000).*
- Teach the need to stop smoking during pregnancy and to not smoke around the infant, that smoking is a risk factor for SIDS. **EBN:** *A study demonstrated that newborns whose mothers smoked have a limited ability to maximize and vary their heart rate, which can result in the infant being unable to maximize cardiac output during stress, which puts the infant at an increased risk for morbidity and possibly mortality (Sherman et al, 2002).* **EB:** *Research has demonstrated that smoking during pregnancy is a risk factor for SIDS (Alm et al, 1998; Pollack, 2001; Schoendorf & Kiely, 1992). Smoke in the environment after birth is considered a risk factor in several studies (Mitchell et al, 1993; Schoendorf & Kiely, 1992; US Department of Health and Human Services, 2004).*
- Recommend that parents with infants in child care make it very clear to the employees that the infant must be placed in the supine position only to sleep, not prone or side-lying. **EB:** *A survey of licensed child care facilities demonstrated that only 14.3% were in compliance with the recommendation that infants be placed in the supine position to sleep (Ford & Linker, 2002).*
- Teach child care employees how best to position infants for sleeping and the dangers of a too soft environment. **EB:** *A study demonstrated that an 60-minute educational experience designed for child care providers was effective in increasing the compliance with guidelines and increasing the number of written sleep position policies at the child care centers (Moon & Oden, 2003).*

▲ Teach parents living in deprived areas of precautions to prevent SIDS. **EB:** *A study in New Zealand demonstrated that SIDS is more common in infants living in deprived areas, although SIDS can occur in infants living in any situation (Mitchell et al, 2000).*

▲ Involve family members in learning and practicing rescue techniques, including treatment of choking, breathing, and cardiopulmonary resuscitation (CPR). Initiate referral to formal training classes. *Family members need adequate preparation to deal with emergency situations and should take part in the AHA Basic Lifesaving Course or the American Red Cross Infant/Child CPR Course (Gotsch et al, 2002).* **EBN:** *A study demonstrated that learning CPR did not reduce anxiety in the parents regarding SIDS but did increase their confidence in dealing with emergencies (Clarke, 1998).*

## evolve WEBSITES FOR EDUCATION

See the EVOLVE website for World Wide Web resources for client education.

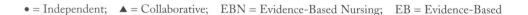

D

## REFERENCES

Alm B, Milerad J, Wennergren G et al: A case-control study of smoking and sudden infant death syndrome in the Scandinavian countries 1992 to 1995. The Nordic Epidemiological SIDS Study, *Arch Dis Child*, 78(4):329, 1998.

Changing concepts of sudden infant death syndrome: implications for infant sleeping environment and sleep position. American Academy of Pediatrics. Task Force on Infant Sleep Position and Sudden Infant Death Syndrome, *Pediatrics* 105(3 Pt 1):650, 2000.

Brooke H, Gibson A, Tappin D et al: Case-control study of sudden infant death syndrome in Scotland, 1992-5, *BMJ* 314(7093): 1516, 1997.

Carpenter RG, Irgens LM, Blair PS et al: Sudden unexplained infant death in 20 regions in Europe: case control study, *Lancet* 363(9404):185-191, 2004.

Clarke K: Research. Infant CPR: the effect on parental anxiety regarding SIDS, *Br J Midwifery*, 6(11):710, 1998.

Committee on Fetus and Newborn. American Academy of Pediatrics: Apnea, sudden infant death syndrome, and home monitoring, *Pediatrics* 111(4 Pt 1):914, 2003.

Ford KM, Linker LA: Compliance of licensed child care centers with the American Academy of Pediatrics' recommendations for infant sleep positions, *J Community Health Nurs* 19(2):83, 2002.

Gilbert R, Rudd P, Berry PJ et al: Combined effect of infection and heavy wrapping on the risk of sudden unexpected infant death, *Arch Dis Child* 67(2):171, 1992.

Gotsch K, Annest JL, Holmgreen P: Nonfatal choking-related episodes among children—United States, 2001, *MMWR Morb Mortal Wkly Rep* 51(42):945, 2002.

Guarnaccia P: Multicultural experiences of family caregiving: a Study of African American, European American, and Hispanic American families, *New Direct Ment Health Serv* 77:45, 1998.

Hauck FR, Herman SM, Donovan M et al: Sleep environment and the risk of sudden infant death syndrome in an urban population: the Chicago infant mortality study, *Pediatrics* 111(5 Part 2):1207-1214, 2003.

Iyasu S, Randall LL, Welty TK et al: Risk factors for sudden infant death syndrome among northern plains Indians, *JAMA* 288(21): 2717, 2002.

James C, Klenka H, Manning D: Sudden infant death syndrome: bed sharing with mothers who smoke, *Arch Dis Child* 88(2): 112, 2003.

Li DK, Petitti DB, Willinger M et al: Infant sleeping position and the risk of sudden infant death syndrome in California, 1997-2000, *Am J Epidemiol* 157(5):446-455, 2003.

Malloy MH, Freeman DH: Age at death, season, and day of death as indicators of the effect of the back to sleep program on sudden infant death syndrome in the United States, 1992-1999, *Arch Pediatr Adolesc Med* 158(4):359, 2004.

Malloy MH, Hoffman H: Home apnea monitoring and sudden infant death syndrome, *Prev Med* 25:645, 1996.

Malloy MS: Trends in postneonatal aspiration deaths and reclassification of sudden infant death syndrome: impact of the "Back to Sleep" program, *Pediatrics* 109(4):661, 2002.

Mesich HM: Mother-infant co-sleeping: understanding the debate and maximizing infant safety, *MCN Am J Matern Child Nurs* 30(1):30-37, 2005.

Mitchell EA, Stewart AW, Crampton P: Deprivation and sudden infant death syndrome, *Soc Sci Med* 51(1):147, 2000.

Mitchell EA, Thompson JM, Ford R et al: Sheepskin bedding and the sudden infant death syndrome. New Zealand Cot Death Study Group, *J Pediatr* 133(5):701, 1998.

Moon RY, Oden RP: Back to sleep: can we influence child care providers? *Pediatrics* 112(4):878-882, 2003.

Persing J, James H, Swanson J et al: Prevention and management of positional skull deformities in infants, *Pediatrics* 112(1 Pt 1): 199-202, 2003.

Person TL, Lavezzi WA, Wolf BC: Cosleeping and sudden unexpected death in infancy, *Arch Pathol Lab Med* 126(3):343, 2002.

Pollack HA: Sudden infant death syndrome, maternal smoking during pregnancy, and the cost-effectiveness of smoking cessation intervention, *Am J Public Health* 91(3):432, 2001.

Ponsonby A, Dwyer T, Cochrane J: Population trends in sudden infant death syndrome, *Semin Perinatol* 26(4):296, 2002.

Ponsonby AL, Dwyer T, Gibbons LE et al: Thermal environment and sudden infant death syndrome: case-control study, *BMJ* 304(6822):277, 1992.

Ponsonby AL, Dwyer T, Couper D et al: Association between use of a quilt and sudden infant death syndrome: case-control study, *BMJ* 316(7126):195, 1998.

Rasinski KA, Kuby A, Bzdusek SA et al: Effect of a sudden infant death syndrome risk reduction education program on risk factor compliance and information sources in primarily black urban communities, *Pediatrics* 11(4 pt 1):E347, 2003.

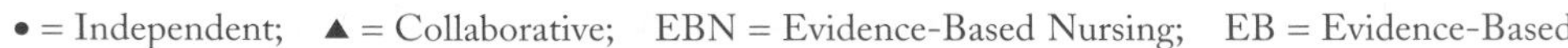

Roberts H, Upton D: Research. New mother's knowledge of sudden infant death syndrome, *Br J Midwifery* 8(3):147, 2000.
Scheers NJ, Rutherford GW, Kemp JS: Where should infants sleep? A comparison of risk for suffocation of infats sleeping in cribs, adult beds, and other sleeping locations, *Pediatrics* 112(4):883-889, 2003.
Schoendorf KC, Kiely JL: Relationship of sudden infant death syndrome to maternal smoking during and after pregnancy, *Pediatrics* 90:905, 1992.
Sherman J, Young A, Sherman MP et al: Prenatal smoking and alterations in newborn heart rate during transition, *J Obstet Gynecol Neonatal Nurs* 31(6):680, 2002.
Taylor JA, Krieger JW, Reay DT et al: Prone sleep position and the sudden infant death syndrome in King County Washington: a case-control study, *J Pediatr* 128(5 Pt 1):626, 1996.
Unger B, Kemp JS, Wilkins D et al: Racial disparity and modifiable risk factors among infants dying suddenly and unexpectedly, *Pediatrics* 111(2):E127, 2003.
US Department of Health and Human Services: *The health consequences of smoking: a report of the Surgeon General,* US Department of Health and Human Services, CDC, 2004.

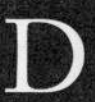

# Ineffective Denial

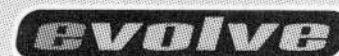

*Ann Keeley and Gail Ladwig*

## NANDA

### Definition

The conscious or unconscious attempt to disavow the knowledge or meaning of an event to reduce anxiety/fear, but leading to the detriment of health

### Defining Characteristics

Delays seeking or refuses health care attention to the detriment of health; does not perceive personal relevance of symptoms or danger; displaces source of symptoms to other organs; displays inappropriate affect; does not admit fear of death or invalidism; makes dismissive gestures or comments when speaking of distressing events; minimizes symptoms; unable to admit impact of disease on life pattern; uses home remedies (self-treatment) to relieve symptoms; displaces fear of impact of condition

### Related Factors (r/t)

Fear of consequences; chronic or terminal illness; actual or perceived fear of possible losses (e.g., job, significant other); refusal to acknowledge substance abuse problem; fear of the social stigma associated with disease

## NOC

### Outcomes (Nursing Outcomes Classification)

#### Suggested NOC Outcomes

Acceptance: Health Status, Anxiety Self-Control, Health Beliefs: Perceived Threat, Symptom Control

**Example NOC Outcome with Indicators**

**Anxiety Self-Control** as evidenced by the following indicators: Eliminates precursors of anxiety/Monitors physical manifestations of anxiety/Controls anxiety response (Rate each indicator of **Anxiety Self-Control:** 1 = never demonstrated, 2 = rarely demonstrated, 3 = sometimes demonstrated, 4 = often demonstrated, 5 = consistently demonstrated [see Section I].)



## Client Outcomes

**Client Will (Specify Time Frame):**

- Seek out appropriate health care attention when needed
- Use home remedies only when appropriate
- Display appropriate affect and verbalize fears
- Remain substance free
- Actively engage in treatment program related to identified "substance" of abuse
- Demonstrate alternate adaptive coping mechanism

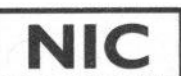

## Interventions (Nursing Interventions Classification)

### Suggested NIC Intervention

Anxiety Reduction

**Example NIC Activities—Anxiety Reduction**

Use a calm, reassuring approach; stay with the patient to promote safety and reduce fear

## Nursing Interventions and Rationales

- Assess the client's understanding of symptoms and illness. **EBN:** *Negative responses to a need for change in behavior related to an alteration in health status can only be understood following a thorough assessment of the client's appraisal framework (Dudley-Brown, 2002).*
- Spend time with the client, allow time for responses. *Nursing presence, one-on-one interaction, connecting with the client's experience, going beyond the scientific data, and knowing what will work and when to act all support the nurse-client relationship and affirm their respective selves. As a result, the client grows in awareness of his or her own being (Doona et al, 1999).*
- Assess whether the use of denial is helping or hindering the patient's care. Provide support for clients who are using denial as a way of coping. **EBN:** *Denial may be used as an adaptive mechanism during times of illness and stress. Patience, understanding, and self-awareness are crucial for providing a safe, trusting environment for patients who are experiencing denial (Stephenson, 2004).*
- Allow the client to express and use denial as a coping mechanism. **EBN:** *This time period of denial may be necessary for the client to develop a construct within which the infor-*

*mation has meaning and can be appraised as not a threat to survival (Norris & Spelic, 2002).*

- Assess for subtle signs of denial (e.g., unrealistic display of optimism, downplaying of symptoms, inability to admit one's own fear). *Minimization and denial are part of the alcoholism pathophysiology (Becke & Walton-Moss, 2001).*
- Avoid confrontation. *Rather than direct confrontation, informing of the reality of consequences of a specific behavior may be more therapeutically assimilated into the client's appraisal framework. Assess individual spiritual coping style (Faltz & Skinner, 2002).*
- Support the client's spiritual coping measures. **EBN:** *Most religious coping is considered positive (Meisenhelder, 2002). Physical and mental health is interrelated with spiritual health (Taylor, 2002).*
- Develop a trusting, therapeutic relationship with the client/family. **EBN:** *In this study of nurse-patient relationships in palliative care it was demonstrated that nurses who develop trusting relationships demonstrate a holistic approach to caring, show their understanding of patients' suffering, are aware of their unvoiced needs, provide comfort without actually being asked, and are reliable, proficient, competent, and dedicated in their care (Mok & Chui, 2004).*
- Encourage individual family members to share their concerns and worries. **EBN:** *This may help reframe the experience in a way that is acceptable. Allows the nurse to identify possible misperceptions and/or questions (Mellon, 2002).*
- Ask appropriate questions using an assessment tool such as FAST to assess whether denial is being used in association with alcoholism or drug use. The client is asked to circle the appropriate response for each question: Less than monthly; Monthly; Weekly; Daily; Almost Daily.
  1. MEN: How often do you have EIGHT or more drinks on one occasion? WOMEN: How often do you have SIX or more drinks on one occasion?
  2. How often during the last year have you been unable to remember what happened the night before because you had been drinking?
  3. How often during the last year have you failed to do what was normally expected of you because of drinking?
  4. In the last year has a relative or friend, or a doctor or other health worker been concerned about your drinking or suggested you cut down?

  **EB:** *The four-item FAST alcohol questionnaire had good sensitivity and specificity, across a range of settings, when the AUDIT alcohol assessment score was used as the gold standard. The FAST questionnaire is quick to administer, because more than 50% of clients are categorized using just one question (Hodgson et al, 2002). Include in questionnaire drug use in addition to drinking (Hinkin et al, 2001). T-ACE and TWEAK are modified to be used with women.* **EBN:** *Alcoholism rates are increasing in women and women may have distinct assessment risk factors (Becker & Walton-Moss, 2001; see Gorski, 2005, for a brief addiction screening tool).*
- Sit at eye level. *Honest caring behaviors on the part of the nurse facilitate acceptance of reality on the part of the client (Haltz & Skinner, 2002).*
- Use touch if appropriate and with permission. Touch the client's hand or arm. *Appropriate expression of caring on the part of the nurse facilitates therapeutic client response (Haltz & Skinner, 2002).*

D

- Explain signs and symptoms of illness; as necessary, reinforce use of prescribed treatment plan. *A straightforward education on the effects of an abused substance is integral to motivation on the part of the client (Becker & Walton-Moss, 2001).*
- Have the client make choices regarding treatment and actively involve him or her in the decision-making process. **EB:** *Interventions that increase the self-efficacy of clients support maintenance of abstinence (Vielva & Iraurgi, 2001).*
- Help the client recognize existing and additional sources of support; allow time for adjustment. *The influence of environment on a positive adaptation is significant (Moser et al, 2001).*
- Encourage the client/family to describe prior crises and methods of coping. **EBN:** *Allows the nurse to identify the family's communication style and adapt his or her interventions. Provides the nurse an opportunity to point out family strengths that may be used (Mellon, 2002).*

▲ If appropriate, refer family to a skilled mental health counselor for help in planning an intervention to observe whether denial has been or is being used as a coping mechanism in other areas of life. *Referral may be necessary to provide the most thorough assessment and treatment choices for the client (Becker & Walton-Moss, 2001).*

- Refer to care plans **Defensive Coping** and **Dysfunctional Family processes: alcoholism**

## Geriatric

- Identify recent losses of the client, because grieving may prolong denial. Encourage the client to take one day at a time. *Elderly clients often have experienced significant, multiple losses in a variety of domains. This may complicate adaptation to an individual change in health status as the resources formerly used for successful adaptation are no longer available (Boyd & Stanley, 2002).*
- Encourage the client to verbalize feelings. **EBN:** *This study indicated that bereaved individuals benefited from individual, family and group therapy to discuss losses (Douglas, 2004).*
- Encourage communication among family members. *Communication problems within families are pivotal in the development of family adjustment to a change in health status and or adaptation to a life change (Hanson, 2002).*
- Recognize denial. *Denial is a defensive avoidance of emotion. It can be beneficial as a coping mechanism, but total denial can be detrimental (Robinson, 1999).*
- Use reality-focusing techniques. Wherever possible, provide realistic feedback, allowing the client to validate his or her perceptions. *Providing validation of actual stressors and available resources aids in a positive adaptation (Pakenham, 2001).*

## Multicultural

- Assess for the influence of cultural beliefs, norms, and values on the client's understanding of and ability to acknowledge health status. **EBN:** *Willingness to acknowledge health status may be based on cultural perceptions (Cochran, 1998; Doswell & Erlen, 1998; Leininger & McFarland, 2002).*
- Discuss with the client those aspects of his or her health behavior/lifestyle that will re-

main unchanged by health status. **EBN:** *Aspects of the client's life that are meaningful and valuable to him or her should be understood and preserved without change (Leininger & McFarland, 2002).*

- Negotiate with the client regarding the aspects of health behavior that will need to be modified as a result of health status. **EBN:** *Give and take with the client will lead to culturally congruent care (Leininger & McFarland, 2002).*
- Assess the role of fatalism on the client's ability to acknowledge health status. **EBN:** *Fatalistic perspectives, which involve the belief that you cannot control your own fate, may influence health behaviors in some Asian, African-American, and Latino populations (Chen, 2001; Harmon et al, 1996; Phillips et al, 1999). A culturally appropriate way to deal with fatalistic views is to communicate to the family that it is also fate that the best care is available (Munet-Vilaro, 2004).*
- Validate the client's feelings of anxiety and fear related to health status. **EBN:** *Validation is the therapeutic communication technique that lets the client know that the nurse has heard and understands what was said, and it promotes the nurse-client relationship (Heineken, 1998).*

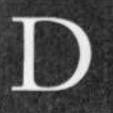

D

### Home Care

- Observe family interaction and roles. Assess whether denial is being used to meet the needs of another family member. *Communication problems within families are pivotal in the development of family adjustment to a change in health status and or adaptation to a life change (Hanson, 2002).*
- ▲ Refer the client and family to psychiatric clinical nurse specialist or medical social services for evaluation and treatment as indicated per physician order. *It may be necessary to involve the entire family to effectively treat the client.*
- ▲ Refer the client/family for follow-up if prolonged denial is a risk. *Prolonged denial almost always interferes with successful treatment. Only when denial subsides does the patient regain control (Robinson, 1999).*
- ▲ Identify an emergency plan, including how to contact hotlines and receive emergency services. *Denial may be abandoned when the need for emergency care is perceived by the client or the family.*
- Encourage communication between family members, particularly when dealing with the loss of a significant person. *Communication problems within families are pivotal in the development of family adjustment to a change in health status and or adaptation to a life change (Hanson, 2002).* **EBN:** *An understanding of the family structure, patterns of communication, health care history, and cultural influences will facilitate effective interventions on the part of the nurse. In the context of some family patterns of communication, defensive coping may be a learned behavior (Hellemann et al, 2002).*

## Client/Family Teaching

- Teach signs and symptoms of illness and appropriate responses (e.g., taking medication, going to the emergency department, calling the physician). Provide a list of names and numbers. *Family members should be involved at all points of care to ensure that the necessary care will be provided in a safe, accurate manner (Harmon, 2001).*

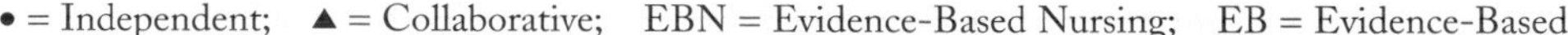

D

- • Teach family members that denial may continue throughout the adjustment to home and not to be confrontational. *Denial is normal especially during phases of adjustment, and reprimanding can lead to increased frustration and further denial (Robinson, 1999).*
- ▲ If the problem is substance abuse, refer to an appropriate community agency (e.g., Alcoholics Anonymous). **EBN:** *Families need assistance in coping with health changes. The nurse is often perceived as the individual who can help them obtain necessary social support (Northouse et al, 2002; Tak & McCubbin, 2002).*
- • Teach families of clients with brain injuries that denial has been associated with damage to the right hemisphere. *The client may exhibit inappropriate affect and anxiety.*
- • Inform family of available community support resources. *Mutual support groups can have a positive effect not only in Western cultures but also in the Eastern cultures (Fung & Chien, 2002).*

## evolve WEBSITES FOR EDUCATION

See the EVOLVE website for World Wide Web resources for client education.

## REFERENCES


Becker KL, Walton-Moss B: Detecting and addressing alcohol abuse in women, *Nurse Pract* 26(10):13, 2001.

Boyd MA, Stanley M: Mental health assessment of the elderly. In Boyd MA, editor: *Psychiatric nursing in contemporary practice,* ed 2, Philadelphia, 2002, Lippincott.

Chen YC: Chinese values, health and nursing, *J Adv Nurs* 36(2):270, 2001.

Cochran M: Tears have no color, *Am J Nurs* 98(6):53, 1998.

Davidhizar R, Newman-Giger J: Patients' use of denial: coping with the unacceptable, *Nurs Stand* 12(43):44, 1998.

Doona M, Chase S, Haggerty L: Nursing presence, *J Holist Nurs* 17(1):54, 1999.

Doswell W, Erlen J: Multicultural issues and ethical concerns in the delivery of revising care interventions, *Nurs Clin North Am* 33(2):353, 1998.

Douglas DH: The lived experience of loss: a phenomenological study, *J Am Psychiatr Nurses Assoc* 10(1):24-32, 2004.

Faltz BG, Skinner MK: Substance abuse disorders. In Boyd MA, editor: *Psychiatric nursing in contemporary practice,* ed 2, Philadelphia, 2002, Lippincott.

Fung WY, Chien WT: The effectiveness of a mutual support group for family caregivers of a relative with dementia, *Arch Psychiatr Nurs* 16(3):134, 2002.

Gorski T: Women at risk: brief screening tools. Available at www.tgorski.com/clin_mod/atp/women_at_risk-brief_sceening_tools.htm#TWEAK, accessed on April 7, 2005.

Harmon MP, Castro FG, Coe K: Acculturation and cervical cancer: knowledge, beliefs, and behaviors of Hispanic women, *Women Health* 24(3):37, 1996.

Harmon SMH: *Family health care nursing,* Philadelphia, 2001, FA Davis.

Heineken J: Patient silence is not necessarily client satisfaction: communication in home care nursing, *Home Healthc Nurse* 16(2): 115, 1998.

Hellemann MS V, Lee KA, Kary FS: Strengths and vulnerabilities of women of Mexican descent in relation to depressive symptoms, *Nurs Res* 51(3):175, 2002.

Hinkin CH, Castellon SA, Dickson-Fuhrman E et al: Screening for drug and alcohol abuse among older adults using a modified version of the CAGE, *Am J Addict* 10:319, 2001.

Hodgson R, Alwyn T, John B et al: The FAST alcohol screening test, *Alcohol Alcohol* 37(1):61, 2002.

Leininger MM, McFarland MR: *Transcultural nursing: concepts, theories, research and practices,* ed 3, New York, 2002, McGraw-Hill.

Meisenhelder JB: Terrorism, posttraumatic stress, and religious coping, *Issues Ment Health Nurs* 23:771, 2002.

Mellon S: Comparisons between cancer survivors and family members on meaning of the illness and family quality of life, *Oncol Nurs Forum* 29(7):1117, 2002.

Mok E, Chui PC: Nurse-patient relationships in palliative care, *J Adv Nurs* 48(5):475-483, 2004.
Moser KM, Sowell RL, Phillips KD: Issues of women dually diagnosed with HIV infection and substance use problems in the Carolinas, *Issues Ment Health Nurs* 22:23, 2001.
Munet-Vilaro F: Delivery of culturally competent care to children with cancer and their families—the Latino experience, *J Pediatr Oncol Nurs* 21(3):155-159, 2004.
Norris J, Spelic SS: Supporting adaption to body image disruption, *Rehabil Nurs* 27(1):8, 2002.
Pakenham KI: Application of a stress and coping model to caregiving in multiple sclerosis, *Psychol Health Med* 6(1):13, 2001.
Phillips JM, Cohen MZ, Moses G: Breast cancer screening and African American women: fear, fatalism, and silence, *Oncol Nurs Forum* 26(3):561, 1999.
Robinson AW: Getting to the heart of denial, *Am J Nurs* 99(5):38-43, 1999
Russell GC: The role of denial in clinical practice, *J Adv Nurs* 18:938, 1993.
Stephenson PS: Understanding denial, *Oncol Nurs Forum* 31(5):985-988, 2004.
Taylor EJ: *Spiritual care: nursing theory, research and practice,* Upper Saddle River, NJ, 2002, Prentice-Hall.
Vielva I, Iraurgi I: Cognitive and behavioural factors as predictors of abstinence following treatment for alcohol dependence, *Addiction* 96:297, 2001.

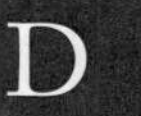


# Impaired Dentition

*Betty J. Ackley*

**NANDA**

## Definition

Disruption in tooth development/eruption patterns or structural integrity of individual teeth

## Defining Characteristics

Excessive plaque; crown or root caries; halitosis; tooth enamel discoloration; toothache; loose teeth; excessive calculus; incomplete eruption for age (may be primary or permanent teeth); malocclusion or tooth misalignment; premature loss of primary teeth; worn down or abraded teeth; tooth fracture(s); missing teeth or complete absence; erosion of enamel; asymmetrical facial expression

## Related Factors (r/t)

Ineffective oral hygiene; sensitivity to heat or cold; barriers to self-care; nutritional deficits; dietary habits; genetic predisposition; selected prescription medications; premature loss of primary teeth; excessive intake of fluorides; chronic vomiting; chronic use of tobacco, coffee, tea, red wine; lack of knowledge regarding dental health; excessive use of abrasive cleaning agents; bruxism

**NOC**

## Outcomes (Nursing Outcomes Classification)

### Suggested NOC Outcomes

Oral Hygiene, Self-Care: Oral Hygiene

### Example NOC Outcome with Indicators

**Oral Hygiene** as evidenced by the following indicators: Cleanliness of teeth/Cleanliness of gums/Cleanliness of dentures/Tongue integrity/Gum integrity (Rate each indicator of **Oral Hygiene:** 1 = severely compromised, 2 = substantially compromised, 3 = moderately compromised, 4 = mildly compromised, 5 = not compromised [see Section I].)

D

## Client Outcomes

### Client Will (Specify Time Frame):

- Have clean teeth, gums healthy pink color, mouth with pleasant odor
- Demonstrate ability to masticate foods without difficulty
- State no pain originating from teeth
- Demonstrate measures can take to improve dental hygiene

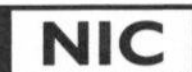

## Interventions (Nursing Interventions Classification)

### Suggested NIC Interventions

Oral Health Maintenance, Oral Health Promotion, Oral Health Restoration

### Example NIC Activities—Oral Health Maintenance

Establish a mouth care routine; arrange for dental check-ups as needed

## Nursing Interventions and Rationales

- ▲ Inspect oral cavity/teeth at least once daily and note any discoloration, presence of debris, amount of plaque buildup, presence of lesions, edema, or bleeding, intactness of teeth. Refer to a dentist or periodontist as appropriate. *Systematic inspection can identify impending problems (Walton et al, 2001).*
- • Monitor the client's nutritional and fluid status to determine if adequate. Recommend the client eat a balanced diet and limit between meal snacks. *Poor nutrition predisposes clients to dental disease (ADA, 2004).*
- • Recommend the client decrease or preferably stop intake of soft drinks. *Sugar containing soft drinks can cause cavities and the low pH of the drink can cause erosion in teeth (ADA, 2004).* **EB:** *Persons who consumed sugared soft drinks three or more times daily had 17%-62% higher rate of dental caries than those who consumed no soft drinks (Heller et al, 2001).*
- ▲ Assess the client for underlying medical condition that may be causing halitosis. **EB:** *Potential sources of blood-borne halitosis are some systemic diseases, metabolic disorders, medication, and certain foods (Tangreman, 2002).* **EB:** *Patients who believe they have oral malodor often have a dry mouth condition instead (Kleinberg et al, 2002).*
- • Determine the client's mental status and manual dexterity; if the client is unable to

care for self, nursing personnel must provide dental hygiene. The nursing diagnosis **Bathing/hygiene Self-care deficit** is then also applicable.

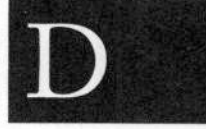

- Determine the client's usual method of oral care. Whenever possible, build on the client's existing knowledge base and current practices to develop an individualized plan of care.
- If the client is free of bleeding disorders and is able to swallow, encourage the client to brush teeth with a soft toothbrush using fluoride-containing toothpaste after every meal and to floss teeth daily. *The toothbrush is the most important tool for oral care; toothbrushing is the most effective method of reducing plaque and controlling periodontal disease (Stiefel et al, 2000; Pearson & Hutton, 2002).*
- If the client is unable to brush own teeth, follow this procedure:
  1. Use a soft bristle baby toothbrush.
  2. Use fluoride toothpaste and tap water or saline as a solution.
  3. Brush teeth in an up-and-down manner.
  4. Suction as needed.
- Avoid using foam sticks to clean teeth; use only to swab out the oral cavity. *Use of this nursing protocol results in improved oral hygiene in a vulnerable population (Stiefel et al, 2000).* **EBN:** *Foam sticks are not effective for removing plaque; the toothbrush is much more effective (DeWalt, 1975; Pearson & Hutton, 2002).*
- Tell the client to direct the toothbrush vertically toward the tooth surfaces. **EB:** *One study demonstrated that brushing with the toothbrush bristles perpendicular to the surface of the teeth has a high efficacy of plaque removal and maintains good gingival condition (Sasahara & Kawamura, 2000).*
- Instruct the client to clean the tongue when performing oral hygiene. Brush tongue with soft toothbrush and follow with a mouth rinse. Use tap water or saline only for a mouth rinse. Avoid the use of hydrogen peroxide, lemon-glycerin swabs, or alcohol-based mouthwashes. *Tongue brushing and mouth rinsing are basic treatment measures for halitosis (Yaegaki et al, 2002).* **EBN:** *Hydrogen peroxide can cause mucosal damage and is extremely foul tasting to clients (Tombes & Gallucci, 1993). Lemon-glycerin swabs can result in decreased salivary amylase and oral moisture, as well as erosion of tooth enamel (Foss-Durant & McAffee, 1997; Poland, 1987).*
- If the client does not have a bleeding disorder, encourage the client to floss daily with approximately 18 inches of floss using a gentle rubbing up and down motion. *Floss is useful to remove plaque buildup between the teeth (Brown & Yoder, 2002; ADA, 2004).*
- ▲ Recommend client see a dentist at prescribed intervals, generally two times per year if teeth are in satisfactory condition. *It is important to see a dentist at regular intervals for preventative dental care (ADA, 2004).*
- If platelet numbers are decreased, or if the client is edentulous, use moistened toothettes or a specially made very soft toothbrush for oral care. *A toothbrush can cause soft tissue injury and bleeding in clients with low numbers of platelets.*
- Provide scrupulous dental care to critically ill clients. *Cultures of the teeth of critically ill clients have yielded significant bacterial colonization, which can cause nosocomial pneumonia (Scannapieco et al, 1992).*
- If teeth are nonfunctional for chewing, modification of oral intake (e.g., edentulous

diet, soft diet) may be necessary. The nursing diagnosis **Imbalanced Nutrition: less than body requirements** may apply.
- If the client is unable to swallow, keep suction nearby when providing oral care.
- See care plan for **Impaired Oral mucous membrane.**

D

## Geriatric

- Consider recommending use of an ultrasonic toothbrush if any impairment of manual dexterity exists. **EB:** *Use of an ultrasonic toothbrush was shown to reduce plaque and bleeding in a study of 12 patients age 65 years and older (Whitmyer et al, 1998).*
- Carefully observe oral cavity and lips for abnormal lesions when providing dental care. *Malignant lesions in the mouth are common in the elderly, especially if there is a history of smoking or alcohol use. The elderly are least likely to see a dentist, and often lesions are painless until they invade other structures (Aubertin, 1997).*
- ▲ Consider professional oral health care for the elderly in nursing homes. **EB:** *Professional oral health care administered by dental hygienists to a group of elderly patients needing daily nursing care was associated with a reduction in prevalence of fever and fatal pneumonia (Adachi, 2002).*
- Ensure that dentures are removed and cleaned regularly, preferably after every meal and before bedtime; select appropriate adhesives to improve breath. *Dentures left in the mouth at night impede circulation to the palate and predispose the client to oral lesions.* **EB:** *Fixodent denture adhesives provide the denture wearer with a noticeable improvement in breath odor (Myatt et al, 2002).*
- ▲ Recognize that halitosis in older adults is a common condition that may have oral or nonoral sources. *Bad breath may reflect serious local or systemic conditions, including gingivitis, periodontal disease, diabetic acidosis, hepatic failure, or respiratory infection. Nonoral sources require treatment of the underlying cause, whereas suspected oral sources require referral for a dental evaluation (Durham et al, 1993).*

## Pregnant Client

- Encourage the expectant mother to eat a healthy, balanced diet that is rich in calcium. *The teeth usually start to form in the gums during the second trimester of pregnancy. To encourage the development of good, strong teeth, expectant mothers should eat a healthy, balanced diet that is rich in calcium (Koop, 2004).*

## Infant Oral Hygiene

- Gently wipe baby's gums with a washcloth or sterile gauze at least once a day. *Wiping gums prevents bacterial buildup in the mouth (Koop, 2004).* **EB:** *Infants of breastfeeding mothers need early and consistent mouth care when the teeth erupt. Early and consistent mouth care is imperative (Valaitis et al, 2000).*
- Never allow child to fall asleep with a bottle containing milk, formula, fruit juice, or sweetened liquids. If child needs a comforter between regular feedings, at night, or during naps, fill a bottle with cool water or give the child a clean pacifier recommended by your dentist or physician. Never give child a pacifier dipped in any sweet liquid. Avoid filling child's bottle with liquids such as sugar water and soft drinks. *Decay in infants and children can destroy the teeth and most often occurs in the upper front*

*teeth, but other teeth may also be affected. Decay occurs when sweetened liquids are given and are left clinging to an infant's teeth for long periods. Many sweet liquids cause problems, including milk, formula, and fruit juice. Bacteria in the mouth use these sugars as food. They then produce acids that attack the teeth. Each time the child drinks these liquids, acids attack for 20 minutes or longer. After many attacks, the teeth can decay. It is not just what is put in the child's bottle that causes decay, but how often—and for how long (ADA, 2004).*

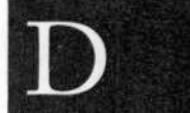


- When multiple teeth appear, brush with small toothbrush with small (pea-size) amount of fluoride toothpaste. Recommend that child either use a fluoride gel or fluoride varnish. *Use of topical fluoride (mouth rinses, gels, or varnishes) in addition to toothpaste containing fluoride resulted in a modest reduction of cavity formation versus use of fluoride toothpaste only (Marinho et al, 2004).*

### Older Children

- ▲ Encourage family to talk with the dentist about dental sealants, which can help prevent cavities in permanent teeth. **EB:** *Sealants should be available to all children regardless of socioeconomic status. In this study, children of low socioeconomic status in this study had a higher rate of caries in primary and permanent teeth than children of higher socioeconomic status (Gillcrist et al, 2001).*
- Recommend the child use dental floss to help prevent gum disease. The dentist will give guidelines on when to start using floss. Talk with your dentist about when to start.
- Recommend to parents that they not permit the child to smoke or chew tobacco, and stress the importance of setting a good example by not using tobacco products themselves.
- Recommend the child drink fluoridated water when possible. **EB:** *Drinking-water fluoridation is associated with an increase in the percentage of 5-year-old children with no experience of tooth decay (Gray & Davies-Slowik, 2001).*
- ▲ If a child has halitosis, consider the presence of parasites in the gastrointestinal system as a cause. **EB:** *Among those children who had evidence of parasites in stool samples at the beginning of the trial, 18 of 28 who were treated with mebendazole recovered from halitosis. Mebendazole therapy seems to offer benefit to those children with parasites as a potential cause of their halitosis (Ermis, 2002).*

### Multicultural

- Assess for the influence of cultural beliefs, norms, and values on the client's understanding of dental care. **EBN:** *What the client considers normal and abnormal dental care may be based on cultural perceptions (Cochran, 1998; Doswell & Erlen, 1998; Leininger & McFarland, 2002).*
- Assess for barriers to access to dental care such as lack of insurance. **EBN:** *Poverty and lack of dental care insurance may prevent the obtainment of dental care (Woolfolk et al, 1999). African Americans and persons of lower socioeconmic status reported more new dental symptoms, were less likely to obtain dental care, and reported more tooth loss (Gilbert, Duncan, & Shelton, 2003).*
- Instruct mothers on the danger of feeding infants bottles filled with soda, juice, or milk when the infant goes to sleep. **EBN:** *Studies have shown that Navajo, African-*

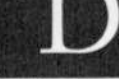

*American, Latino, and some other cultural groups engage in this feeding practice, which is known to cause dental caries in children (Andrews, 2003).*

- Assess for dental anxiety. **EBN:** *Anxiety is a major reason for infrequent dental checkups (Woolfolk et al, 1999).*
- Validate the client's feelings with regard to dental health and access to dental care. **EBN:** *Validation is the therapeutic communication technique that lets the client know that the nurse has heard and understands what was said, and it promotes the nurse-client relationship (Heineken, 1998). Recent studies show that children from racial minority groups had significantly more difficulty in finding access to dental care.(Savage, Lee, Kotch, & Vann, 2004).*
- Introduce the dental home concept to improve families' access to dental care. **EB:** *The dental home is a locus for preventive oral health supervision and emergency care. When culture and ethnicity are barriers to care, the dental home offers a site adapted to care delivery and sensitive to family values (Nowak & Casamassimo, 2002).*

### Home Care

- Assess client patterns for daily and professional dental care and related patterns (e.g., smoking, nail biting). Assess for environmental influences on dental status (e.g., fluoride). **EB:** *Many dental problems are preventable with good dental hygiene and care. Behaviors to preserve oral health in old age are essential (Barmes, 2000).*
- Assess client facilities and financial resources for providing dental care. *Lack of appropriate facilities or financial resources is a barrier to positive dental care patterns. Provision for dental care may be missing from health care plans or unavailable to the uninsured.*
- Request dietary log from the client, adding column for type of food (i.e., soft, pureed, regular).
- Observe typical meal to assess first-hand the impact of impaired dentition on nutrition. *Clients, especially the elderly, are often hesitant to admit nutritional changes that may be embarrassing.*
- Identify mechanical needs for food preparation and ease of ingestion/digestion to meet the client's dental/nutritional needs.
- Assist the client with accessing financial or other resources to support optimum dental and nutritional status.

## Client/Family Teaching

- Teach how to inspect the oral cavity and monitor for problems with the teeth and gums.
- Teach how to implement a personal plan of dental hygiene, including appropriate brushing of teeth and tongue and use of dental floss. **EB:** *Toothbrushing and flossing appropriately, in conjunction with regular professional care, are capable of virtually preventing caries and most periodontal disease and maintaining oral health (Choo et al, 2001).*
- Teach the client the value of having an optimal fluoride concentration in drinking water, and to brush teeth twice daily with fluoride toothpaste. *This recommendation helps achieve maximum protection against dental caries.*

- Teach clients of all ages the need to decrease intake of sugary foods and to brush teeth regularly. **EB:** *One study demonstrated that intake of foods such as caramel, toffees, and sugar lumps increased the number of organisms on the teeth significantly. Just 1 day of withdrawal of normal oral hygiene resulted in an approximately tenfold increase in the number of microorganisms on the teeth (Beighton et al, 1999).*
- Suggest chewing gum with sugar to reduce oral malodor. *Sugarless chewing gum increased methyl mercaptan, one of the principal components of oral malodor (Yaegaki, 2002).*
- Inform individuals who are considering tongue piercing of the potential complications such as chipping and cracking of teeth and possible trauma to the gingiva. If piercing is done, teach the client how to care for the wound and prevent complications. *Often clients are not informed of appropriate care following piercing (De Moor et al, 2000; Knox, 2002).* **EB:** *Complications identified in the literature from tongue piercing include postoperative swelling, infection, and bleeding; damage to the teeth; and trauma to the soft tissues (Knox, 2002).*

D

## evolve WEBSITES FOR EDUCATION

See the EVOLVE website for World Wide Web resources for client education.

## REFERENCES


Adachi M, Ishihara K, Abe S et al: Effect of professional oral health care on the elderly living in nursing homes, *Oral Surg Oral Med Oral Pathol Oral Radiol Endod* 94(2):191-195, 2002.

American Dental Association (ADA): Oral health topics A-Z. Available at www.ada.org/public/topics, accessed on December 22, 2004.

Andrews MM: Transcultural perspectives in the nursing care of children. In Andrews MM, Boyle J, editors: *Transcultural concepts in nursing practice*, Philadelphia, 2003, JB Lippincott.

Aubertin MA: Oral cancer screening in the elderly: the home healthcare nurse's role, *Home Healthc Nurse* 15(9):595, 1997.

Barmes DE: Public policy on oral health and old age: a global view, *J Public Health Dent* 60(4):335, 2000.

Beighton D, Brailsford SR, Lynch E et al: The influence of specific foods and oral hygiene on the microflora of fissures and smooth surfaces of molar teeth: a 5-day study, *Caries Res* 33(5):349, 1999.

Brown CG, Yoder LH: Stomatitis: an overview, *Am J Nurs* 102(Suppl 4):20, 2002.

Choo A, Delac DM, Messer LB: Oral hygiene measures and promotion: review and considerations, *Aust Dent J* 46(3):166, 2001.

Cochran M: Tears have no color, *Am J Nurs* 98(6):53, 1998.

Gilbert GH, Duncan RP, Shelton BJ: Social determinants of tooth loss, *Health Serv Res* 38(6 Pt 2), 2003.

De Moor RJ, De Witte AM, De Bruyne MA: Tongue piercing and associated oral and dental complications, *Endod Dent Traumatol* 16(5):232, 2000.

DeWalt EM: Effect of timed hygienic measures on oral mucosa in a group of elderly subjects, *Nurs Res* 24(2):104, 1975.

Doswell W, Erlen J: Multicultural issues and ethical concerns in the delivery of revising care interventions, *Nurs Clin North Am* 33(2):353, 1998.

Durham TM, Malloy T, Hodges ED: Halitosis: knowing when "bad breath" signals systemic disease, *Geriatrics* 48(8):55, 1993.

Ermis B, Aslan T, Beder L et al: A randomized placebo-controlled trial of mebendazole for halitosis, *Arch Pediatr Adolesc Med* 156(10):995-998, 2002.

Foss-Durant AM, McAffee A: A comparison of three oral care products commonly used in practice, *Clin Nurs Res* 6:1, 1997.

Gillcrist JA, Brumley DE, Blackford JU: Community socioeconomic status and children's dental health, *J Am Dent Assoc* 132(2): 216, 2001.

Gray MM, Davies-Slowik J: Changes in the percentage of 5-year-old children with no experience of decay in Dudley towns since the implementation of fluoridation schemes in 1987, *Br Dent J* 190(1):30, 2001.

Heller K, Burt BA, Eklund SA: Sugared soda consumption and dental caries in the United States, *J Dent Res* 80(10):1949, 2001.

Heineken J: Patient silence is not necessarily client satisfaction: communication in home care nursing, *Home Healthc Nurse* 16(2):115, 1998.

Kleinberg I, Wolff MS, Codipilly DM: Role of saliva in oral dryness, oral feel and oral malodour, *Int Dent J* 52(Suppl 3):236, 2002.
Knox KT: The potential complications of intra-oral and peri-oral piercing, *Dent Health* 41:3, 2002.
Koop CE: Kids' dental health. Available at www.drkoop.com/template.asp?page=newsdetailandap=93andid=508508, accessed on February 25, 2003.
Leininger MM, McFarland MR: *Transcultural nursing: concepts, theories, research and practices*, ed 3, New York, 2002, McGraw-Hill.
Marinho VC, Higgins JP, Sheiham A et al: Combinations of topical fluoride versus single topical fluoride for preventing dental caries in children and adolescents, *Cochrane Database Syst Rev* (1):CD002781, 2004.
Recommendations for using fluoride to prevent and control dental caries in the United States, *MMWR Recomm Rep* 50(RR-14):1-42, 2001.
Myatt GJ, Hunt SA, Barlow AP et al: A clinical study to assess the breath protection efficacy of denture adhesive, *J Contemp Dent Pract* 3(4):1-9, 2002.
Nowak AJ, Casamassimo PS: The dental home: a primary care oral health concept, *J Am Dent Assoc* 133(1):93-8, 2002.
Pearson LS, Hutton JL: A controlled trial to compare the ability of foam swabs and toothbrushes to remove dental plaque, *J Adv Nurs* 39(5):480, 2002.
Poland JM: Comparing Moi-Stir to lemon-glycerin swabs, *Am J Nurs* 87(4):422, 1987.
Roberts J: Developing an oral assessment and intervention tool for older people, *Br J Nurs* 9(18):2033, 2000.
Sasahara H, Kawamura M: Behavioral dental science: the relationship between tooth-brushing angle and plaque removal at the lingual surfaces of the posterior teeth in the mandible, *J Oral Sci* 42(2):79, 2000.
Savage MF, Lee JY, Kotch JB et al: Early preventive dental visits: effects on subsequent utilization and costs, *Pediatrics* 114(4):e418-423, 2004.
Scannapieco FA, Stewart EM, Mylotte JM: Colonization of dental plaque by respiratory pathogens in medical intensive care patients, *Crit Care Med* 20:740, 1992.
Stiefel KA, Damron S, Sowers NJ et al: Improving oral hygiene for the seriously ill patient: implementing research-based practice, *Medsurg Nurs* 9(1):40-43, 2000.
Tombes MB, Gallucci B: The effects of hydrogen peroxide rinses on the normal oral mucosa, *Nurs Res* 42:332, 1993.
Valaitis R, Hesch R, Passarelli C et al: A systematic review of the relationship between breastfeeding and early childhood caries, *Can J Public Health* 91(6):411-417, 2000.
Walton JC, Miller J, Tordecilla L: Elder oral assessment and care, *Medsurg Nurs* 10:1, 2001.
Whitmyer CC, Terezhalmy GT, Miller DL et al: Clinical evaluation of the efficacy and safety of an ultrasonic toothbrush system in an elderly patient population, *Geriatr Nurs* 19(1):29, 1998.
Woolfolk MW, Lang WP, Borgnakke WS et al: Determining dental checkup frequency, *J Am Dental Assoc* 130(5):715, 1999.
Yaegaki K, Coil JM, Kamemizu T et al: Tongue brushing and mouth rinsing as basic treatment measures for halitosis, *Int Dent J* 52(Suppl 3):192-196, 2002.

D

# Risk for delayed Development

*Gail B. Ladwig*

**NANDA**

## Definition

At risk for delay of 25% or more in one or more of the areas of social or self-regulatory behavior or cognitive, language, gross, or fine motor skills

## Risk Factors

### Prenatal

Maternal age <15 or >35 years, substance abuse, infections, genetic or endocrine disorders, unplanned or unwanted pregnancy, lack of late or poor prenatal care, inadequate, illiteracy, poverty

### Individual

Prematurity; seizures; congenital or genetic disorders; positive drug screening test; brain damage (e.g., hemorrhage in postnatal period, shaken baby, abuse, accident); vision impairment; hearing impairment or frequent otitis media; chronic illness; technology dependence; failure to thrive, inadequate nutrition; foster or adopted child; lead poisoning; chemotherapy; radiation therapy; natural disaster; behavior disorders; substance abuse

### Environmental

Poverty, violence

### Caregiver

Abuse, mental illness, mental retardation or severe learning disability

NOC

## Outcomes (Nursing Outcomes Classification)

### Suggested NOC Outcomes

Child Development: 1 Month, 2 Months, 4 Months, 6 Months, 12 Months, 2 Years, 3 Years, 4 Years, Preschool, Middle Childhood, Adolescence; Growth; Neglect Recovery; Knowledge: Infant Care, Parenting

**Example NOC Outcome with Indicators**

**Child Development** as evidenced by the following indicators: Appropriate milestones of physical, cognitive, and psychosocial age appropriate progression (Rate each indicator of **Child Development:** 1 = never demonstrated, 2 = rarely demonstrated, 3 = sometimes demonstrated, 4 = often demonstrated, 5 = consistently demonstrated [see Section I].)

## Client Outcomes

**Client/Parents/Primary Caregiver Will (Specify Time Frame):**

- Describe realistic, age-appropriate patterns of development
- Promote activities and interactions that support age-related developmental tasks

● = Independent; ▲ = Collaborative; EBN = Evidence-Based Nursing; EB = Evidence-Based

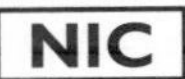

## Interventions (Nursing Interventions Classification)

### Suggested NIC Interventions

Active Listening, Developmental Enhancement: Child, Emotional Support, Kangaroo Care, Self-Care Assistance, Self-Responsibility Facilitation

D

**Example NIC Activities—Developmental Enhancement: Child**

Teach caregivers about normal developmental milestones and associated behaviors; enhance parental effectiveness

## Nursing Interventions and Rationales

- Refer to care plan for **Delayed Growth and development.**

NOTE: Determination of the etiology for delayed development is critical because it will direct the selection of interventions for treating the diagnosis. Parenting skill deficits, lack of consistency between caregivers, and hospitalization versus a chronic medical condition/developmental disability will necessitate different strategies. A hospitalization experience with regressive behaviors can be a transient occurrence as opposed to a chronic situation, which may have more severe and longer delays requiring more in-depth intervention. Parenting skills and consistent expectations between multiple caregivers can be addressed by more intensive education efforts (Seideman & Kleine, 1995; Stutts, 1994).

- Avoid exposure to organic solvents during pregnancy. **EB:** *This study indicates that utero exposure to organic solvents is associated with poorer performance on some specific subtle measures of neurocognitive function, language, and behavior. Reducing exposure in pregnancy is merited until more refined risk assessment is possible. Further studies that address exposure to specific solvents, dose, and gestational timing of exposure are needed (Laslo et al, 2004).*

### Multicultural

- Acknowledge racial/ethnic differences at the onset of care. **EBN:** *Acknowledgment of race/ethnicity issues will enhance communication, establish rapport, and promote treatment outcomes (D'Avanzo et al, 2001; Ludwick & Silva, 2000; Vontress & Epp, 1997).*
- Assess for the influence of cultural beliefs, norms, and values on the client's perceptions of child development. **EBN:** *What the client considers normal and abnormal child development may be based on cultural perceptions (Cochran, 1998; Doswell & Erlen, 1998; Leininger & McFarland, 2002). Latino mothers of children with developmental disabilities viewed their child as not being responsible for the behavior problem (Chavira et al, 2000). Latino mothers of developmentally disabled adults reported their relationship with the educational and service delivery systems to be characterized by poor communication, low effort in providing services, negative attitudes of professionals toward the client-children, and negative treatment of parents by professionals (Shapiro et al, 2004).*

- Use a neutral, indirect style when addressing areas in which improvement is needed, such as a need for verbal stimulation, when working with clients. **EBN:** *Using indirect statements such as "Other mothers have tried" or "I had a client who tried 'X' and it seemed to work very well" will assist in avoiding resentment from the parent (Seideman et al, 1996).*
- Assess whether exposure to community violence is contributing to developmental problems. **EBN:** *Exposure to community violence has been associated with increases in aggressive behavior and depression (Gorman-Smith & Tolan, 1998).*
- Validate the client's feelings and concerns related to child's development. **EBN:** *Validation is the therapeutic communication technique that lets the client know that the nurse has heard and understands what was said, and it promotes the nurse-client relationship (Heineken, 1998).*

D

## Home Care

- Assess for the presence of substances that could cause developmental delay. *Children's access to substances that cause neurological deficits (e.g., lead-based paints) should be identified and removed.*
- Assist family to identify appropriate skill-building activities for child. *Exposure to age-appropriate or lower age games, toys, activities can provide essential stimuli for development. Family members may need to adjust expectations of child's behaviors to be appropriate not only for age but also for any developmental limitations.*
- Provide emotional support for family members' reactions to evidence of developmental delay. *Parents may be distressed by the potential for developmental delay in a child.*
- ▲ If possible, refer family to a program of animal-assisted therapy. **EBN:** *Research suggests that interactions with dogs may assist clients with pervasive developmental disorders (PDDs) to establish bonds with their social environment. Children with PDD were more playful, more focused, and more aware of their social environment in the presence of a therapy dog as opposed to a toy or a stuffed dog (Martin & Farnum, 2002).*

## Client/Family Teaching

- ▲ Encourage mothers to abstain from alcohol and cocaine use during pregnancy; refer to treatment programs for substance abuse. **EB:** *In the largest multisite study of its kind to date, we found that prenatal exposures to both cocaine and opiates were strongly associated with elevated risk of central nervous system/autonomic nervous system (CNS/ANS) manifestations (Das, Poole, & Bada, 2004). Smoking during pregnancy is a well-established determinant of fetal growth and risk of low birth weight. Maternal smoking in pregnancy may influence the development of the fetal respiratory system, as suggested by findings of a relation between maternal smoking in pregnancy and lung function impairment in newborns. A recent study provided suggestive evidence that low birth weight is a predictor of subsequent childhood asthma. Some evidence shows that maternal smoking increases the risk of childhood asthma (Jaakkola & Gissler, 2004).*
- ▲ Provide support groups and education on human immunodeficiency virus (HIV) and caring for infants with this diagnosis. *Developmental delay has been well-documented in infants with HIV (Potterton & Eales, 2001).*

D

- Provide developmental care interventions to preterm infants to improve neurodevelopmental outcomes. **EB:** *Developmental care is effective to improve outcomes (Symington & Pinelli, 2002).*
- Provide neonatal positioning procedures for preterm infants to prevent extremity malalignment, skull deformities, and gross motor delay. *Alignment and shaping of the musculoskeletal system occur with each body position change in a neonatal intensive care unit (NICU)—use of proper positioning strategies promotes skeletal integrity, postural control, and sensorimotor organization (Sweeney & Gutierrez, 2002).*
- Encourage adequate antepartum and postpartum care for both mother and child. *Access to prenatal and postnatal health care promotes optimal growth and development (Bland, 2000).*
- Counsel parents, siblings, and caregivers about the importance of smoking cessation and the necessity of eliminating all secondhand smoke exposure. *This study shows that smoking affects development not only during intrauterine life but also during the early stage of extrauterine life (Bottini et al, 2004).*
- Teach caregivers of children appropriate developmental interactions; use anticipatory guidance to facilitate preparation for developmental milestones. **EB:** *Children with intelligence quotient (IQ) scores of 90 or higher had more developmentally appropriate interaction by caregivers (P = 0.043) and higher scores on six of eight subscales and Total HOME (Home Observation for Measurement of the Environment) (P =0.05) than the group of children with IQ scores of less than 90.* ***Conclusions:*** *Two postnatal factors—home environment and caregiver-child interaction—were associated with full-scale IQ scores of 90 or higher, whereas prenatal and natal factors were not. These potentially malleable postnatal factors can be targeted for change to improve cognitive outcome of inner-city children (Hurt et al, 1998).*

## evolve WEBSITES FOR EDUCATION

See the EVOLVE website for World Wide Web resources for client education.

## REFERENCES

Bland M, Vermillion ST, Soper DE et al: Late third trimester treatment of rectovaginal group B streptococci with benzathine penicillin G, *Am J Obstet Gynecol* 183(2):372, 2000.

Bottini N, Gloria-Bottini F, Magrini A et al: Maternal cigarette smoking, metabolic enzyme polymorphism, and developmental events in the early stages of extrauterine life, *Hum Biol* 76(2):289-297, 2004.

Chavira V, Lopez SR, Blacher J et al: Latina mothers' attributions, emotions, and reactions to the problem behaviors of their children with developmental disabilities, *J Child Psychol Psychiatry* 41(2):245-252, 2000.

Cochran M: Tears have no color, *Am J Nurs* 98(6):53, 1998.

Das A, Poole WK, Bada HS: Repeated measures approach for simultaneous modeling of multiple neurobehavioral outcomes in newborns exposed to cocaine in utero, *Am J Epidemiol* 159(9):891-899, 2004.

D'Avanzo CE et al: Developing culturally informed strategies for substance-related interventions. In Naegle MA, D'Avanzo CE, editors: *Addictions and substance abuse: strategies for advanced practice nursing,* St Louis, 2001, Mosby.

Doswell W, Erlen J: Multicultural issues and ethical concerns in the delivery of revising care interventions, *Nurs Clin North Am* 33(2):353, 1998.

Giger JN, Davidhizar RE: *Transcultural nursing,* ed 2, St Louis, 1995, Mosby.

Gorman-Smith D, Tolan P: The role of exposure to community violence and developmental problems among inner city youth, *Dev Psychopathol* 10(1):101, 1998.

Heineken J: Patient silence is not necessarily client satisfaction: communication in home care nursing, *Home Healthc Nurse* 16(2): 115, 1998.
Hurt H, Malmud E, Braitman LE et al: Inner-city achievers: who are they? *Arch Pediatr Adolesc Med* 152(10):993-997, 1998.
Jaakkola JJ, Gissler M: Maternal smoking in pregnancy, fetal development, and childhood asthma, *Am J Public Health* 94(1):136-40, 2004.
Laslo-Baker D, Barrera M, Knittel-Keren D et al: Child neurodevelopmental outcome and maternal occupational exposure to solvents, *Arch Pediatr Adolesc Med* 158(10):956-961, 2004.
Leininger MM, McFarland MR: *Transcultural nursing: concepts, theories, research and practices,* ed 3, New York, 2002, McGraw-Hill.
Ludwick R, Silva M: Nursing around the world: cultural values and ethical conflicts, *Online J Issues Nurs.* Available at www.nursingworld.org/ojin/ethcol/ethics_4.htm.
Martin F, Farnum J: Animal-assisted therapy for children with pervasive developmental disorders, *West J Nurs Res* 24:657, 2002.
Potterton J, Eales C: Prevalence of developmental delay in infants who are HIV positive, *S Afr J Physiother* 57(3):11, 2001.
Seideman RY, Kleine PF: Theory of transformed parenting: parenting a child with developmental delay/mental retardation, *Nurs Res* 44:38, 1995.
Seideman RY, Jacobson S, Primeaux M et al: Assessing American Indian families, *MCN Am J Matern Child Nurs* 21(6):274, 1996.
Shapiro J, Monzo LD, Rueda R et al: Alienated advocacy: perspectives of Latina mothers of young adults with developmental disabilities on service systems, *Ment Retard* 42(1):37-54, 2004.
Stuart GW, Laraia MT: Therapeutic nurse-patient relationship. In Stuart GW, Laraia MT, editors: *Principles and practice of psychiatric nursing,* St Louis, 2001, Mosby.
Stutts AL: Selected outcomes of technology dependent children receiving home care and prescribed child care services, *Pediatr Nurs* 20:501, 1994.
Sweeney J, Gutierrez T: Musculoskeletal implications of preterm infant positioning in the NICU, *J Perinat Neonat Nurs* 16(1):58, 2002.
Symington A, Pinelli J: Developmental care for promoting development and preventing morbidity in preterm infants, *Cochrane Database Syst Rev* (3):CD001814, 2002.
Vontress CE, Epp LR: Historical hostility in the African American client: implications for counseling, *J Multicult Counseling Dev* 25:170, 1997.

# Diarrhea

evolve

*Betty J. Ackley*

**NANDA**

## Definition

Passage of loose, unformed stools

## Defining Characteristics

Hyperactive bowel sounds, at least three loose liquid stools per day, urgency, abdominal pain, cramping

## Related Factors (r/t)

### Psychological

High stress levels and anxiety

### Situational

Alcohol abuse, toxins, laxative abuse, radiation, tube feedings, adverse effects of medications, contaminants, travel

### Physiological

Inflammation, malabsorption, infectious processes, irritation, parasites

**NOC**

## Outcomes (Nursing Outcomes Classification)

### Suggested NOC Outcomes

Bowel Elimination, Electrolyte and Acid-Base Balance, Fluid Balance, Hydration, Treatment Behavior: Illness or Injury

**Example NOC Outcome with Indicators**

**Bowel Elimination** as evidenced by the following indicators: Elimination pattern/Stool soft and formed/Diarrhea not present/Control of bowel movements/Comfort of stool passage/Painful cramps not present (Rate each indicator of **Bowel Elimination:** 1 = severely compromised, 2 = substantially compromised, 3 = moderately compromised, 4 = mildly compromised, 5 = not compromised [see Section I].)

## Client Outcomes

**Client Will (Specify Time Frame):**

- Defecate formed, soft stool every day to every third day
- Maintain a rectal area free of irritation
- State relief from cramping and less or no diarrhea
- Explain cause of diarrhea and rationale for treatment
- Maintain good skin turgor and weight at usual level
- Contain stool appropriately (if previously incontinent)

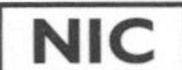

## Interventions (Nursing Interventions Classification)

### Suggested NIC Intervention

Diarrhea Management

**Example NIC Activities—Diarrhea Management**

Evaluate medication profile for gastrointestinal side effects; suggest trial elimination of foods containing lactose

## Nursing Interventions and Rationales

- • Assess pattern of defecation or have the client keep a diary that includes the following: time of day defecation occurs; usual stimulus for defecation; consistency, amount, and frequency of stool; type of, amount of, and time food consumed; fluid intake; history of bowel habits and laxative use; diet; exercise patterns; obstetrical/gynecological, medical, and surgical histories; medications; alterations in perianal sensations; and present bowel regimen. *Assessment of defecation pattern will help direct treatment (Hogan, 1998).*
- • Assess stool consistency and its influence on risk for stool loss. *Several classification systems for stool have been promulgated. They assist the nurse and client to differentiate between normal soft, formed stool, hardened stools associated with constipation, and liquid stools associated with diarrhea (Bliss et al, 2001).* **EBN:** *A study of stool consistency found good reliability when evaluated by professional nurses, student nurses, and clients. Word-only descriptors yielded equivocal consistency when assessed by subjects as did tools that combined words with illustrations of various stool consistencies (Bliss et al, 2001).*
- ▲ Identify cause of diarrhea if possible based on history (e.g., rotavirus exposure, HIV infection, seafood ingestion; medication effect; radiation therapy; protein malnutrition; laxative abuse; stress). See Related Factors (r/t). *Identification of the underlying cause is important because the treatment often depends on it (Thielman & Guerrant, 2004).*
- ▲ If the client has watery diarrhea, a low-grade fever, abdominal cramps, and a history of antibiotic therapy, consider possibility of *Clostridium difficile* infection. C. difficile *infection and pseudomembranous colitis have become increasingly common because of the frequent use of broad-spectrum antibiotics (Thielman & Guerrant, 2004).*
- ▲ If the client has diarrhea associated with antibiotic therapy, consult with primary care practitioner regarding the use of probiotics such as yogurt with active cultures to treat diarrhea (Van Niel et al, 2002) or also use probiotics to prevent diarrhea when first beginning antibiotic therapy. **EB:** *A study demonstrated that ingestion of Lactobacillus could be helpful to treat children with acute infectious diarrhea caused by a virus (Van Niel et al, 2002). Probiotics have been shown to be helpful to prevent antibiotic-associated diarrhea (D'Souza et al, 2002; Teitelbaum & Walker, 2002). A Cochrane review concluded that probiotics are a useful adjunct to rehydration therapy in treating acute infectious diarrhea in both adults and children (Bricker et al, 2005).*
- ▲ Use standard precautions when caring for clients with diarrhea to prevent spread of infectious diarrhea; use gloves and hand washing. C. difficile *has been shown to be contagious and difficult to eradicate because of spore formation (Poutanen & Simor, 2004).*
- ▲ Obtain stool specimens as ordered to either rule out or diagnose an infectious process (e.g., ova and parasites, *C. difficile* infection, bacterial cultures). **EB:** *One study of medical patients demonstrated that more than 30% developed nosocomial diarrhea after admission to a nursing unit, and the majority of cases were caused by* C. difficile *(McFarland, 1995). If the client has infectious diarrhea, avoid using medications that slow peristalsis. If an infectious process is occurring, such as* C. difficile *infection or food poisoning, medication to slow down peristalsis should generally not be given (Bliss et al, 2000). The increase in gut motility helps eliminate the causative factor, and use of antidiarrheal medication could result in a toxic megacolon (Gantz et al, 1998).*

• = Independent; ▲ = Collaborative; EBN = Evidence-Based Nursing; EB = Evidence-Based

D

- Observe and record number and consistency of stools per day; if desired, use a fecal incontinence collector for accurate measurement of output. *Documentation of output provides a baseline and helps direct replacement fluid therapy.*
- Inspect, palpate, percuss, and auscultate abdomen; note whether bowel sounds are frequent.
- Assess for dehydration by observing skin turgor over sternum and inspecting for longitudinal furrows of the tongue. Watch for excessive thirst, fever, dizziness, lightheadedness, palpitations, excessive cramping, bloody stools, hypotension, and symptoms of shock. *Severe diarrhea can cause deficient fluid volume with extreme weakness (Hogan, 1998) and cause death in the very young, chronically ill, and elderly.*
- Observe for symptoms of sodium and potassium loss (e.g., weakness, abdominal or leg cramping, dysrhythmia). Note results of electrolyte laboratory studies. *Stool contains electrolytes; excessive diarrhea causes electrolyte abnormalities that can be especially harmful to clients with existing medical conditions.*
- Monitor and record intake and output; note oliguria and dark, concentrated urine.
- Measure specific gravity of urine if possible. *Dark, concentrated urine, along with a high specific gravity of urine, is an indication of deficient fluid volume.*
- Weigh the client daily and note decreased weight. *An accurate daily weight is an important indicator of fluid balance in the body (Metheny, 2000).*
- Give dilute clear fluids as tolerated (e.g., clear soda, gelatin dessert), serving at lukewarm temperature.

▲ If diarrhea is associated with cancer or cancer treatment, once infectious cause of diarrhea is ruled out, provide medications as ordered to stop diarrhea. *The loss of proteins, electrolytes, and water from diarrhea in a cancer client can lead to rapid deterioration and possibly fatal dehydration (Kornblau et al, 2000).*

▲ If the client has chronic diarrhea causing fecal incontinence at intervals, consider suggesting use of dietary fiber from psyllium or gum Arabic after consultation with primary practitioner. **EBN and EB:** *A study demonstrated that use of a fiber supplement decreased the number of incontinent stools and improved stool consistency in a group of adults (Bliss et al, 2001). The use of soluble dietary fiber is useful for controlling diarrhea and normalizing the intestinal flora (Nakao et al, 2002).*

▲ If diarrhea is chronic and there is evidence of malnutrition, consult with primary care practitioner for a dietary consult and possible use of a hydrolyzed formula (a clear liquid supplement containing increased protein) to maintain nutrition while the gastrointestinal system heals. *A hydrolyzed formula contains protein that is partially broken down to amino acids for people who cannot digest nutrients (Lutz & Przytulski, 2001).*

- Encourage the client to eat small, frequent meals and to consume foods that are easy to digest (e.g., bananas, crackers, pretzels, rice, potatoes, clear soups, applesauce). Encourage the client to avoid milk products, foods high in fiber, and caffeine (dark sodas, tea, coffee, chocolate). *The use of a BRAT diet (bananas, rice, applesauce, and toast) with avoidance of milk products (since a transient lactase deficiency may occur) is commonly recommended, although limited data for supports this (Thielman & Guerrant, 2004).*
- Provide a readily available bedpan, commode, or bathroom.
- If the client has diarrhea and incontinence, consider use of a Perineal Assessment Tool

• = Independent; ▲ = Collaborative; EBN = Evidence-Based Nursing; EB = Evidence-Based

to measure the risk for perineal skin injury. **EBN:** *An instrument entitled the Perineal Assessment Tool has been developed to determine the risk of perineal skin injury. The initial results of the study are encouraging, and further studies are needed (Nix, 2002).*

- Thoroughly cleanse and dry the perianal and perineal skin daily and as needed (PRN) using a cleanser capable of stool. Select a product with a slightly acidic pH designed to preserve its acid mantle, and designed to remove irritants from the skin with minimal physical force. Avoid vigorous scrubbing with water, soap and a washcloth. Consider selection of a product with a moisturizer. *Traditional soaps tend to be alkaline, interfering with the natural acid mantle of the integument and increasing its susceptibility to irritant dermatitis and secondary infection. Brisk scrubbing may exacerbate skin erosion and further increase the risk of irritation and infection (Gray, 2004; Gray, Ratliff, & Donovan, 2002).*
- If the client is receiving a tube feeding, do not assume it is the cause of diarrhea. Perform a complete assessment to rule out other causes such as medication effects, sorbitol in medications, or an infection. *Research has shown that tube feedings do not usually cause diarrhea (Campbell, 1994). However, sorbitol in medication has been linked to diarrhea (Drug Watch, 1994).*
- If the client is receiving a tube feeding, note rate of infusion, and prevent contamination of feeding by rinsing container every 8 hours and replacing it every 24 hours. *Rapid administration of tube feeding and contaminated feedings have been associated with diarrhea.*
- If the client is receiving a tube feeding, suggest formulas that contain a bulking agent such as Jevity or add soluble dietary fiber to the feeding per physicians/dietitians order. **EB:** *Bulking agents including soluble fiber are useful in tube feedings to prevent or treat diarrhea in the tube-fed client (Nakao et al, 2002).*

## Pediatric

▲ Recommend the parents give the child oral rehydration fluids to drink in the amounts specified by the physician, especially during the first 4 to 6 hours to replace fluid losses. Once the child is rehydrated, an orally administered maintenance solution should be used along with food. **EBN and EB:** *Oral rehydration therapy is effective for treating mild to moderate dehydration in children with diarrhea and may help prevent the need for hospitalization with administration of intravenous fluids (Larson, 2000). Reduced osmolarity oral rehydration fluid compared with standard rehydration fluid resulted in lower stool volume, less need for intravenous fluids, and less vomiting (Hahn, Kim, & Garner, 2005). A study demonstrated that treatment with oral rehydration fluids for children were generally as effective as intravenous (IV) fluids, and IV fluids did not shorten the duration of gastroenteritis and are more likely to cause adverse effects than oral rehydration therapy (Banks & Meadows, 2005).*

- Recommend the mother resume breastfeeding as soon as possible.
- Recommend parents not give the child decarbonated soda, fruit juices, gelatin dessert, or instant fruit drink. *These fluids have a high osmolality from carbohydrate contents and can exacerbate diarrhea. In addition they have low sodium concentrations that can aggravate existing hyponatremia (Behrman, Kliegman, & Jenson, 2004).*

▲ Recommend parents give children foods with complex carbohydrates such as potatoes, rice, bread, cereal, yogurt, fruits, and vegetables. The BRAT diet is often advocated: bananas, rice, applesauce, and toast. Avoid fatty foods and foods high in simple sugars *(Behrman, Kliegman, & Jenson, 2004).*



## Geriatric

▲ Evaluate medications the client is taking. Recognize that many medications can result in diarrhea, including digitalis, propranolol, angiotensin-converting enzyme (ACE) inhibitors, histamine-receptor antagonists, nonsteroidal antiinflammatory drugs (NSAIDs), anticholinergic agents, oral hypoglycemia agents, antibiotics, and others. *A drug-associated cause should always be considered when treating diarrhea in the older person; many drugs can result in diarrhea (Ratnaike, 2000).*

▲ Monitor the client closely to detect whether an impaction is causing diarrhea; remove impaction as ordered. *Clients with fecal impaction commonly experience leakage of mucus or liquid stool as a consequence of rectal irritation, distention, and impaired anal sensation (Butcher, 2004).*

▲ Seek medical attention if diarrhea is severe or persists for more than 24 hours, or if the client has symptoms of dehydration or electrolyte disturbances such as lassitude, weakness, or prostration. *Elderly clients can dehydrate rapidly, especially serious is development of hypokalemia with dysrhythmias.*

• Provide emotional support for clients who are having trouble controlling unpredictable episodes of diarrhea. *Diarrhea can be a great source of embarrassment to the elderly and can lead to social isolation and a feeling of powerlessness.*

## Home Care

• Above interventions may be adapted for home care use.

• Assess the home for general sanitation and methods of food preparation. Reinforce principles of sanitation for food handling. *Poor sanitation or mishandling of food may cause bacterial infection or transmission of dangerous organisms from utensils to food.*

• Assess for methods of handling soiled laundry if the client is bed bound or has been incontinent. Instruct or reinforce Universal Precautions with family and bloodborne pathogen precautions with agency caregivers. *The Bloodborne Pathogen Regulations of the Occupational Safety and Health Administration (OSHA) identify legal guidelines for caregivers.*

▲ When assessing medication history, include over-the-counter (OTC) drugs, both general and those currently being used to treat the diarrhea. Instruct clients not to mix OTC medications when self-treating. *Mixing OTC medications can further irritate the gastrointestinal system, intensifying the diarrhea or causing nausea and vomiting.*

▲ Evaluate current medications for indication that specific interventions are warranted. *Blood levels of medications may increase during prolonged episodes of diarrhea, indicating the need for close monitoring of the client or direct intervention.*

▲ Consult with physician regarding need for blood work or stool specimens. *Laboratory tests may be needed to identify presence of a bacterial pathogen or assess for electrolyte imbalance.*

▲ Evaluate need for home health aide or homemaker service referral. *Caregiver may need support for maintaining client cleanliness to prevent skin breakdown (e.g., may benefit from assistance with washing bedclothes).*

▲ Evaluate need for durable medical equipment in the home. *The client may need bedside commode, call bell, or raised toilet seat to facilitate prompt toileting.*

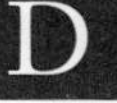

## Client/Family Teaching

- Encourage avoidance of coffee, spices, milk products, and foods that irritate or stimulate the gastrointestinal tract.
- Teach appropriate method of taking ordered antidiarrheal medications; explain side effects.
- Explain how to prevent the spread of infectious diarrhea (e.g., careful hand washing, appropriate handling and storage of food).
- Help the client to determine stressors and set up an appropriate stress reduction plan.
- Teach signs and symptoms of dehydration and electrolyte imbalance.
- Teach perirectal skin care.

## evolve WEBSITES FOR EDUCATION

See the EVOLVE website for World Wide Web resources for client education.

## REFERENCES


Allen SJ, Okoko B, Martinez E, et al: Probiotics for treating infectious diarrhea, *Cochrane Database Syst Rev* (2):CD003048, 2004.

Anastasi J: Diarrhea in acquired immune deficiency syndrome (AIDS), *Ostomy Wound Manage* 39:14, 1993.

Banks JB, Meadows S: Intravenous fluids for children with gastroenteritis, *Am Fam Physician* 71(1):121, 2005.

Behrman RE, Kliegman RM, Jenson HB: *Nelson textbook of pediatrics*, ed 17, Philadelphia, 2004, Saunders.

Bliss DZ, Jung HJ, Savik K et al: Supplementation with dietary fiber improves fecal incontinence, *Nurs Res* 50(4):203, 2001.

Bliss DZ, Johnson S, Savik K et al: Fecal incontinence in hospitalized patients who are acutely ill, *Nurs Res* 49(2):101, 2000.

Bockus S: When your patient needs tube feeding: making the right decision, *Nursing* 93:34, 1993.

Bosley C: Three methods of stool management for patients with diarrhea, *Ostomy Wound Manage* 40:52, 1994.

Bricker E, Garg R, Nelson R et al: Antiobiotic treatment for *Clostridium difficile*–associated diarrhea in adults, *Cochrane Database Syst Rev* (1):CD004610, 2005.

Butcher L: Clinical skills: nursing considerations in patients with faecal incontinence, *Br J Nurs* 13(13):760, 2004.

Campbell C: Research for practice: diarrhea not always linked to tube feedings, *Am J Nurs* 94(4):59, 1994.

Doughty D: Maintaining normal bowel function in the patient with cancer, *J Enterostomal Nurs* 18:90, 1991.

Drug Watch: Sorbitol: missing link to diarrhea, *Am J Nurs* 10:50, 1994.

D'Souza AL, Rajkumar C, Cooke J et al: Probiotics in prevention of antibioitic associated diarrhea: meta-analysis, *BMJ* 324(7350):1361, 2002.

Gantz NM, Gerding DN, Johnson PC: Managing and containing *Clostridium difficile* disease, *Patient Care* 15:171, 1998.

Gray M: Preventing and managing perineal dermatitis: a shared goal for wound and continence care, *J Wound Ostomy Continence Nurs* 31(Suppl 1): S2-S9, 2004.

Gray M, Ratliff C, Donovan A: Perineal skin care for the incontinent patient, *Adv Skin Wound Care* 15:170, 2002.

Hahn S, Kim S, Garner P: Reduced osmolarity oral rehydration solution for treating dehydration caused by acute diarrhea in children, *Cochrane Database Syst Rev* (1):CD002847, 2002.

Haisfield-Wolfe ME, Rund C: A nursing protocol for the management of perineal-rectal skin alterations, *Clin J Oncol Nurs* 4(1): 15, 2000.

Hogan CM: The nurse's role in diarrhea management, *Oncol Nurs Forum* 25(5):879, 1998.

Kornblau S, Benson AB, Catalano R et al: Management of cancer treatment-related diarrhea: issues and therapeutic strategies, *J Pain Symptom Manage* 19(2):118, 2000.

Larson CE: Evidence-based practice: safety and efficacy of oral rehydration therapy for the treatment of diarrhea and gastroenteritis in pediatrics, *Pediatr Nurs* 26(2):177, 2000.

Lutz C, Przytulski K: *Nutrition and diet therapy*, Philadelphia, 2001, FA Davis.

McFarland LV: Epidemiology of infectious and iatrogenic nosocomial diarrhea in a cohort of general medicine patients, *Am J Infect Control* 23:295, 1995.

Metheny N: *Fluid and electrolyte balance: nursing considerations,* ed 4, Philadelphia, 2000, Lippincott.

Nakao M, Ogura Y, Satake S et al: Usefulness of soluble dietary fiber for the treatment of diarrhea during general nutrition in elderly patients, *Nutrition* 18(1):35, 2002.

Nix DH: Validity and reliability of the Perineal Assessment Tool, *Ostomy Wound Manage* 48:2, 2002.

Poutanen SM, Simor AE: Clostridium difficile-associated diarrhea in adults, *CMAJ* 171(1):51, 2004.

Ratnaike RN: Drug-induced diarrhea in older persons, *Clin Geriatr* 8(1):67, 2000.

Rice KH: Oral rehydration therapy: a simple, effective solution, *J Pediatr Nurs* 9:349, 1994.

Teitelbaum JE, Walker WA: Nutritional impact of pre- and probiotics as protective gastrointestinal organisms, *Annu Rev Nutr* 22:107, 2002.

Thielman NM, Guerrant RL: Clinical practice. Acute infectious diarrhea, *New Engl J Med* 350(1):38, 2004.

Van Niel CW, Feudtner C, Garrison MM et al: Lactobacillus therapy for acute infectious diarrhea in children: a meta-analysis, *Pediatrics* 109(4):678, 2002.

# Risk for Disuse syndrome

*Betty J. Ackley*

**NANDA**

## Definition

At risk for a deterioration of body systems as the result of prescribed or unavoidable musculoskeletal inactivity

## Risk Factors

Paralysis; altered level of consciousness; mechanical immobilization; prescribed immobilization; severe pain (NOTE: complications from immobility can include pressure ulcer, constipation, stasis of pulmonary secretions, thrombosis, urinary tract infection and/or retention, decreased strength or endurance, orthostatic hypotension, decreased range of joint motion, disorientation, disturbed body image, and powerlessness.)

## Related Factors (r/t)

See Risk Factors

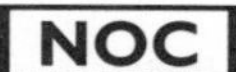

## Outcomes (Nursing Outcomes Classification)

### Suggested NOC Outcomes

Endurance; Immobility Consequences: Physiological; Mobility; Neurological Status: Consciousness; Pain Level

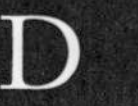


**Example NOC Outcome with Indicators**

**Immobility Consequences: Physiological** as evidenced by the following indicators: Pressure sores/Constipation/Compromised nutrition status/Urinary calculi/Compromised muscle strength (Rate each indicator of **Immobility Consequences: Physiological:** 1 = severe, 2 = substantial, 3 = moderate, 4 = mild, 5 = none [see Section I].)

## Client Outcomes

### Client Will (Specify Time Frame):

- Maintain full range of motion in joints
- Maintain intact skin, good peripheral blood flow, and normal pulmonary function
- Maintain normal bowel and bladder function
- Express feelings about imposed immobility
- Explain methods to prevent complications of immobility

NIC

## Interventions (Nursing Interventions Classification)

### Suggested NIC Interventions

Energy Management; Exercise Therapy: Joint Mobility, Muscle Control

**Example NIC Activities—Energy Management**

Determine the client's physical limitations; determine the client's significant other's perception of causes of fatigue

## Nursing Interventions and Rationales

- Use a functional assessment instrument to evaluate abilities, including instruments such as the Barthel Index, the Katz Index of activities of Daily Living, or the FIM instrument. *There are many instruments available to measure client function, and a baseline measurement of function should be done to determine appropriate level of care and services (Quigly, 2001).*
- Have the client do exercises in bed if not contraindicated (e.g., flexing and extending feet and quadriceps, performing gluteal and abdominal sitting exercises, lifting small weights to maintain muscle strength). *Unused muscles lose 1% to 3% of their strength per day, even in healthy persons. A person who is immobilized for 3 weeks may lose half of his or her muscle strength (Fried & Fried, 2001). In-bed exercises help maintain muscle strength and tone (Kasper & Talbor, 2002).* **EB:** *Strength improvement in response to resisted exercise is possible even in the very elderly and extremely sedentary client with multiple chronic diseases and functional disabilities. Increased strength can help prevent falls (Connelly, 2000).*

▲ If not contraindicated by the client's condition, obtain referral to physical therapy for use of tilt table to provide weight bearing on long bones. *The upright position helps maintain bone strength, increase circulation, and prevent postural hypotension (Kasper et al, 2005).*

D

- Perform range of motion exercises for all possible joints at least twice daily; perform passive or active range of motion exercises as appropriate. *If not used, muscles weaken and shorten; contractures begin forming after 8 hours of immobility (Fletcher, 2005).*
- Use high-top sneakers or specialized boots from the occupational therapy department to prevent footdrop; remove shoes twice daily to provide foot care. *Sneakers or boots help keep the foot in normal anatomical alignment; footdrop can make it difficult or impossible to walk after bed rest.*
- Position the client so that joints are in normal anatomical alignment at all times. *Improper positioning can damage peripheral nerves and blood vessels, as well as cause joint deformities (Fried & Fried, 2001).*
- If client is immobile, consider use of a transfer chair, a chair that becomes a stretcher. *Using a transfer chair where the client is pulled onto a flat surface, and then sat up in the chair can help previously immobile clients get out of bed (Nelson et al, 2003).*
- Assist the client to walk as soon as medically possible. **EB:** *Almost all clients can get out of bed now with use of the stretcher-chair, which converts from a stretcher to a chair. Bed rest is almost always harmful to clients; early mobilization is better than bed rest for most health conditions (Allen et al, 1999).*
- Consider use of a continuous lateral rotation therapy bed. *Continuous lateral rotation therapy has been shown to be effective for prevention of deep vein thrombosis (DVT) in spinal cord injury clients (Von Rueden & Harris, 1995).* **EB:** *Continuous lateral rotation therapy has been shown to be effective for the prevention of pneumonia in transplant clients (Whiteman et al, 1995).* **EBN:** *Implementing kinetic therapy in the ICU resulted in improved oxygenation and decreased length of stay for clients with pulmonary disorders (Powers & Daniels, 2004).*

▲ If at all possible, help the client begin a walking program, using a physical therapist as needed. **EB:** *Early mobilization has been shown to improve the outcome for clients after treatment of medical conditions and procedures (Allen et al, 1999).*

- Be very careful when helping the client into a chair and when transferring. Be sure to lock beds and wheelchairs. Recognize that there is a high probability for falls. **EB:** *Nonambulatory clients have a substantially greater number of serious falls than their ambulatory peers: 87% of falls with injuries involved equipment misuse such as not locking beds and wheelchairs, 82% occurred while seated or transferring, and 54% occurred at chair or bed height only (Thapa et al, 1996).*
- Minimize cardiovascular deconditioning by positioning clients as close to the upright position as possible several times daily. *The hazards of bed rest in the elderly are multiple, serious, quick to develop, and slow to reverse. Decondition of the cardiovascular system occurs within days and involves fluid shifts, fluid loss, decreased cardiac output, decreased peak oxygen uptake, and increased resting heart rate (Fletcher, 2005; Kasper et al, 2005; Resnick, 1998a).*
- When getting the client up after bed rest, do so slowly and watch for signs of postural hypotension, tachycardia, nausea, diaphoresis, or syncope. Take the blood pressure lying, sitting, and standing, waiting 2 minutes between each reading. *Sitting or stand-*

*ing after 3 or 4 days of bed rest results in postural hypotension because of cardiovascular reflex dysfunction (Fletcher, 2005).*

- Obtain assistive devices such as braces, crutches, or canes to help the client reach and maintain as much mobility as possible.
- Turn the client at least every 2 hours and carefully observe skin condition, especially bony prominences. *Turning clients is of paramount importance to prevent all of the complications of bed rest. Routine turning has been demonstrated to reduce the length of stay of critical care patients (Von Reuden & Harris, 1995).*

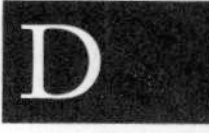

- Provide the client with a pressure-relieving horizontal support surface. For further interventions on skin care, refer to the care plan for **Impaired Skin integrity.**
- ▲ Request a physical therapy referral to help the client learn how to move self in bed including bridging and also how to transfer out of bed (Fried & Fried, 2001).
- ▲ Apply graduated compression stockings as ordered. Ensure proper fit by measuring, remove at least twice, in the morning with bath and in the evening to assess condition of extremity, then reapply. **EBN and EB:** *A meta-analysis of 11 studies with 1752 subjects demonstrated that graduated compression stockings reduced the incidence of DVT in a high-risk orthopedic surgical population and that additional antithrombotic measures along with stockings decreased the incidence even further (Joanna Briggs Institute, 2001). Graduated compression stockings, alone or used in conjunction with other prevention modalities, prevent deep venous thrombosis in hospitalized patients (Amarigiri & Lees, 2000).*
- Monitor peripheral circulation and especially note color, pulse, and calf or thigh swelling; check Homans' sign, but recognize that it is an unreliable sign of DVT. *Because of venous stasis, pressure of mattress against veins, and hypercoagulability of blood, bed rest predisposes the client to deep vein thrombosis (Fried & Fried, 2001; Harper & Lyles, 1988).*
- Have the client cough and deep breathe or use incentive spirometry every 2 hours while awake. *Bed rest compromises breathing because of decreased chest expansion, decreased cilia activity, and pooling of mucous (Fletcher, 2005).*
- Monitor respiratory functions, noting breath sounds and respiratory rate. Percuss for new onset of dullness in lungs. *Immobility results in hypoventilation, which predisposes the client to atelectasis, the pooling of respiratory secretions, and thus pneumonia (Fried & Fried, 2001; Fletcher, 2005).*
- Note bowel function daily. Provide increased fluids, fiber, and natural laxatives such as prune juice as needed. *Constipation is common in immobilized clients because of decreased activity and fluid and food intake.*
- Increase fluid intake to 2000 mL/day within the client's cardiac and renal reserve. *Adequate fluids help prevent kidney stones and constipation and help counteract dehydration associated with bed rest (Rubin, 1988).*
- Encourage intake of a balanced diet with adequate amounts of fiber and protein. *Reduced muscular activity and lowered metabolism generally reduce the appetite of a client on bed rest (Fletcher, 2005; Rubin, 1988).*

## Geriatric

- Help the mostly immobile client achieve mobility as soon as possible, depending on physical condition. *In the elderly, mobility impairment can predict increased mortality and*

D

*dependence; however, this can be prevented by physical exercise (Fletcher, 2005; Hirvensalo, Rantanen, & Heikkinen, 2000).*

- Use the Outcome Expectation for Exercise Scale to determine client's self-efficacy expectations and outcomes expectations toward exercise. **EBN:** *The client's self-efficacy expectations and outcome expectations for exercise will greatly influence his or her willingness to exercise. If the individual has a low outcome, interventions can be implemented to strengthen the expectations and hopefully improve exercise behavior (Resnick, Zimmerman, & Orwig, 2001).*
- For a client who is mostly immobile, minimize cardiovascular deconditioning by positioning the client in an upright position several times daily. *The hazards of bed rest in the elderly are multiple, serious, quick to develop, and slow to reverse. Deconditioning of the cardiovascular system occurs within days and involves fluid shifts, fluid loss, decreased cardiac output, decreased peak oxygen uptake, and increased resting heart rate (Fletcher, 2005; Kasper et al, 2005; Resnick & Daly, 1998).*
- If client is frail, ensure good nutrition, appropriate medications, attention to vision and hearing deficits, and increase social support along with exercise. *Fraility in the elderly can be multifactorial and often can be ameliorated or reversed (Storey & Thomas, 2004).*
- If the client is mostly immobile, encourage him or her to attend a low-intensity aerobic chair exercise class that includes stretching and strengthening chair exercises. **EBN:** *A study of sedentary elderly subjects demonstrated that chair exercises have been shown to increase flexibility and balance (Mills, 1994).*

▲ Refer the client to physical therapy for resistance exercise training as able including abdominal crunch, leg press, leg extension, leg curl, calf press, and more. **EB:** *A study demonstrated that 6 months of resistance exercise for the elderly greatly increased their aerobic capacity, possibly from increased skeletal muscle strength (Vincent et al, 2002). An additional study where clients in an extended care facility were put on a strength, balance, and endurance training program, the client's balance and mobility improved significantly (Rydwik, Kerstin & Akner, 2005). A Cochrane review found that progressive resistance training is effective in increasing strength in older people (Latham et al, 2003).*

▲ If geriatric, the client is scheduled for an elective surgery that will result in admission into ICU and immobility, or recovery from a knee replacement, initiate a prehabilitation program that includes a warm-up, aerobic strength, flexibility, and functional task work. **EBN:** *By increasing the functional capacity of the individual before the stressor of inactivity, the predictable declines in physical activity can be prevented or alleviated (Topp et al, 2002). In a study, clients who performed strength activities preoperatively walked significantly greater distances postoperatively after total hip replacement (Whitney & Parkman, 2002).*

▲ Refer to physical therapy for an individualized strength-training program.

- Monitor for signs of depression: flat affect, poor appetite, insomnia, many somatic complaints. *Depression can commonly accompany decreased mobility and function in the elderly (Fletcher, 2005; Resnick, 1998b).*
- Keep careful track of bowel function in the elderly; do not allow the client to become constipated. *The elderly can easily develop impactions as a result of immobility.*

D

## Home Care

NOTE: Care for all body systems because the immobilized or otherwise at risk client must continue in the home as stated in the previously mentioned interventions. The primary nurse monitors and adjusts the plan of care accordingly per physician orders.

- • Some of the previous interventions may be adapted for home care use.
- ▲ Begin discharge planning as soon as possible with case manager or social worker to assess need for home support systems and community or home health services.
- ▲ Become oriented to all programs of care for the client before discharge from institutional care.
- ▲ Confirm the immediate availability of all necessary assistive devices for home. *Continuity in management of care promotes success in meeting client-centered goals.*
- • Perform complete physical assessment and recent history at initial visit. *A complete assessment validates the status of the client upon discharge and defines client problems needing immediate intervention. Presence of pressure ulcers may indicate need for additional treatment measures.*
- ▲ Refer to physical and occupational therapies for immediate evaluations of the client's potential for independence and functioning in the home setting and for follow-up care. *Early identification of client needs allows for early intervention and prevention of secondary problems.*
- • Allow the client to have as much input and control of the plan of care as possible. *Client perception of control increases self-esteem and motivation to follow medical plan of care.*
- • Assess knowledge of all care with caregivers. Review as necessary. *Having the necessary knowledge and skills to perform care decreases caregiver role strain and supports safety of the client.*
- ▲ Support the family of the client in assumption of caregiver activities. Refer for home health aide services for assistance and respite as appropriate. Refer to medical social services as appropriate.
- ▲ Institute case management of frail elderly to support continued independent living. *Disuse syndrome represents and can lead to increasing needs for assistance in using the health care system effectively. Case management combines nursing activities of the client and family assessment, planning and coordination of care among all health care providers, delivery of direct nursing care, and monitoring of care and outcomes. These activities are able to address continuity of care, mutual goal setting, behavior management, and prevention of worsening health problems (Guttman, 1999).*

## Client/Family Teaching

- • Teach how to perform range of motion exercises in bed if not contraindicated.
- • Teach the family how to turn and position the client and provide all care necessary.

NOTE: Nursing diagnoses that are commonly relevant when the client is on bed rest include **Constipation, Risk for impaired Skin integrity, Disturbed Sensory perception, Disturbed Sleep pattern, Adult Failure to thrive,** and **Powerlessness.**

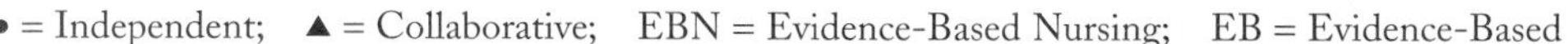

## evolve WEBSITES FOR EDUCATION

See the EVOLVE website for World Wide Web resources for client education.

## REFERENCES

D


Allen C, Glasziou P, Del Mar C: Bed rest: a potentially harmful treatment needing more careful attention, *Lancet* 354(9186):1229, 1999.

Amarigiri SV, Lees TA: Elastic compression stockings for prevention of deep vein thrombosis, *Cochrane Database Syst Rev* (3): CD001484, 2000.

Connelly DM: Resisted exercise training of institutionalized older adults for improved strength and functional mobility: a review, *Top Geriatr Rehabil* 15(3):6, 2000.

Fletcher K: Immobility: geriatric self-learning module, *Medsurg Nurs* 14(1):35, 2005.

Fried KM, Fried GW: Immobility. In Derstine JB, Hargrove SD, editors: *Comprehensive rehabilitation nursing,* Philadelphia, 2001, WB Saunders.

Guttman R: Case management of the frail elderly in the community, *Clin Nurs Spec* 13(4):174, 1999.

Harper CM, Lyles YM: Physiology and complications of bed rest, *J Am Geriatr Soc* 36:1047, 1988.

Hirvensalo M, Rantanen T, Heikkinen E: Mobility difficulties and physical activity as predictors of mortality and loss of independence in the community-living older population, *J Am Geriatr Soc* 48(5):493, 2000.

Joanna Briggs Institute: Best practice: graduated compression stockings for the prevention of post-operative venous thromboembolism, *Evidenced Based Practice Information Sheets for Health Professions* 5:2, 2001.

Kasper DL et al: *Harrison's principles of internal medicine,* ed 16, New York, 2005, McGraw-Hill.

Kasper CE, Talbor LA: Skeletal muscle damage and recovery, *AACN Clin Issues* 13(2):237, 2002.

Latham N, Anderson C, Bennett D et al: Progressive resistance strength training for physical disability in older people, *Cochrane Database Syst Rev* (2):CD002759, 2003.

Mills EM: The effect of low-intensity aerobic exercise on muscle strength, flexibility, and balance among sedentary elderly persons, *Nurs Res* 43:207, 1994.

Nelson A, Owen B, Lloyd JD et al: Safe patient handling and movement, *Am J Nurs* 103(3):32-43, 2003.

Quigley P: Functional assessment. In Derstine JB, Hargrove SD, editors: *Comprehensive rehabilitation nursing,* Philadelphia, 2001, WB Saunders.

Powers J, Daniels D: Turning points: implementing kinetic therapy in the ICU, *Nurs Manage* 35(5):1, 2004.

Resnick B: Predictors of functional ability in geriatric rehabilitation patients, *Rehabil Nurs* 23(1):21, 1998a.

Resnick N: *Geriatric medicine in current medical diagnosis and treatment,* ed 37, Stamford, Conn, 1998b, Appleton and Lange.

Resnick B, Zimmerman S, Orwig D: Model testing for reliability and validity of the outcome expectations for exercise scale, *Nurs Res* 50(5):293, 2001.

Rubin M: The physiology of bed rest, *Am J Nurs* 88:50, 1988.

Rydwik E, Kerstin F, Akner G: Physical training in institutionalized elderly people with multiple diagnoses—a controlled pilot study, *Arch Gerontol Geriatr* 40(1):29, 2005.

Story E, Thomas RL: Understanding and ameliorating fraility in the elderly, *Top Geriatr Rehabil* 20(1):86, 2004.

Tempkin T, Tempkin A, Goodman H: Geriatric rehabilitation, *Nurs Pract Forum* 8(2):59, 1997.

Thapa PB, Brockman KG, Gideon P et al: Injurious falls in nonambulatory nursing home residents: a comparative study of circumstances, incidence, and risk factors, *J Am Geriatr Soc* 44:273, 1996.

Topp R, Ditmyer M, King K: The effect of bedrest and potential of prehabilitation on patients in the intensive care unit, *AACN Clin Issues* 13(2):263, 2002.

Vincent KR, Braith RW, Feldman RA et al: Improved cardiorespiratory endurance following 6 months of resistance exercise in elderly men and women, *Arch Intern Med* 162:673, 2002.

Von Rueden KT, Harris JR: Pulmonary dysfunction related to immobility in the trauma patient, *AACN Clin Issues* 6:212, 1995.

Whiteman K et al: Effects of continuous lateral rotation therapy on pulmonary complications in liver transplant patients, *Am J Crit Care* 4:133, 1995.

Whitney JA, Parkman S: Preoperative physical activity, anesthesia, and analgesia: effects on early postoperative walking after total hip replacement, *Appl Nurs Res* 15(1):19, 2002.


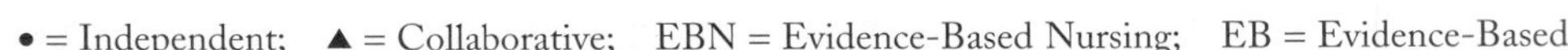

# Deficient Diversional activity

*Betty J. Ackley*

D

## NANDA

### Definition

Decreased stimulation from (or interest or engagement in) recreational or leisure activities

### Defining Characteristics

Usual hobbies cannot be undertaken in hospital; patient's statements regarding boredom and the wish for something to do, to read, and so on

### Related Factors (r/t)

Environmental lack of diversional activity as a result of long-term hospitalization and/or frequent or lengthy treatments

## NOC

### Outcomes (Nursing Outcomes Classification)

#### Suggested NOC Outcomes

Leisure Participation, Play Participation, Social Involvement

**Example NOC Outcome with Indicators**

**Leisure Participation** as evidenced by the following indicators: Expresses satisfaction with leisure activities/Feels relaxed from leisure activities/Enjoys leisure activities (Rate each indicator of **Leisure Participation:** 1 = never demonstrated, 2 = rarely demonstrated, 3 = sometimes demonstrated, 4 = often demonstrated, 5 = consistently demonstrated [see Section I].)

### Client Outcomes

**Client Will (Specify Time Frame):**

- Engage in personally satisfying diversional activities

## NIC

### Interventions (Nursing Interventions Classification)

#### Suggested NIC Interventions

Recreation Therapy, Self-Responsibility Facilitation

**Example NIC Activities—Recreation Therapy**

Assist the client to identify meaningful recreational activities; provide safe recreational equipment

## Nursing Interventions and Rationales



- • Observe for signs of deficient diversional activity: restlessness, unhappy facial expression, and statements of boredom and discontent.
- • Observe ability to engage in activities that require good vision and use of hands. *Diversional activities must be tailored to the client's capabilities.*
- • Discuss activities with clients that are interesting and feasible in the present environment.
- • Encourage the client to share feelings about situation of inactivity away from usual life activities. *Work and hobbies provide structure and continuity to life; the client can feel a sense of loss when unable to engage in usual activities.* **EB:** *A study demonstrated that spinal cord injury clinets who experienced increased frequency of recreational experiences had increased levels of well being (Lee & McCormick, 2004).*
- • Encourage a mix of physical and mental activities (e.g., crafts, videotapes). Provide activities that are entertaining, such as videotapes, joke books, or a "humor room." *Humor can help clients reduce anxiety and survive in a high technology environment (Radziewicz, 1992).*
- • Use "bread therapy"—have clients bake bread with a bread maker two times per day or prn. *Assembling the ingredients is a group activity and can be therapeutic. The smell of bread baking gives a homelike, loving atmosphere to a health care environment.*
- ▲ Arrange animal-assisted therapy, with a dog or cat for the client to interact with and care for. *Studies have demonstrated increased feelings of self-worth, reduced anxiety, reduced blood pressure and triglycerides, and increased relaxation and social functioning in clients involved in animal-assisted therapy (Stanley-Hermans & Miller, 2002).* **EBN:** *A study demonstrated that dog-assisted therapy may alleviate psychological distress in children and parents, help facilitate adaptation to the therapeutic process, and promote well-being during hospitalization (Gagnon et al, 2004).*
- • Encourage the client to schedule visitors so that they are not all present at once or at inconvenient times. *A schedule prevents the client from becoming exhausted from frequent company.*
- • Provide reading material, television, radio, and books on tape.
- • If clients are able to write, have them keep journals; if clients are unable to write, have them record thoughts on tape. *Keeping a journal is diversional and can also help the client deal with the many feelings that result from hospitalization or confinement. A journal can also help the client gain perspective on the situation.*
- ▲ Request recreational or art therapist to assist with providing diversional activities. *Recreational therapists specialize in helping people have fun. Art therapy can be effective for helping people express emotions, as well as provide diversion (Shaw & Wilkinson, 1996).*
- ▲ Request an order for a child life specialist or, if not available, a play therapist for children.
- • Provide a change in scenery; get the client out of the room as possible. *A lack of sensory stimulation has significant adverse effects on clients.*
- • Help the client to experience nature through looking at a nature scene from a window, or walking through a garden if possible. **EBN:** *Exposure to a natural environment can be helpful to promote relaxation, stress recovery, and mental restoration (Cimprich, 1993;*

*Jones & Haight, 2002). Listening to birds, and feeling the sun on their faces can be a wonderful experience for long-term clients (Fioravanti, 2004).*

- Structure the environment as needed to promote optimal comfort and sensory diversity (e.g., have family bring in posters, banners, or a sound system; change lighting; change direction bed faces). *Modification of the environment is sometimes necessary for the well-being of the client.*
- Recommend activities in which the client can watch movement of animals and develop involvement (e.g., bird-watching, keeping a fish tank).
- Work with family to provide music that is enjoyable to the client. **EBN:** *Research has shown that music can help decrease anxiety in hospitalized clients (Evans, 2002; Smolen et al, 2002).*
- Structure the client's schedule around personal wishes for time of care, relaxation, and participation in fun activities. *Increased client control fosters increased client self-esteem.*
- Spend time with the client when possible or arrange for a friendly visitor. *Simply being available for the client as a fellow human being is important and helpful (Gardner, 1992).*

D

## Pediatric

- Provide activities such as video projects, use of computer-based support groups for children, such as Starbright World, a computer network where children interact virtually, sharing their experiences and escaping hospital routines. **EB:** *The use of Starbright Hospital Pals group was shown to reduce distress related to radiation therapy of children with cancer (Klosky et al, 2004). Starbright World was show to significantly reduce loneliness and withdrawn behavior in chronically ill children (Wiener et al, 2002).*
- Provide virtual reality experiences for children, which can be used as distraction techniques such as during chemotherapy treatments. Recommend programs such as Magic Carpet, Sherlock Holmes Mystery, and Seventh Guest. *Virtual reality experiences as a distraction technique can be effective and result in positive clinical outcomes (Schneider & Workman, 2000).*

## Geriatric

- If the client is able, arrange for him or her to attend a group senior citizen exercise session for progressive strength training, even if exercise can only be done while seated. *Strength training can help seniors improve balance, coordination, range of motion, flexibility, and spatial awareness while receiving social support and having fun (Brill, 1999).*
- Encourage involvement in senior citizen activities (e.g., AARP, YMCA, church groups). Arrange transportation to activities as needed.
- Encourage clients to use their ability to help others by volunteering. *Assisting others can help the client grow as a generative human being.*
- Provide an environment that promotes activity (e.g., one that has adequate lighting for crafts, large-print books); allow periods of solitude and privacy. *Periods of solitude are important for emotional well-being in the elderly.*
- Use reminiscence therapy in conjunction with the expression of emotions. Refer to a reminiscence group if available. **EBN and EB:** *Two studies demonstrated that participation in a reminiscence group reduced symptoms of depression (Zauszniewski et al, 2004;*

D

*Jones, 2003). Reminiscence therapy can also increase social interaction, self-esteem, and well-being (Jonsdottir et al, 2001; Taylor-Price, 1995; Burnside, 1990).*

- ▲ Use the Eden Alternative with the elderly; bring in appropriate plants for the elderly client to care for, animals such as birds, fish, dogs, and cats as appropriate for the client, and children to visit. *The Eden Alternative offers a more natural human habitat where the quality of life is improved resulting in less loneliness, helplessness, and boredom (Barba et al, 2002).* **EBN:** *Animal-assisted therapy program for dementia clients resulted in decreased agitation behavior and increased social interactions (Richeson, 2003). A study demonstrated the heart rate and systolic blood pressure decreased significantly when elderly women were interacting with small dogs (Luptak & Nuzzo, 2004).*
- • For clients in assisted living facilities, provide leisure educational programs. **EB:** *A study demonstrated that participation in leisure education programs resulted in increased perception of quality of life (Janssen, 2004).*
- • Provide recreational therapy exercises in the morning for clients with dementia in the extended care facility. **EB:** *A study demonstrated that morning recreational exercises resulted in decreased agitation and passivity and also increased strength and flexibility (Buetttner & Fitzsimmons, 2004).*

## Multicultural

- • Assess for the influence of cultural beliefs, norms, and values on the client's leisure activity interests. **EBN:** *Leisure interests or hobbies may be based on cultural preferences (Cochran, 1998; Doswell & Erlen, 1998; Leininger & McFarland, 2002).*
- • Validate the client's feelings and concerns related to lack of stimulation or interest in leisure activities. **EBN:** *Validation is a therapeutic communication technique that lets the client know that the nurse has heard and understands what was said and promotes the nurse-client relationship (Heineken, 1998).*

## Home Care

NOTE: Many of the previously listed interventions should be administered in the home setting (e.g., modifying the environment to stimulate the client, scheduling visitors to allow for rest and activity). Some adaptations will be necessary.

- • Explore with the client previous interests; consider related activities that are within the client's capabilities. *New activities that build on past interests may attract the client's attention and broaden perception of available activities (e.g., a client who enjoyed gardening but is now immobilized may be tempted by landscaping books to plan next season's garden).*
- ▲ Assess the client for depression. Refer for mental health services as indicated. *Anhedonia, or lack of interest in previously enjoyed activities, is part of the syndrome of depression. Increase in diversional activities is unlikely unless the underlying depression is treated.*
- • Assess the family's ability to respond to the client's psychosocial needs for stimulation. Assist as able. *Individuals and caregivers provide care through the context of their own cultural experiences.*
- ▲ Refer to occupational therapy to assist the client and family with identifying diversional activities within the capability of the client and family. *Some services require the consultation of specialty prepared professionals.*

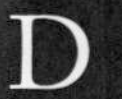

- ▲ Introduce (or continue) friendly volunteer visitors if the client is willing and able to have the company. If transportation is an issue or if the client does not want visitors in the home, consider alternatives (e.g., telephone contacts, computer messaging). *Simply being available for the client as a fellow human being is important and helpful (Gardner, 1992).*
- ▲ In the presence of a psychiatric disorder, refer for psychiatric home health care services for client reassurance and implementation of therapeutic regimen. *Psychiatric home care nurses can address issues relating to the client's depression and its interference with ability to adjust to changes in health status. Behavioral interventions in the home can assist the client to participate more effectively in treatment plan (Patusky et al, 1996).*

## Client/Family Teaching

- Work with the client and family on learning diversional activities that the client is interested in (e.g., knitting, hooking rugs, writing memoirs).
- If the client is in isolation, give the client complete information on why isolation is needed and how it should be accomplished, especially guidelines for visitors. **EBN:** *In one study, 21 clients who were in isolation identified their greatest needs, which were for more information about the isolation regulations and the need for guidelines for visitors so that visitors would be comfortable and continue to visit (Ward, 2000).*

## evolve WEBSITES FOR EDUCATION

See the EVOLVE website for World Wide Web resources for client education.

## REFERENCES


Barba BE, Tesh AS, Courts NF: Promoting thriving in nursing homes, the Eden alternative, *J Gerontol Nurs* 28(3):7 2002.

Brill PA: Effective approach toward prevention and rehabilitation in geriatrics, *Activ Adapt Aging* 23(4):21, 1999.

Buettner LL, Fitzsimmons S: Recreational therapy exercise on the special care unit: impact on behaviors, *Am J Recreation Ther* 3(4):8-24, 2004.

Burnside IM: *The effect of reminiscence groups on fatigue, affect, and life satisfaction in older women,* Austin, 1990, University of Texas (unpublished doctoral dissertation).

Cochran M: Tears have no color, *Am J Nurs* 98(6):53, 1998.

Doswell W, Erlen J: Multicultural issues and ethical concerns in the delivery of revising care interventions, *Nurs Clin North Am* 33(2):353, 1998.

Evans D: The effectiveness of music as an intervention for hospital patients: a systematic review, *J Adv Nurs* 37(1):8, 2002.

Fioravanti MA: Helping patients break the boredom, *RN* 67(1):46-49, 2004.

Gagnon J, Bouchard F, Landry M et al: Implementing a hospital-based animal therapy program for children with cancer: a descriptive study, *Can Oncol Nurs* J 14(4):210-22, 2004.

Gardner DL: Presence. In Bulechek GM, McCloskey JC, editors: *Nursing interventions: essential nursing treatments,* Philadelphia, 1992, WB Saunders.

Giger JN, Davidhizar RE: *Transcultural nursing,* ed 2, St Louis, 1995, Mosby.

Hamilton DB: Reminiscence therapy. In Bulechek GM, McCloskey JC, editors: *Nursing interventions: essential nursing treatments,* Philadelphia, 1992, WB Saunders.

Heineken J: Patient silence is not necessarily client satisfaction: communication in home care nursing, *Home Healthc Nurse* 16(2): 115, 1998.

Janssen MA: The use of leisure education in assisted living facilities, *Am J Recreation Ther* 3(4):25-30, 2004.

Jones ED, Beck-Litle R: The use of reminiscence therapy for the treatment of depression in rural-dwelling older adults, *Issues Ment Health Nurs* 23:3, 2002.

Jones MM, Haight BK: Environmental transformations: an integrative review, *J Gerontol Nurs* 28(3):23, 2002.
Jonsdottir H et al: Group reminiscence among people with end-stage chronic lung diseases, *J Adv Nurs* 35(1):79, 2001.
Klosky JL, Tyc VL, Srivastava DK al: Evaluation of an interactive intervention designed to reduce pediatric distress during radiation therapy procedures, *J Pediatr Psychol* 29(8):621-626.
Kuntz N et al: Therapeutic play and bone marrow transplantation, *J Pediatr Nurs* 11(6):359, 1996.
Leininger MM, McFarland MR: *Transcultural nursing: concepts, theories, research and practices,* ed 3, New York, 2002, McGraw-Hill.
Lee Y, McCormick B: Subjective well-being of people with spinal cord injury: does leisure contribute? *J Rehabil* 70(3), 2004.
Luptak JE, Nuzzo NA: The effects of small dogs on vital signs in elderly women: a pilot study, *Cardiopulm Phys Ther J* 15(1), 2004.
Patusky KL, Rodning C, Martinez-Kratz M: Clinical lessons in psychiatric home care: a case study approach, *J Home Healthc Manage* 9:18, 1996.
Radziewicz RM: Using diversional activities to enhance coping, *Cancer Nurs* 15(4):293, 1992.
Richeson NE: Effects of animal–assisted therapy on agitated behaviors and social interactions of older adults with dementia: an evidence-based therapeutic recreation intervene, *Am J Recreation Ther* (4), 2003.
Rode D et al: Therapeutic use of technology, *Am J Nurs* 98(12):32, 1998.
Schneider SM, Workman ML: Virtual reality as a distraction intervention for older children receiving chemotherapy, *Pediatr Nurs* 26(6):593, 2000.
Shaw R, Wilkinson W: Therapy and rehabilitation: building the pyramids—palliative care patients' perceptions of making art, *Int J Palliat Nurs* 2(4):217, 1996.
Smolen D, Topp R, Singer L: The effect of self-selected music during colonoscopy on anxiety, heart rate, and blood pressure, *Appl Nurs Res* 15(3):126, 2002.
Stanley-Hermanns M, Miller J: Animal-assisted therapy, *Am J Nurs* 102(10):69, 2002.
Stuart GW, Laraia MT: Therapeutic nurse-patient relationship. In Stuart GW, Laraia MT, editors: *Principles and practice of psychiatric nursing,* St Louis, 2001, Mosby.
Taylor-Price C: *The efficacy of structured reminiscence group psychotherapy as an intervention to decrease depression and increase psychological well-being in female nursing home residents,* Starkville, Miss, 1995, Mississippi State University (unpublished doctoral dissertation).
Ward D: Infection control: reducing the psychological effects of isolation, *Br J Nurs* 9(3):162, 2000.
Battles HB, Weiner LS: Effects of an electronic network on the social environment of children with life-threatening illness, *Children's Health Care* 31(1): 47-68, 2002.
Williams MA: The physical environment and patient care, *Am Rev Nurs Res* 6:61, 1988.
Zauszniewski JA, Eggenschwiler K, Preechawong S et al: Focused reflection reminiscence group for elders: implementation and evaluation, *Appl Gerontol* 23(4):429-442, 2004.

# Disturbed Energy field

evolve

*Gail B. Ladwig*

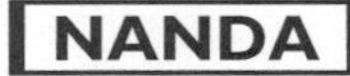


## Definition

Disruption of the flow of energy surrounding a person's being results in disharmony of the body, mind, and/or spirit

## Defining Characteristics

Perceptions of changes in patterns of energy flow, such as: movement (wave, spike, tingling, dense, flowing, sounds [tone, words]); temperature change (warmth, coolness);

visual changes (image, color); disruption of the field (deficit, hole, spike, bulge, obstruction, congestion, diminished flow in energy field)

## Related Factors

Slowing or blocking of energy flows secondary to: pathophysiologic factors; illness (specify); pregnancy; injury; treatment-related factors; immobility; labor and delivery; perioperative experience; chemotherapy; situational factors (personal, environmental); pain; fear; anxiety; grieving; maturational factors; age-related developmental difficulties or crisis (specify)

**NOC**

## Outcomes (Nursing Outcomes Classification)

### Suggested NOC Outcomes

Personal Well-Being, Comfort Level, Spiritual Health

**Example NOC Outcome with Indicators**

**Personal Well-Being** as evidenced by the following indicators: Psychological health/Spiritual life/Ability to relax/Level of happiness (Rate each indicator of **Personal Well-Being:** 1 = not all satisfied, 2 = somewhat satisfied, 3 = moderately satisfied, 4 = very satisfied, 5 = completely satisfied [see Section I].)

## Client Outcomes

### Client Will (Specify Time Frame):

- State sense of well-being
- State feeling of relaxation
- State decreased pain
- State decreased tension
- Demonstrate evidence of physical relaxation (e.g., decreased blood pressure, pulse, respiration rate, muscle tension)

**NIC**

## Interventions (Nursing Interventions Classification)

### Suggested NIC Intervention

Therapeutic Touch (TT)

**Example NIC Activities—Therapeutic Touch**

Focuses awareness on inner self; focuses awareness on the intention to facilitate wholeness and healing at all levels of consciousness

## Nursing Interventions and Rationales

E

- Refer to care plans for **Anxiety, Acute Pain,** and **Chronic Pain.**
- Consider using Therapeutic Touch for clients with anxiety, tension, pain and other conditions that indicate a disruption in the flow of energy. **EBN:** *Representing the largest published sample size of therapeutic touch (TT) outcomes to date, data from this continuous quality improvement (CQI) clinical study suggests that TT, when provided in the clinical setting, promotes comfort, calmness, and well-being among hospitalized patients (Newshan & Schuller-Civitella, 2003).* **EBN:** *This pilot study tested the effectiveness of 6 therapeutic touch treatments on the experience of pain and quality of life for persons with fibromyalgia syndrome. TT may be an effective treatment for relieving pain and improving quality of life in this specific population of persons with fibromyalgia syndrome (Denison, 2004). In this study using gentle touch with clients with cancer, tests showed statistically significant improvements in psychological and physical functioning, with positive effects on quality of life. The most pronounced improvements were seen in ratings for stress and relaxation, severe pain/discomfort, and depression/anxiety, particularly in those with the most severe symptoms on entry. The study found no adverse effects resulting from the treatment (Weze et al, 2004).*
- Consider use of treatments for clients with psychological depression and self-perceived stress. **EB:** *The long-term effects of energetic healing were examined in an experimental design on clients with symptoms of psychological depression and self-perceived stress as measured by the Beck Depression Inventory, Beck Hopelessness, and Perceived Stress scales. Forty-six participants were randomly assigned to one of three groups: hands-on Reiki, distance Reiki, or distance Reiki placebo, and remained blind to treatment condition. Each participant received a 1 to 1.5 hour treatment each week for 6 weeks. On completion of treatment, there was a significant reduction in symptoms of psychological distress in treatment groups as compared with controls these differences continued to be present 1 year later (Shore, 2004).*
- Administer TT as described in following discussion (may also include healing touch and Reiki practice). **EBN:** *Meta-analytic techniques were used to integrate the research-based literature with scientific evidence supporting TT as a nursing intervention in the past decade. The results seem to indicate that TT has a positive, medium effect on physiological and psychological variables (Peters, 1999).* **EBN:** *Studies of healing touch (HT) indicated results in reducing stress, anxiety, and pain; accelerated healing; some improvement in biochemical and physiological markers; and a greater sense of well-being. Participants generally reported improved quality of life physically, emotionally, relationally, and spiritually. HT might also be another treatment option for nurses to provide safe, noninvasive care to promote healing (Wardell & Weymouth, 2004).*

### Guidelines for Therapeutic Touch

- TT may be practiced by anyone with the requisite preparation, desire, and commitment. Required preparation is the completion of a minimum 12–contact hour basic workshop by a TT practitioner who meets the criteria as a Nurse Healer–Professional Associates International, Inc. (NH-PAI)–qualified TT teacher. Health care professionals need to have practiced TT on a consistent basis for at least 1 year under the direction of a mentor (during the mentorship year, at the discretion and under the supervision of a mentor, the health care professional can begin using TT in a health care/hospital setting). A further requirement of the practitioner is the completion of a 14–contact hour intermediate level course of instruction by a qualified TT teacher.

- Those who are not licensed health care professionals may practice TT within their families, religious or spiritual community, and friends. Investigation of state licensing laws and regulations is necessary before accepting fees for practicing TT to ensure lawful practices. Those who are licensed to perform specific or general health-related services, including counseling or massage therapy, need to clarify roles and scope of practice parameters with their respective state regulatory entity or board or an attorney.

E

NOTE: Nurses who are not trained in TT should consider spending quiet time with clients listening to their concerns. **EBN:** *In this study of TT regardless of experimental or control intervention participation, women expressed feelings of calmness, relaxation, security, and comfort and a sense of awareness. The women regarded either nursing intervention as a positive experience. Nurses who are not trained in the administration of TT may use quiet time and dialogue to enhance feelings of calmness and relaxation in patients with breast cancer (Kelly et al, 2004).*

- TT practitioners adhere to a code of ethics in the practice of TT. Keeping client information confidential, using TT only with permission of the client, charging reasonable fees for services, and practicing responsible use of other interventions in conjunction with the TT process are important elements of that code.
- TT is conducted according to the standards for its practice developed by Dolores Krieger and Dora Kunz and in accordance with the above guidelines (NH-PAI, Inc., 2003).
- Administer TT by performing the following steps:
  - Centering in the present moment: Shift awareness from the physical environment to an inner focus on the center within self, a center of calm and balance through which nurses perceive themselves and the client as a unitary whole. *The point of entry into the TT process is the act of centering (Krieger, 1997).* **EBN:** *This study suggests that TT, when provided by the nurse in the clinical setting, can promote feelings of comfort, peace, calm, and security among patients (Hayes & Cox, 1999).*
  - Assessment: Pass palmar surface of hands 2 to 4 inches over the client's body from head to toe. **EBN:** *The key constructs that emerged in this study are associated with feelings such as tingling, warmth, coolness, comfort, peace, calm, and security. The results emphasized the relationship associated with what is known by the mind and instinctively felt by the body (Hayes & Cox, 1999). Validation study cues include heat, decreased or disrupted energy flow, cold, tingling, pulsating, congestion, heaviness, unbalance, decreased flow, and field symmetry (Mornhinweg et al, 1996).*
  - Treatment (unruffling): Use hands to brush or smooth out the energy flow. Sweep the hands downward and out of the field from head to toe, and concentrate on the areas of disturbance that were identified during the assessment. *Unruffling facilitates the vital energy flows that are already in the healee's system (Krieger, 1997).*
  - Direction and modulation of energy: Rest hands on or near the body area where a block of congestion is detected or in other areas of energy imbalance. Facilitate transfer of energy to these areas. *This step corrects energy imbalances (Krieger, 1997).*

- Finish: Finish when it is judged that the appropriate amount of change has taken place (i.e., for an infant, 1-2 minutes; for an adult, 5 to 7 minutes), keeping in mind the importance of gentleness. Or stop procedure when the client indicates it is time to stop. Note whether the client has experienced a relaxation response and any related outcomes. *This final phase allows for rest and evaluation (McCloskey-Dochterman & Bulechek, 2004).*

E

## Pediatric

- Consider using TT or healing touch (HT) for pediatric clients with adjunct therapies to decrease stress, anxiety, and pain. **EBN:** *HT and TT are unique touch techniques with origins in the nursing profession. They are widely available in pediatric hospitals. Practitioners, as well as patients, may notice improved sense of well-being during and after treatments. Additional research is needed to determine the mechanisms by which these effects occur, the optimal duration and frequency of treatments, factors predictive of treatment response, and the overall costs and benefits of including TT and HT in treatment in addition to traditional therapies. These therapies are safe and readily available (Kemper & Kelly, 2004).*
- Teach that when working with the very young, old, or ill, or in the head area, TT should be gentle and used only for short periods. *Exercise caution when using TT with patients who may exhibit an extreme sensitivity to the process (e.g., premature infants, frail elderly, psychotic clients) (Sayer-Adams, 1994).*

## Geriatric

- Consider TT for agitated clients with Alzheimer's disease. **EBN:** *TT may be an effective technique to alleviate agitation in people with Alzheimer's disease (Hawranik, Deatrich, & Johnston, 2004).*

## Multicultural

- Assess for the influence of cultural beliefs, norms, and values on the client's sense of disharmony of mind and spirit. **EBN:** *The client's sense of disharmony may have cultural roots (Cochran, 1998; Doswell & Erlen, 1998; Leininger & McFarland, 2002). Nurses can increase their knowledge about other health systems through assessment and incorporate these into the plan of care for patients as needed (Snyder & Niska, 2003).*
- Assess for the presence of specific culture-bound syndromes that may manifest as disturbances in energy or spirit. **EBN:** *Voodoo death, evil eye, and trance dissociation are some of the culture-bound syndromes that have symptoms of disharmony of mind and spirit (Arnault, 1998).*
- Validate the client's feelings and concerns related to sense of disharmony or energy disturbance. **EBN:** *Validation is a therapeutic communication technique that lets the client know that the nurse has heard and understands what was said, and it promotes the nurse-client relationship (Heineken, 1998).*

## Home Care

- See Guidelines for TT.

▲ Help the client and family accept TT as a healing intervention. *Consultation and collaboration with a specialist may be the best approach to nursing care. Numerous studies have reported positive outcomes of HT as a noninvasive complementary therapy (Umbreit, 2000).*

- • Assist the family with providing an appropriate space in which TT can be administered.
- ▲ Assess clients with bipolar disorder for the occurrence of social rhythm disruption, particularly during periods of stressful life events. Refer for mental health treatment. *Stressful life events, particularly those involving social rhythm disruption, appear to play a role in initiating manic episodes (Malkoff-Schwartz et al, 2000).*
- ▲ In the presence of a psychiatric disorder, refer for psychiatric home health care services for client reassurance and implementation of therapeutic regimen. **EBN:** *Psychiatric home care nurses can address issues relating to the client's bipolar disorder and its interference with ability to adjust to changes in health status. Behavioral interventions in the home can assist the client to participate more effectively in treatment plan (Patusky et al, 1996).*

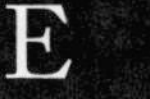

## Client/Family Teaching

- • Teach the TT process to clients and family members. *TT enables caregivers to embrace their compassion and to touch people with effect (Dalglish, 1999).* **EBN:** *Helping patients while using touch therapy related to Ki (a Korean type of energy therapy) was found to be a dynamic process with each participant actively engaged in increasing the activating, potential power of the human being (Chang et al, 2003).*
- • Teach that when working with the very young, old, or ill, or in the head area, TT should be gentle and used only for short periods. *Exercise caution when using TT with patients who may exhibit an extreme sensitivity to the process (e.g., premature infants, frail elderly, psychotic clients) (Sayer-Adams, 1994).*
- • Teach the client how to use guided imagery. *The nurse can facilitate healing by helping the client recontact and reclaim parts of the self (resolve energy disturbance) through guided imagery (Rancour, 1994).*
- • Teach the client to use deep breathing to relax. Ask the client to have the disease, affected organ, or symptom assume an image. After the image has been identified, ask the client to speak with the image to address an unresolved issue. *By describing a previously unacknowledged part of the self, liberated energy can transform resistance, defenses, and disease into self-acceptance, peace, and wholeness (Remen, 1994).*

## evolve WEBSITES FOR EDUCATION

See the EVOLVE website for World Wide Web resources for client education.

## REFERENCES

Arnault DS: Framework for culturally relevant psychiatric nursing. In Varcarolis EM, editor: *Foundations of psychiatric mental health nursing,* ed 3, Philadelphia, 1998, WB Saunders.

Chang SO: The nature of touch therapy related to Ki: practitioners' perspective, *Nurs Health Sci* 5(2):103-114, 2003.

Cochran M: Tears have no color, *Am J Nurs* 98(6):53, 1998.

Dalglish S: Worklife. Therapeutic touch in an acute care community hospital, *Can Nurse* 95(3):57, 1999.

Doswell W, Erlen J: Multicultural issues and ethical concerns in the delivery of revising care interventions, *Nurs Clin North Am* 33(2):353, 1998.

Denison B: Touch the pain away: new research on therapeutic touch and persons with fibromyalgia syndrome, *Holist Nurs Pract* 18(3):142-151, 2004.

Giger JN, Davidhizar RE: *Transcultural nursing,* ed 2, St Louis, 1995, Mosby.
Hayes J, Cox C: The experience of therapeutic touch from a nursing perspective, *Br J Nurs* 8(18):1249, 1999.
Hawranik P, Deatrich J, Johnston P: Therapeutic touch: another approach for the management of agitation, *Can Nurs Home* 15(1):46-48, 2004.
Heineken J: Patient silence is not necessarily client satisfaction: communication in home care nursing, *Home Healthc Nurse* 16(2): 115, 1998.
Kelly AE, Sullivan P, Fawcett J et al: Therapeutic touch, quiet time, and dialogue: perceptions of women with breast cancer, *Oncol Nurs Forum* 31(3):625-631, 2004.
Kemper KJ, Kelly EA: Treating children with therapeutic and healing touch, *Pediatr Ann* 33(4):248-252, 2004.
Krieger D: *Therapeutic touch inner workbook,* Santa Fe, NM, 1997, Bear and Company.
Leininger MM, McFarland MR: *Transcultural nursing: concepts, theories, research and practices,* ed 3, New York, 2002, McGraw-Hill.
Malkoff-Schwartz S, Frank E, Anderson BP et al: Social rhythm disruption and stressful life events in the onset of bipolar and unipolar episodes, *Psychol Med* 30:1005, 2000.
McCloskey Dochterman J, Bulechek G: *Nursing interventions classification (NIC),* ed 4, St Louis, 2004, Mosby.
Mornhinweg G: Energy field disturbance validation study, *Healing Touch Newsletter* 6:11, 1996.
Nurse Healers-Professional Associates International: Guidelines of recommended standards and scope of practice for Therapeutic Touch. Available at www.therapeutic-touch.org/content/guidelines.asp, accessed on January 25, 2005, revised July, 2003.
Newshan G, Schuller-Civitella D: Large clinical study shows value of therapeutic touch program, *Holist Nurs Pract* 17(4):189-192, 2003.
Patusky KL, Rodning C, Martinez-Kratz M: Clinical lessons in psychiatric home care: a case study approach, *J Home Healthc Manage* 9:18, 1996.
Peters RM: The effectiveness of therapeutic touch: a meta-analytic review, *Nurs Sci Q* 12(1):52, 1999.
Rancour P: Interactive guided imagery with oncology patients, *J Holist Nurs* 12:149, 1994.
Remen N: Psychosynthesis and healing, *J Holist Nurs* 12:150, 1994.
Sayer-Adams J: Complementary therapies: therapeutic touch nursing function, *Nurs Stand* 8:25, 1994.
Shore AG: Long-term effects of energetic healing on symptoms of psychological depression and self-perceived stress, *Altern Ther Health Med* 10(3):42-48, 2004.
Snyder M, Niska K: Cultural related complementary therapies: their use in critical care units, *Crit Care Nurs Clin North Am* 15(3): 341-346, 2003.
Umbreit AW: Healing touch: applications in the acute care setting, *AACN Clin Issues* 11(1):105, 2000.
Wardell DW, Weymouth KF: Review of studies of healing touch, *J Nurs Scholarship* 36(2):147-154, 2004.
Weze C, Leathard HL, Grange J: Evaluation of healing by gentle touch in 35 clients with cancer, *Eur J Oncol Nurs* 8(1):40-49, 2004.

# Impaired Environmental interpretation syndrome

*Betty J. Ackley*

**NANDA**

## Definition

Consistent lack of orientation to person, place, time, or circumstances for more than 3 to 6 months, necessitating a protective environment

## Defining Characteristics

Chronic confusional states; consistent disorientation in known and unknown environments; loss of occupation or social functioning resulting from memory decline; slow to respond to questions; inability to follow simple directions/instructions, concentrate, or reason

## Related Factors (r/t)

Depression; dementia (e.g., Alzheimer's, multiinfarct, Pick's disease, AIDS, Parkinson's disease, alcoholism); Huntington's disease

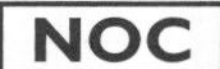


## Outcomes (Nursing Outcomes Classification)

### Suggested NOC Outcomes

Cognitive Orientation; Concentration; Information Processing; Memory; Neurological Status: Consciousness

**Example NOC Outcome with Indicators**

**Concentration** as evidenced by the following indicators: Maintains focus without being distracted/Responds appropriately to visual cues/Responds appropriately to language cues/Draws a circle (on command)/Draws a pentagon (on command) (Rate each indicator of **Concentration:** 1 = severely compromised, 2 = substantially compromised, 3 = moderately compromised, 4 = mildly compromised, 5 = not compromised [see Section I].)

## Client Outcomes

**Client Will (Specify Time Frame):**

- Remain content and free from harm
- Function at maximal cognitive level
- Participate in activities of daily living (ADLs) at the maximum of functional ability

**NIC**

## Interventions (Nursing Interventions Classification)

### Suggested NIC Interventions

Dementia Management; Environmental Management; Reality Orientation; Surveillance: Safety

**Example NIC Activities—Dementia Management**

Encourage the client to verbalize memories of loss, both past and current; help the client to identify personal coping strategies

## Nursing Interventions and Rationales, Client/Family Teaching

Refer to care plan for **Chronic Confusion.**

# Adult Failure to thrive

evolve

*Gail B. Ladwig*

**NANDA**

## Definition



Progressive functional deterioration of a physical and cognitive nature with remarkably diminished ability to live with multisystem diseases, cope with ensuing problems, and manage care

## Defining Characteristics

Anorexia: does not eat meals when offered; states does not have an appetite, is not hungry, or "I don't want to eat"; inadequate nutritional intake: eating less than body requirements; consumption of minimal to no food at most meals (i.e., consumes less than 75% of normal requirements); weight loss (from baseline weight): 5% unintentional weight loss in 1 month or 10% unintentional weight loss in 6 months; physical decline (decline in bodily function): evidence of fatigue, dehydration, incontinence of bowel and bladder; frequent exacerbations of chronic health problems (e.g., pneumonia, urinary tract infections); cognitive decline (decline in mental processing) as evidenced by problems with responding appropriately to environmental stimuli, demonstrated difficulty in reasoning, decision making, judgment, memory, and concentration; decreased perception; decreased social skills; social withdrawal: noticeable decrease from usual past behavior in attempts to form or participate in cooperative and interdependent relationships (e.g., decreased verbal communication with staff, family, friends); decreased participation in activities of daily living (ADLs) that the older person once enjoyed; self-care deficit: no longer looks after or takes charge of physical cleanliness or appearance; difficulty performing simple self-care tasks; neglect of home environment and/or financial responsibilities; apathy as evidenced by lack of observable feeling or emotion in terms of normal ADLs and environment; altered mood state: expresses feelings of sadness, being low in spirit; expresses loss of interest in pleasurable outlets such as food, sex, work, friends, family, hobbies, or entertainment; verbalizes desire for death

## Related Factors (r/t)

Depression, apathy, fatigue

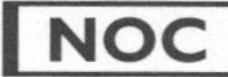


## Outcomes (Nursing Outcomes Classification)

### Suggested NOC Outcomes

Physical Aging; Psychosocial Adjustment: Life Change; Will to Live

F

**Example NOC Outcome with Indicators**

**Will to Live** as evidenced by the following indicators: Expression of determination to live/Expression of hope/Use of strategies to compensate for problems associated with disease (Rate each indicator of **Will to Live:** 1 = severely compromised, 2 = substantially compromised, 3 = moderately compromised, 4 = mildly compromised, 5 = not compromised [see Section I].)

## Client Outcomes

### Client Will (Specify Time Frame):

- Resume highest level of functioning possible
- Express feelings
- Participate in ADLs
- Participate in social interactions
- Consume adequate dietary intake for weight and height
- Maintain usual weight
- Have adequate fluid intake with no signs of dehydration
- Maintain clean personal and home environment

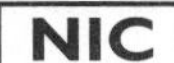

## Interventions (Nursing Interventions Classification)

### Suggested NIC Interventions

Hope Instillation, Mood Management, Self-Care Assistance

**Example NIC Activities—Hope Installation**

Help the client/family to identify areas of hope in life; involve the client actively in own care

## Nursing Interventions and Rationales

### Psychosocial

- Elderly clients who have failure to thrive (FTT) should be evaluated by review of the patient's ADLs, cognitive function, and mood; a targeted history and physical examination; and selected laboratory studies. *Early recognition of dementia is an important factor in obtaining timely and appropriate care (Insel & Badger, 2002).* **EB:** *This retrospective review of the medical record of patients with altered mental status indicated that the patient history and physical examination were most useful in diagnostic terms (Kanich et al, 2002).* **EB:** *Recent attempts to profile patients at an increased risk of dementia suggest that this can be done in skilled hands, especially in people whose symptoms prompt them to seek medical attention (Davis & Rockwood, 2004).*

- Assess for depression using a geriatric depression scale. Be alert for depression in clients newly admitted to nursing homes. **EBN:** *Depression was identified in 52% of the of the homebound elderly adults in this study using the Geriatric Depression Scale (GDS) (Loughlin, 2004).* **EB:** *In this study of medical rehabilitation clients, clients discharged to a nursing home reported higher levels of depressive symptoms than those discharged to live alone (Loeher et al, 2004).*
- ▲ Carefully assess for elder abuse and refer for treatment. **EB:** *Elderly men and women of all socioeconomic and ethnic backgrounds are vulnerable to mistreatment, and most often it goes undetected (Kahan & Paris, 2003).*
- Screen for depression in persons with adult macular degeneration (AMD) and low vision or vision loss. **EB:** *This study of 114 elderly AMD clients indicated that 49 patients met DSM-IV criteria for syndromal depression and that visual acuity was the only variable significantly associated with vision-specific function. Although there are no effective treatments for restoring vision in AMD, depression is treatable. Both psychotherapy and antidepressants are efficacious and may indirectly improve function among older people with vision loss (Casten et al, 2002).*
- Provide reality orientation for clients with mild dementia. **EBN:** *This study shows some evidence that reality orientation is effective in improving cognitive ability (Bates et al, 2004).*
- Provide music for clients with dementia. **EBN:** *In this study of clients with senile dementia when using music therapy scores for "irritability" decreased significantly (Suzukie et al, 2004).*
- ▲ Consider the use of "light therapy." **EB:** *The results of this placebo-controlled study suggest that bright light treatment may be effective among institutionalized older adults, providing nonpharmacological intervention in the treatment of depression (Sumaya et al, 2001).*
- Instill hope and encourage the expression of positive thoughts. **EB:** *The findings from this study of 1002 older disabled women suggest that positive emotions can protect older persons against adverse health outcomes (Penninx et al, 2000).* **EB:** *The data from this study confirm the argument that hopefulness appears to be central to a family's coping with the impact of mental illness. Nurses should be mindful of their capacity to sustain or diminish the hopes of family members (Bland & Darlington, 2002).*
- Provide opportunities for interaction with the natural environments. **EB:** *This demonstrates evidence to support the intuitive belief that interaction with the natural world is a vital part of biopsychosocial-spiritual well-being (Irvine & Warber, 2002).*
- Provide opportunities for visitation from animals. **EBN:** *Animal visitation programs have been used in a wide variety of clinical settings with predominantly positive outcomes reported anecdotally (Johnson et al, 2002).* **EB:** *Pets play a central role in the lives of many elderly people (Ebenstein & Worthan, 2001).*
- Encourage clients to reminiscence and to share and compile life histories. **EBN:** *Research suggests that reminiscence can improve well-being (Reichman et al, 2004; McKee et al, 2003).*
- Encourage clients to pray if they wish. **EB:** *This study indicated prayer could be used as a coping strategy (Ai et al, 2004).*

- Encourage elderly clients to take part in activities and social relationships according to their capacity and wishes. **EBN:** *Review of the literature suggests that thriving is related to helping the elderly person concentrate on activities that they are still able to do (Bergland & Kirkevold, 2001).*
- Help clients to participate in activities by assessing motivation and helping them to identify reasons to participate such as better mobility, more independence, and feelings of well-being. **EBN:** *Motivation has been identified as an important factor in the older adult's ability to perform functional activities (Resnick, 1998).*
- Provide physical touch for clients. Touch the client's hand or arm when speaking with him or her; offer hugs with permission. **EBN:** *Appropriate use of touch by nurses has the potential to significantly improve the health status of older adults (Bush, 2001; Edvardsson et al, 2003).*
- Administer therapeutic touch (TT). **EB:** *Results of this clinical trial of (N = 16) patients in the advanced stages of dementia of the Alzheimer's type (DAT), showed that discomfort levels decreased significantly after five TT sessions, becoming significantly lower than levels in the control group (N = 10) (Giasson et al, 1999).* **EBN:** *TT may be an effective technique to alleviate agitation in people with Alzheimer's disease (Hawranik, Deatrich, & Johnston, 2004).*

F

## Physiological

▲ Assess possible causes for adult FTT and treat any underlying problems such as malnutrition, diarrhea, renal failure, and illnesses that are caused by physical and cognitive changes. **EBN:** *Malnutrition is a frequent and serious problem in the elderly. Today, there is no doubt that malnutrition contributes significantly to morbidity and mortality in the elderly (Chen, 2001).* **EB:** *Physicians who care for elderly patients should be alert to the possible presence of diarrhea and malabsorption if there is unexplained weight loss and FTT. Older patients may not admit to having chronic diarrhea, particularly if they also are incontinent (Holt, 2001).* **EB:** *Retrospective chart review indicated that renal failure was found in 26.4% of the oldest-old admitted to an acute geriatric department. The elderly client with renal failure is more often admitted for failure to thrive (Van den Noortgate et al, 2001).*

▲ Assess for signs of dehydration. Administer 1600 mL/24. Offer fluids regularly to bedridden clients. **EBN:** *Dehydration is the most common fluid and electrolyte imbalance in older adults. Offering fluids and maintaining intake of 1600 mL/day ensures adequate hydration (Hodgkinson et al, 2003).*

- Assess for signs of fatigue and sensory changes that may indicate an infection is present that may be related to undetected diabetes mellitus or human immunodeficiency virus (HIV). **EB:** *In this multicenter study a group of care home residents not known to have diabetes and able to undergo testing, a substantial proportion had undetected diabetes based on a 2-hour postglucose load (Sinclair et al 2001).* **EB:** *Many older adults are sexually active and often demonstrate risky sexual behavior, such as dispensing with the use of condoms, and the isolation that frequently accompanies old age can lead to alcoholism and injectable drug use (Lieberman, 2000).*
- Assess how often the frail elder living at home goes outdoors. (Ask how often do you go outside the house? Examples include shopping, taking a walk, going out to work

in garden.) **EB:** *This study indicated that frail elders living at home in Japan who went outdoors less than once a week might be a high-risk group for functional decline, intellectual activity, and self-efficacy. This may be a useful and simple indicator to predict these changes (Kono et al, 2004).*

- Assess grip strength. **EB:** *This study suggests that grip strength may prove a more useful single marker of frailty for older people of similar age than chronological age alone. Its validity in a clinical setting needs to be tested (Syddall, 2003).*
- Monitor weight loss, leaving 25% or more of food uneaten at most meals, psychiatric/mood diagnoses, and deteriorated ability to participate in activities of daily living. **EBN:** *This study demonstrated the above criteria as significant predictors of protein calorie malnutrition (Crogan et al, 2002). Diagnosis and intervention of malnutrition can prevent loss of function and independence and decrease morbidity and mortality in the elderly (Ennis et al, 2001).*
- Offer nutrient-dense foods such as dairy and fruit products (e.g., vanilla custard, strawberry yogurt, vanilla/apple yogurt, orange/peach juice, apple/berry/grape juice, and applesauce). (These suggested foods were used in the research below in the Netherlands; adopt appropriate foods for the individual tastes of the elderly client.) **EB:** *A randomized intervention study of 161 frail elderly in the Netherlands demonstrated that the group receiving nutrient-dense foods had increased blood nutrient values and decreased homocysteine levels. The results also suggest a beneficial effect on bone mass and density for those consuming enriched foods compared with controls, although this needs further clinical confirmation (De Jong, 2001).*
- Play soothing music during mealtimes to increase the amount of food eaten. **EB:** *One study suggested that dinner music, particularly soothing music, can reduce irritability, fear, panic, and depressed mood and can stimulate the appetite of demented patients in a nursing home. In this study the patients were less irritable, anxious, and depressed during the periods when music was playing (Ragneskog et al, 1996).* **EBN:** *Findings from this study suggest that soothing music selections have beneficial effects on relaxation in community-residing elderly people (Lai, 2004).*
- Decrease noise and increase lighting in the dining area. **EB:** *This case study indicates that lighting enhancement and noise reduction may further improve dietary intake, which, in turn, may promote improved nutritional status (McDaniel et al, 2001).*
- Serve "family style meals." **EBN:** *This study suggests family-style meals may result in modest increases in mealtime participation and communication of residents with dementia (Altus et al, 2002).*
- Provide appropriate nutrition for the client whose obesity may be affecting physical performance and thus has limited ability to perform ADLs, which leads to functional dependence. **EB:** *Malnutrition includes obesity (overnutrition); obesity among older persons is defined as being at least 30% above ideal body weight. Obesity may contribute to the previously mentioned problems (Still et al, 1997).*
- Frail elderly clients should also participate in carefully supervised group exercise, balance and gait programs accompanied by music. (The exercise program used in the research: twice-weekly 45-minute group session; walking, stooping, and chair stands under the supervision of skilled trainers. Exercises were moderate but gradually increased in intensity and included different materials such as balls, ropes, weights, and

elastic bands.) (Another treatment is to use a wheelchair bicycle, combining small group activity therapy and one-on-one bike rides with a staff member.) **EB:** *This intervention study of 161 frail elderly clients in the Netherlands indicated that exercise preserved lean body mass and energy intake, it helped to improve or maintain physical fitness and the functioning vital for independent living (De Jong, 2001).* **EB:** *In long-term care residents with dementia using wheelchair bicycle riding, depression levels were significantly reduced. Improvements were also found in sleep and levels of activity engagement (Buettne & Fitzsimmons, 2002).* **EBN:** *Subjects in these studies reported significantly enhanced mood while exercising to music compared with subjects exercising without music (Murrock, 2002; Van de Winckel, 2004).* **EB:** *Balance exercises led to improvements in static balance function and gait exercises resulted in improvements to dynamic balance and gait functions in the very frail elderly (Shimada, 2003).*

▲ Refer for possible pharmacological intervention. **EB:** *This case report describes one such course of treatment for a patient with multiple myeloma with failure-to-thrive who was successfully treated with modafinil and mirtazapine. By using combination pharmacotherapy, we were able to achieve immediate results in a gravely ill patient (Schillerstrom & Seaman, 2002).*

• Refer to care plans for **Imbalanced Nutrition: less than body requirements, Hopelessness,** and **Disturbed Energy field.**

## Multicultural

• Assess for the influence of cultural beliefs, norms, and values on the family's or caregiver's understanding of FTT. **EBN:** *What the family considers normal and abnormal health behavior may be based on cultural perceptions (Leininger & McFarland, 2002; Cochran, 1998; Doswell & Erlen, 1998; Guaranccia, 1998).*

▲ Refer culturally diverse patients to appropriate social, medical, mental health and long-term care services. **EB:** *In a system providing access to and coordination of comprehensive medical and long-term care services for frail older people, black patients showed a lower mortality rate than white patients (Tan, Eng, & Covinsky, 2003). Being black was associated with moderately high and very high levels of nutritional risk (Sharkey & Schoenberg, 2002).*

• Validate the family's feelings and concerns related to the FTT symptoms. **EBN:** *Validation is therapeutic communication technique that lets the family know that the nurse has heard and understands what was said, and it promotes the nurse-client relationship (Heineken, 1998).*

## Home Care

• Above interventions may be adapted for home care use.

▲ Begin discharge planning as soon as possible with case manager or social worker to assess need for home support systems, assistive devices, and community or home health services.

• Assess clients' willingness to eat; fashion interventions accordingly. **EBN:** *Older adults reported that their willingness to eat influenced appetite, and factors influencing appetite included mood, personal values (independence and integrity); wholesomeness (being in good health); food (preparation, consistency, and freshness); eating environment (pleasantness); and meal companionship (Wikby & Fagerskiold, 2004).*

- Assess and track areas of decreased functioning resulting from failure to thrive. Ensure that all symptomatology is considered for necessary action. *Clients may change response to stressors/needs with changes in environment or interventions.*
- Give permission for role activity changes. Negotiate and clarify role expectations and reevaluate as necessary. *Failure to thrive may require an extended period of recovery. Chronic illness often requires role changes to preserve a functional unit. Comfort level with role activities supports continued recovery.*
- Provide support for family/caregivers. *Support for caregivers decreases caregiver burden.*



- If FTT is due to a dementing illness, refer to care plan for **Chronic Confusion**.
- Assess nutritional status for multiple potential influences of malnutrition, including chronic and acute disorders, loss of self-sufficiency, malabsorption disorders, changes in sense of taste, dental problems, reduced physical activity, problems with appropriate medication use, and economic or psychological factors. **EB:** *Malnutrition is underestimated in older adults, and may result in the need for hospitalization or admission to a skilled nursing facility. A detailed history should include food habits. Interventions include observation of capacity for swallowing foods of varying consistencies; flexibility during meals; provision of variety in meals; and efforts to satisfy nutritional requests (Baldelli et al, 2004).*

▲ Refer to medical social services or mental health counseling, resource identification, and/or community support groups. If necessary, contract with the client to attend sessions. *Counseling support can increase coping ability; group participation provides support and offers new problem-solving strategies to the client.*

▲ Refer to home health aide services for assistance with ADLs throughout the duration of decreased participation. *Maintaining ADLs and the integrity of the environment prevents further decline in status of those areas and decreases frustration as the client recovers and resumes responsibility for them.*

▲ Institute case management of frail elderly to support continued independent living. *Failure to thrive represents and can lead to increasing needs for assistance in using the health care system effectively. Case management combines nursing activities of the client and family assessment, planning and coordination of care among all health care providers, delivery of direct nursing care, and monitoring of care and outcomes. These activities are able to address continuity of care, mutual goal setting, behavior management, and prevention of worsening health problems (Guttman, 1999).*

▲ Refer for homemaker or psychiatric home health care services for respite, client reassurance, and implementation of therapeutic regimen. *Responsibility for a person at high risk for adult failure to thrive may provide high caregiver stress. Respite decreases caregiver stress. The presence of caring individuals is reassuring to both the client and caregivers, especially during periods of client anxiety or inability to follow treatment regimen. Failure to thrive behavior, especially if accompanied by depression, can make use of the interventions described above, modified for the home setting.* **EBN:** *Psychiatric home care nurses can address issues relating to the client's depression and its interference with ability to adjust to changes in health status. Behavioral interventions in the home can assist the client to participate more effectively in treatment plan (Patusky et al, 1996).*

## Client/Family Teaching

- ▲ Refer for medical evaluation when cognitive changes are noticed. **EB:** *The combination of functional imaging and neuropsychological tests can diagnose with high sensitivity and specificity if a patient is suffering cognitive impairment in its early stages, and may aid in predicting the risk of developing dementia (Cabranes et al, 2004).*
- • Encourage family to provide social interaction with the client. **EBN:** *The importance of family involvement, may be effective in enhancing the lives of frail elders (Gosline, 2003).*
- • Instruct the family to monitor the elder persons weight. **EBN:** *Monitoring the elder weight regularly is a surveillance measure of nutritional status (Cowan et al, 2004).*
- ▲ Provide referral for evaluation of hearing and appropriate hearing aids. **EB:** *This study of 60 subjects older than 65 years (mean age: 79 years) living in nursing homes demonstrated that hearing loss affects the communication, sociability, and psychological aspects of quality of life (Tsuruoka et al, 2001).*
- ▲ Refer for psychotherapy and possible medication if the etiology is depression. *Geriatric depression is a common but frequently unrecognized or inadequately treated condition in the elderly population. Nonpharmacological and pharmacological treatment options for managing depression are available (Lapid & Rummans, 2003).*
- ▲ Refer for possible medication therapy when the diagnosis is dementia. **EB:** *In this retrospective cohort study of residents with dementia in nursing homes, there were 1449 users of tacrine and 6119 nonusers of tacrine. Tacrine was associated with lower mortality (Ott & Lapane, 2002).*

F

## evolve WEBSITES FOR EDUCATION

See the EVOLVE website for World Wide Web resources for client education.

## REFERENCES

Ai AL, Peterson C, Tice TN et al: Faith-based and secular pathways to hope and optimism subconstructs in middle-aged and older cardiac patients, *J Health Psychol* 9(3):435-450, 2004.

Altus DE, Engelman KK, Mathews RM: Using family-style meals to increase participation and communication in persons with dementia, *J Gerontol Nurs* 28(9):47-53, 2002.

Baldelli MV, Boiardi R, Ferrari P et al: Evaluation of the nutritional status during stay in the subacute care nursing home, *Arch Gerontol Geriatr* (Suppl 9):39, 2004.

Bates J, Boote J, Beverley C: Psychosocial interventions for people with a milder dementing illness: a systematic review, *J Adv Nurs* 45(6):644-658 (41 ref), 2004.

Bergland A, Kirkevold M: Thriving—a useful theoretical perspective to capture the experience of well-being among frail elderly in nursing homes? *J Adv Nurs* 36(3):426-432, 2001.

Bland R, Darlington Y: The nature and sources of hope: perspectives of family caregivers of people with serious mental illness, *Perspect Psychiatr Care* 38(2):61, 2002.

Buettner LL, Fitzsimmons S: AD-venture program: therapeutic biking for the treatment of depression in long-term care residents with dementia, *Am J Alzheimers Dis Other Demen* 17(2):121-127, 2002.

Bush E: The use of human touch to improve the well-being of older adults: a holistic nursing intervention, *J Holist Nurs* 19(3): 256-270, 2001.

Cabranes JA, De Juan R, Encinas M et al: Relevance of functional neuroimaging in the progression of mild cognitive impairment, *Neurol Res* 26(5):496-501, 2004.

Casten RJ, Rovner BW, Edmonds SE: The impact of depression in older adults with age-related macular degeneration, *J Vis Impair Blindness* 96(6):399, 2002.

Chen CC, Schilling LS, Lyder CH: A concept analysis of malnutrition in the elderly, *J Adv Nurs* 36(1):131-142, 2001.
Cochran M: Tears have no color, *Am J Nurs* 98(6):53, 1998.
Cowan DT, Roberts JD, Fitzpatrick JM: Nutritional status of older people in long term care settings: current status and future directions, *Int J Nurs Stud* (3):225-237, 2004.
Crogan NL, Corbett CF, Short RA: The minimum data set: predicting malnutrition in newly admitted nursing home residents, *Clin Nurs Res* 11(3):341, 2002.
Davis HS, Rockwood K: Conceptualization of mild cognitive impairment: a review, *Int J Geriatr Psychiatry* 19(4):313-319, 2004.
De Jong N: Sensible aging: using nutrient-dense foods and physical exercise with the frail elderly, *Nutr Today* 36(4):202, 2001.
Doswell W, Erlen J: Multicultural issues and ethical concerns in the delivery of revising care interventions, *Nurs Clin North Am* 33(2):353, 1998.
Ebenstein H, Worthan J: The value of pets in geriatric practice: a program example, *J Gerontol Soc Work* 35(2):99-115, 2001.
Edvardsson JD, Sandman P, Rasmussen RH: Meanings of giving touch in the care of older patients: becoming a valuable person and professional, *J Clin Nurs* 12(4):601-609, 2003.
Ennis BW, Saffel-Shrier S, Verson H: Diagnosing malnutrition in the elderly, *Nurse Pract* 26(3):52, 2001.
Giasson M, Leroux G, Tardif H et al: Therapeutic touch, *Infirm Que* 6(6):38-47, 1999.
Gosline MB: Client participation to enhance socialization for frail elders, *Geriatr Nurs* 24(5):286-289, 2003.
Guarnaccia P: Multicultural experiences of family caregiving: a Study of African American, European American, and Hispanic American families, *New Direct Ment Health Serv* 77:45, 1998.
Hawranik P, Deatrich J, Johnston P: Therapeutic touch: another approach for the management of agitation, *Can Nurs Home* 15(1):46-48, 2004.
Heineken J: Patient silence is not necessarily client satisfaction: communication in home care nursing, *Home Healthcare Nurse* 16(2):115, 1998.
Hodgkinson B, Evans D, Wood J: Maintaining oral hydration in older adults: a systematic review, *Int J Nurs Pract* 9(3):S19-S28, 2003.
Holt PR: Diarrhea and malabsorption in the elderly, *Gastroenterol Clin North Am* 30(2):427, 2001.
Insel KC, Badger TA: Deciphering the 4 D's: cognitive decline, delirium, depression and dementia—a review, *J Adv Nurs* 38(4):360, 2002.
Irvine KN, Warber SL: Greening healthcare: practicing as if the natural environment really mattered, *Altern Ther Health Med* 8(5):76, 2002.
Johnson RA, Odendaal JS, Meadows RL: Animal-assisted interventions research: issues and answers, *West J Nurs Res* 24(4):422, 2002.
Kahan FS, Paris BE: Why elder abuse continues to elude the health care system, *Mt Sinai J Med* 70(1):62, 2003.
Kanich W, Brady WJ, Huff JS et al: Altered mental status: evaluation and etiology in the ED, *Am J Emerg Med* 20(7):613-617, 2002.
Kono A, Kai I, Sakato C et al: Frequency of going outdoors: a predictor of functional and psychosocial change among ambulatory frail elders living at home, *J Gerontol A Biol Sci Med Sci* 59(3):275-280, 2004.
Lai H: Music preference and relaxation in Taiwanese elderly people, *Geriatr Nurs* 25(5):286-291, 2004.
Leininger MM, McFarland MR: *Transcultural nursing: concepts, theories, research and practices,* ed 3, New York, 2002, McGraw-Hill.
Lapid MI, Rummans TA: Evaluation and management of geriatric depression in primary care, *Mayo Clin Proc* 78(11):1423-1429, 2003.
Lieberman R: HIV in older Americans: an epidemiologic perspective, *J Midwifery Womens Health* 45(2):176, 2000.
Loeher KE, Bank AL, MacNeill SE: Nursing home transition and depressive symptoms in older medical rehabilitation patients, *Clin Gerontol* 27(1/2):59-70, 2004.
Loughlin A: Depression and social support: effective treatments for homebound elderly adults. *J Gerontol Nurs* 30(5):11-15, 2004.
McDaniel JH et al: Impact of dining room environment on nutritional intake of Alzheimer's residents: a case study, *Am J Alzheimers Dis Other Demen* 16(5):297, 2001.
McKee KJ, Wilson F, Elford H et al: Reminiscence: is living in the past good for wellbeing? *Nurs Residential Care* 5(10):489-491, 2003.
Murrock CJ: The effects of music on the rate of perceived exertion and general mood among coronary artery bypass graft patients enrolled in cardiac rehabilitation phase II, *Rehabil Nurs* 27(6):227, 2002.
Ott BR, Lapane KL: Tacrine therapy is associated with reduced mortality in nursing home residents with dementia, *J Am Geriatr Soc* 50(1):35, 2002.

Patusky KL, Rodning C, Martinez-Kratz M: Clinical lessons in psychiatric home care: a case study approach, *J Home Healthcare Manag* 9:18, 1996.
Penninx BW, Guralnik JM, Bandeen-Roche K et al: The protective effect of emotional vitality on adverse health outcomes in disabled older women, *J Am Geriatr Soc* 48(11):1359-1366, 2000.
Ragneskog H, Brane G, Karlsson I et al: Influence of dinner music on food intake and symptoms common in dementia, *Scand J Caring Sci* 10(1):11-17, 1996.
Resnick B: Functional performance of older adults in a long-term care setting, *Clin Nurs Res* 7(3):230, 1998.
Reichman S, Leonard C, Mintz T et al: Compiling life history resources for older adults in institutions: development of a guide, *J Gerontol Nurs* 30(2):20-28, 55-56, 2004.
Schillerstrom JE, Seaman JS: Modafinil augmentation of mirtazapine in a failure-to-thrive geriatric inpatient, *Int J Psychiatry Med* 32(4):405-410, 2002.
Sharkey JR, Schoenberg NE: Variations in nutritional risk among black and white women who receive home-delivered meals, *J Women Aging* 14(3-4):99-119, 2002.
Shimada H, Uchiyama Y, Kakurai S: Specific effects of balance and gait exercises on physical function among the frail elderly, *Clin Rehabil* 17(5):472-479, 2003.
Sinclair AJ, Gadsby R, Penfold S et al: Prevalence of diabetes in care home residents, *Diabetes Care* 24(6):1066-1068, 2001.
Still C, Apovian C, Jensen G: Failure to thrive in older adults, *Ann Intern Med* 126(8):668, 1997.
Sumaya IC, Rienzi BM, Deegan JF, II et al: Bright light treatment decreases depression in institutionalized older adults: a placebo-controlled crossover study, *J Gerontol A Biol Sci Med Sci* 56(6):M356-M360, 2001.
Suzuki M, Kanamori M, Watanabe M et al: Behavioral and endocrinological evaluation of music therapy for elderly patients with dementia, *Nurs Health Sci* 6(1):11-18, 2004.
Syddall H, Cooper C, Martin F: Is grip strength a useful single marker of frailty? *Age Ageing* 32(6):650-656, 2003.
Tan EJ, Lui LY, Eng C: Differences in mortality of black and white patients enrolled in the program of all-inclusive care for the elderly, *J Am Geriatri Soc* 51(2):246-251, 2003.
Van de Winckel A, Feys H, De Weerdt W et al: Cognitive and behavioural effects of music-based exercises in patients with dementia, *Clin Rehabil* 18(3):253-260, 2004.
Wikby K, Fagerskiold A: The willingness to eat. An investigation of appetite among elderly people, *Scand J Caring Sci* 18:120, 2004.

# Risk for Falls

evolve

*Betty J. Ackley*

**NANDA**

## Definition

Increased susceptibility to falling that may cause physical harm

## Risk Factors

### Adults

History of falls; wheelchair use; 65 years of age or older; female (if elderly); lives alone; lower limb prosthesis; use of assistive devices (e.g., walker, cane)

### Physiological

Presence of acute illness; postoperative conditions; visual difficulties; hearing difficulties; arthritis; orthostatic hypotension; sleeplessness; faintness when turning or extending neck; anemias; vascular disease; neoplasms (i.e., fatigue/limited mobility, urgency and/or incontinence, diarrhea, decreased lower extremity strength, postprandial blood sugar changes, foot problems, impaired physical mobility, impaired balance, difficulty with gait, unilateral neglect, proprioceptive deficits, neuropathy); diminished mental status (e.g., confusion, delirium, dementia, impaired reality testing)

### Medication

Antihypertensive agents; angiotensin-converting enzyme (ACE) inhibitors; diuretics; tricyclic antidepressants; alcohol use; antianxiety agents; opiates; hypnotics or tranquilizers

### Environment

Restraints; weather conditions (e.g., wet floors/ice); throw/scatter rugs; cluttered environment; unfamiliar, dimly lit room; no antislip material in bath and/or shower

### Children (<2 Years of Age)

Male gender when younger than 1 year, lack of auto restraints, lack of gate on stairs, lack of window guard, bed located near window, unattended infant on bed/changing table/sofa, lack of parental supervision

## Related Factors (r/t)

See Risk Factors

**NOC**

## Outcomes (Nursing Outcomes Classification)

### Suggested NOC Outcomes

Fall Prevention Behavior; Knowledge: Child Physical Safety

**Example NOC Outcome with Indicators**

**Fall Prevention Behavior** as evidenced by the following indicators: Uses assistive devices correctly/ Elimination of clutter, spills, glare from floors/Uses safe transfer procedures (Rate each indicator of **Fall Prevention Behavior:** 1 = never demonstrated, 2 = rarely demonstrated, 3 = sometimes demonstrated, 4 = often demonstrated, 5 = consistently demonstrated [see Section I].)

## Client Outcomes

### Client Will (Specify Time Frame):

- Remain free of falls
- Change environment to minimize the incidence of falls
- Explain methods to prevent injury

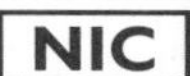

## Interventions (Nursing Interventions Classification)

### Suggested NIC Interventions

Dementia Management; Fall Prevention; Surveillance: Safety

**Example NIC Activities—Fall Prevention**

Assist unsteady individual with ambulation; monitor gait, balance, and fatigue level with ambulation

F

## Nursing Interventions and Rationales

- Determine risk of falling by using an evaluation tool such as the Fall Risk Assessment (Farmer, 2000), The Conley Scale (Conley et al, 1999), or the FRAINT Tool for fall risk assessment (Parker, 2000). *Risk factors for falling include recent history of falls, confusion, depression, altered elimination patterns, cardiovascular/respiratory disease impairing perfusion or oxygenation, postural hypotension, dizziness or vertigo, primary cancer diagnosis, and altered mobility (Farmer, 2000; Hendrich et al, 1995). Predictors of fall risk in the community included atrial fibrillation, neurological problems, living alone, and not adhering to a regular exercise program (Resnick, 1999).*
- Screen all clients for stability and mobility skills (supine to sit, sitting supported and unsupported, sit to stand, standing, walking and turning around, transferring, stooping to floor and recovering, and sitting down). Use tools such as the Balance Scale by Tinetti or the Get Up and Go Scale by Mathais. *It is helpful to determine the client's functional abilities and then plan for ways to improve problem areas or determine methods to ensure safety (MacKnight & Rockwood, 1996; Tinetti, 2003).*
- Recognize that when people attend to another task while walking, such as carrying a cup of water, clothing, or supplies, they are more likely to fall. **EB:** *Those who slow down when given a carrying task are at a higher risk for subsequent falls (Lundin-Olsson et al, 1998).*
- Be careful when getting a mostly immobile client up. Be sure to lock the bed and wheelchair and have sufficient personnel to protect the client from falls. *The most important preventive measure to reduce the risk of injurious falls for nonambulatory residents involves increasing safety measures while transferring, including careful locking of equipment such as wheelchairs and beds before moves (Thapa et al, 1996). These immobile clients commonly sustain the most serious injuries when they fall.*
- Identify clients likely to fall by placing a "Fall Precautions" sign on the doorway and by keying the Kardex and chart. Use a "high-risk fall" armband and room sign to alert staff for increased vigilance and mobility assistance. *These steps alert the nursing staff of the increased risk of falls (McCarter-Bayer, Bayer, & Hall, 2005).*

▲ If necessary to place the client in a wrist or vest restraint with an order from the physician, use increased vigilance and watch for falls. *The risk of falling is highest soon after a client has been placed in a mechanical restraint (Arbesman & Wright, 1999).*

• = Independent; ▲ = Collaborative; EBN = Evidence-Based Nursing; EB = Evidence-Based

F

- ▲ Evaluate the client's medications to determine whether medications increase the risk of falling; consult with physician regarding the client's need for medication if appropriate. *Polypharmacy, or taking more than four medications, has been associated with increased falls. Medications such as benzodiazepines and antipsychotic and antidepressant medications given to promote sleep actually increase the rate of falls (Capezuti, 1999b).* **EB:** *Use of selective serotonin reuptake inhibitors and tricyclic antidepressants resulted in increased incidences of falls (Liu et al, 1998; Thapa et al, 1998).*
- • Thoroughly orient the client to environment. Place the call light within reach and show how to call for assistance; answer call light promptly.
- • Use one quarter– to one half–length side rails only, and maintain bed in a low position. Ensure that wheels are locked on bed and commode. Keep dim light in room at night. *Use of full side rails can result in the client climbing over the rails, leading with the head, and sustaining a head injury. Side rails with widely spaced vertical bars and side rails not situated flush with the mattress have been associated with asphyxiation deaths because of rail and in bed entrapment and should not be used (Capezuti, 2004; Hanger et al, 1999; Todd et al, 1997).*
- • Routinely assist the client with toileting on his or her own schedule. Always take the client to bathroom on awakening, before bedtime, and before administering sedatives (McCarter-Bayer, Bayer, & Hall, 2005; Wilson, 1998). Keep the path to the bathroom clear, label the bathroom, and leave the door open. *The majority of falls are related to toileting. It is more acceptable to fall than to "wet yourself." Studies have indicated that falls are often linked to the need to eliminate in a hurry (Wilson, 1998).*
- ▲ Avoid use of restraints if at all possible. Obtain a physician's order if restraints are necessary. *The use of restraints has been associated with serious injuries including rhabdomyolysis, brachial plexus injury, neuropathy, dysrhythmias, as well as strangulation, asphyxiation, traumatic brain injuries and all the consequences of immobility (Capezuti, 2004). Restraint-free extended care facilities were shown to have fewer residents with ADLs deficiencies and fewer residents with bowel or bladder incontinence than facilities that use restraints (Castle & Fogel, 1998).* **EBN and EB:** *A study demonstrated that there was no increase in falls or injuries in a group of clients that were not restrained, versus a similar group that was restrained in a nursing home (Capezuti et al, 1999b). Restrained elderly clients often experience an increased number of falls, possibly as a result of muscle deconditioning or loss of coordination (Tinetti, Liu, & Ginter, 1992).* **EB:** *A study in two acute care hospitals demonstrated that when restraints were not used, there was no increase in client falls, injuries or therapy disruptions (Mion et al, 2001).*
- • In place of restraints, use the following:
  - Well-staffed and educated nursing personnel with frequent client contact
  - Nursing units designed to care for clients with cognitive or functional impairments
  - Nonskid footwear
  - Alarm systems with ankle, above the knee, or wrist sensors
  - Bed or wheelchair alarms
  - Increased observation of the client
  - Locked doors to unit
  - Low or very low height beds
  - Border-defining pillow/mattress to remind the client to stay in bed

*These alternatives to restraints can be helpful to prevent falls (McCarter-Bayer, Bayer, & Hall, 2005; Capezuti, 2004; Capezuti et al, 1999a).*

- If the client has a new onset of confusion (delirium), recognize that the cause is usually physiological and is a medical emergency. Provide reality orientation when interacting. Have family bring in familiar items, clocks, and watches from home to maintain orientation. *Reality orientation can help prevent or decrease the confusion that increases risk of falling for clients with delirium.* See interventions for **Acute Confusion.**
- If the client has chronic confusion with dementia, use validation therapy that reinforces feelings but does not confront reality. *Validation therapy is effective for clients with dementia (Fine & Rouse-Bane, 1995).* See interventions for **Chronic Confusion.**
- Ask family to stay with the client to prevent the client from accidentally falling or pulling out tubes.
- If the client is unsteady on feet, use a walking belt or two nursing staff members when ambulating the client. *The client can walk independently with a walking belt, but the nurse can rapidly ensure safety if the knees buckle.*
- Place a fall-prone client in a room that is near the nurses' station. *Such placement allows more frequent observation of the client.*
- Help clients sit in a stable chair with arm rests. Avoid use of wheelchairs and geri-chairs except for transportation as needed. *Clients are likely to fall when left in a wheelchair or geri-chair because they may stand up without locking the wheels or removing the footrests. Wheelchairs do not increase mobility; people just sit in them the majority of the time (Lipson & Braun, 1993; Simmons et al, 1995).*
- Ensure that the chair or wheelchair fits the build, abilities, and needs of the client to ensure propulsion with legs or arms and ability to reach the floor, eliminating footrests and minimizing problems with shearing. *The seating system should fit the needs of the client so that the client can move the wheels, stand up from the chair without falling, and not be harmed by the chair. Footrests can cause skin tears and bruising, as well as postural alignment and sitting posture problems (Nelson et al, 2004; Rader et al, 2000).*
- Avoid use of wheelchairs as much as possible because they can serve as a restraint device. Most people in wheelchairs do not move. *Wheelchairs unfortunately serve as a restraint device.* **EB:** *A study has shown that only 4% of residents in wheelchairs were observed to propel them independently and only 45% could propel them, even with cues and prompts. Another study showed that no residents could unlock wheelchairs without help, the wheelchairs were not fitted to residents, and residents were not trained in propulsion (Simmons et al, 1995).*

▲ Refer to physical therapy for strengthening exercises, gait training, and help with balance to increase mobility. **EB:** *Balance, gait training, and strengthening exercises in physical therapy have been shown to be effective for preventing falls (Gillespie et al, 2005; Robertson et al, 2001).*

## Geriatric

- Assess ability to move using the Get Up and Go test. Ask the client to rise from a sitting position, walk 10 feet, turn, and return to the chair to sit. *Performance on this screening exam demonstrates the client's mobility and ability to leave the house safely. If the client completes the test in less than 20 seconds, they usually can live independently. If*



F

*completing the test takes longer than 30 seconds are more likely to be dependant on others, and more likely to sustain a fall (Robertson & Montagnini, 2004).*

- If new onset of falling, check blood pressure and pulse rate supine, sitting, and standing for orthostatic hypotension. *If orthostatic hypotension is present and there is minimal change in the heart rate, most likely the baroreceptors are not working to maintain blood pressure on arising. This is common in the elderly and can be from cardiovascular disease, neurological disease, or a medication effect (Sclater & Kannayiram, 2004).*
- Encourage the client to wear glasses and use walking aids when ambulating.
- Help the client obtain and wear a specially designed hip protector when ambulating. Hip protectors are worn in a specially designed stretchy undergarment containing a pocket on each side for placement of the protector. **EB:** *A Cochrane review suggested that hip protectors were effective for vulnerable clients in institutions (Parker et al, 2004). A study suggested that the use of external hip protectors could reduce hip fractures among older adults at risk (Heikinheimo, Jalonen-Mannikko, Asumaniemi, et al, 2004).*
- If the client experiences dizziness because of orthostatic hypotension when getting up, teach methods to decrease dizziness, such as rising slowly, remaining seated several minutes before standing, flexing feet upward several times while sitting, sitting down immediately if feeling dizzy, and trying to have someone present when standing. *Always have the client dangle at the bedside before trying standing to evaluate for postural hypotension. Watch the client closely for dizziness during increased activity. Postural hypotension can be detected in up to 30% of elderly clients. These methods can help prevent falls (Tinetti, 2003).*

▲ If the client is experiencing syncope, determine symptoms that occur before syncope, and note medications that the client is taking. Refer for medical care. The circumstances surrounding syncope often suggest the cause. *Use of many medications, including diuretics, antihypertensives, digoxin, beta-blockers, and calcium channel blockers can cause syncope. Use of the tilt table can be diagnostic in incidences of syncope (Cox, 2000).*

▲ Observe client for signs of anemia, and refer to primary care practitioner for testing if appropriate. **EB:** *One study demonstrated that elderly clients with mild anemia had a three times increased incidence of falls (Dharmarajan & Norkus, 2004).*

▲ Evaluate client for chronic alcohol intake, as well as mental health and neurologic function. **EBN:** *A study of falls in a community of older adults found that age, gender, neurological disease, mental health, and regular use of alcohol significantly influenced the rate of falls (Resnick & Junlapeeya, 2004).*

▲ Refer to physical therapy for strength training, using free weights or machines. *Strength improvement in response to resisted exercise is possible even in the very elderly, extremely sedentary client, with multiple chronic diseases and functional disabilities. Increased strength can help prevent falls (Connelly, 2000).*

▲ If an elderly woman has symptoms of urge incontinence, refer to a urologist for evaluation and ensure the path to the bathroom is well lit and free of obstructions. *Urge urinary incontinence was associated with an increased incidence of falls in older women (Brown et al, 2000).*

## Home Care

- Some of the above interventions may be adapted for home care use.
- If the client was identified as a fall risk in the hospital, recognize that there is a high

incidence of falls after discharge, and use all measures possible to reduce the incidence of falls. **EBN:** *The rate of falls is substantially increased in the geriatric client who has been recently hospitalized, especially during the first month after discharge (Mahoney et al, 2000).*

- Assess and monitor for acute changes in cognition and behavior. *An acute change in cognition and behavior is the classic presentation of delirium. Delirium is reversible and should be considered a medical emergency. Delirium can become chronic if untreated, and clients may be discharged from hospitals to home care in states of undiagnosed delirium.* **EBN:** *Falls may be a precipitating event or an indication of frailty consistent with acute confusion (Mentes et al, 1999).*
- Assess for additional factors leading to risk for falls. **EB:** *A study of individuals receiving home care services found that risk factors included medical history (neurological and cardiovascular impairments); medication usage (antipsychotic and tricyclic antidepressant medications); and fall history (fall recurrence during the preceding 3 months) (Lewis et al, 2004).*
- Assess home environment for threats to safety: clutter, slippery floors, scatter rugs, unsafe stairs and stairwells, blocked entries, extension cords (across pathway), high beds, pets, and pet excrement. Use antiskid acrylic floor wax, nonskid rugs, use of stair rails, and skid-proof strips near the bed to prevent slippage. Evaluate need for safety devices in bathing area (e.g., hand grip, shower chair, hand-held showerhead). *Clients suffering from impaired mobility, impaired visual acuity, and neurological dysfunction, including dementia and other cognitive functional deficits, are all at risk for injury from common hazards. These recommendations were shown to be effective to reduce falls (Tinetti, 2003).*

▲ Institute a home-based, nurse-delivered exercise program to reduce falls or refer to physical therapy services for client and family education of safe transfers and ambulation and for strengthening exercises (for the client). *A home-based, nurse-delivered exercise program was effective in reducing the number of falls, especially in clients over 80 years of age (Robertson et al, 2001).* **EBN:** *A meta-analysis of studies demonstrated a 4% reduction in the rate of falls in individuals who received fall prevention programs (Hill-Westmoreland et al, 2002).*

▲ Instruct the client and family or caregivers on how to correct identified hazards. Refer to occupational therapy services for assistance if needed. **EB:** *Home visits by a health professional to assess and modify the home environment have been shown to be effective to reduce the number of falls (Gillespie et al, 2005).*

▲ Use a multifactorial assessment along with interventions targeted to the identified risk factors. Key components of the interventions include evaluating need for all medications, balance, gait and strength training, use of strategies to deal with postural hypotension if present, home safety evaluation with needed modifications, and any needed cardiovascular treatment. **EB:** *The use of a multifactorial assessment along with interventions identified has been shown to be very effective in reducing the number of falls (Close et al, 1999; Tinetti et al, 1994).*

- Encourage the client to eat a balanced diet, with particular inclusion of vitamin D and calcium. *Hypovitaminosis D and hypocalcemia are common in older adults, contributing to falls, musculoskeletal complaints, and functional and mobility deficits (Dharmarajan et al, 2001).*
- If the client lives alone or spends a lot of time alone, teach the client what to do if he

or she falls and cannot get up, and make sure he or she has a personal emergency response system or a cellular phone that is available from the floor (Tinetti, 2003). If the client is at risk for falls, use gait belt and additional persons when ambulating. *Gait belts decrease the risk of falls during ambulation.* **EBN:** *Be aware that clients may react ambivalently to a personal emergency response system. A study showed that, while the system alleviated some anxiety about ability to receive help, concern was also expressed about being shocked by hearing strangers enter the home (Porter, 2003).*

F

- Ensure appropriate nonglare lighting in the home. Ask the client to install indoor strip or "runway" type of lighting to baseboards to help clients balance. Install motion-sensitive lighting that turns on automatically when the client gets out of bed to go to the bathroom. *Up to 79% of the elderly have inadequate lighting in their homes predisposing them to falls (Slay, 2002). The disorientation of waking in the dark could affect the client's balance. Caregiver may be alerted by light that the client is awake and out of bed.*
- Have the client wear supportive low-heeled shoes with good traction when ambulating. *Supportive shoes provide the client with better balance and protect the client from instability on uneven surfaces.*
- Consider the use of external hip protectors for clients at risk of falls. **EB:** *A study suggested that the use of external hip protectors could reduce hip fractures among older adults at risk (Heikinheimo et al, 2004).*
- ▲ Refer to physical therapy services for the client and family education of safe transfers and ambulation and for strengthening/balance exercises (for the client) for ambulation and transfers. **EB:** *A program of muscle strengthening and balance training taught by a professional have been shown effective to reduce falls (Gillespie et al, 2005).*
- Provide a signaling device for clients who wander or are at risk for falls. *Orienting a vulnerable client to a safety net relieves anxiety of the client and caregiver and allows for rapid response to a crisis situation.*
- Provide medical identification bracelet for clients at risk for injury from dementia, seizures, or other medical disorders.
- Suggest a T'ai chi class designed for the elderly to selected clients who have sufficient balance to participate. *Functional balance can be improved by tai chi (Geriatrics, 2005).* **EB:** *One study demonstrated that elderly who participated in a T'ai chi class had half the number of falls as elderly clients who did not (Wolf et al, 1996).*

## Client/Family Teaching

- Teach the client how to safely ambulate at home, including using safety measures such as hand rails in bathroom, and need to avoid carrying things or performing other tasks while walking. *In the frail elderly, multitasking results in decreased motor performance and may lead to falls (Hauer et al, 2002).*
- Teach the client the importance of maintaining a regular exercise program such as walking. *Lack of a consistent exercise program was one of the variables associated with a higher incidence of falls (Resnick, 1999).*

## evolve WEBSITES FOR EDUCATION

See the EVOLVE website for World Wide Web resources for client education.

• = Independent; ▲ = Collaborative; EBN = Evidence-Based Nursing; EB = Evidence-Based

## REFERENCES


Arbesman MD, Wright C: Mechanical restraints, rehabilitation therapies, and staffing adequacy as risk factors for falls in an elderly hospitalized population, *Rehabil Nurs* 24(3):122, 1999.

Brown JS, Vittinghoff E, Wyman JF et al: Urinary incontinence: does it increase risk for falls and fractures? Study of Osteoporotic Fractures Research Group, *J Am Geriatr Soc* 48(7):721, 2000.

Capezuti E: Minimizing the use of restrictive devices in dementia patients at risk for falling, *Nurs Clin North Am* 39:625, 2004.

Capezuti E, Talerico KA, Cochran I et al: Individualized interventions to prevent bed-related falls and reduce siderail use, *J Gerontol Nurs* 25(11):26, 1999a.

Capezuti E, Strumpf N, Evans I et al: Outcomes of nighttime physical restraint removal for severely impaired nursing home residents, *Am J Alzheimers Dis Other Demen* 14(3):157, 1999b.

Castle NG, Fogel B: Characteristics of nursing homes that are restraint free, *Gerontologist* 38(2):181, 1998.

Close J, Ellis M, Hooper R et al: Prevention of falls in the elderly trial (PROFET): a randomized controlled trial, *Lancet* 353:93, 1999.

Conley D, Schultz AA, Selvin R: The challenge of predicting patients at risk for falling: development of the Conley Scale, *Medsurg Nurs* 8(6):348, 1999.

Connelly DM: Resisted exercise training of institutionalized older adults for improved strength and functional mobility: a review, *Top Geriatr Rehabil* 15(3):6, 2000.

Cox MM: Uncovering the cause of syncope, *Patient Care* 30:39, 2000.

Dharmarajan TS, Norkus EP: Mild anemia and the risk of falls in older adults from nursing homes and the community, *J Am Med Dir Assoc* 5(6):395, 2004.

Dharmarajan TS, Ahmed S, Russell RO: Recurrent falls from hypocalcemia due to vitamin D deficiency: a preventable problem in home care, *Home Healthc Consult* 8(8):8, 2001.

Farmer BC: Try this: fall risk assessment, *J Gerontol Nurs* 26(7):6, 2000.

Fine JI, Rouse-Bane S: Using validating techniques to improve communication with cognitively impaired older adults, *J Gerontol Nurs* 21:39, 1995.

Functional balance can be improved by tai chi, *Geriatrics* 60(2), 2005.

Gillespie LD, Gillespie WJ, Robertson MC et al: Interventions for preventing falls in elderly people, *Cochrane Database Syst Rev* (3):CD000340, 2005.

Hanger HC, Ball MC, Wood LA: An analysis of falls in the hospital: can we do without bedrails? *J Am Geriatr Soc* 47(5):529, 1999.

Hauer K, Marburger C, Oster P: Motor performance deteriorates with simultaneously performed cognitive tasks in geriatric patients, *Arch Phys Med Rehabil* 83(2):217, 2002.

Heikinheimo R, Jalonen-Mannikko A, Asumaniemi H et al: External hip protectors in home-dwelling older persons, *Aging Clin Exp Res* 16:41, 2004.

Hill-Westmoreland EE, Soeken K, Spellbring AM: A meta-analysis of fall prevention programs for the elderly: how effective are they? *Nurs Res* 51(1):1, 2002.

Lewis BJ et al: *The functional tool book,* Washington, DC, 1994, Learn.

Lipson J, Braun S: *Toward a restraint-free environment: reducing the use of physical and chemical restraint in long-term care and acute settings,* Baltimore, 1993, Health Professions Press.

Lewis CL, Moutoux M, Slaughter M et al: Characteristics of individuals who fell while receiving home health services, *Phys Ther* 84(1):23, 2004.

Liu B, Anderson G, Mittmann N et al: Use of selective serotonin-reuptake inhibitors of tricyclic antidepressants and risk for hip fractures in elderly people, *Lancet* 351(9112):1303, 1998.

Lundin-Olsson L, Nysberg L, Gustafson Y: Attention, frailty, and falls: the effect of a manual task on basic mobility, *J Am Geriatr Soc* 46:758, 1998.

MacKnight C, Rockwood K: Mobility and balance in the elderly: a guide to bedside assessment, *Postgrad Med* 99(3):269, 1996.

Mahoney JE, Palta M, Johnson J et al: Temporal association between hospitalization and rate of falls after discharge, *Arch Intern Med* 160(18):2788, 2000.

McCarter-Bayer A, Bayer F, Hall K: Preventing falls in acute care: an innovative approach, *J Gerontol Nurs* 31(3):25, 2005.

Mentes J, Culp K, Maas M et al: Acute confusion indicators: risk factors and prevalence using MDS data, *Res Nurs Health* 22:95, 1999.

Mion LC, Fogel J, Sandhu S et al: Outcomes following physical restraint reduction programs in two acute care hospitals, *Joint Comm J Qual Improv* 27(11):605, 2001.

Nelson A: Technology to promote safe mobility in the elderly, *Nurs Clin North Am* 39:649, 2004.

Parker MJ, Gillespie LD, Gillespie WJ: Hip protectors for preventing hip fractures in the elderly, *Cochrane Database Syst Rev* (3): CD001255, 2004.
Parker R: Assessing the risk of falls among older inpatients, *Prof Nurse* 15(8):511, 2000.
Porter EJ: Moments of apprehension in the midst of a certainty: Some frail older widows' lives with a personal emergency response system, *Qual Health Res* 13(9):1311, 2003.
Rader J, Jones D, Miller L: The importance of individualized wheelchair seating for frail older adults, *J Gerontol Nurs* 26(11):24, 2000.
Resnick B: Falls in a community of older adults, *Clin Nurs Res* 8(3):251, 1999.
Resnick B, Junlapeeya P: Falls in a community of older adults: findings and implications for practice, *Appl Nurs Res* 17(2):81, 2004.
Robertson MC, Devlin N, Gardner MM et al: Effectiveness and economic evaluation of a nurse delivered home exercise programme to prevent falls. 1: Randomised controlled trial, *BMJ* 322(7288):697, 2001.
Robertson RG, Montagnini M: Geriatric failure to thrive, *Am Family Physician* 70(2):343, 2004.
Sclater A, Kannayiram A: Orthostatic hypotension: a primary care primer for assessment and treatment, *Geriatrics* 59(8), 2004.
Simmons SF, Schnelle JF, MacRae PG et al: Wheelchairs as mobility restraints: predictors of wheelchair activity in nonambulatory nursing home residents, *J Am Geriatr Soc* 43:384, 1995.
Slay DH: Home-based environmental lighting assessments for people who are visually impaired: developing techniques and tools, *J Vis Impair Blindness* 96(2):109, 2002.
Thapa PB, Brockman KG, Gideon P et al: Injurious falls in nonambulatory nursing home residents: a comparative study of circumstances, incidence, and risk factors, *J Am Geriatr Soc* 44:273, 1996.
Thapa PB, Gideon P, Cost TW et al: Antidepressants and the risk of falls among nursing home residents, *N Engl J Med* 339(13): 875, 1998.
Tinetti ME: Preventing falls in elderly persons, *N Engl J Med* 348(1):42, 2003.
Tinetti ME, Liu WL, Ginter SF: Mechanical restraint use and fall-related injuries among residents of skilled nursing facilities, *Ann Intern Med* 116:369, 1992.
Tinetti ME, Baker DI, McAvay G et al: A multifactorial intervention to reduce the risk of falling among elderly people living in the community, *N Engl J Med* 331:821, 1994.
Todd JF, Ruhl CE, Gross TP: Injury and death associated with hospital bed side-rails: reports of the U.S. Food and Drug Administration from 1985 to 1995, *Am J Public Health* 87(10):1675, 1997.
Wilson EB: Preventing patient falls, *AACN Clin Issues* 9(1):100, 1998.
Wolf SL, Barnhart HX, Kutner NG et al: Reducing frailty and falls in older persons: an investigation of tai chi and computerized balance training, *J Am Geriatr Soc* 44:489, 1996.

# Dysfunctional Family processes: alcoholism

evolve

*Gail B. Ladwig*

**NANDA**

## Definition

The state in which the psychosocial, spiritual, and physiological functions of the family unit are chronically disorganized, leading to conflict, denial of problems, resistance to change, ineffective problem solving, and a series of self-perpetuating crises

## Defining Characteristics

### Roles and Relationships

Inconsistent parenting/low perception of parental support, ineffective spouse communication/marital problems, intimacy dysfunction, deterioration in family relationships/disturbed family dynamics, altered role function/disruption of family roles, closed communication systems, chronic family problems, family denial, lack of cohesiveness, neglected obligations, lack of skills necessary for relationships, reduced ability of family members to relate to each other for mutual growth and maturation, family unable to meet security needs of its members, disrupted family rituals, economic problems, family does not demonstrate respect for individuality and autonomy of its members, triangulating family relationships, pattern of rejection

### Behavioral

Refusal to get help/inability to accept and receive help appropriately; inadequate understanding or knowledge of alcoholism; ineffective problem-solving skills; loss of control of drinking; manipulation; rationalization/denial of problems; blaming; inability to meet emotional needs of its members; alcohol abuse; broken promises; criticizing; dependency; impaired communication; difficulty with intimate relationships; enabling to maintain drinking; expression of anger inappropriately; isolation; inability to meet spiritual needs of its members; inability to express or accept wide ranges of feelings; inability to deal with traumatic experiences constructively; inability to adapt to change; immaturity; harsh self-judgment; lying; lack of dealing with conflict; lack of reliability; nicotine addiction; orientation toward tension relief rather than achievement of goals; seeking approval and affirmation; difficulty having fun; agitation; chaos; contradictory, paradoxical communication; diminished physical contact; disturbances in academic performance in children; disturbances in concentration; escalating conflict; failure to accomplish current or past developmental tasks/difficulty with life cycle transitions; family special occasions are alcohol centered; controlling communication/power struggles; self-blaming; stress-related physical illnesses; substance abuse other than alcohol; unresolved grief; verbal abuse of spouse or parent

### Feelings

Insecurity; lingering resentment; mistrust; vulnerability; rejection; repressed emotions; responsibility for alcoholic's behavior; shame/embarrassment; unhappiness; powerlessness; anger/suppressed rage; anxiety, tension, or distress; emotional isolation/loneliness; frustration; guilt; hopelessness; hurt; decreased self-esteem/worthlessness; hostility; lack of identity; fear; loss; emotional control by others; misunderstood; moodiness; abandonment; being different from other people; being unloved; confused love and pity; confusion; failure; depression; dissatisfaction

## Related Factors (r/t)

Abuse of alcohol, genetic predisposition, lack of problem-solving skills, family history of alcoholism, resistance to treatment, biochemical influences, addictive personality

**NOC**

## Outcomes (Nursing Outcomes Classification)

### Suggested NOC Outcomes

Family Coping, Family Functioning, Family Health Status, Substance Addiction Consequences

**Example NOC Outcome with Indicators**

**Family Coping** as evidenced by the following indicators: Confronts/manages family problems/Seeks family assistance when appropriate (Rate each indicator of **Family Coping:** 1 = never demonstrated, 2 = rarely demonstrated, 3 = sometimes demonstrated, 4 = often demonstrated, 5 = consistently demonstrated [see Section I].)

F

## Client Outcomes

### Family/Client Will (Specify Time Frame):

- Develop relationship with nurse that demonstrates at least minimal level of trust
- Demonstrate an understanding of alcoholism as a family illness and the severity of the threat to emotional and physical health of family members
- Develop and state a belief in feasibility and effectiveness of efforts to address alcoholism
- Demonstrate change from dysfunctional patterns by moving from inappropriate to appropriate role relationships, improving cohesion among family members, decreasing conflict and social isolation, and improving coping behaviors
- Maintain improvements

NIC

## Interventions (Nursing Interventions Classification)

### Suggested NIC Interventions

Family Process Maintenance, Substance Use Treatment

**Example Activities—Family Process Maintenance**

Identify effects of role changes on family processes; assist family members to use existing support measures

## Nursing Interventions and Rationales

- When completing a family assessment, assess behaviors of alcohol abuse, loss of control of drinking, denial, nicotine addiction, impaired communication, inappropriate expression of anger, and enabling behaviors. **EBN:** *This study clinically validated the defining characteristics for altered family process alcoholism using subjects (N = 150) who completed Fehring's (1987) Clinical Diagnostic Validation (CDV) (Bartek et al, 1999).*
- Screen clients for at-risk drinking during routine primary care visits. At-risk drinking is defined as consuming an average of two or more drinks per day (chronic drinking), or two or more occasions of consuming five or more drinks in the past month (binge drinking), or, in the past month, one or more occasion of driving after consuming three or more drinks (drinking and driving). **EB:** *At least 1 in 10 patients making routine primary care visits have drinking practices that place them at risk for negative consequences from drinking. In this study, 3439 patients with advance appointments in 23 primary care practices completed a health survey before their visit (Curry et al, 2000).*

- Ask appropriate questions using an assessment tool such as FAST (Fast Alcohol Screening Test) to assess whether denial is being used in association with alcoholism or drug use. The client is asked to circle the appropriate response for each question: Less than monthly, monthly, weekly, daily, almost daily.
  1. **Men:** How often do you have EIGHT or more drinks on one occasion?
     **Women:** How often do you have SIX or more drinks on one occasion?
  2. How often during the last year have you been unable to remember what happened the night before because you had been drinking?
  3. How often during the last year have you failed to do what was normally expected of you because of drinking?
  4. In the last year has a relative or friend, or a doctor or other health worker been concerned about your drinking or suggested you cut down?

  **EB:** *The four-item FAST alcohol questionnaire had good sensitivity and specificity, across a range of settings, when the AUDIT alcohol assessment score was used as the gold standard. The FAST questionnaire is quick to administer, since more than 50% of clients are categorized using just one question (Hodgson et al, 2002). Include drug use in addition to drinking in questionnaire (Hinkin et al, 2001). T-ACE and TWEAK are modified to be used with women.* **EBN:** *Alcoholism rates are increasing in women and women may have distinct assessment risk factors (Becker & Walton-Moss, 2001).*
- Demonstrate high levels of empathy and expectancy of positive outcomes in interactions with family members. *A Swiss campaign used a short intervention approach that focused on an empathic and open discussion of drinking habits. This approach is efficient; takes little time; and, for nondependent patients, can considerably reduce the quantity of alcohol consumed (Stoll & Wick, 2000).*
- Stress individual self-focus as a first step in problem resolution. **EBN:** *Health Beliefs Model Research confirms that client understanding of the severity of the threat to personal and family health and a belief in the feasibility and effectiveness of treatment are important motivating factors in changing health-related behavior (Giuffra, 1993; Damrosch, 1991).*
- Help family to restructure family patterns of interaction and function to support the development of consistency, a predictable environment, emotional nurturance, and positive modeling. **EB:** *Studies indicate that consistency, a predictable environment, emotional nurturance, and positive social modeling may act as ameliorating factors in the dysfunctional environment (Seilhamer et al, 1993).*
- Assist with stabilization and maintenance of positive change in the family. Instruct the alcoholic's family members before the client's discharge to give verbal messages that convey concern about the alcoholic's problem drinking, their observations of the alcoholic's past episodes of drinking, and wishes and support for abstinence. **EB:** *This intervention method can help the alcoholic face the reality of his or her drinking problem and alcohol dependence and thus remain longer in long-range rehabilitation programs, which is a prerequisite for successful recovery from alcohol dependence. Clients' maintenance of abstinence was significantly better only when both they and their family members attended hospital outpatient follow-up sessions and/or self-help group meetings (Ino & Hayasida, 2000).*
- Instill hope and encourage the expression of positive thoughts. **EB:** *The data from this multicenter study confirm the argument that hopefulness appears to be central to a family's*

*coping with the impact of mental illness. Nurses should be mindful of their capacity to sustain or diminish the hopes of family members (Bland & Darlington, 2002).*

- Monitor family closely for return to old patterns of behavior. **EBN:** *This report indicated the presence of family feelings of unhappiness, hurt, frustration, guilt, moodiness, powerlessness, loneliness, mistrust, anger, anxiety, and hopelessness (Bartek et al, 1999).*
- Provide activities that are physical in nature, such as adventure therapy and therapeutic camping, as part of a substance abuse treatment program. **EBN:** *The goal of this therapy is to encourage the adolescents to enhance their self-concept. This is a mental health promotion (MHP) and is considered a strategy to promote health (Epstein, 2004).*



▲ Consider alternative therapies such as acupuncture. *Acupuncture may be helpful in detoxification and is valuable when used in combination with counseling (Serrano, 2003).*

▲ Refer for possible use of medications such as naltrexone and acamprosate to control problem drinking. **EB:** *The results of this randomized, double-blind, placebo-controlled protocol study support the efficacy of pharmacotherapeutic strategies in the relapse prevention of alcoholism. Naltrexone and acamprosate, especially in combination, considerably enhance the potential of relapse prevention (Kiefer et al, 2003).*

- Refer to care plans **Ineffective Denial** and **Defensive Coping**.

## Pediatric

▲ Educate family members about available educational and support programs. **EB:** *A program aimed at early intervention and problem behaviors in preschool children in alcoholic families indicates that prevention programming is more appropriately family based rather than aimed at individuals (Nye et al, 1999).*

▲ Use closed-ended questions when questioning adolescents about drinking behavior. *In this study the numbers of students reporting specific beverage type use were higher when using closed questions compared with an open question. The adolescent drinking amount self-reports seem reasonably reliable and valid both on a population and individual level. (Lintonen, Ahlström, & Metso, 2004).*

- Provide a brief motivational interviewing and cognitive-behavioral-based alcohol intervention group (AIG) program for with young people at risk of developing a problem with alcohol. **EB:** *Participants in the AIG program showed an increase in readiness to reduce their alcohol consumption. They also reduced their frequency of drinking at posttreatment and the first follow-up assessment, whereas the control group reported increases at the second follow-up assessment. This pilot study also showed that young people who are identified as being "at risk" of developing alcohol abuse, and who are also ambivalent about changing drinking behaviors, can be recruited and retained in a treatment programme (Bailey et al, 2004).*
- Encourage parent involvement with adolescents: supervision and emotional support. *The results of this study indicate that inadequate parent involvement may be a form of neglect which leads to influence adolescent alcohol involvement. Neglected adolescents were more likely to develop alcohol use disorders (AUDs) (Duncan et al, 2004).*
- Work at strengthening adolescents' relationships in and out of the home. *Three waves of data from an ethnically diverse community sample of women, assessed over 16 years of*

*age are used to study how various psychosocial factors in adolescence influenced later drinking, depression, and their shared association. Prevention interventions focusing on increasing socially conforming attitudes and on strengthening relationships both in and out of the home during adolescence are likely to be effective in reducing aspects of Alcohol Involvement for women in the general community (Locke & Newcomb, 2004).*

▲ Provide school-based prevention programs using peer leaders at an early age. **EB:** *The results of this study suggest that targeting middle school-aged children and designing programs that can be delivered primarily by peer leaders will increase the effectiveness of school-based substance use prevention programs (Gottfredson et al, 2003).*

▲ Provide a school based drug-prevention program to junior high students. **EB:** *Controlling for gender and alcohol use, students who received the drug prevention program during junior high school were less likely to have violations and points on their driving records relative to control group participants that did not receive the prevention program. Findings indicated that antidrinking attitudes mediated the effect of the intervention on driving violations but not points. These results support the hypothesis that the behavioral effects of competence-enhancement prevention programs can extend to risk behaviors beyond the initial focus of intervention, such as risky driving (Griffin, Botvin, & Nichols, 2004).*

F

## Geriatric

- Include assessment of possible alcohol abuse when assessing elderly family members. **EB:** *Alcohol abuse and alcoholism are common but underrecognized problems among older adults. One third of older alcoholic persons develop a problem with alcohol in later life, whereas the other two thirds grow older with the medical and psychosocial sequelae of early-onset alcoholism (Rigler, 2000).* **EB:** *Alcohol abuse and dependence in older people are important problems, which frequently remain undetected by health services (Beullens & Aertgeerts, 2004).*
- Use CAGE tool with this population and include drug use along with drinking. An affirmative answer to two or more of the following questions is considered a basis for suspicion of alcohol abuse:
  **C:** Have you ever felt you ought to **Cut down** on drinking?
  **A:** Have people **Annoyed** you by criticizing your drinking?
  **G:** Have you ever felt bad or **Guilty** about your drinking?
  **E:** Have you ever had a drink first thing in the morning to steady your nerves or get rid of a hangover **(Eye opener)**?
  **EBN:** *Alcoholism and drug abuse are present in the geriatric population and the CAGE tool is effective in identifying individuals at risk (Hinkin et al, 2001).* **EB:** *Most older adults with drinking problems are encountered in nonaddictions settings, seeking assistance (or referred for assistance) for something other than an alcohol-related problem (Hanson & Gutheil, 2004).* **EB:** *Appropriate screening tool for elderly (Beullens & Aertgeerts, 2004).*

▲ Provide alcohol treatment programs for geriatric clients in primary care settings. **EB:** *In this study older primary care patients were more likely to accept collaborative mental health treatment within primary care than in mental health/substance abuse clinics. These results suggest that integrated service arrangements improve access to mental health and substance abuse services for older adults who underuse these services (Bartels et al, 2004).*

## Multicultural

- Acknowledge racial/ethnic differences at the onset of care. **EBN:** *Acknowledgment of race/ethnicity issues will enhance communication, establish rapport, and promote treatment outcomes (D'Avanzo et al, 2001; Ludwick & Silva, 2000; Vontress & Epp, 1997).*
- Approach families of color with respect, warmth, and professional courtesy. **EBN:** *Instances of disrespect and lack of caring have special significance for families of color (D'Avanzo, 2001; Vontress & Epp, 1997).*
- Give rationale when assessing black families about alcohol use and misuse. **EBN:** *Many blacks may expect Caucasian caregivers to hold negative and preconceived ideas. Giving a rationale for questions asked will help alleviate this perception (D'Avanzo et al, 2001; Vontress & Epp, 1997).*
- Use a family-centered approach when working with Latino, Asian-American, African-American, and Native-American clients. **EBN:** *Latinos may perceive family as a source of support, solver of problems, and source of pride. Asian Americans may regard the family as the primary decision maker and influence on individual family members (D'Avanzo et al, 2001). Native-American families may be extended structures that could exert powerful influences over functioning (Seideman et al, 1996).*
- When working with Asian-American clients, provide opportunities for the family to save face. **EBN:** *This will allow the family to not have to own the shame of the alcohol problem. Asian-American families may avoid situations that bring shame on the family unit (Chen, 2001; D'Avanzo et al, 2001).*
- Some less acculturated Latino families may be unwilling to discuss family issues with health care providers until they perceive a close personal relationship with the provider. **EBN:** *Some Latino families may believe that personal problems should be kept private and may not respond to the health care provider until there is an established personal relationship (Galanti, 2003).*
- Use family strengthening interventions, e.g., behavioral parent training, family skills training, in-home family support, brief family therapy, and family education when working with culturally diverse families. **EB:** *Comprehensive prevention programs combining multiple approaches produced large positive effects when used with different cultural groups and with different ages of children (Kumpfer, Alvarado, & Whiteside, 2003). Increased alcohol use is strongly related to increased separation from family and increased family conflict in both Mexican-American and African-American adolescents (Bray et al, 2001).*
- Work with families in a way that incorporates cultural elements. **EB:** *Activities such as tundra walks and time with elders are supported in treatment were used successfully for substance abuse treatment with Yup'ik and Cup'ik Eskimo (Mills, 2003).*

## Home Care

NOTE: In the community setting, alcoholism as an etiology for dysfunctional family processes must be considered in two categories. The first is when the client suffers personally from the illness; the second is when a significant other suffers from the illness, that is, the client is not the active alcoholic but may be dependent on the alcoholic for caregiving. The following considerations apply to both situations with appropriate adaptation for the circumstances:

- Above interventions may be adapted for home care use.
- Identify client/family expectations of the home care nurse and nurse expectations of the client/family by use of a well-defined contract. Be specific and realistic. Adjust the contract only with clear consent and understanding of the client/family. *A well-defined contract supports success in meeting goals and encourages positive family dynamics. A contract defines conditions under which care can be safely provided and under which care cannot continue. Safety of the staff should never be jeopardized.*
- ▲ Work with family members to support a sense of valued fit on their part; include them in treatment planning, and identify the importance of their roles in the client's care. At the same time, encourage their pursuit of positive outside activities that enhance their sense of belonging. **EBN:** *Sense of belonging (valued fit) has been identified as a buffer to depression among both depressed and nondepressed individuals with a family history of alcoholism. A buffering effect was not found for individuals with a family history of drug abuse (Sargent et al, 2002).*
- ▲ Establish well-defined contingency and emergency plans for the care of the client. **EB:** *Safety of the client between visits is a primary goal of the home care nurse (Stanhope & Lancaster, 1996).*
- Request concrete, measurable tasks of the client and family for caregiving and provide concrete, nonjudgmental instruction to the client/family regarding the interactions of alcohol use with medications, therapeutic regimen. *The client/family will exercise ultimate control over whether or not to continue alcohol use. Clear information, delivered without judgment of the person, may provide the client/family with motivation to modify, if not discontinue, alcohol use.*
- ▲ Observe for abuse of other medications. Notify physician of problems noted. *Cross-addiction is a concern. Clients may substitute the use of other psychoactive medications for alcohol, or may be already addicted to hypnotics and/or pain medications. The presence of other addictions may raise issues with regard to withdrawal and synergistic effects.*
- ▲ If the client is a recovering alcoholic, extreme care must be taken in the use of psychoactive or pain medications. Notify physician if inappropriate medications have been inadvertently ordered. *Addiction to alcohol increases the potential for readdiction, especially if strong pain medications are introduced. In many instances, it is policy to prescribe nothing stronger than extra-strength acetaminophen for recovering alcoholics in need of pain medication. Sleep medications should be avoided.*
- ▲ Refer for medical social work services at outset of care. *The social worker can help identify, set the structure for, and guide appropriate client/family and client/family/nurse interactions that will promote the plan of care throughout the length of the stay.*
- ▲ Provide information regarding available substance use treatment programs and support groups. *A variety of program types are available, from Alcoholics Anonymous (AA) to intensive inpatient treatment, with specialty units available in some areas for older adults.*
- Acknowledge without judging when resolution of alcoholism is not a goal of care. *It is usually not appropriate for terminally ill or hospice clients or their families to change family*

*life patterns. Recognizing this fact nonjudgmentally helps the client or family use remaining energy to complete other end-of-life work.*

▲ Refer for psychiatric home health care services for client reassurance and implementation of therapeutic regimen. **EBN:** *Psychiatric home care nurses can address issues relating to the client's or family member's alcoholism and its interference with ability to adjust to changes in health status. Behavioral interventions in the home can assist the client to participate more effectively in treatment plan (Patusky et al, 1996).*

## Client Family Teaching

F

- Suggest client do a confidential Internet self-screening test for identification of problems and suggestions for treatment if a problem with alcohol is suspected. There are many tools available. The website www.*AlcoholScreening.org helps individuals assess their own alcohol consumption patterns to determine if their drinking is likely to be harming their health or increasing their risk for future harm. Through education and referral, the site urges those whose drinking is harmful or hazardous to take positive action, and informs all adults who consume alcohol about guidelines and caveats for lower-risk drinking (Boston University School of Public Health, 2005).*

## evolve WEBSITES FOR EDUCATION

See the EVOLVE website for World Wide Web resources for client education.

## REFERENCES


AHCPR (Agency for Healthcare Research and Quality): *Evidence report/technology assessment number 3: Pharmacotherapy for alcohol dependence,* AHCPR Pub No 99-E004. Available at www.ahcpr.gov/clinic/index.html#evidence, accessed on January 16, 2000.

Bailey KA, Baker AL, Webster RA et al: Pilot randomized controlled trial of a brief alcohol intervention group for adolescents, *Drug Alcohol Rev* 23(2):157-166, 2004.

Bartek JK, Lindeman M, Hawks JH: Clinical validation of characteristics of the alcoholic family, *Nurs Diagn* 10(4):158, 1999.

Bartels SJ, Coakley EH, Zubritsky C et al: Improving access to geriatric mental health services: a randomized trial comparing treatment engagement with integrated versus enhanced referral care for depression, anxiety, and at-risk alcohol use, *Am J Psychiatry* 161(8):1455-1462, 2004.

Becker KL, Walton-Moss B: Detecting and addressing alcohol abuse in women, *Nurse Pract* 26(10):13, 2001.

Beullens J, Aertgeerts B: Screening for alcohol abuse and dependence in older people using DSM criteria: a review, *Aging Ment Health* 8(1):76-82, 2004.

Bland R, Darlington Y: The nature and sources of hope: perspectives of family caregivers of people with serious mental illness, *Perspect Psychiatr Care* 38(2):61, 2002.

Boston University School of Public Health: Available at www.alcoholscreening.org, accessed on January 18, 2005.

Bray JH, Adams GJ, Getz JG et al: Developmental, family, and ethnic influences on adolescent alcohol usage: a growth curve approach, *J Fam Psychol* 15(2):301-314, 2001.

Chen YC: Chinese values, health and nursing, *J Adv Nurs* 36(2):270, 2001.

Curry SJ, Ludman E, Grothaus L et al: At-risk drinking among patients making routine primary care visits, *Prev Med* 31(5): 595-602, 2000.

Damrosch S: General strategies for motivating people to change their behavior, *Nurs Clin North Am* 26:833, 1991.

D'Avanzo CE et al: Developing culturally informed strategies for substance-related interventions. In Naegle MA, D'Avanzo CE, editors: *Addictions and substance abuse: strategies for advanced practice nursing,* St Louis, 2001, Mosby.

Clark DB, Thatcher DL, Maisto SA: Adolescent neglect and alcohol use disorders in two-parent families, *Child Maltreat* 9(4): 357-370, 2004.
Epstein I: Adventure therapy: a mental health promotion strategy in pediatric oncology, *J Pediatr Oncol Nurs* 21(2):103-110, 2004.
Galanti GA: The Hispanic family and male-female relationships: an overview, *J Transcult Nurs* 14(3):180-185, 2003.
Giuffra MJ: Nursing strategies with alcohol and drug problems in the family. In Naegle MA, editor: *Substance abuse in education in nursing,* vol 3, Pub No 15-2464, New York, 1993, National League for Nursing Press.
Gorski T: *Women at risk brief screening tools.* Available at www.tgorski.com/clin_mod/atp/women_at_risk-brief_sceening_tools.htm#TWEAK, accessed on February 19, 2003.
Gottfredson DC, Wilson DB: Characteristics of effective school-based substance abuse prevention, *Prev Sci* 4(1):27, 2003.
Griffin KW, Botvin GJ, Nichols TR: Long-term follow-up effects of a school-based drug abuse prevention program on adolescent risky driving, *Prev Sci* 5(3):207-212, 2004.
Hanson M, Guthei IA: Motivational strategies with alcohol-involved older adults: implications for social work practice, *Social Work* 49(3):364-373, 2004.
Hinkin CH, Castellon SA, Dickson-Fuhrman E et al: Screening for drug and alcohol abuse among older adults using a modified version of the CAGE, *Am J Addict* 10:319-326, 2001.
Hodgson R, Alwyn T, John B et al: The FAST alcohol screening test, *Alcohol Alcohol* 37(1):61-66, 2002.
Ino A, Hayasida M: Before-discharge intervention method in the treatment of alcohol dependence, *Alcohol Clin Exp Res* 24(3): 373, 2000.
Kiefer F, Jahn H, Tarnaske T et al: Comparing and combining naltrexone and acamprosate in relapse prevention of alcoholism: a double-blind, placebo-controlled study, *Arch Gen Psychiatry* 60(1):92-99, 2003.
Kumpfer KL, Alvarado R, Whiteside HO: Family-based interventions for substance use and misuse prevention, *Subst Use Misuse* 38(11-13):1759-1787, 2003.
Lintonen T, Ahlström S, Metso L: The reliability of self-reported drinking in adolescence, *Alcohol Alcohol* 39(4):362-368, 2004.
Locke TF, Newcomb MD: Adolescent predictors of young adult and adult alcohol involvement and dysphoria in a prospective community sample of women, *Prev Sci* 5(3):151-168, 2004.
Ludwick R, Silva M: Nursing around the world: cultural values and ethical conflicts, *Online J Issues Nurs.* Available at www.nursingworld.org/ojin/ethcol/ethics_4.htm.
Mills PA: Incorporating Yup'ik and Cup'ik Eskimo traditions into behavioral health treatment, *J Psychoactive Drugs* 35(1):85-88, 2003.
Nye CL, Zucker RA, Fitzgerald HE: Early family-based intervention in the path to alcohol problems: rationale and relationship between treatment process characteristics and child and parenting outcomes, *J Stud Alcohol Suppl* 13:10, 1999.
Patusky KL, Rodning C, Martinez-Kratz M: Clinical lessons in psychiatric home care: a case study approach, *J Home Healthc Manag* 9:188, 1996.
Rigler SK: Alcoholism in the elderly, *Am Fam Physician* 61(6):1710, 2000.
Sargent J, Williams RA, Hagerty B et al: Sense of belonging as a buffer against depressive symptoms, *J Am Psychiatr Nurs Assoc* 8(4):120-129, 2002.
Seideman RY, Jacobson S, Primeaux M et al: Assessing American Indian families, *MCN Am J Matern Child Nurs* 21(6):274, 1996.
Seilhamer RA, Jacob T, Dunn NJ: The impact of alcohol consumption on parent-child relationships in families of alcoholics, *J Stud Alcohol* 54:189, 1993.
Serrano R: Solution focused addictions counseling, acupuncture treatment for substance abuse. Available at www.holisticwebs.com/solution/sfac4.html, accessed January 18, 2003.
Stanhope M, Lancaster J, editors: *Community health nursing: promoting health of aggregates, families, and individuals,* ed 4, St Louis, 1996, Mosby.
Stoll B, Wick HD: Short intervention approach: one-way of reducing excessive alcohol consumption, *Abhangigkeiten* Feb 2000.
Vontress CE, Epp LR: Historical hostility in the African American client: implications for counseling, *J Multicult Counseling Dev* 25:170, 1997.

# Readiness for enhanced Family processes

*Gail B. Ladwig*

**NANDA**

## Definition

F

A pattern of family functioning that is sufficient to support the well-being of family members and can be strengthened

## Defining Characteristics

Expresses willingness to enhance family dynamics, family functioning meets physical, social, and psychological needs of family members, activities support the safety and growth of family members, communication is adequate, relationships are generally positive, interdependent with community, family tasks are accomplished, family roles are flexible and appropriate for developmental stages, respect for family members is evident, family adapts to change, boundaries of family members are maintained, energy level of family supports activities of daily living, family resilience is evident, balance exists between autonomy and cohesiveness

**NOC**

## Outcomes (Nursing Outcomes Classification)

### Suggested NOC Outcomes

Family Coping, Family Physical Environment, Health Orientation, Health Promoting Behavior, Health Seeking Behavior, Leisure Participation, Parent-Infant Attachment, Parenting Performance, Psychosocial Adjustment: Life Change, Risk Control, Role Performance, Social Support, Spiritual Health

**Example NOC Outcome with Indicators**

**Family Coping** as evidenced by the following indicators: Confronts/manages family problems/Involves family members in decision making (Rate each indicator of **Family Coping:** 1 = never demonstrated, 2 = rarely demonstrated, 3 = sometimes demonstrated, 4 = often demonstrated, 5 = consistently demonstrated [see Section I].)

## Client Outcomes

**Family/Client Will (Specify Time Frame):**

- Identify ways to cope effectively and use appropriate support systems (family)
- Meet physical, psychosocial, and spiritual needs of members or seeks appropriate assistance (family)

- Demonstrate knowledge of potential environmental, lifestyle, and genetic risks to health and use appropriate measures to decrease possibility of risk (family)
- Focus on wellness, disease prevention, and maintenance (family and individual)
- Seek balance among exercise, work, leisure, rest, and nutrition (family and individual)

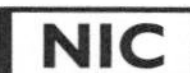


## Interventions (Nursing Interventions Classification)

### Suggested NIC Interventions

Active Listening; Anticipatory Guidance; Attachment Promotion; Coping Enhancement; Decision-Making Support; Environmental Management: Attachment Process; Exercise Promotion; Family Integrity Promotion; Family Involvement Promotion; Family Mobilization; Family Process Maintenance; Health Screening; Mutual Goal Setting; Parent Education: Adolescent, Childrearing Family; Risk Identification; Role Enhancement

**Example NIC Activities—Risk Identification**

Determine community support systems; determine presence and quality of family support

## Nursing Interventions and Rationales

- Assess the family's stress level and coping abilities during the initial nursing assessment. **EBN:** *Nurses need to assess the family's baseline stress level and effectiveness of coping responses and assist the family as a whole as well as individual members in meeting their varying needs. Families differ in their ability to cope with multiple stressors (Rutledge et al, 2000a).*
- Consider the use of family theory as a framework to help guide interventions (e.g., family stress theory, role theory, social exchange theory). **EBN:** *This study demonstrated that use of a family assessment tool is an effective way of appraising families and addressing suffering. Formative evaluations demonstrated improvements in team members' perceptions of their knowledge, family centeredness, and ability to assess and intervene with families (Hogan & Logan, 2004).*
- Use family-centered care, and role modeling for holistic care of families. **EBN:** *Specific techniques of role modeling and reflective practice are suggested as effective approaches to teach family sensitive care in clinical settings where families are part of the care environment (Tomlinson et al, 2002).*
- Discuss with the family members how they have handled previous crises. *Such a discussion gives the nurse clues and information that can help in plan of care. Families that have a broad and diverse array of coping behaviors are more likely than others to meet needs and to have a good outcome (Coleman & Taylor, 1995).*
- Support family empowerment; strength and resourcefulness. **EBN:** *The family can empower itself but it is also possible to empower the family from the outside, such as in child health clinics (Pelkonen, 2002).*

- Spend time with family members; allow them to verbalize their feelings. **EBN:** *Interactions help the client and family feel relieved and allow anxiety levels to decrease. Critical care nurses can provide support for families after the death of a loved one (Coolican & Politoski, 1994).*
- Encourage family members to find meaning in a serious illness like cancer. **EBN:** *The positive dimensions of survivorship in meaning of the illness and family quality of life were seen for patients and family members with cancer (Mellon, 2002).*
- Have family members participate in client conferences that involve all members of the health care team. *Conferences allow for distribution of information, input by all members at one time, and a decrease in anxiety levels of family members.*

F

- ▲ Provide family-centered care to explore and use all available resources appropriate for situation (e.g., counseling, social services, self-help groups, pastoral care). **EBN:** *Meeting the need of families involves various kinds of interventions including those that offer reassurance and provide information. Family-centered care is a philosophical approach to meeting these needs (Rutledge et al, 2000b). Families are profoundly affected by the social contexts of mental illnesses (Rose et al, 2002).*
- ▲ Consider referral for walk-in family therapy. **EB:** *This therapy modality is aimed at providing an immediately accessible, affordable, nonstigmatizing, single-session-focused resource. Follow-up telephone interviews were conducted with 43 clients 3 to 6 months after they received treatment. Generally, former clients reported satisfaction with the service. The majority (67%) indicated some level of improvement, and 43% of participants found their single session sufficient to address their concern*s *(Miller & Slive, 2004).*

## Pediatric

- Provide a parenting class series based on individual and couple changes in meaning/identity, roles, and relationship/interaction during the transition to parenthood. Address mother/father roles, infant communication abilities, and patterns of the first 3 months of life in a mutually enjoyable, possibility-focused way. **EBN:** *This study demonstrated that interventions that enhance mutual parent-child interaction through increased sensitivity to cues and responsiveness to infant needs or signals are important avenues for facilitating secure attachment, father and mother involvement, optimal development, and prevention of child abuse and neglect (Bryan, 2000).*
- Encourage families with adolescents to have family meals. *Data from a 1998 to 1999 school-based survey of 4746 adolescents from ethnically and socioeconomically diverse communities in the Minneapolis/St Paul, Minnesota, metropolitan area suggest that eating family meals may enhance the health and well-being of adolescents. Public education on the benefits of family mealtime is recommended (Eisenberg, 2004).*
- ▲ Consider the use of adventure therapy (AT) for adolescents with cancer. **EBN:** *The goal of this therapy is to encourage the adolescents to enhance their self-concept. The adolescents with cancer who participate in AT also learn about themselves through self-evaluation, self-exploration, self-reevaluation, self-acceptance, and self-realization. This is a mental health promotion (MHP) and is considered a strategy to promote health (Epstein, 2004).*

### Geriatric

- Carefully listen to residents and family members in the long-term care facility. **EBN:** *This study suggests that by listening to residents and family members nurses can improve life for residents and dignify them as individuals (Iwasiw et al, 2002).*
- Support caregivers' awareness of the positive effects of their contribution to the well-being of parents. **EBN:** *This study indicates that family satisfaction of caregivers of elderly parents may be influenced by reciprocity, emotional well-being, and family functioning (Carruth et al, 1997).*
- Teach family members about impact of developmental events (e.g., retirement, death, change in health status, and household composition). *Knowledge regarding normative developmental challenges of aging can reduce the stress such challenges place on families.*
- Encourage social networks, social integration, and social engagement with friends, children, and relatives for the elderly. **EB:** *This longitudinal study indicates that few social ties, poor integration, and social disengagement are risk factors for cognitive decline among community-dwelling elderly persons (Zunzunegui, 2003).*

F

### Multicultural

- Assess for the influence of cultural beliefs, norms, and values on the family's perceptions of normal functioning. **EBN:** *What the family considers normal and abnormal family functioning may be based on cultural perceptions (Leininger, 2002). Latino families who express a higher degree of familism are characterized by positive interpersonal familial relationships, high family unity, social support, interdependence in the completion of daily activities, and close proximity with extended family members (Romero et al, 2004).*
- With the client's consent, facilitate a group meeting for family members to discuss how the family is functioning. **EBN:** *A family meeting opens communication and lets each family member know it is okay to talk about what is happening (Rivera-Andino & Lopez, 2000). Focus groups with African Americans found that families could benefit from help placement of family members in nursing homes and hospital and the process of family decision making (Turner et al, 2004).*
- Facilitate modeling and role playing for the client and family regarding healthy ways to start a discussion about the client's prognosis. **EBN:** *It is helpful for families and the client to practice communication skills in a safe environment before trying them in a real-life situation (Rivera-Andino & Lopez, 2000).*
- Identify and acknowledge the stresses unique to racial/ethnic families. **EBN:** *Financial difficulties and maintaining cultural values are two of the most common family stressors cited by women of color (Majumdar & Ladak, 1998). In this study, women in Turkey perceive themselves as wives sharing everything within the family. Women's decision-making rate was lower than that of men, except for selecting clothes (Erci, 2003).*
- Offer frequent gestures of support to family members. **EBN:** *African-American mothers of seriously ill children identified support from the health care team as their highest source of satisfaction (Miles et al, 1999).*

- Encourage family mealtimes. **EB:** *Frequency of family meals was inversely associated with tobacco, alcohol, and marijuana use; low grade point average; depressive symptoms and suicide involvement of diverse adolescents (Eisenberg et al, 2004).*

### Home Care

- The nursing interventions described previously for **Readiness for enhanced Family processes** should be used in the home environment with adaptations as necessary.
- Provide a videophone network for peer support for frail elderly people living at home. **EB:** *A videophone network appears to be helpful for elderly people in their peer support relationships. It supports and improves the functional independence of frail elderly people at home (Ezumi et al, 2003).*
- Encourage families to assist women caring for husbands with chronic obstructive pulmonary disease (COPD) to provide respite care so the women may have recreation time. **EBN:** *Women caregivers of husbands with COPD were dissatisfied with their lack of recreation, as well as support from friends, families, and health care providers (Bergs, 2002).*

### Client/Family Teaching

- Refer to Client/Family Teaching in **Readiness for enhanced family Coping** for suggestions that may be used with minor adaptations.

## evolve WEBSITES FOR EDUCATION

See the EVOLVE website for World Wide Web resources for client education.

## REFERENCES


Bergs D: "The hidden client"—women caring for husbands with COPD: their experience of quality of life, *J Clin Nurs* 11(5):613, 2002.

Bryan AA: Enhancing parent-child interaction with a prenatal couple intervention, *MCN Am J Matern Child Nurs* 25(3):139, 2000.

Calvert WJ: Protective factors within the family, and their role in fostering resiliency in African American adolescents, *J Cult Divers* 4(4):110, 1997.

Carruth AK, Tate US, Moffett BS et al: Reciprocity, emotional well-being, and family functioning as determinants of family satisfaction in caregivers of elderly parents, *Nurs Res* 46(2):93, 1997.

Coleman W, Taylor E: Family-focused pediatrics: issues, challenges, and clinical methods, *Pediatr Clin North Am* 42(1):119, 1995.

Coolican MB, Politoski G: Donor family programs, *Crit Care Nurs Clin North Am* 6(3):613, 1994.

Eisenberg ME, Olson RE, Neumark-Sztainer D et al: Correlations between family meals and psychosocial well-being among adolescents, *Arch Pediatr Adolesc Med* 158(8):792-796, 2004.

Epstein I: Adventure therapy: a mental health promotion strategy in pediatric oncology, *J Pediatr Oncol Nurs* 21(2):103-110, 2004.

Erci B: Women's efficiency in decision making and their perception of their status in the family, *Public Health Nurs* 20(1):65, 2003.

Ezumi H et al: Peer support via video-telephony among frail elderly people living at home, *J Telemed Telecare* 9(1):30, 2003.

Giger JN, Davidhizar RE: *Transcultural nursing,* ed 2, St Louis, 1995, Mosby.

Iwasiw C, Goldenberg D, Bol N et al: Resident and family perspectives: the first year in a long-term care facility, *J Gerontol Nurs* 29(1):45, 2003.

Hogan DL, Logan J: The Ottawa Model of Research Use: a guide to clinical innovation in the NICU, *Clin Nurse Spec* 18(5):255-261, 2004.

Katz D, Gagnon AJ: Evidence of adequacy of postpartum care for immigrant women, *Can J Nurs Res* 34(4):71, 2002.
Leininger MM, McFarland MR: *Transcultural nursing: concepts, theories, research and practices,* ed 3, New York, 2002, McGraw-Hill.
Majumdar B, Ladak S: Management of family and workplace stress experienced by women of color from various cultural backgrounds, *Can J Public Health* 89(1):48, 1998.
Mellon S: Comparisons between cancer survivors and family members on meaning of the illness and family quality of life, *Oncol Nurs Forum* 29(7):1117, 2002.
Miller JK, Slive A: Breaking down the barriers to clinical service delivery: walk-in family therapy, *J Marital Fam Ther* 30(1):95-103, 2004.
Pilkonen M, Hakulinen T: An empowerment model for family nursing, *Hoitotiede* 14(5):202, 2002 (in Finnish).
Rivera-Andino J, Lopez L: When culture complicates care, *RN* 63(7):47, 2000.
Romero AJ, Robinson TN, Haydel KF et al: Associations among familism, language preference, and education in Mexican-American mothers and their children, *J Dev Behav Pediatr* 25(1):34-40, 2004.
Rose L, Mallinson RK, Walton-Moss B: A grounded theory of families responding to mental illness, *Nurs Res* 24(5):516, 2002.
Rutledge DN, Donaldson NE, Pravikoff DS: Caring for families of patients in acute or chronic health care settings: Part I—Principles, *Online J Clin Innovat* 3(3):1, 2000a.
Rutledge DN, Donaldson NE, Pravikoff DS: Caring for families of patients in acute or chronic care settings: Part II—Interventions, *Online J Clin Innovat* 3(3):1, 2000b.
Stuart GW, Laraia MT: Therapeutic nurse-patient relationship. In Stuart GW, Laraia MT, editors: *Principles and practice of psychiatric nursing,* St Louis, 2001, Mosby.
Tomlinson PS, Thomlinson E, Peden-McAlpine C et al: Clinical innovation for promoting family care in paediatric intensive care: demonstration, role modelling and reflective practice, *J Adv Nurs* 38(2):161, 2002.
Turner WL, Wallace BR, Anderson JR et al: The last mile of the way: understanding caregiving in African American families at the end-of-life, *J Marital Fam Ther* 30(4):427-438, 2004.
Zunzunegui MV, Alvarado BE, Del Ser T et al: Social networks, social integration, and social engagement determine cognitive decline in community-dwelling Spanish older adults, *Gerontol B Psychol Sci Soc Sci* 58(2):S93, 2003.

F

# Interrupted Family processes

*Gail B. Ladwig*

**NANDA**

## Definition

Change in family relationships and/or functioning

## Defining Characteristics

Changes in power alliances, assigned tasks, effectiveness in completing assigned tasks, mutual support, availability for affective responsiveness and intimacy, patterns and rituals, participation in problem solving, participation in decision making, communication patterns, availability for emotional support, satisfaction with family, stress-reduction behaviors, expressions of conflict with and/or isolation from community resources, somatic complaints, expressions of conflict within family

## Related Factors (r/t)

Power shift of family members, family roles shift, shift in health status of a family member, developmental transition and/or crisis, situational transition and/or crisis, informal or formal interaction with community, modification in family social status, modification in family finances

**NOC**

## Outcomes (Nursing Outcomes Classification)

F

### Suggested NOC Outcomes

Family Coping, Family Social Climate, Family Functioning, Family Normalization, Parenting Performance, Psychosocial Adjustment: Life Change, Role Performance

**Example NOC Outcome with Indicators**

**Family Coping** as evidenced by the following indicators: Confronts/manages family problems/Involves family members in decision making (Rate each indicator of **Family Coping:** 1 = never demonstrated, 2 = rarely demonstrated, 3 = sometimes demonstrated, 4 = often demonstrated, 5 = consistently demonstrated [see Section I].)

## Client Outcomes

**Family/Client Will (Specify Time Frame):**

- Express feelings (family)
- Identify ways to cope effectively and use appropriate support systems (family)
- Treat impaired family member as normally as possible to avoid overdependence (family)
- Meet physical, psychosocial, and spiritual needs of members or seeks appropriate assistance (family)
- Demonstrate knowledge of illness or injury, treatment modalities, and prognosis (family)
- Participate in the development of the plan of care to the best of ability (significant person)

**NIC**

## Interventions (Nursing Interventions Classification)

### Suggested NIC Interventions

Family Integrity Promotion, Family Process Maintenance, Family Therapy, Normalization Promotion, Role Enhancement, Support System Enhancement

**Example NIC Activities—Family Integrity Promotion**

Collaborate with family in problem solving; counsel family members on additional effective coping skills for their own use

## Nursing Interventions and Rationales

- Assess the family's stress level and coping abilities during the initial nursing assessment. **EBN:** *Nurses need to assess the family's baseline stress level and effectiveness of coping responses and to assist the family as a whole and individual members in meeting their varying needs. Families differ in their ability to cope with multiple stressors (Rutledge et al, 2000a).*
- Establish rapport with families by providing accurate communication. **EBN:** *This qualitative exploratory study of families in psychiatric settings indicated that family care can be improved by focusing on building rapport and communicating problems and concerns between families and health professionals (Rose, Mallinson, & Walton-Moss, 2004).*
- Use family-centered care and role modeling for holistic care of families. **EBN:** *Specific techniques of role modeling and reflective practice are suggested as effective approaches to teach family-sensitive care in clinical settings where families are part of the care environment (Tomlinson et al, 2002).*

▲ Provide family-centered care to explore and use all available resources appropriate for situation (e.g., counseling, social services, self-help groups, pastoral care). **EBN:** *Meeting the need of families involves various kinds of interventions including those that offer reassurance and provide information. Family-centered care is a philosophical approach to meeting these needs (Rutledge et al, 2000b).*

- Acknowledge the range of emotions and feelings that may be experienced when there is a change of health status in a family member; counsel family members that it is normal to be angry, afraid, and so on. **EBN:** *This study describes the experiences of the patient's family's experiences after the death of patients in the intensive care unit (ICU). The experiences of the family members resembled a vortex: a downward spiral of prognoses, difficult decisions, feelings of inadequacy, and eventual loss despite the members' best efforts, and perhaps no good-byes (Kirchoff et al, 2002).*
- Encourage family members to list their personal strengths. *A list of strengths provides information that family members can refer to for positive feedback.*
- Involve family members in the care and information/patient teaching sessions with the client. *Family-focused activities can help families cope better with the hospital experience (Worthington, 1995).*
- Encourage family to visit the client; adjust visiting hours to accommodate family's schedule (e.g., schedule around work, school, babysitting needs). Assist with sleeping arrangements if family is spending the night; provide a place to lie down, pillows, and blankets.
- Allow and encourage family to assist in the client's care. Allow family presence during invasive procedures and resuscitation. **EBN:** *Families in critical care units (CCUs) play a significant role in the clients care (Johnson et al, 2004).*

▲ Consider use of video home training as a method of early support in problems of family life control. **EBN:** *The findings show that video home training helped the families to gain better control over their family life. The process of videotaping family life, in-depth analysis of the videotapes, recognition of instances of successful interaction, and search for new alternatives gave participants a feeling that it would be possible for them to make their everyday life fluent and functional (Häggman et al, 2003).*

F

## Pediatric

- Allow and encourage family to assist in the client's care. **EBN:** *Families of hospitalized children may wish to participate more actively in the actual physical care of the patient than family members of an adult patient (Rutledge et al, 2000b).*
- ▲ Carefully assess potential for reunifying children placed in foster care with their birth parents. **EB:** *Reunifying children placed in foster care with their birth parents is a primary goal of the child welfare system. Greater efforts should be made to ensure that reunifications are safe and lasting by improving the safety and stability of reunified families, such as instituting better measures of state performance, and continuing to provide monitoring and supports for families after a child is returned home (Wulczyn, 2004).*

## Geriatric

- Teach family members about the impact of developmental events (e.g., retirement, death, change in health status, and household composition). *Knowledge regarding normative developmental challenges of aging can reduce the stress that such challenges place on families.*
- Encourage family members to be involved in the care of relatives who are in residential care settings. **EB:** *This study supports the positive implications of family involvement in residential long-term care (Gaugler et al, 2004).* **EB:** *If family satisfaction is to be achieved, family presence in a nursing home needs to give caregivers a sense of positive involvement and influence over the care of their relative (Tornatore & Grant, 2004).*
- Support group problem solving among family members and include the older member. *Problem solving is an effective method to manage stressors for family members of all ages.*
- ▲ Refer family for counseling with a psychotherapist who is knowledgeable about gerontology.
- Refer to care plan for **Readiness for enhanced family Coping**.

## Multicultural

- Assess for the influence of cultural beliefs, norms, and values on the family's perceptions of normal functioning. **EBN:** *What the family considers normal and abnormal family functioning may be based on cultural perceptions (Leininger & McFarland, 2002; Cochran, 1998; Doswell & Erlen, 1998; Guaranccia, 1998). Latino families who express a higher degree of familism are characterized by positive interpersonal familial relationships, high family unity, social support, interdependence in the completion of daily activities, and close proximity with extended family members (Romero et al, 2004).*
- With the client's consent, facilitate a group meeting for family members to discuss how the family is functioning. **EBN:** *A family meeting opens communication and lets each family member know it is okay to talk about what is happening (Rivera-Andino & Lopez, 2000). Focus groups with African Americans found that families could benefit from help placement of family members in nursing homes and hospital and the process of family decision making (Turner et al, 2004).*
- Facilitate modeling and role-playing for the client and family regarding healthy ways to start a discussion about the client's prognosis. **EBN:** *It is helpful for families and the*

*client to practice communication skills in a safe environment before trying them in a real-life situation (Rivera-Andino & Lopez, 2000).*

- Identify and acknowledge the stresses unique to racial/ethnic families. **EBN:** *Financial difficulties and maintaining cultural values are two of the most common family stressors cited by women of color (Ludwick & Silva, 2000; Majumdar & Ladak, 1998; Vontress & Epp, 1997).*
- Offer frequent gestures of support to family members. **EBN:** *African-American mothers of seriously ill children identified support from the health care team as their highest source of satisfaction (Miles et al, 1999).*
- Encourage the family members to demonstrate and offer caring and support to each other. **EBN:** *The familial characteristics of care and support are associated with fostering resiliency in black families. Resilience is the ability to experience adverse conditions and to successfully overcome them (Calvert, 1997).*
- Validate the family's feelings regarding concerns about current crisis and family functioning. **EBN:** *Validation is a therapeutic communication technique that lets the client know that the nurse has heard and understands what was said, and it promotes the nurse-client relationship (Heineken, 1998).*
- Encourage family mealtimes. **EB:** *Frequency of family meals was inversely associated with tobacco, alcohol, and marijuana use; low grade point average; depressive symptoms and suicide involvement of diverse adolescents (Eisenberg et al, 2004).*

### Home Care

- The nursing interventions described previously for **Compromised family Coping** should be used in the home environment with adaptations as necessary.
- Assist help from the family when communicating with clients in advanced stages of cancer who are no longer able to communicate their illness and symptom needs. **EBN:** *Next of kin play an integral role in fostering optimal quality of life in symptomatic patients who are coping with cancer in the home setting (Lobchuk & Degner, 2002).*

### Client/Family Teaching

- Refer to Client/Family Teaching in **Compromised family Coping** and **Readiness for enhanced family Coping** for suggestions that may be used with minor adaptations.

## evolve WEBSITES FOR EDUCATION

See the EVOLVE website for World Wide Web resources for client education.

## REFERENCES


Calvert WJ: Protective factors within the family, and their role in fostering resiliency in African American adolescents, *J Cult Divers* 4(4):110, 1997.

Cochran M: Tears have no color, *Am J Nurs* 98(6):53, 1998.

Doswell W, Erlen J: Multicultural issues and ethical concerns in the delivery of revising care interventions, *Nurs Clin North Am* 33(2):353, 1998.

Eisenberg ME, Olson RE, Neumark-Sztainer D et al: Correlations between family meals and psychosocial well-being among adolescents, *Arch Pediatr Adolesc Med* 158(8):792-796, 2004.
Gaugler JE, Anderson KA, Zarit SH et al: Family involvement in nursing homes: effects on stress and well-being, *Aging Ment Health* 8(1):65-75, 2004.
Guarnaccia P: Multicultural experiences of family caregiving: a Study of African American, European American, and Hispanic American families, *New Direct Ment Health Serv* 77:45, 1998.
Haggman-Laitila A, Pietila AM, Friis L et al: Video home training as a method of supporting family life control, *J Clin Nurs* 12(1):93, 2003.
Heineken J: Patient silence is not necessarily client satisfaction: communication in home care nursing, *Home Healthc Nurse* 16(2): 115, 1998.
Johnson P: Reclaiming the everyday world: how long-term ventilated patients in critical care seek to gain aspects of power and control over their environment, *Intensive Crit Care Nurs* 20(4):190-199, 2004.
Kirchhoff KT, Walker L, Hutton A et al: The vortex: families' experiences with death in the intensive care unit, *Am J Crit Care* 11(3):200, 2002.
Leininger MM, McFarland MR: *Transcultural nursing: concepts, theories, research and practices,* ed 3, New York, 2002, McGraw-Hill.
Lobchuk MM, Degner LF: Patients with cancer and next-of-kin response comparability on physical and psychological symptom well-being: trends and measurement issues, *Cancer Nurs* 25(5):358, 2002.
Ludwick R, Silva M: Nursing around the world: cultural values and ethical conflicts, *Online J Issues Nurs.* Available at www.nursingworld.org/ojin/ethcol/ethics_4.htm.
Majumdar B, Ladak S: Management of family and workplace stress experienced by women of color from various cultural backgrounds, *Can J Public Health* 89(1):48, 1998.
Miles MS, Wilson SM, Docherty SL: African American mothers' responses to hospitalization of an infant with serious health problems, *Neonatal Netw* 18(8):17, 1999.
Rivera-Andino J, Lopez L: When culture complicates care, *RN* 63(7):47, 2000.
Romero AJ, Robinson TN, Haydel KF et al: Associations among familism, language preference, and education in Mexican-American mothers and their children, *J Dev Behav Pediatr* 25(1):34-40, 2004.
Rose LE: Mallinson RK: Walton-Moss B, Barriers to family care in psychiatric settings, *J Nurs Sch* 36(1):39-47, 2004.
Rutledge DN, Donaldson NE, Pravikoff DS: Caring for families of patients in acute or chronic health care settings: Part I—Principles, *Online J Clin Innovat* 3(3):1, 2000a.
Rutledge DN, Donaldson NE, Pravikoff DS: Caring for families of patients in acute or chronic care settings: Part II—Interventions, *Online J Clin Innovat* 3(3):1, 2000b.
Stuart GW, Laraia MT: Therapeutic nurse-patient relationship. In Stuart GW, Laraia MT, editors: *Principles and practice of psychiatric nursing,* St Louis, 2001, Mosby.
Tomlinson PS, Thomlinson E, Peden-McAlpine C et al: Clinical innovation for promoting family care in paediatric intensive care: demonstration, role modelling and reflective practice, *J Adv Nurs* 38(2):161, 2002.
Tornatore JB, Grant LA: Family caregiver satisfaction with the nursing home after placement of a relative with dementia, *J Gerontol B Psychol Sci Soc Sci* 59(2):S80-S88, 2004.
Turner WL, Wallace BR, Anderson JR et al: The last mile of the way: understanding caregiving in African American families at the end-of-life, *J Marital Fam Ther* 30(4):427-438, 2004.
Vontress CE, Epp LR: Historical hostility in the African American client: implications for counseling, *J Multicult Counseling Dev* 25:170, 1997.
Worthington R: Effective transitions for families: life beyond the hospital, *Pediatr Nurs* 21:8, 1995.
Wulczyn F: Family reunification, *Future Child* 14(1):94-113, 2004.

# Supportive Family role performance*

*Scott C. Lamont*

## Definition

Patterns of family behavior and expression consistent with expectations and normal role functioning of the family unit in support of an ill or incapacitated family member

## Defining Characteristics

Stated or observed desire of family to be part of the therapy provided to a family member, to provide support to that person during therapy, or to help the person endure the therapy (Lamont, 2003); stated or observed desire of family to be present at the time of family member's death

## Related Factors (r/t)

Family member undergoing therapeutic treatments, including cardiopulmonary resuscitation, invasive procedures, discomforting diagnostic tests, induction of or emergence from general anesthesia; health care crisis

**NOC**

## Outcomes (Nursing Outcomes Classification)

### Suggested NOC Outcomes

Anxiety Level, Caregiver-Patient Relationship, Comfort Level, Coping, Family Coping, Family Integrity, Family Functioning, Family Participation in Professional Care, Family Resiliency, Family Support During Treatment, Fear Level, Fear Level: Child, Grief Resolution, Hope, Participation in Health Care Decisions, Role Performance

**Example NOC Outcome with Indicators**

**Family Support During Treatment** as evidenced by the following indicators: Family members express desire to support ill member/Encourage ill member/Provide comforting touch to ill member (Rate each indicator of **Family Support During Treatment:** 1 = never demonstrated, 2 = rarely demonstrated, 3 = sometimes demonstrated, 4 = often demonstrated, 5 = consistently demonstrated [see Section I].)

*Note: **Supportive Family Role Performance** is a wellness-oriented diagnosis that is not currently an official North American Nursing Diagnosis Association International (NANDA-I) nursing diagnosis. However, it is included because the authors believe that the desire of families to provide support to their members is a normal human response to health care crises and that nurses can use interventions to assist families in meeting this role expectation.

## Client Outcomes

### Client Will (Specify Time Frame):

- Express appropriate concern for ill member and ask how they may assist or support (family)
- Request information about process/procedure/therapy and about client condition/ status (family)
- Maintain communication among all members of family unit, including contacting family members not present as desired by ill member, and provide accurate information to other family members (family)
- Identify level of participation/presence and collaboration in determining care desired and appropriate for client needs (individual and family)
- Provide encouragement, comforting touch, and emotional support to ill member (family)
- Seek social and/or spiritual support appropriate for ill member (family and individual)
- Verbalize meaning and significance of health crisis (family and individual)
- State that his or her sense of support is adequate (individual)
- Express feeling supported, able to cope (individual)
- Appear less anxious and/or exhibit improved cooperation with treatment activities (individual)
- State feeling of accomplishment or role fulfillment (family)

NIC

## Interventions (Nursing Interventions Classification)

### Suggested NIC Interventions

Anxiety Reduction, Coping Enhancement, Crisis Intervention, Environmental Management, Family Integrity Promotion, Family Integrity Promotion: Childbearing Family, Family Involvement Promotion, Family Mobilization, Family Presence Facilitation, Family Process Maintenance, Family Support, Security Enhancement, Spiritual Support

**Example NIC Activities—Family Presence Facilitation**

Assess suitability of the physical location for family presence; prepare the family, assuring they have been informed about what to expect, what they will see, hear, and/or smell

## Nursing Interventions and Rationales

- When providing perioperative care for a pediatric client, offer the parents the option to be present during induction and recovery from anesthesia. **EB and EBN:** *A randomized study involving 103 children and their parents comparing parental presence with a sedative to a sedative alone at induction found that although anxiety levels did not differ between the two groups of children, parental anxiety after separation from the child was significantly lower and parental satisfaction with care provided was significantly higher in the* *intervention group than in the control group (Kain et al, 2000). Parent's level of anxiety was also lower post operatively for those who were present in the recovery room compared to those who were not, although there was no difference in children's anxiety levels pre- and postoperatively (Bru et al, 1993). Parents felt that their presence was beneficial to their child, themselves, and staff (Himes, Munyer, & Henly, 2003).*

- • Assess the anxiety level, temperament, and physical health of the child and parents before surgery to guide individualized care and to screen for those who may not benefit from this intervention. **EB:** *Parents had an increased heart rate and skin conductance level until induction when compared to a control group, although anxiety level and blood pressure did not differ between groups and no abnormal electrocardiogram (ECG) changes were noted (Kain et al, 2003). A randomized study found that children older than four years, children who had a calm temperament, and children whose parents had a low trait anxiety level had significantly lower serum cortisol levels with parental presence at induction when compared with control (Kain et al, 1996). Emergence distress in children was predicted by a temperament described as highly dependent or a history of frequent temper tantrums rather than by parental presence or absence at emergence (Tripi et al, 2004).*
- ▲ If you are not already part of the procedural or resuscitation team, introduce yourself to the staff responsible for treating the client and family. *Communication among team members is an important component of providing the option for family presence (Emergency Nurses Association, 2000).*
- • Assess the suitability of the client's physical location for family presence. *Some environments of care may not have adequate room for family members to be present.*
- ▲ Obtain consensus from the staff for the family's presence and the timing of the family's presence. **EB and EBN:** *The practice of family presence during resuscitation and invasive procedures is controversial, with significant differences in opinion between attending physicians, residents, and nurses (Beckman et al, 2002; Fein, Ganesh, & Alpern, 2004; Helmer et al, 2000; Meyers et al, 2000). Physicians and nurses with less experience may be resistant to or uncomfortable with the family's presence (Ellison, 2003; Fein, Ganesh, & Alpern, 2004).*
- • Obtain information about the client's status, response to treatment, and likely ongoing needs and convey this information to the client's family in a timely manner. Assist the family in contacting family members not currently present, if requested. **EBN:** *Families wonder what is happening with regard to their relative's condition and the care they are receiving (Meyers et al, 2000) and fear that information will be withheld from them (Wagner, 2004).*
- • Facilitate family involvement and presence in accordance with the client's and/or family's stated desires. *A qualitative study involving nine emergency room patients found that the patients believed that the positives of having their family present during invasive procedures or cardiopulmonary resuscitation (CPR) outweighed the negative. Some of the positive aspects cited included enhanced comfort and reminding healthcare providers of the client's "personhood" (Eichhorn et al, 2001). However, a recent study found that 21% of surveyed emergency room patients would not want to have any family member present in the event they were being resuscitated (Benjamin, Holger, & Carr, 2004).*
- • Advocate for the family's desire to be present during resuscitation if the prognosis is very grim. **EB:** *The outcomes of both adult and pediatric resuscitation in the emergency room*

*for an arrest outside the hospital are predictably poor (Graves et al, 1997; Schindler et al, 1996). In a survey of parents in the emergency room, respondents presented with several resuscitation scenarios were most likely to want to be present if their child were likely to die during the attempt (Boie et al, 1999). In this respect, nurses' attitudes toward family presence in another survey study were closer to that of the parents in the Boie study than those of physicians (Beckman et al, 2002).*

F

- Introduce yourself and other members of the support team to the family and client. Use the client's name when speaking to the family.
- Make a holistic assessment of the client's and family's emotional, psychosocial, and spiritual support needs, taking into consideration developmental status. *Young children are often fearful of separation from their parents.* **EB and EBN:** *Parental presence during invasive procedures promotes comfort in pediatric clients (MacLean et al, 2003). Parental anxiety is reduced by parents being present during invasive procedures performed on their children (Powers & Rubenstein, 1999).*
- ▲ Determine the psychological burden of the prognosis and participation for the family, and inform the treatment team of the family's emotional reaction to client's condition. **EB:** *A small retrospective study of bereaved relatives a month after the resuscitation attempt on their relative found that there were no reported adverse psychological effects among those members who witnessed the resuscitation, and that all members were satisfied with their choice to remain with the client (Robinson et al, 1998).*
- Treat the family as a cohesive unit and as participants in the client's care. **EB and EBN:** *Timmermans (1997) identified a "holistic framework" held by some health care providers in relation to resuscitation, described as concern about the survival of the individual, but coupled with family members treated as participants in the resuscitation. A majority of parents want to be involved in the decision to be present (Boie, Moore, Brummett, & Nelson, 1999), however, a significant number of nurses and physicians do not share this point of view (Beckman, 2002).*
- If undergoing resuscitation, assure the family that best possible care is being given to their relative. *While conveying accurate information, foster realistic hope.*
- Inform the family of behavior expectations and limits before entering the treatment area. Provide a dedicated staff person to assure that family members are never left unattended at the bedside. *If children will be present in the treatment area, additional support staff may be needed to attend to their needs (Emergency Nurses Association, 2000).* **EB and EBN:** *Several studies have indicated that a major staff concern is the potential that family member actions may interfere with procedures or resuscitative efforts (Ellison, 2003; Fein, Ganesh, & Alpern, 2004; Jarvis, 1998).*
- When family members indicate a wish to be present, accompany them to and from the treatment area, announce their presence to the treatment staff each time the family enters. Escort the family from the bedside if requested by the staff providing direct care. **EBN:** *Nurses reported that they are often asked by family members to be present when their family members undergo resuscitation or invasive procedures (MacLean et al, 2003). Nurses have also reported wanting to have some control over who is at the bedside when providing care (Ellison, 2003).*
- Provide the opportunity for the family to ask questions and to see, touch, and speak to

the client prior to transfers. **EBN:** *One study found that families felt that they have the right and obligation to be present during treatment and provide their relative with support, comfort, and protection (Meyers et al, 2000).*

- Offer families the opportunity to be present during painful or distressing procedures to provide comfort, and demonstrate techniques that the family may employ to enhance the comfort of their ill family member. **EBN:** *Almost all children prefer to have their parents present during stressful procedures and believe that parental presence is helpful in reducing pain experienced (MacLean et al, 2003).*
- Families may request to be present during critical diagnostic procedures such as testing for brainstem death. **EBN:** *Although a relatively new concept, there are reports that family members have occasionally been allowed to witness brainstem death testing, and therefore developing appropriate guidelines to address this circumstance must be developed (Doran, 2004).*

▲ In the event of a client death, offer and/or coordinate family bereavement follow-up at established intervals. **EB:** *Being present during a family member's resuscitation attempt may assist in the grieving process (Robinson et al, 1998).*

- If specific policies regarding family presence are not available for the care area or facility, advocate the development and adoption of such policies. *Studies have shown that nurses are frequently asked about the option of family presence; however, many organizations have not adopted policies to guide nursing practice (MacLean et al, 2003).*

F

## Multicultural

- No specific multicultural studies have been performed for this diagnosis.
- Assess for the influence of cultural beliefs, norms, values, and expectations on the individual's and family's perception of appropriate family support and family presence during treatment. *What the family considers appropriate or expected may be based on cultural perceptions (Leininger & McFarland, 2002).*
- Cultural differences between organizations and their associated professional staff and clients and their families may limit clinician responses to crisis situations. **EBN:** *A survey of 208 nurses found that respondents identified concerns regarding potential culturally associated barriers to meeting family needs (Ellison, 2003).*
- Refer to the care plan for **Readiness for enhanced family Coping.**

## Geriatric

- Current studies have not addressed the specific needs of geriatric clients and their families related to family presence during resuscitation and invasive procedures.
- Older clients may be less likely to prefer having family members present during resuscitation when compared with younger clients. **EB:** *In one study, the mean age of patients who did not wish to have family members present was significantly older than the mean age of patients who did want to have family present (Benjamin, Holger, & Carr, 2004).*
- Refer to the care plans for **Readiness for enhanced Family processes** and **Anticipatory Grieving.**

### Home Care

- An increasing number of invasive procedures are being performed in the home setting. The client and family preferences regarding family presence during these procedures should be assessed.
- Above interventions may be adapted for home care use.
- Refer to the care plan for **Readiness for enhanced Family processes.**

### Client/Family Teaching

F

- Provide education to parents regarding their role and expectations when they are present for induction and recovery from anesthesia. **EBN:** *A study using a quasi-experimental pre- and posttest design found a significant reduction in anxiety and increase in satisfaction with care when provided with an education program before their child's surgery (Chan & Molassiotis, 2002).*
- Prepare the family (and client, if conscious) before entering the treatment area, assuring they have been informed about what to expect, what they will see, hear, and/or smell. *Guidelines for family presence recommended by the Emergency Nurses Association (2000) include preparing the family adequately before allowing them into the treatment area, particularly if the patient has died.*
- Provide information and explanations to the family and client regarding the interventions being performed or anticipated, medical or nursing jargon used during treatment, and expectations of the client's response to treatment. **EBN:** *A study employing mixed methodology found that family members felt that visitation during treatment helped them understand the seriousness of their relative's condition and to know that every possible intervention had been performed (Meyers et al, 2000).*

## evolve WEBSITES FOR EDUCATION

See the EVOLVE website for World Wide Web resources for client education.

## REFERENCES


Beckman AW et al: MR; P50 (Parental Presence during Painful Pediatric Procedures) Research Group: Should parents be present during emergency department procedures on children, and who should make that decision? A survey of emergency physician and nurse attitudes. *Acad Emerg Med* 9(2):154-158, 2002.

Benjamin M, Holger J, Carr M: Personal preferences regarding family member presence during resuscitation, *Acad Emerg Med* 11(7):750-753, 2004.

Boie ET et al: Do parents want to be present during invasive procedures performed on their children in the emergency department? A survey of 400 parents, *Ann Emerg Med* 34(1):70-74, 1999.

Bru G et al: Parental visitation in the post anesthesia care unit: a means to lessen anxiety. *Child Health Care* 22(3):217-226, 1993.

Chan CS, Molassiotis A: The effects of an educational programme on the anxiety and satisfaction level of parents having parent present induction and visitation in a postanaesthesia care unit, *Paediatr Anaesth* 12(2):131-139, 2002.

Doran M: The presence of family during brain stem death testing, *Intensive Crit Care Nurs* 20(2):87-92, 2004.

Eichhorn DJ et al: Family presence during invasive procedures and resuscitation: hearing the voice of the patient, *Am J Nurs* 101(5):48-55, 2001.

Ellison S: Nurses' attitudes toward family presence during resuscitative efforts and invasive procedures, *J Emerg Nurs* 29(6):515-521, 2003.

Emergency Nurses Association: *Presenting the option for family presence,* ed 2, Des Plaines, IL, 2000, The Association.

Fein JA, Ganesh J, Alpern ER: Medical staff attitudes toward family presence during pediatric procedures, *Pediatr Emerg Care* 20(4):224-227, 2004.

Graves JR et al: Survivors of out of hospital cardiac arrest: their prognosis, longevity and functional status, *Resuscitation* 35(2):117-121, 1997.

Helmer SD et al: Family presence during trauma resuscitation: a survey of AAST and ENA members, *J Trauma* 48(6):1015-1022; discussion 1023-1024, 2000.

Himes MK, Munyer K, Henly SJ: Parental presence during pediatric anesthetic inductions, *AANA J* 71(4):293-298, 2003.

Jarvis AS: Parental presence during resuscitation: attitudes of staff on a paediatric intensive care unit. *Intensive Crit Care Nurs* 14(1):3-7, 1998.

Kain ZN et al: Parental presence during induction of anesthesia: physiological effects on parents, *Anesthesiology* 98(1):58-64, 2003.

Kain ZN et al: Parental presence during induction of anesthesia: a randomized controlled trial, *Anesthesiology* 84(5):1060-1067, 1996.

Kain ZN et al: Parental presence and a sedative premedicant for children undergoing surgery: a hierarchical study, *Anesthesiology* 92(4):939-946, 2000.

Lamont SC: Nursing classification language to describe family presence during resuscitation and invasive procedures, *Int J Nurs Terminol Classif* 14(4):S54, 2003.

Leininger MM, McFarland MR: *Transcultural nursing: concepts, theories, research, and practices,* ed 3, New York, 2002, McGraw-Hill.

Maclean SL et al: Family presence during cardiopulmonary resuscitation and invasive procedures: practices of critical care and emergency nurses, *J Emerg Nurs* 29(3):208-221, 2003.

Meyers TA et al: Family presence during invasive procedures and resuscitation, *Am J Nurs* 100(2):32-42, 2000.

Powers KS, Rubenstein JS: Family presence during invasive procedures in the pediatric intensive care unit: a prospective study, *Arch Pediatr Adolesc Med* 153(9):955-958, 1999.

Robinson SM et al: Psychological effect of witnessed resuscitation on bereaved relatives, *Lancet* 352(9128):614-667, 1998.

Schindler MB et al: Outcome of out-of-hospital cardiac or respiratory arrest in children, *N Engl J Med* 335(20):1473-1479, 1996.

Timmermans S: High touch in high tech: the presence of relatives and friends during resuscitative efforts, *Sch Inq Nurs Pract* 11(2):153-168; discussion 169-173, 1997.

Tripi PA et al: Assessment of the risks editors for emergence distress and post operative behavioral changes in children following general anesthesia, *Paediatr Anaesth* 14(3):235-240, 2004.

Wagner JM: Lived experience of critically ill patients' family members during cardiopulmonary resuscitation, *Am J Crit Care* 13(5):416-420, 2004.

# Fatigue

evolve

*Barbara Given and Paula Sherwood*

**NANDA**

## Definition

An overwhelming, sustained sense of exhaustion and decreased capacity for physical and mental work at usual level

## Defining Characteristics

Inability to restore energy even after sleep, lack of energy or inability to maintain usual level of physical activity, increase in rest requirements, tired, inability to maintain usual routines, verbalization of an unremitting and overwhelming lack of energy, lethargic or listless, perceived need for additional energy to accomplish routine tasks, compromised concentration, disinterest in surroundings, introspection, decreased performance, compromised libido, drowsy, feelings of guilt for not keeping up with responsibilities, inability to concentrate, weakness

## Related Factors (r/t)

### Psychological

Stress, anxiety, depression

### Environmental

Humidity, lights, noise, temperature

### Situational

Negative life events, occupation

### Physiological

Sleep deprivation; pregnancy; poor physical condition; disease states (i.e. cancer, HIV, multiple sclerosis); increased physical exertion; malnutrition; anemia; metabolic imbalance.

**NOC**

## Outcomes (Nursing Outcomes Classification)

### Suggested NOC Outcomes

Concentration, Endurance, Energy Conservation, Nutritional Status, Energy, Vitality

**Example NOC Outcome with Indicators**

**Endurance** as evidenced by the following indicators: Performance of usual routine/Activity/Rested appearance/Blood oxygen level within normal limits/Muscle endurance (Rate each indicator of **Endurance:** 1 = severely compromised, 2 = substantially compromised, 3 = moderately compromised, 4 = mildly compromised, 5 = not compromised [see Section I].)

## Client Outcomes

**Client Will (Specify Time Frame):**

- Identify potential factors that aggravate and relieve fatigue
- Describe ways to assess and track patterns of fatigue
- Verbalize increased energy and improved well-being
- Explain energy conservation plan to offset fatigue
- Explain energy restoration plan to offset fatigue

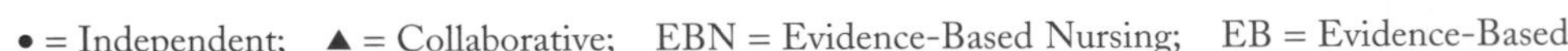

NIC

## Interventions (Nursing Interventions Classification)

### Suggested NIC Intervention

Energy Management (including conservation and restoration)

**Example NIC Activities—Energy Management**

Determine patient's physical limitations; determine significant other's perception of causes of fatigue; determine contributing and aggravating factors

F

## Nursing Interventions and Rationales

- Assess severity of fatigue on a scale of 0 to 10 (average fatigue, worst and best levels); assess frequency of fatigue (number of days per week and time of day), activities and symptoms associated with increased fatigue (i.e., pain), ability to perform ADLs and instrumental activities of daily living (IADLs), interference with social and role function, times of increased energy, ability to concentrate, mood, and usual pattern of activity. Consider use of an instrument such as the Profile of Mood State Short Form Fatigue Subscale, the Multidimensional Assessment of Fatigue, the Lee Fatigue Scale, the Multidimensional Fatigue Inventory, the HIV-Related Fatigue Scale, the Brief Fatigue Inventory, or the Dutch Fatigue Scale to accurately assess fatigue. *These assessments have all been shown to have good internal reliability. The Profile of Mood State Short Form Fatigue Scale was the strongest performer in one study (Meek et al, 2000).* **EBN:** *The Dutch Fatigue Scale, which is based on NANDA-I defining characteristics, is a reliable and valid measurement tool for assessment of fatigue (Tiesinga et al, 2001). The HIV-Related Fatigue EBN Scale is valuable for measuring fatigue in HIV-positive clients (Barroso & Lynn, 2002). The Revised Schwartz Cancer Fatigue Scale and the M.D. Anderson Symptom Inventory are valuable for assessing fatigue in clients with cancer (Cleeland et al, 2000; Schwartz & Meek, 1999).*
- Evaluate adequacy of nutrition and sleep patterns (napping throughout the day, inability to fall asleep or stay asleep). Encourage the client to get adequate rest, limit naps (particularly in the late afternoon or evening), use a routine sleep/wake schedule; and eat a well-balanced diet with at least eight glasses of water a day. Refer to **Imbalanced Nutrition: less than body requirements** or **Disturbed Sleep pattern** if appropriate. *Note: The most commonly suggested treatment for fatigue is rest, although excessive sleep can aggrevate fatigue (Carpenter et al, 2004; Pigeon, Sateia, & Ferguson, 2003). Inadequate nutrition can also contribute to fatigue.*

▲ Determine with help from the primary care practitioner whether there is a physiological or psychological cause of fatigue that could be treated, such as anemia, pain, electrolyte imbalance (i.e., altered potassium levels), hypothyroidism, depression, or medication effect. *The presence of fatigue is associated with biological, psychological, social, and personal factors (Bensing, Hulsman, & Schreurs, 1999). If an etiology for fatigue can be determined, fatigue should be treated according to the underlying cause. Depression and anxiety have been significantly correlated with fatigue in patients with HIV (Phillips et al, 2004).*

▲ Work with the physician to determine if the client has chronic fatigue syndrome. *The Centers for Disease Control and Prevention (CDC) defines chronic fatigue syndrome as "Clinically evaluated, unexplained, persistent, or relapsing chronic fatigue (over 6 months' duration) that is of new or definite onset (has not been lifelong); is not the result of ongoing exertion; is not alleviated by rest; and results in substantial reduction in previous levels of occupational, educational, social, or personal activities. In addition, four or more the following symptoms must concurrently be present for over 6 months: impaired memory or concentration, sore throat, tender cervical or axial lymph nodes, muscle pain, multijoint pain, new headaches, unrefreshing sleep, and postexertion malaise lasting more than 24 hours" (Walker, 1999).*

F

- Encourage the client to express feelings about fatigue, including the client's perception of potential causes of fatigue and possible interventions to alleviate fatigue; use active listening techniques and help identify sources of hope. **EB:** *Chronic fatigue is a disabling illness characterized by persistent fatigue accompanied by rheumatological, cognitive, and infectious appearing symptoms (Craig & Kakumanu, 2002).*
- Encourage the client to keep a journal of activities, symptoms of fatigue, and feelings, including how fatigue impacts the client's normal activities and roles. *The journal helps the client express feelings and monitor progress toward resolving or coping with fatigue, which helps with adjustment (Whitmer, Jakubek, & Barsevick, 1998). The journal can increase the client's awareness of symptoms and sense of control and facilitate communication with health care practitioners (Schumacher et al, 2002).*
- Help the client set small, easily achieved short-term goals such as writing two sentences in a journal daily or walking to the end of the hallway twice daily to increase activity tolerance.
- Help the client identify essential and nonessential tasks and determine which can be delegated. Give the client permission to limit social and role demands if needed (e.g., switch to part-time employment, hire cleaning service). *The nurse can help the client look at life realistically to balance available energy and energy demands.*
- Assist the client with ADLs as necessary; encourage independence and activity without causing exhaustion.
- Encourage walking exercise. **EBN:** *Women undergoing treatment for cancer exercised 90 minutes per week on 3 or more days and reported significantly less fatigue and emotional distress, as well as higher functional ability and quality of life than did women who were less active during treatment (Mock et al, 2001).*

▲ With the physician's approval, refer to physical therapy for carefully monitored aerobic exercise program and possible physical aids, such as a walker or cane. **EBN:** *Aerobic exercise and physical therapy can reduce fatigue in some oncology clients (Stone, 2002).* **EB:** *An exercise program for patients receiving chemotherapy or radiation treatments for breast cancer helped improve levels of fatigue (Mock et al, 2004). An exercise program can also be helpful to the client with other medical conditions, such as heart failure (Gary et al, 2004).* **EB:** *Supervised aerobic exercise training has beneficial effects on physical capacity and fibromyalgia symptoms (Busch et al, 2002).*

- ▲ Patients may desire multiple strategies to relieve fatigue, rather than one single intervention, particularly when there are multiple potential etiologies present. **EB:** *Participants often used multiple strategies to alleviate their fatigue, possibly because of their tendency to attribute it to multiple causes (Seigal, Brown-Bradley, & Lekas, 2004).*
- ▲ Refer the client to diagnosis-appropriate support groups such as National Chronic Fatigue Syndrome Association, Multiple Sclerosis Association, or cancer fatigue websites such as the Oncology Nurses Association. *Support groups can help clients deal with body changes and cope with the frequent depression that accompanies fatigue (Jain & DeLisa, 1998).*
- ▲ For a cardiac client, recognize that fatigue is common following a myocardial infarction (Lee et al, 2000). Refer to cardiac rehabilitation for carefully prescribed and monitored exercise program. *Carefully monitored exercise is thought to decrease symptoms of fatigue in heart patients (Gary et al, 2004).*
- • For fatigue with multiple sclerosis, encourage energy conservation, "recharging efforts," excellent self-care, and consider use of a cooling suit for clients with multiple sclerosis (MS) whose fatigue increases in a warm environment. **EBN:** *Use of a cooling suit by individuals with MS may decrease their sense of fatigue (Flensner & Lindencrona, 2002).*
- • For attentional fatigue, suggest restorative activities using nature such as sitting outside, bird-watching, and gardening (Erickson, 1996; Cimprich, 1993). *Being outside and enjoying nature are restorative activities that can help people recover their strength and think more clearly.*
- ▲ Consider referring for cognitive therapy to help deal with symptoms of fatigue and help change negative thought patterns. *Cognitive therapy can be effective for clients with chronic fatigue syndrome (Walker, 1999; Fisher, 1997), also for clients with HIV (Rose et al, 1998).* **EB:** *Cognitive behavior therapy significantly benefits physical functioning in adult outpatients with chronic fatigue syndrome (Price & Couper, 2002).*
- • For fatigue with cancer, monitor lab values for potential anemia, evaluate treatment regimen (chemotherapy and/or radiation) and tumor burden and suggest energy conservation interventions (Barsevick et al, 2004).
- ▲ If fatigue is associated with cancer or cancer related treatment, assess for other symptoms that may enhance fatigue (i.e., pain or depression). **EB:** *Increased fatigue was seen in breast cancer clients receiving chemotherapy if they were also experiencing unrelieved pain, had nausea with vomiting, or developed mouth sores (Jacobsen et al, 1999). Patients with cancer who reported both pain and fatigue reported three times as many other symptoms as patients who reported neither pain nor fatigue; fatigue was linked to the presence of pain, multiple co-morbid conditions, and site of cancer (Given et al, 2001).*
- ▲ Fatigue in patients with cancer may manifest itself as the inability to direct attention necessary to perform usual activities (attentional fatigue). **EB:** *Reduced performance in cognitive function was observed before treatment and found to persist over time in older women newly diagnosed with breast cancer (Cimprich & Ronis, 2003).*
- ▲ Refer the client to occupational therapy to learn new energy-conserving and energy-restoring ways to perform tasks. *Occupational therapy can help clients learn energy-conserving techniques so that clients can perform ADLs without exhaustion.*

### Geriatric

- Review co-morbid conditions that may contribute to fatigue, such as congestive heart failure (CHF); arthritis; and cancer.
- Identify recent losses; monitor for depression as a possible contributing factor to fatigue. **EBN:** *Thirty elderly women with depression identified symptoms of fatigue and weakness (Ugarriza, 2002).*
- ▲ Review medications for side effects. *Certain medications (e.g., beta-blockers, antihistamines, pain medications, anticonvulsants, chemotherapeutic agents) may cause fatigue in the elderly.*



### Home Care

- Above interventions may be adapted for home care use.
- Assess the client's history and current patterns of fatigue as they relate to the home environment; environmental and behavioral triggers of increased fatigue. *Fatigue may be more pronounced in specific settings for physical, environmental (e.g., stairs required to reach bathroom, patterns of movement around home, cleaning activities that require high energy), or psychological (e.g., rooms associated with loss of loved ones) reasons.*
- ▲ Refer to occupational therapy if substantial intervention is needed to assist the client in adapting to home and daily patterns.
- Assist the client with identifying or creating a safe, restful place within the home that can be used routinely (e.g., a room with familiar, nonthreatening, or nonfrightening belongings). *Withdrawal to a secluded area can allow the client to rest and regain strength.*
  For clients receiving chemotherapy, intervene to:
  - Relieve symptom distress (negative mood, nausea, difficulty sleeping)
  - Encourage as much physical activity as possible
  - Support a positive attitude for the future
  - Support adequate recovery time between treatments

  **EBN:** *The above factors have been identified as contributing to fatigue, particularly during early stages of chemotherapy (Berger & Walker, 2001).*
- ▲ Refer cancer clients to a community-based pain and fatigue management program, such as the I Feel Better program, if available. **EB:** *A program such as I Feel Better was received with enthusiasm and rapid enrollment by cancer clients (Grant et al, 2000).*
- Teach the client/family the importance of and methods for setting priorities for activities, especially those having a high energy demand (e.g., home/family events). Instruct in realistic expectations and behavioral pacing. **EBN:** *The client and/or family may assume a more rapid rate of energy recovery than actually occurs. Assistance may be needed to insure accuracy of expectations for the client. Unrealistic expectations provoke guilt feelings in the client, leading to efforts that can exceed the client's energy capacity (Patusky, 2002).*
- Assess effect of fatigue on the client's relatedness; recognize that the client's fatigue affects the whole family. Initiate the following interventions:
  - Avoid dismissing reports of fatigue; validate the client's experience and foster hope for eventual treatment, if not resolution, of the fatigue.

- Identify with the client ways in which he or she continues to be a valued part of his or her social environment.
- Identify with the client ways in which he or she continues to participate in equitable exchange with others.
- Encourage the client to maintain regular family routines (e.g., meals, sleep patterns) as much as possible.
- Initiate cognitive restructuring to refute the client's guilt-producing and negative thought patterns.
- Assess and intervene with family/friend's contributions to guilt-inducing self-talk.
- Work with the client to inoculate against the negative thinking of others.
- Explore family life and demands to identify accommodations.
- Support the client's efforts at limit setting on the demands of others.
- Assist the client to move toward a state of parallelism by working to identify and relieve sources of physical or emotional discomfort. Degree of involvement, limited by fatigue, need not be changed.

**EBN:** *Based on reports of fatigued women, the above interventions have been suggested as addressing problem areas. Parallelism is a state of comfortable noninvolvement, and was described by some fatigued women as achievable and relatively positive state, given their fatigue (Patusky, 2002). Closeness and acceptance in relationships may decrease the psychological burden and modify the fatigue of chemotherapy recipients (Berger & Walker, 2001).*

▲ Refer for family therapy in the event the client's fatigue interferes with normal family functioning. *Family therapy may be necessary to address underlying problems that may be magnified by the influence of fatigue (Patusky, 2002).*

▲ If fatigue has affected the client's ability to participate in relationships effectively, refer for psychiatric home health care services for client reassurance and implementation of therapeutic regimen. *Psychiatric home care nurses can address issues relating to the client's ability to adjust to changes in health status. Behavioral interventions in the home can assist the client to participate more effectively in the treatment plan (Patusky, 2002).*

## Client/Family Teaching

- Help client to do cognitive reframing: Share information about fatigue and how to live with it, including need for positive self-talk. *Client education legitimizes fatigue and enhances the client's control through self-care and positive self-talk (Fisher, 1997).*
- Teach strategies for energy conservation (e.g., sitting instead of standing during showering, storing items at waist level). *Energy conservation strategies can decrease the amount of energy used (Vanage, Gilbertson, & Mathiowetz, 2001).*
- Teach the client to carry a pocket calendar, make lists of required activities, and post reminders around the house. *Chronic fatigue is often associated with memory loss and sometimes difficulty thinking (Jain & DeLisa, 1998). Fatigue can also result in the inability to direct attention to a certain task, such as cooking or paying bills (i.e., attentional fatigue).*
- Teach the importance of following a healthy lifestyle with adequate nutrition fluids and rest, pain relief, correct insomnia, and appropriate exercise to decrease fatigue (i.e., energy restoration).

- Teach stress-reduction techniques such as controlled breathing, imagery, and use of music.
- See **Anxiety** care plan if appropriate; anxiety is correlated with increased fatigue.

## evolve WEBSITES FOR EDUCATION

See the EVOLVE website for World Wide Web resources for client education.

F

## REFERENCES

Barroso J, Lynn MR: Psychometric properties of the HIV-Related Fatigue Scale, *J Assoc Nurses AIDS Care* 13(1):66, 2002.

Barsevick A, Dudley W, Beck S et al: A randomized clinical trial of energy conservation for patients with cancer-related fatigue, *Cancer* 100(6):1302, 2004.

Berger AM, Walker SN: An explanatory model of fatigue in women receiving adjuvant breast cancer chemo-therapy, *Nurs Res* 50:42, 2001.

Bensing J, Hulsman R, Schreurs K: Gender differences in fatigue: Biopsychosocial factors relating to fatigue in men and women, *Med Care* 37(10):1078, 1999.

Busch A, Schachter CL, Peloso PM et al: Exercise for treating fibromyalgia syndrome, *Cochrane Database Syst Rev* (3):CD003786, 2002.

Carpenter J, Elan J, Ridner S et al: Sleep, fatigue, and depressive symptoms in breast cancer survivors and matched healthy women experiencing hot flashes, *Oncol Nurs Forum* 31(3):591, 2004.

Cimprich B: Development of an intervention to restore attention in cancer patients, *Cancer Nurs* 16(2):83, 1993.

Cimprich B, Ronis D: An environmental intervention to restore attention in women with newly diagnosed breast cancer, *Cancer Nurs* 26(4):284, 2003.

Cleeland CS, Mendoza TR, Wang XS et al: Assessing symptom distress in cancer patients: The MD Anderson Symptom Inventory, *Cancer* 89(7):1634, 2000.

Craig T, Kakumanu S: Chronic fatigue syndrome: evaluation and treatment, *Am Fam Physician* 65(5):1083, 2002.

Erickson JM: Anemia, *Semin Oncol Nurs* 12(1):2, 1996.

Fisher L: Chronic fatigue syndrome, *Prof Nurse* 12(8):578, 1997.

Flensner G, Lindencrona C: The cooling-suit: case studies of its influence on fatigue among eight individuals with multiple sclerosis, *J Adv Nurs* 37(6):541, 2002.

Gary et al: Home-based exercise improves functional performance and quality of life in women with diastolic heart failure, *Heart Lung* 33(4):210, 2004.

Given C, Given B, Azzouz F et al: Predictors of pain and fatigue in the year following diagnosis among elderly cancer patients, *J Pain Symptom Manage* 21(6):456, 2001.

Grant M, Golant M, Rivera L et al: Developing a community program on cancer pain and fatigue, *Cancer Pract* 8(4):187, 2000.

Jacobsen PB, Hann DM, Azzarello LM et al: Fatigue in women receiving adjuvant chemotherapy for breast cancer: characteristics, course, and correlates, *J Pain Symptom Manage* 18(4):233, 1999.

Jain SS, DeLisa JA: Chronic fatigue syndrome: a literature review from a physiatric perspective, *Am J Phys Med Rehabil* 77(2):160, 1998.

Lee H, Kohlman GC, Lee K et al: Fatigue, mood, and hemodynamic patterns after myocardial infarction, *Appl Nurs Res* 13(2):60, 2000.

Meek PM, Nail LM, Barsevick A et al: Psychometric testing of fatigue instruments for use with cancer patients, *Nurs Res* 49(4):181, 2000.

Mock V, Frangakis C, Davidson NE et al: Exercise manages fatigue during breast cancer treatment: a randomized controlled trial, *Psychooncology* Oct 14, 2004.

Mock V, Pickett M, Ropka ME et al: Fatigue and quality of life outcomes of exercise during cancer treatment, *Cancer Pract* 9(3):119, 2001.

Patusky KL: Relatedness theory as a framework for the treatment of fatigued women, *Arch Psychiatr Nurs* 5:224, 2002.

Pigeon W, Sateia M, Ferguson R: Distinguishing between excessive daytime sleepiness and fatigue: toward improved detection and treatment, *J Psychosom Res* 54(1):61, 2003.

Phillips K, Sowell R, Rojas M et al: Physiological and psychological correlates of fatigue in HIV disease, *Biol Res Nurs* 6(1):59, 2004.
Price JR, Couper J: Cognitive behavior therapy for chronic fatigue syndrome in adults, *Cochrane Library* (3):CDOO1027, 2002.
Rose L, Pugh LC, Lears K et al: The fatigue experience: persons with HIV infection, *J Adv Nurs* 28(2):295, 1998.
Schwartz A, Meek P: Additional construct validity of the Schwartz Cancer Fatigue Scale, *J Nurs Meas* 7(1):35, 1999.
Schumacher A, Wewers D, Heinecke A et al: Fatigue as an important aspect of quality of life in patients with acute myeloid leukemia, *Leuk Res* 26(4):355, 2002.
Seigel K, Brown-Bradley C, Lekas H: Strategies for coping with fatigue among HIV-positive individuals fifty years and older, *AIDS Patient Care* 18(5):275, 2004.
Stone P: The measurement, causes and effective management of cancer-related fatigue, *Int J Palliative Nurs* 8(3):120, 2002.
Tiesinga LJ et al: Sensitivity, specificity and usefulness of the Dutch Fatigue Scale, *Nurs Diagn* 12(3):93, 2001.
Ugarriza DN: Elderly women's explanation of depression, *J Gerontol Nurs* 28(5):22, 2002.
Vanage S, Gilbertson K, Mathiowetz V: Effects of an energy conservation course on fatigue impact for persons with progressive multiple sclerosis, *Am J Occup Ther* 57(3):315, 2003.
Walker TL: Chronic fatigue syndrome. Do you know what it means, *Am J Nurs* 99(3):70, 1999.
Whitmer K, Jakubek P, Barsevick A: Use of a daily journal for fatigue management, *Oncol Nurs Forum* 25(6):987, 1998.

F

# Fear

evolve

*Michele Walters*

**NANDA**

## Definition

Response to perceived threat that is consciously recognized as a danger

## Defining Characteristics

Report of apprehension; increased tension; decreased self-assurance; excitement; being scared; jitteriness; dread; alarm; terror; panic

### Cognitive

Identifies object of fear; stimulus believed to be a threat; diminished productivity, learning ability, problem-solving ability

### Behaviors

Increased alertness; avoidance or attack behaviors; impulsiveness; narrowed focus on "it" (i.e., the focus of the fear)

### Physiological

Increased pulse, anorexia, nausea, vomiting, diarrhea, muscle tightness, fatigue, increased respiratory rate and shortness of breath, pallor, increased perspiration, increased systolic blood pressure, pupil dilation, dry mouth

## Related Factors (r/t)

Natural/innate origin (e.g., sudden noise, height, pain, loss of physical support); learned response (e.g., conditioning, modeling from or identification with others); separation from support system in potentially stressful situation (e.g., hospitalization, hospital procedures); unfamiliarity with environmental experience(s); language barrier; sensory impairment; innate releasers (neurotransmitters); phobic stimulus

NOC

## Outcomes (Nursing Outcomes Classification)

F

### Suggested NOC Outcome

Fear Self-Control

**Example NOC Outcome with Indicators**

**Fear Self-Control** as evidenced by the following indicators: Eliminates precursors of fear/Seeks information to reduce fear/Plans coping strategies for fearful situations (Rate each indicator of **Fear Self-Control:** 1 = never demonstrated, 2 = rarely demonstrated, 3 = sometimes demonstrated, 4 = often demonstrated, 5 = consistently demonstrated [see Section I].)

## Client Outcomes

**Client Will (Specify Time Frame):**

- Verbalize known fears
- State accurate information about the situation
- Identify, verbalize, and demonstrate those coping behaviors that reduce own fear
- Report and demonstrate reduced fear

NIC

## Interventions (Nursing Interventions Classification)

### Suggested NIC Interventions

Anxiety Reduction; Coping Enhancement; Security Enhancement

**Example NIC Activities—Anxiety Reduction**

Use a calm reassuring approach; stay with the patient to promote safety and reduce fear

## Nursing Interventions and Rationales

- Assess source of fear with the client. **EB:** *The capacity to experience fear is adaptive, enabling rapid and energetic response to imminent threat or danger (Poulton & Menzies, 2002).*
- Assess for a history of anxiety. **EB:** *Participants in a study of stress responses that were*

*found to have a higher level of anxiety reported higher levels of increased fears (Ronen et al, 2003).*

- Have the client draw the object of their fear. **EBN:** *This can be used as an assessment tool to better understand the experience of the client to facilitate better nursing and professional practice in valuing the experience of others (Locsin et al, 2003).*
- Discuss situation with the client and help distinguish between real and imagined threats to well-being. **EB:** *Fear activation occurs before conscious cognitive analysis of the stimulus can occur (Mineka & Ohman, 2002).*
- Encourage the client to explore underlying feeling that may be contributing to the fear. *Exploring underlying feelings may help the client to confront unresolved conflicts and develop coping abilities (Townsend, 2003).*
- Stay with clients when they express fear; provide verbal and nonverbal (touch and hug with permission and if culturally acceptable) reassurances of safety if safety is within control. **EB:** *Of 376 patients surveyed in 20 family practices throughout Ontario, Canada, 66% believe touch is comforting and healing and view distal touches (on the hand and shoulder) as comforting (Osmun et al, 2000).*
- Explore coping skills used previously by the client to deal with fear; reinforce these skills and explore other outlets. **EBN:** *Recounting previous experiences that were perceived by the client as having been dealt with successfully strengthens effective coping and helps eliminate ineffective coping mechanisms (Northouse et al, 2002).*
- Provide backrubs and massage for clients to decrease anxiety. **EB:** *Massage is effective in reducing distress and pain (Taylor et al, 2003).*
- Use TT and healing touch (HT) techniques. **EBN:** *Nurses may offer TT, quiet time, or dialogue when feelings of calmness and relaxation are desired (Kelly et al, 2004).*
- ▲ Refer for cognitive behavior therapy. **EB:** *This study of 253 persons with neck or back pain, the experimental group who received the standardized six session cognitive behavioral group sessions had significantly better results with regard to fear avoidance beliefs than the comparison group (Linton & Ryberg, 2001).*
- ▲ Animal-assisted therapy can be incorporated into the care of perioperative patients. **EBN:** *In a study done on perioperative clients, interaction with animals was shown to reduce blood pressure and cholesterol, decrease anxiety, and improve a person's sense of well-being (Miller & Ingram, 2000).*
- Encourage clients to express their fears in narrative form. **EB:** *One of the main ways in which people adjust to threats associated with serious illness is through the use of narrative, which helps to make sense of illness (Crossley, 2003).*
- Refer to care plans for **Anxiety** and **Death Anxiety**

## Pediatric

- Instruct parents that nighttime fear is common in children. *Nighttime fears are relatively common in normal children with fear of intruders being the most common (Muris et al, 2001).*
- Explore coping skills used previously by the client to deal with fear. Children generally rate their coping behaviors as helpful. *A variety of coping behaviors reported were seeking support from parents, avoidance, distraction, trying to sleep, and clinging to stuffed animals (Muris et al, 2001).*

- Teach parents to use cognitive-behavioral strategies such as positive coping statements ("I am a brave girl [boy]. I can take care of myself in the dark.") and rewards of bravery tokens for appropriate behavior. *Cognitive-behavioral strategies appear to be effective interventions, but more research is indicated due to methodological limitations (Gordon & King, 2002).*
- Screen for depression in clients who report social/school fears. *Evidence corroborates a significant relationship between depression and childhood social/school fears (Neal et al, 2002).*
- Teach relaxation technique to children to induce calmness. **EB:** *Relaxation training may reduce somatic or psychological symptoms or to support children's ability to cope with emotional reactions (Lohaus & Klein-Hessling, 2002).*

## Geriatric

- Establish a trusting relationship so that all fears can be identified. *An elderly client's response to a real fear may be immobilizing.*
- Monitor for dementia and use appropriate interventions. *Fear may be an early indicator of disorientation or impaired reality testing in elderly clients.*
- Provide a protective and safe environment, use consistent caregivers, and maintain the accustomed environmental structure. *Elderly clients tend to have more perceptual impairments and adapt to changes with more difficulty than younger clients, especially during an illness.*
- Observe for untoward changes if antianxiety drugs are taken. *Advancing age renders clients more sensitive to both the clinical and toxic effects of many agents.*
- Assess for fear of falls in hospitalized patients with hip fractures to determine risk of poor health outcomes. **EBN:** *Fear of falls correlated with poor health outcomes and has a major impact on function, especially with regard to walking (Mckee et al, 2002).*
- Encourage exercises to improve physical skills and levels of mobility to decrease fear of falling. *Improving physical skills and levels of mobility counteract excessive fear during activity performance (Fuzhong et al, 2002).*
- Assist the client in identifying and reducing risk factors of falls, including environmental hazards in and out of the home, the importance of good nutrition and activity, proper foot wear, and how to stand up after a fall. **EB:** *Clients receiving education focused on identifying and reducing risk factors for falls were found to have a significant reduction in their fear of falling (Brouwer et al, 2003).*

## Multicultural

- Assess for the presence of culture-bound anxiety/fear states. **EBN:** *The context in which anxiety/fear is experienced, its meaning, and responses to it are culturally mediated (Charron, 1998; Kavanagh, 1999).*
- Assess for the influence of cultural beliefs, norms, and values on the client's perspective of a stressful situation. **EBN:** *What the client considers stressful may be based on cultural perceptions (Cochran, 1998; Doswell & Erlen, 1998; Leininger & McFarland, 2002).*
- Identify what triggers fear response. **EBN:** *Arab Muslim clients may express a high correlation between fear and pain (Sheets & El-Azhary, 1998).*

- Identify how the client expresses fear. **EBN:** *Research indicates that the expression of fear may be culturally mediated (Shore & Rapport, 1998).*
- Validate the client's feelings regarding fear. **EBN:** *Validation is therapeutic communication technique that lets the client know that the nurse has heard and understands what was said, and it promotes the nurse-client relationship (Heineken, 1998).*
- Assess for fears of racism in culturally diverse clients. **EB:** *Findings suggest that, independent of the effects of gender, age, and household social class, being worried about being a victim of racial harassment could have an important impact on an individual's health experience (Karlsen & Nazroo, 2004).*

F

## Home Care

- Above interventions may be adapted for home care use.
- Assess to differentiate the presence of fear versus anxiety.
- Refer to care plan for **Anxiety.**
- During initial assessment, determine whether current or previous episodes of fear relate to the home environment (e.g., perception of danger in home or neighborhood or of relationships that have a history in the home). *Investigating the source of the fear allows the client to verbalize feelings and the nurse to determine appropriate interventions.*
- Identify with the client what steps may be taken to make the home a "safe" place to be. *Identifying a given area as a safe place reduces fear and anxiety when the client is in that area.*
- ▲ Encourage the client to seek or continue appropriate counseling to reduce fear associated with stress or to resolve alterations in irrational thought processes. *Correcting mistaken beliefs reduces anxiety.*
- ▲ Encourage the client to have a trusted companion, family member, or caregiver present in the home for periods when fear is most prominent. Pending other medical diagnoses, a referral to homemaker/home health aide services may meet this need. *Creating periods when fear and anxiety can be reduced allows the client periods of rest and supports positive coping.*
- ▲ Offer to sit with a terminally ill client quietly as needed by the client or family, or provide hospice volunteers to do the same. *Terminally ill clients and their families often fear the dying process. The presence of a nurse or volunteer lets clients know they are not alone. Fears are reduced, and the dying process becomes more easily tolerated.*

## Client/Family Teaching

- Teach the client the difference between warranted and excessive fear. *Different interventions are indicated for rational and irrational fears.*
- Teach stress management interventions to clients who experience emotions of fear. *Acute stress caused by strong emotions such as fear can sometimes cause sudden death in people with underlying coronary artery disease (Pashkow, 1999).*
- Teach families to share personal stories about an illness using the computer-based psychoeducational application experience journal. *The educational journal was reported to be useful for increasing understanding of familial feelings for families facing pediatric illness (DeMaso et al, 2000).*

- • Teach clients to use guided imagery when they are fearful: have them use all senses to visualize a place that is "comfortable and safe" for them. *Imagery makes use of subjective symbolism bypassing the rational mind and making the areas "safe" that the client may otherwise be reluctant to face (Yip, 2003).*
- ▲ Teach use of appropriate community resources in emergency situations (e.g., hotlines, emergency departments, law enforcement, judicial systems). *Serious emergencies need immediate assistance to ensure the client's safety.*
- ▲ Encourage use of appropriate community resources in nonemergency situations (e.g., family, friends, neighbors, self-help and support groups, volunteer agencies, churches, recreation clubs and centers, seniors, youths, others with similar interests).
- ▲ Teach the client appropriate use of ordered medications.
- ▲ In the event of bioterrorism provide accurate information, and ensure that health care personnel have appropriate training and preparation. *Clear, consistent, accessible, reliable, and redundant information (received from trusted sources) will diminish public uncertainty about the cause of symptoms that might otherwise prompt persons to seek unnecessary treatment. Training for providers is essential (Benedek et al, 2002).*

## evolve WEBSITES FOR EDUCATION

See the EVOLVE websites for World Wide Web resources for client education.

## REFERENCES


Benedek DM, Holloway HC, Becker SM: Emergency mental health management in bioterrorism events, *Emerg Med Clin North Am* 20(2):393, 2002.

Brouwer B, Walker C, Rydahl S et al: Reducing fear of falling in seniors through education and activity programs: a randomized trial, *J Am Geriatr Soc* 51:829-834, 2003.

Charron HS: Anxiety disorders. In Varcarolis EM, editor: *Foundations of psychiatric mental health nursing,* ed 3, Philadelphia, 1998, WB Saunders.

Cochran M: Tears have no color, *Am J Nurs* 98(6):53, 1998.

Crossley ML: "Let me explain": narrative employment and one patient's experience of oral cancer, *Soc Sci Med* 56(3):439, 2003.

DeMaso DR, Gonzalez-Heydrich J et al: The experience journal: a computer-based intervention for families facing congenital heart disease, *J Am Acad Child Adolesc Psychiatr* 39(6):727-734, 2000.

Doswell W, Erlen J: Multicultural issues and ethical concerns in the delivery of revising care interventions, *Nurs Clin North Am* 33(2):353, 1998.

Gordon J, King N: Children's night-time fears: an overview, *Couns Psychol Q* 15(2):121, 2002.

Heineken J: Patient silence is not necessarily client satisfaction: communication in home care nursing, *Home Healthcare Nurs* 16(2): 115, 1998.

Karlsen S, Nazroo JY: Fear of racism and health, *J Epidemiol Community Health* 58(12):1017-1018, 2004.

Kavanagh KH: The role of cultural diversity in mental health nursing. In Fontaine KL, Fletcher JS, editors: *Mental health nursing,* ed 4, Menlo Park, Calif, 1999, Addison-Wesley.

Kelly A, Sullivan P, Fawcett J et al: Therapeutic touch, quiet time and dialogue: perceptions of women with breast cancer, *Oncol Nurs Forum* 31(3):645, 2004.

Leininger MM, McFarland MR: *Transcultural nursing: concepts, theories, research and practices,* ed 3, New York, 2002, McGraw-Hill.

Fuzhong L, McAuley E, Fisher KJ et al: Self-efficacy as a mediator between fear of falling and functional ability in the elderly, *J Aging Health* 14(4):452, 2002.

Linton SJ, Ryberg M: A cognitive-behavioral group intervention as prevention for persistent neck and back pain in a non-patient population: a randomized controlled trial, *Pain* 90(1-2):83, 2001.

Locsin RC, Barnard A, Matua AG: Surviving ebola: understanding experience through artistic expression, *Int Nurs Rev* 50:156-166, 2003.
Lohaus A, Klein-Hessling J: Relaxation in children: effects of extended and intensified training, *Psychol Health* 18(2):237-249, 2003.
McKee KJ, Orbell S, Austin CA et al: Fear of falling, falls efficacy, and health outcomes in older people following hip fracture, *Disabil Rehabil* 24(6):327, 2002.
Miller J, Ingram L: Perioperative nursing and animal-assisted therapy, *AORN J* 72(3):477, 2000.
Mineka S, Ohman A: Phobias and preparedness: the selective, automatic, and encapsulated nature of fear, *Biol Psychiatry* 15(52): 10, 2002.
Muris P, Merckelbach H, Ollendick TH et al: Children's night-time fears: parent-child ratings of frequency, content, origins, coping behaviors and severity, *Behav Res Ther* 39(1):13-28, 2001.
Neal J, Edelmann R, Glachan M: Behavioural inhibition and symptoms of anxiety and depression: is there a specific relationship with social phobia? *Br J Clin Psychol* 41:361, 2002.
Northouse LL, Walker J, Schafenacker A et al: A family-based program of care for women with recurrent breast cancer and their family members, *Oncol Nurs Forum* 29(10):1411-1419, 2002.
Osmun WE, Brown JB, Stewart M et al: Patients' attitudes to comforting touch in family practice, *Can Fam Physician* 46(12): 2411-2416, 2000.
Pashkow F: Is stress linked to heart disease? The evidence grows stronger, *Cleve Clin J Med* 66(2):75, 1999.
Poulton R, Menzies RG: Non-associative fear acquisition: a review of the evidence from retrospective and longitudinal research, *Behav Res Ther* 40(2):127, 2002.
Ronen T, Rahav G, Appel N: Adosescent stress responses to a single acute stress and to continuous external stress: terrorist attacks, *J Loss Trauma* 8(4):261-282, 2003.
Sheets DL, El-Azhary RA: The Arab Muslim client: implications for anesthesia, *AANA J* 66(3):304, 1998.
Taylor A, Galper D, Taylor P et al: Effects of adjunctive Swedish massage and vibration therapy on short-term postoperative outcomes: a randomized, controlled trial, *J Altern Complement Med* 9(1):77-89, 2003.
Townsend M: *Psychiatric mental health nursing: concepts of care*, ed 4, Philadelphia, 2003, FA Davis.
Yip K: The relief of a caregiver's burden through guided imagery, role-playing, humor, and paradoxical intervention, *Am J Psychother* 57(1):109-122, 2003.



# Readiness for enhanced Fluid balance

*Betty J. Ackley*

**NANDA**

## Definition

A pattern of equilibrium between fluid volume and chemical composition of body fluids that is sufficient for meeting physical needs and can be strengthened

## Defining Characteristics

Expresses willingness to enhance fluid balance; stable weight; moist mucous membranes; food and fluid intake adequate for daily needs; straw-colored urine with specific gravity within normal limits; good tissue turgor; no excessive thirst; urine output appropriate for intake; no evidence of edema or dehydration

## Related Factors (r/t)

Motivation to improve hydration status

**NOC**

## Outcomes (Nursing Outcomes Classification)

### Suggested NOC Outcomes

Fluid Balance; Hydration; Nutritional Status: Food and Fluid Intake

F

**Example NOC Outcome with Indicators**

**Fluid Balance** as evidenced by the following indicators: Skin turgor/Moist mucous membranes/Orthostatic hypotension not present/24-hour intake and output balanced/Urine specific gravity (Rate each indicator of **Fluid Balance:** 1 = severely compromised, 2 = substantially compromised, 3 = moderately compromised, 4 = mildly compromised, 5 = not compromised [see Section I].)

## Client Outcomes

### Client Will (Specify Time Frame):

- Maintain light yellow urine output
- Maintain elastic skin turgor, moist tongue, and mucous membranes
- Explain measures that can be taken to improve fluid intake.

**NIC**

## Interventions (Nursing Interventions Classification)

### Suggested NIC Intervention

Fluid Management

**Example NIC Activities—Fluid Management**

Monitor hydration status (e.g., moist mucous membranes, adequacy of pulses, and orthostatic blood pressure) as appropriate; Monitor food/fluid ingested and calculate daily caloric intake, if appropriate

## Nursing Interventions and Rationales

- Discuss normal fluid requirements. *A guideline is 1 to 1.5 mL of fluid per each calorie needed, so an average intake would be between 2000 and 3000 ml/day, or at least 8 cups of fluid (Grodner, Long, & DeYoung, 2004). The Adequate Intake recommendation is 3 liters for the 19 to 30 year old male and 2.2 L for the 19 to 30 year old female. Water balance studies suggest that adult men require 2.5 L per day (Institute of Medicine, 2004).*

- Recommend mainly intake of water, but milk or fruit juice can also be effective in maintaining good fluid balance (Cataldo et al, 2003).
- Recommend the client decrease the use of alcoholic beverages and beverages containing caffeine to provide fluid to the body. *Both alcohol and caffeine act as a diuretic, causing increased loss of fluid in the urine. But drinking fluids with caffeine or alcohol are not associated with increased incidence of dehydration, and consumption of these fluids does contribute to the total body fluid needs of individuals (Institute of Medicine, 2004).*
- Recommend the client avoid intake of carbonated beverages, instead suggest the client drink water. *Most carbonated beverages contain large amounts of sugar, 10 or more teaspoons of sugar, are a significant source of empty calories, and can cause significant damage to the teeth (ADA, 2004).*

F

### Geriatric

- Encourage the elderly client to develop a pattern of drinking water regularly. *Thirst sensations diminish with aging, dehydration can threaten elderly clients (Grodner, Long, & DeYoung, 2004; Mentes, 2004).* **EB:** *A study demonstrated that healthy men age 67 to 75 years were less thirsty and replaced less fluid than did young people during fluid deprivation (Philips et al, 1984).*

### Home Care

- Assess availability of clean drinking water in the home, or assess resources to acquire bottled water. *Willingness to maintain fluid balance may be compromised by a lack of available clean water.*

▲ Assess available and preferred fluids. Refer for social services if resources are needed to purchase adequate fluid. *Affordability of milk or juice may be an obstacle to availability of fluids. Assistance to obtain food stamps may be indicated.*

## Client/Family Teaching

- Teach the client to drink water before and during engaging in activities that can result in dehydration quickly such as the distance runner or the gardener in hot weather. *Maintaining hydration before, during, and after training and competition helps reduce fluid loss, maintain performance, reduce heat stress, heat exhaustion, and possible heart stroke (Von Duvillard et al, 2004).* **EB:** *A study demonstrated that there was a decrease in long-term memory when exercising in a hot environment and not replacing lost fluids, which did not occur if the subject ingested fluids to restore fluid balance (Cian et al, 2001). Another study demonstrated that drinking fluids earlier resulted in a faster rate of plasma and fluid balance restoration, even though similar amounts of fluid were ingested (Kovacs et al, 2002).*
- Caution the athlete client not to drink excessively during competition or training, to follow the dictates of thirst. *There have been at least seven deaths and 250 cases of hyponatremic encephalopathy since the advice of "drink the maximum amount that can be tolerated" (Noakes, 2003). Excessive hydration without adequate sodium intake may result in sodium depletion (Institute of Medicine, 2004; Von Duvillard et al, 2004).*

- Teach clients who work in hot environments or exercise in hot environments to increase intake of both water and use of electrolyte-carbohydrate beverages, the sports drinks are needed when exercise exceeds 1 hour or during prolonged competitive games that require repeated intermittent activity (Welsh et al, 2002). *A review of the literature demonstrated that drinks containing low to moderate levels of electrolytes and carbohydrates may provide significant advantages in industrial situations (Clap et al, 2002).* **EB:** *A study demonstrated that drinking flavored drinks during sports athletic activity compared with water enhanced fluid balance (Minehan et al, 2002).*
- Ask the client to monitor the color of urine to tell if adequately hydrated. *In a hydrated person the urine should be light yellow—the color of lemonade. Urine the color of apple juice indicates slight dehydration (Cataldo et al, 2003).* **EBN:** *A research study on elderly veterans demonstrated that urine color correlated significantly with urine osmolality, serum sodium, and blood urea nitrogen (BUN)/creatinine ratio (Wakefield et al, 2002).*

## evolve WEBSITES FOR EDUCATION

See the EVOLVE website for World Wide Web resources for client education.

## REFERENCES

American Dental Association: Oral health topics A-Z. Available at www.ada.org/public/topics, accessed on March 5, 2005.

Cataldo CB, DeBruyne LK, Whitney EN: *Nutrition and diet therapy,* ed 6, Belmont, Calif, 2003, Thomson Wadsworth.

Cian C, Barraud PA, Melin B et al: Effects of fluid ingestion on cognitive function after heat stress or exercise-induced dehydration, *Int J Psychophysiol* 42(3):243, 2001.

Clap AJ, Bishop PA, Smith JF et al: A review of fluid replacement for workers in hot jobs, *AIHA J* 63(2):190, 2002.

Grodner M, Long S, DeYoung S: *Foundations and clinical applications of nutrition: a nursing approach,* ed 3, St. Louis, 2004, Mosby.

Institute of Medicine: Applications of dietary reference intakes for electrolytes and water, *National Academy of Sciences*, National Academies Press, 2004.

Kovacs EM, Schmahl RM, Senden JM et al: Effect of high and low rates of fluid intake on post-exercise rehydration, *Int J Sport Nutr ExercMetab* 12(1):14, 2002.

Mentes JC: Hydration management. Iowa City (IA): University of Iowa Gerontological Nursing Interventions Research Center, Research Dissemination Core, 2004.

Minehan MR, Riley MD, Burke LM: Effect of flavor and awareness of kilojoule content of drinks on preference and fluid balance in team sports, *Int J Sport Nutr Exerc Metab* 12(1):81, 2002.

Noakes TD: Overconsumption of fluids by athletes, *BMJ* 327(7407):113, 2003.

Philips PA, Rolls BJ, Ledingham JG et al: Reduced thirst after water deprivation in healthy elderly men, *N Engl J Med* 311(12): 753, 1984.

Von Duvillard SP, Braun WA, Markofski M et al: Fluids and hydration in prolonged endurance performance. *Nutrition* 20(7-8): 651, 2004.

Wakefield B, Mentes J, Diggelmann L et al: Monitoring hydration status in elderly veterans, *West J Nurs Res* 24(2):132, 2002.

Welsh RS, Davis JM, Burke JR et al: Carbohydrates and physical/mental performance during intermittent exercise to fatigue, *Med Sci Sports Exerc* 34(4):723, 2002.

# Deficient Fluid volume

evolve

*Betty J. Ackley*

**NANDA**

## Definition

Decreased intravascular, interstitial, and/or intracellular fluid (refers to dehydration, water loss alone without change in sodium level)

F

## Defining Characteristics

Decreased urine output; increased urine concentration; weakness; sudden weight loss (except in third-spacing); decreased venous filling; increased body temperature; decreased pulse volume/pressure; change in mental state; elevated hematocrit; decreased skin/tongue turgor; dry skin/mucous membranes; thirst; increased pulse rate; decreased blood pressure

## Related Factors (r/t)

Active fluid volume loss; failure of regulatory mechanisms

**NOC**

## Outcomes (Nursing Outcomes Classification)

### Suggested NOC Outcomes

Electrolyte and Acid-Base Balance; Fluid Balance; Hydration; Nutritional Status: Food and Fluid Intake

**Example NOC Outcome with Indicators**

**Fluid Balance** as evidenced by the following indicators: Skin turgor/Moist mucous membranes/Orthostatic hypotension not present/24-hour intake and output balanced/Urine specific gravity (Rate each indicator of **Fluid Balance:** 1 = severely compromised, 2 = substantially compromised, 3 = moderately compromised, 4 = mildly compromised, 5 = not compromised [see Section I].)

## Client Outcomes

**Client Will (Specify Time Frame):**

- Maintain urine output more than 1300 mL/day (or at least 30 mL/hr)
- Maintain normal blood pressure, pulse, and body temperature
- Maintain elastic skin turgor; moist tongue and mucous membranes; and orientation to person, place, and time

• = Independent; ▲ = Collaborative; EBN = Evidence-Based Nursing; EB = Evidence-Based

- Explain measures that can be taken to treat or prevent fluid volume loss
- Describe symptoms that indicate the need to consult with health care provider

NIC

## Interventions (Nursing Interventions Classification)

### Suggested NIC Interventions

Fluid Management; Hypovolemia Management; Shock Management: Volume

F

**Example NIC Activities—Fluid Management**

Monitor hydration status (e.g., moist mucous membranes, adequacy of pulses, and orthostatic blood pressure) as appropriate; Administer intravenous fluids at room temperature

## Nursing Interventions and Rationales

- Watch for early signs of hypovolemia, including restlessness, weakness, muscle cramps, headaches, inability to concentrate and postural hypotension. *Late signs include oliguria, abdominal or chest pain, cyanosis, cold clammy skin, and confusion (Kasper et al, 2005).* **EB:** *A study of healthy volunteers who experienced a fluid restriction of up to 37 hours reported symptoms of headache, decreased alertness, and inability to concentrate (Shirreffs et al, 2004).*
- Monitor for the existence of factors causing deficient fluid volume (e.g., vomiting, diarrhea, difficulty maintaining oral intake, fever, uncontrolled type 2 diabetes, diuretic therapy). *Early identification of risk factors and early intervention can decrease the occurrence and severity of complications from deficient fluid volume. The gastrointestinal system is a common site of abnormal fluid loss (Metheny, 2000).*
- Monitor daily weight for sudden decreases, especially in the presence of decreasing urine output or active fluid loss. Weigh the client on the same scale with the same type of clothing at same time of day, preferably before breakfast. *Body weight changes reflect changes in body fluid volume (Kasper et al, 2005; Suhayda & Walton, 2002). A 1-pound weight loss reflects a fluid loss of about 500 mL (Metheny, 2000).*
- Monitor total fluid intake and output every 8 hours (or every hour for the unstable client). Recognize that urine output is not always an accurate indicator of fluid balance. *A urine output of less than 30 mL/hr is insufficient for normal renal function and indicates hypovolemia or onset of renal damage (Metheny, 2000). Urine output can be unreliable to indicate fluid balance because if the client is hypothermic or elderly or has renal dysfunction, the client may be unable to concentrate urine leading to falsely high urine output (Schulman, 2002).*
- Watch trends in output for 3 days; include all routes of intake and output and note color and specific gravity of urine. *Monitoring for trends for 2 to 3 days gives a more valid picture of the client's hydration status than monitoring for a shorter period (Metheny, 2000). Dark-colored urine with increasing specific gravity reflects increased urine concentration.*
- Monitor vital signs of clients with deficient fluid volume every 15 minutes to 1 hour for the unstable client (every 4 hours for the stable client). Observe for tachycardia,

tachypnea, decreased pulse pressure first, then hypotension, decreased pulse volume, and increased or decreased body temperature. *A decreased pulse pressure is an earlier indicator of shock than is the systolic blood pressure (Mikhail, 1999). Decreased intravascular volume results in hypotension and decreased tissue oxygenation. The temperature will be decreased as a result of decreased metabolism, or it may be increased if there is infection or hypernatremia present (Metheny, 2000).*

- Check orthostatic blood pressures with the client lying, sitting, and standing. *A 20 mm Hg drop when upright or an increase of 15 beats/min in the pulse rate are seen with deficient fluid volume (Kasper et al, 2005). If the systolic blood pressure drops 20 mm Hg and the pulse rate does not change, the baroreceptors in the body are not working, and the cause can be cardiovascular, neurologic or a medication effect (Sclater & Kannayiram, 2004).*
- Monitor for inelastic skin turgor, thirst, dry tongue and mucous membranes, longitudinal tongue furrows, speech difficulty, dry skin, sunken eyeballs, weakness (especially of upper body), headache, and confusion. *These are symptoms of decreased body fluids (Metheny, 2000).*
- Provide frequent oral hygiene, at least twice a day (if mouth is dry and painful, provide hourly while awake). *Oral hygiene decreases unpleasant tastes in the mouth and allows the client to respond to the sensation of thirst.*
- Provide fresh water and oral fluids preferred by the client (distribute over 24 hours [e.g., 1200 mL on days, 800 mL on evenings, and 200 mL on nights]); provide prescribed diet; offer snacks (e.g., frequent drinks, fresh fruits, fruit juice); instruct significant other to assist the client with feedings as appropriate. *The oral route is preferred for maintaining fluid balance (Metheny, 2000). Distributing the intake over the entire 24-hour period and providing snacks and preferred beverages increases the likelihood that the client will maintain the prescribed oral intake.*
- Provide free water with tube feedings as appropriate (50 to 100 mL every 4 hours) or 30 mL/kg of body weight (Suhayda & Walton, 2002). *This provides water for replacement of intravascular or intracellular volume as necessary. Tube feeding has been found to increase the risk for dehydration (Sheehy et al, 1999; Lavizzo-Mourey et al, 1988).*
- Institute measures to rest the bowel when the client is vomiting or has diarrhea (e.g., restrict food or fluid intake when appropriate, decrease intake of milk products).

▲ Hydrate the client with ordered intravenous (IV) solutions if prescribed. *The most common cause of deficient fluid volume is gastrointestinal (GI) loss of fluid. At times it is preferable to allow the GI system to rest before resuming oral intake. Hydration should be maintained.* Refer to care plan for **Diarrhea** or **Nausea**.

▲ Provide oral replacement therapy as ordered and tolerated with a hypotonic glucose-electrolyte solution when the client has acute diarrhea or nausea/vomiting. Provide small, frequent quantities of slightly chilled solutions. *Maintenance of oral intake stabilizes the ability of the intestines to digest and absorb nutrients; glucose-electrolyte solutions increase net fluid absorption while correcting deficient fluid volume. Use diluted carbohydrate-electrolyte solutions such as sports replacement drinks, cola, and ginger ale, which are often tolerated better than other solutions, sometimes even with vomiting and diarrhea (Suhayda & Walton, 2002).* **EB:** *A study demonstrated that decreasing the osmolality of standard glucose-electrolyte oral replacement solutions improves the absorption of water, and stool volume (Farthing, 2002).*

- ▲ Administer antidiarrheals and antiemetics as appropriate. *The goal is to stop the loss that results from vomiting or diarrhea.*
- ▲ If the client requires IV fluid replacement, maintain patent IV access, set an appropriate IV infusion flow rate, and administer at a constant flow rate as ordered. *Isotonic intravenous fluids such as 0.9% normal saline or lactated Ringer's allow replacement of intravascular volume (Metheny, 2000).*
- • Assist with ambulation if the client has postural hypotension. *Postural hypotension can cause dizziness, which places the client at higher risk for injury.*



## Critically Ill

- • If a trauma client, check manual blood pressure until the systolic is 110. Do not rely on automatic blood pressure measurements. **EB:** *A study demonstrated that automatic blood pressure measurements were consistently higher than manual, and the manual blood pressures better represented the injury severity, degree of acidosis, and resuscitation volume needed (Davis et al, 2003).*
- • Monitor central venous pressure, right atrial pressure, and pulmonary wedge pressure for decreases. *Hemodynamic parameters are sensitive indicators of intravascular fluid volume, and hemodynamic measurements are especially needed in the client with cardiac or renal problems (Kasper et al, 2005; Metheny, 2000).*
- • Monitor serum and urine osmolality, serum sodium, BUN/creatinine ratio, and hematocrit for elevations. *These are all measures of concentration and will be elevated with decreased intravascular volume (Kasper et al, 2005).*
- • Utilize a sublingual capnometry device if available to determine level of tissue hypoxia caused by lack of fluid volume. *Recognizing decreased perfusion during resuscitation from blood loss can help avoid onset of multiple organ failure (Boswell & Scalea, 2003).*
- ▲ Insert a foley catheter if ordered and measure urine output hourly. Notify physician if less than 30 mL/hour. *A decrease in urine output is seen with increasing severity of shock in the client with normal kidneys (Docherty & McIntyre, 2002).*
- ▲ When ordered, initiate a fluid challenge of crystalloids (0.9% normal saline or lactated Ringer's) for replacement of intravascular volume; monitor the client's response to prescribed fluid therapy and fluid challenge, especially noting central venous pressure and pulmonary capillary wedge pressure readings, vital signs, urine output, blood lactate concentrations, and lung sounds. *A fluid challenge can help the client with deficient fluid volume regain intravascular volume quickly, but the client must be carefully observed to ensure that he or she does not go into fluid volume overload (Kruse et al, 2003). In trauma clients, if there is no clinical improvement after 2L of crystalloids, then generally a blood transfusion should be initiated (Kasper et al, 2005; Jordan, 2000).*
- • Position the client flat with legs elevated when hypotensive, if not contraindicated. *This position enhances venous return, thus contributing to the maintenance of cardiac output.*
- ▲ Monitor trends in serum lactic acid levels and base deficit obtained from blood gasses as ordered. *A trend of increasing lactic acid levels and increasing base deficit can help identify occult hypoperfusion, which results in decreased survival and increased incidence of organ failure (Schulman, 2002).*
- ▲ Consult physician if signs and symptoms of deficient fluid volume persist or worsen.

*Prolonged deficient fluid volume increases the risk for development of complications, including shock, multiple organ failure, and death.*

## Pediatric

- Monitor the child for signs of deficient fluid volume, including capillary refill time, skin turgor, and respiratory pattern along with other symptoms. **EB:** *A meta-analysis of the literature identified these factors as more significant in identifying dehydration, but these are still imprecise and it is difficult to determine the exact degree of dehydration (Steiner, DeWalt, & Byerley, 2004).*
- ▲ Reenforce the physician's recommendation for the parents to give the child oral rehydration fluids to drink in the amounts specified, especially during the first 4 to 6 hours to replace fluid losses. Once the child is rehydrated, an orally administered maintenance solution should be used along with food. **EBN and EB:** *Oral rehydration therapy is effective for treating mild to moderate dehydration in children with diarrhea and may help prevent the need for hospitalization with administration of IV fluids (Larson, 2000). Reduced osmolarity oral rehydration fluid compared with standard rehydration fluid resulted in lower stool volume, less need for IV fluids, and less vomiting (Hahn, Kim, & Garner, 2005).* **EB:** *A study demonstrated that treatment with oral rehydration fluids for children were generally as effective as intravenous fluids, and IV fluids did not shorten the duration of gastroenteritis and are more likely to cause adverse effects than oral rehydration therapy (Banks & Meadows, 2005).*
- Recommend the mother resume breastfeeding as soon as possible.
- Recommend parents not give the child decarbonated soda, fruit juices, gelatin dessert, or instant fruit drink mix. *These fluids have a high osmolality due to carbohydrate contents and can exacerbate diarrhea. In addition they have low sodium concentrations, which can aggravate existing hyponatremia (Behrman, Kliegman, & Jenson, 2004).*
- Recommend parents give children foods with complex carbohydrates such as potatoes, rice, bread, cereal, yogurt, fruits, and vegetables. The BRAT diet is often advocated: bananas, rice, applesauce, and toast. Avoid fatty foods and foods high in simple sugars *(Behrman, Kliegman, & Jenson, 2004).*

## Geriatric

- Monitor elderly clients for deficient fluid volume carefully, noting new onset of weakness, dizziness, or dry mouth with longitudinal furrows. *The elderly are predisposed to deficient fluid volume because of decreased fluid in body, decreased thirst sensation, and decreased ability to concentrate urine (Suhayda & Walton, 2002; Bennett, 2000).*
- Evaluate the risk for dehydration using the Dehydration Risk Appraisal Checklist (Mentes, 2004).
- Check skin turgor of elderly client on the forehead, sternum, or inner thigh; also look for the presence of longitudinal furrows on the tongue and dry mucous membranes. *Elderly people commonly have decreased skin turgor from normal age-related loss of elasticity; therefore checking skin turgor on the arm is not reflective of fluid volume (Bennett, 2000; Suhayda & Walton, 2002). The presence of longitudinal furrows or dry mucous membranes is a good indication of dehydration in the elderly (Bennett, 2000).*

- Encourage fluid intake by offering fluids regularly to cognitively impaired clients. *The elderly have a decreased thirst sensation (Metheny, 2000), and short-term memory loss may impede the client's memory of fluid intake, or the client may be unable to obtain fluids as needed (Amella, 2004).*
- Incorporate regular hydration into daily routines (e.g., extra glass of fluid with medication or social activities). Consider use of a beverage cart and a hydration assistant to routinely offer increased beverages to clients in extended care. **EBN and EB:** *A nursing study demonstrated that institution of a beverage cart with a trained hydration assistant resulted in increased number of bowel movements, less use of laxatives, decreased number of falls, less urinary tract infections, respiratory infections, and skin breakdown (Robinson & Rosher, 2002). A study demonstrated that verbal prompting and offering preference fluids resulted in increased fluid intake among nursing home residents (Simmons et al, 2001).*
- If client is identified as having chronic dehydration, flag the food tray to indicate to caregivers they should finish 75% to 100% of their food and fluids (Mentes, 2004).
- Note the color of urine and compare against a urine color chart to monitor adequate fluid intake. **EBN:** *A research study on elderly veterans demonstrated that urine color correlated significantly with urine osmolality, serum sodium, and BUN/creatinine ratio (Wakefield et al, 2002).*
- Monitor elderly clients for excess fluid volume during the treatment of deficient fluid volume: listen to lung sounds, watch for edema, and note vital signs. *The elderly client has a decreased ability to adapt to rapid increases in intravascular volume and can quickly develop fluid overload (Allison & Lobo, 2004).*

## Home Care

- Determine if it is appropriate to intervene for deficient fluid volume or to allow the client to die comfortably without fluids as desired. *Deficient fluid volume may be a symptom of impending death in terminally ill clients. The deficit may result in a mild euphoria and a more comfortable death (Bennett, 2000).* **EB:** *A study of witnessed death by hospice nurses demonstrated that clients who voluntarily refused fluids and food usually die a "good" death within two weeks (Ganzini et al, 2003).*
- Teach family members how to monitor output in the home (e.g., use of commode "hat" in the toilet, urinal, or bedpan, or use of catheter and closed drainage). Instruct them to monitor both intake and output. *An accurate measure of fluid intake and output is an important indicator of client fluid status (Metheny, 2000).*
- When weighing the client, use same scale each day. Be sure scale is on a flat, not cushioned, surface. Do not weigh the client with scale placed on any kind of rug. Use bed or chair scales for clients who are unable to stand. *An accurate daily weight is an excellent reflection of fluid balance (Metheny, 2000).*

▲ Teach family about complications of deficient fluid volume and when to call physician.

▲ If the client is receiving intravenous fluids, there must be a responsible caregiver in the home. Teach caregiver about administration of fluids, complications of IV administration (e.g., fluid volume overload, speed of medication reactions), and when to call for assistance. Assist caregiver with administration for as long as necessary to maintain client safety. *Administration of intravenous fluids in the home is a high-technology procedure and requires sufficient professional support to ensure safety of the client.*

▲ Identify an emergency plan, including when to call 911. *Some complications of deficient fluid volume cannot be reversed in the home and are life threatening. Clients progressing toward hypovolemic shock will need emergency care.*

## Client/Family Teaching

- Instruct the client to avoid rapid position changes, especially from supine to sitting or standing.
- Teach the client and family about appropriate diet and fluid intake.
- Teach the client and family how to measure and record intake and output accurately.
- Teach the client and family about measures instituted to treat hypovolemia and to prevent or treat fluid volume loss.
- Instruct the client and family about signs of deficient fluid volume that indicate they should contact health care provider.



## evolve WEBSITES FOR EDUCATION

See the EVOLVE websites for World Wide Web resources for client education.

## REFERENCES


Allison SP, Lobo, DN: Fluid and electrolytes in the elderly, *Curr Opin Clin Nutr Metab Care* 7(1):27, 2004.

Amella EJ: Feeding and hydration issues for older adults with dementia, *Nurs Clin North Am* 39:607, 2004.

Banks JB, Meadows S: Intravenous fluids for children with gastroenteritis, *Am Family Physician* 71(1):121, 2005.

Bennett JA: Dehydration: hazards and benefits, *Geriatr Nurs* 21(2):84, 2000.

Behrman RE, Kliegman RM, Jenson HB: *Nelson textbook of pediatrics*, ed 17, Philadelphia, 2004, WB Saunders.

Boswell SA, Scalea TM: Sublingual capnometry: an alternative to gastric tonometry for the management of shock resuscitation, *AACN Clin Issues* 14(2):176, 2003.

Davis JW, Davis IC, Bennink LD et al: Are automated blood pressure measurements accurate in trauma patients? *J Trauma* 55(5): 860, 2003.

Docherty B, McIntyre L: Nursing considerations for fluid management in hypovolaemia, *Prof Nurse* 17(9):545, 2002.

Farthing MJ: Oral rehydration: an evolving solution, *J Pediatr Gastroenterol Nutr* 34(Suppl 1):S64, 2002.

Ganzini L, Goy ER, Miller LL et al: Nurses' experiences with hospice patients who refuse food and fluids to hasten death, *N Engl J Med* 349(4):359, 2003.

Hahn S, Kim S, Garner P: Reduced osmolarity oral rehydration solution for treating dehydration caused by acute diarrhea in children, *Cochrane Database Syst Rev* (1):CD002847, 2002.

Jordan KS: Fluid resuscitation in acutely injured patients, *J Intravenous Nurs* 23(2):81, 2000.

Kasper DL et al, editors: *Harrison's principles of internal medicine,* ed 16, New York, 2005, McGraw-Hill.

Kruse JA, Fink MP, Carlson RW: *Saunders manual of critical care,* Philadelphia, 2003, WB Saunders.

Larson CE: Evidence-based practice: safety and efficacy of oral rehydration therapy for the treatment of diarrhea and gastroenteritis in pediatrics, *Pediatr Nurs* 26(2):177, 2000.

Lavizzo-Mourey RM, Johnson J, Stolley P: Risk factors for dehydration among elderly nursing home residents, *J Am Geriatr Soc* 36(3):213, 1988.

Mentes JC: Hydration management. Iowa City: University of Iowa Gerontological Nursing Interventions Research Center, Research Dissemination Core, 2004.

Metheny N: *Fluid and electrolyte balance: nursing considerations,* ed 4, Philadelphia, 2000, JB Lippincott.

Mikhail J: Resuscitation endpoints in trauma, *AACN Clin Issues* 10(1):10, 1999.

Robinson SB, Rosher RB: Can a beverage cart help improve hydration? *Geriatr Nurs* 23:4, 2002.
Sclater A, Kannayiram A: Orthostatic hypotension: a primary care primer for assessment and treatment, *Geriatrics* 59(8):22, 2004.
Schulman C: End points of resuscitation: choosing the right parameters to monitor, *Dimens Crit Care Nurs* 21(1):2, 2002.
Sheehy CM, Perry PA, Cromwell SL: Dehydration: biological considerations, age-related changes, and risk factors in older adults, *Biol Res Nurs* 1(1):30, 1999.
Shirreffs SM, Merson SJ, Fraser SM et al: The effects of fluid restriction on hydration status and subjective feelings in man, *Br J Nutr* 91(6):951, 2004.
Simmons SF, Alessi C, Schnelle JF: An intervention to increase fluid intake in nursing home residents: prompting and preference compliance, *J Am Geriatr Soc* 49(7):926, 2001.
Steiner MJ DeWalt DA, Byerley JS: Is this child dehydrated? *JAMA* 291(22):2764, 2004.
Suhayda R, Walton JC: Preventing and managing dehydration, *Medsurg Nurs* 11(6):267, 2002.
Wakefield B, Mentes J, Diggelmann L et al: Monitoring hydration status in elderly veterans, *West J Nurs Res* 24(2):132, 2002.

F

# Excess Fluid volume

evolve

*Betty J. Ackley*

**NANDA**

## Definition

Increased isotonic fluid retention

## Defining Characteristics

Jugular vein distention; decreased hemoglobin and hematocrit; weight gain over short period; changes in respiratory pattern, dyspnea or shortness of breath; orthopnea; abnormal breath sounds (rales or crackles); pulmonary congestion; pleural effusion; intake exceeds output; S3 heart sound; change in mental status; restlessness; anxiety; blood pressure changes; pulmonary artery pressure changes; increased central venous pressure; oliguria; azotemia; specific gravity changes; altered electrolytes; edema, may progress to anasarca; positive hepatojugular reflex

## Related Factors (r/t)

Compromised regulatory mechanism, excess fluid intake, excess sodium intake

**NOC**

## Outcomes (Nursing Outcomes Classification)

### Suggested NOC Outcomes

Electrolyte and Acid-Base Balance, Fluid Balance, Hydration

**Example NOC Outcome with Indicators**

**Fluid Balance** as evidenced by the following indicators: Peripheral edema/Neck vein distention/Adventitious breath sounds/Body weight increase/Intake and output imbalance (Rate each indicator of **Fluid Balance:** 1 = severe, 2 = substantial, 3 = moderate, 4 = mild, 5 = none [see Section I].)

WNL, Within normal limits.

## Client Outcomes

### Client Will (Specify Time Frame):

- Remain free of edema, effusion, anasarca; weight appropriate for the client
- Maintain clear lung sounds; no evidence of dyspnea or orthopnea
- Remain free of jugular vein distention, positive hepatojugular reflex, and gallop heart rhythm
- Maintain normal central venous pressure, pulmonary capillary wedge pressure, cardiac output, and vital signs
- Maintain urine output within 500 mL of intake with normal urine osmolality and specific gravity
- Explain measures that can be taken to treat or prevent excess fluid volume, especially fluid and dietary restrictions and medications
- Describe symptoms that indicate the need to consult with health care provider

NIC

## Interventions (Nursing Interventions Classification)

### Suggested NIC Interventions

Fluid Management, Fluid Monitoring

**Example NIC Activities—Fluid Monitoring**

Weigh daily and monitor trends; maintain accurate intake and output record

## Nursing Interventions and Rationales

- Monitor location and extent of edema; use a millimeter tape in the same area at the same time each day to measure edema in extremities. *Generalized edema (e.g., in the upper extremities and eyelids) is associated with decreased oncotic pressure as a result of nephrotic syndrome. Measuring the extremity with a millimeter tape is more accurate than using the 1+ to 4+ scale (Metheny, 2000). Heart failure and renal failure are usually associated with dependent edema because of increased hydrostatic pressure; dependent edema will cause swelling in the legs and feet of ambulatory clients and the presacral region of clients on bed rest.* **EBN:** *Dependent edema was found to demonstrate the greatest sensitivity as a defining characteristic for excess fluid volume (Rios et al, 1991).*

F

- Monitor daily weight for sudden increases; use same scale and type of clothing at same time each day, preferably before breakfast. *Body weight changes reflect changes in body fluid volume. Clinically, it is extremely important to get an accurate body weight of a client with fluid imbalance (Metheny, 2000).* **EB:** *A study demonstrated that body weight could safely be used to monitor for fluid overload when administering hyperhydration with high dose chemotherapy (Mank et al, 2003).*
- Monitor lung sounds for crackles, monitor respirations for effort, and determine the presence and severity of orthopnea. *Pulmonary edema results from excessive shifting of fluid from the vascular space into the pulmonary interstitial space and alveoli. Pulmonary edema can interfere with the oxygen/carbon dioxide exchange at the alveolar-capillary membrane (Metheny, 2000), resulting in dyspnea and orthopnea.*
- With head of bed elevated 30 to 45 degrees, monitor jugular veins for distention in the upright position; assess for positive hepatojugular reflex. *Increased intravascular volume results in jugular vein distention, even in a client in the upright position, and also a positive hepatojugular reflex.*
- Monitor central venous pressure, mean arterial pressure, pulmonary artery pressure, pulmonary capillary wedge pressure, and cardiac output; note and report trends indicating increasing pressures over time. *Increased vascular volume with decreased cardiac contractility increases intravascular pressures, which are reflected in hemodynamic parameters. Over time, this increased pressure can result in uncompensated heart failure (Kasper et al, 2005).*
- Monitor vital signs; note decreasing blood pressure, tachycardia, and tachypnea. Monitor for gallop rhythms. If signs of heart failure are present, see the care plan for **Decreased Cardiac output.** *Heart failure results in decreased cardiac output and decreased blood pressure. Tissue hypoxia stimulates increased heart and respiratory rates.*
- Monitor serum osmolality, serum sodium, BUN/creatinine ratio, and hematocrit for decreases. *These are all measures of concentration and will decrease (except in the presence of renal failure) with increased intravascular volume. In clients with renal failure, the BUN will increase because of decreased renal excretion (Kasper et al, 2005).*
- Monitor intake and output; note trends reflecting decreasing urine output in relation to fluid intake. *Accurately measuring intake and output is very important for the client with fluid volume overload.*
- Monitor the client's behavior for restlessness, anxiety, or confusion; use safety precautions if symptoms are present. *When excess fluid volume compromises cardiac output, the client may experience cerebral tissue hypoxia, and the client may demonstrate restlessness and anxiety (Kasper et al, 2005). When the excess fluid volume results in hyponatremia, symptoms such as agitation, irritability, inappropriate behavior, confusion, and seizures may occur (Kasper et al, 2005; Kruse et al, 2003).*
- Monitor for the development of conditions that increase the client's risk for excess fluid volume. *Common causes are heart failure, renal failure, and liver failure, all of which result in decreased glomerular filtration rate and fluid retention. Other causes are increased intake of oral or intravenous fluids in excess of the client's cardiac and renal reserve levels, increased levels of antidiuretic hormone, or movement of fluid from the interstitial space to the intravascular space (Kasper et al, 2005). Early detection allows the institution of specific treatment measures before the client develops pulmonary edema.*

- ▲ Assist with continuous renal replacement therapy (CRRT) as ordered if the client is critically ill and excessive fluid must be removed. *CRRT is indicated for severe volume overload, refractory heart failure, oliguric renal failure, metabolic acidosis, and azotemia with uremic symptoms (Kempher, 2003; Kruse et al, 2003).*
- ▲ Provide a restricted-sodium diet as appropriate if ordered. *Restricting the sodium in the diet will favor the renal excretion of excess fluid. Take care to avoid hyponatremia. Decreasing sodium can be just as important as restricting fluid intake with fluid overload (Kasper et al, 2005).*
- ▲ Monitor serum albumin level and provide protein intake as appropriate. *Serum albumin is the main contributor to serum oncotic pressure, which favors the movement of fluid from the interstitial space into the intravascular space. When serum albumin is low, peripheral edema may be severe.*
- ▲ Administer prescribed diuretics as appropriate; check blood pressure before administration to ensure is adequate. If IV administration of a diuretic, note and record urine output following the dose.
- ▲ Monitor for side effects of diuretic therapy: orthostatic hypotension (especially if the client is also receiving ACE inhibitors), hypovolemia and electrolyte imbalances (hypokalemia and hyponatremia). Observe for hyperkalemia in clients receiving a potassium-sparing diuretic, especially with the concurrent administration of an ACE inhibitor (Kasper et al, 2005).
- ▲ Implement fluid restriction as ordered, especially when serum sodium is low; include all routes of intake. Schedule fluids around the clock, and include the type of fluids preferred by the client. *Fluid restriction may decrease intravascular volume and myocardial workload. Overzealous fluid restriction should not be used because hypovolemia can worsen heart failure. Client involvement in planning will enhance participation in the necessary fluid restriction.*
- • Maintain the rate of all IV infusions carefully. *This is done to prevent inadvertent exacerbation of excess fluid volume.*
- • Turn clients with dependent edema frequently (i.e., at least every 2 hours). *Edematous tissue is vulnerable to ischemia and pressure ulcers (Casey, 2004).*
- • Provide for scheduled rest periods. *Bed rest can induce diuresis related to diminished peripheral venous pooling, resulting in increased intravascular volume and glomerular filtration rate (Metheny, 2000).*
- • Promote a positive body image and good self-esteem. *Visible edema may alter the client's body image.* Refer to the care plan for **Disturbed Body image**.
- ▲ Consult with physician if signs and symptoms of excess fluid volume persist or worsen. *Because excess fluid volume can result in pulmonary edema, it must be treated promptly and aggressively (Kasper et al, 2005).*

## Geriatric

- • Recognize that the presence of risk factors for excess fluid volume is particularly serious in the elderly. *Sodium and fluid overload is common in hospitalized elderly clients and can result in increased morbidity and mortality in surgical clients (Allison & Lobo, 2004).*

## Home Care

- • Assess client and family knowledge of disease process causing excess fluid volume.
- ▲ Teach about disease process and complications of excess fluid volume, including when to contact physician. *Knowledge of disease and complications promotes early detection of and intervention for pending problems.*
- • Assess client and family knowledge and compliance with medical regimen, including medications, diet, rest, and exercise. Assist family with integrating restrictions into daily living. *Knowledge promotes compliance. Assistance with integration of cultural values, especially those related to foods, with medical regimen promotes compliance and decreased risk of complications.*
- • If the client is confined to bed rest or has difficulty reclining, follow previously mentioned positioning recommendations.
- ▲ Teach and reinforce knowledge of medications. Instruct the client not to use over-the-counter (OTC) medications (e.g., diet medications) without first consulting the physician.
- ▲ Instruct the client to make primary physician aware of medications ordered by other physicians. *There is potential for undesirable interaction among multiple medications, especially when use of over-the-counter and other prescribed medications is not monitored.*
- ▲ Identify emergency plan for rapidly developing or critical levels of excess fluid volume when diuresing is not safe at home. *When out of control, excess fluid volume can be life threatening.*
- ▲ Teach about signs and symptoms of both excess and deficient fluid volume and when to call physician. *Fluid volume balance can change rapidly with aggressive treatment.*

## Client/Family Teaching

- • Describe signs and symptoms of excess fluid volume and actions to take if they occur.
- ▲ Teach client on diuretics to weigh self daily in the morning, and notify the physician if there is a 3 pound or more change in weight (Karch, 2004).
- ▲ Teach the importance of fluid and sodium restrictions. Help the client and family to devise a schedule for intake of fluids throughout entire day. Refer to dietitian concerning implementation of low-sodium diet.
- ▲ Teach how to take diuretics correctly: take one dose in the morning and second dose (if taken) no later than 4 p.m. Adjust potassium intake as appropriate for potassium-losing or potassium-sparing diuretics. Note the appearance of side effects such as weakness, dizziness, muscle cramps, numbness and tingling, confusion, hearing impairment, palpitations or irregular heartbeat, and postural hypotension.
- • Caution the athlete client not to drink excessively during competition or training, to follow the dictates of thirst. *There have been at least seven deaths and 250 cases of hyponatremic encephalopathy since the advice of "drink the maximum amount that can be tolerated" (Noakes, 2003). Excessive hydration without adequate sodium intake may result in sodium depletion (Institute of Medicine, 2004; Von Duvillard et al, 2004).*

- For the client undergoing hemodialysis, spend time with the client to detect any factors that may interfere with the client's compliance with the fluid restriction or restrictive diet. **EBN:** *The nurse who knows the client well is able to develop individualized interventions to help the client adhere to the restriction (Morgan, 2001).*

## evolve WEBSITES FOR EDUCATION

See the EVOLVE website for World Wide Web resources for client education.

F

## REFERENCES

Allison SP, Lobo, DN: Fluid and electrolytes in the elderly, *Curr Opin Clin Nutr Metab Care* 7(1):27, 2004.
Byers J, Goshorn J: How to manage diuretic therapy, *Am J Nurs* 95(2):38, 1995.
Casey G: Edema: causes, physiology and nursing management, *Nur Stand* 18(51):45, 2004.
Cody R, Kubo S, Pickworth K: Diuretic treatment for the sodium retention of congestive heart failure, *Arch Intern Med* 154:1905, 1994.
DePriest J: Reversing oliguria in critically ill patients, *Postgrad Med* 102(3):245, 1997.
Dunbar SB, Jacobson LH, Deaton C: Heart failure: strategies to enhance patient self-management, *AACN Clin Issues* 9(2):244, 1998.
Kasper DL et al, editors: *Harrison's principles of internal medicine,* ed 16, New York, 2005, McGraw-Hill.
Kempher KJ: Continuous renal replacement therapy for management of overhydration in heart failure, *AACN Clin Issues* 14(4): 512, 2003.
Kruse JA, Finnk MP, Carlson RW: *Saunders manual of critical care,* Philadelphia, 2003, WB Saunders.
Mank A, Semin-Goossens A, Lelie J et al: Monitoring hyperhydration during high-dose chemotherapy: body weight or fluid balance? *Acta Haematol* 109(4):163, 2003.
Mentes JC: Hydration management. Iowa City: University of Iowa Gerontological Nursing Interventions Research Center, Research Dissemination Core, 2004.
Metheny N: *Fluid and electrolyte balance: nursing considerations,* ed 4, Philadelphia, 2000, JB Lippincott.
Rios H et al: Validation of defining characteristics of four nursing diagnoses using a computerized data base, *J Prof Nurs* 7:293, 1991.

# Risk for deficient Fluid volume

*Betty J. Ackley*

**NANDA**

### Definition

At risk for experiencing vascular, cellular, or intracellular dehydration

### Risk Factors

Factors influencing fluid needs (e.g., hypermetabolic state); extremes of age; extremes of weight; excessive losses of fluid through normal routes (e.g., diarrhea); loss of fluids through abnormal routes (e.g., indwelling tubes); deviations affecting access, intake, or absorption of fluids (e.g., physical immobility); knowledge deficiency regarding fluid volume; medication (e.g., diuretics)

## Related Factors (r/t)

See Risk Factors

NOC

## Outcomes (Nursing Outcomes Classification)

F

### Suggested NOC Outcomes

Fluid Balance; Hydration; Knowledge: Treatment Regimen

**Example NOC Outcome with Indicators**

**Fluid Balance** as evidenced by the following indicators: Skin turgor/Moist mucous membranes/Orthostatic hypotension not present/24-hour intake and output balanced/Urine specific gravity (Rate each indicator of **Fluid Balance:** 1 = severely compromised, 2 = substantially compromised, 3 = moderately compromised, 4 = mildly compromised, 5 = not compromised [see Section I].)

## Client Outcomes

**Client Will (Specify Time Frame):**

- Maintain urine output of more than 1300 mL/day (or at least 30 mL/hr)
- Maintain normal blood pressure, pulse, and body temperature
- Maintain elastic skin turgor; moist tongue and mucous membranes; and orientation to person, place, and time
- Explain measures that can be taken to treat or prevent fluid volume loss
- Describe symptoms that indicate the need to consult with health care provider

NIC

## Interventions (Nursing Interventions Classification)

### Suggested NIC Interventions

Fluid Management; Fluid Monitoring, Hypovolemia Management

**Example NIC Activities—Fluid Management**

Monitor hydration status (e.g., moist mucous membranes, adequacy of pulses, and orthostatic blood pressure) as appropriate

## Nursing Interventions and Rationales

- Watch for early signs of hypovolemia, including restlessness, weakness, muscle cramps, headaches, inability to concentrate and postural hypotension. *Late signs include oliguria, abdominal or chest pain, cyanosis, cold clammy skin, and confusion (Kasper et al, 2005).* **EB:** *A study of healthy volunteers who experienced a fluid restriction of up to 37 hours reported symptoms of headache, decreased alertness, and inability to concentrate (Shirreffs et al, 2004).*

- Monitor for the existence of factors causing deficient fluid volume (e.g., vomiting, diarrhea, difficulty maintaining oral intake, fever, uncontrolled type 2 diabetes, diuretic therapy). *Early identification of risk factors and early intervention can decrease the occurrence and severity of complications from deficient fluid volume. The GI system is a common site of abnormal fluid loss (Metheny, 2000).*
- Monitor daily weight for sudden decreases, especially in the presence of decreasing urine output or active fluid loss. Weigh the client on the same scale with the same type of clothing at same time of day, preferably before breakfast. *Body weight changes reflect changes in body fluid volume (Kasper et al, 2005; Suhayda & Walton, 2002). A 1-pound weight loss reflects a fluid loss of about 500 mL (Metheny, 2000).*
- Monitor total fluid intake and output every 8 hours (or every hour for the unstable client). Recognize that urine output is not always an accurate indicator of fluid balance. *A urine output of less than 30 mL/hr is insufficient for normal renal function and indicates hypovolemia or onset of renal damage (Metheny, 2000). Urine output can be unreliable to indicate fluid balance because if the client is hypothermic or elderly or has renal dysfunction, the client may be unable to concentrate urine leading to falsely high urine output (Schulman, 2002).*
- Check orthostatic blood pressures with the client lying, sitting, and standing. *A 20 mm Hg drop when upright or an increase of 15 beats/min in the pulse rate is seen with deficient fluid volume (Kasper et al, 2005). If the systolic blood pressure drops 20 mm Hg and the pulse rate does not change, the baroreceptors in the body are not working, and the cause can be cardiovascular, neurologic, or a medication effect (Sclater & Kannayiram, 2004).*
- Monitor for inelastic skin turgor, thirst, dry tongue and mucous membranes, longitudinal tongue furrows, speech difficulty, dry skin, sunken eyeballs, weakness (especially of upper body), headache, and confusion. *These are symptoms of decreased body fluids (Metheny, 2000).*
- Use appropriate preoperative fasting guidelines as ordered: "allow the consumption of clear liquids up to two hours before elective surgery, a light breakfast (tea and toast, for example) six hours before the procedure, and a heavier meal eight hours beforehand" (Crenshaw & Winslow, 2002, p 36). **EBN and EB:** *Research has demonstrated that pulmonary aspiration is a rare complication of anesthesia, and prolonged fasting before surgery can lead to dehydration, headache, and hypoglycemia (Smith et al, 1997; Hung, 1992). A study demonstrated that most patients received instructions of nothing by mouth (NPO) after midnight for preoperative fasting, resulting in some patients with afternoon surgeries fasting up to 20 hours from liquids, and 37 hours from solids (Crehshaw & Winslow, 2002).*
- Refer to care plan for **Deficient Fluid volume.**

## Geriatric

- Monitor elderly clients for deficient fluid volume carefully, noting new onset of weakness, dizziness, or dry mouth with longitudinal furrows. *The elderly are predisposed to*



F

*deficient fluid volume because of decreased fluid in body, decreased thirst sensation, and decreased ability to concentrate urine (Suhayda & Walton, 2002; Bennett, 2000).*

- Evaluate the risk for dehydration using the Dehydration Risk Appraisal Checklist (Mentes, 2004).
- Check skin turgor of elderly client on the forehead, sternum, or inner thigh; also look for the presence of longitudinal furrows on the tongue and dry mucous membranes. *Elderly people commonly have decreased skin turgor from normal age-related loss of elasticity; therefore checking skin turgor on the arm is not reflective of fluid volume (Bennett, 2000; Suhayda & Walton, 2002). The presence of longitudinal furrows or dry mucous membranes is a good indication of dehydration in the elderly (Bennett, 2000).*
- Encourage fluid intake by offering fluids regularly to cognitively impaired clients. *The elderly have a decreased thirst sensation (Metheny, 2000), and short-term memory loss may impede the client's memory of fluid intake, or the client may be unable to obtain fluids as needed (Amella, 2004).*
- Incorporate regular hydration into daily routines (e.g., extra glass of fluid with medication or social activities). Consider use of a beverage cart and a hydration assistant to routinely offer increased beverages to clients in extended care. **EBN and EB:** *A nursing study demonstrated that institution of a beverage cart with a trained hydration assistant resulted in increased number of bowel movements, less use of laxatives, decreased number of falls, less urinary tract infections, respiratory infections, and skin breakdown (Robinson and Rosher, 2002). A study demonstrated that verbal prompting and offering preference fluids resulted in increased fluid intake among nursing home residents (Simmons et al, 2001).*
- Aim for 1500 mL of oral liquids per day unless contraindicated by a medical condition such as congestive heart failure.
- Allow adequate time for eating and drinking at meals. *Meals can provide two thirds of daily fluids if clients are encouraged to consume liquids and have sufficient time to do so (Bennett, 2000).*
- Note the color of urine and compare against a urine color chart to monitor adequate fluid intake. **EBN:** *A research study on elderly veterans demonstrated that urine color correlated significantly with urine osmolality, serum sodium, and BUN to creatinine ratios (Wakefield et al, 2002).*

### Home Care

- Assess availability of clean drinking water in the home, or assess resources to acquire bottled water. *Willingness to maintain fluid balance may be compromised by a lack of available clean water.*
- ▲ Assess available and preferred fluids. Refer for social services if resources are needed to purchase adequate fluid. *Affordability of milk or juice may be an obstacle to availability of fluids. Assistance to obtain food stamps may be indicated.*

## Client/Family Teaching

- Teach clients who work in hot environments or exercise in hot environments to increase intake of both water and use of electrolyte-carbohydrate beverages. *A review of the literature demonstrated that drinks containing low to moderate levels of electrolytes and carbohydrates may provide significant advantages in industrial situations (Clap et al, 2002).*

## evolve WEBSITES FOR EDUCATION

See the EVOLVE website for World Wide Web resources for client education.

## REFERENCES


Amella EJ: Feeding and hydration isues for older adults with dementia, *Nurs Clin North Am* 39:607, 2004.

Bennett JA: Dehydration: hazards and benefits, *Geriatr Nurs* 21(2):84, 2000.

Clap AJ, Bishop PA, Smith JF et al: A review of fluid replacement for workers in hot jobs, *AIHA J* 63(2):190, 2002.

Crenshaw JT, Winslow EH: Preoperative fasting: old habits die hard, *Am J Nurs* 102(5):36, 2002.

Hung P: Preoperative fasting, *Nurs Times* 88:48, 1992.

Kasper DL et al, editors: *Harrison's principles of internal medicine,* ed 16, New York, 2005, McGraw-Hill.

Mentes JC: Hydration management. Iowa City: University of Iowa Gerontological Nursing Interventions Research Center, Research Dissemination Core, 2004.

Metheny N: *Fluid and electrolyte balance: nursing considerations,* ed 4, Philadelphia, 2000, Lippincott.

Robinson SB, Rosher RB: Can a beverage cart help improve hydration? *Geriatr Nurs* 23(4):208, 2002.

Schulman C: End points of resuscitation: choosing the right parameters to monitor, *Dimens Crit Care Nurs* 21(1):2, 2002.

Sclater A, Kannayiram A: Orthostatic hypotension: a primary care primer for assessment and treatment, *Geriatrics* 59(8):22, 2004.

Shirreffs SM, Merson SJ, Fraser SM et al: The effects of fluid restriction on hydration status and subjective feelings in man, *Br J Nutr* 91(6):951, 2004.

Simmons SF, Alessi C, Schnelle JF: An intervention to increase fluid intake in nursing home residents: prompting and preference compliance, *J Am Geriatr Soc* 49(7):926, 2001.

Smith AF, Vallance H, Slater RM: Shorter preoperative fluid fasts reduce postoperative emesis, *BMJ* 314(7092):1486, 1997.

Suhayda R, Walton JC: Preventing and managing dehydration, *Medsurg Nurs* 11(6):267, 2002.

Wakefield B, Mentes J, Diggelmann L et al: Monitoring hydration status in elderly veterans, *West J Nurs Res* 24(2):132, 2002.


# Risk for imbalanced Fluid volume

*Terri Foster and Betty J. Ackley*

**NANDA**

### Definition

At risk for a decrease, increase, or rapid shift from one to the other of intravascular, interstitial, and/or intracellular fluid (refers to body fluid loss, gain, or both)

### Risk Factors

Major invasive procedures

**NOC**

### Outcomes (Nursing Outcomes Classification)

#### Suggested NOC Labels

Fluid Balance, Electrolyte and Acid-Base Balance, Hydration

**Example NOC Outcome with Indicators**

Maintains **Fluid Balance** as evidenced by the following indicators: BP/Peripheral pulses palpable/Skin turgor/Moist mucous membranes/Serum electrolytes/Hematocrit/Peripheral edema/Neck vein distention/Body weight stable/24-hour intake and output balanced/Urine specific gravity/ Adventitious breath sounds (Rate each indicator of **Fluid Balance:** 1 = severely compromised, 2 = substantially compromised, 3 = moderately compromised, 4 = mildly compromised, 5 = not compromised [see Section I])

## Client Outcomes

- Lung sounds clear, respiratory rate 12 to 20, and free of dyspnea postoperatively
- Urine output greater than 30 mL/hr (Beyea, 2002)
- Blood pressure, pulse rate, temperature and pulse oximetry within expected range (Beyea, 2002)
- Laboratory values within expected range (Beyea, 2002)
- Nonedematous extremities and dependent areas
- Mental orientation unchanged from preoperative status

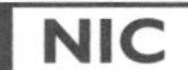

## Interventions (Nursing Interventions Classification)

### Suggested NIC Interventions

Acid-base Management, Acid-base Monitoring, Autotransfusion, Bleeding Precautions, Bleeding Reduction: Wound, Electrolyte Management, Fluid Management, Fluid Monitoring, Hemodynamic Regulation, Hypervolemia Management, Hypovolemia Management, Intravenous Therapy, Invasive Hemodynamic Monitoring, Shock Management: Volume, Vital Signs Monitoring

**Example NIC Activities—Fluid Management**

Maintain accurate intake and output record; monitor vital signs

## Nursing Interventions and Rationales

- Monitor vital signs of clients with deficient fluid volume q15 min/hr if unstable and q4hr if stable. Observe for tachycardia, tachypnea, and decreased pulse pressure which will occur first, followed by hypotension, decreased pulse volume, and increased or decreased body temperature. *Decreased intravascular volume results in hypotension and decreased tissue oxygenation. A decrease in temperature is a result of decreased metabolism, and an increase in temperature is a result of presence of infection or hypernatremia (Metheny, 2000).*
- Check the client's orthostatic blood pressures. *A 15 mm Hg drop in blood pressure when upright or an increase of 15 beats/min in pulse rate is seen with deficient fluid volume (Metheny, 2000).*

- Monitor for non-elastic skin turgor, thirst, dry tongue and mucous membranes, longitudinal tongue furrows, difficulty speaking, dry skin, sunken eyeballs, weakness (especially upper body), headache, and confusion which are symptoms of decreased body fluids (Metheny, 2000). **EB:** *A study of healthy volunteers who experienced a fluid restriction of up to 37 hours reported symptoms of headache, decreased alertness, and inability to concentrate (Shirreffs et al, 2004).*
- Provide frequent oral hygiene—at least twice daily. If the client's mouth is dry and painful, provide oral hygiene hourly while awake. *Oral hygiene decreases unpleasant tastes in the mouth and allows the client to respond to the sensation of thirst.*
- Initiate measures to rest the bowel when the client is vomiting or has diarrhea, i.e., restrict food or fluid intake when appropriate, decrease intake of milk products, and so on. Hydrate the client with any prescribed (ordered) intravenous solutions. *The most common cause of deficient fluid volume is gastrointestinal loss of fluid. At times it is preferable to allow the gastrointestinal system to rest before resuming oral intake. Hydration should be maintained.* Refer to care plan for **Diarrhea** or **Nausea.**
- Provide oral replacement therapy as ordered and tolerated, with a hypotonic glucose-electrolyte solution when the client has acute diarrhea or nausea/vomiting. Provide small, frequent qualities of slightly chilled solutions. *Use carbohydrate-electrolyte solutions such as sports replacement drinks, cola, and ginger ale, which are often tolerated better than other solutions when vomiting and diarrhea are occurring (Suhayda & Walton, 2002).* **EB:** *A study demonstrated that decreasing the osmolality of standard glucose-electrolyte oral replacement solutions improves the absorption of water, and stool volume (Farthing, 2002).*
- Maintain patent intravenous access, if the client requires intravenous fluid replacement. *Isotonic intravenous fluids such as 0.9% normal saline or lactated Ringer's allow replacement of intravascular volume (Metheny, 2000).*
- Monitor for the existence of factors causing deficient fluid volume, i.e., vomiting, diarrhea, difficulty maintaining oral intake, fever, uncontrolled type 2 diabetes, diuretic therapy, preoperative bowel prep, and so on. *Early identification of risk factors and early intervention can decrease the occurrence and severity of complications due to deficient fluid volume. The gastrointestinal system is a common site of abnormal fluid loss (Metheny, 2000).*

▲ When ordered, administer a fluid challenge giving a specified amount of IV fluid, such as 0.9% normal saline rapidly IV, for replacement of intravascular volume and monitor client's response noting vital signs, lung sounds, and urine output, and pulmonary capillary wedge pressure or central venous pressures if applicable. *A fluid challenge can help reverse deficient fluid volume rapidly, but the client must be carefully observed to ensure he/she does not go into fluid volume overload (Kruse et al, 2003).*

- Keep all IV fluids on a volumetric pump. *This is done to ensure that IVs do not "run in" and fluid-overload the client and so that client receives sufficient fluids.*
- Monitor intake and output. *Assessment, accurate documentation of intake and output, and management of fluid and electrolyte imbalances is crucial to prevent serious problems*

*(Kumar, 2001). The main goal of fluid management should be to ensure adequate oxygen delivery through the optimization of blood oxygenation, perfusion pressure, and circulating volume (Kreimeier, 2000).*

- ▲ Measure urine output hourly. If urine output is <30 mL/hr or 0.5 mL/kg/hr, notify the physician. *Urine output may not always be an accurate indicator of fluid balance. Urine output less than 30 mL/hr is insufficient for normal renal function and indicates hypovolemia or onset of renal damage (Metheny, 2000). Urine output can be unreliable as an indicator of fluid balance because hypothermic or elderly clients, or clients with renal dysfunction may not be able to concentrate urine, leading to a falsely high urine output (Schulman, 2002). Assessment, accurate documentation of intake and output, and management of fluid and electrolyte imbalances is crucial to prevent serious problems (Kumar, 2001).*
- Observe for trends in output for 3 days; include all routes of intake and output and note color and specific gravity of urine. *Monitoring for trends for 2 to 3 days gives a more valid picture of the client's hydration status than monitoring over a shorter period (Metheny, 2000). Dark-colored urine with increasing specific gravity reflects increased urine concentration.*
- Monitor daily weight for sudden decreases, especially in the presence of decreasing urine output or active fluid loss. Weigh the client on the same scale, in the same type clothing, at the same time of day, preferably before breakfast. *Body weight changes reflect changes in body fluid volume (Suhayda & Walton, 2002). A 1-pound weight loss reflects a fluid loss of about 500 mL (Metheny, 2000).*
- Monitor trends in serum lactic acid levels and base deficit, obtained from blood gasses as ordered. *A trend of increasing lactic acid levels and increasing base deficit can help identify occult hypoperfusion, which results in decreased survival and increased incidence of organ failure (Schulman, 2002).*

## Surgical Clients

- Perform a preoperative assessment to identify clients with increased risk for hemorrhage or hypovolemia such as those with recent traumatic injury, abnormal bleeding or clotting times, complicated renal/liver disease, major organ transplant, history of aspirin, nonsteroidal antiinflammatory usage, or anticoagulant therapy, history of hemophilia, von Willebrand's disease, or disseminated intravascular coagulation. *Use of laxatives, preoperative dehydration, infection, abnormal drainage, or hemorrhage can lead to hypotension during anesthesia induction if not corrected preoperatively.*
- Monitor for signs of intraoperative hypovolemia (e.g., decreased urinary output, decreased central venous pressure, hypotension, increased pulse, and/or increased respirations). *Hypovolemia can occur in the surgical client due to NPO status, hemorrhage, or third spacing. Urine output less than 30 mL/hr, is insufficient for normal renal function and indicates hypovolemia or onset of renal damage (Metheny, 2000).* **EB:** *In a study of 100 clients who underwent major elective surgery with an anticipated blood loss of more than 500 mL, it was concluded that goal-directed fluid administration leads to an earlier return of bowel function, a lower incidence of postoperative nausea and vomiting, and a decrease in length of postoperative hospital stay (Gan et al, 2002).*
- Monitor for signs of intraoperative hypervolemia, (i.e., dyspnea, coarse crackles, increased pulse and respirations, decreased urinary output, all of which could progress to

pulmonary edema). *Surgical clients with preexisting chronic kidney or liver disease, or congestive heart failure may be prone to hypervolemia. Increased fluid intake, can potentially increase postoperative cardiac morbidity, predispose the client to pneumonia and respiratory failure, cause urinary retention due to increased excretory demands on the kidney and resultant diuresis, inhibition of gastrointestinal motility resulting in prolonged postoperative ileus, decreased tissue oxygenation resulting in poor wound healing and postoperative thrombosis formation due to coagulation being enhanced (Holte et al, 2002).*

- Monitor for signs of intraoperative third spacing. *Third spacing can occur due to surgery itself. It may be necessary to replace fluid intraoperatively (Holte et al, 2002).*
- In the critically ill surgical client with a pulmonary artery catheter, monitor pressures, especially wedge pressure. *Pulmonary artery pressures are helpful for determining fluid balance, including preload and afterload, and they can help to guide fluid administration and administration of vasoactive IV drips such as dopamine. Hemodynamic parameters are sensitive indicators of intravascular fluid volume and hemodynamic measurements are especially needed in the client with cardiac or renal problems (Metheny, 2000).* **EB:** *Use of the Starling curve in combination with central venous pressures or esophageal Doppler cardiac output measurements "optimize" cardiac function by allowing better fluid regimens. Fluids must be individually titrated based on each client's dynamic changes in appropriately monitored variables (Mitchell et al, 2003).*
- Monitor clients undergoing laparoscopic or hysteroscopic procedures for the development of pulmonary edema when Dextran is used as the irrigation fluid. *The manufacturer of Dextran recommends vigilance for pulmonary edema when laparoscopic/hysteroscopic procedures last longer than 45 minutes, when more than 250 mL of Dextran 70 is absorbed, when large areas of endometrium are resected, or when IV fluid administration is greater then maintenance rate (Cooper & Brady, 2000).*
- Monitor Dextran infusion and recovery rates every 15 minutes. *Frequent monitoring of infusion/recovery rates keeps the nurse cognizant of absorption rates (Cooper & Brady, 2000).*
- If large amounts of hypotonic irrigation solutions (e.g., glycine) are used during surgery, carefully keep track of fluid inflow and outflow. *If there is a deficit of 1000 mL or more in outflow, request an order for a serum sodium (Kriplani et al, 1998) and also a serum osmolality (Metheny, 2000).* **EB:** *In a study of 697 women who underwent a hysteroscopy 5% experienced excessive hypotonic fluid absorption (Belloni, 2001). Research has shown that when a fluid deficit of 1000 mL occurs and the procedure is halted, the occurrence of serious sequelae were rare (Belloni, 2001). When large amounts of hypotonic, electrolyte-free fluids used for distention are absorbed, hyponatremic hypervolemia can occur (Cooper & Brady, 2000).*
- Monitor clients undergoing TURP (transurethral resection of the prostate) procedures for symptoms of TURP syndrome: headache, visual changes, agitation, lethargy, vomiting, muscle twitching, bradycardia, diminished pupillary reflexes, hypertension, and respiratory distress (Metheny, 2000). *Considerable fluid absorption occurs during TURP procedures (Kukreja et al, 2002).*
- Monitor clients undergoing percutaneous nephrolithotomy (PCNL) procedures for excessive fluid absorption and volume overload. *Clients with borderline cardiorespiratory or renal status can experience clinically significant volume overload during*

*PCNL procedures, especially if they also experience excessive bleeding and large perforations. The volume of fluid absorbed has been shown to increase with the amount of irrigation fluid used and the length of the procedure (Kukreja et al, 2002).*

- If the client is undergoing endometrial ablation under general anesthesia, watch for symptoms of decreased body temperature, decreased oxygen saturation, dilated pupils, and tremulousness (Metheny, 2000). *Serious fluid overload and dilutional hyponatremia can develop in surgeries such as trans-urethral resections of the prostate, transcervical resection of the endometrium, or a hysteroscopy as a result of the absorption of large amounts of irrigation solution into circulation which can cause permanent morbidity or death (Rose, 2001). Nonelectronic (saline cannot be used), isotonic irrigating solution must be used to ensure electrical current is transmitted and to keep the are clear for visualization (Rothrock, 2003).*
- Observe the surgical client for signs of hyperkalemia, i.e., cardiac dysrhythmias, heart block, asystole, abdominal distention, and weakness. *Hyperkalemia can occur intraoperatively due to massive blood transfusions, tissue breakdown from surgery, shifting of potassium from the cells in to the extracellular fluid, decreased potassium excretion due to renal failure or hypovolemia, crush injuries, or burns (Rothrock, 2003).*
- Observe the clients who have undergone bilateral thyroid surgery for hypocalcemia. *Due to surgery on the thyroid, the parathyroids may become edematous and decrease function, decreasing absorption of calcium (Kumar, 2001).*
- Observe surgical clients closely for signs of hypokalemia. *Hypokalemia commonly causes dysrhythmias. Stress and/or gastrointestinal fluid loss in surgical clients make them susceptible to hypokalemia.*
- Recognize that the surgical client may develop hyponatremia related to inappropriate antidiuretic hormone (ADH) secretion, which can be caused by trauma, thrombosis, abscesses, hemorrhages, or hematomas (Leite, 2001). *ADH, which acts on the kidneys to control water loss/retention, is an important factor in surgical clients under stress (Kumar, 2001).*
- Monitor the surgical client for signs and symptoms of hyponatremia: nausea, confusion, disorientation, twitching, seizures, and/or hypotension. *Risk factors for hyponatremia include prolonged surgery, large tissue resection, and excessive height of the irrigation reservoir, which, in turn, causes the fluid to be introduced into the body under high pressure (Rose, 2001).* **EB:** *In a study of 12 clients who underwent surgical procedures lasting more than 4 hours, metabolic acidosis was found to occur in relation to chloride administration, which was probably from the normal saline IV, because there was no increase in plasma volume (Water et al, 1999).*
- Accurately measure blood loss intraoperatively. *Weighing sponges is a reliable means of estimating blood loss and gauging replacement needs (Rothrock, 2003). Estimates of intraoperative blood loss can be inaccurate and lead to inappropriate fluid management (Kreimeier, 2000).* **EB:** *Maximizing cardiac output as a result of optimizing fluid management leads to improved surgical outcomes (McFall et al, 2004).*

## Home Care

- Determine if it is appropriate to intervene for deficient fluid volume or to allow the client to die comfortably without fluids as desired. *Deficient fluid volume may be a symptom of impending death in terminally ill clients. The deficit may result in a mild euphoria and a more comfortable death (Bennett, 2000).* **EB:** *A study of witnessed death by Hospice nurses demonstrated that clients who voluntarily refused fluids and food usually die a "good" death within two weeks (Ganzini et al, 2003).*

- Family members should be taught how to monitor output in the home (i.e., commode "hat" in toilet, urinal, bedpan, use of catheter, and so on). *An accurate measurement of fluid intake and output is an important indicator of client fluid status (Metheny, 2000).*

## Geriatric

F

- Be especially vigilant when monitoring vital signs and fluids in elderly surgical clients. *The elderly have depressed homeostatic mechanisms to regulate fluid balance during surgery, and many have renal insufficiency or heart failure, which can result in increased morbidity and sometimes mortality postoperatively (Metheny, 2000).*
- Assess preoperatively for symptoms of dehydration, i.e., weakness, dizziness, dry mouth with longitudinal tongue furrows. *The elderly are predisposed to deficient fluid volume because of decreased fluid in the body, decreased thirst sensation, and decreased ability to concentrate urine (Suhayda & Walton, 2002; Bennett, 2000).*
- Check skin turgor of the elderly client on the forehead, sternum, or inner thigh; also look for the presence of longitudinal tongue furrows and dry mucous membranes. *Elderly people commonly have decreased skin turgor from normal age-related loss of elasticity, therefore checking skin turgor on the arm is not reflective of fluid volume (Suhayda & Walton, 2002; Bennett, 2000). The presence of longitudinal furrows or dry mucous membranes is a good indication of dehydration in the elderly (Bennett, 2000).*
- Encourage fluid intake regularly to cognitively impaired clients. *The elderly have a decreased thirst sensation (Metheny, 2000), and short-term memory loss may impede the client's memory of fluid intake.*
- Incorporate regular hydration into daily routines, such as providing an extra glass of fluid with medication or during social activities. Consider using a beverage cart and a hydration assistant to routinely offer beverages to clients in extended care facilities. **EBN and EB:** *A nursing study demonstrated that institution of a beverage cart with a trained hydration assistant resulted in increased number of bowel movements, decreased laxative use, decreased number of falls, decreased urinary tract infections, respiratory infections and skin breakdown (Robinson & Rosher, 2002). A study demonstrated that verbal prompting and offering preference fluids resulted in increased fluid intake among nursing home residents (Simmons et al, 2001).*
- Note the color of urine and compare against a urine color chart to monitor adequate fluid intake. **EBN:** *A research study on elderly veterans demonstrated that urine color correlated significantly with urine osmolality, serum sodium, and BUN/creatinine ratio (Wakefield et al, 2002).*
- Monitor elderly clients for excess fluid volume during the treatment of deficient fluid volume: listen to lung sounds, watch for edema, and note vital signs. *The elderly client has a decreased ability to adapt to rapid increases in intravascular volume and can quickly develop fluid overload (Allison & Lobo, 2004).*

### Pediatric

- Monitor pediatric surgical clients closely for signs of fluid loss. *Small losses can be life-threatening to these clients (Kumar, 2001). Mild dehydration although difficult to determine often presents with dry mouth, malaise, and history of decreased urinary output. Moderate dehydration presents as loss of appetite, oliguria, and lethargy. Severe dehydration presents with tachycardia, mottled cool skin, capillary refill >5 seconds, anuria, and hypotension (Aker, 2002).*
- Administer fluids preoperatively until NPO status must be initiated, so that fluid deficit is decreased. **EB:** *Recommendations for pediatric NPO times have been revised to allow "clear" liquids up to 2 hours preoperative for pediatric clients <6 months age and up to 3 hours preoperative for pediatric clients 6 months and older (Aker, 2002).*

## evolve WEBSITES FOR EDUCATION

See the EVOLVE website for World Wide Web resources for client education.

## REFERENCES


Aker J: Pediatric fluid management, *Curr Rev Pain* 24(7):73-84, 2002.

Allison SP, Lobo, DN: Fluid and electrolytes in the elderly, *Curr Opin Clin Nutr Metab Care* 7(1):27, 2004.

Belloni C: Intraoperative complications of 697 consecutive operative hysteroscopies, *Minerva Ginecol* 53(1):13, 2001.

Bennett JA: Dehydration: hazards and benefits, *Geriatr Nurs* 21(2):84, 2000.

Beyea S: Perioperative nursing data set: the perioperative nursing vocabulary, ed 2, *Fluid/Electrolyte/Acid-Base Balances,* Denver, 2002, The Association of Perioperative Nursing.

Cooper JM, Brady RM: Intraoperative and early postoperative complications of operative hysteroscopy, *Obstet Gynecol Clin North Am* 23(2):347-365, 2000.

Farthing MJ: Oral rehydrations: an evolving solution, *J Pediatr Gastroenterol Nutr* 34(Suppl 1):S64, 2002.

Fortunato N: *Berry & Kohn's operating room technique*, ed 9, St. Louis, 2002, Mosby.

Gan TJ, Soppitt A, Maroof M et al: Goal-directed intraoperative fluid administration reduces length of hospital stay after major surgery, *Anesthesiology* 97(4):820, 2002.

Ganzini L, Goy ER, Miller LL et al: Nurses' experiences with hospice patients who refuse food and fluids to hasten death, *N Engl J Med* 349(4):359, 2003.

Holte K, Sharrock NE, Kehlet H: Pathophysiology and clinical implications of perioperative fluid excess, *Br J Anaesth* 89(4):622-632, 2002.

Kreimeier U: Pathophysiology of fluid imbalance, *Crit Care* 4(Suppl 2):S3-S7, 2000.

Kukreja RA, Desai MR, Sabnis RB et al: Fluid absorption during percutaneous nephrolithotomy: does it matter? *J Endourol* 16(4): 221-224, 2002.

Kumar N: Monitoring fluids and electrolytes in the surgical patient. Available at www.advancefornurses.com/ls1.html?issue=22, accessed on March 5, 2001.

Leite W: Fluid and electrolyte disorders—part I: disorders of sodium balance. Available at www.medstudents.com.br/cirur/cirur1.htm, accessed on March 5, 2001.

McFall MR, Woods GA, Wakeling HG: The use of oesophageal Doppler cardiac output measurement to optimize fluid management during colorectal surgery (readers response to editor), *Eur J Anaesthesiol* 21(7):581, 2004.

Metheny N: *Fluid and electrolyte balance: nursing considerations,* ed 4, Philadelphia, 2000, Lippincott.

Mitchell G, Hucker T, Venn R et al: Pathophysiology and clinical implications of perioperative fluid excess (reader comments to article published in 2002), *Br J Anaesth* 90(3):395, 2003.

Rose BD: Hyponatremia following transurethral resection or laparoscopic irrigation. Available at www.uptodateonline.com, accessed October 2001.

Rothrock J: *Alexander's care of the patient in surgery,* ed 12, St Louis, 2003, Mosby.

Schulman C: End points of resuscitation: choosing the right parameters to monitor, *Dimens Crit Care Nurs* 21:1, 2002.

Shirreffs SM, Merson SJ, Fraser SM et al: The effects of fluid restriction on hydration status and subjective feelings in man, *Br J Nutr* 91(6):951, 2004.

Simmons SF, Alessi C, Schnelle JF: An intervention to increase fluid intake in nursing home residents: prompting and preference compliance, *J Am Geriatr Soc* 49(7):926, 2001.

Suhayda R, Walton JC: Preventing and managing dehydration, *Medsurg Nurs* 11(6):267, 2002.

Wakefield B, Mentes J, Diggelmann L et al: Monitoring hydration status in elderly veterans, *West J Nurs Res* 24(2):132, 2002.

Waters JH, Miller LR, Clack S et al: Cause of metabolic acidosis in prolonged surgery, *Crit Care Med* 27(10):2142, 1999.




# Impaired Gas exchange

evolve

*Betty J. Ackley*

## NANDA

### Definition

Excess or deficit in oxygenation and/or carbon dioxide elimination at the alveolar-capillary membrane

### Defining Characteristics

Visual disturbances; decreased carbon dioxide; dyspnea; abnormal arterial blood gas levels; hypoxia; irritability; somnolence; restlessness; hypercapnia; tachycardia; cyanosis; abnormal skin color (pale, dusky); hypoxemia; hypercarbia; headache on awakening; abnormal rate, rhythm, depth of breathing; diaphoresis; abnormal arterial pH; nasal flaring

### Related Factors (r/t)

Ventilation-perfusion imbalance; alveolar-capillary membrane changes

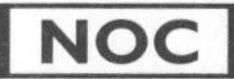


### Outcomes (Nursing Outcomes Classification)

**Suggested NOC Outcomes**

Respiratory Status: Gas Exchange, Ventilation

**Example NOC Outcome with Indicators**

Achieves appropriate **Respiratory Status: Gas Exchange** as evidenced by the following indicators: Cognitive status/Partial pressure of oxygen/Partial pressure of carbon dioxide/Arterial pH/Oxygen saturation (Rate each indicator of **Respiratory Status:** 1 = severely compromised, 2 = substantially compromised, 3 = moderately compromised, 4 = mildly compromised, 5 = not compromised [see Section I].)

## Client Outcomes

**Client Will (Specify Time Frame):**

- Demonstrate improved ventilation and adequate oxygenation as evidenced by blood gas levels within normal parameters for that client
- Maintain clear lung fields and remain free of signs of respiratory distress
- Verbalize understanding of oxygen supplementation and other therapeutic interventions

NIC

## Interventions (Nursing Interventions Classification)

G

### Suggested NIC Interventions

Acid-Base Management; Airway Management

**Example NIC Activities—Acid-Base Management**

Monitor for symptoms of respiratory failure (e.g., low $Pao_2$ and elevated $Paco_2$ levels and respiratory muscle fatigue); monitor determinants of tissue oxygen delivery (e.g., $Pao_2$, $Sao_2$, and hemoglobin levels, and cardiac output) if available

## Nursing Interventions and Rationales

- Monitor respiratory rate, depth, and effort, including use of accessory muscles, nasal flaring, and abnormal breathing patterns. *Increased respiratory rate, use of accessory muscles, nasal flaring, abdominal breathing, and a look of panic in the client's eyes may be seen with hypoxia.*
- Auscultate breath sounds every 1 to 2 hours. The presence of crackles and wheezes may alert the nurse to airway obstruction, which may lead to or exacerbate existing hypoxia. *In severe exacerbations of chronic obstructive pulmonary disease (COPD), lung sounds may be diminished or distant with air trapping (Zampella, 2003).*
- Monitor the client's behavior and mental status for the onset of restlessness, agitation, confusion, and (in the late stages) extreme lethargy. *Changes in behavior and mental status can be early signs of impaired gas exchange (Simmons & Simmons, 2004). In the late stages the client becomes lethargic and somnolent.*
- Monitor oxygen saturation continuously using pulse oximetry. Note blood gas results as available. *An oxygen saturation of less than 90% (normal: 95% to 100%) or a partial pressure of oxygen of less than 80 mm Hg (normal: 80 to 100 mm Hg) indicates significant oxygenation problems (Berry & Pinard, 2002; Grap, 2002). The goal of inpatient therapy for the COPD client is to maintain the oxygen saturation greater than 90% and partial pressure of oxygen at or above 80 mm Hg to maintain cellular oxygenation (Celli & MacNee, 2004).*
- Observe for cyanosis of the skin; especially note color of the tongue and oral mucous membranes. *Central cyanosis of the tongue and oral mucosa is indicative of serious hypoxia and is a medical emergency. Peripheral cyanosis in the extremities may or may not be serious (Kasper et al, 2005).*
- Position clients in semi-Fowler's position, with an upright posture at 45 degrees if possible. **EB:** *Research done on clients on a ventilator demonstrated that being in a 45 de-*

*gree upright position increased oxygenation and ventilation (Speelberg & Van Beers, 2003). Research on healthy subjects demonstrated that sitting upright resulted in higher tidal volumes and minute ventilation versus sitting in a slumped posture (Landers et al, 2003).*

- If the client has unilateral lung disease, alternate semi-Fowler's position in an upright posture with a lateral position (with 10- to 15-degree elevation and "good lung down" for 60 to 90 minutes). This method is contraindicated for clients with pulmonary abscess or hemorrhage or interstitial emphysema. *Gravity and hydrostatic pressure cause the dependent lung to become better ventilated and perfused, which increases oxygenation (Lasater-Erhard, 1995).*
- If the client has bilateral lung disease, position the client in either semi-Fowler's or a side-lying position, which increases oxygenation as indicated by pulse oximetry (or, if the client has a pulmonary catheter, venous oxygen saturation).
- Turn the client every 2 hours. Monitor mixed venous oxygen saturation closely after turning. If it drops below 10% or fails to return to baseline promptly, turn the client back into the supine position and evaluate oxygen status. If the client does not tolerate turning, consider use of a kinetic bed that rotates the client from side to side in a turn of at least 40 degrees. **EBN:** *Turning is important to prevent complications of immobility, but in critically ill clients with low hemoglobin levels or decreased cardiac output, turning on either side can result in desaturation (Winslow, 1992). Critically ill clients should be turned carefully and watched closely (Gawlinksi & Dracup, 1998). Use of the kinetic bed was shown to decrease development of atelectasis and ventilator associated pneumonia in critically ill clients (Ahrens, 2004).*
- If the client is obese or has ascites, consider positioning the client in reverse Trendelenburg's position at 45 degrees for periods as tolerated. **EBN:** *A study demonstrated that use of reverse Trendelenburg's position at 45 degrees resulted in increased tidal volumes and decreased respiratory rates in a group of intubated clients with obesity, abdominal distention, and ascites (Burns et al, 1994).*

▲ If the client has adult respiratory distress syndrome, or difficulty maintaining oxygenation, consider positioning the client prone with the upper thorax and pelvis supported, allowing the abdomen to protrude. Monitor oxygen saturation and turn back to supine position if desaturation occurs. **EBN and EB:** *Oxygenation levels have been shown to improve in the prone position, probably due to decreased shunting and better perfusion of the lungs (Curley, Thompson, & Arnold, 2000; Mure et al, 1997; Vollman & Bander, 1996).*

- If the client is acutely dyspneic, consider having the client lean forward over a bedside table, if tolerated. *Leaning forward can help decrease dyspnea, possibly because gastric pressure allows better contraction of the diaphragm (Celli, 1998). This is called the tripod position and is used during times of distress (Zampella, 2003).*
- Help the client deep breathe and perform controlled coughing. Have the client inhale deeply, hold the breath for several seconds, and cough two or three times with the mouth open while tightening the upper abdominal muscles as tolerated. *This technique can help increase sputum clearance and decrease cough spasms (Celli, 1998). Controlled coughing uses the diaphragmatic muscles, which makes the cough more forceful and effective.*

  NOTE: If the client has excessive fluid in the respiratory system, see the interventions for **Ineffective Airway clearance.**

- ▲ Monitor the effects of sedation and analgesics on the client's respiratory pattern; use judiciously. *Both analgesics and medications that cause sedation can depress respiration at times. However, these medications can be very helpful for decreasing the sympathetic nervous system discharge that accompanies hypoxia.*
- • Schedule nursing care to provide rest and minimize fatigue. *The hypoxic client has limited reserves; inappropriate activity can increase hypoxia.*
- ▲ Administer humidified oxygen through an appropriate device (e.g., nasal cannula or Venturi mask per the physician's order); aim for an oxygen ($O_2$) saturation level of 90%. Watch for onset of hypoventilation as evidenced by increased somnolence. *There is a fine line between ideal or excessive oxygen therapy; increasing somnolence is caused by retention of carbon dioxide ($CO_2$) leading to $CO_2$ narcosis (Simmons & Simmons, 2004).*

G

- • Assess nutritional status including serum albumin level and body mass index (BMI). *Weight loss in a client with COPD has a negative effect on the course of the disease; it can result in loss of muscle mass in the respiratory muscles, including the diaphragm, which can lead to respiratory failure (Berry & Baum, 2001; Celli & MacNee, 2004).* **EB:** *Being underweight, less than 21 BMI, has been associated with increased mortality in COPD clients (Schols et al, 1995).*
- • Assist the client to eat small meals frequently and use dietary supplements as necessary. For some clients, drinking 30 ml of a supplement such as Ensure or Pulmocare every hour while awake can be helpful. **EB:** *Improved nutrition can help increase muscle aerobic capacity and exercise tolerance (Palange et al, 1995).*
- • If the client is severely debilitated from chronic respiratory disease, consider the use of a wheeled walker to help in ambulation. **EB:** *Use of a wheeled walker has been shown to result in significant decrease in disability, hypoxemia, and breathlessness during a 6-minute walk test (Honeyman, Barr, & Stubbing, 1996).*
- ▲ Watch for signs of psychological distress including anxiety, agitation, and insomnia. Refer for counseling as needed. **EBN:** *One study demonstrated a clear association between hospitalization for COPD and psychological distress (Andenaes et al, 2004).*
- ▲ Refer the COPD client to a pulmonary rehabilitation program. **EB:** *Pulmonary rehabilitation has been shown to relieve dyspnea and fatigue, and enhance clients' sense of control over their disease. Rehabilitation is an important component of the management of COPD (Lacasse et al, 2002). Pulmonary rehabilitation was effective in reducing the utilization of health care resources (California Pulmonary Rehabilitation Collaborative Group, 2004).* NOTE: If the client becomes ventilator dependent, see the care plan for **Impaired spontaneous Ventilation.**

## Geriatric

- ▲ Use central nervous system (CNS) depressants carefully to avoid decreasing respiration rate. *An elderly client is prone to respiratory depression.*
- ▲ Maintain low-flow oxygen therapy. *An elderly client is susceptible to oxygen-induced respiratory depression.*

## Home Care

- • Assess the home environment for irritants that impair gas exchange. Help the client to adjust the home environment as necessary (e.g., install an air filter to decrease the level of dust).

- ▲ Refer the client to occupational therapy as necessary to assist the client in adaptation to the home and environment and in energy conservation.
- • Assist the client with identifying and avoiding situations that exacerbate impairment of gas exchange (e.g., stress-related situations, exposure to pollution of any kind, proximity to noxious gas fumes such as chlorine bleach). *Irritants in the environment decrease the client's effectiveness in accessing oxygen during breathing.*
- • Refer to GOLD and ACP-ASIM/ACCP guidelines for management of home care and indications of hospital admission criteria (Chojnowski, 2003).
- • Instruct the client to keep the home temperature above 68° F (20° C) and to avoid cold weather. *Cold air temperatures cause constriction of the blood vessels and increased moisture, which impairs the client's ability to absorb oxygen.*
- • Instruct the client to limit exposure to persons with respiratory infections.
- • Instruct the family in the complications of the disease and the importance of maintaining the medical regimen, including when to call a physician.
- • Assess nutritional status. Instruct the client to eat several small meals and use dietary supplements as necessary. For some clients, drinking 30 mL of a supplement such as Ensure or Pulmocare every hour while awake can be helpful. *Weight loss in a client with COPD has a negative effect on the course of the disease; it can result in loss of muscle mass in the respiratory muscles, including the diaphragm, which can lead to respiratory failure (Berry & Baum, 2001).*
- ▲ Refer the client for home health aide services as necessary for assistance with activities of daily living. *Clients with decreased oxygenation have decreased energy to carry out personal and role-related activities.*
- • When respiratory procedures are being implemented, explain equipment and procedures to family members, and provide needed emotional support. *Family members assuming responsibility for respiratory monitoring often find this stressful. They may not have been able to assimilate fully any instructions provided by hospital staff (McNeal, 2000).*
- • When electrically based equipment for respiratory support is being implemented, evaluate home environment for electrical safety, proper grounding, and so on. Ensure that notification is sent to the local utility company, the emergency medical team, and police and fire departments. *Notification is important to provide for priority service (McNeal, 2000).*
- ▲ Assess family role changes and coping ability. Refer the client to medical social services as appropriate for assistance in adjusting to chronic illness. *Inability to maintain the level of social involvement experienced before illness leads to frustration and anger in the client and may create a threat to the family unit.* **EBN:** *Clients with chronic lung problems were described as negative, helpless, confused, and socially obstreperous by family members in one study (Leidy & Traver, 1996).*
- • Support the family of the client with chronic illness. *Severely compromised respiratory functioning causes fear and anxiety in clients and their families. Reassurance from the nurse can be helpful.*

## Client/Family Teaching

- Teach the client how to perform pursed-lip breathing and controlled diaphragmatic breathing, and how to use the tripod position. Have the client watch the pulse oximeter to note improvement in oxygenation with these breathing techniques. *Controlled-breathing techniques can help reduce anxiety and decrease panic and dyspnea (Celli, 1998).* **EB:** *Pursed lip breathing reduces end expiratory volume and breathlessness (Bianchi et al, 2004).*
- Teach the client energy conservation techniques and the importance of alternating rest periods with activity. See nursing interventions for **Fatigue. EBN:** *Fatigue is a common symptom of COPD and needs to be assessed and managed (Theander & Unosson, 2004).*

G

▲ Teach the importance of not smoking:
  ■ Be very clear in approach, and ask the client to set a date for smoking cessation.
  ■ Recommend pharmacological support or else contraindicated (nicotine replacement therapy or antidepressant).
  ■ Refer the client to smoking-cessation programs.
  ■ Encourage clients who relapse to keep trying to quit.

  *Clinicians need to address smoking cessation at every entry into the health care system (U.S. Public Health Service, 2003).* **EB:** *Giving up smoking can slow the course of disease, and some clients may regain some lung function (Anthonisen et al, 1994; Willemse et al, 2004). A combination of psychosocial and pharmacological interventions was more effective than either intervention alone to stop smoking behavior (van der Meer et al, 2003).*

▲ Instruct the family regarding home oxygen therapy if ordered (e.g., delivery system, liter flow, safety precautions). *Long-term oxygen therapy can improve survival, exercise ability, sleep and ability to think in hypoxemic clients. Client education improves compliance with prescribed use of oxygen (Celli & MacNee, 2004).*

- Teach the client the need to receive a yearly influenza vaccine. **EB:** *A review of the literature demonstrated that receiving the vaccine may reduce exacerbations of COPD (Poole et al, 2000).*
- Teach the client relaxation techniques to help reduce stress responses and panic attacks resulting from dyspnea. **EBN:** *Relaxation therapy can help reduce dyspnea and anxiety (Gift, Moore, & Soeken, 1992).*
- Teach the client to use music, along with a rest period to decrease dyspnea and anxiety **EBN:** *A study demonstrated that use of music along with a resting period were effective in relieving anxiety and exercise induced dyspnea in clients with COPD (Sidani et al, 2004).*

## evolve WEBSITES FOR EDUCATION

See the EVOLVE website for World Wide Web resources for client education.

## REFERENCES

Ahrens T, Kollef M, Stewart J et al: Effect of kinetic therapy on pulmonary complications, *Am J Crit Care* 13(5):376, 2004.

Andenaes R, Kalfoss MH, Wahl A: Psychological distress and quality of life in hospitalized patients with chronic obstructive pulmonary disease, *J Adv Nurs* 46(5):523, 2004.

Anthonisen NR, Connett JE, Kiley JP et al: Effects of smoking intervention and the use of an inhaled anticholinergic bronchodilator on the rate of decline of $FEV_1$. The Lung Health Study, *JAMA* 272(19):1497, 1994.
Berry BE, Pinard AE: Assessing tissue oxygenation, *Crit Care Nurse* 22(3):22, 2002.
Berry JK, Baum CL: Malnutrition in chronic obstructive pulmonary disease: adding insult to injury, *AACN Clin Issues* 12(2):210, 2001.
Bianchi R, Gigliotti F, Romagnoli I et al: Chest wall kinematics and breathlessness during pursed-lip breathing in patients with COPD, *Chest* 125(2):459, 2004.
Burns SM, Egloff MB, Ryan B et al: Effect of body position on spontaneous respiratory rate and tidal volume in patients with obesity, abdominal distention and ascites, *Am J Crit Care* 3:102, 1994.
California Pulmonary Rehabilitation Collaborative Group: Effects of pulmonary rehabilitation on dyspnea, quality of life and healthcare costs in California, *J Cardiopulm Rehabil* 24(1):52, 2004.
Celli BR: Pulmonary rehabilitation for COPD, *Postgrad Med* 103(4):159, 1998.
Celli BR, MacNee W, ATS/ERS Task Force: Standards for the diagnosis and treatment of patients with COPD: a summary of the ATS/ERS position paper, *Eur Respir J* 23(6):932, 2004.
Chojnowski D: "GOLD" standards for acute exacerbation in COPD, *Nurs Practitioner* 28(5):26, 2003.
Curley MA, Thompson JE, Arnold JH: The effects of early and repeated prone positioning in pediatric patients with acute lung injury, *Chest* 118(1):156, 2000.
Gawlinski A, Dracup K. Effect of positioning on $Svo_2$ in the critically ill patient with a low ejection fraction, *Nurs Res* 47(5):293, 1998.
Grap MJ. Protocols for practice: applying research at the bedside: pulse oximetry, *Crit Care Nurse* 22(3):69, 2002.
Honeyman P, Barr P, Stubbing DG: Effect of a walking aid on disability, oxygenation, and breathlessness in patients with chronic airflow limitation, *J Cardiopulm Rehabil* 16:63, 1996.
Kasper DL: *Harrison's principles of internal medicine*, ed 16, New York, 2005, McGraw Hill.
Lacasse Y, Brosseau L, Milne S et al: Pulmonary rehabilitation for chronic obstructive pulmonary disease, *Cochrane Database Syst Rev* (3):CD003793, 2002.
Landers M, Barker G, Wallentine S et al: A comparison of tidal volume breathing frequency, and minute ventilation between two sitting postures in healthy adults, *Physiother Theory Pract* 19(2):109-119, 2003.
Lasater-Erhard M: The effect of patient position on arterial oxygen saturation, *Crit Care Nurse* 15(5):31, 1995.
Leidy NK, Traver GA: Adjustment and social behavior in older adults with chronic obstructive pulmonary disease: the family's perspective, *J Adv Nurs* 23:252, 1996.
McNeal GJ: *AACN guide to acute care procedures in the home,* Philadelphia, 2000, Lippincott.
Mure M, Martling CR, Lindahl SG: Dramatic effect on oxygenation in patients with severe acute lung insufficiency treated in the prone position, *Crit Care Med* 25(9):1539, 1997.
Palange P, Forte S, Felli A et al: Nutritional state and exercise tolerance in patients with COPD, *Chest* 107:1206, 1995.
Poole PJ, Chacko E, Wood-Baker RW et al: Influenza vaccine for patients with chronic obstructive pulmonary disease, *Cochrane Database Syst Rev* (4):CD002733, 2000.
Schols AM, Soeters PB, Mostert R et al: Physiologic effects of nutritional support and anabolic steroids in patients with chronic obstructive pulmonary disease. A placebo-controlled randomized trial, *Am J Respir Crit Care Med* 152(4 Pt 1):1268, 1995.
Simmons P, Simmons M: Informed nursing practice: the administration of oxygen to patients with COPD, *Medsurg Nurs* 13(2):82, 2004.
Speelberg B, Van Beers F: Artificial ventilation in the semi-recumbent position improves oxygenation and gas exchange, *Chest* 124(4):S203, 2003.
Theander K, Unosson M: Fatigue in patients with chronic obstructive pulmonary disease, *J Adv Nurs* 45(2):172, 2004.
U.S. Public Health Service: Treating Tobacco Use and Dependence—Clinician's Packet. A How-To Guide for Implementing the Public Health Service Clinical Practice Guideline. Available at www.surgeongeneral.gov/tobacco/clinpack.html, accessed on March 2003.
van der Meer RM, Wagena EJ, Ostelo RW et al: Smoking cessation for chronic obstructive pulmonary disease, *Cochrane Database Syst Rev* (2):CD002999, 2003.
Vollman KM, Bander JJ: Improved oxygenation utilizing a prone positioner in patients with acute respiratory distress syndrome, *Int Care Med* 22(10):1105, 1996.
Willemse BW, ten Hacken NH, Rutgers B et al: Smoking cessation improves both direct and indirect airway hyperresponsiveness in COPD, *Eur Respir J* 24(3):391, 2004.
Winslow EH: Turn for the worse, *Am J Nurs* 92:16C, 1992.
Winslow EH: High Fowler's won't always ease breathing, *Am J Nurs* 96:59, 1996.
Zampella MA: COPD: managing flare-ups, *RN* 14:14, 2003.

# Grieving[2]

evolve

*Betty J. Ackley and Gail B. Ladwig*

NANDA

## Definition

State in which an individual or group of individuals reacts to an actual or perceived loss, which may be loss of a person, object, function, status, relationship, or body part

NOTE: Grieving is not an official North American Nursing Diagnosis Association International (NANDA-I) nursing diagnosis, but it is included because the authors believe that grieving is part of the normal human response to loss and that nurses can use interventions to help the client grieve. Grieving is a wellness-oriented nursing diagnosis.

G

## Defining Characteristics

Verbal expression of distress at loss; anger; sadness; crying; difficulty in expressing loss; alterations in eating habits, sleep patterns, dream patterns, activity levels, or libido; reliving of past experiences; interference with life function; alterations in concentration or pursuit of tasks

## Related Factors (r/t)

Actual or perceived object loss, which may include loss of people, possessions, job, status, home, ideals, or parts and processes of the body

NOC

## Outcomes (Nursing Outcomes Classification)

### Suggested NOC Outcomes

Grief Resolution; Hope; Mood Equilibrium; Psychosocial Adjustment: Life Change

**Example NOC Outcome with Indicators**

**Grief Resolution** with plans for a positive future as evidenced by the following indicators: Resolves feelings about loss/Verbalizes acceptance of loss/Describes meaning of loss or death/Reports decreased preoccupation with loss/Expresses positive expectations about the future (Rate each indicator of **Grief Resolution:** 1 = never demonstrated, 2 = rarely demonstrated, 3 = sometimes demonstrated, 4 = often demonstrated, 5 = consistently demonstrated [see Section I].)

## Client Outcomes

**Client Will (Specify Time Frame):**

- Express feelings of guilt, fear, anger, or sadness
- Identify problems associated with grief (e.g., changes in appetite, insomnia, loss of libido, decreased energy, alteration in activity level)

[2]Grieving is not a NANDA-I–approved nursing diagnosis.

- Plan for the future one day at a time
- Function at normal developmental level and perform activities of daily living

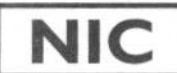

## Interventions (Nursing Interventions Classification)

### Suggested NIC Interventions

Grief Work Facilitation; Grief Work Facilitation: Perinatal Death

**Example NIC Activities—Grief Work Facilitation**

Encourage client to verbalize memories of the loss, both past and current; assist client to identify personal coping strategies



## Nursing Interventions and Rationales

- Use a grief instrument such as the Hogan Grief Reaction Checklist (HGRC) to evaluate the client with regard to the six factors in the normal trajectory of the grieving process: Despair, Panic Behavior, Blame and Anger, Detachment, Disorganization, and Personal Growth. **EB:** *The HGRC was developed empirically from data collected from bereaved adults who had experienced the death of a loved one (Hogan, Greenfield, & Schmidt, 2001).*
- Allow family members to participate in care of the body of the deceased if desired. Help survivors say goodbye in the most loving and caring way possible. **EBN:** *One study revealed a theme of a need to remember and to hold onto the memory. Participants in this study found comfort in knowing they were not alone (Hentz, 2002).*
- Allow the family "holding" behaviors, including taking photographs of the deceased or clipping a piece of hair. *Memory keepsakes facilitate the grief process (Buxbaum & Brant, 2001).*
- Help the bereaved client survive during times of acute grief. Ensure that the client maintains sufficient nutrition and help the client determine a routine to make it through each day. *It is common for a newly bereaved person to eat minimally for several days (Rodebaugh, Schwindt, & Valentine, 1999), but after that it is important that the person eat to maintain health.* **EB:** *One study indicated that bereaved individuals, regardless of whether they had counseling for grief resolution, had a moderate risk for poor nutrition (Johnson, 2002).*
- Encourage the client to share memories and tell stories of the person or object of loss by making comments such as, "Tell me about your wife [husband, parent]." Conduct an in-depth personal interview to learn about the client and loved one or loss. *A personal history can help a nurse understand the unique loss that the person has experienced, the meaning of the loss to the individual, and the strengths the person brings to the situation (The Centre for Grief Education, 2005).* **EB:** *The goal in the aftermath of September 11, 2001, was to allow the victims to tell their stories. By sharing their stories, individuals start the process of moving from helpless victim to proactive survivor (Pessin et al, 2002).*
- Consider the use of a "grief map." *This allows the individual to conceptualize each*

*phenomenon of grief and to visualize progress through the issues associated with the feelings.* **EB:** *The grief map provides a constructive multidimensional framework for dealing with the phenomena of the grieving process and for rebuilding life following major loss. It provides individuals with a means of describing their experiences (Clark, 2001).*

G

- Actively listen to the client's expression of grief; do not interrupt, do not tell your own story, and do not offer meaningless platitudes such as, "It will be better this way." *These behaviors do not help and can often hurt (Hoffman, 1997).*
- Encourage the client to "cry out" his or her grief and express feelings, including sadness and anger. **EB:** *In a content analysis of the narratives of 85 mourners, nine unique meaning constructs emerged, the most prominent of which spoke to the theme of feeling the absence of the deceased (Gamino, Hogan, & Sewell, 2002).*
- If the client or family members are expressing anger, try not to react in anger. Instead, allow feelings to be expressed, listen to the expressions of anger, and accept their right to those feelings. Try lowering your voice and slowing your rate of speech as you respond to the client and/or family. *It is not therapeutic to respond to anger with anger. Instead, strive to be therapeutic, helping the client and/or family express the anger and gain control of themselves by modeling calm behavior (Clements et al, 2004; Rueth & Hall, 1999).*
- Help the client identify previous successful personal coping strategies. Use music if appropriate. **EBN:** *One study revealed the theme of a need to remember and to hold onto the memory (Hentz, 2002). Four case studies demonstrated the usefulness of music therapy in assisting palliative care clients and families to cope with grief and loss (Hilliard, 2001b),* **EB:** *A study demonstrated that participation of grieving children in music therapy–based bereavement groups served to reduce grief symptoms among subjects evaluated in the home (Hillard, 2001a).*
- Encourage the client to follow comforting grief rituals such as interacting with nature, lighting votive candles, saying a rosary, prayer, or whatever ritual brings spiritual comfort in dealing with the loss. *These traditional methods of grieving can help the client find meaning in the loss (Eisenhandler, 2004).*
- Help the client realize that feelings of "why me" or "if only" may come with grieving. *Feelings of guilt may accompany grieving and are to be expected (American Family Physician, 2003).*
- Warn the grieving client that when driving, he or she may experience overwhelming grief. **EB:** *A review of data from two interview studies demonstrated that people often grieve actively while driving and feelings of grief can be overwhelming (Rosenblat, 2004).*

▲ Refer the client for spiritual counseling if desired. **EB:** *A study demonstrated that those people who professed stronger spiritual beliefs seemed to resolve their grief more rapidly and completely after the death of a close person than did people with no spiritual beliefs (Walsh et al, 2002).*

- Provide information about the grief process, including the stages of grieving: denial, anger, bargaining, and acceptance (*American Family Physician,* 2003; Kubler-Ross, 1969), or the six stages of grieving: "Recognizing the loss, reacting to the separation, recollecting and reexperiencing the deceased and the relationship, relinquishing the old attachments of the deceased and the old assumptive world, readjustment to move into the new world without forgetting the old, and reinvestment into the current world and life" (Clements et al, 2004, p. 150).

- Help the client realize that spasms of grief can come at any time, that most people don't go through the stages in a predictable fashion, and that the grieving process takes time and is painful. *This information helps normalize the grief experience and provides clients with hope that they can survive (Rodebaugh, Schwindt, & Valentine, 1999).*
- Help the client determine the best way and place to find social support. Encourage the client to continue to use supports for 1 to 2 years. **EB:** *Social support has been shown to help bereaved individuals as they reconstruct their lives and find new meaning in life (Hogan & Schmidt, 2002).*

▲ Assess for causes of dysfunctional grieving (e.g., sudden death, highly dependent or ambivalent relationship with the deceased, lack of coping skills, lack of social support, previous physical or mental health problems, death of a child, death of a wife, death of a loved one by suicide). Refer for counseling, starting 2 to 8 weeks after the loss and for up to 3 months following bereavement (Steen, 1998). Refer to the care plan for **Dysfunctional Grieving.** *Life circumstances can interfere with normal grieving (Steen, 1998).*

G

- Assess for signs of depression: feelings of worthlessness, inability to eat or sleep, or sleeping all the time. *Depression can occur in nearly half of all grieving people, and 10% of people who are grieving suffer major depression (Steen, 1998).*
- Encourage family members to set aside time to talk with one another about the loss without criticizing or belittling one another's feelings. *Help families to grieve as a system, not just as individual mourners (Steen, 1998).* **EBN:** *A study analyzing the grief and coping of mothers who had lost children under age 7 years found that the spouse, remaining children, grandparents, next of kin, friends, and colleagues were the main sources of support (Laakso & Paunonen-Ilmonen, 2002).*

▲ Identify available community resources, including bereavement groups at local hospitals and hospice centers. Volunteers who provide bereavement support can also be effective. *Support groups can have positive effects on bereavement outcomes. Group counseling is an effective intervention because it addresses the issue of disenfranchised grief (Barlow & Morrison, 2002).*

▲ Recognize times when you as a nurse are affected by loss and need grief resolution. Attend a grief resolution group, ask for help from pastoral services, speak with a kind friend who is supportive, or seek counseling. *Nursing staff can experience unresolved grief from the death of a client or may suffer other losses that require grief resolution so that they can function effectively and be able to give to others.*

## Pediatric/Parent

- Treat the child with respect, give them the opportunity to talk about their concerns, and answer questions honestly. *Children know much more than adults realize. They are very observant and generally know if a parent or loved one is dying, or cause of death, even if they have not been told (Schuurman, 2005).*
- Listen to the child's expression of grief. *The best thing to be done to help a child is to listen to them, with our ears, eyes, hearts, and souls, and recognize that we do not have to have answers (Schuurman, 2005).*
- Consider giving the child a "Memory Bag" to have after experiencing a sudden death; contents include a teddy bear, a coloring book on working through grief for different

ages, a journal for children to write in, and crayons. *The memory bags give children permission to grieve and feel the loss they experience so deeply (Foley, 2004).*

- Help parents recognize that the child does not have to be "fixed," instead he or she needs support going through an experience of grieving just as adults. *The role of the nurse, parent, and friends is to support and assist, not to help a child "get over it" (Schuurman, 2005).*
- Ask the child if he or she would like a photo of the deceased person or a lock of hair to keep. *Memory keepsakes facilitate the grief process (Buxbaum & Brant, 2001).*
- Encourage children to listen to music that they enjoy. **EB:** *The investigator concluded that participation of grieving children in music therapy–based bereavement groups served to reduce grief symptoms among the subjects as evaluated in the home (Hilliard, 2001a).*

G

- ▲ Refer grieving children and parents to a program to help facilitate grieving if desired, especially if the death was traumatic. **EB:** *A study demonstrated that treatment for children and parents with grief associated with trauma helped decrease symptoms of posttraumatic stress disorder (PTSD) (Cohen, 2004).* **EBN:** *A program desired for grieving children involving riding horses was shown to increase self-confidence and self-esteem (Glazer, Clark, & Stein, 2004).*
- Help the adolescent determine sources of support and how to use them effectively. **EBN:** *In a study of adolescents dealing with the death of a loved one, the most important factors that helped adolescents cope with the grief were self-help and support from parents, relatives, and friends (Rask, Kaunonen, & Paunonen-Ilmonen, 2002).*
- ▲ Encourage parents to seek mental health services as needed, learn stress reduction, and take good care of their health. *Research has demonstrated that the loss of a child for a mother results in an increased loss of life within 18 years either due to disease or suicide (Lawson, 2003).* **EBN:** *A study analyzing the grief and coping of mothers who had lost children under age 7 years found that the spouse, remaining children, grandparents, next of kin, friends, and colleagues were the main sources of support (Laakso & Paunonen-Ilmonen, 2002).*

## Geriatric

- ▲ Use reminiscence therapy in conjunction with the expression of emotions. Refer to a reminiscence group if available. **EBN and EB:** *Two studies demonstrated that participation in a reminiscence group reduced symptoms of depression (Jones, 2003; Zauszniewski et al, 2004).*
- Identify previous losses and assess the client for depression. *Losses and changes associated with aging often occur in rapid succession without adequate recovery time (Hegge & Fischer, 2000).* **EBN:** *Having more than two concurrent losses increases the incidence of unresolved grief (Herth, 1990). The grieving elderly widow may develop depression that results in poor nutrition, noncompliance with medication regimens, decreasing cognition, and multiple health problems (Fischer & Hegge, 2000).*
- Monitor an older adult who has been treated for bereavement-related depression for relapse or recurrence. **EB:** *In a 2-year study, 36% of older adults treated for bereavement-related depression experienced relapse or recurrence (Pasternak et al, 1997).*
- Evaluate the social support system of the elderly client. If the support system is mini-

mal, help the client determine how to increase available support. **EBN:** *The elderly who have poor grieving outcomes often do not live with family members and have a minimal support system. The support of family, especially children, and friends is a common way for elderly widows to cope with a loss (Hegge & Fischer, 2000).*

- Provide support for the family when the loss is associated with dementia of the family member. *Psychosocial death is a significant dimension of the dementia of the Alzheimer's-type disease process. Grieving occurs throughout the illness of the parent (Furlini, 2001).*

## Multicultural

- Assess for the influence of cultural beliefs, norms, and values on the client's grief and mourning practices. **EBN:** *Grief and mourning practices may be based on cultural conventions (Clements et al, 2003; Leininger & McFarland. 2002; Cochran, 1998; Doswell & Erlen, 1998). Some African Americans may place great emphasis on attendance at funerals; many Native-American tribes hold long, somber wakes, during which food and memorial gifts are distributed; Chinese and Japanese families may have specific funeral rituals that must be followed precisely to ensure safe passage of their loved ones into the next world; Latinos may hold wakes, use prayer during a novena, and light candles in honor of the dead; and in West Indian/Caribbean cultures, death arrangements might be made by a kinsman of the deceased (McQuay, 1995).*
- Assess for the influence of cultural beliefs, norms, and values on the client's expressions of grief. **EBN:** *African Americans may be expected to act "strong" and go about the business of life after a death; Native Americans may not talk about the death because of beliefs that such talk will detract from spirituality and bring bad luck; Latinos may wear black and act subdued during their* luto *(mourning) period; and Southeast Asian families may wear white when mourning (Lewis & McBride, 2004; McQuay, 1995).*
- Identify whether the client had been notified of the deceased's health status and was able to be present at the deathbed. **EBN:** *Not being present during terminal illness and death can disrupt the grieving process (McQuay, 1995).*
- Validate the client's feelings regarding the loss. **EBN:** *Validation is a therapeutic communication technique that lets the client know that the nurse has heard and understood what was said, and it promotes the nurse-client relationship (Heineken, 1998). Patients who were from an ethnic minority group were significantly more likely to report that interviews about death, dying, and bereavement were helpful (Emanuel et al, 2004). Storytelling was at the heart of every African-American widow's description of her bereavement experience. Nurses can engage the older African-American widow in storytelling as an effective therapeutic intervention and as a means to gain in-depth understanding and cultural insight into the meaning of the widow's grief experience (Rodgers, 2004).*
- Teach patients to recognize grief responses. **EBN:** *Recognition of grief patterns will allow patients to manage their responses more effectively and may prevent adverse outcomes to their physical and mental health (Van & Meleis, 2003).*

## Home Care

NOTE: Grieving may be encountered as the client comes to terms with his or her own loss or death, or as the family reacts to the client's death.

- • The interventions described previously may be adapted for home care use.
- • Listen actively as the client grieves his or her own death, or real or perceived loss. Normalize the client's expressions of grief for himself or herself. Demonstrate a caring and hopeful approach. *Active listening supports the client without intrusive advice giving. Normalizing lets the client know that his or her responses are appropriate ways of preparing for death.* **EBN:** *Caring for and with the client, and projecting hopefulness, has been shown to inspire hope in bereavement counseling (Cutcliffe, 2004).*
- • If the agency has served the deceased as a client, allow the primary caregivers to attend the services. *Families experiencing the loss of a loved one perceive staff attendance at services as a significant statement of caring and support.*
- • Plan the first home visit within 10 days after the loss by the client; be guided by the type of loss and the family's schedule following the loss. *Support is a contributing factor to completion of grief work. The nurse can provide support and guidance.*
- • If the loss is of a loved one, allow the client to express feelings about the loss through interaction with the home environment (e.g., looking at pictures, keeping special chairs or clothing). *Symbols of the lost loved one can be comforting and allow the bereaved to accept the loss in stages. Support and normalize the family grieving process.*
- • Do not react with shock or disbelief at family members' reports (e.g., feeling like the deceased is still there). *A wide range of behaviors and perceptions occurs during the grieving response.*
- ▲ Refer the client to medical social services as necessary for losses not related to death. *Support is helpful to grief work for all types of losses. Social workers can assist the client with planning for financial changes as a result of job losses and help with community referrals as appropriate.*
- ▲ Refer the bereaved to hospice bereavement programs. *Relief of the suffering of clients and families (i.e., physical, emotional, and spiritual) is the goal of hospice care (Krisman-Scott & McCorkle, 2002).*
- ▲ Refer the bereaved spouse to an Internet self-help group if desired. Palliative home care resources include a number of available websites (Smith-Stoner & Oliver, 2003). **EBN:** *An Internet-based self-help group can assist the bereaved spouse in coping, receiving support, developing a sense of family, sharing information, and helping others (Bacon, Condon, & Fernsler, 2000).*
- • Assess caregiver reaction to bereavement issues and caregiver burden. Suggest preventive intervention for potential bereavement maladjustment if indicated. **EB:** *A study demonstrated that bereavement maladjustment is more likely with caregivers who are over 61 years old, who perceive a substantial emotional burden, and who have been unable to continue working. Preventive interventions could reduce health and social costs (Ferrario et al, 2004).*
- • Modify expectations of the client's response according to the degree of anticipation of the loved one's death. *If the loved one died at an old age or of a natural cause, the client may have experienced anticipatory grieving; the current reaction may be less than expected. If the loved one died of accidental or criminal causes, the grief reaction may be magnified. Grief may be prolonged, and a referral for supportive counseling is more likely to be needed.*
- ▲ After loss of a pregnancy, encourage the client to follow through on a counseling re-

ferral. **EBN and EB:** *Parents with a history of perinatal loss are at higher risk for depressive symptoms and pregnancy-specific anxiety during subsequent pregnancies, particularly before the third trimester. Mothers had a higher level of symptoms than fathers (Armstrong, 2002; Franche & Mikail, 1999).*

## evolve WEBSITES FOR EDUCATION

See the EVOLVE website for World Wide Web resources for client education.

## REFERENCES


American Psychiatric Association: *Diagnostic and statistical manual of mental disorders,* ed 4, Washington, DC, 2000, The Association.

Armstrong DS: Emotional distress and prenatal attachment in pregnancy after perinatal loss, *J Nurs Scholarsh* 34:339, 2002.

Bacon ES, Condon EH, Fernsler JI: Young widows' experience with an internet self-help group, *J Psychosoc Nurs Ment Health Serv* 38(7):24, 2000.

Barlow CA, Morrison H: Survivors of suicide. Emerging counseling strategies, *J Psychosoc Nurs Ment Health Serv* 40(1):28, 2002.

Buxbaum L, Brant JM: When a parent dies from cancer, *Clin J Oncol Nurs* 5(4):135, 2001.

Centre for Grief Education: Commonly asked questions about grief. Available at www.grief.org.au/support.html, accessed on March 7, 2005.

Clark S: Mapping grief: an active approach to grief resolution, *Death Stud* 25(6):531, 2001.

Clements PT, DeRanieri JT, Vigil GJ et al: Life after death: grief therapy after the sudden traumatic death of a family member, *Perspect Psychiatr Care* 40(4):149, 2004.

Cochran, M: Tears have no color, *Am J Nurs* 98(6):53, 1998.

Cohen JA, Mannarino AP, Knudsen K: Treating childhood traumatic grief: a pilot study, *J Am Acad Child Adolesc Psychiatry* 43(10):1225, 2004.

Cutcliffe JR: The inspiration of hope in bereavement counseling, *Issues Ment Health* 25:165, 2004.

Doswell W, Erlen J: Multicultural issues and ethical concerns in the delivery of nursing care interventions, *Nurs Clin North Am* 33(2):353, 1998.

Eisenhandler SA: The arts of consolation: commemoration and folkways of faith, *Generations* 28(2), 2004.

Emanuel EJ, Fairclough DL, Wolfe P et al: Talking with terminally ill patients and their caregivers about death, dying, and bereavement: is it stressful? Is it helpful? *Arch Intern Med* 164(18):1999, 2004.

Ferrario SR, Cardillo V, Vicario F et al: Advanced cancer at home: caregiving and bereavement, *Palliative Med* 18:129, 2004.

Fischer C, Hegge M: The elderly woman at risk, *Am J Nurs* 100(6):54, 2000.

Foley T: Encouraging the inclusion of children in grief after a sudden death: memory bags, *J Emerg Nurs* 30:341, 2004.

Franche R, Mikail S: The impact of perinatal loss on adjustment to subsequent pregnancy, *Soc Sci Med* 48:1613, 1999.

Furlini L: The parent they knew and the "new" parent: daughters' perceptions of dementia of the Alzheimer's type, *Home Health Care Serv Q* 20(1):21, 2001.

Gamino LA, Hogan NS, Sewell KW: Feeling the absence: a content analysis from the Scott and White grief study, *Death Stud* 26(10):793, 2002.

Glazer HR, Clark MD, Stein DS: The impact of hippotherapy on grieving children, *J Hospic Palliat Nurs* 6(3):171-175, 2004.

Hegge M, Fischer C: Grief responses of senior and elderly widows: practice implications, *J Gerontol Nurs* 26(2):35, 2000.

Heineken J: Patient silence is not necessarily client satisfaction: communication in home care nursing, *Home Healthc Nurse* 16(2): 115, 1998.

Hentz P: The body remembers: grieving and a circle of time, *Qual Health Res* 12(2):161, 2002.

Herth K: Relationship of hope, coping styles, concurrent losses, and setting to grief resolution in the elderly widow(er), *Res Nurs Health* 13:109, 1990.

Hilliard RE: The effects of music therapy–based bereavement groups on mood and behavior of grieving children: a pilot study, *J Music Ther* 38(4):291, 2001a.

Hilliard RE: The use of music therapy in meeting the multidimensional needs of hospice patients and families, *J Palliat Care* 17(3):161, 2001b.

Hoffman C: Volunteers providing bereavement support, *Caring* 16(11):48, 1997.

Hogan NS, Greenfield DB, Schmidt LA: Development and validation of the Hogan Grief Reaction Checklist, *Death Stud* 25(1):1, 2001.
Hogan NS, Schmidt LA: Testing the grief to personal growth model using structural equation modeling, *Death Stud* 26(8):615, 2002.
Information from your family doctor: grieving: facing illness, death, and other losses, *Am Fam Physician* 67(5):1053, 2003.
Johnson CS: Nutritional considerations for bereavement and coping with grief, *J Nutr Health Aging* 6(3):171, 2002.
Jones ED: Reminiscence therapy for older women with depression. Effects of nursing intervention classification in assisted-living long-term care, *J Gerontol Nurs* 29(7):26, 2003.
Krisman-Scott MA, McCorkle R: The tapestry of hospice, *Holist Nurs Pract* 16(2):32, 2002.
Kubler-Ross E: *On death and dying,* New York, 1969, Macmillan.
Laakso H, Paunonen-Ilmonen M: Mothers' experience of social support following the death of a child, *J Clin Nurs* 11(2):176, 2002.
Leininger MM, McFarland MR: *Transcultural nursing: concepts, theories, research and practices,* ed 3, New York, 2002, McGraw-Hill.
Lawson W: Grieving mothers suffer early deaths, *Psychology Today* 36(3):18, 2003.
McQuay JE: Cross-cultural customs and beliefs related to health crises, death, and organ donation/transplantation: a guide to assist health care professionals understand different responses and provide cross-cultural assistance, *Crit Care Nurs Clin North Am* 7(3):581, 1995.
Pasternak RE, Prigerson H, Hall M et al: The posttreatment illness course of depression in bereaved elders, *Am J Geriatr Psychiatry* 5:54, 1997.
Pessin N, Lindy DC, Hicks K et al: Sharing stories, healing shattered lives, *Caring* 21(1):6, 2002.
Rask K, Kaunonen M, Paunonen-Ilmonen M: Adolescent coping with grief after the death of a loved one, *Int J Nurs Pract* 8(3): 137, 2002.
Rodebaugh LS, Schwindt RG, Valentine FM: How to handle grief, *Nursing* 29(10):52, 1999.
Rodgers LS: Meaning of bereavement among older African American widows, *Geriatr Nurs* 25(1):10-16, 2004
Rosenblatt PC: Grieving while driving, *Death Stud* 28(7):679, 2004.
Rueth TW, Hall SE: Dealing with the anger and hostility of those who grieve, *Am J Hosp Palliat Care* 16(6):743, 1999.
Schuurman DL: The club no one wants to join: a dozen lessons I've learned from grieving children and adolescents, Centre for Grief Education. Available at www.grief.org.au/child_support.html, accessed on March 7, 2005.
Smith-Stoner M, Oliver M: Ten palliative home care resources, *Home Healthc Nurs* 21(11):731, 2003.
Solari-Twadell PA, Bunkers SS, Wang CE et al: The pinwheel model of bereavement, *Image J Nurs Sch* 27(4):323, 1995.
Steen KF: A comprehensive approach to bereavement, *Nurse Pract* 23(3):54, 1998.
Van P, Meleis AI: Coping with grief after involuntary pregnancy loss: perspectives of African American women, *J Obstet Gynecol Neonatal Nurs* 32(1):28-39, 2003.
Walsh K, King M, Jones L et al: Spiritual beliefs may affect outcome of bereavement: prospective study, *BMJ* 324(7353):1551, 2002.
Zauszniewski JA, Eggenschwiler K, Preechawong S et al: Focused reflection reminiscence group for elders: implementation and evaluation, *Appl Gerontol* 23(4):429, 2004.

# Anticipatory Grieving

evolve

*Betty J. Ackley*

**NANDA**

## Definition

Intellectual and emotional responses and behaviors by which individuals, families, and communities work through the process of modifying self-concept based on the perception of potential loss

• = Independent; ▲ = Collaborative; EBN = Evidence-Based Nursing; EB = Evidence-Based

## Defining Characteristics

Expression of distress at potential loss; sorrow; guilt; denial of potential loss; anger; altered communication patterns; potential loss of significant object (e.g., people, possessions, job, status, home, ideals, parts and processes of the body); denial of significance of the loss; bargaining; alteration in eating habits, sleep patterns, dream patterns, activity level, or libido; difficulty taking on new or different roles; resolution of grief before the reality of loss

## Related Factors (r/t)

Perceived or actual impending loss of people, objects, possessions, job, status, home, ideals, or parts and processes of the body

NOC

## Outcomes (Nursing Outcomes Classification)

### Suggested NOC Outcomes

Coping; Family Coping; Grief Resolution; Psychosocial Adjustment: Life Change

**Example NOC Outcome with Indicators**

**Grief Resolution** with plans for a positive future as evidenced by the following indicators: Resolves feelings about loss/Verbalizes acceptance of loss/Describes meaning of loss or death/Reports decreased preoccupation with loss/Expresses positive expectations about the future (Rate each indicator of **Grief Resolution:** 1 = never demonstrated, 2 = rarely demonstrated, 3 = sometimes demonstrated, 4 = often demonstrated, 5 = consistently demonstrated [see Section I].)

## Client Outcomes

**Client Will (Specify Time Frame):**

- Express feelings of guilt, anger, or sorrow
- Identify problems associated with anticipatory grief (e.g., changes in activity, eating, or libido)
- Seek help in dealing with anticipated problems
- Plan for the future one day at a time

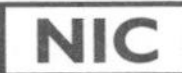

## Interventions (Nursing Interventions Classification)

### Suggested NIC Interventions

Grief Work Facilitation; Grief Work Facilitation: Perinatal Death

**Example NIC Activities—Grief Work Facilitation**

Encourage client to verbalize memories of the loss, both past and current; assist client to identify personal coping strategies

## Nursing Interventions and Rationales

- Actively listen to the client's and/or family's expression of grief; do not interrupt, do not tell your own story, and do not offer meaningless platitudes such as, "It will be better this way." *Just being with the client and/or family and listening can be the most helpful thing the nurse does (Furman, 2000; Davidson, 2003).*
- If grief results from the impending death of a loved one:
  - Allow family members to stay with the loved one during the dying process if desired and help them determine appropriate times to take breaks if appropriate
  - Spend time in the room with the dying client and family
  - Check in frequently when you are not able to stay at the bedside
  - Talk openly about the dying process and changes in condition that indicate death is near
  - Caution families that the dying person can often hear, and encourage them to reminisce about the good times
  - Encourage family members to touch the dying client if they are comfortable doing so

  *These are methods of providing support both to the client and to the family, to help with the bereavement process (Davidson, 2003). What the nurse says is not that important, what the nurse does is very important.*
- Encourage family members to listen carefully to messages given by the dying loved one; they may hear symbolic or obscure language referring to the dying process. *As a client approaches death, he or she develops an understanding of how his or her death will unfold. The client communicates this awareness in symbolic language (Callanan, 1994).*
- Ask the client if he or she is suffering, and take whatever measures possible to relieve suffering. *Suffering is more than pain; it is the client's point of view of the world. Sometimes just asking about suffering can help relieve suffering by acknowledging its existence (Ufema, 2004a).*
- If the dying client or family is denying the seriousness of his or her condition, do not negate the denial. Instead listen to clients so that they feel they have been understood, and know that they are supported in dealing with their situation. *Denial protects clients from hopelessness and may be their coping mechanism to deal with reality. Never take away a client's hope, and hope is available no matter how poor the prognosis (Ufema, 2004b).*
- Help the dying client maintain hope by focusing on the moment, reviewing his or her assets, making decisions regarding care, and maintaining important relationships. *Hope maintains a connection to the world, and at the end of life, hope is for a peaceful death.*
- Help family members to let the loved one go if appropriate; give the loved one permission to die. *Sometimes dying people wait until they know their family members are strong enough to accept the loss before they allow themselves to die (Callanan, 1994).*
- Use therapeutic communication with open-ended questions such as, "What are your thoughts and fears?" **EB:** *In a retrospective cohort study, individuals who had experienced the death of a family member were asked to rate the quality of the dying experience after the family member's death (Curtis et al, 2002).*
- Keep family members informed about the client's condition. **EBN:** *Lack of communication from health care providers contributes to the anxiety and distress reported by families. A study of the experience of clients' families after a client's death in the intensive care unit*

*(ICU) demonstrated that families' information about the client is often lacking or inadequate. (Kirchhoff et al, 2002).*

- Encourage the client to "cry out" grief and express feelings, including sadness or anger. *Grief is work and is best treated as an active process in which the grieving client expresses and feels the grief.*
- Encourage the client to take care of any unfinished business if appropriate. Have the client make an advance directive with support. *A large number of Americans would prefer to rely more on family and friends rather than their physicians with regard to end-of-life care and decisions (Foster & McLellan, 2002).* **EB:** *In a study of dying clients and their families and caregivers, respondents showed consensus on the importance of naming someone to make decisions, knowing what to expect about one's physical condition, having financial affairs in order, having treatment preferences in writing, and knowing that one's physician is comfortable talking about death and dying (Steinhauser et al, 2001).*
- Help the dying client build memories. This can be done a number of ways, including the following:
  - Writing love letters: to be opened on family birthdays or other special days after death
  - Making audiotape or videotape recordings: to share memories and say goodbye
  - Writing a journal: to be read by children and loved ones
  - Planning his or her own funeral
  - Writing his or her own obituary
  - Leaving a legacy to designate money for favorite causes

  *These are creative ways to nurture family relationships by leaving mementos for loved ones (Brant, 1998).*
- Determine the need for sedation during the dying process if desired by the client. **EB:** *Sedation can be helpful to decrease the physical and psychological stress of dying but there are ethical concerns regarding the practice. A study demonstrated that use of sedation in palliative care is increasing (Muller-Busch, Andres, & Jehser, 2003).*
- ▲ Assess for spiritual distress and refer the client for spiritual counseling if desired and appropriate. *Spiritual support can help clients; the nurse should approach the client with a nonjudgmental, listening ear and refer to the appropriate spiritual leader.*
- Help the client and/or family determine how best to obtain social support. **EB:** *Social support is shown to assist the bereaved individuals as they reconstruct their lives and find new meaning in life (Hogan & Schmidt, 2002).* **EBN:** *In a study of adolescents dealing with the death of a loved one, the most important factors that helped adolescents cope with the grief were self-help and support from parents, relatives, and friends (Rask, Kaunonen, & Paunonen-Ilmonen, 2002).*
- Identify problems with eating or sleeping, and intervene with suggestions as appropriate. *A grieving client can feel stunned and helpless and may be unable to consume food for a period of time. One study indicated that bereaved individuals, irrespective of whether they had counseling for grief resolution or not, had a moderate risk for poor nutrition. The implication is that food issues need to be included in grief resolution interventions (Johnson, 2002).*
- Encourage the caregiver of a dying person to live one day at a time and recognize that mourning is occurring while caring for the loved one. Help the caregiver express

feelings of loss and encourage the caregiver to practice self-care. Refer to the care plan for **Caregiver role strain** if appropriate. **EBN:** *Caregivers grieve as they care for the dying person. They can develop an increased intimacy and involvement in the relationship, which can help them have a positive bereavement outcome (Costello, 1999).*

### Pediatric/Parent

- Treat the child with respect, give them the opportunity to talk about their concerns, and answer questions honestly. *Children know much more than adults realize. They are very observant and generally know if a parent or loved one is dying, or cause of death, even if they have not been told (Schuurman, 2005).*
- Listen to the child's expression of grief. *The best thing to be done to help a child is to listen to them, with our ears, eyes, hearts, and souls, and recognize that we do not have to have answers (Schuurman, 2005).*
- Help parents recognize that the child does not have to be "fixed," instead they need support going through an experience of grieving just as adults. *The role of the nurse, parent, and friends is to support and assist, not to help the child "get over it" (Schuurman, 2005).*
- Ask the child if he or she would like a lock of hair to keep. *Memory keepsakes facilitate the grief process (Buxbaum & Brant, 2001).*
- Encourage children to listen to music that they enjoy. **EB:** *The investigator concluded that participation of grieving children in music therapy–based bereavement groups served to reduce grief symptoms among the subjects as evaluated in the home (Hilliard, 2001).*
- Help the adolescent determine sources of support and how to utilize them effectively. **EBN:** *In a study of adolescents dealing with the death of a loved one, the most important factors that helped adolescents cope with the grief were self-help and support from parents, relatives, and friends (Rask, Kaunonen, & Paunonen-Ilmonen, 2002).*

### Geriatric

- Assist the client with end-of-life decisions and advance directives. **EB:** *One study found that older adults should be asked specific questions about their end-of-life choices and the reasons for these choices. A thorough understanding of an individual's end-of-life preferences may help health professionals working with older adults develop client-centered care plans for the end of life (Vig, Davenport, & Pearlman, 2002).*
- In extended care facilities, consider use of nurse "Bereavement Leaders" who are responsible to help dying clients and their families in the process of bereavement. *The use of a nurse trained in facilitating bereavement for client and family can result in improved outcomes for everyone, the client, the family and the nursing staff (Davidson, 2003).*

### Multicultural

- Assess for the influence of cultural beliefs, norms, and values on the client's grief and mourning practices. **EBN:** *Grief and mourning practices may be based on cultural conventions (Clements et al, 2003; Leininger & McFarland, 2002; Cochran, 1998; Doswell & Erlen, 1998). Some African Americans may place great emphasis on attendance at funerals;*

*many Native-American tribes hold long, somber wakes, during which food and memorial gifts are distributed; Chinese and Japanese families may have specific funeral rituals that must be followed precisely to ensure safe passage of their loved ones into the next world; Latinos may hold wakes, use prayer during a novena, and light candles in honor of the dead; and in West Indian/Caribbean cultures, death arrangements might be made by a kinsman of the deceased (McQuay, 1995).*

- Encourage discussion of the grief process. **EBN:** *Patients who were from an ethnic minority group were significantly more likely to report that interviews about death, dying, and bereavement were helpful (Emanuel et al, 2004). Storytelling was at the heart of every African-American widow's description of her bereavement experience. Nurses can engage the older African-American widow in storytelling as an effective therapeutic intervention and as a means to gain in-depth understanding and cultural insight into the meaning of the widow's grief experience (Rodgers, 2004).*
- Assess for the influence of cultural beliefs, norms, and values on the client's expressions of grief. **EBN:** *African Americans may be expected to act "strong" and go about the business of life after a death; Native Americans may not talk about the death because of beliefs that such talk will detract from spirituality and bring bad luck; Latinos may wear black and act subdued during their* luto *(mourning) period; and Southeast Asian families may wear white when mourning (McQuay, 1995).*
- Teach patients to recognize grief responses. **EBN:** *Recognition of grief patterns will allow patients to manage their responses more effectively and may prevent adverse outcomes to their physical and mental health (Van & Meleis, 2003).*

G

## Home Care

NOTE: Hospice care encourages clients and families to experience the client's final days in the setting of choice. All of the previously mentioned interventions can and should be applied in the home setting when that is the setting selected.

- Listen actively. Normalize the client's and family's expressions of grief for a loved one who is expected to die. Demonstrate a caring and hopeful approach. *Active listening supports the client and family without intrusive advice giving. Normalizing lets the client and family know that their responses are appropriate ways of preparing for death.* **EBN:** *Caring for and with the client, and projecting hopefulness, has been shown to inspire hope in bereavement counseling (Cutcliffe, 2004).*

▲ When the client has a history of loss of a pregnancy, assess the client's need for a counseling referral during subsequent pregnancies. **EBN:** *Parents with a history of perinatal loss are at higher risk for depressive symptoms and pregnancy-specific anxiety during subsequent pregnancies, particularly before the third trimester. Mothers had a higher level of symptoms than fathers (Armstrong, 2002; Franche & Mikail, 1999).*

## Palliative Care

▲ When the potential loss is of a loved one, refer the grieving client to hospice volunteer services for support. *Social support has been identified as the most important predictor of a positive bereavement experience (Cooley, 1992). Relief of suffering of clients and fam-*

G

*ilies (i.e., physical, emotional, and spiritual) is the goal of hospice care (Krisman-Scott & McCorkle, 2002).*

- Evaluate symptomatology of client in anticipation of planning for terminal care. Raise the issue with client and family; discuss advance care directives; determine wishes for remaining at home and contingency plans for terminal hospitalization. **EB:** *Characteristics of COPD clients most likely to die within 6 to 12 months include severe, irreversible airflow obstruction, severely impaired and declining exercise capacity, older age, cardiovascular or other comorbid disease, and recent acute care hospitalization. When these characteristics apply, planning for death should be implemented (Hansen-Flaschen, 2004).*
- Assess caregiver reaction to bereavement issues and caregiver burden. Suggest preventive intervention for potential bereavement maladjustment if indicated. **EB:** *A study demonstrated that bereavement maladjustment is more likely with caregivers who are over 61 years old, who perceive a substantial emotional burden, and who have been unable to continue working. Periodic assessments and preventive interventions could anticipate caregiver needs, and reduce health and social costs (Ferrario et al, 2004; Kurtz et al, 2004).*
- Encourage caregivers to ventilate feelings and concerns about their perceptions of the client's suffering, of loss and feelings of inadequacy, and of any physical or psychological symptoms they are having. Implement interventions in response to expressed powerlessness. Refer to care plan for **Powerlessness. EB:** *Caregivers in the palliative home care situation often feel helpless and powerless (Milberg, Strang, & Jakobsson, 2004).*
- Assist client to optimize retention of as many usual activities and family/friends contacts as possible. Explain all elements of care to client. Refer to care plan for **Powerlessness. EBN:** *Clients in palliative care feel a loss of their sense of living. Maintaining as much as possible of the existence before illness and ensuring that client receives information about what is happening helps mitigate feelings of powerlessness (Appelin & Bertero, 2004).*
- Focus on spiritual needs of client to ensure a continued sense of connectedness. Refer to care plan for **Spiritual Distress. EBN:** *Clients receiving palliative care become strongly aware of their relatedness with others and with elements of their lives (Appelin & Bertero, 2004).*

## Client/Family Teaching

- Teach caregivers that they are doing anticipatory grieving as they care for loved ones, which is part of the reason care can be so difficult. The grief can become more acute as death approaches. *Anticipatory grieving allows adaptation to the loss to begin before the loved one's death (Costello, 1999).*
- Teach families how to provide mouth care and other comfort measures for the dying client as desired. *Providing hands on care can be helpful for the families of dying clients (Davidson, 2003).*

## evolve WEBSITES FOR EDUCATION

See the EVOLVE website for World Wide Web resources for client education.

## REFERENCES


Appelin G, Bertero C: Patients' experiences of palliative care in the home: a phenomenological study of a Swedish sample, *Cancer Nurs* 27(1):65, 2004.

Armstrong DS: Emotional distress and prenatal attachment in pregnancy after perinatal loss, *J Nurs Scholarsh* 34:339, 2002.

Brant JM: The art of palliative care: living with hope, dying with dignity, *Oncol Nurs Forum* 25(6):995, 1998.

Buxbaum L, Brant JM: When a parent dies from cancer, *Clin J Oncol Nur* 5(4):135, 2001.

Brown MA, Powell-Cope G: Themes of loss and dying in caring for a family member with AIDS, *Res Nurs Health* 16:179, 1993.

Callanan M: Farewell messages: dealing with death, *Am J Nurs* 94(5):19, 1994.

Carpenito JL: *Nursing diagnosis: applications to clinical practice,* ed 5, Philadelphia, 1993, JB Lippincott.

Clements PT, Vigil GJ, Manno MS et al: Cultural perspectives of death, grief, and bereavement, *J Psychosoc Nurs Ment Health Serv* 41(7):18-26, 2003.

Cochran M: Tears have no color, *Am J Nurs* 98(6):53, 1998.

Cohen JA, Mannarino AP, Knudsen K: Treating childhood traumatic grief, *J Am Acad Child Adolesc Psychiatry* 43(10):1225, 2004.

Cooley ME: Bereavement care: a role for nurses, *Cancer Nurs* 15:125, 1992.

Costello J: Anticipatory grief: coping with the impending death of a partner, *Int J Palliat Nurs* 5(5):223, 1999.

Curtis JR, Patrick DL, Engelberg RA et al: A measure of the quality of dying and death. Initial validation using after-death interviews with family members, *J Pain Symptom Manage* 24(1):17, 2002.

Cutcliffe JR: The inspiration of hope in bereavement counseling, *Issues Ment Health* 25:165, 2004.

Davidson KM: Evidence-based protocol: family bereavement support before and after the death of a nusing home resident, *J Gerontol Nurs* 29(1):10, 2003.

Doswell W, Erlen J: Multicultural issues and ethical concerns in the delivery of nursing care interventions, *Nurs Clin North Am* 33(2):353, 1998.

Emanuel EJ, Fairclough DL, Wolfe P et al: Talking with terminally ill patients and their caregivers about death, dying, and bereavement: is it stressful? Is it helpful? *Arch Intern Med* 164(18):1999, 2004.

Ferrario SR, Cardillo V, Vicario F et al: Advanced cancer at home: caregiving and bereavement, *Palliative Med* 18:129, 2004.

Foster LW, McLellan LJ: Translating psychosocial insight into ethical discussions supportive of families in end-of-life decision-making, *Soc Work Health Care* 35(3):37, 2002.

Franche R, Mikail S: The impact of perinatal loss on adjustment to subsequent pregnancy, *Soc Sci Med* 48:1613, 1999.

Furman J: Taking a holistic approach to the dying time, *Nursing* 30(6):46, 2000.

Glazer HR, Clark MD, Stein DS: The impact of hippotherapy on grieving children, *J Hosp Palliat Nurs* 6(3):161, 2004.

Hansen-Flaschen J: Chronic obstructive pulmonary disease: the last year of life, *Respir Care* 49(1):90, 2004.

Hilliard RE: The effects of music therapy–based bereavement groups on mood and behavior of grieving children: a pilot study, *J Music Ther* 38(4):291, 2001.

Hogan NS, Schmidt LA: Testing the grief to personal growth model using structural equation modeling, *Death Stud* 26(8):615, 2002.

Johnson CS: Nutritional considerations for bereavement and coping with grief, *J Nutr Health Aging* 6(3):171, 2002.

Kirchhoff KT, Walker L, Hutton A et al: The vortex: families' experiences with death in the intensive care unit, *Am J Crit Care* 11(3):200, 2002.

Krisman-Scott MA, McCorkle R: The tapestry of hospice, *Holist Nurs Pract* 16(2):32, 2002.

Kurtz ME, Kurtz JC, Given CW et al: Depression and physical health among family caregivers of geriatric patients with cancer: a longitudinal view, *Med Sci Monit* 10(8):CR447, 2004.

Laakso H, Paunonen-Ilmonen M: Mothers' experience of social support following the death of a child, *J Clin Nurs* 11(2):176, 2002.

Lawson W: Grieving mothers suffer early deaths, *Psychology Today* 36(3):18, 2003.

Leininger MM, McFarland MR: *Transcultural nursing: concepts, theories, research and practices,* ed 3, New York, 2002, McGraw-Hill.

McQuay JE: Cross-cultural customs and beliefs related to health crises, death, and organ donation/transplantation: a guide to assist health care professionals understand different responses and provide cross-cultural assistance, *Crit Care Nurs Clin North Am* 7(3):581, 1995.

Milberg A, Strang P, Jakobsson M: Next of kin's experience of powerlessness and helplessness in palliative home care, *Support Care Cancer* 12:120, 2004.

Muller-Busch HC, Andres I, Jehser: Sedation in paplliative care: a critical analysis of 7 years experience, *BMC Palliat Care* 2(1):2, 2003.

Rask K, Kaunonen M, Paunonen-Ilmonen M: Adolescent coping with grief after the death of a loved one, *Int J Nurs Pract* 8(3): 137, 2002.
Rodgers LS: Meaning of bereavement among older African American widows, *Geriatr Nurs* 25(1):10-16, 2004.
Schuurman DL: The club no one wants to join: a dozen lessons I've learned from grieving children and adolescents, Centre for Grief Education. Available at www.grief.org.au/child_support.html, accessed on March 10, 2005.
Steinhauser KE, Christakis NA, Clipp EC et al: Preparing for the end of life: preferences of patients, families, physicians, and other care providers, *J Pain Symptom Manage* 22(3):727, 2001.
Ufema J: Unwelcome script change, *Nursing* 34(11):28, 2004a.
Ufema J: Power of suggestion, *Nursing* 34(10):10, 2004b.
Van P, Meleis AI: Coping with grief after involuntary pregnancy loss: perspectives of African American women, *J Obstet Gynecol Neonatal Nurs* 32(1), 28-39, 2003.
Vig EK, Davenport NA, Pearlman RA: Good deaths, bad deaths, and preferences for the end of life: a qualitative study of geriatric outpatients, *J Am Geriatr Soc* 50(9):1541, 2002.



# Dysfunctional Grieving

evolve

*Betty J. Ackley*

**NANDA**

## Definition

Extended unsuccessful use of intellectual and emotional responses by which individuals, families, and communities attempt to work through the process of modifying self-concept based on the perception of loss

NOTE: It is now recognized that sometimes what was previously diagnosed as **Dysfunctional Grieving** might instead be **Chronic Sorrow,** in which grief lingers and is reactivated at intervals (Eakes, Burke, & Hainsworth, 1998). Refer to the nursing diagnosis **Chronic Sorrow** if appropriate.

## Defining Characteristics

Repetitive use of ineffectual behaviors associated with attempts to reinvest in relationships; crying; sadness; reliving of past experiences with little or no reduction (diminishment) of intensity of grief; labile affect; expression of unresolved issues; interference with life functioning; verbal expression of distress at loss; idealization of lost object (e.g., people, possessions, job, status, home, ideals, parts and processes of the body); difficulty in expressing loss; denial of loss; anger; alterations in eating habits, sleep patterns, dream patterns, activity level, libido, concentration, and/or pursuit of tasks; developmental regression; expression of guilt; prolonged interference with life functioning; onset or exacerbation of somatic or psychosomatic responses

## Related Factors (r/t)

Actual or perceived object loss (e.g., of people, possessions, job, status, home, ideals, parts and processes of the body)

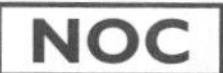

## Outcomes (Nursing Outcomes Classification)

### Suggested NOC Outcomes

Coping; Family Coping; Grief Resolution; Psychosocial Adjustment: Life Change

#### Example NOC Outcome with Indicators

**Grief Resolution** with plans for a positive future as evidenced by the following indicators: Resolves feelings about loss/Verbalizes acceptance of loss/Describes meaning of loss or death/Reports decreased preoccupation with loss/Expresses positive expectations about the future (Rate each indicator of **Grief Resolution:** 1 = never demonstrated, 2 = rarely demonstrated, 3 = sometimes demonstrated, 4 = Often demonstrated, 5 = consistently demonstrated [see Section I].)

G

## Client Outcomes

### Client Will (Specify Time Frame):

- Express appropriate feelings of guilt, fear, anger, or sadness
- Identify problems associated with grief (e.g., changes in appetite, insomnia, nightmares, loss of libido, decreased energy, alteration in activity levels)
- Seek help in dealing with grief-associated problems
- Plan for the future one day at a time
- Identify personal strengths
- Function at a normal developmental level and perform activities of daily living after an appropriate length of time

NIC

## Interventions (Nursing Interventions Classification)

### Suggested NIC Interventions

Grief Work Facilitation; Grief Work Facilitation: Perinatal Death; Guilt Work Facilitation

#### Example NIC Activities—Grief Work Facilitation

Encourage client to verbalize memories of the loss, both past and current; assist client to identify personal coping strategies

## Nursing Interventions and Rationales

- Assess the client's state of grieving. Use a tool such as the Hogan Grief to Personal Growth Model or the Grief Experience Inventory. **EB:** *These are commonly used measures of grief that have been shown to measure grief effectively (Gamino, Sewell, & Easterling, 2000; Hogan & Schmidt, 2002).*
- Assess for the causes of dysfunctional grieving (suddenness, interpersonal violence,

trauma, suicide, homicide, also highly dependent or ambivalent relationship with the deceased, inadequate coping skills, lack of social support, or previous physical or mental health problems. *Life circumstances can interfere with normal grieving and can be risk factors for dysfunctional grieving (Clements, 2004; Gamino, Sewell, & Easterling, 2000).*

- Identify problems of eating and sleeping; ensure that basic human needs are being met. **EB:** *One study indicated that bereaved individuals, regardless of whether they had counseling for grief resolution, had a moderate risk for poor nutrition (Johnson, 2002).*
- Develop a trusting relationship with the client by using therapeutic communication techniques. **EB:** *In a study of fathers who had lost infants before birth, fathers sought understanding from both the hospital personnel and their partners, as well as from relatives. Being able to protect their partner and to grieve in their own way was important to the fathers (Samuelsson, Radestad, & Segesten, 2001).*

G

- Establish a defined time to meet and discuss feelings about the loss and to perform grief work. Encourage the client to "cry out" grief and to talk about feelings of anger, sadness, and guilt. *Grief is work and is best treated as an active process in which the bereaved expresses and feels the grief. The grieving person will need to tell the story of their loss (Clements, 2004).*

▲ Assess for spiritual distress and refer the client to the appropriate spiritual leader. *Intrinsic spirituality can help the client grieve (Gamino, Sewell, & Easterling, 2000).* **EBN:** *The nurse should approach the client with a nonjudgmental, listening ear and refer the client to the appropriate spiritual leader.*

- Help the client recognize that, although sadness will occur at intervals for the rest of his or her life, it will become bearable. *The sadness associated with chronic sorrow is permanent, but as the grief resolves, there can be times of satisfaction and even happiness (Teel, 1991).* **EBN:** *Grief has a lasting nature; it changes and softens but never ends (Clements, 2004).*
- Help the client complete the following "guilt work" exercises:
  - Identify "if onlys" and put them into perspective.
  - Deal with "I didn't do" by looking at what was accomplished.
  - Forgive himself or herself; say to the client, "You are being awfully hard on yourself; try not to hurt yourself over something you could not have controlled." *The client may need to resolve guilt before successfully grieving and moving on with life.*
  - Help the client review past experiences, role changes, and coping skills. **EBN:** *In one study, getting over the loss was not a focus for many of the participants. The theme of a need to remember and to hold onto the memory was evident (Hentz, 2002).*
  - Encourage the client to keep a journal and write about the bereavement experience. **EB:** *Writing projects can be helpful for clients who are grieving, especially for those experiencing the unique bereavement of suicidal death (Range, Kovac, & Marion, 2000).*
  - Help the client to identify his or her own strengths to use in dealing with loss, reinforce these strengths, and consider the use of music. **EB:** *In a clinical controlled trial, single-session music therapy interventions with hospice clients demonstrated significant results in three client problem areas: pain control, physical comfort, and relaxation (Krout, 2001).*
  - If the client or family members are expressing anger, try not to react in anger. In-

stead, allow feelings to be expressed, listen to the expressions of anger, and accept their right to those feelings. Try lowering your voice and slowing your rate of speech as you respond to the client and/or family. *It is not therapeutic to respond to anger with anger. Instead, strive to be therapeutic, helping the client and/or family members express the anger and gain control of themselves by modeling calm behavior (Clements, 2004; Rueth & Hall, 1999).*

- ■ Expect the client to meet responsibilities; give positive reinforcement. Help the client to identify areas of hope in life and to determine their purposes if possible. **EBN:** *A significant positive relationship has been found between the level of grief resolution and the level of hope (Herth, 1990). Grieving people who have little purpose in life often experience more anger than individuals with more purpose.*

▲ Identify available community resources, including bereavement groups at local hospitals and hospice centers. **EBN:** *Bereaved individuals can benefit from grief resolution support groups (Douglas, 2004).*

▲ Determine whether the client is experiencing depression, suicidal tendencies, or other emotional disorders. Refer the client for counseling as appropriate. **EB:** *Counseling, including the use of relaxation therapy, desensitization, and biofeedback in addition to traditional psychotherapy, has been shown to be helpful (Arnette, 1996). Depression syndromes occur in almost one half of all grieving people, and 10% suffer major depression (Steen, 1998). Cognitive behavior therapy can be helpful for traumatic grief (Jacobs & Prigerson, 2000).*

G

## Pediatric/Parent

• Treat the child with respect, give them the opportunity to talk about their concerns, and answer questions honestly. *Children know much more than adults realize. They are very observant and generally know if a parent or loved one is dying, or the cause of death, even if they have not been told (Schuurman, 2005).*

• Listen to the child's expression of grief. *The best thing to be done to help a child is to listen to them, with our ears, eyes, hearts, and souls, and recognize that we do not have to have answers (Schuurman, 2005).*

• Help parents recognize that the child does not have to be "fixed," instead they need support going through an experience of grieving just as adults. *The role of the nurse, parent, and friends is to support and assist, not to help them "get over it" (Schuurman, 2005).*

• Encourage children to listen to music that they enjoy. **EB:** *The investigator concluded that participation of grieving children in music therapy–based bereavement groups served to reduce grief symptoms among the subjects as evaluated in the home (Hilliard, 2001).*

▲ Refer grieving children and parents to a program to help facilitate grieving if desired, especially if the death was traumatic. **EB:** *A study demonstrated that treatment for children and parents with grief associated with trauma helped decrease symptoms of post-traumatic stress disorder (PTSD) (Cohen, 2004).* **EBN:** *A program designed for grieving children involving riding horses was shown to increase self-confidence and self-esteem (Glazer, Clark, & Stein, 2004).*

• Help the adolescent determine sources of support and how to use them effectively. **EBN:** *In a study of adolescents dealing with the death of a loved one, the most important* *factors that helped adolescents cope with the grief were self-help and support from parents, relatives, and friends (Rask, Kaunonen, & Paunonen-Ilmonen, 2002).*

- Encourage parents to seek mental health services as needed, learn stress reduction, find sources of support, and take good care of their health. *Research has demonstrated that the loss of a child for a mother results in an increased loss of life within 18 years either due to disease or suicide (Lawson, 2003).* **EBN:** *A study analyzing the grief and coping of mothers who had lost children under age 7 years found that the spouse, remaining children, grandparents, next of kin, friends, and colleagues were the main sources of support (Laakso & Paunonen-Ilmonen, 2002).*
- If client is an adolescent exposed to a peer's suicide, watch for symptoms of traumatic grief, as well as PTSD, which include numbness, preoccupation with the deceased, functional impairment, and poor adjustment to the loss. **EB:** *A study demonstrated that adolescents in this situation were a high risk for depression, anxiety disorder, substance abuse, conduct disorder, attention deficit/hyperactivity disorder (ADHD), and depression (Melhem et al, 2004).*

G

### Geriatric

- Use reminiscence therapy in conjunction with the expression of emotions. Refer to a reminiscence group if available. **EBN and EB:** *Two studies demonstrated that participation in a reminiscence group reduced symptoms of depression (Zauszniewski et al, 2004; Jones, 2003).*
- Identify previous losses and assess the client for depression. *Losses and changes associated with aging often occur in rapid succession without adequate recovery time (Hegge & Fischer, 2000).* **EBN:** *Having more than two concurrent losses increases the incidence of unresolved grief (Herth, 1990). The grieving elderly widow may develop depression that results in poor nutrition, noncompliance with medication regimens, decreasing cognition, and multiple health problems (Fischer & Hegge, 2000).*
- Monitor an older adult who has been treated for bereavement-related depression for relapse or recurrence. **EB:** *In a 2-year study, 36% of older adults treated for bereavement-related depression experienced relapse or recurrence (Pasternak et al, 1997).*
- Evaluate the social support system of the elderly client. If the support system is minimal, help the client determine how to increase available support. **EBN:** *The elderly who have poor grieving outcomes often do not live with family members and have a minimal support system. The support of family, especially children. and friends is a common way for elderly widows to cope with a loss (Hegge & Fischer, 2000).*

### Multicultural

- Assess for the influence of cultural beliefs, norms, and values on the client's grief and mourning practices. **EBN:** *Grief and mourning practices may be based on cultural conventions (Clements et al, 2003; Leininger & McFarland. 2002; Cochran, 1998; Doswell & Erlen, 1998). Some African Americans may place great emphasis on attendance at funerals; many Native-American tribes hold long, somber wakes, during which food and memorial gifts are distributed; Chinese and Japanese families may have specific funeral rituals that must be followed precisely to ensure safe passage of their loved ones into the next world; Lati-*

*nos may hold wakes, use prayer during a novena, and light candles in honor of the dead; and in West Indian/Caribbean cultures, death arrangements might be made by a kinsman of the deceased (McQuay, 1995).*

- Assess for the influence of cultural beliefs, norms, and values on the client's expressions of grief. **EBN:** *African Americans may be expected to act "strong" and go about the business of life after a death; Native Americans may not talk about the death because of beliefs that such talk will detract from spirituality and bring bad luck; Latinos may wear black and act subdued during their* luto *(mourning) period; and Southeast Asian families may wear white when mourning (American Psychological Association, 2000; McQuay, 1995).*
- Encourage discussion of the grief process. **EBN:** *Patients who were from an ethnic minority group were significantly more likely to report that interviews about death, dying, and bereavement were helpful (Emanuel et al, 2004). Storytelling was at the heart of every African-American widows description of her bereavement experience. Nurses can engage the older African-American widow in storytelling as an effective therapeutic intervention and as a means to gain in-depth understanding and cultural insight into the meaning of the widow's grief experience (Rodgers, 2004).*
- Identify whether the client had been notified of the health status of the deceased and was able to be present during illness and death. **EBN:** *Not being present during terminal illness and death can disrupt the grieving process (McQuay, 1995).*
- Validate the client's feelings regarding the loss. **EBN:** *Validation is a therapeutic communication technique that lets the client know that the nurse has heard and understood what was said, and it promotes the nurse-client relationship (Heineken, 1998).*
- Teach patients to recognize grief responses. **EBN:** *Recognition of grief patterns will allow patients to manage their responses more effectively may prevent adverse outcomes to their physical and mental health (Van & Meleis, 2003).*

## evolve WEBSITES FOR EDUCATION

See the EVOLVE website for World Wide Web resources for client education.

## REFERENCES


American Psychiatric Association: *Diagnostic and statistical manual of mental disorders,* ed 4, Washington, DC, 2000, The Association.

Armstrong DS: Emotional distress and prenatal attachment in pregnancy after perinatal loss, *J Nurs Scholarsh* 34:339, 2002.

Arnette JD: Physiological effects of chronic grief: a biofeedback treatment approach, *Death Stud* 20:59, 1996.

Bateman A, Broderick D, Gleason L et al: Dysfunctional grieving, *J Psychosoc Nurs Ment Health Serv* 30(12):5, 1992.

Clements PT, DeRanieri JT, Vigil GJ et al: Life afer death: grief therapy after the sudden traumatic death of a family member, *Perspect Psychiatr Care* 40(4):149, 2004.

Cochran M: Tears have no color, *Am J Nurs* 98(6):53, 1998.

Cohen JA, Mannarino AP, Knudsen K: Treating childhood traumatic grief: a pilot study, *J Am Acad Child Adolesc Psychiatry* 43(10):171, 2004.

Constantino RE, Sekula LK, Rubinstein EN: Group intervention for widowed survivors of suicide, *Suicide Life Threat Behav* 31(4):428, 2001.

Doswell W, Erlen J: Multicultural issues and ethical concerns in the delivery of nursing care interventions, *Nurs Clin North Am* 33(2):353, 1998.

Douglas DH: The lived experience of loss: a phenomenological study, *J Am Psychiatr Nurses Assoc* 10(1):24, 2004.

Eakes GG, Burke ML, Hainsworth MA: Theory: middle-range theory of chronic sorrow, *Image J Nurs Sch* 30:179, 1998.
Emanuel EJ, Fairclough DL, Wolfe P et al: Talking with terminally ill patients and their caregivers about death, dying, and bereavement: is it stressful? Is it helpful? *Arch Intern Med* 164(18):1999, 2004.
Fischer C, Hegge M: The elderly woman at risk, *Am J Nurs* 100(6):54, 2000.
Franche R, Mikail S: The impact of perinatal loss on adjustment to subsequent pregnancy, *Soc Sci Med* 48:1613,1999.
Gamino LA, Sewell KW, Easterling LW: Scott and White Grief Study—phase 2: toward an adaptive model of grief, *Death Stud* 24:633, 2000.
Glazer HR, Clark MD, Stein DS: The impact of hippotherapy on grieving children, *J Hosp Palliat Nurs* 6(3):171, 2004.
Hegge M, Fischer C: Grief responses of senior and elderly widows: practice implications, *J Gerontol Nurs* 26(2): 35, 2000.
Heineken J: Patient silence is not necessarily client satisfaction: communication in home care nursing, *Home Healthc Nurse* 16(2): 115, 1998.
Hentz P: The body remembers: grieving and a circle of time, *Qual Health Res* 12(2):161, 2002.
Herth K: Relationship of hope, coping styles, concurrent losses, and setting to grief resolution in the elderly widow(er), *Res Nurs Health* 13:109, 1990.
Hilliard RE: The effects of music therapy–based bereavement groups on mood and behavior of grieving children: a pilot study, *J Music Ther* 38(4):291, 2001.
Hogan NS, Schmidt LA: Testing the grief to personal growth model using structural equation modeling, *Death Stud* 26(8):615, 2002.
Jacobs S, Prigerson H: Psychotherapy of traumatic grief: a review of evidence for psychotherapeutic treatments, *Death Stud* 24:479, 2000.
Johnson CS: Nutritional considerations for bereavement and coping with grief, *J Nutr Health Aging* 6(3):171, 2002.
Jones ED: Reminiscence therapy for older women with depression: effects of nursing intervention classification in assisted-living long-term care, *J Gerontol Nurs* 29(7):26, 2003.
Krout RE: The effects of single-session music therapy interventions on the observed and self-reported levels of pain control, physical comfort, and relaxation of hospice patients, *Am J Hosp Palliat Care* 18(6):383, 2001.
Laakso H, Paunonen-Ilmonen M: Mothers' experience of social support following the death of a child, *J Clin Nurs* 11(2):176, 2002.
Lange A, van de Ven JP, Schrieken B et al: Interapy, treatment of post-traumatic stress through the Internet: a controlled trial, *J Behav Ther Exp Psychiatry* 32(2):73, 2001.
Lawson W: Grieving mothers suffer early deaths, *Psychology Today*, 36(3):18, 2003.
Leininger MM, McFarland MR: *Transcultural nursing: concepts, theories, research and practices,* ed 3, New York, 2002, McGraw-Hill.
McQuay JE: Cross-cultural customs and beliefs related to health crises, death, and organ donation/transplantation: a guide to assist health care professionals understand different responses and provide cross-cultural assistance, *Crit Care Nurs Clin North Am* 7(3):581, 1995.
Melhem NM, Day N, Shear MK et al: Traumatic grief among adolescents exposed to a peer's suicide, *Am J Psychiatry* 161(8):1411, 2004.
Pasternak RE, Prigerson H, Hall M et al: The posttreatment illness course of depression in bereaved elders, *Am J Geriatr Psychiatry* 5:54, 1997.
Patusky KL, Rodning C, Martinez-Kratz M: Clinical lessons in psychiatric home care: a case study approach, *J Home Health Case Manage* 9:18, 1996.
Range LM, Kovac SH, Marion MS: Does writing about the bereavement lessen grief following sudden, unintentional death? *Death Stud* 24:115, 2000.
Rask K, Kaunonen M, Paunonen-Ilmonen M: Adolescent coping with grief after the death of a loved one, *Int J Nurs Pract* 8(3): 137, 2002.
Rodgers, LS: Meaning of bereavement among older African American widows, *Geriatr Nurs* 25(1):10-16, 2004.
Rueth TW, Hall SE: Dealing with the anger and hostility of those who grieve, *Am J Hosp Palliat Care* 16(6):743, 1999.
Samuelsson M, Radestad I, Segesten K: A waste of life: fathers' experience of losing a child before birth, *Birth* 28(2):124, 2001.
Schuurman DL: The club no one wants to join: a dozen lessons I've learned from grieving children and adolescents, Centre for Grief Education. Available at www.grief.org.au/child_support.html, accessed on March 7, 2005.
Steen KF: A comprehensive approach to bereavement, *Nurse Pract* 23(3):54, 1998.
Teel CS: Chronic sorrow: analysis of the concept, *J Adv Nurs* 16:1311, 1991.
Van P, Meleis AI: Coping with grief after involuntary pregnancy loss: perspectives of African American women, *J Obstet Gynecol Neonatal Nurs* 32(1), 28-39, 2003.

Zauszniewski JA, Eggenschwiler K, Preechawong S et al: Focused reflection reminiscence group for elders: implementation and evaluation, *Appl Gerontol* 23(4):429, 2004.

# Risk for dysfunctional Grieving

*Betty J. Ackley*

G

**NANDA**

## Definition

At risk for extended, unsuccessful use of intellectual and emotional responses and behaviors by an individual, family, or community following a death or perception of loss

## Risk Factors

### General

Preloss neuroticism; preloss psychological symptoms; frequency of major life events; predisposition for anxiety and feelings of inadequacy; past psychiatric or mental health treatment

### Perinatal

Later gestational age at time of loss, limited time since perinatal loss and subsequent conception; length of life of infant, absence of other living children, congenital anomaly, number of past perinatal losses, marital adjustment problems, viewing of ultrasound images of the fetus

## Related Factors (r/t)

See Risk Factors

**NOC**

## Outcomes (Nursing Outcomes Classification)

### Suggested NOC Outcomes

Coping; Family Coping; Grief Resolution; Psychosocial Adjustment: Life Change

**Example NOC Outcome with Indicators**

**Grief Resolution** with plans for a positive future as evidenced by the following indicators: Resolves feelings about loss/Verbalizes acceptance of loss/Describes meaning of loss or death/Reports decreased preoccupation with loss/Expresses positive expectations about the future (Rate each indicator of **Grief Resolution:** 1 = never demonstrated, 2 = rarely demonstrated, 3 = sometimes demonstrated, 4 = Often demonstrated, 5 = consistently demonstrated [see Section I].)

## Client Outcomes

**Client Will (Specify Time Frame):**

- Express appropriate feelings of guilt, fear, anger, or sadness
- Identify problems associated with grief (e.g., changes in appetite, insomnia, nightmares, loss of libido, decreased energy, alteration in activity levels)
- Seek help in dealing with grief-associated problems
- Plan for the future one day at a time
- Identify personal strengths
- Function at a normal developmental level and perform activities of daily living (ADLs) after an appropriate length of time

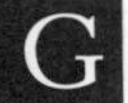

**NIC**

## Interventions (Nursing Interventions Classification)

### Suggested NIC Interventions

Grief Work Facilitation; Grief Work Facilitation: Perinatal Death; Guilt Work Facilitation

**Example NIC Activities—Grief Work Facilitation**

Encourage client to verbalize memories of the loss, both past and current; assist client to identify personal coping strategies

## Nursing Interventions and Rationales, Client Teaching

Refer to care plan for **Dysfunctional Grieving.**

# Delayed Growth and development

evolve

*Gail B. Ladwig*

**NANDA**

## Definition

Deviations from age-group norms

## Defining Characteristics

Altered physical growth; delay or difficulty in performing skills (motor, social, expressive) typical of age group; inability to perform self-care or self-control activities appropriate for age; flat affect; listlessness; decreased response time

## Related Factors (r/t)

Prescribed dependence, indifference; separation from significant others; environmental and stimulation deficiencies; effects of physical disability; inadequate caretaking; inconsistent responsiveness; multiple caretakers

**NOC**

## Outcomes (Nursing Outcomes Classification)

### Suggested NOC Outcomes

Child Development: 2 Months, 4 Months, 6 Months, 12 Months, 2 Years, 3 Years, 4 Years, Preschool, Middle Childhood, Adolescence; Growth; Mobility; Neurological Status; Physical Maturation: Female, Male; Knowledge Parenting

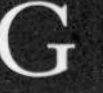


**Example NOC Outcome with Indicators**

**Growth** as evidenced by the following indicators: Weight percentiles for age, sex, and height (Rate each indicator of **Growth:** 1 = severe deviation from normal range, 2 = substantial deviation from normal range, 3 = moderate deviation from normal range, 4 = mild deviation from normal range, 5 = no deviation from normal range [see Section I].)

## Client Outcomes

**Client/Parents/Primary Caregiver Will (Specify Time Frame):**

- Describe realistic, age-appropriate patterns of growth and development
- Promote activities and interactions that support age-related developmental tasks
- Display consistent, sustained achievement of age-appropriate behaviors (social, interpersonal, and/or cognitive) and/or motor skills
- Achieve realistic developmental and/or growth milestones based on existing abilities, extent of disability, and functional age
- Exhibit limited temporary behavioral regression that reverses shortly after episode of illness or hospitalization
- Attain steady gains in growth patterns

**NIC**

## Interventions (Nursing Interventions Classification)

### Suggested NIC Interventions

Active Listening; Body Image Enhancement; Developmental Enhancement: Adolescent, Child; Emotional Support; Kangaroo Care; Nutrition Therapy; Nutritional Monitoring; Positioning; Self-Care Assistance; Self-Responsibility Facilitation

**Example NIC Activities—Nutritional Monitoring**

Monitor trends in weight loss and gain; monitor food preferences and choices

## Nursing Interventions and Rationales

NOTE: Determination of the etiological basis for delayed growth and development is critical because it will direct the selection of interventions for treating the client. Parenting skill deficits, lack of consistency between caregivers, hospitalization, and a chronic medical condition or developmental disability will necessitate different strategies. A hospitalization experience with regressive behaviors can be a transient occurrence, whereas a chronic situation may result in more severe and longer delays requiring more in-depth intervention. Parenting skills and consistent expectations by multiple caregivers can be addressed by more intensive education efforts (Seideman & Kleine, 1995; Stutts, 1994).



- ▲ To determine risk for or actual deviations in normal development, consider the use of a screening tool. *Some tools are the Brigance Infant and Toddler Screens and the Pregnancy Risk Assessment Monitoring System (PRAMS).* **EB:** *The Brigance Infant and Toddler Screens are shown to be accurate, valid, and reliable tools that can be administered by a range of professionals using either parental interview or direct elicitation and observation, or both (Glascoe, 2002).* **EB:** *PRAMS is a surveillance project of the Centers for Disease Control and Prevention (CDC) and state health departments. PRAMS collects state-specific, population-based data on maternal attitudes and experiences prior to, during, and immediately following pregnancy (CDC, 2004).*
- • Provide skin-to-skin contact for newborns and moms. Place the naked baby prone on the mother's bare chest at birth or soon afterwards (<24 hour). **EBN:** *This study demonstrated statistically significant and positive effects of early skin-to-skin contact on breastfeeding at 1 to 3 months postbirth (Anderson et al, 2004).*
- • Regularly compare height and weight measurements for the child or adolescent with established age-appropriate norms and previous measurements. **EB:** *Growth charts are not intended to be used as a sole diagnostic instrument. Instead, growth charts are tools that contribute to forming an overall clinical impression for the child being measured. The revised growth charts provide an improved tool for evaluating the growth of children in clinical and research settings (CDC, 2002).*
- ▲ Initiate referrals for a more comprehensive growth and/or development evaluation if indicated. *Presence of a risk factor alone does not always obviate the need for referrals. The number and weight of risk factors and normal differences of each child must be considered (Curry & Duby, 1994).*
- ▲ Identify coexisting health or medical conditions that may be contributing to the alteration in growth and/or development, and refer the client to a specialist in the appropriate health care discipline for management. **EB:** *A specific cause can be determined in the majority of children with global developmental delay. Certain routine screening tests are indicated and, depending on history and examination findings, additional specific testing may be performed (Shevell et al, 2003).*
- • Examine parental/caregiver expectations of future learning, ability, and developmental achievements of children with developmental disabilities. **EBN:** *Initiation of measures to support or enhance family and child motivation and ability increases achievement (Edwards-Beckett, 1994).*
- • Prepare children for hospitalization; include hospital tours, film, books and play therapy, interventions all designed to increase knowledge and promote understanding of the hospitalization process. *Children cope more effectively with the stresses of hospitalization if they have an understanding of the hospitalization process before being admitted to hospital. The most effective programs used a multicomponent approach, which combined information provision and coping skills training (Mitchell, Johnston, & Keppell, 2004).*

- Provide support groups and education on human immunodeficiency virus (HIV) and caring for infants with this diagnosis. *Developmental delay has been well-documented infants with HIV (Potterton & Eales, 2001).*
- Provide meaningful stimulation for hospitalized infants and children. *Stimulation is essential to the development of gross and fine motor adaptive skills, language, and personal-social functioning in infants and children. Disruption of this process for infants, even those without preexisting developmental delays, can occur in the absence of intervention. Hospitalized infants are often subjected to understimulation or an overabundance of meaningless stimulation (Slusher & McClure, 1995).*
- Provide opportunities for mother-infant skin-to-skin contact (kangaroo care, or KC) for preterm infants. **EB:** *One study showed that the neurodevelopmental profile was more mature for infants receiving KC. Results underscore the role of early skin-to-skin contact in the maturation of the autonomic and circadian systems in preterm infants (Feldman & Eidelman, 2003).*

G

- ▲ Engage the child in appropriate play activities. Refer the child to a play/recreational therapist (if available) for supplemental strategies. **EB:** *Play is essential for learning in children. Toys should be safe, affordable, and developmentally appropriate. Children do not need expensive toys (Glassy & Romano, 2003).*
- Enlist and encourage involvement of the parents and/or family as participants in care, particularly for hospitalized infants, toddlers, preschoolers, or school-age children, whenever possible without exceeding the parent's/family's emotional and physical limits. *Frequent and consistent parent/family contact and care diminish normal separation anxiety. Most infants and toddlers find this presence comforting and as a result are better able to cope with the situation and stress (Craft & Willadsen, 1992).*
- Model age-appropriate and cognitively appropriate caregiver skills by doing the following:
  - Communicating with the child in a manner appropriate to cognitive level of development
  - Giving the child tasks and responsibilities appropriate to age or functional age level
  - Instituting the use of safety devices such as assistive equipment
  - Encouraging the child to perform ADLs as appropriate

  *These actions illustrate parenting and child-rearing skills and behaviors for parents and family members (McCloskey & Bulechek, 1992).*
- Provide an environment that promotes additional sleep and rest opportunities. **EB:** *Reduced quality of sleep can have important implications for the developing child as it can impair growth, learning, and emotional development (Boyle & Copley, 2004).*
- Provide developmental care interventions to preterm infants to improve neurodevelopmental outcomes (Symington & Pinelli, 2002).
- Provide neonatal positioning procedures for preterm infants to prevent extremity malalignment, skull deformities, and gross motor delay. *Alignment and shaping of the musculoskeletal system occur with each body position change in a neonatal intensive care unit (NICU); use of proper positioning strategies promotes skeletal integrity, postural control, and sensorimotor organization (Sweeney & Gutierrez, 2002).*

G

## Multicultural

- Acknowledge racial/ethnic differences at the onset of care. **EBN:** *Acknowledgment of race/ethnicity issues will enhance communication, establish rapport, and promote treatment outcomes (D'Avanzo et al, 2001; Ludwick & Silva, 2000; Vontress & Epp, 1997).*
- Assess for the influence of cultural beliefs, norms, and values on the client's perceptions of child development. **EBN:** *What the client considers normal and abnormal child development may be based on cultural perceptions (Cochran, 1998; Doswell & Erlen, 1998; Leininger & McFarland, 2002).*
- Use a neutral, indirect style in addressing areas in which improvement is needed (such as a need for verbal stimulation) when working with Native American clients. **EBN:** *Using indirect statements such as "Other mothers have tried . . ." or "I had a client who tried 'X' and it seemed to work very well," will assist in avoiding resentment of the parent (Seideman et al, 1996).*
- Assess whether exposure to community violence is contributing to developmental problems. **EBN:** *Exposure to community violence has been associated with increases in aggressive behavior and depression in children (Gorman-Smith & Tolan, 1998).*
- Assess and identify for possible environmental conditions, which may be contributing factor to altered growth and development. **EB:** *Insecticide exposures were widespread among minority women in New York City during pregnancy and high levels were associated with lower birth weight and length (Whyatt et al, 2004).*
- Validate the client's feelings and concerns related to the child's development. **EBN:** *Validation is a therapeutic communication technique that lets the client know that the nurse has heard and understood what was said, and it promotes the nurse-client relationship (Heineken, 1998).*
- Provide information on the effects of environmental risk exposure on growth and development. **EB:** *Minority children with prenatal environmental tobacco smoke exposure were twice as likely to be classified as significantly cognitively delayed, when compared with unexposed children (Rauh et al, 2004). Data suggest that environmental exposure may lead to delayed growth and pubertal development in African-American and Mexican-American girls (2003).*

## Home Care

- The interventions described previously may be adapted for home care use.
- Assess for the presence of substances that could cause developmental delay. Children's access to substances that cause neurological deficits (e.g., lead-based paints) should be identified and eliminated.

▲ Refer maternal drug users to home intervention programs. **EB:** *Ongoing maternal drug use was associated with worse developmental outcomes among a group of drug-exposed infants. A home intervention led to higher scores on the Bayley Scales of Infant Development among drug-exposed infants (Schuler, Nair, & Kettinger, 2003).*

- Help the family to identify appropriate skill-building activities for the child. *Exposure to age-appropriate or lower-age games, toys, and activities can provide essential stimuli for development. Family members may need to adjust their expectations of the child's behaviors to be appropriate not only for age but also for any developmental limitations.*

- Provide emotional support for family members in their reactions to evidence of developmental delay. *Parents may be distressed by the potential for developmental delay in a child.*
- ▲ If possible, refer the family to a program of animal-assisted therapy. **EBN:** *Research suggests that interactions with dogs may assist clients with pervasive developmental disorders (PDDs) to establish bonds with their social environment. Children with PDDs were more playful, more focused, and more aware of their social environment in the presence of a therapy dog than in the presence of a toy or a stuffed dog (Martin & Farnum, 2002).*

## Client/Family Teaching



- Provide parents and/or caregivers realistic expectations for attainment of growth and development milestones. Clarify expectations and correct misconceptions. **EBN:** *Learning about the growth and developmental differences between children with congenital heart defect (CHD) and normal children may help parents of the former to detect problems associated with delayed growth and development earlier. These children and their families should have the opportunity to participate in a long-term, follow-up program that provides information and encourages developmental progress (Chen, Li, & Wang, 2004).*
- Have parents and/or caregivers rehearse coping strategies for approaching developmental milestones and acknowledge positive actions and behaviors. *As children progress to another developmental stage such as adolescence, families are challenged to master developmental tasks that seem enigmatic. Anticipating and preparing can strengthen their ability to deal with situations and enhance achievement (Reisch & Forsyth, 1992).*
- Teach methods of providing meaningful stimulation for infants and children. *Stimulation is essential to the development of gross and fine motor adaptive skills, language, and personal-social functioning in infants and children (Slusher & McClure, 1995).*
- Instruct the client with regard to age-appropriate activities and play, nutrition, discipline, and safety, and how to support growth and development. *Parents are then better equipped to promote the growth and development of the child (McCloskey & Bulechek, 1992).* **EBN:** *The use of baby walkers is controversial. Some studies suggested that they may delay walking by 11 to 26 days; other studies were inconclusive. There was no support that they aided walking. Further work is required to determine if they are an independent causal factor in accidents (Burrows & Griffiths, 2002).*
- ▲ Elicit the involvement of parents and caregivers in social support groups and parenting classes.
- ▲ Furnish information about community resources. *Support groups and other opportunities to obtain guidance serve to empower parents and clarify and reinforce knowledge and parenting skills (Kinney, Mannetter, & Carpenter, 1992; McCloskey & Bulechek, 1992).*

## evolve WEBSITES FOR EDUCATION

See the EVOLVE website for World Wide Web resources for client education.

## REFERENCES

Boyle J, Copley M: Children's sleep: problems and solutions, *J Fam Health Care* 14(3):61-63, 2004.

Burrows P, Griffiths P: Do baby walkers delay onset of walking in young children? *Br J Community Nurs* 7(11): 581, 2002.

Centers for Disease Control and Prevention (CDC): National Center for Health Statistics, 2002. Available at www.cdc.gov/nchs/about/major/nhanes/growthcharts/background.htm, accessed on January 16, 2005.

Centers for Disease Control and Prevention (CDC): Reproductive Health Information Source, 2004. Available at www.cdc.gov/reproductivehealth/srv_prams.htmm, accessed on January 16. 2005.

Chen C, Li C, Wang J: Growth and development of children with congenital heart disease, *J Adv Nurs* 47(3):260-269, 2004.

Cochran M: Tears have no color, *Am J Nurs* 98(6):53, 1998.

Craft MJ, Willadsen JA: Interventions related to family, *Nurs Clin North Am* 27:517-540, 1992.

Curry DM, Duby JC: Developmental surveillance by pediatric nurses, *Pediatr Nurs* 20:40, 1994.

D'Avanzo CE et al: Developing culturally informed strategies for substance-related interventions. In Naegle MA, D'Avanzo CE, editors: *Addictions and substance abuse: strategies for advanced practice nursing,* St Louis, 2001, Mosby.

Doswell W, Erlen J: Multicultural issues and ethical concerns in the delivery of nursing care interventions, *Nurs Clin North Am* 33(2):353, 1998.

Edwards-Beckett J: Caregivers' expectations of future learning of dependents with a developmental disability, *J Pediatr Nurs* 9:27, 1994.

Feldman R, Eidelman A: Skin-to-skin contact (kangaroo care) accelerates autonomic and neurobehavioural maturation in preterm infants, *Dev Med Child Neurol* 45(4):274, 2003.

Glascoe FP: The Brigance Infant and Toddler Screen: standardization and validation, *J Dev Behav Pediatr* 23(3):145, 2002.

Glassy D, Romano J: Selecting appropriate toys for young children: the pediatrician's role, *Pediatrics* 111(4 pt 1):911, 2003.

Gorman-Smith D, Tolan P: The role of exposure to community violence and developmental problems among inner city youth, *Dev Psychopathol* 10(1):101, 1998.

Heineken J: Patient silence is not necessarily client satisfaction: communication in home care nursing, *Home Healthc Nurse* 16(2):115, 1998.

Kinney CK, Mannetter R, Carpenter MA: Support groups. In Bulechek GM, McCloskey JC, editors: *Nursing interventions: essential nursing treatment,* Philadelphia, 1992, WB Saunders.

Leininger MM, McFarland MR: *Transcultural nursing: concepts, theories, research and practices,* ed 3, New York, 2002, McGraw-Hill.

Ludwick R, Silva M: Nursing around the world: cultural values and ethical conflicts, *Online J Issues Nurs,* August 14, 2000. Available at www.nursingworld.org/ojin/ethicol/ethics_4.htm, accessed on June 19, 2003.

Martin F, Farnum J: Animal-assisted therapy for children with pervasive developmental disorders, *West J Nurs Res* 24:657, 2002.

McCloskey JC, Bulechek GM, editors: *Nursing interventions classification (NIC),* St Louis, 1992, Mosby.

Mitchell M, Johnston L, Keppell M: Preparing children and their families for hospitalisation: a review of the literature, *Neonat Paediatr Child Health,* 7(2):5-15, 2004

Potterton J, Eales C: Prevalence of developmental delay in infants who are HIV positive, *S Afr J Physiother* 57(3):11, 2001.

Rauh VA, Whyatt RM, Garfinkel R et al: Developmental effects of exposure to environmental tobacco smoke and material hardship among inner-city children, *Neurotoxicol Teratol* 26(3):373-285, 2004.

Reisch SK, Forsyth DM: Preparing to parent the adolescent: a theoretical overview, *J Child Adolesc Psychiatr Ment Health Nurs* 5:31, 1992.

Schuler ME, Nair P, Kettinger L: Drug-exposed infants and developmental outcome: effects of a home intervention and ongoing maternal drug use, *Arch Pediatr Adolesc Med* 157(2):133, 2003.

Seideman RJ, Kleine PF: A theory of transformed parenting: parenting a child with developmental delay/mental retardation, *Nurs Res* 44:38, 1995.

Seideman RY, Jacobson S, Primeaux M et al: Assessing American Indian families, *MCN Am J Matern Child Nurs* 21(6):274-179, 1996.

Selevan SG, Rice DC, Hogan KA et al: Blood lead concentration and delayed puberty in girls, *N Engl J Med* 348(16):1527-1536, 2003.

Shevell M, Ashwal S, Donley D et al: Practice parameter: evaluation of the child with global developmental delay: report of the Quality Standards Subcommittee of the American Academy of Neurology and The Practice Committee of the Child Neurology Society, *Neurology* 60(3):367-380, 2003.

Slusher IL, McClure MJ: Infant stimulation during hospitalization, *J Pediatr Nurs* 7:276, 1995.

Stutts AL: Selected outcomes of technology-dependent children receiving home care and prescribed child care services, *J Pediatr Nurs* 20:501, 1994.

Sweeney J, Gutierrez T: Musculoskeletal implications of preterm infant positioning in the NICU, *J Perinat Neonatal Nurs* 16(1):58, 2002.

Symington A, Pinelli J: Developmental care for promoting development and preventing morbidity in preterm infants, *Cochrane Database Syst Rev* (3):CD001814, 2002.
Vontress CE, Epp LR: Historical hostility in the African American client: implications for counseling, *J Multicult Counseling Dev* 25:170, 1997.
Whyatt RM, Rauh V, Barr DB et al: Prenatal insecticide exposures and birth weight and length among an urban minority cohort, *Environ Health Perspect* 112(10):1125, 2004.

# Risk for disproportionate Growth

*Gail B. Ladwig*

G

**NANDA**

## Definition

At risk for growth above the 97th percentile or below the third percentile for age, crossing two percentile channels; disproportionate growth

## Risk Factors

### Prenatal

Congenital/genetic disorders, maternal malnutrition, multiple gestation, teratogen exposure, substance use/abuse, maternal infection

### Individual

Infection, prematurity, malnutrition, organic and inorganic factors, caregiver and/or individual maladaptive feeding behaviors, anorexia, insatiable appetite, chronic illness, substance abuse

### Environmental

Deprivation, teratogen exposure, lead poisoning, poverty, violence, natural disasters

### Caregiver

Abuse, mental illness, mental retardation, or severe learning disability

**NOC**

## Outcomes (Nursing Outcomes Classification)

### Suggested NOC Outcomes

Body Image; Child Development: 2 Months, 4 Months, 6 Months, 12 Months, 2 Years, 3 Years, 4 Years, Preschool, Middle Childhood, Adolescence; Growth; Knowledge: Infant Care, Preconception Maternal Health, Pregnancy; Physical Maturation: Female, Male; Weight: Body Mass

**Example NOC Outcome with Indicators**

**Growth** as evidenced by the following indicators: Weight percentiles for age, sex, and height (Rate each indicator of **Growth:** 1 = severe deviation from normal range, 2 = substantial deviation from normal range, 3 = moderate deviation from normal range, 4 = mild deviation from normal range, 5 = no deviation from normal range [see Section I].)

## Client Outcomes

**Client/Parents/Primary Caregiver Will (Specify Time Frame):**

- State information related to possible teratogenic agents
- State information related to adequate nutrition
- Seek help from appropriate professionals for nutritional needs

G

NIC

## Interventions (Nursing Interventions Classification)

### Suggested NIC Interventions

Behavior Modification; Counseling; Nutrition Therapy; Nutritional Monitoring; Teaching: Infant Nutrition, Toddler Nutrition; Parent Education: Child-Rearing Family

**Example NIC Activities— Parent Education: Child-Rearing Family**

Review nutritional requirements for specific age groups; inform parents of community resources

## Nursing Interventions and Rationales

NOTE: Management of a risk diagnosis necessitates the use of approaches incorporating primary and secondary prevention. Primary prevention interventions, which include activities such as nutrition counseling, focus on thwarting the development of a disease or condition. Secondary prevention is achieved through screening, monitoring, and surveillance (Shortridge & Valanis, 1992).

▲ Consider the use of formula milk for preterm and low-birth-weight infants. *In preterm and low-birth-weight infants, feeding with formula milk, compared with unfortified term human milk, leads to a greater rate of growth in the short term (Henderson, Anthony, & McGuire, 2004).*

▲ Assess and limit exposure to all drugs (prescription, "recreational," and over-the-counter) and give the mother information on known teratogenic agents (Table III-1). **EB:** *No drug can be considered safe during pregnancy. Consequently, a pregnant woman should never take a medication that has not been prescribed for her own benefit or that of her fetus. It should be emphasized that any drug has the potential for causing a birth defect, so no listing of known teratogens is ever complete (see Polifka & Friedman, 1999, for a good clinically oriented review; Florida Birth Defects Registry, 2005).* **EBN:** *The consumption of alcohol during pregnancy can harm the fetus irreparably. Preventive measures can be helpful in decreasing or stopping the use of alcohol during pregnancy. Alcohol is a definite teratogen (Eustace, Kang, & Coombs, 2003).*

TABLE III-1

## Teratogenic Agents

| Drug | Risk/Effect |
|---|---|
| ACE inhibitors (captopril, enalapril, and so on) | Appear to be teratogenic when used in the second and third trimesters, causing fetal calvarial hypoplasia, oligohydramnios, and renal anomalies. |
| Alcohol | Risk for FAS, alcohol-related birth defects, or alcohol-related neurodevelopmental abnormalities. FAS may be characterized by microcephaly, IUGR, and/or developmental delay. Chronic alcoholism is considered most harmful. Binge drinking may also confer significant risk. No safe limit for prenatal alcohol consumption has been established. |
| Anticonvulsants (hydantoin, valproic acid, carbamazepine, and primidone [Mysoline]) | Effects may include cardiac defects, microcephaly, IUGR, hypoplastic nails, depressed nasal bridge, cleft lip, hip dislocation, hypoplastic nose, low-set ears, small mandible; risk increases with number of anticonvulsants used concurrently. |
| Antineoplastics (alkylating agents) | Case reports show 10% to 50% of cases were malformed for different drugs in this class, including busulfan, chlorambucil, cyclophosphamide, and mechlorethamine. The malformation rate for first trimester exposure is quoted at 11.6%. Problems seen include IUGR, cleft palate, agenesis of kidney, malformations of digits, cardiac anomalies, and cloudy corneas. |
| Antineoplastics (antimetabolites) | Only case reports are available, but an average of 40% of cases were malformed. This class includes aminopterin, 5-fluorouracil, methotrexate, and methylaminopterin, which are strong folic acid antagonists. First-trimester exposure produces risk for cleft lip and palate, low-set ears, cranial anomalies, and anencephaly. Fetal abnormalities with cyclophosphamide and vinblastine have also been noted. |
| Cocaine | Can cause vascular disruption anomalies (e.g., intestinal atresia, limb reductions), IUGR, microcephaly, genitourinary tract defects, irritability, and muscular rigidity in the newborn. |
| Fluconazole | Fetal anomalies have been observed only when high-dose parenteral therapy is used (e.g., treatment of the mother for coccidiomycosis meningitis). |
| Diethylstilbestrol | In female offspring, increases risk for cancer, uterine and cervical malformations, reduced fertility, preterm deliveries, perinatal mortality, and SABs; in male offspring, may cause cysts of epididymis, cryptorchidism, hypogonadism, and diminished spermatogenesis. |
| Lithium | Small increase in risk for cardiac defects (Ebstein's anomaly in particular). Important in this drug to consider benefits and risk potentials. |

*Continued*

TABLE III-1

## Teratogenic Agents—cont'd

| Drug | Risk/Effect |
|---|---|
| Methimazole | Antithyroid drug that may increase the risk for prematurity, small-for-gestational-age infants, and scalp defects. |
| Methylene blue | Reported to cause intestinal atresias when injected into amniotic fluid during amniocentesis. |
| Penicillamine | Increases risk for connective tissue defects, cerebral palsy, and hydrocephalus. |
| Retinoids (isotretinoin, etretinate, acitretin) | Use of systemic retinoids increases risk for SAB; deformities of cranium, ears, face, limbs, and liver; hydrocephalus; microcephalus; heart defects; and cognitive defects without dysmorphology. Quoted risk for adverse outcome with use of isotretinoin is 38%. These agents have a prolonged teratogen risk because they are stored in adipose tissue and can persist for months. |
| Tetracyclines | Use from the twentieth gestational week on causes dental staining. |
| Thalidomide | High risk for limb defects, facial hemangiomas, microtia, and ocular and renal anomalies. Now back on the market. |
| Warfarin (Coumadin) and indandione (anisindione) anticoagulants | Increased risk for SAB, stillbirth, and prematurity as well as fetal warfarin syndrome (CNS defects, nasal hypoplasia, skull defects, abnormal ears, malformed eyes, microcephaly, skeletal deformities, mental retardation, and so on). Malformations are reported in 16% of exposed fetuses, hemorrhages in 3%, and stillbirths in 8%. |

*ACE,* angiotensin-converting enzyme; *CNS,* central nervous system; *FAS,* fetal alcohol syndrome; *IUGR,* intrauterine growth retardation; *SAB,* spontaneous abortion.

▲ Reduce the risk of TORCH infections (i.e., toxoplasmosis, other infections, rubella, cytomegalovirus [CMV] infection, and herpes simplex) as follows:
- Varicella-zoster and rubella viruses: Vaccinate nonimmune women before conception.
- CMV: Practice meticulous hand washing and secretion control and limit exposure to large numbers of infants and children.
- *Toxoplasma gondii:* Avoid exposure to cat litter and avoid work in garden or areas where cat feces may be present; do not feed undercooked meats to cats.
- Parvovirus: Limit contact with persons with known fifth disease.
- Herpes virus: Practice meticulous hand washing and secretion control, especially in contact with young infants.

**EB:** *Infection with any of the aforementioned agents can cause fetal harm resulting in serious damage to the central nervous system and other organs (Florida Birth Defects Registry, 2005).*

▲ Promote a team approach toward preconception and pregnancy glucose control for women with diabetes. **EB:** *Offspring of women with diabetes mellitus type 1 or type 2 have a two- to fourfold increased risk of birth defects. Available data suggest that excellent preconception and first-trimester glucose control in the mother can greatly reduce, if not eliminate, this risk. The increased risk for fetal structural birth defects in women with gestational diabetes is of lesser magnitude, but fetal morbidity may still be high in the second and third trimesters if gestational diabetes is not under good control. Programs with a team approach have been the most successful (Florida Birth Defects Registry, 2005).*

- ▲ Women with phenylketonuria (PKU) should be referred to a nutritionist experienced in the dietary implications of phenylalanine restriction. *Because 40% of all pregnancies are unplanned, women with PKU are urged to maintain phenylalanine restriction throughout their childbearing years.* **EB:** *Women with PKU (in whom the disorder was identified first at birth but who have become adults) who do not maintain strict dietary control may have blood phenylalanine levels above 20 mg/dL. Phenylalanine crosses the placenta at this high level and causes direct fetal damage, although the activity of the enzyme phenylalanine hydroxylase may be normal in the fetus. Phenylalanine has been found to be one of the most potent teratogens, with more than 90% of fetuses affected with microcephaly and developmental delay when maternal serum levels are above 25 mg/dL. Dietary restriction of phenylalanine should thus be started before conception, and birth outcomes can be normal with such restriction. Initiation of phenylalanine restriction in the first trimester improves developmental outcome, but this is often too late to avoid structural birth defects and brain damage in the fetus (Florida Birth Defects Registry, 2005).*
- • Provide for adequate nutrition and nutritional monitoring in clients with developmental disorders. **EB:** *When nutrition therapy is given in the early stages of diagnosis and treatment of cerebral palsy, growth delays may be prevented or remediated (Sanders et al, 1990). Nutrient needs may be altered as a result of long-term medication for conditions such as epilepsy, recurrent urinary or respiratory tract infections, chronic constipation, and behavioral problems (American Dietetic Association, 2003).*
- ▲ Adequate intake of vitamin D is set at 200 international units (IU)/day by the National Academy of Sciences. Because adequate sunlight exposure is difficult to determine, a supplement of 200 IU/day is recommended for the following groups to prevent rickets and vitamin D deficiency in healthy infants and children:
  - All breast-fed infants unless they are weaned to at least 500 mL/day of vitamin D–fortified formula or milk.
  - All non-breast-fed infants who are ingesting less than 500 mL/day of vitamin D–fortified formula or milk.
  - Children and adolescents who do not receive regular sunlight exposure, do not ingest at least 500 mL/day of vitamin D–fortified milk, or do not take a daily multivitamin supplement containing at least 200 IU of vitamin D.

  **EB:** *Cases of rickets in infants attributable to inadequate vitamin D intake and decreased exposure to sunlight continue to be reported in the United States. Rickets is an example of extreme vitamin D deficiency. A state of deficiency occurs months before rickets is obvious on physical examination. The new recommendation by the National Academy of Sciences for adequate intake of vitamin D to prevent vitamin D deficiency in normal infants, children, and adolescents is 200 IU/day (Gartner and Greer, 2003).*
- ▲ All women of childbearing age who are capable of becoming pregnant should take

400 mcg of folic acid daily. **EB:** *Periconceptional use of folic acid reduces the incidence of neural tube defects (NTDs). In fact, up to 70% of NTDs could be prevented if all women who can become pregnant consumed 400 mcg of folic acid from at least 1 month before conception through the first trimester of pregnancy (Florida Birth Defects Registry, 2005).*

- ▲ Provide for adequate nutrition for clients with active intestinal inflammation. **EB:** *Nutrition is clearly disturbed by active intestinal inflammation. Appetite is reduced, yet energy substrates are diverted into the inflammatory process; thus weight loss is characteristic. The nutritional disturbance represents part of a profound defect of somatic function. Linear growth and pubertal development in children are notably retarded, body composition is altered, and significant psychosocial disturbance may be present. Increasing evidence shows that an aggressive nutritional program may in itself be sufficient to reduce the mucosal inflammatory response. Recent research suggests that enteral nutrition alone may reduce the levels of many proinflammatory cytokines to normal values and allow mucosal healing (Murch & Walker-Smith, 1998).*
- ▲ Provide for adequate nutrition for pediatric and adolescent clients on long-term oral glucocorticoid therapy (e.g., those treated for chronic severe asthma). **EB:** *Growth may be inhibited by long-term use of these agents; however, recent studies suggest that use of the inhaled form of such agents does not affect long-term growth (Agertoft, 2000).*
- ▲ Provide tube feedings per physician's orders when appropriate for clients with neuromuscular impairment. **EB:** *Infants with isolated neonatal swallowing dysfunction have a good long-term prognosis. Nasogastric feedings followed by a gastrostomy is recommended in those without gastroesophageal reflux. Jejunal feedings are necessary in some. Although most infants improve over time, they may need nutritional support for 3 years or more (Heuschkel et al, 2003).*
- • Refer to the care plan for **Delayed Growth and development.**

G

## Multicultural

- • Assess for the influence of cultural beliefs, norms, values, and expectations on parents' perceptions of normal growth and development. **EBN:** *How the parent views normal growth and development may be based on cultural perceptions (Cochran, 1998; Doswell & Erlen, 1998; Leininger & McFarland, 2002). One Mexican-American pediatrician reported that the primary complaint of his Mexican-American parents is that their children do not eat enough despite being obviously overweight (Garcia, 2004). Research findings suggest that nutrition education efforts targeting Latino mothers of young children can be culturally reframed to identify positive eating behaviors rather than focusing on a child's weight (Crawford et al, 2004).*
- • Assess for the influence of acculturation. **EB:** *Acculturation to the United States is a risk factor for obesity-related behaviors among Asian-American and Hispanic adolescents (Unger et al, 2004).*
- • Negotiate with clients regarding which aspects of healthy nutrition can be modified while still honoring cultural beliefs. **EBN:** *Give and take with clients will lead to culturally congruent care (Leininger & McFarland, 2002).*
- • Assess whether the parents are concerned about the amount of food eaten. **EBN:** *Some cultures may add semisolid food within the first month of life because of concerns that the*

*infant is not getting enough to eat and the perception that "big is healthy" (Bentley et al, 1999; Higgins, 2000).*

- Assess the influence of family support on patterns of nutritional intake. **EBN:** *Women are the keepers and transmitters of culture in families. Female family members can play a dominant role in how children and infants are fed (Cesario, 2001; Pillitteri, 1999).*
- Encourage parental efforts at increasing physical activity and decreasing dietary fat for their children. **EB:** *Physical activity and dietary fat consumption were inversely related among African-American girls (Thompson et al, 2004). Interventions to increase physical activity among preadolescent African-American girls may benefit from a parental component to encourage support and self-efficacy for daughters' physical activity (Adkins et al, 2004).*
- Encourage limiting television viewing to <2 hr/day for children and discourage the consumption of sweetened soft drinks. **EB:** *Longer hours of child television viewing and higher soft-drink intake was associated with the occurrence of overweight for Hispanic children (Ariza et al, 2004; Giammattei et al, 2003).*



## Home Care

- The interventions described previously may be adapted for home care use.
- Provide aids to assist in compliance with the care plan (e.g., prepare medication schedules and put a week's medication in daily containers).
- Provide sufficient outside supports (e.g., written notices, calendars, planned ride shares) to assist with follow-through of the agreed-upon actions. *Cues play a significant role in stimulating completion of desired health actions.*

▲ Include a health promotion focus for clients with disabilities, with the goals of reducing secondary conditions (e.g., obesity, hypertension, pressure sores), maintaining functional independence, providing opportunities for leisure and enjoyment, and enhancing overall quality of life. *Greater emphasis on health promotion for persons with disabilities must take place in the community to accomplish the listed goals (Rimmer, 1999). New enablement models and functional assessment measures are available to evaluate rehabilitation and forecast future needs (Chiriboga, Ottenbacher, & Haber, 1999).*

- Encourage a mindset and program of self-care management. **EBN:** *Partnership based on respect and caring can focus the older adult on fostering health while aging. An exploration of the beliefs held by the older adult about aging provide an opportunity to introduce positive role models and images of aging, alternative ways of dealing with adversity, and new views of the self as reasonably healthy. Actions such as scheduled socialization can be introduced to build a repertoire of skills that support the self-concept (Leenerts, Teel, & Pendleton, 2002).*
- Establish a written contract with the client to follow the agreed-upon health care regimen. *Written agreements reinforce the verbal agreement and serve as a reference.*
- Meet with the client following completion of the proposed actions to review the contract and determine the next course of action. Do this until the client is able to initiate and follow through independently. *Successful completion of contracts promotes improved self-esteem and positive coping.*
- Using self-care management precepts, instruct the client in the multiple possible situations to which he or she may need to respond; include the use of role playing. In-

struct the client in generating hypotheses from available evidence rather than solely from experience. **EBN:** *A study of people with long-standing type 1 diabetes found that the need to react to unanticipated blood glucose levels could be frequent. When the situation contained familiar elements, clients were able to respond rapidly and expertly. When the situation was unfamiliar, decision making could be less accurate; clients would formulate a guess based on past experience and seek clues to confirm that guess, rather than generate a decision based on available evidence (Paterson & Thorne, 2000).*

## Client/Family Teaching

G

- • Provide anticipatory guidance for parents and caregivers regarding expectations for normal patterns of growth. Clarify expectations and correct misconceptions. *Parents and caregivers with this knowledge will be able to recognize and report early deviations in normal growth, which allows for more timely intervention.*
- ▲ Refer clients to a registered dietitian for nutritional counseling. *Help from qualified professionals is often needed to meet the nutritional needs of clients with deviations in normal growth.*
- ▲ Teach families the importance of taking measures to prevent lead poisoning: Wash the hands before preparing the child's food. Wash the child's hands before serving food. Wash bottle nipples and pacifiers frequently, especially if they fall on the floor. Wash the child's toys often. Stomp the feet before coming into the house to clean shoes of outside soil that may carry lead from exterior house paint. Damp mop often along baseboards, around door frames, under windowsills, and around iron radiators. Wash windowsills and window wells often. (The window well is the depression behind the windowsill into which the window fits when it is closed.) Move the crib away from window wells. Always damp mop before sweeping or vacuuming. Home vacuum cleaners do not trap lead dust; they blow it into the air. *The child's exposure to ingested lead can be lowered by following these instructions (Stapleton, 2003).*

## evolve WEBSITES FOR EDUCATION

See the EVOLVE website for World Wide Web resources for client education.

## REFERENCES

Adkins S, Sherwood NE, Story M et al: Physical activity among African-American girls: the role of parents and the home environment, *Obes Res* (Suppl 12):38S-45S, 2004.

American Dietetic Association: Nutrition in comprehensive program planning for persons with developmental disabilities (1996-1999), *J Am Diet Assoc* 97:189, 1997. Available www.eatright.org/adap0297b.html, accessed on April 18, 2003.

Ariza AJ, Chen EH, Binns HJ et al: Risk factors for overweight in five- to six-year-old Hispanic-American children: a pilot study, *J Urban Health* 81(1):150-161, 2004.

Bentley M, Gavin L, Black MM et al: Infant feeding practices of low-income, African-American, adolescent mothers: an ecological, multigenerational perspective, *Soc Sci Med* 49(8):1085-1100, 1999.

Cesario S: Care of the Native American woman: strategies for practice, education, and research, *J Gynecol Neonat Nurs* 30(1):13, 2001.

Chiriboga DA, Ottenbacher K, Haber DA: Disability in older adults. 3. Policy implications, *Behav Med* 24:171, 1999.

Cochran M: Tears have no color, *Am J Nurs* 98(6):53, 1998.

Crawford PB, Gosliner W, Anderson C et al: Counseling Latina mothers of preschool children about weight issues: suggestions for a new framework, *J Am Diet Assoc* 104(3):387-394, 2004.

Doswell W, Erlen J: Multicultural issues and ethical concerns in the delivery of nursing care interventions, *Nurs Clin North Am* 33(2):353, 1998.

Eustace LW, Kang DH, Coombs D: Fetal alcohol syndrome: a growing concern for health care professionals, *J Obstet Gynecol Neonatal Nurs* 32(2):215-221, 2003.

Florida Birth Defects Registry (Professional): Prevention strategies index: strategies to prevent birth defects: limit all drug exposures (prescriptions, "recreational," and over-the-counter). Available at www.flbdr.hsc.usf.edu/professional/index.html, accessed on January 16, 2005.

Garcia RS: No come nada, *Health Aff* 23(2):215-219, 2004.

Gartner M, Greer F: Prevention of rickets and vitamin D deficiency: new guidelines for vitamin D intake, *Pediatrics* 111(4):908, 2003. Available at www.aap.org/policy/s010116.html, accessed on April 18, 2003.

Giammattei J, Blix G, Marshak HH et al: Television watching and soft drink consumption: associations with obesity in 11- to 13-year-old schoolchildren, *Arch Pediatr Adolesc Med* 157(9):882-886, 2003.

Henderson G, Anthony MY, McGuire W: Formula milk versus term human milk for feeding preterm or low birth-weight infants, *Cochrane Database Syst Rev* (4):CD002971, 2001.

Heuschkel RB, Fletcher K, Hill A et al: Isolated neonatal swallowing dysfunction: a case series and review of the literature, *Dig Dis Sci* 48(1):30-35, 2003.

Higgins B: Puerto Rican cultural beliefs: influence on infant feeding practices in western New York, *J Transcult Nurs* 11(1):19, 2000.

Leenerts MH, Teel CS, Pendleton MK: Building a model of self-care for health promotion in aging, *J Nurs Scholarsh* 34:355, 2002.

Leininger MM, McFarland MR: *Transcultural nursing: concepts, theories, research and practices,* ed 3, New York, 2002, McGraw-Hill.

Murch SH, Walker-Smith JA: Nutrition in inflammatory bowel disease, *Baillieres Clin Gastroenterol* 12(4):719, 1998.

Paterson B, Thorne S: Expert decision making in relation to unanticipated blood glucose levels, *Res Nurs Health* 23:147, 2000.

Pillitteri A: Nutritional needs of the newborn. In Pillitteri A, editor: *Maternal and child health nursing: care of the childbearing and childrearing family,* Philadelphia, 1999, Lippincott Williams & Wilkins.

Polifka JE, Friedman JM: Clinical teratology: identifying teratogenic risks in humans, *Clin Genet* 56:409, 1999.

Agertoft L, Pedersen S: Effect of long-term treatment with inhaled budesonide on adult height in children with asthma, *N Engl J Med* 343(15):1064-1069, 2000.

Rimmer JH: Health promotion for people with disabilities: the emerging paradigm shift from disability prevention to prevention of secondary conditions, *Phys Ther* 79:495, 1999.

Sanders K, Cox K, Cannon R et al: Growth response to enteral feeding by children with cerebral palsy, *JPEN J Parenter Enteral Nutr* 14(1):23-26, 1990.

Shortridge L, Valanis B: The epidemiological model applied in community health nursing. In Stanhope M, Lancaster J, editors: *Community health nursing: process and practice for promoting health,* ed 3, St Louis, 1992, Mosby.

Stapleton R: Help prevent childhood lead poisoning: a resource for parents. Available at www.nolead.home.mindspring.com/whatcani.htm#whatcanido, accessed on April 18, 2003.

Thompson D, Jago R, Baranowski T et al: Covariability in diet and physical activity in African-American girls, *Obes Res* 12 (Suppl):46S-54S, 2004.

Unger JB, Reynolds K, Shakib S et al: Acculturation, physical activity, and fast-food consumption among Asian-American and Hispanic adolescents, *J Community Health* 29(6):467-481, 2004.

# Ineffective Health maintenance

evolve

*Gail B. Ladwig*

H

**NANDA**

## Definition

Inability to identify, manage, or seek out help to maintain health

## Defining Characteristics

History of lack of health-seeking behavior; reported or observed lack of equipment, financial, and/or other resources; reported or observed impairment of personal support systems; expressed interest in improving health behaviors; demonstrated lack of knowledge regarding basic health practices; demonstrated lack of adaptive behaviors to internal and external environmental changes; reported or observed inability to take responsibility for meeting basic health practices in any or all functional pattern areas

## Related Factors (r/t)

Ineffective family coping; perceptual-cognitive impairment (complete or partial lack of gross and/or fine motor skills); lack of or significant alteration in communication skills (written, verbal, and/or gestural); unachieved developmental tasks; lack of material resources; dysfunctional grieving; disabling spiritual distress; inability to make deliberate and thoughtful judgments; ineffective individual coping

**NOC**

## Outcomes (Nursing Outcomes Classification)

### Suggested NOC Outcomes

Health Beliefs: Perceived Resources; Health-Promoting Behavior; Health-Seeking Behavior

**Example NOC Outcome with Indicators**

**Health-Seeking Behavior** as evidenced by the following indicators: Completes health-related tasks/Performs self-screening when indicated/Seeks assistance from health professionals when indicated (Rate each indicator of **Health-Seeking Behavior:** 1 = never demonstrated, 2 = rarely demonstrated, 3 = sometimes demonstrated, 4 = often demonstrated, 5 = consistently demonstrated [see Section I].)

## Client Outcomes

### Client Will (Specify Time Frame):

- Discuss fear of or blocks to implementing health regimen
- Follow mutually agreed on health care maintenance plan
- Meet goals for health care maintenance

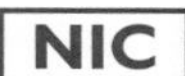

## Interventions (Nursing Interventions Classification)

### Suggested NIC Interventions

Health Education, Health System Guidance, Support System Enhancement

**Example NIC Activities—Health Education**

Prioritize identified learner needs based on client preference, skills of nurse, resources available, and likelihood of successful goal attainment; emphasize immediate or short-term positive health benefits to be gained from positive lifestyle behaviors rather than long-term benefits or negative effects of noncompliance

## Nursing Interventions and Rationales

H

- • Assess the client's feelings, values, and reasons for not following the prescribed plan of care. See Related Factors. *A factor to assess when examining client responsibility is the level of dissatisfaction with current lifestyle and readiness for change (Clark, 1996).* **EB:** *Health values saliency, sensitively designed health information, and health status perception, as well as socioeconomic status, should be considered for successful promotion of healthy lifestyle among the adult Japanese male population studied in this research (Shi, Nakamura, & Takano, 2004).*
- • Assess for family patterns, economic issues, and cultural patterns that influence compliance with a given medical regimen. *Responsiveness to clients enables the nurse to gain an understanding of clients' lives and to cultivate their connections to a responsive community, encouraging clients to avoid getting into "receiving" behaviors (Smith-Battle, 1997).*
- • Help the client determine how to arrange a daily schedule that incorporates the new health care regimen (e.g., taking pills before meals).
- ▲ Refer the client to social services for financial assistance if needed. **EB:** *Information-seeking behavior is a strategy that many people use as a means of dealing with and reducing stress when coping with an illness such as cancer (van der Molen, 1999).*
- ▲ Identify support groups related to the disease process (e.g., Reach to Recovery for a woman who has had a mastectomy).
- • Help the client to choose a healthy lifestyle and to have appropriate diagnostic screening tests. **EBN:** *One study found that women who adopt a healthy lifestyle and practice preventive healthy behaviors can reduce the risks of some cancers and other diseases such as heart disease and sexually transmitted infections (Furniss, 2000).*
- • Assist the client in reducing stress. **EBN:** *In a convenience sample of 24 men and women who were admitted to a regional hospital in Victoria, Australia, with a provisional diagnosis of myocardial infarction (MI), stress was the most commonly cited cause of illness (King, 2002).*
- • Identify complementary healing modalities such as herbal remedies, acupuncture, healing touch, yoga, or cultural shamans that the client uses in addition to or instead of the prescribed allopathic regimen. **EB:** *Expenditures for alternative medicine professional services increased by 45% from 1990 to 1997. Total visits to alternative medical practitioners exceeded total visits to all U.S. primary care practitioners (Eisenberg et al,*

*1998). A widening recognition of the mind-body-spirit connection in Western medicine has resulted in a growing interest in ancient health practices such as yoga (Herrick & Ainsworth, 2000).*

- ▲ Refer the client to community agencies for appropriate follow-up care (e.g., day treatment or adult day health program). **EBN:** *Increased social support has been related to a reduction in mortality rates and incidence of physical and mental illness (Callaghan & Morrissey, 1993).* **EB:** *One study showed a positive response when a community youth setting, such as the Girl Scouts, was used for interventions to prevent disordered eating behaviors (Neumark-Sztainer et al, 2000).*
- • Obtain or design educational material that is appropriate for the client; use pictures if possible. **EBN:** *Verbal reinforcement of personalized written instructions appears to be the best intervention. In one study, compliance was better with the use of computer-generated, personalized instructions than with the use of handwritten instructions (Hayes, 1998).*
- • Ensure that follow-up appointments are scheduled before the client is discharged; discuss a way to ensure that appointments are kept. **EBN:** *The client brings to the learning situation a unique personality, established social interaction patterns, cultural norms and values, and environmental influences (Bohny, 1997).*

H

## Geriatric

- ▲ Assess sensory deficits and psychomotor skills. Supply the appropriate assistive devices. **EB:** *This study suggests that older individuals with disabilities view certain assistive devices as important in maintaining independence. The top five most important devices were eyeglasses, canes, wheelchairs, walkers, and telephones. Controlling for the number of people using the device, the top five most important devices were oxygen tanks, dentures, 3-in-1 commodes, computers, and wheelchairs (Mann et al, 2004).*
- • Discuss "symptoms of daily living" in addition to the major illness. **EBN:** *Older adults are unlikely to report day-to-day symptoms such as headaches because they do not view them as illnesses. However, these day-to-day complaints may foretell more serious problems (Musil et al, 1988).*
- • Recognize resistance to change in lifelong patterns of personal health care. **EBN:** *The client brings to the learning situation a unique personality, established social interaction patterns, cultural norms and values, and environmental influences (Bohny, 1997).*
- • Discuss with the client and support person realistic goals for changes in health maintenance. **EB:** *The emotional and instrumental support provided by a family member or friend and size of social support network were found to be unique predictors of health goal attainment The importance of personalized goals and social support in designing health interventions for older adults is identified (VonDras & Madey, 2004).*
- • Instruct the client in the symptoms of MI and the need for timeliness in seeking care. **EBN:** *Women, especially those of advanced age, delay longer before seeking treatment for signs and symptoms of acute MI. Effective treatment is time dependent; mortality and morbidity rise with increased prehospital delay (Lefler, 2002).*
- • Consider the age of the client when suggesting screening for disease. **EB:** *Even if one assumes that the mortality reduction with screening persists in the elderly, 80% of the benefit is achieved before age 80 years for colon cancer, before age 75 years for breast cancer,*

*and before age 65 years for cervical cancer. The small benefit of screening in the elderly may be outweighed by the harms: anxiety, additional testing, and unnecessary treatment (Rich & Black, 2000).*

## Multicultural

- Assess influence of cultural beliefs, norms, and values on the client's ability to modify health behavior. **EBN:** *What the client considers normal and abnormal health behavior may be based on cultural perceptions (Cochran, 1998; Doswell & Erlen, 1998; Leininger & McFarland, 2002).*
- Discuss with the client those aspects of health behavior and lifestyle that will remain unchanged by health status. **EBN:** *Aspects of the client's life that are meaningful and valuable to him or her should be understood and preserved. Negotiate with the client regarding the aspects of health behavior that will need to be modified.* **EBN:** *Give and take with the client will lead to culturally congruent care (Leininger & McFarland, 2002).*
- Assess the effect of fatalism on the client's ability to modify health behavior. **EBN:** *Fatalistic perspectives, which involve the belief that one cannot control one's own fate, may influence health behaviors in some Asian, African-American, and Latino populations (Chen, 2001; Harmon, Castro, & Coe, 1996; Phillips, Cohen, & Moses, 1999).*
- Validate the client's feelings regarding the impact of health status on current lifestyle. **EBN:** *Validation is a therapeutic communication technique that lets the client know that the nurse has heard and understood what was said, and it promotes the nurse-client relationship (Heineken, 1998).*
- Assess access to health services. **EB:** *Compared with Caucasians, African-American women reported significantly less access to health services for bone mineral density testing and prescription and nonprescription osteoporosis therapy (Mudano et al, 2003).*

## Home Care

- The interventions described previously may be adapted for home care use.
- Assessment of urologic, developmental, psychosocial, and sleep-related etiologies is important in evaluating the presence of enuresis as an unachieved developmental task. *A specific etiology of enuresis is difficult to establish, and all possible sources should be evaluated (Fritz et al, 2004).*
- ▲ Provide aids to assist in compliance with the plan of care (e.g., prepare medication schedules and put a week's medication in daily containers).
- Provide sufficient outside supports (e.g., written notices, calendars, planned ride shares) to assist with follow-through on the agreed-on actions. *Cues play a significant role in stimulating completion of desired health actions.*
- ▲ Include a health promotion focus for the client with disabilities, with the goals of reducing secondary conditions (e.g., obesity, hypertension, pressure sores), maintaining functional independence, providing opportunities for leisure and enjoyment, and enhancing overall quality of life. **EB:** *Greater emphasis on health promotion for persons with disabilities must take place in the community to accomplish the listed goals (Rimmer, 1999). New enablement models and functional assessment measures are available to evaluate rehabilitation and forecast future needs (Chiriboga, Ottenbacher, & Haber, 1999).*
- Encourage a mind-set and program of self-care management. **EBN:** *Partnership based*

*on respect and caring can help the older adult to foster health while aging. An exploration of the beliefs held by the older adult about aging provides an opportunity to introduce positive role models. Actions such as scheduled socialization can be introduced to build a repertoire of skills that support the self-concept (Leenerts, Teel, & Pendleton, 2002).*

- Establish a written contract with the client to follow the agreed-upon health care regimen. *Written agreements reinforce the verbal agreement and serve as a reference.*
- Meet with the client following completion of the proposed actions to review the contract and determine the next course of action. Do this until the client is able to initiate and follow through independently. *Successful completion of contracts promotes improved self-esteem and positive coping.*
- Using self-care management precepts, instruct the client about multiple possible situations to which he or she may need to respond; include the use of role playing. Instruct in generating hypotheses from available evidence rather than solely from experience. **EBN:** *A study of people with long-standing type 1 diabetes found that the need to react to unanticipated blood glucose levels could be frequent. When the situation contained familiar elements, clients were able to respond rapidly and expertly. When the situation was unfamiliar, decision making could be less accurate; clients would formulate a guess based on past experience and seek clues to confirm that guess, rather than generate a decision based on available evidence (Paterson & Thorne, 2000).*

H

## Client/Family Teaching

- Provide the family with lists of addresses where information can be obtained from the Internet. (Most libraries have Internet access with printing capabilities.) *Internet-based technologies have emerged as potentially powerful tools to enable meaningful communication and proactive partnership in care for various medical conditions (Patel, 2001).* **EBN:** *A study of 469 Internet postings of clients with implantable defibrillators showed that the clients used the Internet for practical information seeking and support in coping (Dickerson, Flaig, & Kennedy, 2000).*
- Have the client and family demonstrate at least twice any procedures to be done at home. *Practicing a procedure exposes problems, enhances skill level, and promotes confidence in performing new behaviors.*
- Teach the client about the symptoms associated with discontinuation of a selective serotonin reuptake inhibitor (SSRI) and consider dosage tapering. **EBN:** *Based on emerging research findings, nurses are urged to become more aware of SSRI discontinuation syndrome. To ameliorate or avoid the associated symptoms, client education is recommended, and dosage tapering is encouraged whenever possible (Finfgeld, 2002).*
- Explain nonthreatening aspects before introducing more anxiety-producing possible side effects of the disease or medical regimen. *An individual's perception of barriers and benefits has consistently been most predictive of subsequent behavior (Fenn, 1998).*
- Treat tobacco use as a chronic problem. Acknowledge the pleasure associated with smoking. Encourage the client to work towards a goal of permanent abstinence. Advise the client about possible relapse. **EBN:** *In a convenience sample of 20 pregnant women, the women were able to abstain from smoking during pregnancy but relapsed after the birth of the baby. Recognition of the chronic nature of the problem and the development of*

*long-term care delivery systems are needed to assist clients in achieving the goals of permanent abstinence and better personal and family health (Buchanan, 2002).* **EB:** *This study suggested that an acknowledgment of the attractive, pleasurable aspects of smoking may be seen as unacceptable and irresponsible but doing so could well provide an opportunity to relate to the everyday and multiple practices of smoking and encourage cessation (McKie et al, 2003).*

## evolve WEBSITES FOR EDUCATION

See the EVOLVE website for World Wide Web resources for client education.

## REFERENCES


Bohny B: A time for self-care: role of the home healthcare nurse, *Home Healthc Nurse* 15(4):281, 1997.

Buchanan L: Implementing a smoking cessation program for pregnant women based on current clinical practice guidelines, *J Am Acad Nurse Pract* 14(6):243, 2002.

Callaghan P, Morrissey G: Social support and health: a review, *J Adv Nurs* 18(2):203-210, 1993.

Chen YC: Chinese values, health and nursing, *J Adv Nurs* 36(2):270, 2001.

Chiriboga DA, Ottenbacher K, Haber DA: Disability in older adults. 3. Policy implications, *Behav Med* 24: 171, 1999.

Clark C: *Wellness practitioner: concepts, research and strategies,* New York, 1996, Springer.

Cochran M: Tears have no color, *Am J Nurs* 98(6):53, 1998.

Dickerson SS, Flaig DM, Kennedy MC: Therapeutic connection: help seeking on the Internet for persons with implantable cardioverter defibrillators, *Heart Lung* 29(4):248, 2000.

Doswell W, Erlen J: Multicultural issues and ethical concerns in the delivery of nursing care interventions, *Nurs Clin North Am* 33(2):353, 1998.

Eisenberg DM, Davis RB, Ettner SL et al: Trends in alternative medicine use in the United States 1990-1997, *JAMA* 280(18): 1569-1575, 1998.

Fenn M: Health promotion: theoretical perspectives and clinical applications, *Holist Nurs Pract* 12(2):1, 1998.

Finfgeld DL: Selective serotonin reuptake inhibitor. Discontinuation syndrome, *J Psychosoc Nurs Ment Health Serv* 40(12):8, 2002.

Fritz G, Rockney R, Bernet W et al: Practice parameters for the assessment and treatment of children and adolescents with enuresis, *J Am Acad Child Adolesc Psychiatry* 43(12):1540, 2004.

Furniss K: Tomatoes, Pap smears, and tea? Adopting behaviors that may prevent reproductive cancers and improve health, *J Obstet Gynecol Neonatal Nurs* 29(6):641, 2000.

Harmon MP, Castro FG, Coe K: Acculturation and cervical cancer: knowledge, beliefs, and behaviors of Hispanic women, *Women Health* 24(3):37, 1996.

Hayes K: Randomized trial of geralogy-based medication instruction in the emergency department, *Nurs Res* 47(4):211, 1998.

Heineken J: Patient silence is not necessarily client satisfaction: communication in home care nursing, *Home Healthcare Nurse* 16(2):115, 1998.

Herrick CM, Ainsworth AD: Invest in yourself: yoga as a self-care strategy, *Nurs Forum* 35(2):32, 2000.

King R: Illness attributions and myocardial infarction: the influence of gender and socio-economic circumstances on illness beliefs, *J Adv Nurs* 37(5):431, 2002.

Leenerts MH, Teel CS, Pendleton MK: Building a model of self-care for health promotion in aging, *J Nurs Sch* 34:355, 2002.

Lefler L: The advanced practice nurse's role regarding women's delay in seeking treatment with myocardial infarction, *J Am Acad Nurse Pract* 14(10):449, 2002.

Leininger MM, McFarland MR: *Transcultural nursing: concepts, theories, research and practices,* ed 3, New York, 2002, McGraw-Hill.

McKie L, Laurier E, Taylor RJ et al: Eliciting the smoker's agenda: implications for policy and practice, *Soc Sci Med* 56(1):83-94, 2003.

Mudano AS, Casebeer L, Patino F et al: Racial disparities in osteoporosis prevention in a managed care population, *South Med J* 96(5):445-51, 2003.

Musil CM, Ahn S, Haug M et al: Health problems and health actions among community-dwelling older adults: results of a health diary study, *Appl Nurs Res* 11(3):138, 1998.
Neumark-Sztainer D, Sherwood NE, Coller T et al: Primary prevention of disordered eating among preadolescent girls: feasibility and short-term effect of a community-based intervention, *J Am Diet Assoc* 100(12):1466-1473, 2000.
Patel AM: Using the internet in the management of asthma, *Curr Opin Pulm Med* 7(1):39, 2001.
Paterson B, Thorne S: Expert decision making in relation to unanticipated blood glucose levels, *Res Nurs Health* 23:147, 2000.
Phillips JM, Cohen MZ, Moses G: Breast cancer screening and African American women: fear, fatalism, and silence, *Oncol Nurs Forum* 26(3):561, 1999.
Rich JS, Black WC: When should we stop screening? *Eff Clin Pract* 3(2):78, 2000.
Rimmer JH: Health promotion for people with disabilities: the emerging paradigm shift from disability prevention to prevention of secondary conditions, *Phys Ther* 79:495, 1999.
Shi H, Nakamura K, Takano T: Health values and health-information-seeking in relation to positive change of health practice among middle-aged urban men, *Prev Med* 39(6):1164-1171, 2004.
Smith-Battle L: The responsive use of self in community health nursing practice, *ANS Adv Nurs Sci* 10(2):75, 1997.
van der Molen B: Relating information needs to the cancer experience. 1. Information as a key coping strategy, *Eur J Cancer Care (Engl)* 8(4):238, 1999.
VonDras DD; Madey SF: The attainment of important health goals throughout adulthood: an integration of the theory of planned behavior and aspects of social support, *Int J Aging Hum Dev* 59(3):205-234, 2004.



# Health-seeking behaviors (specify)

*Gail B. Ladwig*

**NANDA**

## Definition

Active seeking (by a person in stable health) of ways to alter personal health habits and/or environment to move toward higher level of health
NOTE: *Stable health* is defined as the achievement of age-appropriate illness-prevention measures; report of good or excellent health from the client; and control of signs and symptoms of disease, if present.

## Defining Characteristics

Expressed or observed desire to seek higher level of wellness, demonstrated or observed lack of knowledge of health-promoting behaviors, stated or observed unfamiliarity with wellness community resources, expressed concern about effect of current environmental conditions on health status, expressed or observed desire for increased control of health practice

## Related Factors (r/t)

Role change; change in developmental level (e.g., marriage, parenthood, empty-nest status, retirement); lack of knowledge regarding need for preventive health behaviors, appropriate health screenings, optimal nutrition, weight control, regular exercise program, stress management, supportive social network, and responsible role participation

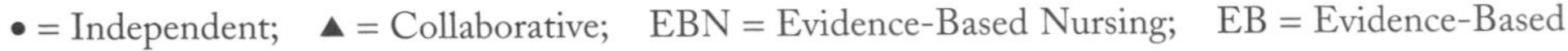

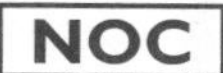

## Outcomes (Nursing Outcomes Classification)

### Suggested NOC Outcomes

Adherence Behavior, Health Beliefs, Health Orientation, Health-Promoting Behavior, Health-Seeking Behavior

### Example NOC Outcome with Indicators

**Health-Seeking Behavior** as evidenced by the following indicators: Completes health-related tasks/Performs self-screening when indicated/Seeks assistance from health professionals when indicated (Rate each indicator of **Health-Seeking Behavior:** 1 = never demonstrated, 2 = rarely demonstrated, 3 = sometimes demonstrated, 4 = often demonstrated, 5 = consistently demonstrated [see Section I].)

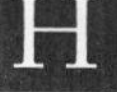

## Client Outcomes

### Client Will (Specify Time Frame):

- Maintain ideal weight and be knowledgeable about nutritious diet
- Demonstrate ways to fit newly prescribed change in health habits into lifestyle
- List community resources available for assistance with achieving wellness
- List ways to include wellness behaviors in current lifestyle

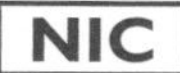

## Interventions (Nursing Interventions Classification)

### Suggested NIC Interventions

Health Education; Health System Guidance; Support System Enhancement

### Example NIC Activities—Health Education

Prioritize identified learner needs based on client preference, skills of nurse, resources available, and likelihood of successful goal attainment; emphasize immediate or short-term positive health benefits to be gained by positive lifestyle behaviors rather than long-term benefits or negative effects of noncompliance

## Nursing Interventions and Rationales

- Discuss the client's beliefs about health and his or her ability to maintain health. **EBN:** *One study indicated that understanding the transitions of women with chronic illness will enable nurses to move beyond the biomedically orientated concepts of nursing practice toward a holistic approach (Kralik, 2002).*
- Identify barriers and benefits to being healthy. *An individual's perception of barriers and benefits has consistently been most predictive of behavior changes (Fenn, 1998).*
- Identify environmental and social factors that the client perceives as health promoting. **EBN:** *Exposure to a health-promoting environment had statistically significant direct and indirect effects (Conrad et al, 1996).*

### Nutritional

- Determine the client's height and weight. Compare results with the standard weight for age and height.
- Assess the role that stress plays in overeating and weight-cycling. *Women who weight-cycle are triggered to overeat by unpleasant feelings or stress, whereas normal-weight subjects tend to overeat in social situations (Smith-Battle, 1997).*
- Encourage client to use the new nutritional guidelines as developed by the U.S. Department of Agriculture (USDA).

#### Adequate Nutrients Within Calorie Needs

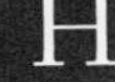


- Consume a variety of nutrient-dense foods and beverages within and among the basic food groups while choosing foods that limit the intake of saturated and *trans* fats, cholesterol, added sugars, salt, and alcohol.
- Meet recommended intakes within energy needs by adopting a balanced eating pattern, such as the USDA Food Guide or the Dietary Approaches to Stop Hypertension (DASH) Eating Plan.

#### Weight Management

- To maintain body weight in a healthy range, balance calories from foods and beverages with calories expended.
- To prevent gradual weight gain over time, make small decreases in food and beverage calories and increase physical activity.

#### Food Groups to Encourage

- Consume a sufficient amount of fruits and vegetables while staying within energy needs. Two cups of fruit and two and a half cups of vegetables per day are recommended for a reference 2000-calorie intake, with higher or lower amounts depending on the calorie level.
- Choose a variety of fruits and vegetables each day. In particular, select from all five vegetable subgroups (dark green, orange, legumes, starchy vegetables, and other vegetables) several times a week.
- Consume 3-ounce (or more) equivalents of whole-grain products per day, with the rest of the recommended grains coming from enriched or whole-grain products. In general, at least half the grains should come from whole grains.
- Consume 3 cups per day of fat-free or low-fat milk or equivalent milk products.

#### Fats

- Consume less than 10% of calories from saturated fatty acids and less than 300 mg/day of cholesterol, and keep *trans* fatty acid consumption as low as possible.
- Keep total fat intake between 20% to 35%, with most fats coming from sources of polyunsaturated and monounsaturated fatty acids, such as fish, nuts, and vegetable oils.
- When selecting and preparing meat, poultry, dry beans, and milk or milk products, make choices that are lean, low-fat, or fat-free.

- Limit intake of fats and oils high in saturated and/or *trans* fatty acids, and choose products low in such fats and oils.

Carbohydrates

- Choose fiber-rich fruits, vegetables, and whole grains often.
- Choose and prepare foods and beverages with little added sugars or caloric sweeteners, such as amounts suggested by the USDA Food Guide and the DASH Eating Plan.
- Reduce the incidence of dental caries by practicing good oral hygiene and consuming sugar-and starch-containing foods and beverages less often.

Sodium and Potassium

- Consume less than 2,300 mg (approximately 1 teaspoon of salt) of sodium per day.
- Choose and prepare foods with little salt. At the same time, consume potassium-rich foods, such as fruits and vegetables.



Alcoholic Beverages

- Those who choose to drink alcoholic beverages should do so sensibly and in moderation (defined as the consumption of up to one drink/day for women and up to two drinks/day for men).
- Alcoholic beverages should not be consumed by some individuals, including those who cannot restrict their alcohol intake, women of childbearing age who may become pregnant, pregnant and lactating women, children and adolescents, individuals taking medications that can interact with alcohol, and those with specific medical conditions.
- Alcoholic beverages should be avoided by individuals engaging in activities that require attention, skill, or coordination, such as driving or operating machinery.

NOTE: *The* USDA Dietary Guidelines for Americans 2005 *contains additional recommendations for specific populations. It is available at www.health.gov/dietaryguidelines/dga2005/recommendations.htm.*

### Exercise

- Engage in regular physical activity and reduce sedentary activities to promote health, psychological well-being, and a healthy body weight.
  - To reduce the risk of chronic disease in adulthood: Engage in at least 30 minutes of moderate-intensity physical activity, above usual activity, at work or home on most days of the week.
  - For most people, greater health benefits can be obtained by engaging in physical activity of more vigorous intensity or longer duration.
  - To help manage body weight and prevent gradual, unhealthy body weight gain in adulthood: Engage in approximately 60 minutes of moderate- to vigorous-intensity activity on most days of the week while not exceeding caloric intake requirements.
  - To sustain weight loss in adulthood: Participate in at least 60 to 90 minutes of daily moderate-intensity physical activity while not exceeding caloric intake requirements. Some people may need to consult with a health care provider before participating in this level of activity.
  - Achieve physical fitness by including cardiovascular conditioning, stretching exer-

cises for flexibility, and resistance exercises or calisthenics for muscle strength and endurance. NOTE: *The* USDA Dietary Guidelines for Americans 2005 *contains additional recommendations for specific populations. It is available at www.health.gov/dietaryguidelines/dga2005/recommendations.htm.*

- ▲ Advise the client to consult with a physician for testing to determine the ability to tolerate a specific regimen. *Previous bone injuries or inflammatory disease may rule out jogging and aerobic exercises.*
- Explore with the client weightlifting options to increase muscle strength and stamina.
- Encourage exercise for cancer survivors *In this study findings suggest that exercise improved psychological and social well-being in some women survivors of cancer (Christopher et al, 2004).*
- Help the client focus on the enjoyment of exercise. Set up a support and reward system. *An individual's perception of barriers and benefits has consistently been most predictive of subsequent behavior (Fenn, 1998).*

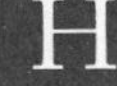

- Consider using music with exercise. **EBN:** *In a study of 30 coronary artery bypass clients, one group reported a significantly enhanced mood while exercising to music and another group reported a significantly decreased mood without music. Enhancement of mood might lead to increased compliance with a regular exercise routine (Murrock, 2002).*
- Encourage aerobic exercises that increase heart rate within the prescribed limit. Encourage the client to exercise at least three times per week for 20 or more minutes using exercises that the client prefers (e.g., walking, jogging, aerobics, swimming, bicycling, yoga, tai chi). **EBN:** *Yoga and tai chi are stretching exercises that promote energy and muscle balance. A widening recognition of the mind-body-spirit connection in Western medicine has resulted in a growing interest in ancient health practices such as yoga (Herrick & Ainsworth, 2000).* **EB:** *Regular exercise such as brisk walking resulted in reduction of body weight and body fat among overweight and obese postmenopausal women (Irwin et al, 2003).* **EB:** *Progressive resistive exercise or a combination of progressive resistive exercise and aerobic exercise appear to be safe and may be beneficial for adults living with human immunodeficiency virus/acquired immune deficiency syndrome (HIV/AIDS) (O'Brien et al, 2004).*

## Stress Management

- Ask the client to define stress in terms of lifestyle events and assign events a value on a scale from 1 to 5. *This exercise helps to distinguish between anxiety as a personality trait and anxiety as a coping response to threatening events.*
- Determine ways in which the client relieves stress and evaluate their effectiveness. *Stress management techniques are of two types, those that focus on body systems and those that focus on handling stress differently through behavioral responses (Clark, 1996).*
- Determine the client's social support network. **EBN:** *Exposure to a health-promoting environment had statistically significant direct and indirect effects (Conrad et al, 1996).*
- Teach stress-relieving techniques (e.g., deep and slow breathing, progressive muscle relaxation, meditation, imagery, problem solving). **EB:** *Body-mind training resulted in an improved capability for physical and mental relaxation as indicated from lower-amplitude electromyograph traces, higher-amplitude alpha brain waves, and decrease in state anxiety in individuals with chronic toxic encephalopathy (Engel & Andersen, 2000).*

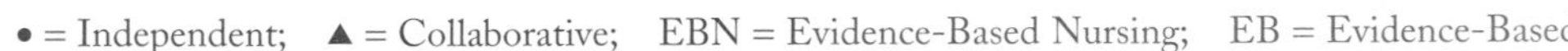

## Smoking, Drinking, Self-Medication

- • Discuss the risk-taking behaviors of smoking, drinking, and self-medication.
- • Discuss the frequency of risk-taking habits. *People move through a series of behaviors—precontemplation, preparation, action, and maintenance—in their effort to change or adopt a new behavior (Fenn, 1998).*
- ▲ Refer a client who smokes to Smoke Enders or a similar community-based program. Discuss ways in which the client can deal with a change in behavior. **EB:** *Although complete cessation of smoking is preferred, sustained reduction is likely to decrease the risk of disease and is a valuable public health outcome (Wakefield et al, 1992).*
- ▲ Refer a client who drinks alcohol excessively to Alcoholics Anonymous (AA). Identify a support person to help the client into the organization. **EBN:** *The period after treatment for alcohol abuse is a major life transition that requires extensive coping efforts, social support, and environmental control (Murphy, 1993).*

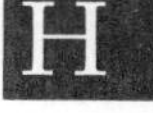

- ▲ Identify patterns of self-medication with over-the-counter medications and herbal remedies, and excessive use of prescribed medications. *Medications and herbal preparations are most effective when taken as intended. Combining remedies predisposes the client to unwanted side effects.*
- • Refer to the care plans for **Dysfunctional Family processes: alcoholism, Ineffective Denial,** and **Defensive Coping.**

## Health-Seeking Behaviors

- • Teach stress-relieving techniques (e.g., deep and slow breathing, progressive muscle relaxation, exercise, meditation, power strategies, problem solving, imagery, verbalization of feelings, spiritual practice [prayer]). *Stress management addresses the sources of tension through physical performance, emotional expression, transcendent spiritual experiences, social relationships, and the surrounding environment.*
- • Recognize and allow the client to discuss the choice of complementary therapies available, such as spiritual practice, relaxation, imagery, exercise, lifestyle, diet (e.g., macrobiotic, vegetarian), and nutritional supplementation. **EBN:** *A study of cancer clients found that the clients unanimously believed that complementary therapies helped to improve their quality of life by assisting them in coping more effectively with stress, decreasing the discomforts of treatment and illness, and giving them a sense of control (Sparber et al, 2000).* **EB:** *One study demonstrated that the use of complementary/alternative medicine for cancer care is widespread. Clients clearly express a need for complementary/alternative medical treatments and are willing to pay for them (Lewith, Broomfield, & Prescott, 2002).*

## Health Screening, Appropriate Health Care

- • Assess the frequency of illness-preventing practices, such as routine physical examinations, dental examinations, influenza immunization, breast self-examinations (BSEs) and mammograms as recommended for women, testicular self-examinations (TSEs) and prostate examinations for men, and screening for familial diseases such as glaucoma and elevated cholesterol level. See the care plan for **Ineffective Health maintenance. EB:** *Immunization against influenza is an effective intervention that reduces serologically confirmed cases by 60% to 70% (Hull et al, 2002). Reducing uncer-*

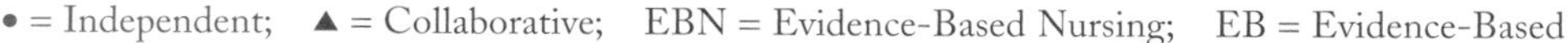

*tainty about how to perform breast self-examination is seen as a key to promoting self-examination (Babrow & Kline, 2000).*

- Provide a phone call to remind the client of appointments. **EB:** *At an adolescent clinic in Australia the use of telephone reminders (intention-to-treat analysis) significantly reduced the nonattendance rate from 20% to 8% (Sawyer, Zalan, & Bond, 2002).*

## Pediatric

- Provide appropriate nutrition for children (see Box III-4). *Every child needs appropriate amounts of calories, proteins, minerals, and vitamins to grow. The best way to ensure kids get what they need while maintaining or losing weight is to provide a variety of nutritious foods that are low in fat and sugar (American Dietetic Association, 2003).*

▲ Follow the recommended guidelines for childhood immunizations as laid out by the Centers for Disease Control and Prevention (CDC) (see Appendix C).

H

## Geriatric

- Assess the client's awareness of deficits that may result from normal aging (e.g., changes in sleep patterns or frequency of urination, loss of visual acuity in night driving, loss of hearing, dietary changes, memory changes, loss of significant others). **EBN:** *If symptoms of health problems are not viewed as an illness, older adults are unlikely to report them to the health care provider. Annual checkups focusing on disease symptoms may fail to uncover day-to-day complaints that foretell more serious problems (Musil, 1998).*

### BOX III-4 PEDIATRIC NUTRITION GUIDELINES

- Aim for five servings of fruits and vegetables each day. You can gradually build up to this amount. Eat fruit with each meal for a week.
- Reduce fat. Opt for low-fat substitutes such as the following:
  - Low-fat dairy skim or 1% milk (after age 2), cheese with 2 to 6 g of fat per ounce
  - Lean meats and poultry (95% lean ground beef or turkey); remove visible fat from meat and skin from poultry
  - Low-fat or fat-free salad dressings, mayonnaise, and margarine
  - Desserts, such as angel food cake, low-fat ice cream or frozen yogurt, animal crackers, vanilla wafers, gingersnaps, or graham crackers
- Eat sugary foods in moderation. If your child eats a healthy diet, one sweet a day is fine.
- Drink water or skim or 1% milk (after age 2) instead of high-calorie, sugary drinks.
- Check ingredients on nutrition labels. Foods with sugar listed as one of the first three or four ingredients may be high in sugar and should be eaten in moderation.
- Eat healthy snacks. Keep healthy foods on hand for snacks. Good snack ideas include the following:
  - Fresh fruit
  - Cereal with low-fat milk
  - Low-fat cheese with low-fat crackers
  - Graham crackers with low-fat hot chocolate
  - Raw vegetables with low-fat dip
  - Applesauce

- • Identify coping mechanisms that promote wellness and place control of life choices back with the client. Discuss ways to prepare for retirement security. *An active sense of accountability for one's own well-being provides the necessary motivation to pursue a health-enhancing lifestyle (Walker, 1993).*
- ▲ Find suitable housing that provides support, safety, protection, meals, and social events. Consider in-home care by adult children when possible. *Informal care reduces home health care use and delays nursing home entry. Informal care by adult children is a common form of long-term care for older adults and can reduce medical expenditures if it substitutes for formal care (Van Houtven & Norton, 2004).*
- ▲ Give the client information about community resources for the elderly (e.g., services providing transportation to appointments, Meals-on-Wheels, home visitation services, pets, American Association of Retired Persons [AARP], Elder Hostel, Internet addresses). *The aging process occurs throughout the life span. The elderly client hopes to be independent and useful for as long as possible without being a burden on others. The website www.healthfinder.org/justforyou/justforyou.asp?KeyWordID=172&branch=1 offers health information for seniors on a variety of topics.*
- ▲ Assess the environment for signs of elder abuse and report as appropriate. **EBN:** *Activities categorized as mistreatment include force-feeding; overmedication/undermedication; withholding of care or needed therapies; and failure to provide health devices such as dentures, glasses, or ambulatory support devices (Rosenblatt, 1997).*
- ▲ Teach health-protecting behaviors to the elderly: monitoring cholesterol intake, exercising, having the stool checked for occult blood, or undergoing a mammogram, Papanicolaou test (Pap smear), or prostate or skin evaluation. **EBN:** *Because common reasons given for not engaging in health screenings are advanced age, absence of direction by primary health care providers, and lack of interest in following up abnormal findings, consider hosting a wellness day in a continuing care retirement community (Resnick, 2000).*
- • Teach the importance of exercise. **EB:** *One study suggested that educating older adults about the benefits of exercise increases the likelihood of their initiating and adhering to an exercise program (Boyette et al, 2002). Muscle weakness in old age is associated with physical disability and an increased risk of falls. Progressive resistance strength (PRT) training exercises (i.e., movements performed against a specific external force that is regularly increased during training). PRT appears to be an effective intervention to increase strength in older people and has a positive effect on some functional limitations (Latham et al, 2003).*
- ▲ Form collaborative multidisciplinary partnerships with nurse-managed clinics for health promotion and chronic disease care management for community-residing older adults. **EBN:** *In one study, senior citizens who participated in a community-based health promotion program reported better general health, performance of roles, and social functioning. Participants required 4.2 doctor visits per year compared with 7.1 office visits for a national comparison group, and 1.6 hospital days per year compared with 2.1 hospital days for the same reference population (Nuñez et al, 2003).*
- • Consider the age of the client when suggesting screening for disease. **EB:** *Even if one assumes that the mortality reduction with screening persists in the elderly, 80% of the benefit is achieved before age 80 years for colon cancer, before age 75 years for breast cancer, and before age 65 years for cervical cancer. The small benefit of screening in the elderly*

*may be outweighed by the harms: anxiety, additional testing, and unnecessary treatment (Rich & Black, 2000).*

## Multicultural

- Assess for the influence of cultural beliefs, norms, and values on the client's beliefs about health behavior. **EBN:** *What the client considers normal and abnormal health behavior may be based on cultural perceptions (Cochran, 1998; Doswell & Erlen, 1998; Leininger & McFarland, 2002). Religion and spirituality are associated with health-seeking behaviors of African-American women (Dessio et al, 2004). Factors underlying health care use among Hispanics included seriousness of symptoms, which had the most effect on visits to the doctor with more serious symptoms leading to prompter visits (Larkey et al, 2001).*
- Acknowledge and praise those aspects of the client's behavior and lifestyle that are health promoting. **EBN:** *Aspects of the client's life that are meaningful and valuable to him or her should be understood and preserved without change (Leininger & McFarland, 2002).*
- Negotiate with the client the aspects of health behavior that will require further modification. **EBN:** *Give and take with the client will lead to culturally congruent care (Leininger & McFarland, 2002).*
- Validate the client's feelings regarding the affect of health behavior on current lifestyle. **EBN:** *Validation is a therapeutic communication technique that lets the client know that the nurse has heard and understood what was said, and it promotes the nurse-client relationship (Heineken, 1998).*
- Use a community focus intervention. **EB:** *Korean-American women with access to a peer-group educational program and low-cost mammography had significantly improved attitudes and knowledge about breast cancer screening (Kim & Sarna, 2004).*

## Home Care

NOTE: All the previously listed nursing interventions are applicable to the home care setting. For more information, see Home Care interventions in the care plan for **Ineffective Health maintenance.**

## Client/Family Teaching

- Discuss the role of environmental and social factors in supporting a healthy family life. *The people are the community. Reciprocal relationships to build community education with a view to prevention is key to enhancing health (Davis, 1998).*

▲ Use written, verbal, and video instruction to provide information about health-seeking opportunities and wellness and provide the family with lists of addresses and where information can be found. Suggest use of the Internet. (Most libraries have Internet access with printing capabilities.) **EBN:** *In a study using an intervention including an educational video and written instructions designed to reduce prehospital delays in clients with chest pain, a significant increase was seen in the use of ambulances in the intervention group but not in the control group (Blank & Smithline, 2002).* **EBN:** *In a study involving a convenience sample subjects found Internet documents under the broad heading of quality health care were easy to use, and they indicated that the Internet resources would help them assess the quality of care they receive from physicians, nurses, and others (Oermann,*

*Lesley, & Kuefler, 2002).* **EB:** *This review recommends the use of both verbal and written health information when communicating about care issues with patients and/or significant others on discharge from hospital to home. The combination of verbal and written health information enables the provision of standardized care information to patients and/or significant others, which appears to improve knowledge and satisfaction. (Johnson, Sandford, & Tyndall, 2003).*

▲ Teach the importance of receiving flu vaccine. Offer vaccinations in convenient locations free of charge, and discuss perceived barriers with patients. **EBN:** *Given the potential negative consequences of contracting the influenza, prevention is the best strategy. Helping to clarify the advantages and disadvantages from the patient's perspective may decrease decisional conflict and increase vaccination rates (Mayo & Cobbler, 2004).*

• Identify physical and emotional threats to family security (e.g., domestic violence, child abuse, school violence). *According to Maslow's Hierarchy of Needs, wellness and health-promoting behaviors can be undertaken only when personal and social safety and security issues are resolved.*

▲ Teach woman how to monitor ovarian health: monthly self-monitoring using a symptom checklist including personal and family risks and early symptoms of gastrointestinal (GI) problems. *Critical review of general health-seeking models showed a need for expansion to include the early and atypical symptom period associated with ovarian cancer and the role of self and primary care in the diagnostic process. Organization of risks and symptom information assists in interpretation of disparate streams of data and gives a recommended outcome: high personal risk level + high family risk level + high early and persistent symptoms presence = high need for a prompt gynecological evaluation (Koldjeski et al, 2004).*

H

## evolve WEBSITES FOR EDUCATION

See the EVOLVE website for World Wide Web resources for client education.

## REFERENCES

American Dietetic Association, 2003. Available at www.wellpoint.com/health_parenting/balanceddiet.html, accessed on January 19, 2005.

Babrow AS, Kline KN: From "reducing" to "coping with" uncertainty: reconceptualizing the central challenge in breast self-exams, *Soc Sci Med* 51(12):1805, 2000.

Blank FS, Smithline HA: Evaluation of an educational video for cardiac patients, *Clin Nurs Res* 11(4):403, 2002.

Boyette LW, Lloyd A, Boyette JE et al: Personal characteristics that influence exercise behavior of older adults, *J Rehabil Res Dev* 39(1):95, 2002.

Christopher KA, Morrow LL: Evaluating a community-based exercise program for women cancer survivors, *Appl Nurs Res* 17(2): 100-108, 2004.

Clark C: *Wellness practitioner: concepts, research and strategies,* New York, 1996, Springer.

Cochran M: Tears have no color, *Am J Nurs* 98(6):53, 1998.

Conrad KM et al: The work site environment as a cue to smoking reduction, *Res Nurs Health* 19(1):21, 1996.

Davis R: Community caring: an ethnographic study within an organizational culture, *Public Health Nurs* 14(2):92, 1998.

Dessio W, Wade C, Chao M et al: Religion, spirituality, and healthcare choices of African-American women: results of a national survey, *Ethn Dis* 14(2):189-197, 2004.

Doswell W, Erlen J: Multicultural issues and ethical concerns in the delivery of nursing care interventions, *Nurs Clin North Am* 33(2):353, 1998.

Engel L, Andersen L: Effects of body-mind training and relaxation stretching on persons with chronic toxic encephalopathy, *Patient Educ Couns* 39(2-3):155, 2000.
Fenn M: Health promotion: theoretical perspectives and clinical applications, *Holist Nurs Pract* 12(2):1, 1998.
Heineken J: Patient silence is not necessarily client satisfaction: communication in home care nursing, *Home Healthc Nurse* 16(2): 115, 1998.
Herrick CM, Ainsworth AD: Invest in yourself: yoga as a self-care strategy, *Nurs Forum* 35(2):32, 2000.
Hull S, Hagdrup N, Hart B et al: Boosting uptake of influenza immunisation: a randomised controlled trial of telephone appointing in general practice, *Br J Gen Pract* 52(482):712, 2002.
Irwin ML, Yasui Y, Ulrich CM et al: Effect of exercise on total and intra-abdominal body fat in postmenopausal women: a randomized controlled trial, *JAMA* 289(3):323-330, 2003.
Johnson A, Sandford J, Tyndall J: Written and verbal information versus verbal information only for patients being discharged from acute hospital settings to home, *Cochrane Database Syst Rev* (4):CD003716, 2003.
Kim YH, Sarna L: An intervention to increase mammography use by Korean American women, *Oncol Nurs Forum* 31(1):105-110, 2004.
Koldjeski D, Kirkpatrick MK, Everett L et al: Health seeking related to ovarian cancer, *Cancer Nurs* 27(5):370-378, 2004.
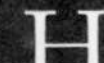
Kralik D: The quest for ordinariness: transition experienced by midlife women living with chronic illness, *J Adv Nurs* 39(2):146, 2002.
Larkey LK, Hecht ML, Miller K et al: Hispanic cultural norms for health-seeking behaviors in the face of symptoms, *Health Educ Behav* 28(1):65-80, 2001.
Latham N, Anderson C, Bennett D et al: Progressive resistance strength training for physical disability in older people, *Cochrane Database Syst Rev* (2):CD002759, 2003.
Leininger MM, McFarland MR: *Transcultural nursing: concepts, theories, research and practices,* ed 3, New York, 2002, McGraw-Hill.
Lewith GT, Broomfield J, Prescott P: Complementary cancer care in Southampton: a survey of staff and patients, *Complement Ther Med* 10(2):100, 2002.
Mayo AM, Cobler S: Flu vaccines and patient decision making: what we need to know, *J Am Acad Nurse Pract* 16(9):402-410, 2004.
Murphy S: Coping strategies of abstainers from alcohol up to 3 years post treatment, *Image J Nurs Sch* 25:32, 1993.
Murrock CJ: The effects of music on the rate of perceived exertion and general mood among coronary artery bypass graft clients enrolled in cardiac rehabilitation phase II [includes commentary by ET Miller], *Rehabil Nurs* 27(6):227, 2002.
Musil C: Health problems and health actions among community dwelling older adults: results of a health diary study, *Appl Nurs Res* 11(3):138, 1998.
Nuñez DE, Armbruster C, Phillips WT et al: Community-based senior health promotion program using a collaborative practice model: the Escalante Health Partnerships, *Public Health Nurs* 20(1):25, 2003.
O'Brien K, Nixon S, Glazier R et al: Progressive resistive exercise interventions for adults living with HIV/AIDS, *Cochrane Database Syst Rev* (4):CD004248, 2004.
Oermann MH, Lesley M, Kuefler SF: Using the Internet to teach consumers about quality care, *Jt Comm J Qual Improv* 28(2):83, 2002.
Resnick B: Hosting a wellness day: promoting health in the old-old, *Clin Excell Nurse Pract* 4(6):326, 2000.
Rich JS, Black WC: When should we stop screening? *Eff Clin Pract* 3(2):78, 2000.
Rosenblatt D: Elder mistreatment, *Crit Care Nurs Clin North Am* 9(2):183, 1997.
Sawyer SM, Zalan A, Bond LM: Telephone reminders improve adolescent clinic attendance: a randomized controlled trial, *J Paediatr Child Health* 38(1):79, 2002.
Smith-Battle L: The responsive use of self in community health nursing practice, *Adv Nurs Sci* 10(2):75, 1997.
Sparber A, Wootton JC, Bauer L et al: Use of complementary medicine by adult patients participating in cancer clinical trials, *Oncol Nurs Forum* 27(4):623, 2000.
U.S. Department of Agriculture (USDA): *The Dietary Guidelines for Americans, 2005.* Available at www.health.gov/dietaryguidelines/dga2005/recommendations.htm, accessed on January 20, 2005.
Van Houtven CH, Norton EC: Informal care and health care use of older adults, *J Health Econ* 23(6):1159-1180, 2004.
Wakefield MA, Wilson D, Owen N et al: Workplace smoking restrictions, occupational status and reduced cigarette consumption, *J Occup Med* 34:693-697, 1992.
Walker S: Wellness for elders, *Holist Nurs Pract* 38:7, 1993.

# Impaired Home maintenance

*Gail B. Ladwig*

**NANDA**

## Definition

Inability to independently maintain a safe and growth-promoting immediate environment

## Defining Characteristics

### Subjective

Household members express difficulty in maintaining their home in a comfortable fashion, household members describe outstanding debts or financial crises, household requests assistance with home maintenance

### Objective

Disorderly surroundings; unwashed or unavailable cooking equipment, clothes, or linen; accumulation of dirt, food wastes, or hygienic wastes; offensive odors; inappropriate household temperature; overtaxed family members (e.g., exhausted, anxious); lack of necessary equipment or aids; presence of vermin or rodents; repeated hygienic disorders, infestations, or infections

## Related Factors (r/t)

Individual/family member with disease or injury, unfamiliarity with neighborhood resources, lack of role modeling, lack of knowledge, insufficient family organization or planning, inadequate support systems, impaired cognitive or emotional functioning, insufficient finances

**NOC**

## Outcomes (Nursing Outcomes Classification)

### Suggested NOC Outcomes

Family Functioning; Parenting: Psychosocial Safety; Parenting Performance; Role Performance; Self-Care: Instrumental Activities of Daily Living (IADLs)

**Example NOC Outcome with Indicators**

**Family Functioning** as evidenced by the following indicators: Regulates behavior of members/Obtains adequate resources to meet needs of family members (Rate each indicator of **Family Functioning:** 1 = never demonstrated, 2 = rarely demonstrated, 3 = sometimes demonstrated, 4 = often demonstrated, 5 = consistently demonstrated [see Section I].)

## Client Outcomes

**Client Will (Specify Time Frame):**

- Wear clean clothing, eat nutritious meals, and have a sanitary and safe home
- Have the resources to cope physically and emotionally with the chronic illness process
- Use community resources to assist with treatment needs

NIC

## Interventions (Nursing Interventions Classification)

### Suggested NIC Intervention

Home Maintenance Assistance

H

**Example NIC Activities—Home Maintenance Assistance**

Provide information on how to make home safe and clean; help family use social support network

## Nursing Interventions and Rationales

- Establish a plan of care with the client and family based on the client's needs and the caregiver's capabilities. **EBN:** *Broad categories of health promotion identified in a study of persons with chronic illness were physical activity, nutritional strategies, life adjustment, maintenance of a positive attitude, and interpersonal support (Stuifbergen, 1997). Health care workers need to provide support when the client and family are facing difficult decisions (Hurley and Volicer, 2002).*
- Assess the concerns of family members, especially the primary caregiver, about long-term home care. **EB:** *Caregiver characteristics significantly associated with yielding up care to another included older age, greater use of respite services, fewer social activities, poorer mental health, and greater depression. Dementia severity was the key predictor of the decision to relinquish care (Bond & Clark, 2002).*
- Set up a system of relief for the main caregiver in the home and plan for sharing of household duties. **EB:** *The level of burden was affected directly by behavioral problems in the care receiver, frequency of getting a break, caregiver self-esteem, and caring for the client at odd hours (Chappell & Reid, 2002).*
- Encourage social relationships with family and friends, even if by phone. **EB:** *Telephone support was considered important by caregivers of elderly persons (Colantonio et al, 2001).*
- ▲ Initiate referral to community agencies as needed, including housekeeping services, Meals-on-Wheels, wheelchair-compatible transportation services, and oxygen therapy services. **EBN:** *Barriers to health promotion in people with chronic illness are fatigue, time, inadequate safety measures, and lack of accessible facilities (Stuifbergen, 1997).*
- ▲ Obtain adaptive equipment and telemedical equipment, as appropriate, to help family members continue to maintain the home environment. **EBN:** *Telemedical equipment available for the home includes infusion pumps, pulse oximeters, 12-lead EKG machines, and telestethoscopes (McNeal, 1998).*
- Consider the use of permethrin-impregnated mattress liners to control dust mites. **EB:** *A trial of permethrin-impregnated bedding significantly reduced house dust mites in*

• = Independent; ▲ = Collaborative; EBN = Evidence-Based Nursing; EB = Evidence-Based

*mattresses for at least 27 months. Allergen concentrations were significantly lowered at 15 months after intervention. No adverse side effects were reported (Cameron & Hill, 2002).*

- ▲ Refer the client to social services to help with debt consolidation or financial concerns. *Financial help ranges from Medicaid and private insurance to aid from specific foundations such as the Shriners Burn Center for Children. Hospital discharge planners are an important resource for coordinating agencies.*
- ▲ Ask the family to identify support people who can help with home maintenance. *Churches, nursing home health agencies, and hospice organizations are sources for reliable in-home support. Community health agencies can evaluate whether the home is safe enough for providing health care to a chronically ill person, can provide direct care, and can assist with resource coordination. Consider supportive housing for clients with mental illness.* **EB:** *Supportive housing programs, which provide independent housing along with health and social services, hold great promise for mentally ill individuals who are homeless (Culhane, Metreaux, & Hadley, 2002).*

H

## Geriatric

- ▲ Explore community resources to assist with home care (e.g., senior centers, Department of Aging, hospital discharge planners, the Internet, or church parish nurse). *Promoting the health of the population has always required an organic relationship to the community and knowledge of specific subpopulations (Smith-Battle, 1997). An Internet resource is the website of geriatrician Robert S. Stall, M.D. Available at www.acsu.buffalo.edu/~drstall.*
- • Visit the client's home to assess safety features (e.g., no throw rugs, safety bars in the bathroom, stair borders that distinguish each step, adequate nonglare lighting). **EB:** *The eye retina changes with age, which makes it easier to perceive red and yellow tones. With age, some glare occurs in bright light, and contrast and shadows blur. A 5-year study documented that increasing age was a strong predictor of visual impairment in an older Australian population (Foran, Mitchell, & Wang, 2003).* **EBN:** *Bath grab bars can minimize the effects of many age-related deficits that may contribute to bath-related falls. One study indicated that they are underutilized and their use needs to be supported (Lockett, Aminzadeh, & Edwards, 2002).*
- • Encourage regular eye examinations. *Early detection of eye changes is imperative to prevent irreversible damage (Age Net, 2003).*
- • The following interventions should be considered for those with low or failing sight:
  - Reduce glare:
    - Use nonglare light bulbs.
    - Remove wax from floors to reduce glare.
    - Encourage the client to wear sunglasses.
    - Use sheer curtains or blinds.
  - Use proper lighting:
    - Use night lights in the bedroom, bathroom, and hallways.
    - Use dimmer switches and three-way bulbs to control light.
    - Put bright lights at the top and bottom of a staircase.
    - Use consistent lighting to minimize shadows.

- Enhance color contrast:
  - Use colored tape to define steps.
  - Paint walls and staircase to contrast with floor.
  - Put glow-in-the-dark tape on light switches and door knobs.
  - Use colored dishes.
- Encourage the client to use low-vision aids:
  - Use magnifiers to improve near vision.
  - Hang magnifiers around the neck for convenience when sewing, doing crafts, or reading.
  - Request large-print medication labels, books, and phones.
  - Use handrails on stairs.
  - Keep flashlights in a convenient location.

*Vision loss can cause less hardship if adaptive strategies and aids are used. Use of aids increases safety and promotes a sense of independence (Age Net, 2003).*

H

▲ During the home visit, be alert for signs of elder abuse. Report any findings. **EBN:** *Activities categorized as mistreatment include force feeding; overmedication/undermedication; withholding care or needed therapies; failure to provide safety precautions; and failure to provide health devices such as dentures, glasses, or ambulatory devices (Rosenblatt, 1997).*

- See the care plan for **Risk for Injury.**

## Multicultural

- Acknowledge the stresses unique to racial/ethnic communities. **EBN:** *Targeted alcohol and tobacco marketing, high levels of unemployment, lack of health insurance, and racism are stresses unique to culturally diverse communities and often accompany poor housing (D'Avanzo et al, 2001; Ludwick & Silva, 2000; Zambrana, Dorrington, & Hayes-Bautista, 1995). One in 10 Latino children lives in a "severely distressed neighborhood," compared with 1 in 63 non-Hispanic Caucasian children (Annie E. Casey Foundation, 1994). Minority adults who moved to low-poverty neighborhoods were less likely to be exposed to violence and disorder, experience health problems, abuse alcohol, receive cash assistance, and were more likely to report satisfaction with neighborhood resources, experience higher housing quality, and be employed, when compared with minority adults who remained in high-poverty neighborhoods (Fauth, Leventhal, & Brookes-Dunn, 2004).*
- Identify what services and information are currently available in the community to assist with housing needs. **EBN:** *This identification will assist in focusing efforts and promote the wise use of valuable resources (National Heart, Lung, and Blood Institute, 1998).*
- Approach families of color with respect, warmth, and professional courtesy. **EBN:** *Instances of disrespect and lack of caring have special significance for individuals of color (D'Avanzo et al, 2001; Vontress & Epp, 1997).*

## Home Care

NOTE: By definition, this nursing diagnosis consists of primarily community-based interventions. Home care and public health nursing are two community resources that can help the family to restore or improve home management. The previous interventions incorporate these resources.

## Client/Family Teaching

- Teach the caregiver the need to set aside some personal time every day to meet his or her own needs. **EBN:** *The most prominent needs were found to be the need for security and the need to provide security to the child. Family needs and need for relief were also identified (Hallström, Runesson, & Elander, 2002).*
- Encourage family members to perform home maintenance activities (e.g., cooking, cleaning, fire prevention). *When one family member becomes ill and requires home care, the roles of other family members may change.*
- ▲ Identify support groups within the community to assist families in the caregiver role. **EBN:** *Caregivers' participation in support groups provides effective assistance to caregivers of clients with schizophrenia (Chou, Liu, & Chu, 2002).*
- Provide support when the family must move their family member to an assisted living facility (ALF). **EBN:** *Secondary data analysis in one study showed that all elements of a crisis were evident among caregivers in the process of moving a relative to an ALF. Perceived lack of family support in conjunction with physical and psychological exhaustion were crisis mediators (Liken, 2001).*
- ▲ Provide written instructions for medication management and side effects, written instructions for equipment brought to the home, and resource phone numbers for emergency needs. **EBN:** *Verbal reinforcement of personalized written instructions appears to be the best intervention. In one study, the use of computer-generated, personalized instructions improved adherence compared with the use of handwritten instructions (Hayes, 1998).*
- ▲ Promote food safety. Instruct client to avoid microbial food-borne illness by:
  - ■ Clean hands, food contact surfaces, and fruits and vegetables. Meat and poultry should not be washed or rinsed.
  - ■ Separate raw, cooked, and ready-to-eat foods while shopping, preparing, or storing foods.
  - ■ Cook foods to a safe temperature to kill microorganisms.
  - ■ Chill (refrigerate) perishable food promptly and defrost foods properly.
  - ■ Avoid raw (unpasteurized) milk or any products made from unpasteurized milk, raw or partially cooked eggs, or foods containing raw eggs, raw or undercooked meat and poultry, unpasteurized juices, and raw sprouts.

  *The* Dietary Guidelines for Americans 2005 *contains additional recommendations for specific populations. It is available at www.health.gov/dietaryguidelines/dga2005/recommendations.htm.*

## evolve WEBSITES FOR EDUCATION

See the EVOLVE website for World Wide Web resources for client education.

## REFERENCES

Age Net: Visual changes. Available at agenet.agenet.com/?Url=link.asp?DOC/36, accessed on February 25, 2003.

Annie E. Casey Foundation: *Kids count data book: state profiles of child well-being,* ed 5, Baltimore, 1994, The Foundation.

Bond MJ, Clark MS: Predictors of the decision to yield care of a person with dementia, *Aust J Ageing* 21(2):86, 2002.

Cameron MM, Hill N: Permethrin-impregnated mattress liners: a novel and effective intervention against house dust mites (Acari: Pyroglyphididae), *J Med Entomol* 39(5):755, 2002.

Chappell NL, Reid RC: Burden and well-being among caregivers: examining the distinction, *Gerontologist* 42(6):772, 2002.
Chou K, Liu S, Chu H: The effects of support groups on caregivers of patients with schizophrenia, *Int J Nurs Stud* 39(7):713, 2002.
Colantonio A, Kositsky AJ, Cohen C et al: What support do caregivers of elderly want? Results from the Canadian Study of Health and Aging, *Can J Public Health* 92(5):376, 2001.
Culhane DP, Metreaux S, Hadley T: Supportive housing for homeless people with severe mental illness, *LDI Issue Brief* 7(5):1, 2002.
D'Avanzo CE et al: Developing culturally informed strategies for substance-related interventions. In Naegle MA, D'Avanzo CE, editors: *Addictions and substance abuse: strategies for advanced practice nursing,* St Louis, 2001, Mosby.
Fauth RC, Leventhal T, Brooks-Gunn J: Short-term effects of moving from public housing in poor to middle-class neighborhoods on low-income, minority adults' outcomes, *Soc Sci Med* 59(11), 2271-2284, 2004.
Foran S, Mitchell P, Wang JJ: Five-year change in visual acuity and incidence of visual impairment: the Blue Mountains Eye Study, *Ophthalmology* 110(1):41, 2003.
Hallström I, Runesson I, Elander G: International pediatric nursing. Observed parental needs during their child's hospitalization, *J Pediatr Nurs* 17(2):140, 2002.
Hayes K: Randomized trial of geragogy-based medication instruction in the emergency department, *Nurs Res* 47(4):211, 1998.
Hurley AC, Volicer L: Alzheimer disease: "It's okay, Mama, if you want to go, it's okay," *JAMA* 288(18):2324, 2002.
Liken MA: Caregivers in crisis: moving a relative with Alzheimer's to assisted living, *Clin Nurs Res* 10(1):52, 2001.
Lockett D, Aminzadeh F, Edwards N: Development and evaluation of an instrument to measure seniors' attitudes toward the use of bathroom grab bars, *Public Health Nurs* 19(5):390, 2002.
Ludwick R, Silva M: Nursing around the world: cultural values and ethical conflicts, *Online J Issues Nurs,* August 14, 2000, available online at http://www.nursingworld.org/ojin/ethcol/ethics_4.htm, accessed June 19, 2003.
Mann WC, Llanes C, Justiss MD et al: Frail older adults' self-report of their most important assistive device, *Occup The J Res* 24(1):4-12, 2004.
McNeal G: Telecommunication techniques in high-tech home care, *Adv Pract Nurse* 10(3):279, 1998.
National Heart, Lung, and Blood Institute of the National Institutes of Health: *Salud para su corazón: bringing heart health to Latinos—a guide for building community programs,* NIH Pub No. 98-3796, Washington, DC, 1998, US Department of Health and Human Services.
Rosenblatt D: Elder mistreatment, *Crit Care Nurs Clin North Am* 9(2):183, 1997.
Smith-Battle L: The responsive use of self in community health nursing practice, *ANS Adv Nurs Sci* 10(2):75, 1997.
Stuifbergen A: Health promotion: an essential component of rehabilitation for persons with chronic disabling conditions, *ANS Adv Nurs Sci* 19(4):1, 1997.
Vontress CE, Epp LR: Historical hostility in the African American client: implications for counseling, *J Multicult Counseling Dev* 25:170, 1997.
Zambrana RE, Dorrington C, Hayes-Bautista D: Family and child health: a neglected vision. In Zambrana RE, editor: *Understanding Latino families,* Thousand Oaks, Calif, 1995, Sage.

H

## Hopelessness

evolve

*Ann Keeley*

**NANDA**

### Definition

Subjective state in which individual sees limited or no alternatives or personal choices available and is unable to mobilize energy on his or her own behalf

### Defining Characteristics

Passivity; decreased verbalization; decreased affect; verbal cues (e.g., saying "I can't," or sighing, "I'll never . . ." or "There is no future"); closing of eyes; anorexia; decreased response to stimuli; increased/decreased sleep; lack of initiative; lack of involvement in care; passively allowing care; shrugging in response to speaker; turning away from speaker; reporting feeling lost, unable to cope, abandoned

## Related Factors (r/t)

Abandonment, prolonged activity restriction creating isolation, loss of beliefs in transcendent values/God, long-term stress, failing or deteriorating chronic physiological and/or psychological condition, negative life review, perception of demands that overwhelm personal resources

**NOC**

## Outcomes (Nursing Outcomes Classification)

### Suggested NOC Outcomes

Decision Making; Hope; Mood Equilibrium; Nutritional Status: Food and Fluid Intake; Quality of Life; Sleep

**Example NOC Outcome with Indicators**

Has a presence of **Hope** as evidenced by the following indicators: Expresses expectation of a positive future/Expresses faith/Expresses will to live (Rate indicator of **Hope:** 1 = never demonstrated, 2 = rarely demonstrated, 3 = sometimes demonstrated, 4 = often demonstrated, 5 = consistently demonstrated [see Section I].)

## Client Outcomes

**Client Will (Specify Time Frame):**

- Verbalize feelings, participate in care
- Make positive statements (e.g., "I can" or "I will try")
- Set goals
- Make eye contact, focus on speaker
- Maintain appropriate appetite for age and physical health
- Sleep appropriate length of time for age and physical health
- Express concern for another
- Initiate activity

**NIC**

## Interventions (Nursing Interventions Classification)

### Suggested NIC Intervention

Hope Instillation

**Example NIC Activities—Hope Instillation**

Assist client/family to identify areas of hope in life; demonstrate hope by recognizing client's intrinsic worth and viewing client's illness as only one facet of the individual; expand client's repertoire of coping mechanisms

## Nursing Interventions and Rationales

- ▲ Monitor and document the potential for suicide. (Refer the client for appropriate treatment if a potential for suicide is identified.) Refer to the care plan for **Risk for Suicide** for specific interventions. *Hopelessness associated with depression is an indicator of higher risk for suicidality (Szanto et al, 2003).*
- Explore the client's definition of hope. **EBN:** *As individuals experience the effects of a life event or illness, their definition of hope may change. It is important for the nurse to be clear what the client's current definition includes. This intervention needs to occur with each encounter (Kylma, Vehvilainen-Julkunen, & Lahdevirta, 2001).*
- Assist in identifying sources of hope. **EBN:** *Depending on the population being served, there may be specific interventions more helpful in promoting hope (Cutcliffe & Grant, 2001).* **EBN:** *A therapeutic relationship will help identify problems and measures to cope with fatigue (Potter, 2004).*
- Assist the client in identifying reasons for living.
- Provide realistic feedback. **EBN:** *Accurate information allows the nurse-client relationship to redefine hope in the present (Kylma, Vehvilainen-Julkunen, & Lahdevirta, 2001).*
- Assess for pain and respond with appropriate measures for pain relief. *Fear of pain and inability to cope with pain are significant risk factors for hopelessness (Duggleby, 2001).*
- Assist with problem solving and decision making. *Cognitive behavioral therapy (CBT) is a useful intervention when working on issues of hope (Collins, 2003).*
- Determine appropriate approaches based on the underlying condition or situation that is contributing to feelings of hopelessness. *Understanding the source of the hopelessness, be it a victimizing relationship or a physical alteration, will indicate the approaches that may be most beneficial to the client (Schreiber, 2001).* **EB:** *Women with advanced breast cancer and their families benefit from specific strategies of intervention (Kershaw et al, 2004).* **EBN:** *Strategies that address meaning and hope in individuals with advanced cancer promote psychosocial well being (Lin, 2003).*
- Assist the client in looking at alternatives and setting goals that are important to him or her. *Use of the nurse's knowledge along with the client's experience within the context of a supportive relationship stimulates an unfolding of possibilities (Kylma, Vehvilainen-Julkunen, & Lahdevirta, 2001).* **EB:** *When health professionals work with women with advanced beast cancer and their family caregivers, they should help them replace avoidant coping strategies (Kershaw, 2004).*
- In dealing with possible long-term deficits, work with the client to set small, attainable goals. Working on mutually agreed upon goals that are meaningful to the client will support hopefulness (Duggleby, 2001). **EBN:** *Women with post-breast cancer lymphedema required individual attention to their specific needs and abilities (Radina, 2004).*
- Spend one-on-one time with the client. Use empathy; try to understand what the client is saying and communicate this understanding to the client. *Hope is constructed in exploring the possibilities. As a person experiences the understanding of another, he or she may explore with that person (the nurse) the possibilities in his or her life (Wang, 2000). Physical presence and active listening inspire hope in the client (Duggleby, 2001). The interview process itself can be therapeutic (Overcash, 2004).*

- Encourage decision making in the daily schedule. *Hopelessness may be an outgrowth of a perceived loss of control and/or self-efficacy. As changes occur, the nurse interacts with the client to evaluate their impact on life goals and assists in making adaptations that support hopefulness (Kylma, Vehvilainen-Julkunen, & Lahdevirta, 2001).*
- Encourage expression of feelings and acknowledge acceptance of them. *Hope is ultimately dependent on external validation in the form of positive interpersonal relationships (Cutcliffe & Grant, 2001). The therapeutic relationship is an essential component of interventions to address hopelessness (Collins, 2003).*
- Give the client time to initiate interactions. After an appropriate amount of time is allowed, approach the client in an accepting and nonjudgmental manner. *The establishing of new relationships and control over events within them is constructive within the context of nurturing hopefulness (Kylma, Vehvilainen-Julkunen, & Lahdevirta, 2001). The therapeutic relationship is an essential component of interventions to address hopelessness (Collins, 2003).*
- Encourage the client to participate in group activities. *Group activities provide social support and help the client to identify alternative ways to problem solve. Group experiences allow the opportunity to care for others and to be cared for (Kylma, Vehvilainen-Julkunen, & Lahdevirta, 2001).* **EBN:** *Women with cancer in church groups report a positive response Ferrell, 2003).*
- Teach alternative coping strategies. **EB:** *Quality of life is enhanced in women with coronary syndrome X when they incorporate exercise and relaxation therapy into their coping behaviors (Tyni-Lenne, 2002).*
- Review the client's strengths with the client. Have the client list his or her own strengths on a note card and carry this list for future reference. *Working with the client to identify positive experiences and personal strengths facilitates the development of hopefulness (Kylma, Vehvilainen-Julkunen, & Lahdevirta, 2001). CBT is a useful intervention when working on issues of hope and hopelessness (Collins, 2003).*
- Communicate clearly what the illness trajectory and/or course of treatment will involve. Efforts must be taken to eliminate as much uncertainty as possible (Kylma, Vehvilainen-Julkunen, & Lahdevirta, 2001). *People coping with nonhealing ulcers benefit from assistance minimizing symptoms and normalizing their existence (Hopkins, 2004). Women who have had breast cancer surgery and their family caregivers have specific needs for different types of information and interventions based on the stage of their cancer (Nikoletti, 2003).*
- Use humor as appropriate. *Humor is an effective intervention for hopelessness (Duggleby, 2001).* **EBN:** *Research with children with cancer found that there was a positive correlation between humor and psychosocial adjustment (Dowling, 2003).* **EB:** *Use of a specific humor intervention in hospital rehabilitation units produced a positive outcome in promoting psychosocial adjustment and healing (Scholl, 2003).*
- Involve family and significant others in the plan of care. *Significant caring relationships foster hope (Duggleby, 2001). Social support is a significant variable related to hope (Ehrenberger et al, 2002).* **EBN:** *Families of children who are technologically dependent benefit from an organized intervention for home care (Montagnino, 2004).*
- Encourage the family and significant others to express care, hope, and love for the cli-

H

ent. *Caring relationships have a positive influence on the presence of hope (Cutcliffe & Grant, 2001; Duggleby, 2001).* **EBN:** *Patients with non–small cell cancer feel a need for support from family (Kuo, 2002).*

- Assess for signs and symptoms of depression. *Hopelessness as one symptom of depression is indicative of a greater likelihood of suicidality (Szanto, 2003).*
- ▲ Consider use of integrative therapies such as omega-3 fatty acids, *Hypericum perforatum* (St. John's Wort), *S*-adenosylmethionine, folate, 5-hydroxytryptophan, acupuncture, exercise, and light therapy **EB:** *Data from double-blind, placebo-controlled trials support each of these as treatment interventions for depression. An evidence-based integrative medicine approach brings together treatment options with proven efficacy and the public's desire for complementary and alternative medicine treatments (Freeman, Helgason, & Hill, 2004).*
- Use touch to demonstrate caring, if culturally appropriate and with the client's permission, and encourage the family to do the same. **EBN:** *Therapeutic touch (TT) produced positive, desired outcomes in women with breast cancer (Kelly et al, 2004). Women with fibromyalgia experienced a positive outcome with therapeutic touch as an intervention (Denison, 2004).*
- Facilitate access to resources to support a positive spirituality. *Spiritual beliefs and practices that are practiced within a positive framework facilitate hope (Duggleby, 2001). Women with cancer who are involved in religious activities and groups report a more positive adaptation (Ferrell, 2003).*
- For additional interventions, see the care plans for **Spiritual distress, Readiness for enhanced Spiritual well-being,** and **Disturbed Sleep pattern.**

H

## Geriatric

- Assess for clinical signs and symptoms of depression; differentiate depression from organic dementia. *In the elderly, the differentiation of depression and dementia is critical prior to establishing a plan of care.*
- ▲ If depression is suspected, confer with the primary physician regarding referral for mental health services. *In older adults, hopelessness and suicidal wishes are present with high levels of depressive symptoms suggestive of higher risk of suicidality (Szanto et al, 2003).*
- Take threats of self-harm or suicide seriously. *The elderly have the highest rate of completed suicide of all age groups (Szanto, 2003).*
- Identify significant losses that may be leading to feelings of hopelessness. *Helping clients to cope with grief and make more psychological energy available to them will support their hopefulness.* **EB:** *Specific intervention for individuals with HIV coping with bereavement issues produced improvement (Sikkema, 2004).*
- Discuss stages of emotional responses to multiple losses. **EB:** *Specific intervention for HIV individuals coping with bereavement issues produced improvement (Sikkema, 2004).*
- Use reminiscence and life-review therapies to identify past coping skills. *Older people in residential facilities benefit from this therapy (Wang, 2004). Life review produced a positive outcome when used with individuals with right hemisphere cerebral vascular accidents (Davis, 2004).*
- Express hope to the client and give positive feedback whenever appropriate. *The nurse's*

*communication of caring for the client facilitates movement in the direction of hope. The therapeutic relationship has a positive effect on the alleviation of hopelessness (Collins, 2003).*

- Identify the client's past and current sources of spirituality. Help the client explore life and identify those experiences that are noteworthy. The client may want to read the Bible or other religious text or have it read to him or her. **EBN:** *Spirituality is a significant factor in quality of life of women with ovarian cancer (Ferrell, 2003). Spirituality is positively related to self-transcendence in middle-age adults. Self-transcendence is identified as a resource for well-being (Ellermann, 2001).*
- Encourage visits from children. *Social relationships foster hopefulness (Duggleby, 2001).*

▲ Administer medications as ordered and evaluate for possible drug interactions that may produce and/or exacerbate observed symptoms. *The elderly have compromised ability to metabolize medications and are often taking a variety of drugs with side effects that may produce observed symptoms.*

- Position the client by a window, take the client outside, or encourage activities such as gardening (if ability allows). *Environmental changes can foster hope (Cutcliffe & Grant, 2001).*
- Provide esthetic forms of expression such as dance, music, literature, and pictures. **EBN:** *In this study of a Swedish population age 65 to 89 years aesthetic experiences were related to feelings of timelessness and spacelessness, and served as sources of gratification (Wikstrom, 2004).*
- If possible, have the client perform daily regular exercise adapted to his or her abilities. *Exercise has been demonstrated to be an effective treatment for depression.*

H

## Multicultural

- Assess for the influence of cultural beliefs, norms, and values on the client's feelings of hopelessness. **EBN:** *The client's expressions of hopelessness may be based on cultural perceptions (Cochran, 1998; Doswell & Erlen, 1998; Leininger & McFarland, 2002).* **EB:** *A recent study found perceived racism was associated with higher levels of hopelessness for African-American boys (Nyborg & Curry, 2003).*
- Assess the effect of fatalism on the client's expression of hopelessness. **EBN:** *Fatalistic perspectives, which involve the belief that one cannot control one's own fate, may influence health behaviors in some Asian, African-American, and Latino populations (Chen, 2001; Harmon, Castro, & Coe, 1996; Phillips, Cohen, & Moses, 1999).*
- Assess for depression and refer to appropriate services. **EBN:** *A study examining somatization and depression in older Taiwanese-American adults with depressive symptoms reported hopelessness as a symptom (Suen & Tusaie, 2004). A study of expression of depression in African Americans and Latinas found that severity of depression was predicted by feelings of hopelessness (Myers et al, 2002).*
- Encourage spirituality as a source of support for hopelessness. **EBN:** *African Americans and Latinos may identify spirituality, religiousness, prayer, and church-based approaches as coping resources (Samuel-Hodge et al, 2000; Bourjolly, 1998; Mapp & Hudson, 1997).*
- Validate the client's feelings regarding the impact of health status on current lifestyle. **EBN:** *Validation is a therapeutic communication technique that lets the client know that the nurse has heard and understood what was said, and it promotes the nurse-client relationship (Heineken, 1998).*

## Home Care

- • Assess for isolation within the family unit. Encourage the client to participate in family activities. If the client cannot participate, encourage him or her to be in the same area and watch family activities. If possible, move the client's bed or primary sitting place to an active household area. *Significant caring relationships foster hope (Duggleby, 2001). Participation in events increases energy and promotes a sense of belonging. Hope is facilitated by meaningful interpersonal relationships (Cutcliffe & Grant, 2001).*
- ▲ If depression is suspected, confer with the primary health care provider regarding referral for mental health services. *Hopelessness connected associated with depression is an indicator of higher suicidality (Szanto, 2003).*
- • Reminisce with the client about his or her life. *The process of remembering past pleasant activities and sharing them in a supportive environment inspires hope (Duggleby, 2001). Use of the self in the context of an interpersonal relationship with the client will facilitate hope (Cutcliffe & Grant, 2001). Older people in residential facilities benefit from this therapy (Wang, 2004). Life review produced a positive outcome when used with individuals with right hemisphere cerebral vascular accidents (Davis, 2004).*
- • Identify areas in which the client can have control. Allow the client to set achievable goals in these areas. Assist the client when necessary to negotiate desirable outcomes. *Mobilization of resources to promote self-efficacy promotes hope (Kylma, Vehvilainen-Julkenen, & Lahdevirta, 2001).*
- • Clearly explain potential benefits and risks of a proposed intervention. *Clear, direct communication of the potential of an intervention to overcome a threat, along with honest discussion of negative aspects, empowers the client and promotes hope (Pinikahana & Happell, 2002).*
- • If illness precipitated the hopelessness, discuss knowledge of and previous experience with the disease. Help the client to identify past coping strengths. *Uncertainty is a danger when it results in pessimism. Knowledge of the disease and previous positive coping experience with the illness provide hope for the future (Richer & Ezer, 2002).*
- ▲ Provide plant or pet therapy if possible. *Caring for pets or plants helps to redefine the client's identity and makes him or her feel needed and loved. Pet therapy has been reported to have a positive effect on a variety of client populations (Hooker, 2002).*
- ▲ Provide a safe environment so that the client cannot harm himself or herself. (See also the no-suicide contract in the following section.) Provide one-to-one contact when necessary. Refer the client for immediate mental health treatment if needed. *Hopelessness is an accurate indicator of suicidal risk. A safe environment reassures the client.*
- ▲ If it is consistent with the client's religious beliefs, refer for spiritual counseling by clergy of the client's choice.
- ▲ In the presence of a psychiatric disorder, refer for psychiatric home health care services for client reassurance and implementation of a therapeutic regimen.

## Client/Family Teaching

- • Provide information regarding the client's condition, treatment plan, and progress. *Clear, direct communication of the potential of an intervention to overcome a threat along with honest discussion of negative aspects empowers the client and promotes hope (Pinikahana & Happell, 2002).*

- Provide positive reinforcement, praise, and acknowledgment of the challenges of caregiving to family members. *Nurses provide much-needed support and encouragement to caregivers (Dibartolo, 2002).*
- Teach the use of stress-reduction techniques, relaxation, and imagery. Many cassette tapes on relaxation and meditation are available. Assist the client and caregivers with relaxation based on their preference from the initial assessment. *Stress management techniques are effective interventions for clients and their caregivers (Ducharme & Trudeau, 2002).* **EB:** *Women with coronary syndrome X benefited from physical training and relaxation therapy (Tynk-Lenne, 2002).*
- Encourage families to express love, concern, and encouragement, and allow the client to verbalize feelings.

▲ Refer the client to self-help groups such as I Can Cope and Make Today Count. **EBN:** *Self-help and/or professionally led curriculum-based support programs for families are effective in reducing stress and facilitating coping and hope (Northouse et al, 2002).*

▲ Refer the family to community support groups targeted to the specific needs of the family caregivers. *Support groups provide validation of feelings, information, and an opportunity for sharing of creative strategies among participants (Fung & Chien, 2002).*

H

## evolve WEBSITES FOR EDUCATION

See the EVOLVE website for World Wide Web resources for client education.

## REFERENCES


Bourjolly JN: Differences in religiousness among black and white women with breast cancer, *Soc Work Health Care* 28(1):21, 1998.

Chan SW, Leung JK: Cognitive behavioural therapy for clients with schizophrenia: implications for mental health nursing practice, *J Clin Nurs* 11(2):214-224, 2002.

Chen YC: Chinese values, health and nursing, *J Adv Nurs* 36(2):270, 2001.

Cochran M: Tears have no color, *Am J Nurs* 98(6):53, 1998.

Collins S, Cutcliffe JR: Addressing hopelessness in people with suicidal ideation: building upon the therapeutic relationship utilizing a cognitive behavioral approach, *J Psychiatr Ment Health Nurs* 10:175-185, 2003.

Cutliffe JR: Hope, counseling and complicated bereavement reactions, *J Adv Nurs* 28(4):754, 1998.

Cutcliffe JR, Grant G: What are the principles and processes of inspiring hope in cognitively impaired older adults within a continuing care environment? *J Psychiatr Ment Health Nurs* 8:427, 2001.

Davis MC: Life review therapy as an intervention to manage depression and enhance life satisfaction in individuals with right hemisphere cerebral vascular accidents, *Issues Ment Health Nurs* 25(5):503-515, 2004.

Denison B: Touch the pain away: new research on therapeutic touch and persons with fibromyalgia syndrome, *Holistic Nurs Pract* 18(3):142-151, 2004.

Dibartolo MC: Exploring self-efficacy and hardiness in spousal caregivers of individuals with dementia, *J Gerontol Nurs* 28(4):24, 2002.

Doswell W, Erlen J: Multicultural issues and ethical concerns in the delivery of nursing care interventions, *Nurs Clin North Am* 33(2):353, 1998.

Dowling JS, Hockenberry M, Gregory RL: Sense of humor, childhood cancer stressors, and outcomes of psychosocial adjustment, immune function, and infection, *J Pediatr Oncol Nurs* 20(6):271-292, 2003.

Ducharme F, Trudeau D: Qualitative evaluation of a stress management intervention for elderly caregivers at home: a constructivist approach, *Issues Ment Health Nurs* 23:691, 2002.

Duggleby W: Hope at the end of life, *J Hospice Palliat Nurs* 3(2):51, 2001.

Ellermann CR, Reed PG: Self-transcendence and depression in middle-age adults, *West J Nurs Res* 23(7):689-713, 2001.

Ehrenberger HE, Alligood MR, Thomas SP et al: Testing a theory of decision-making derived from King's systems framework in women eligible for a cancer clinical trial, *Nurs Sci Q* 15(2):156, 2002.

Ferrell, FR, Smith SL, Juarez G et al: Meaning of illness and spirituality in ovarian cancer survivors, *Oncol Nurs Forum* 30(2):249-257, 2003.

Fritsch S, Donaldson D, Spirito A et al: Personality characteristics of adolescent suicide attempters, *Child Psychiatry Hum Dev* 30(4):219, 2000.

Fung W, Chien W: The effectiveness of a mutual support group for family caregivers of a relative with dementia, *Arch Psychiatr Nurs* 16(3):134, 2002.

Harmon MP, Castro FG, Coe K: Acculturation and cervical cancer: knowledge, beliefs, and behaviors of Hispanic women, *Women Health* 24(3):37, 1996.

Heineken J: Patient silence is not necessarily client satisfaction: communication in home care nursing, *Home Healthc Nurse* 16(2): 11, 1998.

Hooker SD, Freeman LH, Stewart P: Pet therapy research: a historical review, *Holist Nurs Pract* 17(1):17-23, 2002.

Kelly AE, Sullivan P, Fawcett J et al: Therapeutic touch, quiet time, and dialogue: perceptions of women with breast cancer, *Oncol Nurs Forum* 31(3):625-631, 2004.

Kylma J, Vehvilainen-Julkunen K, Lahdevirta J: Hope, despair and hopelessness in living with HIV/AIDS: a grounded theory study, *J Adv Nurs* 33(6):764, 2001.

Kuo TT, Ma FC: Symptoms, distresses and coping strategies in patients with non-small-cell lung cancer, *Cancer Nurs* 25(4):309-317, 2002.

Leininger MM, McFarland MR: *Transcultural nursing: concepts, theories, research and practices,* ed 3, New York, 2002, McGraw-Hill.

Malone KM, Oquendo MA, Haas GL et al: Protective factors against suicidal acts in major depression: reasons for living, *Am J Psychiatry* 157(7):1084, 2000.

Mapp I, Hudson R: Stress and coping among African American and Hispanic parents of deaf children, *Am Ann Deaf* 142(1):48, 1997.

Montagnino BA, Maurico RV: The child with a tracheostomy and gastrostomy: parental stress and coping in the home: a pilot study, *Pediatr Nurs* 30(5):373-401, 2004.

Myers HF, Lesser I, Rodriguez N et al: Ethnic differences in clinical presentation of depression in adult women, *Cultur Divers Ethnic Minor Psychol* 8(2):138-156, 2003.

Nicoletti S, Kristjanson LJ, Tataryn, D et al: Information needs and coping styles of primary family caregivers of women following breast cancer surgery, *Oncol Nurs Forum* 30(6):987-996, 2003.

Northouse LL, Walker J, Schafenacker A et al: A family-based program of care for women with recurrent breast cancer and their family members, *Oncol Nurs Forum* 29(10):1411, 2002.

Nyborg VM, Curry JF: The impact of perceived racism: psychological symptoms among African American boys, *J Clin Child Adolesc Psychol* 32(2):258-266, 2003.

Overcash JA: Using narrative research to understand the quality of life of older women with breast cancer, *Oncol Nurs Forum* 31(6): 1153-1159, 2004.

Phillips JM, Cohen MZ, Moses G: Breast cancer screening and African American women: fear, fatalism, and silence, *Oncol Nurs Forum* 26(3):561, 1999.

Pinikahana J, Happell B: Exploring the complexity of compliance in schizophrenia, *Issues Ment Health Nurs* 23: 513, 2002.

Purnell LD, Pualanka BJ: *Guide to culturally competent health care*. Philadelphia, 2004, FA Davis.

Radina ME, Armer JM, Culbertson S et al: Post-breast cancer lymphedema: understanding women's knowledge of their condition, *Oncol Nurs Forum* 31(1):97-104, 2004.

Richer MC, Ezer H: Living in it, living with it, and moving on: dimensions of meaning during chemotherapy, *Oncol Nurs Forum* 29(1):113, 2002.

Samuel-Hodge CD, Headen SW, Skelly AH et al: Influences on day-to-day self-management of type 2 diabetes among African American women: spirituality, the multi-caregiver role, and other social context factors, *Diabetes Care* 23(7):928, 2000.

Scholl JC, Ragan SL: The use of humor in promoting positive provider-patient interactions in a hospital rehabilitation unit, *Health Commun* 15(3):319-330, 2003.

Schneider SM., Prince-Paul M, Allen MJ et al: Virtual reality as a distraction intervention for women receiving chemotherapy, *Oncol Nurs Forum* 31(1):81-88, 2004.

Schreiber R: Wandering in the dark: women's experiences with depression, *Health Care Women Int* 22(1/2):85, 2001.

Sikkema KJ, Hansen NB, Kochman A et al: Outcomes from a randomized controlled trial of a group intervention for HIV positive men and women coping with AIDS-related loss and bereavement, *Death Stud* 28(3):187-209, 2004.
Suen LJ, Tusaie K: Is somatization a significant depressive symptom in older Taiwanese Americans, *Geriatr Nurs* 25(3):157-163, 2004.
Szanto K, Gildengers A, Mulsant B et al: Identification of suicidal ideation and prevention of suicidal behaviour in the elderly, *Drugs Aging* 19(1):11-24, 2002.
Tyni-Lenne R, Stryjan S, Eriksson B et al: Beneficial therapeutic effects of physical training and relaxation therapy in women with coronary syndrome X, *Physiother Res Int* 7(1):35-43, 2003.
Valente SM: Adolescent suicide: assessment and intervention, *J Child Adolesc Psychiatr Ment Health Nurs* 2:34, 1989.
Wang CH: Developing a concept of hope from a human science perspective, *Nurs Sci Q* 13(3):248, 2000.
Wang J: The comparative effectiveness among institutionalized and non-institutionalized elderly people in Taiwan of reminiscence therapy as a psychological measure, *J Nurs Res* 12(3):237-244, 2004.
Wikstrom B: Older adults and the arts: the importance of aesthetic forms of expression in later life, *J Gerontol Nurs* 30(9):30-36, 2004.



# Hyperthermia

evolve

*Marcia LaHaie*

**NANDA**

## Definition

Body temperature elevated above normal range

NOTE: Elevated body temperature can be either fever or hyperthermia. Fever is a normal response in which the core body temperature increases at least 1.5° to 2.0° F (0.8° to 1.1° C) above an individual's normal temperature (>100.5° F [>38° C]). This elevation is in response to a chemical signal (endogenous pyrogen) released as part of an inflammatory response, such as in infection or tissue injury. Because there is a proportional enhancement of the immune system for each degree of temperature elevation, fever is believed to be adaptive to 104° F (40° C) (Kluger, 1991; Kluger et al, 1996). Hyperthermia is an abnormal increase in core body temperature, usually above 104° F (40° C), that occurs as a result of disorders of temperature control (Dinarello, Cannon, & Wolf, 1988). Causes include brain trauma, heat stroke, drugs (e.g., cocaine, "Ecstasy"), or malignant hyperthermia of anesthesia. Hyperthermia is not adaptive (Holtzclaw, 1992) and should be treated as a medical emergency.

## Defining Characteristics

- Fever: core body temperature elevated at least 1.5° to 2.0° F (0.8° to 1.1° C) above individual's normal temperature (>100.5° F [>38° C])
- Hyperthermia: body temperature above 104° F (40° C) with flushed or hot skin, increased respiratory rate, and tachycardia

## Related Factors (r/t)

- Fever: infection, tissue injury, illness or trauma, dehydration, blood transfusion, medication, neoplasm, increased metabolic rate
- Hyperthermia: exposure to hot environment, vigorous activity, inappropriate clothing,

inability or decreased ability to perspire, brain injury, medication, anesthesia, severe illness, trauma

**NOC**

## Outcomes (Nursing Outcomes Classification)

### Suggested NOC Outcomes

Thermoregulation; Thermoregulation: Newborn

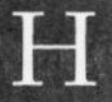

**Example NOC Outcome with Indicators**

**Thermoregulation** as evidenced by the following indicators: Body temperature WNL/Skin temperature IER/No skin color changes/Hydration adequate/Reported thermal comfort (Rate each indicator of **Thermoregulation:** 1 = severely compromised, 2 = substantially compromised, 3 = moderately compromised, 4 = mildly compromised, 5 = not compromised [see Section I].)

IER, In expected range; WNL, within normal limits.

## Client Outcomes

### Client Will (Specify Time Frame):

- Maintain oral temperature within adaptive levels (below 104° F [40° C]) or lower, depending on the presence of cardiopulmonary illness and client comfort
- Remain free of dehydration

**NIC**

## Interventions (Nursing Interventions Classification)

### Suggested NIC Interventions

Fever Treatment, Malignant Hyperthermia Precautions, Temperature Regulation

**Example NIC Activities—Fever Treatment**

Institute use of a continuous core temperature–monitoring device as appropriate; monitor for decreasing levels of consciousness

## Nursing Interventions and Rationales

- ▲ Assess an afebrile hospitalized client's temperature per institutional policy, upon assessment of signs or symptoms of infection, if the client has chills, or at least once a day between 5 PM and 7 PM. *Temperature screening of afebrile clients can be based on daily circadian rhythm patterns (Beaudry, VandenBosch, & Anderson, 1995). Shivering indicates a rising body temperature.*
- • Measure and record a febrile client's temperature at least every 4 to 6 hours or whenever a change in condition occurs (e.g., chills, change in mental status). *Recognizing the pattern of a fever can help determine the source (Cunha, 1996; Holtzclaw, 1992). Temperature can be measured with acceptable accuracy using an electronic probe in the mouth or via*

*the external auditory canal (tympanic membrane) (Schmitz et al, 2000). Although inconvenient, rectal temperature measurement is highly accurate (Schmitz et al, 1995; Varney et al, 2002). A glass (mercury) thermometer is highly accurate in temperature measurement (Latman et al, 2001), but its use involves increased time (6 to 7 minutes), risk of mercury contamination, and risk of rectal perforation (rare), and is culturally undesirable. Axillary measurements are inaccurate and should not be used (Schmitz et al, 1995). Where equipment is available in intensive care unit (ICU) settings, temperature measurement by intravascular or bladder thermistor is a highly accurate method (Nierman, 1991). Measurement of brain temperature may be available for neurosurgical patients and is highly accurate, but the relationship of brain temperature to core temperature has not yet been accurately determined (Mcilvoy, 2004).* **EBN:** *There was no significant difference between average oral and average tympanic temperatures in adult surgical clients (Gilbert, Barton, & Counsell, 2002).*



- • Use the same site and method (device) for temperature measurement for a given client so that temperature trends are assessed accurately. **EBN:** *A difference in the site (oral, rectal, axillary, or pulmonary) of temperature measurement results in a significant difference in temperature reading (Schmitz et al, 1995).*
- ▲ Notify the physician of temperature according to institutional standards or written orders, or when temperature reaches 100.5° F (38° C). Also notify the physician of the presence of a change in mental status. *A change in mental status may indicate the onset of septic shock.*
- ▲ Administer antipyretic medication per physician orders, when infection-induced fever is above 104° F (40° C), and when the client cannot tolerate the increase in metabolic demand, such as the acutely ill or in advanced cardiac or respiratory disease (Mackowiak & Plaisance, 1998). *Elimination of fever will interfere with its enhancement of the immune response (Klein & Cunha, 1996). Temperature elevation is accompanied by an increase in oxygen consumption and metabolic rate. The antipyretic acetaminophen is preferred over aspirin. Acetaminophen was better than aspirin for reducing fever in endotoxemia and did not affect the humoral response of the subjects (Pernerstorfer et al, 1999). Although effective, nonsteroidal antipyretic drugs can cause GI toxicity (Plaisance, 2000), as well as interfere with platelet function.*
- ▲ Assess fluid loss and facilitate oral intake or administer intravenous fluids to accomplish fluid replacement. *Increased metabolic rate and diaphoresis associated with fever cause loss of body fluids.*
- • When diaphoresis is present, assist the client with bathing and changing into dry clothing. *Bathing and clothing changes increase comfort and decrease the possibility of continued shivering caused by water evaporation from the skin.*
- • Do not use external cooling measures such as ice packs, tepid water baths, or removal of blankets and clothing for fever management; these measures cause shivering and are ineffective. *External cooling induces both cutaneous vasoconstriction and shivering (Kurz et al, 1995). If the client's temperature drops in response to external cooling measures, the hypothalamus resets the body temperature at a higher level, which results in more shivering (Klein & Cunha, 1996). Shivering leads to significantly increased oxygen consumption (Holtzclaw, 1993).*
- ▲ Cooling blanket use is indicated for temperature reduction if the client's fever is above

105° F (40.6° C) and cannot be controlled with antipyretics (Styrt & Sugarman, 1990) and if a high body temperature is related to hyperthermia, a disorder of temperature regulation. (Morgan, 1990).

- When using a cooling blanket, choose a convective airflow system, set the temperature regulator to 1° to 2° F (0.6° to 1.1° C ) below the client's current temperature, and wrap the client's extremities with towels to prevent shivering. **EBN:** *Blankets that use convective airflow for cooling may be more effective than those that cool by conductive water flow (Creechan, Vollman, & Kravutske, 2001). Higher blanket temperatures are as effective as lower temperatures in reducing fever and cause less discomfort (Caruso et al, 1992). To prevent shivering when a hypothermia blanket is used for fever reduction, wrap the client's extremities in towels (Caruso et al, 1992).*
- Use a nonsteroidal antipyretic (e.g., acetaminophen) instead of or in conjunction with a cooling blanket to improve fever reduction and decrease the duration of cooling blanket use. *Although external cooling and use of antipyretic were equally effective in decreasing body temperature in critically ill patients, there was a 5% increase in energy expenditure with the use of the external cooling versus a 8% decrease of energy expenditure with the use of an antipyretic (Gozzoli et al, 2004).*

H

## Geriatric

- An increase in oral temperature of 1.5° to 2.0° F (0.8° to 1.1° C) above baseline or above 99° F (37.2° C) should be considered a fever in the elderly. *Baseline temperature is lower in the elderly (Downton, Andrews, & Puxty, 1987). The upward limit for normal temperature (oral) in the elderly is 99° F (37.2° C) (Darowski, Weinbert, & Guz, 1991). Febrile response to infection was found to be reduced with increasing age, and baseline temperatures were generally lower in older clients (Roghmann, Warner, & Mackowiak, 2001).*
- Rectal temperature may be more accurate to diagnose fever in elderly clients. However, nursing judgment must be used to determine if rectal temperature measurement is acceptable to the client, especially a client with mental changes or dementia. **EBN:** *Rectal thermometry identified fevers in elderly clients that were missed by the oral and tympanic routes (Varney et al, 2002). A rectal temperature of 99.5° F (37.5° C) is the upper limit of normal for this route in the elderly (Darowski, Weinbert, & Guz, 1991).*
- Assess for other signs and symptoms of infection in addition to or in the absence of fever in the elderly. Suspect infection when there has been a decline in function, including new or increased confusion, incontinence, falling, decreased mobility, or failure to cooperate (Berman, Hogan, & Fox, 1987). *The temperature response is blunted in the elderly because of changes in physiology resulting from aging (Norman & Yoshikawa, 1996). The onset of pyrexia in the elderly with infections can be delayed several hours; the delay was more than 12 hours for 12% of clients (McAlpine et al, 1986).*

▲ Help the client seek medical attention immediately if fever is present. To diagnose the fever source, assess for possible precipitating factors, including changes in medication, environmental changes, and recent medical interventions or infectious exposures. *Fever in the elderly, especially the very old, is much more likely than in younger persons to be an indication of a serious bacterial infection (Norman & Yoshikawa, 1996). The elderly are more susceptible to environmentally and medication-induced hyperthermia due to the greater incidence of underlying chronic medical conditions that impair thermal regulation or prevent removal from a hot environment (e.g., cardiovascular disease, neurological and psychiatric disorders, obesity, and use of anticholenergic and diuretic drugs) (Brody, 1994).*

- In hot weather, encourage elderly clients to drink 8 to 10 glasses of fluid per day (within their cardiac and renal reserves) regardless of whether they are thirsty. Assess for the need for and presence of fans or air conditioning. *The elderly are more susceptible to a hot environment than are younger adults because of a decreased sensitivity to heat, decreased sweat gland function, and decreased thirst (Brody, 1994). The number of geriatric deaths rises as environmental temperatures increase in the hot summer months (Worfolk, 2000; Bull & Morton, 1978).*
- In hot weather, monitor the elderly client for signs of heat stroke: temperature of 100° F (37.8° C) to 102° F (38.9° C), orthostatic blood pressure drop, weakness, restlessness, mental status changes, faintness, thirst, nausea, and vomiting. If signs are present, move the client to a cool place, have the client lie down, give sips of water, check orthostatic blood pressure, spray with lukewarm water, cool with a fan, and seek medical assistance immediately. *The elderly are predisposed to heat exhaustion and should be watched carefully for its occurrence; if it is present, it should be treated promptly (Worfolk, 2000).*

## Home Care

- Some of the interventions described previously may be adapted for home care use.
- Assess whether the client or family has a thermometer. Instruct as needed in the type of thermometer (non–mercury-containing preferred; sublingual or tympanic location rather than skin patches) and how to use and read it accurately. *An accurate temperature reading is one indicator of the client's condition.*
- Teach the client and family that handwashing is the most effective way to prevent the transmission of viral and bacterial infections that may cause fever. However, it is not necessary to specifically purchase antibacterial household cleaning products as these products have not been shown to decrease the incidence of infection among household members (Larson et al, 2004).
- ▲ Teach the client and family to use acetaminophen rather than aspirin or ibuprofen for fever reduction at home to prevent possible adverse effects. (NOTE: The maximum daily dose of acetaminophen is 4000 mg/day in a healthy adult. In clients with liver dysfunction, doses greater than 2000 mg/day, if taken on a regular basis, may be harmful. A client with kidney dysfunction should take acetaminophen no more often than every 6 hours.)
- Help the client and caregivers prevent and monitor for heat stroke/hyperthermia during times of high outdoor temperatures. Preventive measures include minimizing time spent outdoors, use of air conditioning or fan, increasing fluid intake, and taking frequent rest periods.
- To prevent heat-related injury in athletes, laborers, and military personnel, instruct

them to acclimate gradually to the higher temperatures, increase fluid intake, wear vapor-permeable clothing, and take frequent rests (Bross, Nash, & Carlton, 1994).

▲ In the event of temperature elevation above the adaptive range, institute measures to decrease temperature (e.g., get the client out of the sun and into a cool place, remove excess clothing, have the client drink fluids, spray the client with lukewarm water, and fan with cool air) (Bross, Nash, & Carlton, 1994). Seek medical attention immediately if temperature is at or above 104° F (40° C). *Hyperthermia is an acute and possibly life-threatening symptom. The client cannot stay at home safely.*

▲ If the client is in hospice or is terminally ill, follow the client's wishes and the physician's orders in determining the management of fever. *The goal of terminal care is to provide comfort and dignity during the dying process.*

## Client/Family Teaching

- Teach that infection-induced fever enhances the immune system (the beneficial effect occurs at oral temperatures of less than 104° F (40° C), so the client can participate in the decision of whether to treat the fever. If treatment is elected or appropriate, instruct in the use of acetaminophen as the most effective means for fever reduction with fewer potential side effects than other antipyretics. *Fevers of less than 104° F (40° C) enhance immune system functioning (Roberts, 1991). Acetaminophen effectively reduces fever (Koch-Weser, 1976) and has less potential for detrimental effects (Aronoff & Neilson, 2001).*
- Teach the client that shivering with infection-induced fever has detrimental effects and that activities that can cause shivering (e.g., blanket removal, lowering of room temperature, tepid water baths, ice packs) should be avoided. *External cooling measures result in shivering and discomfort (Styrt & Sugarman, 1990).*
- Instruct to increase fluids to prevent heat-induced hyperthermia and dehydration in the presence of fever, but to avoid liquids that contain alcohol, caffeine, or large amounts of sugar. *Liberal fluid intake replaces fluid lost through perspiration and respiration. The presence of alcohol, caffeine, and sugar in fluids can promote diuresis, unless the client regularly consumes that type of beverage.*
- Teach the client to stay in a cooler environment during periods of excessive outdoor heat or humidity. If the client does go out, instruct him or her to avoid vigorous physical activity, wear lightweight, loose-fitting clothing, and wear a hat to minimize sun exposure. *Such methods reduce exposure to high environmental temperatures, which can cause heat stroke and hyperthermia.*

## evolve WEBSITES FOR EDUCATION

See the EVOLVE website for World Wide Web resources for client education.

## REFERENCES

Aronoff DM, Neilson EG: Antipyretics: mechanisms of action and clinical use in fever suppression, *Am J Med* 111:304, 2001.

Beaudry M, VandenBosch T, Anderson J: Research utilization: once a day temperatures for afebrile patients, *Clin Nurs Spec* 10:21, 1995.

Berman P, Hogan DB, Fox RA: The atypical presentation of infection in old age, *Age Ageing* 16:201, 1987.
Brody GM: Hyperthermia and hypothermia in the elderly, *Clin Geriatr Med* 10(1):213, 1994.
Bross MH, Nash BT Jr, Carlton FB Jr: Heat emergencies, *Am Fam Physician* 50(2):389, 1994.
Bull G, Morton J: Environment, temperature, and death rates, *Age Ageing* 7:210, 1978.
Caruso CC, Hadley BJ, Shukla R et al: Cooling effects and comfort of four cooling blanket temperatures in humans with fever, *Nurs Res* 41(2):68, 1992.
Creechan T, Vollman K, Kravutske ME: Cooling by convection vs cooling by conduction for treatment of fever in critically ill adults, *Am J Crit Care* 10(1):52, 2001.
Cunha BA: The clinical significance of fever patterns, *Infect Dis Clin North Am* 10:33, 1996.
Darowski A, Weinbert JR, Guz A: Normal rectal, auditory, sublingual, and axillary temperature in febrile patients in a warm environment, *Age Ageing* 20:113, 1991.
Dinarello C, Cannon J, Wolf S: New concepts on the pathogenesis of fever, *Rev Infect Dis* 10(1):161, 1988.
Downton JH, Andrews K, Puxty JAH: Silent pyrexia in the elderly, *Age Ageing* 16:41, 1987.
Gilbert M, Barton AJ, Counsell CM: Comparison of oral and tympanic temperatures in adult surgical patients, *Appl Nurs Res* 15:42, 2002.
Gozzoli V, Treggiari MM, Kleger GR et al: Randomized trial of the effect of antipyresis by metamizol, propacetamol or external cooling on metabolism, hemodynamics and inflammatory response, *Intensive Care Med* 30(3):401, 2004.
Harchelroad F: Acute thermoregulatory disorders, *Clin Geriatr Med* 9:621, 1993.
Holtzclaw BJ: The febrile response in critical care: state of the science, *Heart Lung* 21(5):482, 1992.
Klein NC, Cunha BA: Treatment of fever, *Infect Dis Clin North Am* 10:211, 1996.
Kluger MJ: Fever: role of pyrogens and cryogens, *Physiol Rev* 71:93, 1991.
Kluger MJ, Kozak W, Conn CA et al: The adaptive value of fever, *Infect Dis Clin North Am* 10:1, 1996.
Koch-Weser J: Drug therapy. Acetaminophen, *N Engl J Med* 295:1297, 1976.
Kurz A, Sessler DI, Christensen R et al: Heat balance and distribution during core-temperature plateau in anesthetized humans, *Anesthesiology* 83:491, 1995.
Latman NS, Hans P, Nicholson L et al: Evaluation of clinical thermometers for accuracy and reliability, *Biomed Instrum Technol* 35:259, 2001.
Larson EL, Lin SX, Gomez-Picardo C et al: Effect of antibacterial home cleaning and handwashing products on infectious disease symptoms: a randomized, double-blinded trial, *Ann Intern Med* 140(5):321, 2004.
Mackowiak P, Plaisance KI: Benefits and risks of antipyretic therapy, *Ann N Y Acad Sci* 856:214, 1998.
McAlpine CH, Martin BJ, Lennox IM et al: Pyrexia in infection in the elderly, *Age Ageing* 15:230, 1986.
Mcilvoy L: Comparison of brain temperature to core temperature: a review of the literature, *J Neurosci Nurs* 36(1):23, 2004.
Morgan SP: A comparison of three methods of managing fever in the neurologic patient, *J Neurosci Nurs* 22:19, 1990.
Nierman D: Core temperature measurement in the intensive care unit, *Crit Care Med* 19:818, 1991.
Norman DC, Grahn D, Yoshikawa TT: Fever and aging, *J Am Geriatr Soc* 33:859, 1985.
Norman DC, Yoshikawa TT: Fever in the elderly, *Infect Dis Clin North Am* 10:93, 1996.
Pernerstorfer T, Schmid R, Bieglmayer C et al: Acetaminophen has greater antipyretic efficacy in endotoxemia: a randomized, double-blind, placebo-controlled trial, *Clin Pharmacol Ther* 66:51, 1999.
Plaisance KI: Toxicities of drugs used in the management of fever, *Clin Infect Dis* 31(suppl 5):S219, 2000.
Roberts NJ: The immunological consequences of fever. In Mackowiak PA, editor: *Fever: basic mechanisms and management,* New York, 1991, Raven Press.
Roghmann MC, Warner J, Mackowiak PA: The relationship between age and fever magnitude, *Am J Med Sci* 322:68, 2001.
Schmitz T, Bair N, Falk M et al: A comparison of five methods of temperature measurement in febrile intensive care patients, *Am J Crit Care* 4:286, 1995.
Smitz S, Giagoultsis T, Dewe W et al: Comparison of rectal and infrared ear temperatures in older hospital inpatients, *J Am Geriatr Soc* 48(1):63, 2000.
Styrt B, Sugarman B: Antipyresis and fever, *Arch Intern Med* 150:1589, 1990.
Varney SM, Manthey DE, Culpepper VE et al: A comparison of oral, tympanic, and rectal temperature measurement in the elderly, *J Emerg Med* 22:153, 2002.
Worfolk JB: Heat waves: their impact on the health of elders, *Geriatr Nurs* 21:70, 2000.

# Hypothermia

*Betty J. Ackley*

NANDA

## Definition

Body temperature below normal range

## Defining Characteristics

Pallor, reduction in body temperature below normal range, shivering, cool skin, cyanotic nailbeds, hypertension and then hypotension, piloerection, slow capillary refill, tachycardia

H

## Related Factors (r/t)

Exposure to cool or cold environment, use of medications causing vasodilation, malnutrition, inadequate clothing, illness or trauma, evaporation from skin in cool environment, decreased metabolic rate, damage to hypothalamus, consumption of alcohol, aging, inability or decreased ability to shiver, inactivity

NOC

## Outcomes (Nursing Outcomes Classification)

### Suggested NOC Outcomes

Thermoregulation; Thermoregulation: Newborn

**Example NOC Outcome with Indicators**

**Thermoregulation** as evidenced by the following indicators: Body temperature WNL/Skin temperature IER/No skin color changes /Hydration adequate/Reported thermal comfort (Rate each indicator of **Thermoregulation:** 1 = severely compromised, 2 = substantially compromised, 3 = moderately compromised, 4 = mildly compromised, 5 = not compromised [see Section I].)

IER, In expected range; WNL, within normal limits.

## Client Outcomes

### Client Will (Specify Time Frame):

- Maintain body temperature within normal range
- Identify risk factors of hypothermia
- State measures to prevent hypothermia
- Identify symptoms of hypothermia and actions to take when hypothermia is present

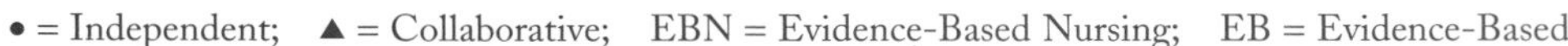

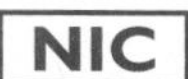

## Interventions (Nursing Interventions Classification)

### Suggested NIC Interventions

Hypothermia Treatment; Temperature Regulation; Temperature Regulation: Intraoperative; Vital Signs Monitoring

**Example NIC Activities—Temperature Regulation**

Institute use of a continuous core temperature–monitoring device, as appropriate; promote adequate fluid and nutritional intake

## Nursing Interventions and Rationales



- Remove the client from the cause of the hypothermic episode (e.g., cold environment, cold or wet clothing). Ensure that the client is in a warm environment. *The goal is to eliminate the causative or contributing factor and begin the warming process.*
- Watch the client for signs of hypothermia: shivering, slurred speech, clumsy movements, fatigue, confusion. As hypothermia progresses, the skin becomes pale, numb and waxy. Muscles are tense, fatigue and weakness progress, and gradually there can be loss of consciousness with loss of a pulse and breathing (Elliott, 2004).
- Cover the client with warm blankets and apply a covering to the head and neck to conserve body heat. *Layering of dry clothing including wearing a hat can be effective in warming a client with mild hypothermia (Elliott, 2004).*
- Take the temperature at least hourly; if more than mild hypothermia is present (temperature lower than 95° F [35° C]), use a continuous temperature-monitoring device.
- Use a pulmonary artery catheter temperature-measuring device if available; if not, consider using a bladder catheter that measures temperature. **EBN:** *Measurement of the pulmonary artery temperature is considered the gold standard in assessing core body temperature. If a pulmonary artery catheter is not appropriate for the client, temperature measurement with a temperature-sensitive indwelling urinary catheter can be effective and provide a reliable indication of core temperature (Erickson & Meyer, 1994; Fallis, 2002).*
- If the client is awake, measure the oral temperature, instead of the tympanic or axillary temperature. **EBN:** *Oral temperature measurement provides a more accurate temperature than tympanic measurement (Fisk & Arcona, 2001; Giuliano et al, 2000; Lee, McKenzie, & Cathcart, 1999). Axillary temperatures are often inaccurate (Fulbrook, 1997). The oral temperature is usually accurate even in an intubated client (Fallis, 2002). The SolarTherm and DataTherm devices correlated strongly with core body temperatures obtained from a pulmonary artery catheter (Smith, 2004).*
- Monitor the client's vital signs every hour and as appropriate. Note changes associated with hypothermia, such as initially increased pulse rate, respiratory rate, and blood pressure with mild hypothermia, and then decreased pulse rate, respiratory rate, and blood pressure with moderate to severe hypothermia. *With mild hypothermia, there is activation of the sympathetic nervous system, which can increase the values of vital signs.*

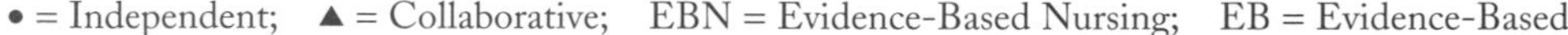

*As hypothermia progresses, decreased circulating volume develops, which results in decreased cardiac output and depressed oxygen delivery. Hypoxia, metabolic acidosis, and intrinsic irritability of a cold myocardium result in various dysrhythmias (Edwards, 1999; Ruffolo, 2002; Smith & Yamat, 2000).*

- Attach electrodes and a cardiac monitor. Watch for dysrhythmias. *With hypothermia the client is prone to dysrhythmias because of the cold myocardium; dysrhythmias may include atrial fibrillation, ventricular fibrillation, or asystole (McCullough & Arora, 2004; Ruffolo, 2002).*
- Monitor for signs of coagulopathy (e.g., oozing of blood from any open areas or from intravascular catheter sites or mucous membranes). Also note results of clotting studies as available. *Coagulopathy is a common occurrence during hypothermia in trauma clients (McCullough & Arora, 2004; Ruffolo, 2002).*

H

- For mild hypothermia (core temperature of 95° F [35° C ]), rewarm client passively:
  - ■ Set room temperature to 70° to 75° F (21° to 24° C).
  - ■ Keep the client dry, remove any damp or wet clothing.
  - ■ Layer clothing and blankets and cover the client's head; use insulated metallic blankets.
  - ■ Offer warm fluids and no alcohol or caffeine.

  *For mild hypothermia, allow the client to rewarm at his or her own pace. Heat is regained through the body's ability to generate heat. Passive rewarming is not encouraged for clients with temperatures lower than 82.4° F (28° C) because it is a slow process and may increase the risk of cardiac arrest in these circumstances (McCullough & Arora, 2004; Cochrane, 2001).*

▲ For moderate hypothermia (core temperature 89.6° to 82.4° F [32° to 28° C]) use active external rewarming methods. The rewarming rate should not exceed 1.8° F (1° C) per hour. Methods include the following:
  - ■ Forced-air warming systems
  - ■ Carbon-fiber blanket
  - ■ Electric blankets
  - ■ Radiant heat lights

  **EB:** *A study of four forced-air warming systems demonstrated the Bair Hugger system to was more effective in hear transfer from the periphery of the body to the core (Giesbrecht, Ducharme, & McGuire, 1994). Another study compared the effectiveness of the Bair Hugger versus a thermostat electric undermattress, the Bair Hugger raised the temperature faster (Janke, Pilkington, & Smith, 1996). Resistive heating using a carbon-fiber blanket was shown to be much more effective to rewarm hypothermic subjects than use of metallic-foil blankets (Greif et al, 2000). The carbon-fiber resistive heating blanket was shown to be more effective than regular blankets to maintain the client's core body temperatures during transport (Kober et al, 2001).*

▲ For severe hypothermia (core temperature below 82.4° F [28° C]) use active core-rewarming techniques:
  - ■ Recognize that continuous arteriovenous extracorporeal blood rewarming is most effective. NOTE: this requires cardiopulmonary bypass and not all facilities have this capability.

- ■ Administer heated and humidified oxygen through the ventilator as ordered.
- ■ Administer heated intravenous (IV) fluids at prescribed temperature.
- ■ Perform peritoneal lavage, bladder irrigations.

*Severe hypothermia is associated with acidosis, coma, ventricular fibrillation, apnea, thrombocytopenia, platelet dysfunction, impaired clotting, and increased mortality in trauma clients and requires prompt core body rewarming (Eddy, Morris, & Cullinane, 2000; McCullough & Arora, 2004).*

- • Check blood pressure frequently when rewarming; watch for hypotension. *As the body warms, formerly vasoconstricted vessels dilate, which results in hypotension (Edwards, 1999).*
- ▲ Administer IV fluids, using a rapid infuser IV fluid warmer as ordered. *Fluids are often needed to maintain adequate fluid volume. If the client develops untreated fluid depletion, hypotension with decreased cardiac output and acute renal failure can result (Edwards, 1999). A rapid infuser warmer is needed to keep IV fluids warmed sufficiently to be effective in raising the body temperature (Ruffolo, 2002).*
- • Determine the factors leading to the hypothermic episode; see Related Factors. *It is important to assess risk factors and precipitating events to prevent another incident of hypothermia and to direct treatment.*
- ▲ Request a social service referral to help the client obtain the heat, shelter, and food needed to maintain body temperature. *A preventive approach that includes adequate food and fluid intake, shelter, heat, and clothing decreases the risk of hypothermia.*
- ▲ Encourage proper nutrition and hydration. Request a referral to a dietitian to identify appropriate dietary needs. *Insufficient calorie and fluid intake predispose the client to hypothermia.*

H

## Pediatric

- • Recognize that pediatric clients have a decreased ability to adapt to temperature extremes. Take the following actions to maintain body temperature in the infant/child:
  - ■ Keep the head covered.
  - ■ Use blankets to keep the client warm.
  - ■ Keep the client covered during procedures, transport, and diagnostic testing.
  - ■ Keep the room temperature at 72° F (22.2° C).

  *These measures can help prevent hypothermia in the child, which is a very possible occurrence, especially in the pediatric trauma client (Bernardo & Henker, 1999). The combination of a relatively larger body surface area, smaller body fluid volume, less well-developed temperature control mechanisms, and smaller amount of protective body fat limits the infant's and child's ability to maintain normal temperatures (Hockenberry, 2005).*
- • For the preterm or low-birth-weight newborn, use specially designed bags, skin-to-skin care and transwarmer mattresses to keep preterm infants warm. **EB:** *These methods can help keep the vulnerable newborn warm in the delivery room, there is a need for more studies in this area (McCall et al, 2005).*

## Geriatric

- • Assess neurological signs frequently, watching for confusion and decreased level of

consciousness. *Older adults are less likely to shiver or complain of feeling cold. Early signs of hypothermia are subtle (McCullough & Arora, 2004).*
- Recognize that the elderly can develop indoor hypothermia from air conditioning or ice baths. Clients present with vague complaints of mental and/or other skill deterioration (McCullough & Arora, 2004).

### Home Care

NOTE: Hypothermia is not a symptom that appears in the normal course of home care. When it occurs, it is a clinical emergency and the client/family should access emergency medical services immediately.

- Some of the interventions described earlier may be adapted for home care use.
- Before a medical crisis occurs, confirm that the client or family has a thermometer and can read it. Instruct as needed. Verify that the thermometer registers accurately. *An accurate temperature is one indicator of the client's condition.*
- Instruct the client or family to take the temperature when the client displays cyanosis, pallor, or shivering.
- ▲ Monitor temperature every hour, as noted previously. If the temperature of the client begins dropping below the normal range, apply layers of clothing or blankets, or adjust environmental heat to the comfort level. Do not overheat. Contact a physician. *Passive rewarming is the only method of rewarming that is appropriate for home care under normal circumstances.*
- ▲ If temperature continues to drop, activate the emergency system and notify a physician. *Hypothermia is a clinically acute condition that cannot be managed safely in the home.*
- ▲ If the client is in hospice care or is terminally ill, follow advance directives, client wishes, and the physician's orders. Keep the client free of pain. *The goal of terminal care is to provide dignity and comfort during the dying process.*

## Client/Family Teaching

- Teach the client and family signs of hypothermia and the method of taking the temperature (age-appropriate).
- Teach the client methods to prevent hypothermia: wearing adequate clothing, including a hat and mittens; heating the environment to a minimum of 68° F (20° C); and ingesting adequate food and fluid. *Simple measures such as layering clothes, wearing a hat, and avoiding extremes in temperature prevent significant heat loss (Elliott, 2004; Laskowski-Jones, 2000).*
- ▲ Teach the client and family about medications such as sedatives, opioids, and anxiolytics that predispose the client to hypothermia (as appropriate). *If the client has had hypothermia in the past, using alternative medications is an option if there is no contraindication (Elliott, 2004).*

## evolve WEBSITES FOR EDUCATION

See the EVOLVE website for World Wide Web resources for client education.

## REFERENCES


Bernardo LM, Henker R: Thermoregulation in pediatric trauma: an overview, *Int J Trauma Nurs* 5(3):101, 1999.

Cochrane DA: Hypothermia: a cold influence on trauma, *Int J Trauma Nurs* 7(1):8, 2001.

Eddy VA, Morris JA, Cullinane DC: Hypothermia, coagulopathy, and acidosis, *Surg Clin North Am* 80(3):845, 2000.

Edwards S: Hypothermia, *Prof Nurse* 14(4):253, 1999.

Erickson RS, Meyer LT: Accuracy of infrared ear thermometry and other temperature methods in adults, *Am J Crit Care* 3(1):40, 1994.

Elliott F: You'd better watch out, *Occup Health Saf* 73(11):76, 2004.

Fallis WM: Monitoring urinary bladder temperature in the intensive care unit: state of the science, *Am J Crit Care* 11(1):38, 2002.

Fisk J, Arcona S: Comparing tympanic membrane and pulmonary artery catheter temperatures, *Dimens Crit Care Nurs* 20(2):44, 2001.

Fulbrook P: Core body temperature measurement: a comparison of axilla, tympanic membrane and pulmonary artery blood temperature, *Intensive Crit Care Nurs* 13(5):266, 1997.

Giesbrecht GG, Ducharme MB, McGuire JP: Comparison of forced-air patient warming systems for perioperative use, *Anesthesiology* 80(3):671, 1994.

Giuliano KK, Giuliano AJ, Scott SS et al: Temperature measurement in critically ill adults: a comparison of tympanic and oral methods, *Am J Crit Care* 9(4):254, 2000.

Greif R, Rajek A, Laciny S et al: Resistive heating is more effective than metallic-foil insulation in an experimental model of accidental hypothermia: a randomized controlled trial, *Ann Emerg Med* 35(4):337, 2000.

Hockenberry MJ: *Wong's essentials of pediatric nursing*, ed 7, St. Louis, 2005, Mosby.

Janke EF, Pilkington SN, Smith DC: Evaluation of two warming systems after cardiopulmonary bypass, *Br J Anaesth* 77(2):268, 1996.

Kober A, Scheck T, Fulesdi B et al: Effectiveness of resistive heating compared with passive warming in treating hypothermia associated with minor trauma: a randomized trial, *Mayo Clin Proc* 76(4):369, 2001.

Laskowski-Jones L: Responding to winter emergencies, *Nursing* 30(1):34, 2000.

Lee VK, McKenzie NE, Cathcart M: Ear and oral temperatures under usual practice conditions, *Res Nurs Pract* 1(1):8, 1999.

McCall E, Alderdice F, Halliday H et al: Interventions to prevent hypothermia at birth in preterm and/or low birth weight babies, *Cochrane Database Syst Rev* (1):CD004210, 2005.

McCullough L, Arora S: Diagnosis and treatment of hypothermia, *Am Fam Physician* 70(12):2325, 2004.

Ruffolo DC: Hypothermia in trauma: the cold, hard facts, *RN* 65(2):46, 2002.

Smith CE, Yamat RA: Avoiding hypothermia in the trauma patient, *Curr Opin Anaesthesiol* 13:167, 2000.

Smith LS: Temperature measurement in critical care adults: a comparison of thermometry and measurement routes, *Biol Res Nurs* 6(2):117, 2004.

WorfolkJB: Heat waves: their impact on the health of elders, *Geriatr Nurs* 21(2):70, 2000.


I

# Disturbed personal Identity

*Gail B. Ladwig*

**NANDA**

## Definition

Inability to distinguish between self and nonself

## Defining Characteristics

Withdrawal from social contact, change in ability to determine relationship of the body to the environment, inappropriate or grandiose behavior (Carpenito, 1993)

## Related Factors (r/t)

Situational crisis, psychological impairment, chronic illness, pain

**NOC**

## Outcomes (Nursing Outcomes Classification)

### Suggested NOC Outcomes

Identity, Anxiety Self-Control

**Example NOC Outcome with Indicators**

**Identity:** Verbalizes affirmations of personal identity/Exhibits congruent verbal and nonverbal behavior about self/Differentiates self from environment and other human beings (Rate each indicator of **Identity:** 1 = never demonstrated, 2 = rarely demonstrated, 3 = sometimes demonstrated, 4 = often demonstrated, 5 = consistently demonstrated [see Section I].)

I

## Client Outcomes

**Client Will (Specify Time Frame):**

- Show interest in surroundings
- Respond to stimuli with appropriate affect
- Perform self-care and self-control activities appropriate for age
- Acknowledge personal strengths
- Engage in interpersonal relationships
- Verbalize willingness to change lifestyle and use appropriate community resources

**NIC**

## Interventions (Nursing Interventions Classification)

### Suggested NIC Interventions

Self-Esteem Enhancement, Decision-Making Support

**Example NIC Activities—Self-Esteem Enhancement**

Monitor client's statements of self-worth; encourage client to identify strengths

## Nursing Interventions and Rationales

- Assess carefully for a history of abuse. **EB:** *The results obtained in this study through blind and independent assessment suggest that special trauma characteristics (i.e., childhood trauma perpetrated by a family member) rather than sheer cumulative effects of trauma may have greater implications for the development of pathological dissociation (Plattner et al, 2003).* **EB:** *This quantitative sample comprised a nonpsychiatric group (N = 39) of Australian adults reporting sexual abuse histories. The study revealed that current levels of posttraumatic and dissociative symptomatology were significantly higher in the group reporting* *sexual abuse by a perpetrator in a relationship of trust, guardianship, or authority (Leahy, Pretty, & Tenenbaum, 2004).*

- Assess for any history of seizure disorder; adhere to the diagnostic criteria for dissociative disorder in the *Diagnostic and Statistical Manual of Mental Disorders,* Fourth Edition (DSM-IV) and conduct a structured clinical interview. **EB:** *Misdiagnosis of persons with seizures and dissociative symptoms can be avoided by careful adherence to DSM-IV dissociative disorder criteria, the use of video-electroencephalographic monitoring, and systematic assessment of dissociative symptoms with the Structured Clinical Interview for DSM-IV (SCID-D) (Bowman & Coons, 2000).*
- Avoid labeling the client with terms such as multiple personality disorder (MPD). **EB:** *In one study more clients attempted suicide after being diagnosed with MPD than before diagnosis; the reverse was true for other clients hospitalized with a mood disorder (Fetkewicz, Sharma, & Merskey, 2000).*
- Spend time communicating with the client. **EBN:** *In a qualitative study, psychological well-being was found to be enhanced by humanistic and personal interaction with the nurse (Richardson, 2002).*
- Work with the client on setting personal goals. **EB:** *With the aid of a variety of psychotherapeutic methods, patients develop for themselves, in conjunction with their therapists, a concept for treatment, a guideline defining where they are and setting goals that are as realistic and concrete as possible. As a result the clinic's therapeutic program is more effective (Gierig & Hlsewiesche, 2002).*
- Address the client by name. Let the client know who is approaching and orient the client to the surroundings. *These interventions help the client with loss of ego boundaries to identify boundaries between him- or herself and the environment (Haber et al, 1992).*
- Provide communication, clear rules and aims, and safety procedures. **EBN:** *One study demonstrated that with these interventions the use of seclusion for aggressive client behavior was substantially reduced (Mistral et al, 2002).*
- Work with the client to utilize their senses to deescalate problem behavior. **EBN:** *Sensory-based approaches and multisensory rooms are valuable resources as cultures of care shift to become more responsive and collaborative. This article explores the importance and efficacy of trauma-informed approaches that are sensory supportive, address the individual needs of the person, and strengthen the therapeutic relationship (Champagne & Stromberg, 2004).*
- Give the client permission to share his or her experiences. *The client has always lived in secrecy and is not sure how much it is safe to reveal or who believes that the client's illness is an actual illness.* **EB:** *An average of 6.8 years elapses between the time clients are first assessed and the time they receive an accurate diagnosis (Frye, 1990).*
- Use touch only after a thorough assessment and as appropriate. *Touch, which conveys caring, is an appropriate way of communicating unless it makes the person touched feel uncomfortable (Wells-Federman et al, 1995).* **EBN:** *Some clients may touch people to identify separateness from others; other clients experience fusion with others when they touch (Haber et al, 1992).*

▲ Have all team members approach the client in a consistent manner. *Consistency promotes trust, which is necessary to establish a therapeutic relationship that helps the client develop interpersonal relationships.*

- Provide time for one-on-one interactions to establish a therapeutic relationship. **EBN:** *Nursing presence, one-on-one interaction, connecting with the client's experience, going beyond the scientific data, and knowing what will work and when to act all support the nurse-client relationship and affirm the respective selves of nurse and client. As a result, the client grows in awareness of his or her own being (Doona, Chase, & Haggerty, 1999).*
- Encourage the client to verbalize feelings about self and body image. Have the client make a list of strengths. **EB:** *These verbalizations help the client recognize the self; listing strengths promotes self-exploration. In one study 48 women in a psychiatric outpatient clinic completed a survey whose results indicated a correlation between borderline personality and body weight/body image issues that were not necessarily a result of larger size (Sansone, Wiederman, & Monteith, 2001).*
- Hold the client responsible for age-appropriate behavior. Involve the client in the planning of self-care. *Involving clients in care gives them a sense of control and helps clients gain ego strength (Preston, 1994).*

I

- Give positive feedback when appropriate self-control is used. **EB:** *When given positive feedback, the boys in one study were able to relax their defensive posture and offer more realistic self-assessment (Diener & Milich, 1997).*

▲ Encourage participation in group therapy for building relationship skills and getting feedback from others with regard to behavior. **EB:** *Findings suggest that social skills training resulted in greater improvement in certain measures of social adjustment than supportive group therapy (Marder et al, 1996).* **EBN:** *An adaptive narcissistic client's need to depend on other people to feel whole suggests that group therapy could be a powerful tool for treating those who suffer profound wounds to self-esteem (Kurek-Ovshinsky, 1991).*

- Encourage the client to use a daily diary to set achievable and realistic goals and to monitor successes. *Journal writing has been found to improve physical and mental health measurably (Wells-Federman et al, 1995).*

▲ Refer for rational emotive therapy to help dispel underlying irrational thinking. **EBN:** *Rational emotive behavior therapy proposes that psychological disturbance is largely created and maintained through irrational philosophies consisting of internal absolutistic demands. This therapy strives to produce sustained and profound cognitive, emotive, and behavioral change through active, vigorous disputation of underlying irrational philosophies (Sacks, 2004).*

## Geriatric

▲ Monitor for signs of depression, grief, and withdrawal and make an appropriate referral. *The disturbed personal identity may mask underlying depression.*

- Address the client by his or her full name preceded by the proper title (i.e., Mr., Mrs., Ms., Miss); use a nickname or first name only if suggested by the client, and do not use terms of endearment (e.g., "honey"). **EBN:** *Research findings emphasize the importance of relationship-oriented experiences as part of assessment and intervention strategies for individuals with depression (Hagerty & Williams, 1999).*
- Practice reality orientation principles; ask specifically how the client feels about events that are happening. **EB:** *Reality orientation therapy has benefits for both the cognition and behavior of dementia sufferers (Spector et al, 2000).*
- Ask the client about important past experiences. **EBN:** *Factors that influence self-*

*efficacy beliefs are personal expectations, personality, role models, verbal encouragement, progress, past experiences, spirituality, physical sensations, individualized care, social supports, and goals (Resnick, 2002).*

▲ If the client's symptoms are associated with a stroke, refer the client for longer rehabilitation that includes physical programs addressing psychological as well as neuromuscular issues. **EB:** *Clients who have had a stroke find the body unreliable, and the body appears separate from the self. These feelings may last a year or longer (Ellis-Hill, Payne, & Ward, 2000).*

## Multicultural

- Assess for the influence of cultural beliefs, norms, and values on the family's perceptions of infant/child behavior. **EBN:** *What the family considers normal infant/child behavior may be based on cultural perceptions (Cochran, 1998; Doswell & Erlen, 1998; Guarnaccia, 1998; Leininger & McFarland, 2002).*
- Use a neutral, indirect style when addressing areas in which improvement is needed, such as a need for verbal or oral stimulation, when working with Native-American clients. **EBN:** *Using indirect statements such as "Other mothers have tried . . ." or "I had a client who tried 'X,' and it seemed to work very well" help avoid resentment on the part of the parent (Seideman et al, 1996).*
- Acknowledge and praise parenting strengths noted. **EBN:** *This practice will increase trust and foster a working relationship with the parent (Seideman et al, 1996).*
- Use therapeutic communication techniques that emphasize acceptance, offer the self, validate the client's concerns, and convey respect when discussing infant/child behavior. **EBN:** *Validation is a therapeutic communication technique that lets the client know that the nurse has heard and understood what was said, and it promotes the nurse-client relationship (Heineken, 1998). Studies show that even when language is not a barrier, some ethnic clients may be reluctant to discuss their beliefs and practices because of fear of criticism or ridicule (Evans & Cunningham, 1996).*

## Home Care

- The interventions described previously may be adapted for home care use.
- Assess the client's immediate support system and family for relationship patterns and content of communication. *Knowledge of relationship dynamics in the client's environment assists the nurse in individualizing care.*
- Encourage the family to provide support and feedback regarding the client's identity and ego boundaries. *The family is a socially significant cultural group that generates behavior, defines roles, and promotes values.*

▲ If the client is involved in counseling or self-help groups, monitor and encourage attendance. Help the client identify the value of group participation after each group encounter. *Discussion of group participation identifies group feedback and support, and reinforces support for change.*

▲ If the client is taking prescribed psychotropic medications, assess for understanding of possible side effects and the reasons for taking medication. Teach as necessary.

▲ Assess medications for effectiveness and side effects and monitor for compliance. *Clients with poor ego strength may have difficulty adhering to a medication regimen.*

• = Independent; ▲ = Collaborative; EBN = Evidence-Based Nursing; EB = Evidence-Based

- ▲ If the client is homebound, refer for psychiatric home health care services for client reassurance and implementation of a therapeutic regimen. **EBN:** *Psychiatric home care nurses can address issues relating to the client's identity, reality testing, and reaction to identity disturbance. Behavioral interventions in the home can help the client to participate more effectively in the treatment plan (Patusky, Rodning, & Martinez-Kratz, 1996).*

## Client/Family Teaching

- • Teach stress reduction and relaxation techniques. These techniques can be used when the client becomes anxious about the loss of self.
- ▲ Refer to community resources or other self-help groups appropriate for the client's underlying problem (e.g., Adult Children of Alcoholics, parent effectiveness group). **EBN:** *Group therapy provides an arena in which clients can experience the interdependent mode of adaptation without assaults to self-esteem (Kurek-Ovshinsky, 1991).*
- ▲ Refer to appropriate treatment as soon as signs of depression are noted. **EB:** *Effective acute-phase depression treatment reduced somatic distress and improved self-rated overall health (Simon et al, 1998). Results of a study using clinical significance methodology and encompassing 4761 clients undergoing standard psychotherapy in the United States revealed that between 15 and 19 treatment sessions were required for a 50% recovery rate (Hansen et al, 2003).*
- • Be a role model for family members: talk to, not around, the client; give choices to the client when family members may be listening; always address the client by name; and do not interrupt when the client is attempting to communicate. **EBN:** *Validation is a therapeutic communication technique that lets the client know that the nurse has heard and understood what was said, and it promotes the nurse-client relationship (Heineken, 1998).*

I

## evolve WEBSITES FOR EDUCATION

See the EVOLVE website for World Wide Web resources for client education.

## REFERENCES

Bowman ES, Coons PM: The differential diagnosis of epilepsy, pseudoseizures, dissociative identity disorder, and dissociative disorder not otherwise specified, *Bull Menninger Clin* 64(2):164, 2000.

Carpenito LJ: *Nursing diagnosis: application to clinical practice,* ed 5, Philadelphia, 1993, JB Lippincott.

Cochran M: Tears have no color, *Am J Nurs* 98(6):53, 1998.

Champagne T, Stromberg N: Sensory approaches in inpatient psychiatric settings: innovative alternatives to seclusion and restraint, *J Psychosoc Nurs Ment Health Serv* 42(9):34-44, 2004.

Diener MB, Milich R: Effects of positive feedback on the social interactions of boys with attention deficit hyperactivity disorder: a test of the self-protective hypothesis, *J Clin Child Psychol* 26(3):256, 1997.

Doona M, Chase S, Haggerty L: Nursing presence: as real as Milky Way bar, *J Holist Nurs* 17(1):54, 1999.

Doswell W, Erlen J: Multicultural issues and ethical concerns in the delivery of nursing care interventions, *Nurs Clin North Am* 33(2):353, 1998.

Ellis-Hill CS, Payne S, Ward C: Self-body split: issues of identity in physical recovery following a stroke, *Disabil Rehabil* 22(16): 725, 2000.

Evans CA, Cunningham BA: Caring for the ethnic elder, *Geriatr Nurs* 17(3):105, 1996.

Fetkewicz J, Sharma V, Merskey H: A note on suicidal deterioration with recovered memory treatment, *J Affect Disord* 58(2):155, 2000.

Frye B: Art and multiple personality disorder: an expressive framework for occupational therapy, *Am J Occup Ther* 44:1013, 1990.

Gierig L, Hlsewiesche D: [Group of orientations: an systemic-draw-oriented beginning including the expression-centered method] [German], *Ergother Rehabil* 41(7):15-18, 2002.
Guarnaccia P: Multicultural experiences of family caregiving: a study of African American, European American, and Hispanic American families, *New Direct Ment Health Serv* 77:45, 1998.
Haber J et al: *Psychiatric nursing,* ed 4, St Louis, 1992, Mosby.
Hagerty BM, Williams RA: The effects of sense of belonging, social support, conflict, and loneliness on depression, *Nurs Res* 48(4):215, 1999.
Hansen NB, Lambert MJ: An evaluation of the dose-response relationship in naturalistic treatment settings using survival analysis, *Ment Health Serv Res* 5(1):1, 2003.
Heineken J: Patient silence is not necessarily client satisfaction: communication in home care nursing, *Home Healthc Nurse* 16(2): 115, 1998.
Kurek-Ovshinsky C: Group psychotherapy in an acute inpatient setting: techniques that nourish self-esteem, *Issues Ment Health Nurs* 12:81, 1991.
Leininger MM, McFarland MR: *Transcultural nursing: concepts, theories, research and practices,* ed 3, New York, 2002, McGraw-Hill.
Leahy T, Pretty G, Tenenbaum G: Perpetrator methodology as a predictor of traumatic symptomatology in adult survivors of childhood sexual abuse, *J Interpers Violence* 19(5):521-40, 2004.
Marder SR, Wirshing WC, Mintz J et al: Two-year outcome of social skills training and group psychotherapy for outpatients with schizophrenia, *Am J Psychiatry* 153(12):1585, 1996.
Mistral W, Hall A, McKee P: Using therapeutic community principles to improve the functioning of a high care psychiatric ward in the UK, *Int J Ment Health Nurs* 11(1):10, 2002.
Patusky KL, Rodning C, Martinez-Kratz M: Clinical lessons in psychiatric home care: a case study approach, *J Home Health Case Manag* 9:18, 1996.
Plattner B, Silvermann MA, Redlich AD et al: Pathways to dissociation: intrafamilial versus extrafamilial trauma in juvenile delinquents, *J Nerv Ment Dis* 191(12):781-788, 2003.
Preston K: Rehabilitation nursing: a client-centered philosophy, *Am J Nurs* 94:66, 1994.
Resnick B: Geriatric rehabilitation: the influence of efficacy beliefs and motivation, *Rehabil Nurs* 27(4):152, 2002.
Richardson J: Health promotion in palliative care: the patients' perception of therapeutic interaction with the palliative nurse in the primary care setting, *J Adv Nurs* 40(4):432, 2002.
Sacks SB: Rational emotive behavior therapy: disputing irrational philosophies, *J Psychosoc Nurs Ment Health Serv* 42(5):22-31, 2004.
Sansone RA, Wiederman MW, Monteith D: Obesity, borderline personality symptomatology, and body image among women in a psychiatric outpatient setting, *Int J Eat Disord* 29(1):76, 2001.
Seideman RY, Jacobson S, Primeaux M et al: Assessing American Indian families, *MCN Am J Matern Child Nurs* 21(6):274, 1996.
Simon GE, Katon W, Rutter C et al: Impact of improved depression treatment in primary care on daily functioning and disability, *Psychol Med* 28(3):693, 1998.
Spector A, Orrell M, Davies S et al: Reality orientation for dementia, *Cochrane Database Syst Rev* (4):CD001119, 2000.
Wells-Federman CL, Stuart EM, Deckro JP et al: The mind-body connection: the psychophysiology of many traditional nursing interventions, *Clin Nurse Spec* 9:59, 1995.

I

## Functional urinary Incontinence

evolve

*Mikel Gray*

**NANDA**

### Definition

Impairment or loss of continence due to functional deficits, including altered mobility, dexterity, or cognition, or environmental barriers

• = Independent; ▲ = Collaborative; EBN = Evidence-Based Nursing; EB = Evidence-Based

## Defining Characteristics

The relationship between functional limitations and urinary incontinence remains controversial (Hunskaar et al, 1999). Although functional impairment clearly exacerbates the severity of urinary incontinence, the underlying factors that contribute to these functional limitations themselves also contribute to abnormal lower urinary tract function and impaired continence

## Related Factors (r/t)

Cognitive disorders (delirium, dementia, severe or profound retardation); neuromuscular limitations impairing mobility or dexterity; environmental barriers to toileting

**NOC**

## Outcomes (Nursing Outcomes Classification)

I

### Suggested NOC Outcomes

Urinary Continence, Urinary Elimination

**Example NOC Outcome with Indicators**

**Urinary Continence** as evidenced by the following indicators: Recognizes urge to void/Responds in timely manner to urge/Voids in appropriate receptacle/Underclothing remains dry during day/Underclothing or bedding remains dry during night (Rate each indicator of **Urinary Continence:** 1 = never demonstrated, 2 = rarely demonstrated, 3 = sometimes demonstrated, 4 = often demonstrated, 5 = consistently demonstrated [see Section I].)

## Client Outcomes

**Client Will (Specify Time Frame):**

- Eliminate or reduce incontinent episodes
- Eliminate or overcome environmental barriers to toileting
- Use adaptive equipment to reduce or eliminate incontinence related to impaired mobility or dexterity
- Use portable urinary collection devices or urine containment devices when access to the toilet is not feasible

**NIC**

## Interventions (Nursing Interventions Classification)

### Suggested NIC Interventions

Urinary Habit Training, Urinary Incontinence Care

**Example NIC Activities—Urinary Habit Training**

Keep continence specification record for 3 days to establish voiding pattern; establish interval for toileting of preferably not less than 2 hours

## Nursing Interventions and Rationales

- Perform a history taking and physical assessment focusing on bothersome lower urinary tract symptoms, cognitive status, functional status (particularly physical mobility and dexterity), frequency and severity of leakage episodes, and alleviating and aggravating factors. *The history provides clues to the causes, the severity of the condition, and its management (Reuben et al, 1999; Vickerman, 2002).* **EBN:** *Results of physical assessment, functional evaluation (mobility toileting skills, physical examination), and evaluation of cognitive status (Folstein Mini-Mental State Examination) and psychological status (Geriatric Depression Scale) for a group of 90 homebound elders participating in a clinical trial revealed that functional impairments are associated with frequent and severe incontinence. Although these problems were perceived as particularly bothersome (despite multiple comorbid health issues), elders in this group remained optimistic about potential benefits of treatment (Folstein et al, 1975; McDowell et al, 1996).*
- ▲ Consult with the client and family, the client's physician, and other health care professionals concerning treatment of incontinence in the elderly client undergoing detailed geriatric evaluation. **EBN:** *Geriatric assessment units are designed to evaluate and assist clients and their families to deal with multiple problems experienced by geriatric clients, including urinary incontinence. In a study of 128 older adults recruited into a randomized clinical trial of behavioral treatment for urinary incontinence, although treatment was recommended for two thirds, nearly one third received no incontinence treatment recommendation. The recommendation for no treatment was based on a complex assessment of the client's physical health, comorbid conditions, and cognitive and psychological status (Silverman et al, 1997).*
- ▲ Teach the patient, the patient's care providers, or the family to complete a voiding diary (bladder log) by recording voiding frequency, the frequency of urinary incontinent episodes, and their association with urgency (a sudden and strong desire to urinate that is difficult to defer) over a 3- to 7-day period. An electronic voiding diary may be kept whenever feasible. In addition to these parameters, the patient may be asked to record voided volume and fluid intake. *The voiding diary provides a more objective record of lower urinary tract function than the oral history and it often provides a modest therapeutic effect by alerting the patient to factors that promote urinary incontinence episodes (Sampselle, 2003). An electronic voiding diary provides an efficient and possibly more accurate method for documenting these parameters (Quinn et al, 2003).*
- ▲ Assess the patient for potentially reversible or modifiable causes of acute/transient urinary incontinence (e.g., urinary tract infection; atrophic urethritis; constipation or impaction; use of sedatives or narcotics interfering with the ability to reach the toilet in a timely fashion, antidepressants or psychotropic medications interfering with efficient detrusor contractions, parasympatholytics, or alpha-adrenergic antagonists; polyuria caused by uncontrolled diabetes mellitus or insipidus). *Transient or acute incontinence may be relieved or eliminated by treating the underlying cause (Reilly, 2002).*
- Assess the client in an acute care or rehabilitation facility for risk factors for functional incontinence. **EBN:** *Risk factors for urinary incontinence among elderly women admitted to an acute care facility include confusion, use of a wheelchair or assistive device for walking, and dependence on others for ambulation prior to admission (Palmer et al, 2002).*
- Assess the client for coexisting or premorbid urinary incontinence. *Research involving*

*clients recovering from a stroke indicates that a history of premorbid urinary incontinence predicts a higher risk for persistent urinary leakage and poorer functional outcomes at 6 and 12 months (Jawad, Ward, & Jones, 1999; Thommessen, Bautz-Holter, & Laake, 1999).*

- Assess the home, acute care, or long-term care environment for accessibility to toileting facilities, paying particular attention to the following:
  - Distance of the toilet from the bed, chair, and living quarters
  - Characteristics of the bed, including presence of side rails and distance of the bed from the floor
  - Characteristics of the pathway to the toilet, including barriers such as stairs, loose rugs on the floor, and inadequate lighting
  - Characteristics of the bathroom, including patterns of use, lighting, height of the toilet from the floor, presence of handrails to assist transfers to the toilet, and breadth of the door and its accessibility for a wheelchair, walker, or other assistive device

  *Functional continence requires access to a toilet; environmental barriers blocking this access can produce functional incontinence (Wells, 1992).*

I

- Assess the client for mobility, including the ability to rise from chair and bed, transfer to the toilet, and ambulate, and the need for physical assistive devices such as a cane, walker, or wheelchair. *Functional continence requires the ability to gain access to a toilet facility, either independently or with the assistance of devices to increase mobility (Jirovec & Wells, 1990; Wells, 1992).*
- ▲ Assess the patient for dexterity, including the ability to manipulate buttons, hooks, snaps, loop and pile closure, and zippers as needed to remove clothing. Consult a physical or occupational therapist to promote optimal toilet access as indicated. *Functional continence requires the ability to remove clothing to urinate (Lekan-Rutledge, 2004; Maloney & Cafiero, 1999; Wells, 1992).*
- Evaluate cognitive status with a Neecham Confusion Scale (Neelan et al, 1992) in cases of acute cognitive change or with a Folstein Mini-Mental State Examination (Folstein et al, 1975) or other tool as indicated. *Functional continence requires sufficient mental acuity to respond to sensory input from a filling urinary bladder by locating the toilet, moving to it, and emptying the bladder (Maloney & Cafiero, 1999; McDowell et al, 1996).*
- Remove environmental barriers to toileting in the acute care, long-term care, or home setting. Assist the client in removing loose rugs from the floor and improving lighting in hallways and bathrooms. *Functional continence requires ready access to a urinal (Lekan-Rutledge, 2004; Wells, 1992).*
- Provide an appropriate, safe urinary receptacle such as a three-in-one commode, female or male hand-held urinal, no-spill urinal, or containment device when toileting access is limited by immobility or environmental barriers. *These receptacles provide access to a substitute toilet and enhance the potential for functional continence (Rabin, 1998; Wells, 1992).*
- ▲ Help the client with limited mobility to obtain evaluation by a physical therapist and to obtain assistive devices as indicated; assist the client in selecting shoes with a nonskid sole to maximize traction when arising from a chair and transferring to the

toilet. *A physical therapist is an important member of the interdisciplinary team needed to manage urinary incontinence in the client with functional impairments (Maloney & Cafiero, 1999).*

- Assist the client in altering the wardrobe to maximize toileting access. Select loose-fitting clothing with stretch waistbands rather than buttoned or zippered waist; minimize buttons, snaps, and multilayered clothing; and substitute a loop and pile closure or other easily loosened systems for buttons, hooks, and zippers in existing clothing.
- Begin a prompted voiding program or patterned urge response toileting program for the elderly client in the home or a long-term care facility who has functional incontinence and dementia:
  - Determine the frequency of current urination using an alarm system or check-and-change device.
  - Record urinary elimination and incontinent patterns in a bladder log to use as a baseline for assessment and evaluation of treatment efficacy.
  - Begin a prompted toileting program based on the results of this program; toileting frequency may vary from every 1.5 to 2 hours to every 4 hours.
  - Praise the client when toileting occurs with prompting.
  - Refrain from any socialization when incontinent episodes occur; change the client and make her or him comfortable.

  **EBN:** *Prompted voiding or patterned urge response toileting executed during waking hours has been shown to markedly reduce or eliminate functional incontinence in selected clients in long-term care facilities and in the community setting (Colling et al, 1992; Eustice, Roe, & Patterson, 2000; Engberg et al, 2002). It has not been shown to be effective for the reduction of nighttime voiding frequency or nocturnal enuresis in nursing home residents (Ouslander et al, 2001).*

## Geriatric

- Institute aggressive continence management programs for the cognitively intact, community-dwelling client in consultation with the client and family. *Uncontrolled incontinence can lead to institutionalization of an elderly person who prefers to remain in a home care setting (O'Donnell et al, 1992).*
- Monitor the elderly client in a long-term care facility, acute care facility, or home for dehydration. *Dehydration can exacerbate urine loss, produce acute confusion, and increase the risk of morbidity and morality, particularly in the frail elderly client (Colling, Owen, & McCreedy, 1994).*

## Home Care

- The interventions described previously may be adapted for home care use.
- Assess current strategies used to reduce urinary incontinence, including limitation of fluid intake, restriction of bladder irritants, prompted or scheduled toileting, and use of containment devices. *Many elderly clients and care providers use a variety of self-management techniques to control urinary incontinence, such as fluid limitation, avoidance of social contacts, and use of absorptive materials, that may or may not be effective for reducing urinary leakage or beneficial to general health (Johnson, 2000).*

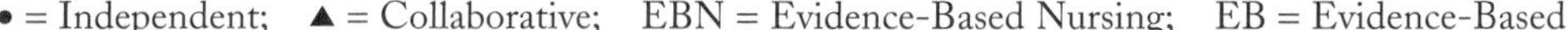

- Encourage a mind-set and program of self-care management. **EBN:** *Addressing self-care activities through exercise, diet, fluid intake, and use of protective devices helps the client to exercise control over incontinence (Leenerts, Teel, & Pendleton, 2002).*
- Implement a bladder-training program, including self-monitoring activities (e.g., reducing caffeine intake, adjusting amount and timing of fluid intake, decreasing long voiding intervals while awake, instituting dietary changes to promote bowel regularity); bladder training; and pelvic muscle exercise. **EBN:** *In one study of women age 55 years or older with involuntary urine loss associated with stress, urge, or mixed incontinence, clients responded to the aforementioned interventions with a 61% decrease in the severity of urinary incontinence at 2 years after intervention. Self-monitoring and bladder training accounted for most of the improvement (Dougherty et al, 2002).*
- For a memory-impaired elderly client, implement an individualized scheduled toileting program (on a schedule developed in consultation with the caregiver, approximately every 2 hours, with toileting reminders provided and existing patterns incorporated, such toileting before or after meals). **EBN:** *Functional incontinence in memory-impaired elderly clients decreased significantly with the described intervention. The client must be able to cooperate for the intervention to be followed (Jirovec & Templin, 2001).*
- Teach the family the general principles of bladder health, including avoidance of bladder irritants, adequate fluid intake, and a routine schedule of toileting. Refer to the care plan for **Impaired Urinary elimination**).
- Teach prompted voiding to the family and client for the client with mild to moderate dementia (refer to previous description) (Colling, 1996; McDowell et al, 1999).
- Teach the principles of perineal skin care to the patient or care provider, including routine cleansing following incontinent episodes, daily cleaning and drying of perineal skin, and the use of moisture barriers as indicated. *Routine cleansing and daily cleaning with appropriate products help maintain the integrity of perineal skin and prevent secondary cutaneous infections (Gray, 2004; Gray, Ratliff, & Donovan, 2002).*
- Advise the client about the advantages of using disposable or reusable insert pads, pad-pant systems, or replacement briefs specifically designed for urinary incontinence (or double urinary and fecal incontinence) as indicated. **EBN:** *Many absorptive products used by community-dwelling elders are not designed to absorb urine, prevent odor, and protect the perineal skin (McClish et al, 1999). Disposable or reusable absorptive devices specifically designed to contain urine or double incontinence are more effective than household products, particularly in cases of moderate to severe incontinence (Gallo & Staskin, 1997; Shirran & Brazelli, 2000).*
- Assist the family with arranging care in a way that allows the client to participate in family or favorite activities without embarrassment. Elicit discussion of the client's concerns about the social or emotional burden of incontinence. **EBN and EB:** *Careful planning can allow the dignity and integrity of family patterns to be retained. Urinary incontinence has a demonstrated influence on subjective well-being and quality of life, with depression, loneliness, or sadness possible (Fultz & Herzog, 2001). Discussing emotional concerns helps the client to develop a sense of control over incontinence (Leenerts, Teel, & Pendleton, 2002).*

▲ Refer to occupational therapy for help in obtaining assistive devices and adapting the home for optimal toilet accessibility.

- ▲ Consider the use of an indwelling catheter for continuous drainage in the client who is both homebound and bed bound and is receiving palliative or end-of-life care (requires a physician's order). *An indwelling catheter may increase client comfort, ease care provider burden, and prevent urinary incontinence in bed-bound clients receiving end-of-life (palliative) care (Gray & Campbell, 2001).*
- ▲ When an indwelling catheter is in place, follow prescribed maintenance protocols for managing the catheter, drainage bag, perineal skin, and urethral meatus. Teach infection control measures adapted to the home care setting. *Proper care reduces the risk of catheter-associated urinary tract infection.* **EBN:** *Multivariate analysis of data for a group of 106 home care clients demonstrated that frequent catheter changes increased the risk of a symptomatic urinary tract infection by approximately 12-fold compared with catheter changes every 4 weeks or less often (White & Ragland, 1995).*
- • Assist the client in adapting to the catheter. Encourage discussion of the client's response to the catheter. **EBN:** *Clients living with a catheter are often keenly aware of its presence; adaptation is served by normalizing the experience. Instruction could include the fact that the client will be more aware of some sensations and sounds (e.g., urine sloshing in the bag, the weight of the bag, pressure or pain when urine flow has been altered). Rehearsing emptying of the bag when away from home will support resumption of activities. Discussion of the client's response will assist him or her in dealing with embarrassment or frustration (Wilde, 2002).*

I

## Client/Family Teaching

- • Work with the client, family, and their extended support systems to assist with needed changes in the environment and wardrobe, and other alterations required to maximize toileting access.
- • Work with the client and family to establish a reasonable, manageable prompted voiding program using environmental and verbal cues to remind caregivers of voiding intervals, such as television programs, meals, and bedtime.
- • Teach the family to use an alarm system for toileting or to carry out a check-and-change program and to maintain an accurate log of voiding and incontinence episodes.

## evolve WEBSITES FOR EDUCATION

See the EVOLVE website for World Wide Web resources for client education.

## REFERENCES

Colling J: Noninvasive strategies to manage urinary incontinence among care-dependent persons, *J Wound Ostomy Continence Nurs* 23:302, 1996.

Colling J, Owen TR, McCreedy MR: Urine volumes and voiding patterns among incontinent nursing home residents, *Geriatr Nurs* 15:188, 1994.

Colling J, Ouslander J, Hadley BJ et al: The effects of patterned urge response toileting (PURT) on urinary incontinence among nursing home residents, *J Am Geriatr Soc* 40:135, 1992.

Dougherty MC, Dwyer JW, Pendergast JF et al: A randomized trial of behavioral management for continence with older rural women, *Res Nurs Health* 25:3, 2002.

Engberg S, Sereika SM, McDowell BJ et al: Effectiveness of prompted voiding in treating urinary incontinence in cognitively impaired homebound older adults, *J Wound Ostomy Continence Nurs* 29(5):252-265, 2002.

Eustice S, Roe B, Paterson J: Prompted voiding for the management of urinary incontinence in adults, *Cochrane Database Syst Rev* CD002113, 2000.

Folstein MF, Folstein SE, McHugh PR: Mini-mental state: a practical method of grading the cognitive state of patients for the clinician, *J Psychiatr Res* 12(3):189, 1975.

Fultz NH, Herzog AR: Self-reported social and emotional impact of urinary incontinence, *J Am Geriatr Soc* 49:892, 2001.

Gallo M, Staskin DR: Patient satisfaction with a reusable undergarment for urinary incontinence, *J Wound Ostomy Continence Nurs* 24:226, 1997.

Gray M: Preventing and managing perineal dermatitis: a shared goal for wound and continence care, *J Wound Ostomy Continence Nurs* 31(1 Suppl):S2-S9, 2004.

Gray M, Campbell F: Urinary tract disorders. In Ferrell B, Coyle N, editors: *Textbook of palliative nursing,* Oxford, England, 2001, Oxford University Press.

Gray M, Ratliff C, Donovan A: Perineal skin care for the incontinent patient, *Adv Skin Wound Care* 15:170, 2002.

Hunskaar S et al: Epidemiology and natural history of urinary incontinence. In Abrams P, Khoury S, Wein A, editors. *Incontinence,* Plymouth, England, 1998, Health Publication, Plymbridge Distributors.

Jawad SH, Ward AB, Jones P: Study of the relationship between premorbid urinary incontinence and stroke functional outcome, *Clin Rehabil* 13(5):447, 1999.

Jirovec MM, Templin T: Predicting success using individualized scheduled toileting for memory-impaired elders at home, *Res Nurs Health* 24:1, 2001.

Jirovec MM, Wells TJ: Urinary incontinence in nursing home residents with dementia: the mobility-cognition paradigm, *Appl Nurs Res* 3:112, 1990.

Johnson ST: From incontinence to confidence, *Am J Nurs* 100(2):69, 2000.

Leenerts MH, Teel CS, Pendleton MK: Building a model of self-care for health promotion in aging, *J Nurs Sch* 34:355, 2002.

Lekan-Rutledge D: Urinary incontinence strategies for frail elderly women, *Urol Nurs* 24(4):281-302, 2004.

Maloney C, Cafiero M: Implementing an incontinence program in long-term care settings: a multidisciplinary approach, *J Gerontol Nurs* 25:47, 1999.

McClish DK, Wyman JF, Sale PG et al: Use and costs of incontinence pads in female study volunteers, *J Wound Ostomy Continence Nurs* 26(4):207, 1999.

McDowell BJ, Engberg S, Sereika S et al: Effectiveness of behavioral therapy to treat incontinence in homebound older adults, *J Am Geriatr Soc* 47(3):309, 1999.

McDowell BJ, Engberg SJ, Rodriguez E et al: Characteristics of urinary incontinence in homebound older adults, *J Am Geriatr Soc* 44(8):963, 1996.

Neelan VJ et al: Use of the NEECHAM confusion scale to assess acute confusional states of hospitalized older patients. In Funk SG et al, editors: *Key aspects of elder care: managing falls, incontinence and cognitive impairment,* New York, 1992, Springer.

O'Donnell BF, Drachman DA, Barnes HJ et al: Incontinence and troublesome behaviors predict institutionalization in dementia, *J Geriatr Psychiatry Neurol* 5:45, 1992.

Ouslander JG, Greendale GA, Uman G et al: Effects of oral estrogen and progestin on the lower urinary tract among female nursing home residents, *J Am Geriatr Soc* 49(6):803-807, 2001.

Palmer MH, Baumgarten M, Langenberg P et al: Risk factors for hospital acquired incontinence in elderly female hip fracture patients, *J Gerontol A Biol Sci Med Sci* 57(10):M672, 2002.

Rabin JM: Clinical use of the FemAssist device in female urinary incontinence, *J Med Syst* 22:257, 1998.

Quinn P, Goka J, Richardson H: Assessment of an electronic daily diary in patients with overactive bladder, *BJU Int* 91(7):647-652, 2003.

Reilly N: Assessment and management of acute or transient urinary incontinence. In Doughty D, editor: *Urinary and fecal incontinence: nursing management,* ed 2, St Louis, 2002, Mosby.

Resnick NM, Beckett LA, Branch LG et al: Short term variability of self-report of incontinence in older persons, *J Am Geriatr Soc* 42:202, 1994.

Reuben DB: A randomized clinical trial of outpatient comprehensive geriatric assessment coupled with an intervention to increase adherence to recommendations, *J Am Geriatr Soc* 47(3):269, 1999.

Sampselle CM: Bladder matters. Teaching women to use a voiding diary: what 'mind over bladder' can accomplish, *Am Nurs* 103(11):62-64, 2003.

Shirran E, Brazelli M: Absorbent products for the containment of urinary and/or fecal incontinence, *Cochrane Database Syst Rev* CD0011406, 2000.

Silverman M, McDowell BJ, Musa D et al: To treat or not to treat: issues in decisions not to treat older persons with cognitive impairment, depression, and incontinence, *J Am Geriatr Soc* 45(9):1094, 1997.
Thommessen B, Bautz-Holter E, Laake K: Predictors of outcome of rehabilitation of elderly stroke patients in a geriatric ward, *Clin Rehabil* 13(2):123, 1999.
Vickerman J: Thorough assessment of functional incontinence, *Nurs Times* 98(28):58, 2002.
Wells TJ: Managing incontinence through managing the environment, *Urol Nurs* 12:48, 1992.
White MC, Ragland KE: Urinary catheter related infections among home care patients, *J Wound Ostomy Continence Nurs* 22:286, 1995.
Wilde MH: Urine flowing: a phenomenological study of living with a urinary catheter, *Res Nurs Health* 25:14, 2002.

# Reflex urinary Incontinence

*Mikel Gray*

I

**NANDA**

## Definition

Involuntary loss of urine at somewhat predictable intervals when a specific bladder volume is reached (North American Nursing Diagnosis Association International [NANDA-I], 2005). Involuntary loss of urine caused by a defect in the spinal cord between the nerve roots at or below the first cervical segment and those above the second sacral segment. Urine elimination occurs at unpredictable intervals; micturition may be elicited by tactile stimuli, including stroking of inner thigh or perineum (Gray, 2003).

## Defining Characteristics

Urinary incontinence caused by neurogenic detrusor overactivity; disruption of spinal pathways leads to absent or diminished awareness of the desire to void or the occurrence of an overactive detrusor contraction; incomplete bladder emptying caused by dyssynergia of striated sphincter mechanism, which produces functional outlet obstruction of bladder; reflex urinary incontinence may be associated with sweating and acute elevation in blood pressure and pulse rate in clients with spinal cord injury. Refer to the care plan for **Autonomic dysreflexia**

## Related Factors (r/t)

Paralyzing spinal disorder affecting spinal segments C1 to S2

**NOC**

## Outcomes (Nursing Outcomes Classification)

### Suggested NOC Outcomes

Urinary Continence, Urinary Elimination

**Example NOC Outcome with Indicators**

**Urinary Continence** as evidenced by the following indicators: Absence of urinary leakage between catheterizations or containment of micturition by condom catheter and drainage bag/Absence of urinary tract infection (absence of leukocytes and absence of bacterial growth or >100,000 colony-forming units per milliliter)/Underclothing dry during day/Underclothing or bedding dry during night (Rate each indicator of **Urinary Continence:** 1 = never demonstrated, 2 = rarely demonstrated, 3 = sometimes demonstrated, 4 = often demonstrated, 5 = consistently demonstrated [see Section I].)

## Client Outcomes

### Client Will (Specify Time Frame):

- Follow prescribed schedule for bladder evacuation
- Demonstrate successful use of triggering techniques to stimulate voiding
- Have intact perineal skin
- Remain clear of symptomatic urinary tract infection
- Demonstrate how to apply containment device or insert indwelling catheter or be able to provide caregiver with instructions for performing these procedures
- Demonstrate awareness of risk of autonomic dysreflexia, its prevention, and management

I

NIC

## Interventions (Nursing Interventions Classification)

### Suggested NIC Interventions

Urinary Catheterization: Intermittent; Urinary Elimination Management; Urinary Incontinence Care

**Example NIC Activities—Urinary Elimination Management**

Monitor urinary elimination including frequency, consistency, odor, volume, and color as appropriate; teach client signs and symptoms of urinary tract infection

## Nursing Interventions and Rationales

- Assess the client's neurological status, including the type of neurological disorder, the functional level of neurological impairment, its completeness (effect on motor and sensory function), and the ability to perform bladder management tasks, including intermittent catheterization, application of a condom catheter, and so on. *In clients with a single, well-circumscribed neurological lesion, knowledge of the level of the lesion strongly correlates with bladder function. In contrast, this correlation is weak in clients with multilevel cord trauma due to secondary bleeding or swelling (Weld, Graney, & Dmochowski, 2000).*
- Knowledge of functional impairments related to a spinal cord injury, including upper extremity function, is essential because it determines the client's ability to manage the bladder by self-catheterization (Gray, 2000).

- Perform a focused assessment of the urinary system, including perineal skin integrity. *Urinary and fecal incontinence associated with neurogenic bladder and bowel dysfunction in the client with a paralyzing disorder predisposes the perineal skin to irritant dermatitis and secondary infection, particularly when a urine containment device such as an adult containment brief or condom catheter is used (Gray 2004; Gray, Ratliff, & Donovan, 2002).*
- Complete a bladder log to determine the pattern of urine elimination, incontinence episodes, and current bladder management program. *The bladder log provides an objective record of urine elimination that confirms the accuracy of the historical report, and a baseline for assessment and evaluation of treatment efficacy (Gray, 2000).*

▲ Consult with the physician concerning current bladder function and the potential of the bladder to produce upper urinary tract distress (hydronephrosis, vesicoureteral reflux, febrile urinary tract infection, or compromised renal function). **EBN:** *Both nursing and medical research demonstrate that reflex incontinence is typically accompanied by detrusor striated sphincter dyssynergia, which increases the risk of upper urinary tract distress (Gray et al, 1991; Killorin et al, 1992; Weld et al, 2000).*

▲ Determine a bladder management program in consultation with the client, family, and rehabilitation team. **EBN:** *The bladder management program profoundly affects the client and significant others; it is determined by holistic assessment that addresses the potential of the bladder to create upper urinary tract distress, the potential for incontinence and related complications, client and family preference, and the perceived impact of the bladder management program on the client's lifestyle (Anson & Gray, 1993; Gray, Rayome, & Anson 1995).*

▲ In consultation with the rehabilitation team, counsel the client and family concerning the merits and potential risks associated with each possible bladder management program, including spontaneous voiding, intermittent self-catheterization, reflex voiding with condom catheter containment, and indwelling catheterization. *All bladder management programs carry some risk of urinary incontinence or serious urinary system complications (Wyndaele et al, 2001).* **EBN:** *Spontaneous voiding and intermittent catheterization carry greater risk of urine loss than condom catheter containment or indwelling catheter, but these latter strategies carry higher risk for serious urinary system complications, including upper urinary tract distress, when evaluated over a period of years (Anson & Gray, 1993; Gray, Rayome, & Anson, 1995).*

- Teach the client with reflex incontinence to consume an adequate amount of fluids on a daily basis (approximately 30 mL/kg of body weight). *Evidence from a systematic literature review reveals that dehydration exacerbates urine loss and increases the risk of related complications, including constipation and urinary tract infection. Increasing fluid intake has also been associated with a diminished risk for bladder cancer, which is particularly important for the patient managed by long-term indwelling catheterization (Gray & Krissovich, 2003).*
- Advise clients that while consumption of cranberry products or cranberry tablets is in no way harmful or contraindicated, it does not reduce the risk for urinary tract infection. **EB:** *A randomized clinical trial involving a small number of patients with spinal cord injury and neurogenic bladder dysfunction found that consumption of 400 mg of cranberry tablets showed that it does not reduce the risk for urinary tract infection as has*

*been demonstrated in community-dwelling women without neurogenic bladder dysfunction (Linsenmeyer et al, 2004).*

• Teach the client with reflex urinary incontinence that is managed by spontaneous voiding to self-administer an alpha-adrenergic blocking medication as directed and to recognize and manage potential side effects. *Clients who spontaneously urinate may take an alpha-adrenergic blocking drug to reduce urethral resistance during voiding (Linsenmeyer, Horton, & Benevento, 2002).*

▲ Begin intermittent catheterization using a modified clean or sterile technique based on facility policies. *Modified clean intermittent catheterization may be used in an inpatient setting with appropriate staff and client education.*

▲ Teach intermittent catheterization as the client approaches discharge as directed. Instruct the client and at least one family member, spouse, or partner in the performance of catheterization using clean technique. Teach the client with quadriplegia how to instruct others to perform this procedure. **EBN:** *Both nursing and medical research demonstrates that intermittent catheterization is a safe and effective bladder management strategy for persons with reflex urinary incontinence. Inclusion of a family member, spouse, or significant other is particularly helpful for the client with limited upper extremity dexterity and reflex urinary incontinence (Anson & Gray, 1993; Chai et al, 1995; Gray, Rayome, & Anson, 1995; Shekelle et al, 1999). Additional research now supports the safety and effectiveness of intermittent catheterization among children with spinal cord injuries and reflex urinary incontinence (Generao et al, 2004).*

I

▲ Teach the client managed by intermittent catheterization to self-administer antispasmodic (parasympatholytic) medications as directed, and to recognize and manage potential side effects. *Antimuscarinic medications enhance catheterized volumes and reduce the frequency of incontinence episodes in persons with reflex incontinence owing to spinal cord injury or multiple sclerosis (Ethans et al, 2004).*

▲ Consult with the physician and occupational therapist concerning the use of a neuroprosthesis or other device designed to improve hand use for the quadriplegic client with partial hand function. *Use of a neuroprosthetic device designed to improve hand function increases clients' independence when performing multiple functions, including bladder management. The high initial costs associated with these devices may be offset by reductions in costs related to partially dependent bladder management over a period of approximately 5 years (Creasey et al, 2000).*

▲ For a male client with reflex incontinence who cannot manage the condition effectively with spontaneous voiding, does not choose to perform intermittent catheterization, or cannot perform catheterization, teach the client and his family to obtain, select, and apply a condom catheter with drainage bag. Assist them in choosing a product that adheres to the penile shaft without allowing seepage of urine onto surrounding skin or clothing, contains a material and adhesive that does not produce hypersensitivity reactions on the skin, and includes a leg bag that is easily concealed under the clothing and does not cause irritation to the skin of the thigh. *Multiple components of the condom catheter affect the product's ability to contain urinary leakage, protect underlying skin, and preserve the client's dignity (Joseph et al, 1998; Watson, 1989; Watson & Kuhn, 1990).*

• Teach the client who uses a condom catheter to remove the condom device, inspect the skin, cleanse the penis thoroughly, and reapply a new catheter every day. *The risk of urinary tract infection increases if a condom catheter is worn for longer than 24 hours (Hirsh, Fainstein, & Musher, 1979).*

- Teach the client whose incontinence is managed by a condom catheter to routinely inspect the skin with each catheter change for evidence of lesions caused by pressure from the containment device or by exposure to urine. *Skin breakdown is a common complication associated with routine use of the condom catheter (Anson & Gray, 1993).*
- Teach the client managed by intermittent or indwelling catheter to recognize signs of significant urinary tract infection and to seek care promptly when these signs occur. The signs of significant infection are the following:
  - Discomfort over the bladder or during urination
  - Acute onset of urinary incontinence
  - Fever
  - Markedly increased spasticity of muscles below the level of the spinal lesion
  - Malaise, lethargy
  - Hematuria
  - Autonomic dysreflexia (hyperreflexia) (Siroky, 2002)

  *Intermittent catheterization is typically associated with asymptomatic bacteriuria, and the indwelling catheter is routinely associated with asymptomatic colonization. Antibiotic treatment of asymptomatic bacteriuria has not proven helpful (Morton et al, 2002; Murphy & Lampert, 2003), but prompt management of significant infection is necessary to prevent urosepsis or related complications (Siroky, 2002).*

## Geriatric

▲ If difficulties are encountered in client teaching, refer the elderly client to a nurse who specializes in care of the aging client with urinary incontinence.

## Home Care

- The interventions described previously may be adapted for home care use. Teach the client what the complications of reflex incontinence are and when to report changes to a physician or primary nurse. *Early detection allows for rapid diagnosis and treatment before irreversible damage to the renal parenchyma occurs (Burns, Rivas, & Ditunno, 2001).*

▲ If the client is taught intermittent self-catheterization, arrange for contingency care in the event that the client is unable to perform self-catheterization. *Although self-catheterization has proved to be an effective and safe bladder management strategy, acute illness or surgery may render the client unable to perform self-catheterization and temporarily reliant on others to carry out this critical task (Joseph et al, 1998).*

- Assess and instruct the client and family in care of the catheter and supplies in the home. *Proper care of supplies reduces the risk of infection (Joseph et al, 1998).*
- Encourage a mind-set and program of self-care management. **EBN:** *Addressing self-care activities through exercise, diet, fluid intake, and protective devices helps the client to exercise control over incontinence (Leenerts, Teel, & Pendleton, 2002).*
- Assist the family with arranging care in a way that allows the client to participate in family or favorite activities without embarrassment. Elicit discussion of the cli-

ent's concerns about the social or emotional burden of incontinence. **EBN and EB:** *Careful planning can help the client retain dignity and maintain the integrity of family patterns. Urinary incontinence has a demonstrated influence on subjective well-being and quality of life, with depression, loneliness, or sadness possible (Fultz & Herzog, 2001). Discussing emotional concerns helps the client to develop a sense of control over incontinence (Leenerts, Teel, & Pendleton, 2002).*

▲ If medications are ordered, instruct the family or caregivers and the client in medication administration, use, and side effects. *Adherence to a medication regimen increases its chances of success and decreases the risk of losing the regimen as an option for care when other alternatives are unacceptable.*

## Client/Family Teaching

- Teach the client with a spinal injury the signs of autonomic dysreflexia, its relationship to bladder fullness, and management of the condition. Refer to the care plan for **Autonomic dysreflexia.**
- Teach the client and several significant others the techniques of intermittent catheterization, indwelling catheter care and removal, or condom catheter management as appropriate.
- Teach the client and family techniques to clean catheters used for intermittent catheterization, including washing with soap and water and allowing to air dry, and using microwave cleaning techniques.

I

## evolve WEBSITES FOR EDUCATION

See the EVOLVE website for World Wide Web resources for client education.

## REFERENCES


Anson C, Gray ML: Secondary complications after spinal cord injury, *Urol Nurs* 13:107, 1993.

Burns AS, Rivas DA, Ditunno JF: The management of neurogenic bladder and sexual dysfunction after spinal cord injury, *Spine* 26(Suppl 24):S129, 2001.

Chai T, Chung AK, Belville WD et al: Compliance and complications of clean intermittent catheterization in the spinal cord injured patient, *Paraplegia* 33:161, 1995.

Creasey GH, Kilgore KL, Brown-Triolo DL et al: Reduction of costs of disability using neuroprostheses, *Assist Technol* 12(1):67, 2000.

Dougherty MC, Dwyer JW, Pendergast JF et al: A randomized trial of behavioral management for continence with older rural women, *Res Nurs Health* 25:3, 2002.

Ethans KD, Nance PW, Bard RJ et al: Efficacy and safety of tolterodine in people with neurogenic detrusor overactivity, *J Spinal Cord Med* 27(3):214-218, 2004.

Fultz NH, Herzog AR: Self-reported social and emotional impact of urinary incontinence, *J Am Geriatr Soc* 49:892, 2001.

Generao SE, Dall'era JP, Stone AR et al: Spinal cord injury in children: long-term urodynamic and urological outcomes, *J Urol* 172(3):1092-1094, 2004.

Gray M: Preventing and managing perineal dermatitis: a shared goal for wound and continence care, *J Wound Ostomy Continence Nurs* 31(Suppl 1):S2-S9, 2004.

Gray M: Reflex urinary incontinence. In: Doughty DB, editor: *Urinary and fecal incontinence: nursing management,* ed 2, St Louis, 2000, Mosby.

Gray M, Krissovich M: Does fluid intake influence the risk for urinary incontinence, urinary tract infection and bladder cancer? *J Wound Ostomy Continence Nurs* 30(3):126-131, 2003.

Gray M, Ratliff C, Donovan A: Perineal skin care for the incontinent patient, *Adv Skin Wound Care* 15:170, 2002.

Gray M, Rayome RG, Anson C: Incontinence and clean intermittent catheterization following spinal cord injury, *Clin Nurs Res* 4:6, 1995.
Gray ML et al: Urethral pressure gradient in the prediction of upper urinary tract distress following spinal cord injury, *J Am Paraplegia Soc* 14:105, 1991.
Hirsh DD, Fainstein V, Musher DM: Do condom catheter collecting systems cause urinary tract infection? *JAMA* 242:340, 1979.
Joseph AC et al: Nursing clinical practice guideline: neurogenic bladder management, *SCI Nurs* 15(2):21, 1998.
Killorin W, Gray M, Bennett JK et al: Evaluative urodynamics and bladder management in the prediction of upper urinary infection in male spinal cord injury, *Paraplegia* 30:437, 1992.
Leenerts MH, Teel CS, Pendleton MK: Building a model of self-care for health promotion in aging, *J Nurs Scholarsh* 34:355, 2002.
Linsenmeyer TA, House JG, Millis SR: The role of abnormal congenitally displaced ureteral orifices in causing reflux following spinal cord injury, *J Spinal Cord Med* 27(2):116-119, 2004.
Linsenmeyer TA, Horton J, Benevento J: Impact of alpha$_1$-blockers in men with spinal cord injury and upper tract stasis, *J Spinal Cord Med* 25(2):124, 2002.
Morton SC, Shekelle PG, Adams JL et al: Antimicrobial prophylaxis for urinary tract infection in persons with spinal cord dysfunction, *Arch Phys Med Rehabil* 83(1):129, 2002.
Murphy DP, Lampert V: Current implications of drug resistance in spinal cord injury, *Am J Phys Med Rehabil* 82(1):72, 2003.
Pannek J, Sommerfeld HJ, Botel U et al: Combined intravesical and oral oxybutynin chloride in adult patients with spinal cord injury, *Urology* 55(3):358, 2000.
Shekelle PG, Morton SC, Clark KA et al: Systematic review of risk factors for urinary tract infection in adults with spinal cord dysfunction, *J Spinal Cord Med* 22(4):258, 1999.
Siroky MB: Pathogenesis of bacteriuria and infection in the spinal cord injured patient, *Am J Med* 113(suppl 1A):67S, 2002.
Watson R: A nursing trial of urinary sheath systems on male hospitalized patients, *J Adv Nurs* 14:467, 1989.
Watson R, Kuhn M: The influence of component parts on the performance of urinary sheath systems, *J Adv Nurs* 15:417, 1990.
Weld KJ, Graney MJ, Dmochowski RR: Clinical significance of detrusor sphincter dyssynergia in patients with post traumatic spinal cord injury, *Urology* 56:565, 2000.
Weld KJ, Wall BM, Mangold TA et al: Influences on renal function in chronic spinal cord injured patients, *J Urol* 164(5):1490, 2000.
Wyndaele JJ, Madersbacher H, Kovindha A: Conservative treatment of the neuropathic bladder in spinal cord injured patients, *Spinal Cord* 39(6):294, 2001.



# Stress urinary Incontinence

*Mikel Gray*

**NANDA**

## Definition

State in which the individual experiences urine loss of less than 50 mL accompanied by increased intraabdominal pressure
NOTE: The value of less than 50 mL for the volume of urine loss may be exceeded by women and men with severe stress incontinence caused by incompetence of the urethral sphincter mechanism. This is sometimes classified as *total incontinence.* In this book, however, *total incontinence* will be used to refer exclusively to incontinence due to extraurethral causes, and all forms of stress incontinence are reviewed under this diagnosis, regardless of severity.

## Defining Characteristics

Observed urine loss with physical exertion (sign of stress incontinence); reported loss of urine associated with physical exertion or activity (symptom of stress incontinence); urine loss associated with increased abdominal pressure (urodynamic stress urinary incontinence) (Abrams et al, 2002)

## Related Factors (r/t)

Urethral hypermobility/pelvic organ prolapse (familial predisposition, multiple vaginal deliveries, delivery of infant large for gestational age, forceps-assisted or breech delivery, obesity, changes in estrogen levels at climacteric, extensive abdominopelvic or pelvic surgery); urethral sphincter mechanism incompetence (multiple urethral suspensions in women, radical prostatectomy in men, uncommon complication of transurethral prostatectomy or cryosurgery of prostate, spinal lesion affecting sacral segments 2 to 4 or cauda equina, pelvic fracture)

NOC



## Outcomes (Nursing Outcomes Classification)

### Suggested NOC Outcomes

Urinary Continence, Urinary Elimination

**Example NOC Outcome with Indicators**

**Urinary Continence** as evidenced by the following indicators: Experiences no urine loss with physical activity or exertion, coughing, sneezing, or other maneuvers that precipitously raise abdominal pressure/Voids in appropriate receptacle/Able to move to toilet after strong desire to urinate is perceived/Underclothing remains dry during day/Underclothing or bedding remains dry during night (Rate each indicator of **Urinary Continence:** 1 = never demonstrated, 2 = rarely demonstrated, 3 = sometimes demonstrated, 4 = often demonstrated, 5 = consistently demonstrated [see Section I].)

## Client Outcomes

**Client Will (Specify Time Frame):**

- Report fewer stress incontinence episodes and/or a decrease in the severity of urine loss
- Experience reduction in grams of urine loss measured objectively by a pad test
- Experience reduction in frequency of urinary incontinence episodes as recorded on voiding diary (bladder log)
- Identify containment devices that assist in management of stress incontinence

NIC

## Interventions (Nursing Interventions Classification)

### Suggested NIC Intervention

Pelvic Muscle Exercises, Urinary Incontinence Care

**Example NIC Activities—Urinary Incontinence Care**

Explain etiology of problem and rationale for actions; modify clothing and environment to provide easy access to toilet

## Nursing Interventions and Rationales

- Take a focused history addressing duration of urinary leakage and related lower urinary tract symptoms, including daytime voiding frequency, urgency, frequency of nocturia, frequency of urinary leakage, and factors provoking urine loss. *A careful description of bothersome lower urinary tract symptoms helps identify the cause of urine loss and optimal treatment options (Addison, 1999).* **EBN:** *A historical report of urine loss with physical exertion correlates well with objective findings of stress urinary incontinence on physical examination or urodynamic testing. In contrast, the symptom of urge incontinence, when reported as an isolated finding, is a poor predictor of consistent urge incontinence. Querying clients about the symptom of urge incontinence, in combination with daytime voiding frequency and nocturia, greatly improves the predictive power of a nursing history in the evaluation of urinary incontinence.*
- Perform a focused physical assessment, beginning with perineal skin assessment. *Urinary incontinence, particularly when combined with fecal incontinence or use of larger containment devices such as adult containment briefs, increases the risk for irritant dermatitis and secondary monilial or bacterial infection (Gray, 2004; Gray, Ratliff, & Donovan, 2002).*
- Attempt to reproduce the sign of stress urinary incontinence by asking the patient to perform Valsalva maneuver or to cough while observing the urethral meatus for urine loss. **EBN:** *Urine loss, the sign of stress urinary incontinence, can be reproduced by asking the patient to perform provocative maneuvers (cough or perform Valsalva maneuver) during physical examination. Mild to moderate stress urinary incontinence can be reproduced by asking the patient to perform these maneuvers while standing and holding a paper towel in front of the urethral meatus (Miller et al, 1998a). More recent research has demonstrated that urine loss volumes less than 1 mL can be detected using this technique (Neumann et al, 2004). Among patient with moderately severe to severe cases, associated with urethral sphincter mechanism incompetence, the sign of stress urinary incontinence can be elicited even when the patient is lying in a supine position and has as little as 10 mL of urine in the bladder vesicle. Nevertheless, it is strongly recommended that the patient be tested in both supine and upright positions and with a moderately filled bladder (Walter et al, 2004).*
- Perform a focused pelvic examination, including visual inspection of the vaginal mucosa, observation of urethral hypermobility and related pelvic floor descent (prolapse), and digital assessment of pelvic floor muscle strength. **EBN:** *Digital assessment of pelvic muscle strength is completed by asking the female patient to contract the pelvic floor muscles after placing one to two gloved fingers in the vaginal vault (Brink et al, 1989, 1992). Pelvic floor muscle strength can be similarly evaluated in men during the digital rectal examination. A review of more contemporary studies has revealed mixed evidence*

*concerning the relationship of a digital assessment of pelvic floor muscle strength with dynamic manometric measurements, but it remains a well-accepted technique for determining the overall strength of the pelvic floor muscles and the patient's ability to identify, contract, and relax this muscle group (Morin et al, 2004; Isherwood et al, 2000).*

- • Determine the client's current use of containment devices; evaluate the devices for their ability to adequately contain urine loss, protect clothing, and control odor. Assist the client in identifying containment devices specifically designed to contain urinary leakage. **EBN:** *Clients, particularly women, tend to select feminine hygiene pads for urine containment. These devices, designed to contain menstrual flow, are not well-suited to address urine loss (McClish et al, 1999).*
- • Teach the patient to complete a voiding diary (bladder log) by recording voiding frequency, the frequency of urinary incontinent episodes and their association with urgency (a sudden and strong desire to urinate that is difficult o defer) over a 3- to 7-day period. An electronic voiding diary may be kept whenever feasible. In addition to these parameters, the patient may be asked to record voided volume and fluid intake. *The voiding diary provides a more objective record of lower urinary tract function than the oral history, and it often provides a modest therapeutic effect by alerting the patient to factors that promote urinary incontinence episodes (Sampselle, 2003). An electronic voiding diary provides an efficient and possibly more accurate method for documenting these parameters (Quinn et al, 2003).*
- ▲ With the client and in close consultation with the physician, review treatment options, including behavioral management; drug therapy; use of a pessary, vaginal device, or urethral insert; and surgery. Outline their potential benefits, efficacy, and side effects. *Multiple treatments have been used to manage stress incontinence; behavioral management options should be offered initially (Burns, 2000).*
- ▲ Assess the client's pelvic muscle strength immediately prior to initiating a pelvic floor muscle rehabilitation using pressure manometry, a digital evaluation technique, or urine stop test. **EBN:** *A baseline of pelvic muscle strength is needed for initial assessment and for evaluation of treatment efficacy. Digital vaginal examination, a urine stream interruption test, or measurement of pelvic floor muscle contraction strength by a fluid-filled balloon are valid and reliable techniques for assessing pelvic floor muscle strength and contractile function (Brink et al, 1992; Sampselle & DeLancey, 1992; Worth, Dougherty, & McKey, 1986).*
- • Begin a pelvic floor muscle rehabilitation program. *Pelvic floor muscle rehabilitation is effective in the treatment of stress and mixed urinary incontinence (Bo, Talseth, & Holme, 1999; Hay-Smith et al, 2004).*
- • Teach the client undergoing pelvic muscle rehabilitation to identify, contract, and relax the pelvic floor muscles without contracting distant muscle groups (e.g., abdominal muscles) using tactile, audible, or visual biofeedback techniques. *Pelvic muscle rehabilitation is enhanced by the use of biofeedback (Berghmans et al, 1996; Bump et al, 1991).*
- • Incorporate principles of exercise physiology into a pelvic muscle rehabilitation program using the following strategies:
  - ■ Begin a graded exercise program, usually starting with 5 to 10 repetitions and ad-

vancing gradually to no more than 35 to 50 repetitions every day or every other day based on baseline and ongoing evaluation of maximal strength and endurance.
- ■ Continue exercise sessions over a period of 3 to 6 months.
- ■ Integrate muscle training into activities of daily living.
- ■ Assess progress every 2 weeks during the first month and every 4 to 6 weeks thereafter.

**EBN:** *Pelvic muscle rehabilitation alleviates or cures stress incontinence using a combination of techniques, including biofeedback and strength training. Application of principles of physiotherapy maximizes the value of pelvic muscle rehabilitation (Brink et al, 1992; Dougherty et al, 1991, 1992; Johnson, 2001; Nygaard et al, 1996).*

- • Alternatively, female patient may be taught to pelvic muscle rehabilitation using weighted vaginal cones. **EBN:** *Weighted vaginal cones help women increase pelvic floor muscle tone and function and alleviate stress urinary incontinence (Laycock et al, 2001). A systematic review of existing research suggests that the efficacy of weighted cones may be comparable to that achieved by pelvic muscle rehabilitation, but more comparative studies are needed before a definitive conclusion can be reached (Hebrison et al, 2004).*
- ▲ Begin transvaginal or transrectal electrical stimulation therapy in selected persons with stress incontinence in consultation with the client and physician. *Electrical stimulation alleviates stress incontinence in selected clients, probably by strengthening the pelvic muscles and possibly through a biofeedback effect (Sand et al, 1995).*
- • Teach the principles of bladder training to women with stress urinary incontinence:
  - ■ Assist the client in completing a voiding diary over a period of a minimum of 3 days or up to 7 days.
  - ■ Review the results with the client, determining typical voiding frequency and establishing goals for voiding frequency.
  - ■ Using baseline voiding frequency, as determined by the diary, teach the client to urinate by the clock when awake, typically every 30 to 120 minutes.
  - ■ Encourage adherence to the program with timing devices, as well as verbal encouragement and support, and address individual reasons for schedule interruption.
  - ■ Gradually increase the time between urinations to the negotiated goal. Time intervals between voiding are typically increased in increments of 15 to 30 minutes for clients with a baseline frequency of less than every 60 minutes and increments of 25 to 30 minutes for clients with a baseline frequency of more than every 60 minutes.

  **EBN:** *Bladder training reduces the frequency and severity of urinary leakage in women with stress incontinence, urge incontinence, and mixed incontinence. Research suggests that the results of bladder training in ambulatory, community-dwelling women is comparable to that achieved through pelvic floor muscle rehabilitation (Theofrastus et al, 2002; Elser et al, 1999; Wyman et al, 1998).*
- ▲ Teach the client to self-administer alpha-adrenergic agonist medications, imipramine, and topical estrogens as directed. *Pharmacotherapeutic agents alleviate or temporarily cure stress incontinence in selected women (Andersson, 2000; Radley et al, 2000).*
- ▲ Refer the female patient with stress urinary incontinence and pelvic organ prolapse who wishes to employ a pessary, vaginal device, or urethral insert to manage stress incontinence to a nurse specialist or gynecologist with expertise in the placement and

I

maintenance of these devices. *Pessaries, vaginal devices, and urethral inserts alleviate or correct stress incontinence; however, they may cause serious complications unless inserted correctly and monitored closely (Frazer et al, 2000). When fitted by an individual with adequate expertise, approximately 90% of bothersome symptoms associated with pelvic organ prolapse and 50% of lower urinary tract symptoms resolved, although occult stress urinary incontinence is uncovered in approximately 21% (Clemons et al, 2004).*

- Discuss potentially reversible or controllable risk factors with the client with stress incontinence and assist the client to formulate a strategy to alleviate or eliminate these conditions. *Although research supports a strong familial predisposition to stress incontinence among women, other risk factors associated with the condition, including obesity and chronic coughing from smoking, are reversible (Mushkat, Bukovsky, & Langer, 1996; Skoner, Thompson, & Caron, 1994).*
- ▲ Provide information about support resources such as the Simon Foundation for Continence or the National Foundation for Continence.
- ▲ Refer the client with persistent stress incontinence to a continence service, physician, or nurse who specializes in the management of this condition. **EBN:** *Complex stress incontinence can be successfully managed by a multidisciplinary approach (McDowell et al, 1996).*

I

### Geriatric

- Evaluate the elderly client's functional and cognitive status to determine the effect of functional limitations on the frequency and severity of urine loss and on plans for management.

### Home Care

- The interventions described previously may be adapted for home care use.
- Elicit discussion of the client's concerns about the social or emotional burden of stress incontinence. **EBN and EB:** *Urinary incontinence has a demonstrated influence on subjective well-being and quality of life, with depression, loneliness, or sadness possible (Fultz & Herzog, 2001). Discussing emotional concerns helps the client to develop a sense of control over incontinence (Leenerts, Teel, & Pendleton, 2002).*
- Encourage a mind-set and program of self-care management. **EBN:** *Addressing self-care activities through exercise, diet, fluid intake, and protective devices helps the client to exercise control over incontinence (Leenerts, Teel, & Pendleton, 2002).*
- Implement a bladder-training program, including self-monitoring activities (reducing caffeine intake, adjusting amount and timing of fluid intake, decreasing long voiding intervals while awake, making dietary changes to promote bowel regularity), bladder training, and pelvic muscle exercise. **EBN:** *In one study of women age 55 years or older with involuntary urine loss associated with stress, urge, or mixed incontinence, clients responded to the aforementioned interventions with a 61% decrease in the severity of urinary incontinence at 2 years after intervention. Self-monitoring and bladder training accounted for most of the improvement (Dougherty et al, 2002).*
- ▲ Consider the use of an indwelling catheter for continuous drainage in the client with severe stress urinary incontinence who is homebound, bed-bound, and receiving palliative or end-of-life care (requires a physician's order). *An indwelling catheter may in-*

*crease client comfort, ease caregiver burden, and prevent urinary incontinence in bed-bound clients receiving end-of-life care.*

- ▲ When an indwelling catheter is in place, follow the prescribed maintenance protocols for managing the catheter, drainage bag, and perineal skin and urethral meatus. Teach infection control measures adapted to the home care setting. *Proper care reduces the risk of catheter-associated urinary tract infection.*
- • Assist the client in adapting to the catheter. Encourage discussion of the client's response to the catheter. **EBN:** *Clients living with a catheter are keenly aware of its presence; adaptation is served by normalizing the experience. Instruction could include the fact that the client will be more aware of some sensations and sounds (e.g., urine sloshing in the bag, the weight of the bag, pressure or pain when urine flow has been altered). Rehearsing emptying of the bag when away from home will support resumption of activities. Discussion of the client's response will help him or her to deal with embarrassment or frustration (Wilde, 2002).*
- • Begin a program of pelvic muscle rehabilitation in the homebound elderly client who is motivated to adhere to the program and has adequate cognitive function to understand and follow instructions. **EBN:** *Homebound elders are capable of completing a program of pelvic muscle rehabilitation and achieving clinically relevant relief from stress and urge urinary incontinence.*

I

## Client/Family Teaching

- • Teach the client to perform pelvic muscle exercise using an audiotape or videotape if indicated
- • Teach the client the importance of avoiding dehydration and instruct the client to consume fluid at the rate of 30 mL/kg of body weight daily (0.5 ounce/pound/day).
- • Teach the client the importance of avoiding constipation by a combination of adequate fluid intake, adequate intake of dietary fiber, and exercise.
- • Teach the client to apply and remove support devices such as a urethral insert.
- • Teach the client to select and apply urine containment devices.

## evolve WEBSITES FOR EDUCATION

See the EVOLVE website for World Wide Web resources for client education.

## REFERENCES


Abrams P, Cardozo L, Fall M et al: The standardization of terminology of lower urinary tract function: report from the Standardisation Sub-committee of the International Continence Society, *Am J Obstet Gynecol* 187(1):116, 2002.

Addison R: Assessment of stress incontinence, *Nurs Times* 95(45):10, 1999.

Andersson KE: Drug therapy for urinary incontinence, *Best Pract Res Clin Obstet Gynecol* 14(2):291, 2000.

Berghmans LC, Frederiks CM, de Bie RA et al: Efficacy of biofeedback when included with pelvic muscle exercise treatment for stress incontinence, *Neurourol Urodyn* 15:37, 1996.

Bo K, Talseth T, Holme I: Single blind, randomized controlled trial of pelvic floor exercises, electrical stimulation, vaginal cones, and no treatment of genuine stress incontinence in women, *BMJ* 318:487, 1999.

Brink CA et al: Pelvic muscle exercise for elderly incontinence women. In Funk SG et al, editors: *Key aspects of elder care: managing falls, incontinence and cognitive impairment,* New York, 1992, Springer.

Brink CA, Sampselle CM, Wells TJ et al: A digital test for pelvic muscle strength in older women with urinary incontinence, *Nurs Res* 38(4):196-199, 1989.
Bump RC, Hurt WG, Fantl JA et al: Assessment of Kegel pelvic muscle exercise performance after brief verbal instruction, *Am J Obstet Gynecol* 165(2):322, 1991.
Burns PA: Stress incontinence. In Doughty DB, editor: *Urinary and fecal incontinence: nursing management,* ed 2, St Louis, 2000, Mosby.
Clemons JL, Aguilar VC, Tillinghast TA et al: Patient satisfaction and changes in prolapse and urinary symptoms in women who were fitted successfully with a pessary for pelvic organ prolapse *Am Obstet Gynecol* 190(4):1025-1029, 2004.
Dougherty MC et al: Graded exercise: effect of pressures developed by the pelvic muscles. In Funk SG et al, editors: *Key aspects of elder care: managing falls, incontinence and cognitive impairment,* New York, 1992, Springer.
Dougherty MC, Dwyer JW, Pendergast JF et al: A randomized trial of behavioral management for continence with older rural women, *Res Nurs Health* 25:3, 2002.
Dougherty MC, Bishop KR, Mooney RA et al: Variation in intravaginal pressure measurements, *Nurs Res* 40:282, 1991.
Elser DM, Wyman JF, McClish DK et al: The effect of bladder training, pelvic floor muscle training, or combination training on urodynamic parameters in women with urinary incontinence. Continence Program for Women Research Group, *Neurourol Urodyn* 18(5):427, 1999.
Frazer M et al: Mechanical devices for urinary incontinence in women, *Cochrane Database System Rev* (4), 2000.
Fultz NH, Herzog AR: Self-reported social and emotional impact of urinary incontinence, *J Am Geriatr Soc* 49:892, 2001.
Gray M: Preventing and managing perineal dermatitis: a shared goal for wound and continence care, *J Wound Ostomy Continence Nurs* 31(Suppl 1): S2-S9, 2004.
Gray M, Ratliff C, Donovan A: Perineal skin care for the incontinent patient, *Adv Skin Wound Care* 15:170, 2002.
Hay-Smith EJC et al: Pelvic floor muscle training for urinary incontinence in women, *Cochrane Database Syst Rev* (1):CD001407, last updated July 2004.
Herbison P, Plevnik S, Mantle J: Weighted vaginal cones for urinary incontinence, *Cochrane Database Syst Rev* (2):CD002114, last updated July 2004.
Isherwood PJ, Rane A: Comparative assessment of pelvic floor strength using a perineometer and digital examination, *BJOG* 107(8):1007-11, 2000.
Johnson VY: How the principles of exercise physiology influence pelvic floor muscle training, *J Wound Ostomy Continence Nurs* 28(3):150, 2001.
Laycock J, Brown J, Cusack C et al: Pelvic floor reeducation for stress incontinence: comparing three methods, *Br J Community Nurs* 6(5):230, 2001.
Leenerts MH, Teel CS, Pendleton MK: Building a model of self-care for health promotion in aging, *J Nurs Scholarsh* 34:355, 2002.
McClish DK, Wyman JF, Sale PG et al: Use and costs of incontinence pads in female study volunteers, *J Wound Ostomy Continence Nurs* 26(4):207, 1999.
McDowell BJ, Burgio KL, Dombrowski M et al: An interdisciplinary approach to the assessment and behavioral treatment of urinary incontinence in geriatric outpatients, *Kango Kenkyu* 29(5):425, 1996.
Miller JM, Ashton-Miller JA, Delancey JO: Quantification of cough-related urine loss using the paper towel test, *Obstet Gynecol* 91(5 pt 1):705, 1998a.
Miller JM, Ashton-Miller JA, DeLancey JO: A pelvic muscle precontraction can reduce cough-related urine loss in selected women with mild SUI, *J Am Geriatr Soc* 46(7):870-874, 1998b.
Morin M, Dumoulin C, Bourbonnais D et al: Pelvic floor maximal strength using vaginal digital assessment compared to dynamometric measurements, *Neurourol Urodyn* 23(4):336-341, 2004.
Mushkat Y, Bukovsky I, Langer R: Female urinary stress incontinence—does it have familial prevalence? *Am J Obstet Gynecol* 174: 617, 1996.
Neumann P, Blizzard L, Grimmer K et al: Expanded paper towel test: an objective test of urine loss for stress incontinence, *Neurourol Urodyn* 23(7):649-655, 2004.
Nygaard IE, Kreder KJ, Lepic MM et al: Efficacy of pelvic floor muscle exercise in women with stress, urge and mixed urinary incontinence, *Am J Obstet Gynecol* 174:120, 1996.
Quinn P, Goka J, Richardson H: Assessment of an electronic daily diary in patients with overactive bladder, *BJU Int* 91(7):647-652, 2003.
Radley SC et al: Alpha adrenergic drugs for urinary incontinence in women, *Cochrane Database System Rev* (4), 2000.
Sampselle CM: Bladder matters. Teaching women to use a voiding diary, *Am J Nurs* 103(11): 62-4, 2003.

Sampselle CM, DeLancey JOL: The urine stream interruption test and pelvic muscle function, *Nurs Res* 41:73, 1992.
Sand PK, Richardson DA, Staskin DR et al: Pelvic floor electrical stimulation in the treatment of genuine stress incontinence: a multicenter placebo controlled trial, *Am J Obstet Gynecol* 173:72, 1995.
Skoner MM, Thompson WD, Caron VA: Factors associated with risk of stress urinary incontinence in women, *Nurs Res* 43:301, 1994.
Theofrastous JP, Wyman JF, Bump RC et al: Effects of pelvic floor muscle training on strength and predictors of response in the treatment of urinary incontinence, *Neurourol Urodyn* 21(5):486-490, 2002.
Walter AJ, Thornton JA, Steele AC: Further characterization of the supine empty stress test for predicting low valsalva leak point pressures, *Int Urogynecol J* 15(5):298-301, 2004.
Wilde MH: Urine flowing: a phenomenological study of living with a urinary catheter, *Res Nurs Health* 25:14, 2002.
Worth AM, Dougherty MC, McKey PL: Development and testing of the circumvaginal muscle (CVM) rating scale, *Nurs Res* 35: 166, 1986.
Wyman JF, Fantl JA, McClish DK et al: Comparative efficacy of behavioral interventions in the management of female urinary incontinence. Continence Program for Women Research Group, *Am J Obstet Gynecol* 179(4):999, 1998.

# Total urinary Incontinence

evolve



*Mikel Gray*

NANDA

## Definition

State in which the individual experiences continuous and unpredictable loss of urine
NOTE: In this book, the diagnosis **Total urinary Incontinence** will be used to refer to continuous urine loss due to an extraurethral cause, and the diagnosis **Stress urinary Incontinence** will be used to refer to leakage caused by urethral sphincter incompetence, regardless of severity.

## Defining Characteristics

Continuous urine flow varying from dribbling incontinence superimposed on an otherwise identifiable pattern of voiding to severe urine loss without identifiable micturition episodes

## Related Factors (r/t)

Ectopia (ectopic ureter opens into vaginal vault or cutaneously; bladder ectopia with exstrophy/epispadias complex); fistula (opening from bladder or urethra to vagina or skin that bypasses urethral sphincter mechanism, allowing continuous urine loss)

NOC

## Outcomes (Nursing Outcomes Classification)

### Suggested NOC Outcomes

Tissue Integrity: Skin and Mucous Membranes; Urinary Continence; Urinary Elimination

**Example NOC Outcome with Indicators**

**Tissue Integrity: Skin and Mucous Membranes** as evidenced by the following indicators: Tissue lesion free/Skin intact (Rate each indicator of **Tissue Integrity: Skin and Mucous Membranes:** 1 = extremely compromised, 2 = substantially compromised, 3 = moderately compromised, 4 = mildly compromised, 5 = not compromised [see Section I].)

## Client Outcomes

### Client Will (Specify Time Frame):

- Experience urine loss that is adequately contained, with clothing remaining unsoiled and odor controlled
- Maintain intact perineal skin
- Maintain dignity, hide urine containment device in clothing, and minimize bulk and noise related to device



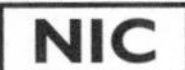

## Interventions (Nursing Interventions Classification)

### Suggested NIC Intervention

Urinary Incontinence Care

**Example NIC Activities—Urinary Incontinence Care**

Provide protective garments as needed; cleanse genital skin at regular intervals

## Nursing Interventions and Rationales

- • Obtain a history of the duration and severity of urine loss, prior management, and aggravating or alleviating features. *Urinary incontinence from an extraurethral source (fistula or ectopia) is often confused with other forms of incontinence. Total incontinence should be suspected whenever the client reports continuous urine loss irrespective of physical exertion or associated urgency (Flores-Carreras et al, 2001).*
- • Perform a focused physical assessment, including inspection of the perineal skin, examination of the vaginal vault, reproduction of the sign of stress incontinence (refer to the care plan for **Stress urinary Incontinence**), and testing of bulbocavernosus reflex and perineal sensations. *The physical examination will provide evidence supporting the diagnosis of extraurethral or another type of incontinence (stress, urge, or reflex) and provide the basis for further evaluation and/or treatment (Gray & Haas, 2000).*
- ▲ Consult a physician concerning the results of colposcopy, cystourethroscopy, intravenous urogram, cystogram, Pyridium pad test, or pelvic examination. *Evaluation of the location and characteristics of a urinary fistula or ectopic ureter requires direct visualization or identification based on an imaging study of the urinary system (Flores-Carreras et al, 2001).*
- • Assist the client in selecting and applying a urine containment device(s). Review types of containment products with the client, including advantages and potential compli-

cations associated with each type of product. *Urine containment products include a variety of absorptive pads, incontinence briefs, underpads for bedding, absorptive inserts that fit into specially designed undergarments, and condom catheters. Careful selection of an absorptive product and education concerning its use maximizes its effectiveness in controlling urine loss in a particular individual (Dunn et al, 2002; Shirran & Brazelli, 2000).*

- • Evaluate disposable versus reusable products for urine containment, considering the setting (home care versus acute care versus long-term care), preferences of the client and caregiver(s), and immediate versus long-term costs. *The economic and related impact of routine use of urine containment devices is significant, regardless of the setting. Economic factors as well as client and caregiver preferences affect the success and ultimate cost of a reusable versus disposable urine containment device (Dunn et al, 2002; Shirran & Brazelli, 2000).* **EBN:** *A study comparing a single reusable device with the "usual" containment device of a group of 175 community-dwelling subjects, which was most often a disposable pad, revealed that reusable garments provide comfort and perceived protection from visible urine loss equivalent to those of disposable pads (Gallo & Staskin, 1997).*
- • Cleanse the perineal skin regularly using a cleanser capable of removing irritants, including urine, stool, and materials. Select a product with a slightly acidic pH close to that of normal skin, with a water base and surfactant designed to remove irritants from the skin with minimal physical force. Avoid vigorous scrubbing with water, soap and a washcloth. Consider selection of a product with a moisturizer. *Traditional soaps tend to be alkaline, interfering with the natural acid mantle of the integument and increasing its susceptibility to irritant dermatitis and secondary infection. Brisk scrubbing may exacerbate skin erosion and further increase the risk of irritation and infection (Gray 2004; Gray, Ratliff, & Donovan, 2002).*
- • Apply a moisture barrier containing dimethicone or zinc oxide to patients with severe urinary incontinence or those with double urinary and fecal incontinence. *Clients with very severe incontinence and those with double fecal and urinary incontinence (particularly when the stool is liquified) typically require a product with vigorous moisture barrier qualities. Petrolatum based products containing dimethicone or zinc oxide are preferred (Gray, 2004; Gray, Ratliff, & Donovan, 2002).*
- • When cleansing a client with a moisture barrier containing zinc oxide, avoid vigorous scrubbing or use of a traditional washcloth to remove the paste. Instead, cleanse fecal materials away from the skin, leaving a clean layer of zinc oxide paste when cleansing after a single episode or gently removing the paste with mineral oil. *Pastes containing zinc oxide are difficult to remove, and it is not necessary to completely remove the product every time the perineal skin is cleansed. When deep cleansing and inspection of the underlying skin are indicated, mineral oil can be used to remove the paste without the need for brisk scrubbing.*
- ▲ Consult the physician concerning use of a moisture barrier with active healing ingredients when perineal dermatitis exists. In addition, an antifungal powder may be applied underneath the ointment when perineal dermatitis is complicated by monilial infection. Teach the client to use the product sparingly when applying to affected areas. **EBN:** *Xenaderm contains active ingredients (Balsam Peru, trypsin, and castor oil) that have been shown more effective than placebo for the management of partial thickness wounds in patients with urinary or fecal incontinence (Gray & Jones, 2004). A thin layer of an*

I

*antifungal powders may be layered beneath the ointment, but application of excessive may paradoxically retain moisture and diminish its effectiveness (Evans & Gray, 2003; Gray, Ratliff, & Donovan, 2002).*

▲ Consult the physician concerning placement of an indwelling catheter when severe urine loss is complicated by urinary retention, when careful fluid monitoring is indicated, when perineal dryness is required to promote healing of a stage 3 or 4 pressure ulcer, during periods of critical illness, or in the terminally ill client when use of absorbent products produces pain or distress. *Although not routinely indicated, the indwelling catheter provides an effective, transient management technique for carefully selected clients (Treatment of Pressure Ulcers Guideline Panel, 1994; Urinary Incontinence Guideline Panel, 1996).*

▲ Refer the client with "intractable" or extraurethral incontinence to a continence service or specialist for further evaluation and management of urine loss. *The successful management of complex, severe urinary incontinence requires specialized evaluation and treatment from a health care provider with special expertise.*

I

### Geriatric

- Provide privacy and support when changing incontinent devices in elderly clients. *Elderly, hospitalized clients frequently express feelings of shame, guilt, and dependency when undergoing urinary containment device changes (Biggerson et al, 1993).*
- Avoid brisk scrubbing and use of a washcloth when cleansing the skin of an aging client. *Brisk washing with a washcloth tends to strip superficial layers of skin, which potentially exacerbates erosion or damage to subcutaneous connective tissues (Gray, Ratliff, & Donovan, 2002).*
- Employ meticulous infection control procedures when using an indwelling catheter.

### Home Care

- The interventions described previously may be adapted for home care use.
- Encourage a mind-set and program of self-care management. **EBN:** *Addressing self-care activities through exercise, diet, fluid intake, and protective devices helps the client to exercise control over incontinence (Leenerts, Teel, & Pendleton, 2002).*
- Assist the family with arranging care in a way that allows the client to participate in family or favorite activities without embarrassment. Elicit discussion of the client's concerns about the social or emotional burden of incontinence. **EBN and EB:** *Careful planning can help the client retain dignity and maintain the integrity of family patterns. Urinary incontinence has a demonstrated influence on subjective well-being and quality of life, with depression, loneliness, or sadness possible (Fultz & Herzog, 2001). Discussing emotional concerns helps the client to develop a sense of control over incontinence (Leenerts, Teel, & Pendleton, 2002).*

▲ Consider the use of an indwelling catheter for continuous drainage in the client with severe urinary incontinence who is homebound, bed-bound, and receiving palliative or end-of-life care (requires a physician's order). *An indwelling catheter may increase client comfort, ease caregiver burden, and prevent urinary incontinence in bed-bound clients receiving end-of-life care.*

- ▲ When an indwelling catheter is in place, follow the prescribed maintenance protocols for managing the catheter, drainage bag, and perineal skin and urethral meatus. Teach infection control measures adapted to the home care setting. *Proper care reduces the risk of catheter-associated urinary tract infection.*
- • Assist the client in adapting to the catheter. Encourage discussion of the client's response to the catheter. **EBN:** *Clients living with a catheter are keenly aware of its presence; adaptation is served by normalizing the experience. Instruction could include the fact that the client will be more aware of some sensations and sounds (e.g., urine sloshing in the bag, the weight of the bag, pressure or pain when urine flow has been altered). Rehearsing emptying of the bag when away from home will support resumption of activities. Discussion of the client's response will help him or her to deal with embarrassment or frustration (Wilde, 2002).*

## Client/Family Teaching

- • Teach the family to obtain, apply, and dispose of or clean and reuse urine containment devices.
- • Teach the family a routine perineal skin care regimen, including daily or every other day hygiene and cleansing with containment product changes.
- • Teach the client and family to recognize and manage perineal dermatitis, ammonia contact dermatitis, and monilial rash.
- • Teach the client to maintain adequate fluid intake (30 mL/kg of body weight per day).
- • Teach the client and family to recognize and manage urinary tract infection.

## evolve WEBSITES FOR EDUCATION

See the EVOLVE website for World Wide Web resources for client education.

## REFERENCES


Biggerson AB et al: Elderly women's feelings about being incontinent, using napkins and being helped by nurses to change napkins, *J Clin Nurs* 2:165, 1993.

Dougherty MC, Dwyer JW, Pendergast JF et al: A randomized trial of behavioral management for continence with older rural women, *Res Nurs Health* 25(1):3, 2002.

Dunn S, Kowanko I, Paterson J et al: Systematic review of the effectiveness of urinary continence products, *J Wound Ostomy Continence Nurs* 29(3):129, 2002.

Evans EC, Gray M: What interventions are effective for the prevention and treatment of cutaneous candidiasis? *J Wound Ostomy Continence Nurs* 30(1):11, 2003.

Flores-Carreras O, Cabrera JR, Galeano PA et al: Fistulas of the urinary tract in obstetric surgery, *Int Urogynecol J Pelvic Floor Dysfunct* 12:203, 2001.

Fultz NH, Herzog AR: Self-reported social and emotional impact of urinary incontinence, *J Am Geriatr Soc* 49:892, 2001.

Gallo M, Staskin DR: Patient satisfaction with a reusable undergarment for urinary incontinence, *J Wound Ostomy Continence Nurs* 24(4):226, 1997.

Gray M: Preventing and managing perineal dermatitis: a shared goal for wound and continence care, *J Wound Ostomy Continence Nurs* 31(Suppl 1):S2-S9, 2004.

Gray M, Haas J: Assessment of the patient with urinary incontinence. In Doughty DB, editor: *Urinary and fecal incontinence: nursing management,* St Louis, 2000, Mosby.

Gray M, Jones D: The effect of different formulations of equivalent active ingredients on the performance of two topical wound treatment products, *Ostomy Wound Manage* 50(3):34-44, 2004.

Gray M, Ratliff C, Donovan A: Perineal skin care for the incontinent patient, *Adv Skin Wound Care* 15:170, 2002.
Leenerts MH, Teel CS, Pendleton MK: Building a model of self-care for health promotion in aging, *J Nurs Scholarsh* 34:355, 2002.
Shirran E, Brazelli M: Absorbent products for the containment of urinary and/or fecal incontinence, *Cochrane Database System Rev* CD0011406, 2000.
Treatment of Pressure Ulcers Guideline Panel: *Treatment of pressure ulcer: clinical practice guideline,* Rockville, Md, 1994, Agency for Health Care Policy and Research.
Urinary Incontinence Guideline Panel: *Urinary incontinence in adults: clinical practice guideline,* ed 2, Rockville, Md, 1996, Agency for Health Care Policy and Research.
Wilde MH: Urine flowing: a phenomenological study of living with a urinary catheter, *Res Nurs Health* 25:14, 2002.

# Urge urinary Incontinence

*Mikel Gray*

**NANDA**

## Definition

State in which the individual experiences involuntary passage of urine occurring with precipitous desire to urinate. *Urge incontinence* is defined within the context of overactive bladder syndrome. The overactive bladder is characterized by bothersome urgency (a sudden and strong desire to urinate that is not easily deferred) (Abrams et al, 2002). Overactive bladder is typically associated with frequent daytime voiding and nocturia, and approximately 37% will experience urge urinary incontinence (Stewart et al, 2003).

## Defining Characteristics

Diurnal urinary frequency (voiding more than once every 2 hours while awake); nocturia (awakening three or more times per night to urinate; voiding more than eight times within a 24-hour period as recorded on a voiding diary (bladder log); bothersome urgency (a sudden and strong desire to urinate that is not easily deferred); symptom of urge incontinence (urine loss associated with desire to urinate); enuresis (involuntary passage of urine while asleep)

## Related Factors

- Neurological disorders (brain disorders, including cerebrovascular accident, brain tumor, normal pressure hydrocephalus, traumatic brain injury)
- Inflammation of bladder (calculi; tumor, including transitional cell carcinoma and carcinoma in situ; inflammatory lesions of the bladder; urinary tract infection)
- Bladder outlet obstruction (see **Urinary retention**)
- Stress urinary incontinence (mixed urinary incontinence; these conditions often coexist but relationship between them remains unclear)
- Idiopathic causes (implicated factors include depression, sleep apnea/hypoxia)

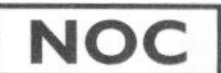

## Outcomes (Nursing Outcomes Classification)

### Suggested NOC Outcomes

Tissue Integrity, Skin and Mucous Membranes, Urinary Continence, Urinary Elimination

**Example NOC Outcome with Indicators**

**Urinary Continence** as evidenced by the following indicators: Responds in timely manner to urge/Voids in appropriate receptacle/Has adequate time to reach toilet between urge and evacuation of urine/Underclothing remains dry during day/Underclothing or bedding remains dry during night (Rate each indicator of **Urinary Continence:** 1 = never demonstrated, 2 = rarely demonstrated, 3 = sometimes demonstrated, 4 = often demonstrated, 5 = consistently demonstrated [see Section I].)

I

## Client Outcomes

### Client Will (Specify Time Frame):

- Report relief from urge urinary incontinence or a decrease in the incidence or severity of incontinent episodes
- Identify containment devices that assist in the management of urge urinary incontinence

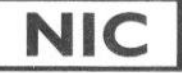

## Interventions (Nursing Interventions Classification)

### Suggested NIC Interventions

Urinary Habit Training, Urinary Incontinence Care

**Example NIC Activities—Urinary Habit Training**

Keep continence specification record for 3 days to establish voiding pattern; establish interval for toileting of preferably not less than 2 hours

## Nursing Interventions and Rationales

- Take a nursing history focusing on duration of urinary incontinence, diurnal frequency, nocturia, severity of symptoms, and alleviating and aggravating factors. *A focused history helps determine the cause of urinary incontinence and guides its subsequent management.* **EBN:** *Querying the client about the isolated symptom of urge incontinence shows a poor correlation with a diagnosis of detrusor overactivity incontinence. However, the agreement between urodynamic testing and the clinical diagnosis obtained by the history rises sharply when the client reports three symptoms: diurnal frequency, urge-related urine loss, and nocturia (Gray et al, 2001).*
- Perform a focused physical assessment, beginning with perineal skin assessment. *Uri-*

*nary incontinence, particularly when combined with fecal incontinence or use of larger containment devices such as adult containment briefs, increases the risk for irritant dermatitis and secondary monilial or bacterial infection (Gray, 2004; Gray, Ratliff, & Donovan, 2002).*

- Perform a focused pelvic examination including visual inspection of the vaginal mucosa, observation of urethral hypermobility and related pelvic floor descent (prolapse), and digital assessment of pelvic floor muscle strength. Refer the woman with moderately severe to severe vaginal wall prolapse (descent to or beyond the introitus) to a female urologist or urogynecologist. *Severe pelvic organ prolapse complicates the management of urge urinary incontinence and predisposes the female patient to urinary retention (Romanzi, 2002). Baseline of pelvic muscle strength is needed for initial assessment and for evaluation of treatment efficacy. It also provides an opportunity for the nurse to determine whether the patient is able to identify, isolate, contract, and relax the pelvic floor muscles.*

I

▲ Complete a urinalysis, examining for the presence of nitrites, leukocytes, glucose, or hemoglobin (red blood cells). *The presence of nitrites and leukocytes raises a suspicion of urinary tract infection, the presence of glucosuria raises the risk of undiagnosed or poorly controlled diabetes mellitus, and the presence of red blood cells in the absence of signs of infection raises a suspicion of a bladder tumor. Each condition may produce acute urinary incontinence requiring treatment of the underlying cause (Fourcroy, 2001).*

- Teach the patient to complete a voiding diary (bladder log) by recording voiding frequency, the frequency of urinary incontinent episodes and their association with urgency (a sudden and strong desire to urinate that is difficult o defer) over a 3- to 7-day period. An electronic voiding diary may be kept whenever feasible. In addition to these parameters, the patient may be asked to record voided volume and fluid intake. *The voiding diary provides a more objective record of lower urinary tract function than the oral history and it often provides a modest therapeutic effect by alerting the patient to factors that promote urinary incontinence episodes (Sampselle, 2003). An electronic voiding diary provides an efficient and possibly more accurate method for documenting these parameters (Quinn et al, 2003).*

▲ Review all medications the patient is receiving, paying particular attention to sedatives, narcotics, diuretics, antidepressants, psychotropic drugs, and cholinergics. Consult the physician or nurse practitioner about altering or eliminating these medications if they are suspected of affecting incontinence. *The side effects of multiple medications may produce or exacerbate urge incontinence (Fourcroy, 2001).*

- Assess the client for urinary retention (see the care plan for **Urinary retention**). *Urinary retention associated with bladder outlet obstruction may be a contributing cause of urge incontinence (Chai, Gray, & Steers, 1998). Urinary retention associated with poor detrusor contraction strength has been described in frail elderly clients (Resnick & Yalla, 1987). Regardless of its cause, retention significantly affects the management of this condition (Gray, 2000).*
- Assess the client for functional limitations (environmental barriers, limited mobility or dexterity, impaired cognitive function; refer to the care plan for **Functional urinary Incontinence**). *Functional limitations affect the severity and management of urge urinary incontinence (Ouslander, 2002).*

- ▲ Consult the physician concerning diabetic management and pharmacotherapy for urinary tract infection when indicated. *In specific cases, urgency and an increased risk of urge incontinence may be related to urinary tract infection (Molander et al, 2000) or polyuria from undiagnosed or poorly managed diabetes mellitus (Samsioe et al, 1999).*
- ▲ Assess for signs and symptoms of atrophic vaginal changes in the perimenopausal or postmenopausal woman, including vaginal dryness, tenderness to touch, mucosal dryness, friability, and discomfort with gentle palpation. Specifically query the woman with atrophic vaginitis concerning associated lower urinary tract symptoms (usually voiding frequency, urgency, and dysuria). Refer the woman with atrophic vaginal changes and bothersome lower urinary tract symptoms to a gynecologist, urologist, or women's health nurse practitioner for further evaluation and management. *The relationship between atrophic vaginitis and urge incontinence risk remains unclear. However, several studies have observed that oral estrogen replacement may slightly increase the frequency of urinary incontinence episodes in postmenopausal women (Brown et al, 1999; Molander et al, 2000). Topical or intravaginal estrogen, particularly rings or tablets, may provide an alternative for relieving bothersome symptoms associated with atrophic vaginitis without the associated risks of oral preparations (Crandall, 2002). In addition, systematic reviews of existing evidence suggest that local hormone replacement therapy may reduce the risk of urinary tract infection in elder women (Rozenberg, 2004; Crandall, 2002).*
- • Teach the principles of bladder training to women with urge urinary incontinence.
  - ■ Assist the client in completing a voiding diary over a period of a minimum of 3 days or up to 7 days.
  - ■ Review the results with the client, determining typical voiding frequency and establishing goals for voiding frequency.
  - ■ Using baseline voiding frequency, as determined by the diary, teach the client to urinate by the clock when awake, typically every 30 to 120 minutes.
  - ■ Encourage adherence to the program with timing devices and verbal encouragement and support, and address individual reasons for schedule interruption.
  - ■ Gradually increase the time between urinations to the negotiated goal. Time intervals between voiding are typically increased in increments of 15 to 30 minutes for clients with a baseline frequency of less than every 60 minutes and increments of 25 to 30 minutes for clients with a baseline frequency of more than every 60 minutes.

  **EBN:** *Bladder training reduces the frequency and severity of urinary leakage in women with urge, stress or mixed urinary incontinence. Research suggests that the results of bladder training in ambulatory, community-dwelling women is comparable to that achieved through pelvic floor muscle rehabilitation (Theofrastus et al, 2002; Elser et al, 1999; Wyman et al, 1998). Bladder training has also been shown to augment the efficacy of pharmacotherapy for patients with urge urinary incontinence (Mattiasson et al, 2003).*
- • Review with the client the types of beverages consumed, focusing on the intake of bladder irritants, including caffeine and alcohol. *A growing body of evidence supports limitation of caffeine as an effective means of reducing voiding frequency (Gray, 2001). Although epidemiological studies have failed to establish a statistically significant relationship between alcohol consumption and urinary incontinence risk (Bortolotti et al, 2000), alcohol is known to act as a diuretic and sedative and clinical observations support its potential to transiently increase the risk of urine loss when consumed in significant quantities.*

- Review with the client the volume of fluids consumed and gradually adjust the fluid intake to meet the Adequate Intake recommendation of 3 L for the 19- to 30-year-old male and 2.2 L for the 19- to 30-year-old female. Water balance studies suggest that adult men require 2.5 L/day (Institute of Medicine, 2004). *Dehydration is postulated to exacerbate the symptoms of urgency (Pearson, 1992, 1993), and excessive fluid intake increases voided volume and urinary frequency (Fitzgerald & Brubaker, 2003). Increasing fluid intake in women with urinary incontinence may reduce the risk of urinary tract infection without increasing the frequency or severity of urine loss (Dougherty et al, 2002).*
- Instruct in techniques of urge suppression. Teach the client to identify, isolate, contract, and relax the pelvic floor muscles. When a strong or precipitous urge to urinate is perceived, teach the client to avoid running to the toilet. Instead, she or he should perform repeated, rapid pelvic muscle contractions until the urge is relieved. Relief is followed by micturition within 5 to 15 minutes, using nonhurried movements when locating a toilet and voiding. **EB:** *Randomized controlled trials comparing urge suppression techniques to pharmacotherapy or bladder training have shown it to be an effective method for reducing urge urinary incontinence episodes (Burgio & Engel, 2002).*

I

- ▲ Begin transvaginal or transrectal electrical stimulation using a low-frequency current (5 to 20 Hz) in consultation with the physician. *Electrical stimulation is an effective treatment for urge incontinence; in one randomized clinical trial it was found to completely eliminate symptoms of urge incontinence in 49% of a group of 121 subjects (Brubaker, et al, 1997).*
- ▲ Teach the client to self-administer antimuscarinic (anticholinergic) drugs as directed. Teach dosage and administration of the medication and the importance of combining pharmacotherapy with scheduled voiding, adequate fluid intake, restriction of bladder irritants, and urge suppression techniques. *Antimuscarinic drugs increase bladder capacity, reduce the frequency of incontinence episodes, and diminish voiding frequency. However, they do not cure bladder dysfunction or reduce the time between perception of a strong urge and onset of an overactive detrusor contraction. The efficacy of pharmacotherapy for urge incontinence and overactive bladder dysfunction is enhanced when combined with behavioral interventions (Burgio, 2002; Burgio, Locher, & Goode, 2000).*
- ▲ Assist the client in selecting, obtaining, and applying a containment device for urine loss as indicated (refer to the care plan for **Total urinary Incontinence**).
- ▲ Provide the client with information about incontinence support groups such as the National Association for Continence and the Simon Foundation for Continence. *Self-help groups provide social support and a forum for sharing strategies for the management of all types of urinary incontinence (Irwin, 2000).*

## Geriatric

- Assess the functional and cognitive status of the elderly client with urge incontinence. *Functional limitations affect the severity and management of urge urinary incontinence (Ouslander, 2002).*
- Plan care in long-term or acute care facilities based on knowledge of the elderly client's established voiding patterns, paying particular attention to patterns of nocturia.
- ▲ Carefully monitor the elderly client for potential adverse effects of antispasmodic

medications, including a severely dry mouth interfering with the use of dentures, eating, or speaking, or confusion, nightmares, constipation, mydriasis, or heat intolerance. *Elderly persons are particularly susceptible to adverse effects associated with antispasmodic medications (Ghoneim & Hassouna, 1997).*

## Home Care

- The interventions described previously may be adapted for home care use.
- Teach the importance of avoiding dehydration or excessive fluid consumption and the paradoxical relationship between dehydration and symptoms of urgency.
- Teach the family and client to identify and correct environmental barriers to toileting within the home.
- Encourage a mind-set and program of self-care management. **EBN:** *Addressing self-care activities through exercise, diet, fluid intake, and protective devices helps the client to exercise control over incontinence (Leenerts, Teel, & Pendleton, 2002).*
- Implement a bladder-training program as appropriate, including self-monitoring activities (reducing caffeine intake, adjusting amount and timing of fluid intake, decreasing long voiding intervals while awake, making dietary changes to promote bowel regularity), bladder training, and pelvic muscle exercise. **EBN:** *In one study of women age 55 years or older with involuntary urine loss associated with stress, urge, or mixed incontinence, clients responded to the aforementioned interventions with a 61% decrease in the severity of urinary incontinence at 2 years after intervention. Self-monitoring and bladder training accounted for most of the improvement (Dougherty et al, 2002).*
- Help the client and family to identify and correct environmental barriers to toileting within the home.

## Client/Family Teaching

- Teach the client and family to recognize foods and beverages that are likely to irritate the bladder.
- Teach the family and client to recognize and manage side effects of antispasmodic medications used to treat urge incontinence.
- Help the client and family to recognize and manage side effect of anticholinergic medications used to manage irritative lower urinary tract symptoms.

## evolve WEBSITES FOR EDUCATION

See the EVOLVE website for World Wide Web resources for client education.

## REFERENCES

Abrams P, Cardozo L, Fall M et al: The standardisation of terminology of lower urinary tract function: report from the Standardization Sub-committee of the International Continence Society, *Am J Obstet Gynecol* 187(1): 116-126, 2002.

Bortolotti A, Bernardini B, Colli E et al: Prevalence and risk factors for urinary incontinence in Italy, *Eur Urol* 37(1):30, 2000.

Brown JS, Grady D, Ouslander JG et al: Prevalence of urinary incontinence and associated risk factors in postmenopausal women. Heart & Estrogen/Progestin Replacement Study (HERS) Research Group, *Obstet Gynecol* 94:66, 1999.

Brubaker L, Benson JT, Bent A et al: Transvaginal electrical stimulation for female urinary incontinence *Am J Obstet Gynecol* 177(3):536-540, 1997.
Burgio KL: Influence of behavior modification on overactive bladder, *Urology* 60(5 Suppl 1):72, 2002.
Burgio KL, Locher JL, Goode PS: Combined behavioral and drug therapy for urge incontinence in older women, *J Am Geriatr Soc* 48(4):370, 2000.
Chai TC, Gray ML, Steers WD: The incidence of a positive ice water test on bladder outlet obstructed patients: evidence for altered innervation, *J Urol* 160:34-38, 1998.
Crandall C: Vaginal estrogen preparations: a review of safety and efficacy for vaginal atrophy, *J Womens Health* 11(10):857-877, 2002.
Dougherty MC, Dwyer JW, Pendergast JF et al: A randomized trial of behavioral management for continence with older rural women, *Res Nurs Health* 25(1):3, 2002.
Elser DM, Wyman JF, McClish DK et al: The effect of bladder training, pelvic floor muscle training, or combination training on urodynamic parameters in women with urinary incontinence. Continence Program for Women Research Group, *Neurourol Urodyn* 18(5):427, 1999.
Eriksen B: A randomized, open, parallel group study on the preventive effect of an estradiol-releasing vaginal ring (Estring) on recurrent urinary tract infections in postmenopausal women, *Am J Obstet Gynecol* 180:1072, 1999.
Fitzgerald MP, Brubaker L: Variability of 24-hour voiding diary variables among asymptomatic women, *J Urol* 169(1):207, 2003.
Fourcroy JL: Overactive bladder: a practical overview of diagnosis and treatment, *Adv Nurse Practit* 9(3):59, 2001.
Ghoneim GM, Hassouna M: Alternatives for the pharmacologic management of urge and stress urinary incontinence in the elderly, *J Wound Ostomy Continence Nurs* 24:311, 1997.
Gray M: Urinary retention: management in the acute care setting, Part 2, *Am J Nurs* 100:36, 2000.
Gray M: Caffeine and urinary incontinence, *J Wound Ostomy Continence Nurs* 28:66, 2001.
Gray M: Preventing and managing perineal dermatitis: a shared goal for wound and continence care, *J Wound Ostomy Continence Nurs* 31(Suppl 1):S2-S9, 2004.
Gray M, McClain R, Peruggia M et al: A model for predicting motor urge urinary incontinence, *Nurs Res* 50:116, 2001.
Gray M, Ratliff C, Donovan A: Perineal skin care for the incontinent patient, *Adv Skin Wound Care* 15:170, 2002.
Irwin B: User support groups in continence care, *Nurs Times* 96(Suppl 31):24, 2000.
Leenerts MH, Teel CS, Pendleton MK: Building a model of self-care for health promotion in aging, *J Nurs Scholarsh* 34:355, 2002.
Mattiasson A, Blaakaer J, Hoye K et al: Tolterodine Scandinavian Study Group, Simplified bladder training augments the effectiveness of tolterodine in patients with an overactive bladder, *BJU Int* 91(1):54-60, 2003.
Molander U, Arvidsson L, Milsom I et al: A longitudinal cohort study of elderly women with urinary tract infection, *Maturitas* 34: 127, 2000.
Moore KN, Gray ML, Rayome RG: Electric stimulation and urinary incontinence: research and alternatives, *Urol Nurs* 15: 94, 1995.
Institute of Medicine: Food and Nutrition Board: *Dietary reference intakes for water, potassium, sodium chloride and sulfate,* Washington, DC, 2004, The National Academies Press.
Ouslander JG: Geriatric considerations in the diagnosis and management of overactive bladder, *Urology* 60(5 suppl 1):50, 2002.
Pearson BD: Urine control by elders: noninvasive strategies. In Funk SG et al editors: *Key aspects of elder care: managing falls, incontinence and cognitive impairment,* New York, 1992, Springer.
Pearson BD: Liquidate a myth: reducing liquids is not advisable for elderly with urine control problems, *Urol Nurs* 13:86, 1993.
Quinn P, Goka J, Richardson H: Assessment of an electronic daily diary in patients with overactive bladder, *BJU Int* 91(7):647-652, 2003.
Resnick NM, Beckett LA, Branch LG et al. Short term variability of self report of incontinence in older persons, *J Am Geriatr Soc* 42:202, 1994.
Resnick NM, Yalla SV: Detrusor hyperactivity with impaired contractile function. An unrecognized but common cause of incontinence in elderly patients, *JAMA* 257:3076, 1987.
Sampselle CM: Teaching women to use a voiding diary, *Am J Nurs* 103(11):62-64, 2003.
Stewart WF, Van Rooyen JB, Cundiff GW et al: Prevalence and burden of overactive bladder in the United States, *World J Urol* 20(6): 327-336, 2003.
Samsioe G, Heraib F, Lidfeldt J et al: Urogenital symptoms in women aged 50-59 years, *Gynecol Endocrinol* 13:113, 1999.
Theofrastous JP, Wyman JF, Bump RC et al: Effects of pelvic floor muscle training on strength and predictors of response in the treatment of urinary incontinence, *Neurourol Urodyn* 21(5):486-490, 2002.

Wyman JF, Fantl JA, McClish DK et al: Continence Program for Women Research Group, Comparative efficacy of behavioral interventions in the management of female urinary incontinence. *Am J Obstet Gynecol* 179(4):999, 1998.
Zorn BH, Montgomery H, Pieper K et al: Urinary incontinence and depression, *J Urol* 162:82, 1999.

# Risk for urge urinary Incontinence

*Mikel Gray*

**NANDA**

## Definition

At risk for involuntary loss of urine associated with a sudden, strong sensation or urinary urgency

## Risk Factors

Overactive bladder dysfunction with associated detrusor overactivity, inflammation from urinary tract infection, inflammatory lesion, bladder to lower ureteral stone, bladder outlet obstruction, dietary risk factors, consumption of caffeine

Overactive bladder is a symptom syndrome characterized by bothersome urgency (a sudden and strong desire to urinate that is not easily deferred) typically associated with day and nighttime voiding frequency (more than eight urinations per day) (Abrams et al, 2002). Although urge urinary incontinence affects approximately 37% of patients with overactive bladder, 63% (Stewart et al, 2003) have an identifiable condition that is not adequately described by this diagnosis. It is hoped that *risk for urge urinary incontinence* will evolve in a manner that more clearly describes the underlying syndrome, overactive bladder.

**NOC**

## Outcomes (Nursing Outcomes Classification)

### Suggested NOC Outcomes

Tissue Integrity: Skin and Mucous Membranes; Urinary Continence; Urinary Elimination

**Example NOC Outcome with Indicators**

**Urinary Continence** as evidenced by the following indicators: Responds in timely manner to urge/Voids in appropriate receptacle/Has adequate time to reach toilet between urge and evacuation of urine/Underclothing remains dry during day/Underclothing or bedding remains dry during night (Rate each indicator of **Urinary Continence:** 1 = never demonstrated, 2 = rarely demonstrated, 3 = sometimes demonstrated, 4 = often demonstrated, 5 = consistently demonstrated [see Section I].)

## Client Outcomes

**Client Will (Specify Time Frame):**

- Report relief from urge urinary incontinence or a decrease in the incidence or severity of incontinent episodes
- Identify containment devices that assist in the management of urge urinary incontinence

**NIC**

## Interventions (Nursing Interventions Classification)

### Suggested NIC Interventions

Urinary Habit Training; Urinary Incontinence Care

**Example NIC Activities—Urinary Habit Training**

Keep continence specification record for 3 days to establish voiding pattern; establish interval for toileting of preferably not less than 2 hours

I

## Nursing Interventions and Rationales

- Take a nursing history focusing on the following lower urinary tract symptoms: daytime voiding frequency, nocturia, presence of bothersome urgency (precipitous desire to urinate that interferes with activities of daily living [ADLs]), and presence of urine loss. *Bothersome lower urinary tract symptoms are strongly correlated with urge incontinence in adult women (Alling-Moller, Lose, & Jorgensen, 2000).* **EBN:** *Diurnal voiding frequency (voiding every 2 hours or less often), nocturia (arising to void more than once each night for younger clients and more than twice each night for adults age 65 years and older), and bothersome urgency are associated with urge incontinence (Gray et al, 2001).*
- Query the client about specific risk factors for urge urinary incontinence, such as childhood enuresis, depression, prostate enlargement with bladder outlet obstruction, and neurological disorders, including stroke or parkinsonism. *Bladder outlet obstruction and neurological disorders affecting modulatory areas in the brain are strongly associated with detrusor overactivity, bothersome lower urinary tract symptoms, and an increased risk for urge incontinence (Mostwin, 2002). Childhood enuresis may be a risk factor for overactive bladder symptoms in adults (Kuh, Cardozo, & Hardy, 1999; Malmsten et al, 1997).*
- Assess the client's functional status, focusing on mobility, dexterity, and cognitive status. *The risk of urinary incontinence rises with increased impairment of mobility; clients who are bedridden are at greatest risk, followed by clients who are confined to a wheelchair, those relying on a walker, and those walking with minimal assistance (Aggazzotti et al, 2000). Cognitive impairment, particularly when accompanied by disoriented perception of time, is associated with an increased risk of urge urinary incontinence in the aging client (Griffiths et al, 2002).*
- ▲ Complete a urinalysis, focusing on the presence of nitrites, leukocytes, glucose, or hemoglobin (red blood cells). *The presence of nitrites and leukocytes raises a suspicion of urinary tract infection, the presence of glucosuria raises a risk of undiagnosed or poorly controlled diabetes mellitus, and the presence of red blood cells in the absence of signs of infection*

*raises a suspicion of a bladder tumor. Each condition increases the risk of urgency symptoms and urge incontinence (Fourcroy, 2001).*

- Teach the patient to complete a voiding diary (bladder log) by recording voiding frequency, the frequency of urgency episodes over a 3- to 7-day period. An electronic voiding diary may be kept whenever feasible. In addition to these parameters, the patient may be asked to record voided volume and fluid intake. *The voiding diary provides a more objective record of lower urinary tract function than the oral history and it often provides a modest therapeutic effect by alerting the patient to factors that promote urinary incontinence episodes (Sampselle, 2003). An electronic voiding diary provides an efficient and possibly more accurate method for documenting these parameters (Quinn et al, 2003).*
- Advise all patients to reduce or eliminate intake caffeinated beverages or over-the-counter medications of dietary aids containing caffeine. *Caffeine acts as a bladder irritant, increasing voiding frequency, urgency, and urge urinary incontinence episodes among those with this condition. Reducing the intake of caffeine alleviates these lower urinary tract symptoms (Gray, 2001).*
- Advise community-dwelling men that moderate consumption of beer may reduce the risk of developing overactive bladder dysfunction and the associated risk for urge urinary incontinence. **EB:** *A longitudinal study of community-dwelling men found that moderate consumption of beer reduced the risk for developing overactive bladder (Dallosso et al, 2004a). Because this effect was not associated with intake of other alcoholic beverages, it seems likely that the protective effect is attributable to some other element of beer than its alcoholic content.*
- Advise community-dwelling women that intake of a balanced diet, and supplementation of vitamin D to ensure meeting daily recommended allowances may reduce the risk for of developing overactive bladder dysfunction and the associated risk for urge urinary incontinence. **EB:** *A longitudinal study of community-dwelling women found that deficits in a number of nutrients was modestly associated with the risk for developing overactive bladder dysfunction and the associated risk for urge urinary incontinence. Among these, vitamin D deficiency emerged as the strongest potential risk factor (Dallosso et al, 2004b).*
- Additional bladder irritants, including aspartame, carbonated drinks, decaffeinated coffee or tea, citrus juices, highly spiced foods, chocolates, and vinegar-containing foods, may be eliminated from the diet and added back singly to determine their impact on lower urinary tract symptoms and urgency. *Evidence is limited in support of the role of these substances as potential bladder irritants in clients at risk of urge urinary incontinence, but they do play a more significant role for those with interstitial cystitis (Interstitial Cystitis Association, 1999; Bade, Peeters, & Mensink, 1997).*
- Review with the client the volume of fluids consumed and gradually adjust the fluid intake to meet the Adequate Intake recommendation of 3 L for the 19- to 30-year-old male and 2.2 L for the 19- to 30-year-old female. Water balance studies suggest that adult men require 2.5 L per day (Institute of Medicine, 2004). *Dehydration is postulated to exacerbate symptoms of urgency (Pearson, 1992, 1993), and excessive fluid intake increases voided volume and urinary frequency. Consumption of fluids within the recommended daily allowance may reduce the risk of urinary tract infection without increasing the frequency or severity of urine loss (Dougherty, 1999).*

- ▲ Review all medications the client is receiving, paying particular attention to sedatives, narcotics, diuretics, antidepressants, psychotropic drugs, and cholinergics. Consult the physician about altering or eliminating these medications if they are suspected of affecting incontinence. *The side effects of multiple medications may produce or exacerbate urge incontinence (Fourcroy, 2001).*
- ▲ Consult the physician concerning diabetic management and pharmacotherapy for urinary tract infection when indicated. *In specific cases, urgency and an increased risk of urge incontinence may be related to urinary tract infection (Molander et al, 2000) or polyuria from undiagnosed or poorly managed diabetes mellitus (Samsioe et al, 1999).*
- ▲ Assess for signs and symptoms of atrophic vaginal changes in the perimenopausal or postmenopausal woman, including vaginal dryness, tenderness to touch, dryness of mucosa on touch with friability, and discomfort with gentle palpation. Specifically query the client with atrophic vaginitis concerning storage lower urinary tract symptoms (voiding frequency, urgency, or dysuria). Refer the client with atrophic vaginal changes and bothersome lower urinary tract symptoms to a gynecologist, urologist, or women's health nurse practitioner for further evaluation and management. *The relationship between atrophic vaginitis and urge incontinence risk remains unclear. However, several studies have found that oral estrogen replacement slightly increases the frequency of urinary incontinence episodes (Brown et al, 1999; Molander et al, 2000).* **EB:** *A modest body of evidence suggests that intravaginal or topical estrogen replacement therapy reduces bothersome symptoms associated with atrophic urogenital changes, including urgency and dysuria. Local estrogen therapy also may reduce the risk for urinary tract infection in postmenopausal women (Rozenberg, 2004; Thacker, 2004).*
- • Teach patients techniques of bladder training and pelvic muscle rehabilitation focusing on urge suppression. **EBN:** *An interdisciplinary research team, including a nurse researcher, has demonstrated that public education of community-dwelling middle-age and elderly women reduces the risk for incontinence and voiding frequency (Diokno et al, 2004).*
- • Provide the client with information about incontinence support groups such as the National Association for Continence and the Simon Foundation for Continence. *Self-help groups provide social support and a forum for sharing strategies for management of all types of urinary incontinence (Irwin, 2000).*

## Geriatric

- • Assess the functional and cognitive status of an elderly client with irritative lower urinary tract symptoms or urge incontinence.
- ▲ Advise a male client with bothersome lower urinary tract symptoms to see his physician or nurse practitioner, because these symptoms may be related to prostate enlargement.
- ▲ Carefully monitor the elderly client for potential adverse effects of anticholinergic medications, including severe dry mouth interfering with the use of dentures, eating, or speaking, or the occurrence of confusion, nightmares, constipation, mydriasis, or heat intolerance. *Elderly persons are particularly susceptible to adverse effects associated with anticholinergic medications.*

### Home Care

- The interventions described previously may be adapted for home care use.
- Encourage a mindset and program of self-care management. **EBN:** *Addressing self-care activities through exercise, diet, fluid intake, and protective devices helps the client take control of incontinence (Leenerts, Teel, & Pendleton, 2002).*
- Implement a bladder-training program, including self-monitoring activities (reducing caffeine intake, adjusting amount and timing of fluid intake, decreasing long voiding intervals while awake, making dietary changes to promote bowel regularity), bladder training, and pelvic muscle exercise. **EBN:** *In one study of women age 55 years or older with involuntary urine loss associated with stress, urge, or mixed incontinence, clients responded to the aforementioned interventions with a 61% decrease in the severity of urinary incontinence at 2 years after intervention. Self-monitoring and bladder training accounted for most of the improvement (Dougherty et al, 2002).*
- Teach the client and family to recognize foods and beverages that are likely to irritate the bladder.
- Teach the importance of avoiding dehydration or excessive fluid consumption and the paradoxical relationship between dehydration and symptoms of urgency.
- Teach the family and client to recognize and manage side effects of anticholinergic medications used to treat irritative lower urinary tract symptoms.
- Teach the family and client to identify and correct environmental barriers to toileting within the home.
- Assist the family with arranging care in a way that allows the client to participate in family or favorite activities without embarrassment. Elicit discussion of the client's concerns about the social or emotional burden of incontinence. **EBN and EB:** *Careful planning can help the client retain dignity and maintain the integrity of family patterns. Urinary incontinence has a demonstrated influence on subjective well-being and quality of life, with depression, loneliness, or sadness possible (Fultz & Herzog, 2001). Discussing emotional concerns helps the client to develop a sense of control over incontinence (Leenerts, Teel, & Pendleton, 2002).*

I

### Client/Family Teaching

- Teach the client and family to recognize foods and beverages that are likely to irritate the bladder.
- Teach the importance of avoiding dehydration or excessive fluid consumption and the paradoxical relationship between dehydration and symptoms of urgency.

## evolve WEBSITES FOR EDUCATION

See the EVOLVE website for World Wide Web resources for client education.

## REFERENCES

Abrams P, Cardozo L, Fall M et al: The standardisation of terminology of lower urinary tract function: report from the Standardization Sub-committee of the International Continence Society, *Am J Obstet Gynecol* 187(1):116-126, 2002.

Aggazzotti G, Pesce F, Grassi D et al: Prevalence of urinary incontinence among institutionalized patients: a cross-sectional epidemiologic study in a midsized city in northern Italy, *Urology* 56(2):245, 2000.
Alling-Moller LA, Lose G, Jorgensen T: Risk factors for lower urinary tract symptoms in women 40 to 60 years of age, *Obstet Gynecol* 96:466, 2000.
Bade JJ, Peeters JM, Mensink HJ: Is the diet of patients with interstitial cystitis related to their disease? *Eur Urol* 32:179, 1997.
Brown JS, Grady D, Ouslander JG et al: Prevalence of urinary incontinence and associated risk factors in postmenopausal women, *Obstet Gynecol* 94:66, 1999.
Burgio KL, Locher JL, Goode PS et al: Behavioral vs. drug treatment for urge urinary incontinence in older women: a randomized controlled trial, *JAMA* 280:1995, 1998.
Dallosso HM, Matthews RJ, McGrother CW et al: The association of diet and other lifestyle factors with the onset of overactive bladder: a longitudinal study in men, *Public Health Nutr* 7(7):885-891, 2004a.
Dallosso HM, McGrother CW, Matthews RJ et al: Nutrient composition of the diet and the development of overactive bladder: a longitudinal study in women, *Neurourol Urodyn* 23(3):204-10, 2004b.
Diokno AC, Sampselle CM, Herzog AR et al: Prevention of urinary incontinence by behavioral modification program: a randomized, controlled trial among older women in the community, *J Urol* 171(3):1165-1171, 2004.
Dougherty MC: *Establishing goals and lifestyle management,* WOCN Continence Conference, Austin, Tex, February 1999.
Dougherty MC, Dwyer JW, Pendergast JF et al: A randomized trial of behavioral management for continence with older rural women, *Res Nurs Health* 25(1):3, 2002.
Eriksen B: A randomized, open, parallel group study on the preventive effect of an estradiol-releasing vaginal ring (Estring) on recurrent urinary tract infections in postmenopausal women, *Am J Obstet Gynecol* 180:1072, 1999.
Fourcroy JL: Overactive bladder: a practical overview of diagnosis and treatment, *Adv Nurse Practit* 9(3):59, 2001.
Fultz NH, Herzog AR: Self-reported social and emotional impact of urinary incontinence, *J Am Geriatr Soc* 49:892, 2001.
Gray M: Caffeine and urinary incontinence, *J Wound Ostomy Continence Nurs* 28:66, 2001.
Gray M, McClain R, Peruggia M et al: A model for predicting motor urge urinary incontinence, *Nurs Res* 50:116, 2001.
Griffiths DJ, McCracken PN, Harrison GM et al: Urge incontinence and impaired detrusor contractility in the elderly, *Neurourol Urodyn* 21(2): 126, 2002.
Interstitial Cystitis Association: *Interstitial cystitis and diet,* Rockville, Md, 1999, The Association.
Irwin B: User support groups in continence care, *Nurs Times* 96(Suppl 31):24, 2000.
Kuh D, Cardozo L, Hardy R: Urinary incontinence in middle aged women: childhood enuresis and other lifetime risk factors in a British prospective cohort, *J Epidemiol Community Health* 53(8):453, 1999.
Leenerts MH, Teel CS, Pendleton MK: Building a model of self-care for health promotion in aging, *J Nurs Scholarsh* 34:355, 2002.
Malmsten UG, Milsom I, Molander U et al: Urinary incontinence and lower urinary tract symptoms: an epidemiological study of men aged 45 to 99 years, *J Urol* 158(5):1733, 1997.
Molander U, Arvidsson L, Milsom I et al: A longitudinal cohort study of elderly women with urinary tract infection, *Maturitas* 34: 127, 2000.
Mostwin JL: Pathophysiology: the varieties of bladder overactivity, *Urology* 60(5 Suppl 1):22, 2002.
National Academy of Sciences, Food and Nutrition Board: *Recommended daily allowances,* ed 9, Washington, DC, 1980, The Academy.
Pearson BD: Urine control by elders: noninvasive strategies. In Funk SG et al, editors: *Key aspects of elder care: managing falls, incontinence and cognitive impairment,* New York, 1992, Springer.
Pearson BD: Liquidate a myth: reducing liquids is not advisable for elderly with urine control problems, *Urol Nurs* 13:86, 1993.
Quinn P, Goka J, Richardson H: Assessment of an electronic daily diary in patients with overactive bladder, *BJU Int* 91(7):647-652, 2003.
Resnick NM, Beckett LA, Branch LG et al: Short term variability of self report of incontinence in older persons, *J Am Geriatr Soc* 42:202, 1994.
Rozenberg S, Pastijn A, Gevers R et al: Estrogen therapy in older patients with recurrent urinary tract infections: a review, *Int J Fertil Womens Med* 49(2):71-74, 2004.
Samsioe G, Heraib F, Lidfeldt J et al: Urogenital symptoms in women aged 50-59 years. Women's Health in Lund Area (WHILSA) Study Group, *Gynecol Endocrinol* 13:113, 1999.
Sampselle CM: Teaching women to use a voiding diary, *Am J Nurs* 103(11): 62-64, 2003.
Stewart WF, Van Rooyen JB, Cundiff GW: Prevalence and burden of overactive bladder in the United States, *World J Urol* 20(6): 327-336, 2003.
Thacker HL: Estrogen ring use for genitourinary atrophy and menopausal symptomatology, *Geriatrics* 59(5):34, 36-7, 2004.

Wyman JF, Fantl JA, McClish DK et al: Comparative efficacy of behavioral interventions in the management of female urinary incontinence. Continence Program for Women Research Group, *Am J Obstet Gynecol* 179:999, 1998.

# Disorganized Infant behavior

*Mary A. Fuerst-DeWys*

**NANDA**

## Definition

Disintegrated physiological and neurobehavioral responses to the environment

A state of being of the infant/child displaying altered regulation, and modulation of the physiological and behavior subsystems of functioning (i.e., autonomic, motor, state, self-regulatory, and attention-interaction systems) that impairs the infant's ability of achieving homeostasis and interacting with the environment in organized, adaptive way (Wyngarden, DeWys, & Padnos, 1999)

I

## Defining Characteristics

### Physiological/Autonomic

*Cardiorespiratory:* bradycardia <100, tachycardia >180, tachypnea >60, dysrhythmias; irregular respirations, pauses, apnea, nasal flaring, chest retractions; skin color: rapid change, pale, mottled, dusky, perioral/periorbital duskiness cyanotic; stress cues: gaze averting, hiccoughing, coughing, sneezing, sighing, drawn face, slack jaw, open mouth, tongue thrust); oxygen desaturation (Wyngarden, DeWys, & Padnos, 1999)

*Visceral:* feeding intolerances, coughing, gagging, emesis, vomiting, hiccoughing, bowel straining, bowel movement with stress (Wyngarden, DeWys, & Padnos, 1999)

*Neuromotor:* tremors, tremulous, excessive startles, twitches, jitteriness, seizures, coughing, sneezing

### Motor System

*Hyper/increased tone:* frantic/disorganized movements, arching, finger splays, rapid extensions and flexions arm/legs, facial grimaces

*Hypo/decreased tone:* flaccid/limp, drawn face, body squirming, incoordinated and purposeless movements (Wyngarden, DeWys, & Padnos, 1999)

### State-Organization System

*Diffuse/disorganized sleep:* difficulty falling asleep, maintaining quiet/deep sleep, frequent awakening, frequent body movements, irregular respirations, whimpering

*Diffuse/disorganized arousal and awake state:* hyperaroused, irritable, fussy, restless, infrequent quiet awake state, dull facial expression, glassy eyes, floating eyes, worried/panicked look, hyperaroused, irritable, restless

*Rapid state oscillations:* difficulty transitioning between states, jumps from sleep to cry and cry to sleep (Wyngarden, DeWys, & Padnos, 1999)

### Self-Regulation System

*Deficient and/or ineffective self-regulatory capabilities:* common behaviors include hands to mouth, hand grasping/clasping, foot/leg bracing, sucking efforts, tucking body, hyper-attending to visual and/or auditory stimuli used effectively to regain or maintain control (Wyngarden, DeWys, & Padnos, 1999)

### Attention-Interaction System

*Attention:* difficulty achieving and maintaining focus attention to orient to visual and auditory sensory stimuli

*Interaction:* difficulty engaging in social interactions; easily stressed communicating avoidance/stress behaviors (e.g., gaze aversion, arching, fussing, irritable, turning away, finger splays leading to physiologic/autonomic indices); easily stressed with more than one type of sensory stimuli (visual, auditory, tactile, movement) (Wyngarden, DeWys, & Padnos, 1999)



## Related Factors (r/t)

### Prenatal

Congenital or genetic disorders; congenital infections; perinatal asphyxia; central nervous system insult; maternal illness (uncontrolled diabetes, mental illness); maternal substance exposure (drugs, alcohol); poor maternal nutrition; excessive maternal smoking

### Postnatal

Immature central nervous system; prematurity; small for gestational age (SGA); malnutrition; neurological and/or neuromotor problems; oral motor problems resulting in feeding problems/intolerances; internal stress (pain, gastrointestional, respiratory problems, and so on); external stress (invasive and painful procedures, inadequately pain medicated, medical illness, environmental stressors, and so on)

### Individual

Medical illness; immature physiological and/or neurological systems; prematurity; unclear cues communicating "hunger," "satiety," attention and consoling needs; sensory integration problems resulting in over- and/or underreactions to sensations (sights/visual, sounds/auditory, touch/tactile, and vestibular/movement); separated from parents; isolation during quiet awake times; imbalance between nurturing touch and task/procedure touch (Wyngarden, DeWys, & Padnos, 1999)

### Environmental

Transition to extrauterine life creates challenges for preterm infants struggling to maintain previously organized patterns of functioning and experiencing noncontigent, nonreciprocal stimulation within the environment; imbalance between sensory overstimulation and sensory deprivation; hospitalization, care practices noncontigent with infant's state and behavior cues; frequent sleep interruptions (Wyngarden, DeWys, & Padnos, 1999)

### Caregiver

Misreading or insensitive to infant's cues; cue deficient knowledge; mismatch between infant/child cues and contingent responding; lack of warmth and pleasure in caregiver's voice; negative mood; unable to successfully console and relieve the infant's distress; does not engage with and display interest in the infant; environmental stimulation contribution (Wyngarden, DeWys, & Padnos, 1999)

NOC

## Outcomes (Nursing Outcomes Classification)

### Suggested NOC Outcomes

Child Development: 2 Months, 4 Months, 6 Months; Growth; Neurological Status; Newborn Adaptation; Nutritional Status: Food and Fluid Intake; Preterm Infant Organization; Sleep; Thermoregulation: Newborn; Vital Signs



**Example NOC Outcome with Indicators**

**Preterm Infant Organization** as evidenced by the following indicators: $O_2$ saturation greater than 85%/Skin color/Feeding tolerance/Relaxed muscle tone/Smooth synchronous movement/Flexed posture/Hands brought to mouth/Appropriate time-out signals/Self-consolability/Deep sleep/Quiet-alert interactive state/Attentiveness to stimuli/Sustained alertness during interaction/Interaction with caregiver (Rate each indicator of **Preterm Infant Organization:** 1 = severely compromised, 2 = substantially compromised, 3 = moderately compromised, 4 = mildly compromised, 5 = not compromised [see Section I].)

## Client Outcomes

### Client Will (Specify Time Frame):

### Infant/Child

- Display clear behavior cues that communicate approach/engagement and stress/avoidance engagement needs (Wyngarden, DeWys, & Padnos, 1999)
- Display organized and physiologic/autonomic stability: cardiorespiratory, visceral, and neuromotor
- Display organized motor system: balance between flexion and extension, smooth, synchronous, and purposeful movements (Wyngarden, DeWys, & Padnos, 1999)
- Display state organizational stability: robust sleep and awake states, ability to maintain organized sleep and awake states, smooth transition between sleep and awake states (Wyngarden, DeWys, & Padnos, 1999)
- Demonstrate progress to and effective self-regulation: displays range of self-regulatory behaviors that facilitate regulation (Wyngarden, DeWys, & Padnos, 1999)
- Demonstrate ability to effectively orally feed
- Demonstrate ability to process, organize, and respond to sensory information sights/vision, sounds/auditory, touch/tactile), movement/vestibular in an adaptive way
- Demonstrate ability to engage in pleasurable parent/caregiver and infant/child interactions

### Parents/Significant Other

- Recognize infant/child behaviors as a unique way of communicating needs and goals
- Recognize infant behaviors used to communicate stress/avoidance and disengagement and approach/engagement
- Recognize and support infant's/child's drive and coping behaviors used to self-regulate
- Demonstrate ways to facilitate state modulation and organization
- Read and sensitively respond to infant/child behavior cues and needs
- Recognize how their style of interactions can positively or negatively affect the infant's/child's responses and allow the infant/child to take lead and by following their lead will foster adaptive communication patterns
- Structure and modify the environment in response to infant/child's behaviors, personal, nurturing, medical, and sensory needs (Wyngarden, DeWys, & Padnos, 1999)
- Identify appropriate positioning and handling techniques that enhance motor organization, comfort, and normal development and prevent positioning-acquired abnormalities (Wyngarden, DeWys, & Padnos, 1999)
- Promote infant/child's attention capabilities to orient and process sensory information (visual, auditory, tactile, vestibular/movement) (Wyngarden, DeWys, & Padnos, 1999)
- Engage in pleasurable parent-infant/child interactions that encourage bonding and attachment (Wyngarden, DeWys, & Padnos, 1999)
- Identify available community resources that provide early intervention services, community health nursing, parenting information, and parent-to-parent support (Wyngarden, DeWys, & Padnos, 1999)

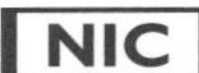

NIC

## Interventions (Nursing Interventions Classification)

### Suggested NIC Interventions

Developmental Care; Patient Education: Infant; Positioning; Sleep Enhancement

**Example NIC Activities—Development Care**

Teach parents to recognize infant states and cues and respond in sensitive way; identify and support infant's self-regulatory activities (e.g., hand-to-mouth, sucking, use of visual or auditory stimulus)

## Nursing Interventions and Rationales

- Identify infant's/child's behavioral organization as their unique way of communicating in five subsystems of functioning (i.e., physiological/autonomic, motor, state, self-regulation, attention-interactional). *The infant's principal method of communicating goals, needs, and limits for stress and stability is by behavior; therefore the infant's own behaviors provide a guide for individualizing care and interactions and promoting development (Als, 1982).*
- Provide individualized developmental care for low-birth-weight, preterm infants that positively influences neurodevelopmental functioning and parenting competence and reduces the severity of medical illnesses. **EB:** *Studies confirm individualized develop-*

*mental care for medically high-risk infants reduces intraventricular hemorrhage, need for mechanical ventilation, and severity of chronic lung disease, and improves neurodevelopmental outcomes (Als, 1994, 1986), and in low-risk preterm infants supports neurobehavioral outcomes by preventing frontal lobe and attentional difficulties seen in later ages (Buehler, 1995). A three-center, randomized, controlled trial of individualized developmental care for very-low-birth-weight preterm infants found improvement in medical, neurodevelopmental, parenting; earlier transition to full oral feeding; reduced discharge ages and hospital charges; improved weight, length, and head circumference; enhanced appreciation of the infant; and lower family stress (Als et al, 2003).*

- Recognize behavior used to communicate stress/avoidance/disengagement and approach/engagement. *The ability to read and interpret infant/child behavior provides a framework for responding to an infant/child contingently in a way that communicates the infant's/child's importance and ability to affect their environment (Als, 1982; Blackburn & Vandenberg, 1991).*
- Identify and support the infant's/child/s use of self-regulatory/consoling and habituation behaviors needed for mastering the environment. *A continuous interaction takes place between the infant and the environment; behaviors such as hand-to-mouth or hand-to-face, hand grasping, foot and leg bracing, sucking on fingers or fists, auditory and visual fixations, and postural changes are used to maintain or regain a balanced adaptation between the self and the environment. Supporting infant behaviors enhances the co-regulatory fit between the infant and the environment (Als, 1986).* **EBN:** *Study results indicated using a decision tree to modify developmental interventions based on physiologic and behavior cues when providing appropriate infant stimulation (Burns et al, 1994).*
- Demonstrate way to facilitate state organization and control. *Pace type, intensity, and timing of stimulation contingent with infant state and behavior cues. Provide care and stimulation contingent with the state of the infant that is critical to facilitation state organization (Fajardo et al, 1990).* **EBN:** *Study identified the importance of effective developmental handling during caregiving promoted behavioral state organization (Becker, 1997).*
- Cluster care whenever possible allowing for longer periods of uninterrupted sleep. *Introduce one intervention at a time and observe infant responses, taking care not to overstimulate during clustered care (Als, 1994; D'Apolito, 1991).*
- Correlate stress/disorganization behaviors to internal factors (e.g., pain, hunger, discomfort) and/or external factors (e.g., lights, noise, handling). *Noise is one of the common stresses in hospital intensive care units (ICUs), resulting in sensory overload with the potential for alteration in development (DePaul & Chambers, 1995; Elander & Hellstrom, 1995). Infant colic characterized by increased irritability, diminished ability to be soothed, and excessive restlessness reflects immature neurobehavior development, disorganized sleep-wake regulation, and internal factors (Keefe et al, 1996). Intrauterine cocaine exposure can result in disorganized behavior patterns of infants (DeWys, 1992).*
- Structure and organize the environment. *A developmental care approach designed to reduce environmental and procedural stress and facilitate motor and sleep-wake organization results in improved behavioral organization during the preterm periods (Als, 1994, 1998; Becker et al, 1991; Buehler et al, 1995; D'Apolito, 1991; Newman, 1986). Patterns of sound, light, and care tasks should minimize stress, conserve energy, and protect the*

*developing neonate from inappropriate environmental stimuli (Blackburn & Vandenberg, 1991; D'Apolito, 1991).*

- Identify appropriate position and handling techniques that enhance motor organization, comfort, and normal development and prevent positioning-acquired abnormalities. *Developmentally correct positioning (e.g., positioning in flexion, frequent positioning changes, using comforting physical containment as appropriate, opportunities for sucking and finger grasping) can provide comfort, decrease stress, conserve energy, enhance sleep, and facilitate normal development of the preterm infant (Aita, 2003; D'Apolito, 1991; McGrath, 1996; Sweeney, 2002).* **EBN and EB:** *Several studies found infants cared for in a neonatal intensive care unit (NICU) with an individualized developmental care approach showed improved motor system functioning compared to infants cared for in the same NICU before the approach was adopted (Mouridan, 1994; Als, 1986). Some research has indicated that use of a prone position improves quality of sleep and decreases stress for ventilated preterm infants (Chang, Anderson, & Lin, 2002). However, recent research indicates that the development of posture and mobility in newborns requires an optimal balance between active and passive muscle tone. Although prone positioning is physiologically more beneficial for the preterm infant, extended use of prone position can lead to short- and long-term postural and associated developmental problems (Monterosso, Kristjanson, & Cole, 2002). Consider swaddling in supine position for sleep as physical containment decreases startles in quiet sleep (QS) and increases duration of rapid eye movement (REM) sleep that helps infants return to sleep by not intervening. Safe swaddling for sleep in supine allows for good hip flexion/abduction and ample chest excursion and prevents sudden infant death syndrome (SIDS) associated with prone sleep positions. Handle infant slowly and gently, observing for cues of stress/stability; prepare for care/events by providing ongoing support during care and after; stay with infant during recovery; time care to avoid overstimulation and promote energy conservation (Fleisher et al, 1995).*
- Provide lots of opportunities for physical closeness, loving touch, massaging, cuddling, skin-to-skin (kangaroo care), and rocking. *Infant massage has been found to be a therapeutic tool that improves developmental outcomes, decreases stress, increases weight gain, improves motor function, aids sleep, increases alert-awake periods, improves pain tolerance, leads to improved feeding tolerance in stable preterm, improves attachment, and helps parents understand their infant's cues and enhances feeling of confidence (Beachy, 2003; Manious, 2002).*
- Include skin-to-skin (kangaroo care) experiences that promote preterm infant's adaptability to external environment. **EBN and EB:** *Parents have been found to be more sensitive, to show more positive affect, touch, and adaptation to infant cues when participating in skin-to-skin (kangaroo care) (Feldman, 2002). Kangaroo care provides an environment that supports autonomic stability and fosters improvement in basic physiological functions (Ludington-Hoe & Swinth, 1996). Infants have been found to benefit with cardiorespiratory stabilization, improved oxygenation, thermoregulation, increased weight gain, earlier feeding, easier breastfeeding, less crying, increases in quiet sleep, and decreases in length of stay (Chwo et al, 2002; Ludington-Hoe et al, 1999). Skin-to-skin contact (kangaroo care) has been found to increase a favorable perception of the infant by the caregiver, and result in parents who feel more competent in caring for their infant (Tessier et al, 1998).*
- Encourage parents' competence by appraising their parenting strengths and capabilities when caring for their infants. *Parent-to-parent programs that use experienced NICU*

*parents to support new parents to cope more effectively with the NICU help parents function comfortably and competently in the parental role (Lindsey et al, 1993).* **EBN:** *New NICU mothers who had participated in the NICU parent-to-parent support program had less anxiety during the first 4 months postdischarge by comparison, self-esteem increased, and mothers also had better maternal-infant relationships and more nurturing home environments at 12 months postdischarge (Roman et al, 1995). Parents must be supported and welcomed as active collaborators in their infant's care (Lawhon, 2002). This study found that when mothers evaluated their caregiving from birth through their infant's first year of life, they cited their most frequent source of confidence and competence was their infant's contentedness of mood and soothability, both of which identify that infant's responsiveness may be particularly salient to a mother's caregiving evaluation (Pridham, 2001).*

- Identify and support infant's/child's attention capabilities. *In organized quiet, alert states, infants are able to focus their attention and interact with their environments in a purposeful way (Burns et al, 1994). It is important to promote transition to alertness without effecting physiological and behavioral costs of disorganized arousal.* **EBN:** *In a study on correlating behavioral state organization of the very-low-birth-weight infants, results demonstrated a positive effect of developmental handling for behavioral state organization and recognizing that alertness may be promoted without the physiological and behavior effects of disorganized arousal (Becker, 1997).*
- Provide opportunities for parent/caregiver to engage in pleasurable parent-infant interactions contingent with infant cues responses; begin slowly and introduce one sensory stimulus at a time—looking, then slowly begin talking softly, adding gentle touch, if infant remains stable, swaddle and slowly pick up. Assess and respond contingently to infant cues. *Engagement and disengagement are infant cues signaling responses to internal and external stimuli (Blackburn, 1978). Contingent stimulation provides opportunity for the infant to explore and learn about their environment and the relationship of people and events. The parent/caregiver becomes the mediator between and infant and the environment (Blackburn, 1983). Pleasurable and rewarding parent-infant interactions will build a trusting relationship that is the core of bonding and attachment.*
- Provide pleasurable sensory motor experiences (i.e., visual, auditory, tactile, vestibular/movement, prioproceptive) that enhance development of sensory pathways. *Healthy 33- to 34-week postconceptual age infants who received 15 minutes of auditory, visual, tactile, and vestibular stimulation each day were found to improve state modulation and their ability to maintain quiet-alert state that enhances parent-infant interactions and feedings (White-Traut et al, 1996). Observe how the infant responds to different sensations. Does he/she "overreact" or "underreact"? And which sensation? Modify sensory experiences as appropriate. By using the decision tree as guide to modify sensory stimulation can promote behavioral organization, positive patterns of maternal-infant interactions, and conserve the energy for growth (Burns et al, 1993).*
- Have knowledge of community-based follow-up programs for preterm and infants at risk and their families discharged from the NICU. *Medical and developmental conditions requiring very close follow-up should be communicated to parents, either through referrals given prior to discharge or who to contact for early intervention services. Health care providers need to be aware and support parents who may feel isolated and in various stages of grieving. Seamless communication between NICU staff and community agencies enhance*

*parent's feelings of confidence during the difficult transition from NICU discharge to home (Sherman, 2002).*

## Multicultural

- Assess for the influence of cultural beliefs, norms, and values on the family's perceptions of infant/child behavior. **EBN:** *What the family considers normal infant/child behavior may be based on cultural perceptions (Cochran, 1998; Doswell & Erlen, 1998; Guarnaccia, 1998; Leininger & McFarland, 2002). A recent study found that Latino mothers overwhelmingly preferred treatment options other than medication because they understood medication to be addictive, dulling of cognitive processes, and inappropriate for behavior problems (Arcia, Fernandez, & Jaquez, 2004). A recent study examined parent and teacher agreement using a child behavior checklist. The predominantly African-American parents generally rated more children as having problem behaviors than did teachers.*
- Use a neutral, indirect style when addressing areas where improvement is needed (such as a need for verbal or oral stimulation) when working with Native-American clients. **EBN:** *Using indirect statements such as "Other mothers have tried . . ." or "I had a client who tried 'X,' and it seemed to work very well" will assist in avoiding resentment from the parent (Seideman et al, 1996).*
- Acknowledge and praise parenting strengths noted. **EBN:** *This will increase trust and foster a working relationship with the parent (Seideman et al, 1996).*
- Use therapeutic communication techniques that emphasize acceptance, offer the self, validate the client's concerns, and convey respect when discussing the infant/child behavior. **EBN:** *Validation is therapeutic communication technique that lets the client know that the nurse has heard and understands what was said, and it promotes the nurse-client relationship (Heineken, 1998). Studies show that even when language is not a barrier, some ethnic clients may be reluctant to discuss their beliefs and practices because of fear of criticism or ridicule (Evans & Cunningham, 1996).*

## Home Care

- The above interventions may be adapted for home care use.
- Educate families in preparing home environment. *Patterns of sound, light, and caregiving tasks should minimize stress, conserve energy, and protect the developing neonate from inappropriate environmental stimuli (Blackburn & Vandenberg, 1991; VandenBerg, 1999).*
- Prepare families for realistic challenges of caring for preterm and at risk infants prior to discharge. Differences include understanding "corrected" age, feeding skills, poor endurance/tire easily, shorter sleep-wake cycles, less alert and more fussy when awake, fuss before returning to sleep, overstimulation, and so on. *Help parents identify their infant's characteristics, developmental capabilities and limitations, interventions that will support optimal growth and development, and their supportive network when helping parents ease the transition from NICU to home (VandenBerg, 1999). It is important for parents to know the typical transition period from hospital to home is up to 4 months from due date (Gorski, 1988).*
- Encourage families to teach friends/visitors to recognize and respond to infant's unique behavioral cues. *It is important for families to feel comfortable obtaining support from their regular support systems; therefore supportive persons need to be taught how to in-*

*teract in the environment in a way that supports both the family and the infant. The ability to read and interpret infant behavior provides a framework for responding to infants in a way that communicates both the infant's/child's importance and the message that he or she is able to affect his or her environment (Als, 1982; Blackburn & Vandenberg, 1991).*

- Provide information of community resources, developmental follow-up services, and parent-to-parent support programs. *Findings of following healthy preterm infants of varying gestational age suggested the need for appropriate anticipatory guidance and support for families, including close development monitoring. Including those born as little as 3 weeks early is advocated. Parents benefit from knowledge and expectations of their infant's autonomic sensitivity, lower threshold to motor system disorganization, potential difficulties with self-calm, and more tentative and fragile ability to orient and attend to environmental and social stimuli. Additional anticipatory guidance should include knowledge about prevention of overstimulation and exhaustion of these more sensitive infants (Mouradian, Als, & Coster, 2000).*

I

## Family Teaching

- Assist families/support systems in recognizing and responding to infant's unique behavioral cues. *Demonstrating and modeling appropriate interactional skills is an integral component of family education and will improve family-infant interactions (McGrath & Conliffe-Torres, 1996). Assisting parents with recognizing infant states and state modulation and self-consoling strategies provides caregivers with greater sense of competence (Nursing Child Assessment Satellite Training, 1994).*
- Give anticipatory guidance to parents about what infant/child behaviors are possible in given situations.
- Model calming interventions to provide parents with tools for positive interactions with their infant/child (Karl, 1999).
- Nurture parents so that they in turn can nurture their infant/child. *The psychological trauma to parents when their infant is hospitalized in the NICU cannot be underestimated (Doering, 1999). The most difficult and overlooked aspects of care of the high-risk neonate is effective, timely, and compassionate information delivery to parents and family by the medical staff (Sherman, 2002).*
- Establish a nurturing environment in which parents can interact with their infant/child (Goulet et al, 1998).
- Have knowledge of community early intervention services and follow-up programs for preterm and at-risk infants and families.

## evolve WEBSITES FOR EDUCATION

See the EVOLVE website for World Wide Web resources for client education.

## REFERENCES

Aita M, Snider L: The art of developmental care in the NICU: a concept analysis, *J Adv Nurs* 41(3):223, 2003.

Als H: A synactive model of neonatal behavioral organization: framework for the assessment and support of the neurobehavioral development of the premature infant and his parents in the environment of the neonatal intensive care unit, *Phys Occup Ther Pediatr* 6:3, 1986.

Als H: Toward a synactive theory of development: promise for the assessment and support of infant individuality, *Infant Ment Health J* 3:229, 1982.

Als H: Developmental care in the newborn intensive care unit, *Curr Opin Pediatr* 10:138, 1998.

Als H, Gilkerson L, Duffy FH et al: A three-center, randomized, controlled trial of individualized developmental care for very low birth weight preterm infants: medical, neurodevelopmental, parenting, and caregiving effects, *J Dev Behav Pediatr* 24(6):399: 2003.

Als H, Lawhon G, Brown E et al: Individualized behavioral and environmental care for the very low birth weight preterm infant at high risk for bronchopulmonary dysplasia: neonatal intensive care unit and developmental outcome, *Pediatrics* 78: 1123, 1986.

Als H, Lawhon G, Duffy FH et al: Individualized developmental care for the very low birth weight preterm infant: medical and neurofunctional effects, *JAMA* 272: 853:1994.

Anderson J, Auster-Liebhaber J: Developmental therapy in the neonatal intensive care unit, *Phys Occup Ther Pediatr* 4:89, 1984.

Beachy JM: Premature infant massage in the NICU, *Neonatal Netw* 22(3):39-45, 2003.

Becker PT, Brazy JE, Grunwald PC: Behavioral state organization of very low birth weight infants: effects of developmental handling during caregiving, *Infant Behav Dev* 20(4):503, 1997.

Becker PT, Grunwald PC, Moorman J et al: Outcomes of developmentally supportive nursing care for very low birth weight infants, *Nurs Res* 40:150, 1991.

Blackburn S: Fostering behavior development of high-risk infants, *J Obstet Gynecol Neonatal Nurs* 12:76-86, 1983.

Blackburn S: State related behaviors and individual differences. In Barnard KE, editor: *Nursing child assessment satellite training: learning resource manual,* Seattle, 1978, University of Washington.

Blackburn S, Vandenberg K: Assessment and management of neonatal development. In Kenner C et al, editors: *Comprehensive neonatal nursing: a physiologic approach,* Toronto, 1991, WB Saunders.

Buehler DM, Als H, Duffy FH et al: Effectiveness of individualized developmental care for low-risk preterm infants: behavioral and electrophysiologic evidence, *Pediatrics* 96(5):923, 1995.

Burns K, Cunningham N, White-Traut R et al: Infant stimulation: modification of an intervention based on physiologic and behavioral cues, *J Obstet Gynecol Neonatal Nurs* 23:581, 1994.

Chang Y, Anderson G, Lin C: Effects of prone and supine positions on sleep state and stress responses in mechanically ventilated preterm infants during the first postnatal week, *J Adv Nurs* 40(2):161, 2002.

Chwo MJ, Anderson GC, Good M et al: A randomized controlled trial of early kangaroo care for preterm infants: effects on temperature, weight, behavior, and acuity, *J Nurs Res* 10(2):129, 2002.

Cochran M: Tears have no color, *Am J Nurs* 98(6):53, 1998.

D'Apolito K: What is an organized infant? *Neonatal Netw* 10(1):23, 1991.

DePaul D, Chambers SE: Environmental noise in the neonatal intensive care unit: implications for nursing practice, *J Perinatal Neonatal Nurs* 8:71, 1995.

DeWys M, McComish-Fry J: Infants states and cues: facilitating effective parent-infant interactions. In *Caring for infants: a resource manual for caring for infant trainers,* East Lansing, Mich, 1992, Michigan State University Board of Trustees.

Doswell W, Erlen J: Multicultural issues and ethical concerns in the delivery of revising care interventions, *Nurs Clin North Am* 33(2):353, 1998.

Elander G, Hellstrom G: Reduction of noise levels in intensive care units for infants: evaluation of an intervention program, *Heart Lung* 24:376, 1995.

Evans CA, Cunningham BA: Caring for the ethnic elder, *Geriatr Nurs* 17(3):105, 1996.

Fajardo B, Browning M, Fisher D et al: Effect of nursery environment on state regulation in very-low-birth-weight premature infants, *Infant Behav Dev* 13:287, 1990.

Feldman R, Eidelman AI, Sirota L et al: Comparison of skin-to-skin (kangaroo) and traditional care: parenting outcomes and preterm infant behavior, *Pediatrics* 110(1):16, 2002.

Fleisher B, VandenBerg K, Constantinou J et al: Individualized developmental care for very low birthweight premature infants, *Clin Pediatr* 34:523-529, 1995.

Goulet C, Bell L, St-Cyr D et al: A concept analysis of parent-infant attachment, *J Adv Nurs* 28(5):1071, 1998.

Guarnaccia, P: Multicultural experiences of family caregiving: a study of African American, European American, and Hispanic American families, *New Direct Ment Health Serv* 77:45, 1998.

Heineken J: Patient silence is not necessarily client satisfaction: communication in home care nursing, *Home Healthc Nurse* 16(2): 115, 1998.

Karl D: The interactive newborn bath: using infant neurobehavior to connect parents and newborns, *MCN Am J Matern Child Nurse* 24(6):280, 1999.

Keefe MR, Kotzer AM, Froese-Fretz A et al: A longitudinal comparison of irritable and nonirritable infants, *Nurs Res* 45:4, 1996.

Lawhon G: Facilitation of parenting the premature infant within the newborn intensive care unit, *J Perinat Neonatal Nurs* 16(1): 71, 2002.
Leininger MM, McFarland MR: *Transcultural nursing: concepts, theories, research and practices,* ed 3, New York, 2002, McGraw-Hill.
Lindsey JK, Roman LA, DeWys M et al: Creative caregiving in the NICU: parent-to-parent support, *Neonatal Netw* 12(4):37-44, 1993.
Ludington SM: Energy conservation during skin-to-skin contact between preterm infants and their mothers, *Heart Lung* 19(5 pt 1):445, 1990.
Ludington-Hoe SM, Swinth JY: Developmental aspects of kangaroo care, *J Obstet Gynecol Neonatal Nurs* 25(8): 691, 1996.
Ludington-Hoe SM, Anderson GC, Simpson S et al: Birth-related fatigue in 34-36–week preterm neonates: rapid recovery with very early kangaroo (skin-to-skin) care, *J Obstet Gynecol Neonatal Nurs* 28(1):94, 1999.
Mainous R: Infant massage as a component of developmental care: past, present, and future, *Holist Nurs Pract* 16(5):1, 2002.
McGrath J, Conliffe-Torres S: Integrating family-centered developmental assessment and intervention into routine care in the neonatal intensive care unit, *Nurs Clin North Am* 31(2):367, 1996.
Monterosso L, Kristjanson L, Cole J: Neuromotor development and the physiologic effects of positioning in very low birth weight infants, *J Obstet Gynecol Neonatal Nurs* 31(2):128, 2002.
Mouradian LE, Als H: The influence of neonatal intensive care unit caregiving practices on motor functioning of preterm infants, *Am J Occup Ther* 48(6):527 1994.
Mouradian LE, Als H, Coster WJ: Neurobehavioral functioning of healthy preterm infants of varying gestational ages, *J Dev Behav Pediatr* 21(6):408-427, 2000.
Newman L: Social and sensory environment of low birth weight infants in a special care nursery, *J Nerv Ment Dis* 169:448, 1986.
Nursing Child Assessment Satellite Training: *NCAST caregiver/parent-child interaction feeding manual,* Seattle, 1994, University of Washington School of Nursing.
Pridham K, Chin-Yu L, Brown R: Mothers' evaluation of their caregiving for premature and full-term infants through the first: contributing factors, *Res Nurs Health* 24:157, 2001.
Roman LA, Lindsey JK, Boger RP et al: Parent-to-parent support initiated in the neonatal intensive care unit, *Res Nurs Health* 18: 385-393, 1995.
Seideman RY, Jacobson S, Primeaux M et al: Assessing American Indian families, *MCN Am J Matern Child Nurs* 21(6):274, 1996.
Sherman MP, et al: Follow-up of the NICU patient. Medicine: Instant Access to the Minds of Medicine. Available at www.emedicine.com/ped/topic2600.htm, accessed on May 28, 2005.
Sweeney J, Gutierrez T: Musculoskeletal implications of preterm infant positioning in the NICU, *J Perinatal Neonatal Nurs* 16(1): 58, 2002.
Tessier R, Cristo M, Velez S et al: Kangaroo mother care and the bonding hypothesis, *Pediatrics* 102(2):e17, 1998.
White-Traut R: Environmental factors and alternative therapies in nursing, *Voice* 4(9):1, 1996.
White-Traut RC, Nelson MN, Silvestri JM et al: Patterns of physiological and behavioral response of intermediate care preterm infants to intervention, *Pediatr Nurs* 19:625, 1993.
Wyngarden K, DeWys M, Padnos M: Learnings from the field: the impact of using two new nursing diagnoses, organized infant behavior and disorganized infant behavior (abstract), Classification of nursing diagnoses: Proceedings of the thirteenth conference, NANDA, 1999.

I

# Risk for disorganized Infant behavior

*Mary A. Fuerst-DeWys and T. Heather Herdman*

**NANDA**

## Definition

Disintegrated physiological and neurobehavioral responses to the environment

A state of being of the infant/child displaying altered regulation, and modulation of the physiological and behavior subsystems of functioning (i.e., autonomic, motor, state, self-regulatory, and attention-interaction systems) that impairs the infant's ability of achieving homeostasis and interacting with the environment in organized, adaptive way (Wyngarden, DeWys, & Padnos, 1999)

## Defining Characteristics

### Physiological/Autonomic

*Cardiorespiratory:* bradycardia <100, tachycardia >180, tachypnea >60, dysrhythmias; irregular respirations, pauses, apnea, nasal flaring, chest retractions skin color: rapid change, pale, mottled, dusky, perioral/periorbital duskiness cyanotic; stress cues: gaze averting, hiccoughing, coughing, sneezing, sighing, drawn face, slack jaw, open mouth, tongue thrust); oxygen desaturation (Wyngarden, DeWys, & Padnos, 1999)
*Viseral:* feeding intolerances, coughing, gagging, emesis, vomiting, hiccoughing, bowel straining, bowel movement with stress (Wyngarden, DeWys, & Padnos, 1999)
*Neuromotor:* tremors, tremulous, excessive startles, twitches, jitteriness, seizures, coughing, sneezing



### Motor System

*Hyper/increased tone:* frantic/disorganized movements, arching, finger splays, rapid extensions and flexions arm/legs, facial grimaces
*Hypo/decreased tone:* flaccid/limp, drawn face, body squirming, incoordinated and purposeless movements (Wyngarden, DeWys, & Padnos, 1999)

### State-Organization System

*Diffuse/disorganized sleep:* difficulty falling asleep, maintaining quiet/deep sleep, frequent awakening, frequent body movements, irregular respirations, whimpering
*Diffuse/disorganized arousal and awake state:* hyperaroused, irritable, fussy, restless, infrequent quiet awake state, dull facial expression, glassy eyes, floating eyes, worried/panic look, hyperaroused, irritable, restless
*Rapid state oscillations:* difficulty transitioning between states, jumps from sleep to cry and cry to sleep (Wyngarden, DeWys, & Padnos, 1999)

### Self-Regulation System

*Deficient and/or ineffective self-regulatory capabilities:* common behaviors include: hands to mouth, hand grasping/clasping, foot/leg bracing, sucking efforts, tucking body, hyperattending to visual and/or auditory stimuli used effectively to regain or maintain control (Wyngarden, DeWys, & Padnos, 1999)

### Attention-Interaction System

*Attention:* difficulty achieving and maintaining focus attention to orient to visual and auditory sensory stimuli
*Interaction:* difficulty engaging in social interactions; easily stressed communicating avoidance/stress behaviors (e.g., gaze aversion, arching, fussing, irritable, turning away, finger splays leading to physiologic/autonomic indices); easily stressed with more than one type of sensory stimuli (visual, auditory, tactile, movement) (Wyngarden, DeWys, & Padnos, 1999)

## Related Factors (r/t)

### Prenatal

Congenital or genetic disorders; congenital infections; perinatal asphyxia; central nervous system insult; maternal illness (uncontrolled diabetes, mental illness); maternal substance exposure (drugs, alcohol); poor maternal nutrition; excessive maternal smoking

### Postnatal

Immature central nervous system; prematurity; small for gestational age (SGA); malnutrition; neurological and/or neuromotor problems; oral motor problems resulting in feeding problems/intolerances; internal stress (pain, gastrointestional, respiratory problems, and so on); external stress (invasive and painful procedures, inadequately pain medicated, medical illness, environmental stressors, and so on)



### Individual

Medical illness; immature physiological and/or neurological systems; prematurity; unclear cues communicating "hunger," "satiety," attention and consoling needs; sensory integration problems resulting in over- and/or underreactions to sensations (sights/visual, sounds/auditory, touch/tactile, and vestibular/movement); separated from parents; isolation during quiet awake times; imbalance between nurturing touch and task/procedure touch (Wyngarden, DeWys, & Padnos, 1999)

### Environmental

Transition to extrauterine life creates challenges for preterm infants struggling to maintain previously organized patterns of functioning and experiencing noncontigent, nonreciprocal stimulation within the environment; imbalance between sensory overstimulation and sensory deprivation; hospitalization, care practices noncontigent with infant's state and behavior cues; frequent sleep interruptions (Wyngarden, DeWys, & Padnos, 1999)

### Caregiver

Misreading or insensitive to infant's cues; cue-deficient knowledge; mismatch between infant/child cues and contingent responding; lack of warmth and pleasure in caregiver's voice; negative mood; unable to successfully console and relieve the infant's distress; does not engage with and display interest in the infant; environmental stimulation contribution (Wyngarden, DeWys, & Padnos, 1999)

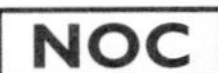


## Outcomes (Nursing Outcomes Classification)

### Suggested NOC Outcomes

Child Development: 2 Months, 4 Months, 6 Months; Growth; Neurological Status; Newborn Adaptation; Nutritional Status: Food and Fluid Intake; Preterm Infant Organization; Sleep; Thermoregulation: Newborn; Vital Signs

**Example NOC Outcome with Indicators**

**Preterm Infant Organization** as evidenced by the following indicators: $O_2$ saturation greater than 85%/Skin color/Feeding tolerance/Relaxed muscle tone/Smooth synchronous movement/Flexed posture/Hands brought to mouth/Appropriate time-out signals/Self-consolability/Deep sleep/Quiet-alert interactive state/Attentiveness to stimuli/Sustained alertness during interaction/Interaction with caregiver (Rate each indicator of **Preterm Infant Organization:** 1 = severely compromised, 2 = substantially compromised, 3 = moderately compromised, 4 = mildly compromised, 5 = not compromised [see Section I].)

## Client Outcomes

### Client Will (Specify Time Frame):

### Infant/Child

- Display clear behavior cues that communicate approach/engagement and stress/avoidance engagement needs (Wyngarden, DeWys, & Padnos, 1999)
- Display organized and physiologic/autonomic stability: cardiorespiratory, visceral, and neuromotor
- Display organized motor system: balance between flexion and extension, smooth, synchronous, and purposeful movements (Wyngarden, DeWys, & Padnos, 1999)
- Display state organizational stability: robust sleep and awake states, ability to maintain organized sleep and awake states, smooth transition between sleep and awake states (Wyngarden, DeWys, & Padnos, 1999)
- Demonstrate progress to and effective self-regulation: displays range of self-regulatory behaviors that facilitate regulation (Wyngarden, DeWys, & Padnos, 1999)
- Demonstrate ability to effectively orally feed
- Demonstrate ability to process, organize, and respond to sensory information sights/vision, sounds/auditory, touch/tactile), movement/vestibular in an adaptive way
- Demonstrate ability to engage in pleasurable parent/caregiver and infant/child interactions

### Parents/Significant Other

- Recognize infant/child behaviors as a unique way of communicating needs and goals
- Recognize infant behaviors used to communicate stress/avoidance and disengagement and approach/engagement
- Recognize and support infant's/child's drive and coping behaviors used to self-regulate
- Demonstrate ways to facilitate state modulation and organization
- Read and sensitively respond to infant/child behavior cues and needs
- Recognize how their style of interactions can positively or negatively affect the infant's/child's responses and allow the infant/child to take lead and by following their lead will foster adaptive communication patterns
- Structure and modify the environment in response to infant/child's behaviors, personal, nurturing, medical, and sensory needs (Wyngarden, DeWys, & Padnos, 1999)
- Identify appropriate positioning and handling techniques that enhance motor organization, comfort, and normal development and prevent positioning-acquired abnormalities (Wyngarden, DeWys, & Padnos, 1999)

- Promote infant/child's attention capabilities to orient and process sensory information (visual, auditory, tactile, vestibular/movement) (Wyngarden, DeWys, & Padnos, 1999)
- Engage in pleasurable parent-infant/child interactions that encourage bonding and attachment (Wyngarden, DeWys, & Padnos, 1999)
- Identify available community resources that provide early intervention services, community health nursing, parenting information, and parent-to-parent support (Wyngarden, DeWys, & Padnos, 1999)

**NIC**

## Interventions (Nursing Interventions Classification)

### Suggested NIC Interventions

Developmental Care; Patient Education: Infant; Positioning; Sleep Enhancement

**Example NIC Activities—Development Care**

Teach parents to recognize infant states and cues and respond in sensitive way; identify and support infant's self-regulatory activities (e.g., hand-to-mouth, sucking, use of visual or auditory stimulus)

I

## Nursing Interventions and Rationales

- Identify infant's/child's behavioral organization as their unique way of communicating in five subsystems of functioning: physiological/autonomic, motor, state, self-regulation, attention-interactional. *The infant's principal method of communicating goals, needs, and limits for stress and stability is by behavior; therefore the infant's own behaviors provide a guide for individualizing care and interactions and promoting development (Als, 1982).*
- Provide individualized developmental care for low-birth-weight, preterm infants that positively influences neurodevelopmental functioning and parenting competence and reduces the severity of medical illnesses. **EB:** *Studies confirm individualized developmental care for medically high-risk infants reduces intraventricular hemorrhage, need for mechanical ventilation, and severity of chronic lung disease, and improves neurodevelopmental outcomes (Als, 1986, 1994), and in low-risk preterm infants supports neurobehavioral outcomes by preventing frontal lobe and attentional difficulties seen in later ages (Buehler, 1995). A three-center, randomized, controlled trial of individualized developmental care for very-low-birth-weight preterm infants found improvement in medical, neurodevelopmental, parenting; earlier transition to full oral feeding; reduced discharge ages and hospital charges; improved weight, length, and head circumference; enhanced appreciation of the infant; and lower family stress (Als et al, 2003).*
- Recognize behavior used to communicate stress/avoidance/disengagement and approach/engagement. *The ability to read and interpret infant/child behavior provides a framework for responding to an infant/child contingently in a way that communicates the infant's/child's importance and ability to affect their environment (Als, 1982; Blackburn & Vandenberg, 1991).*
- Identify and support the infant's/child's use of self-regulatory/consoling and habituation behaviors needed for mastering the environment. *A continuous interaction takes*

*place between the infant and the environment; behaviors such as hand-to-mouth or hand-to-face, hand grasping, foot and leg bracing, sucking on fingers or fists, auditory and visual fixation, and postural changes are used to maintain or regain a balanced adaptation between the self and the environment. Supporting infant behaviors enhances the coregulatory fit between the infant and the environment (Als, 1986).* **EBN:** *Study results indicated when providing appropriate infant stimulation using a decision tree to modify developmental interventions based on physiologic and behavior cues (Burns et al, 1994).*

- Demonstrate way to facilitate state organization and control. *Pace type, intensity, and timing of stimulation contingent with infant state and behavior cues. Provide care and stimulation contingent with the state of the infant that is critical to facilitation state organization (Fajardo et al, 1990).* **EBN:** *Study identified the importance of effective developmental handling during caregiving promoted behavioral state organization (Becker, 1997).*
- Cluster care whenever possible allowing for longer periods of uninterrupted sleep. *Introduce one intervention at a time and observe infant responses, taking care not to overstimulate during clustered care (Als, 1994; D'Apolito, 1991).*
- Correlate stress/disorganization behaviors to internal factors (e.g., pain, hunger, discomfort) and/or external factors (e.g., lights, noise, handling). *Noise is one of the common stresses in hospital ICUs, resulting in sensory overload with the potential for alteration in development (DePaul & Chambers, 1995; Elander & Hellstrom, 1995). Infant colic characterized by increased irritability, diminished ability to be soothed, and excessive restlessness reflects immature neurobehavior development and disorganized sleep-wake regulation and internal factors (Keefe et al, 1996). Intrauterine cocaine exposure can result in disorganized behavior patterns of infants (DeWys, 1992).*
- Structure and organize the environment. *A developmental care approach designed to reduce environmental and procedural stress and facilitate motor and sleep-wake organization results in improved behavioral organization during the preterm periods (Als, 1994, 1998; Becker et al, 1991; Buehler et al, 1995; D'Apolito, 1991; Newman, 1986). Patterns of sound, light, and care tasks should minimize stress, conserve energy, and protect the developing neonate from inappropriate environmental stimuli (Blackburn & Vandenberg, 1991; D'Apolito, 1991).*
- Identify appropriate position and handling techniques that enhance motor organization, comfort, and normal development and prevent positioning-acquired abnormalities. *Developmentally correct positioning (e.g., positioning in flexion, frequent positioning changes, using comforting physical containment as appropriate, opportunities for sucking and finger grasping) can provide comfort, decrease stress, conserve energy, enhance sleep and facilitate normal development of the preterm infant (Aita, 2003; D'Apolito, 1991; McGrath, 1996; Sweeney, 2002).* **EBN and EB:** *Several studies found infants cared for in an NICU with an individualized developmental care approach showed improved motor system functioning compared to infants cared for in the same NICU before the approach was adopted (Mouridan, 1994; Als, 1986). Some research has indicated that use of a prone position improves quality of sleep and decreases stress for ventilated preterm infants (Chang, Anderson, & Lin, 2002). However, recent research indicates that the development of posture and mobility in newborns requires an optimal balance between active and passive muscle tone. Although prone positioning is physiologically more beneficial for the preterm infant, extended use of prone position can lead to short- and long-term postural and associ-*

*ated developmental problems (Monterosso, Kristjanson, & Cole, 2002). Consider swaddling in supine position for sleep as physical containment decreases startles in quiet sleep (QS) and increases duration of REM sleep that helps infants return to sleep by not intervening. Safe swaddling for sleep in supine allows for good hip flexion/abduction and ample chest excursion and prevents SIDS associated with prone sleep positions. Handle infant slowly and gently, observing for cues of stress/stability; prepare for care/events by providing ongoing support during care and after; stay with infant during recovery; time care to avoid overstimulation and promote energy conservation (VandenBerg, 1996).*

- Provide lots of opportunities for physical closeness, loving touch, massaging, cuddling, skin-to-skin (kangaroo care), and rocking. *Infant massage has been found to be a therapeutic tool that improves developmental outcomes, decreases stress, increases weight gain, improves motor function, aids sleep, increases alert-awake periods, improves pain tolerance, leads to improved feeding tolerance in stable preterm, improves attachment, and helps parents understand their infant's cues and enhances feeling of confidence (Beachy, 2003; Manious, 2002).*
- Include skin-to-skin (kangaroo care) experiences that promote preterm infant's adaptability to external environment. **EBN and EB:** *Parents have been found to be more sensitive, to show more positive affect, touch, and adaptation to infant cues when participating in skin-to-skin (kangaroo care)(Feldman, 2002). Kangaroo care provides an environment that supports autonomic stability and fosters improvement in basic physiological functions (Ludington-Hoe & Swinth, 1996). Infants have been found to benefit with cardiorespiratory stabilization, improved oxygenation, thermoregulation, increased weight gain, earlier feeding, easier breastfeeding, less crying, increases in quiet sleep, and decreases in length of stay (Chwo et al, 2002; Ludington-Hoe et al, 1999). Skin-to-skin contact (kangaroo care) has been found to increase a favorable perception of the infant by the caregiver, and result in parents who feel more competent in caring for their infant (Tessier et al, 1998).*
- Encourage parents' competence by appraising their parenting strengths and capabilities when caring for their infants. Parent-to-parent programs that use experienced NICU parents to support new parents to cope more effectively with the NICU help parents function comfortably and competently in the parental role (Lindsey et al, 1993). **EBN:** *New NICU mothers who had participated in the NICU parent-to-parent support program had less anxiety during the first 4 months post discharge by comparison, self-esteem increased and mothers also had better maternal-infant relationships and more nurturing home environments at 12 months post discharge (Roman et al, 1995). Parents must be supported and welcomed as active collaborators in their infant's care (Lawhon, 2002). This study found when mothers evaluated their caregiving from birth through their infant's first year of life, they cited their most frequent source of confidence and competence was their infant's contentedness of mood and soothability, both of which identify that infant responsiveness may be particulary salient to a mother's caregiving evaluation (Pridham, 2001).*
- Identify and support infant/child's attention capabilities. *In organized quiet, alert states, infants are able to focus their attention and interact with their environments in a purposeful way (Burns et al, 1994). It is important to promote transition to alertness without effecting physiological and behavioral costs of disorganized arousal.* **EBN:** *In a study on correlating behavioral state organization of the very-low-birth-weight infants, results demonstrated a positive effect of developmental handling for behavioral state organization and*

*recognizing that alertness may be promoted without the physiological and behavior effects of disorganized arousal (Becker, 1997).*

- Provide opportunities for parent/caregiver to engage in pleasurable parent-infant interactions contingent with infant cues responses; begin slowly and introduce one sensory stimulus at a time—looking, then slowly begin talking softly, adding gentle touch, if infant remains stable, swaddle and slowly pick up. Assess and respond contingently to infant cues. *Engagement and disengagement are infant cues signaling responses to internal and external stimuli (Blackburn, 1978). Contingent stimulation provides opportunity for the infant to explore and learn about their environment and the relationship of people and events. The parent/caregiver becomes the mediator between and infant and the environment (Blackburn, 1983). Pleasurable and rewarding parent-infant interactions will build a trusting relationship that is the core of bonding and attachment.*
- Provide pleasurable sensory motor experiences (i.e., visual, auditory, tactile, vestibular/movement, prioproceptive) that enhance development of sensory pathways. *Healthy 33- to 34-week postconceptual age infants who received 15 minutes of auditory, visual, tactile, and vestibular stimulation each day were found to improve state modulation and their ability to maintain quiet-alert state that enhances parent-infant interactions and feedings (White-Traut et al, 1996). Observe how the infant responds to different sensations. Does he/she "overreact" or "underreact"? And which sensation? Modify sensory experiences as appropriate. By using the decision tree as guide to modify sensory stimulation can promote behavioral organization, positive patterns of maternal-infant interactions, and conserve the energy for growth (Burns et al, 1993).*
- Have knowledge of community-based follow-up programs for preterm and infants at risk and their families discharged from the NICU. *Medical and developmental conditions requiring very close follow-up should be communicated to parents, either through referrals given prior to discharge, who to contact for early intervention services. Health care providers need to be aware and support parents who may feel isolated and in various stages of grieving. Seamless communication between NICU staff and community agencies enhance parent's feelings of confidence during the difficult transition from NICU discharge to home (Sherman, 2002).*

## Multicultural

- Assess for the influence of cultural beliefs, norms, and values on the family's perceptions of infant/child behavior. **EBN:** *What the family considers normal infant/child behavior may be based on cultural perceptions (Cochran, 1998; Doswell & Erlen, 1998; Guarnaccia, 1998; Leininger & McFarland, 2002).*
- Use a neutral, indirect style when addressing areas where improvement is needed, such as a need for verbal or oral stimulation, when working with Native-American clients. **EBN:** *Using indirect statements such as "Other mothers have tried . . ." or "I had a client who tried 'X,' and it seemed to work very well" will assist in avoiding resentment from the parent (Seideman et al, 1996).*
- Acknowledge and praise parenting strengths noted. **EBN:** *This will increase trust and foster a working relationship with the parent (Seideman et al, 1996).*
- Use therapeutic communication techniques that emphasize acceptance, offer the self, validate the client's concerns, and convey respect when discussing the infant/child

behavior. **EBN:** *Validation is therapeutic communication technique that lets the client know that the nurse has heard and understands what was said, and it promotes the nurse-client relationship (Heineken, 1998). Studies show that even when language is not a barrier, some ethnic clients may be reluctant to discuss their beliefs and practices because of fear of criticism or ridicule (Evans & Cunningham, 1996).*

### Home Care

- The above interventions may be adapted for home care use.
- Educate families in preparing home environment. *Patterns of sound, light, and caregiving tasks should minimize stress, conserve energy, and protect the developing neonate from inappropriate environmental stimuli (Blackburn & Vandenberg, 1991; Vandenberg, 1999).*
- Prepare families for realistic challenges of caring for preterm and at risk infants prior to discharge. Differences include understanding "corrected" age, feeding skills, poor endurance/tire easily, shorter sleep-wake cycles, less alert and more fussy when awake, fuss before returning to sleep, overstimulation, and so on. *Help parents identify their infant's characteristics, developmental capabilities and limitations, interventions that will support optimal growth and development, and their supportive network when helping parents ease the transition from NICU to home (VandenBerg, 1999). It is important for parents to know the typical transition period from hospital to home is up to 4 months from due date (Gorski, 1988).*
- Encourage families to teach friends/visitors to recognize and respond to infant's unique behavioral cues. *It is important for families to feel comfortable obtaining support from their regular support systems; therefore, supportive persons need to be taught how to interact in the environment in a way that supports both the family and the infant. The ability to read and interpret infant behavior provides a framework for responding to infants in a way that communicates both the infant's/child's importance and the message that he or she is able to affect his or her environment (Als, 1982; Blackburn & Vandenberg, 1991).*
- Provide information of community resources, developmental follow-up services, and parent-to-parent support programs. *Findings of following healthy preterm infants of varying gestational age suggested the need for appropriate anticipatory guidance and support for families, including close development monitoring. Including those born as little as 3 weeks early is advocated. Parents benefit from knowledge and expectations of their infant's autonomic sensitivity, lower threshold to motor system disorganization, potential difficulties with self-calm, and more tentative and fragile ability to orient and attend to environmental and social stimuli. Additional anticipatory guidance should include knowledge about prevention of overstimulation and exhaustion of these more sensitive infants (Mouradian, Als, & Coster, 2000).*

## Family Teaching

- Assist families/support systems in recognizing and responding to infant's unique behavioral cues. *Demonstrating and modeling appropriate interactional skills is an integral component of family education and will improve family-infant interactions (McGrath & Conliffe-Torres, 1996). Assisting parents with recognizing infant states and state modulation and self-consoling strategies provides caregivers with greater sense of competence (Nursing Child Assessment Satellite Training, 1994).*
- Give anticipatory guidance to parents about what infant/child behaviors are possible in given situations.

- Model calming interventions to provide parents with tools for positive interactions with their infant/child (Karl, 1999).
- Nurture parents so that they in turn can nurture their infant/child. *The psychological trauma to parents when their infant is hospitalized in the NICU cannot be underestimated (Doering, 1999). The most difficult and overlooked aspects of care of the high-risk neonate is effective, timely, and compassionate information delivery to parents and family by the medical staff (Sherman, 2002).*
- Establish a nurturing environment in which parents can interact with their infant/child (Goulet et al, 1998).
- Have knowledge of community early intervention services and follow-up programs for preterm and at risk infants and families.

## evolve WEBSITES FOR EDUCATION



See the EVOLVE website for World Wide Web resources for client education.

## REFERENCES


Aita M, Snider L: The art of developmental care in the NICU: a concept analysis, *J Adv Nurs* 41(3):223, 2003.

Als H: A synactive model of neonatal behavioral organization: framework for the assessment and support of the neurobehavioral development of the premature infant and his parents in the environment of the neonatal intensive care unit, *Phys Occup Ther Pediatr* 6:3, 1986.

Als H: Toward a synactive theory of development: promise for the assessment and support of infant individuality, *Infant Ment Health* J 3:229, 1982.

Als H: Developmental care in the newborn intensive care unit, *Curr Opin Pediatr* 10:138, 1998.

Als H, Lawhon G, Brown E et al: Individualized behavioral and environmental care for the very low birth weight preterm infant at high risk for bronchopulmonary dysplasia: neonatal intensive care unit and developmental outcome, *Pediatrics* 78:1123, 1986.

Als H, Lawhon G, Duffy FH et al: Individualized developmental care for the very low birth weight preterm infant: medical and neurofunctional effects, *JAMA* 272:853, 1994.

Als H, Gilkerson L, Duffy FH et al. A three-center, randomized, controlled trial of individualized developmental care for very low birth weight preterm infants: medical, neurodevelopmental, parenting, and caregiving effects, *J Dev Behav Pediatr* 24(6):399, 2003.

Anderson J, Auster-Liebhaber J: Developmental therapy in the neonatal intensive care unit, *Phys Occup Ther Pediatr* 4:89, 1984.

Beachy JM: Premature infant massage in the NICU, *Neonatal Netw* 22(3):39-45, 2003.

Becker PT, Brazy JE, Grunwald PC: Behavioral state organization of very low birth weight infants: effects of developmental handling during caregiving, *Infant Behav Dev* 20(4):503-514, 1997.

Becker PT, Grunwald PC, Moorman J et al: Outcomes of developmentally supportive nursing care for very low birth weight infants, *Nurs Res* 40(3):150, 1991.

Blackburn S: Fostering behavior development of high-risk infants, *J Obstet Gynecol Neonatal Nurs* 12:76-86:1983.

Blackburn S: State related behaviors and individual differences. In Barnard KE, editor: *Nursing child assessment satellite training: earning resource manual,* Seattle, 1978, University of Washington.

Blackburn S, Vandenberg K: Assessment and management of neonatal development. In Kenner C et al, editors: *Comprehensive neonatal nursing: a physiologic approach,* Toronto, 1991, WB Saunders.

Buehler DM, Als H, Duffy FH et al: Effectiveness of individualized developmental care for low-risk preterm infants: behavioral and electrophysiologic evidence, *Pediatrics* 96(5):923, 1995.

Burns K, Cunningham N, White-Traut R et al: Infant stimulation: modification of an intervention based on physiologic and behavioral cues, *J Obstet Gynecol Neonatal Nurs* 23(7):581, 1994.

Chang Y, Anderson G, Lin C: Effects of prone and supine positions on sleep state and stress responses in mechanically ventilated preterm infants during the first postnatal week, *J Adv Nurs* 40(2):161, 2002.

Chwo MJ, Anderson GC, Good M et al: A randomized controlled trial of early kangaroo care for preterm infants: effects on temperature, weight, behavior, and acuity, *J Nurs Res* 10(2):129, 2002.

Cochran M: Tears have no color, *Am J Nurs* 98(6):53, 1998.
D'Apolito K: What is an organized infant? *Neonatal Netw* 10(1):23, 1991.
DePaul D, Chambers SE: Environmental noise in the neonatal intensive care unit: implications for nursing practice, *J Perinatal Neonatal Nurs* 8:71, 1995.
DeWys M, McComish-Fry J: Infants states and cues: facilitating effective parent-infant interactions. In *Caring for infants: a resource manual for caring for infant trainers,* East Lansing, Mich, 1992, Michigan State University Board of Trustees.
Doswell W, Erlen J: Multicultural issues and ethical concerns in the delivery of revising care interventions, *Nurs Clin North Am* 33(2):353, 1998.
Elander G, Hellstrom G: Reduction of noise levels in intensive care units for infants: evaluation of an intervention program, *Heart Lung* 24:376, 1995.
Evans CA, Cunningham BA: Caring for the ethnic elder, *Geriatr Nurs* 17(3):105, 1996.
Fajardo B et al: Effect of nursery environment on state regulation in very-low-birth-weight premature infants, *Infant Behav Dev* 13:287, 1990.
Feldman R, Eidelman AI, Sirota L et al: Comparison of skin-to-skin (kangaroo) and traditional care: parenting outcomes and preterm infant behavior, *Pediatrics* 110(1):16, 2002.
Goulet C, Bell L, St-Cyr D et al: A concept analysis of parent-infant attachment, *J Adv Nurs* 28(5):1071, 1998.
Guarnaccia, P: Multicultural experiences of family caregiving: a study of African American, European American, and Hispanic American families, *New Direct Ment Health Serv* 77:45, 1998.
Heineken J: Patient silence is not necessarily client satisfaction: communication in home care nursing, *Home Healthcare Nurse* 16(2):115, 1998.
Karl D: The interactive newborn bath: using infant neurobehavior to connect parents and newborns, *MCN Am J Matern Child Nurse* 24(6):280, 1999.
Keefe MR, Kotzer AM, Froese-Fretz A et al: A longitudinal comparison of irritable and nonirritable infants, *Nurs Res* 45:4, 1996.
Lawhon G: Facilitation of parenting the premature infant within the newborn intensive care unit, *J Perinat Neonatal Nurs* 16(1): 71, 2002.
Leininger MM, McFarland MR: *Transcultural nursing: concepts, theories, research and practices,* ed 3, New York, 2002, McGraw-Hill.
Lindsey JK, Roman LA, DeWys M et al: Creative caregiving in the NICU: parent-to-parent support, *Neonatal Netw* 12(4):37-44, 1993.
Ludington SM: Energy conservation during skin-to-skin contact between preterm infants and their mothers, *Heart Lung* 19(5 pt 1):445, 1990.
Ludington-Hoe SM, Swinth JY: Developmental aspects of kangaroo care, *J Obstet Gynecol Neonatal Nurs* 25(8): 691, 1996.
Ludington-Hoe SM, Anderson GC, Simpson S et al: Birth-related fatigue in 34-36–week preterm neonates: rapid recovery with very early kangaroo (skin-to-skin) care, *J Obstet Gynecol Neonatal Nurs* 28(1): 94, 1999.
Mainous R: Infant massage as a component of developmental care: past, present, and future, *Holist Nurs Pract* 16(5):1, 2002.
McGrath J, Conliffe-Torres S: Integrating family-centered developmental assessment and intervention into routine care in the neonatal intensive care unit, *Nurs Clin North Am* 31(2):367, 1996.
Monterosso L, Kristjanson L, Cole J: Neuromotor development and the physiologic effects of positioning in very low birth weight infants, *J Obstet Gynecol Neonatal Nurs* 31(2):128, 2002.
Mouradian LE, Als H: The influence of neonatal intensive care unit caregiving practices on motor functioning of preterm infants, *Am J Occup Ther* 48(6):527-33, 1994.
Mouradian LE, Als H, Coster WJ: Neurobehavioral functioning of healthy preterm infants of varying gestational ages, *J Dev Behav Pediatr* 21(6):408-427, 2000.
Newman L: Social and sensory environment of low birth weight infants in a special care nursery, *J Nerv Ment Dis* 169:448, 1986.
Nursing Child Assessment Satellite Training: *NCAST caregiver/parent-child interaction feeding manual,* Seattle, 1994, University of Washington School of Nursing.
Pridham K, Lin CY, Brown R: Mothers' evaluation of their caregiving for premature and full-term infants through the first year: contributing factors, *Res Nurs Health* 24(3):157-169, 2001.
Roman LA, Lindsey JK, Boger RP et al: Parent-to-parent support initiated in the neonatal intensive care unit, *Res Nurs Health* 18: 385, 1995.
Seideman RY, Jacobson S, Primeaux M et al: Assessing American Indian families, *MCN Am J Matern Child Nurs* 21(6):274, 1996.
Sherman MP et al: Follow-up of the NICU patient, Medicine: Instant Access to the Minds of Medicine. Available at www.emedicine.com/ped/topic2600.htm, accessed on May 28, 2005.
Sweeney J, Gutierrez T: Musculoskeletal implications of preterm infant positioning in the NICU, *J Perinatal Neonatal Nurs* 16(1): 58, 2002.

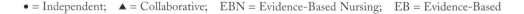

I

Tessier R, Cristo M, Velez S et al: Kangaroo mother care and the bonding hypothesis, *Pediatrics* 102(2):e17, 1998.
White-Traut R: Environmental factors and alternative therapies in nursing, *Voice* 4(9):1, 1996.
White-Traut RC, Nelson MN, Silvestri JM et al: Patterns of physiological and behavioral response of intermediate care preterm infants to intervention, *Pediatr Nurs* 19:625, 1993.
Wyngarden K, DeWys M, Padnos M: Learnings from the field: the impact of using two new nursing diagnoses, organized infant behavior and disorganized infant behavior (abstract), Classification of nursing diagnoses: proceedings of the thirteenth conference, NANDA, 1999.
VandenBerg KA: What to tell parents about the developmental needs of their baby at discharge, *Neonatal Netw* 18(1):57:1999.

# Readiness for enhanced organized Infant behavior

*Mary A. Fuerst-DeWys and T. Heather Herdman*

NANDA

I

## Definition

A pattern of regulation and modulation of the physiological and behavioral subsystems of functioning (i.e., autonomic, motor, state-organizational, self-regulation, and attentional-interactional systems) that is satisfactory but that can be improved, resulting in higher levels of integration in response to environmental stimuli

A pattern of stable regulation and modulation of the physiological and behavioral sub-systems (i.e., autonomic, motor, state-organization, self-regulation, and attentional-interactional) to function harmoniously, which allows the infant/child to interact with the environment in an organized way; the organized infant/child is able to process external sensory stimuli without disrupting his/her physiological and behavioral functioning; if their balance is disrupted, they are more adaptable by being able to regain system balance through self-regulatory behaviors (Wyngarden, DeWys, & Padnos, 1999)

## Defining Characteristics

Definite sleep-wake states; use of some self-regulatory behaviors; response to visual/auditory stimuli; stable physiological measures

### Physiological/Autonomic

*Cardiorespiratory:* stable heart rate, respiratory rate and skin color
*Viseral:* digestion stable, absence of feeding intolerances/problems, regular elimination patterns
*Neuromotor:* absence/minimal startles, tremors, twitches, jitterness

### Motor System

*Posture and tone:* balanced of flexion, extension, and rotation, able to lie in safe, tucked position, does not stiffen or become rigid or stiff
*Movements:* smooth, symmetrical, and purposeful movements, no extensions

### State-Organization System

*State:* displays full range of states from deep sleep (state I) to robust crying (state VI)

*Clarity:* ability to maintain a state for period of time from deep sleep to quiet, alert state (ideal state for learning and interacting with caregivers)
*Modulation:* smooth transition/oscillation between states (awakens gradually, falls asleep easily)
*Habituation:* ability to decrease motor activity resulting in a sleep state with the presence of repetitive stimuli

### Self-Regulation System

*Range:* exhibits repertoire of self-regulatory/coping behaviors (postural change, hand clasp/grasp, hand holding, foot bracing, sucking, visual and auditory attending, habituation, and so on)
*Effective:* adequately uses self-regulatory behaviors to maintain a balance between physiologic and behavior function when exposed to environmental stimuli; if balance state is disrupted, is able to return to state of balance with assistance from the caregiver; continually learning and adding new behaviors to repertoire

### Attention-Interaction System

*Attention:* ability to *focus* attention and *orient* to visual and auditory sensory stimuli; able to *sustain and increase attention* periods; able to *shift* attention from one stimulus to another; able to *inhibit* distractions
*Interaction:* ability to engage in reciprocal interactions (mutual gazing, eye contact, turning to voice, smiling, vocalizing); elicits attention behaviors, enjoys social play; is able to smoothly engage and disengage easily without becoming overstimulated (Wyngarden, DeWys, & Padnos, 1999)

## Related Factors (r/t)

Refer to **Disorganized Infant behavior** as appropriate, although with Readiness for Enhanced Organized, related factors will be minimal (Wyngarden, DeWys, & Padnos, 1999).

**NOC**

## Outcomes (Nursing Outcomes Classification)

### Suggested NOC Outcomes

Child Development: 2 Months, 4 Months, 6 Months; Growth; Neurological Status; Newborn Adaptation; Nutritional Status: Food and Fluid Intake; Preterm Infant Organization; Sleep; Thermoregulation: Newborn; Vital Signs

**Example NOC Outcome with Indicators**

**Preterm Infant Organization** as evidenced by the following indictors: $0_2$ saturation greater than 85%/Skin color/Feeding tolerance/Relaxed muscle tone/Smooth synchronous movement/Flexed posture/Hands brought to mouth/Appropriate time-out signals/Self-consolability/Deep sleep/Quiet-alert interactive state/Attentiveness to stimuli/Sustained alertness during interaction/Interaction with caregiver (Rate each indicator of **Preterm Infant Organization**: 1 = severely compromised, 2 = substantially compromised, 3 = moderately compromised, 4 = mildly compromised, 5 = not compromised [see Section I].)

## Client Outcomes

### Client Will (Specify Time Frame):

#### Infant/Child

- Display stable vital signs and skin color
- Display smooth, synchronous, and purposeful body movements
- Display range of clear sleep and awake states
- Display smooth transitions between sleep and wake states
- Demonstrate range of effective self-consoling behaviors
- Demonstrate smooth visceral/digestive functioning without feeding intolerances
- Ability to effectively attend and interact with the environment with minimal stress
- Enjoys engaging in reciprocal social play experiences
- Displays pleasure with sensory-motor experiences
- Is not "over-" or "underreactive" to sensory-motor experiences (visual, auditory, tactile, movement, body awareness)
- Continues to demonstrate progressive growth and development

#### Parents/Significant Other

- Demonstrate ways to structure and modify the environment that enhances the infant/child's own adaptive capacity for achieving optimal physiologic and neurobehavioral functioning
- Identify their infant/child's behaviors that signal "stress/avoidance" or "approach"
- Demonstrate ways to facilitate motor organization and development by appropriate handling and positioning techniques
- Demonstrate care that is contingent with the state of the infant/child
- Demonstrate additional ways to facilitate state organization/development
- Support and expand infant's/child's self-regulatory skills
- Demonstrate ways to help infant/child achieve an attentive state that allows them to orient to visual and auditory sensory stimuli
- Support and expand infant/child's calm alert periods, the ideal state for learning and interacting
- Demonstrate ways to engage the infant/child in social interactions and allow the infant/child to lead the interaction and respond contingently to their approach/engagement and avoidance/disengagement cues
- Demonstrate ways to provide pleasurable and developmentally appropriate sensory-motor experiences (visual, auditory, tactile, movement, body awareness)

**NIC**

## Interventions (Nursing Interventions Classification)

### Suggested NIC Interventions

Developmental Care, Environmental Management, Kangaroo Care, Newborn Monitoring, Nonnutritive Sucking, Positioning, Sleep Enhancement

**Example NIC Activities—Developmental Care**

Provide water mattress and sheepskin as appropriate; use smallest diaper to avoid hip abduction

### Nursing Interventions and Rationales

Refer to care plans for **Disorganized Infant behavior** and **Risk for disorganized Infant behavior.**

NOTE: Interventions should be based on individual response of the infant/child to each intervention. Interventions appropriate of one infant/child may not be appropriate for another. In addition, a particular intervention that seems appropriate for one infant/child at a particular time may not be as effective with the same infant/child at another time. Carefully observe for the desired adaptive response or expected outcomes and continually reevaluate. Nursing care that is responsive and contingent with the state of the infant is ideal; however, if stressful events occur, provide appropriate interventions to minimize stress and facilitate self-regulation.

I

## REFERENCES

Wyngarden K, DeWys M, Padnos M: Learnings from the field: the impact of using two new nursing diagnoses, organized infant behavior and disorganized infant behavior (abstract), Classification of nursing diagnoses: proceedings of the thirteenth conference, NANDA, 1999.

# Ineffective Infant feeding pattern

*Mary A. DeWys*

**NANDA**

### Definition

Impaired ability to suck or coordinate the suck-swallow response

### Defining Characteristics

Inability to coordinate sucking, swallowing, and breathing; inability to initiate or sustain an effective suck

### Related Factors (r/t)

Prolonged NPO; anatomic abnormality; neurological impairment/delay; coordination of suck-swallow-breathe; tongue thrusting; biting; gagging; abnormal muscle tone—increased and/or decreased; depressed oral reflexes; inappropriate positioning; altered parent/caregiver interaction; prolonged tube feedings; oral hypersensitivity/oral aversion; jaw instability; disorganized tongue and/or jaw movements; preterm birth; hypersensitivity (tactile defensiveness); poor lip closure; altered sensory processing—over- or underreaction to sensory stimuli (i.e., sights, sounds, tactile, movement, body awareness); negative environmental stimuli; sensory overload; swallowing difficulties; cardiorespiratory problems; poor sleep-wake regulation; poor endurance; gastrointestional problems; gastroesophageal reflux disease (GERD); unclear cues—"hunger" and "satiety"

NOC

## Outcomes (Nursing Outcomes Classification)

### Suggested NOC Outcomes

Breastfeeding Establishment: Infant, Maternal; Breastfeeding: Maintenance; Growth; Hydration; Knowledge: Breastfeeding; Neurological Status: Oral Motor Control, Cranial Sensory/Motor Function; Nutritional Status: Food and Fluid Intake

**Example NOC Outcome with Indicators**

**Breastfeeding Establishment: Infant** as evidenced by the following indicators: Proper alignment and latch on/Proper areolar grasp/Proper areolar compression/Correct suck and tongue placement/ Swallowing a minimum of 5 to 10 minutes per breast/Minimum eight feedings per day/Urinations per day appropriate for age/Weight gain appropriate for age (Rate each indicator of **Breastfeeding Establishment: Infant:** 1 = not adequate, 2 = slightly adequate, 3 = moderately adequate, 4 = substantially adequate, 5 = totally adequate [see Section I].)

I

## Client Outcomes

### Infant Will (Specify Time Frame):

- Consume adequate calories to sustain temperature, to provide "catch-up" growth for preterm infants, and to facilitate optimal growth and development
- Have opportunity for skin-to-skin (kangaroo care) experience
- Have opportunity for "trophic" enteral feedings prior to oral feedings
- Progress to safe, self-regulated oral feedings
- Progress to and maintain stable neurobehavioral organization (i.e., motor, state, self-regulation, attention-interaction) behavior subsystems of functioning
- Coordinate suck-swallow with breathing with minimal stress behaviors
- Able to demonstrate self-regulated feeding behaviors
- Display clear behavior cues related to "hunger," "satiety," approach/engagement, avoidance/disengagement
- Display alertness and evidence of pleasure with feedings
- Progress to and ability to engage in mutually positive parent/caregiver-infant/child interactions during feedings

### Parent/Family Will:

- Recognize necessity of consuming adequate calories for optimal growth and development
- Learn to read and respond contingently to infant's behavior cues (e.g., "hunger, "satiety," approach/engagement, stress/avoidance/disengagement)
- Learn strategies that promote organized infant behavior (e.g., physiologic/autonomic, motor, state)
- Learn appropriate positioning and handling techniques
- Learn effective ways to relieve stress behaviors during nippling
- Learn ways to help infant coordinate suck-swallow with breathing

- Engage in mutually positive interactions with infant during feeding experiences
- Recognize ways to facilitate effective feedings, including: feed in quiet alert state; appropriate length of feeding; burping; prepare/structure environment; signs of sensory overload; self-regulation using semidemand protocols, allow pauses between sucking bursts; avoid pulling and twisting nipple during pauses; allow infant to resume sucking when ready; provide oral support (cheek and/or jaw) as needed; use appropriate nipple hole size and flow rate

## NIC

## Interventions (Nursing Interventions Classification)

### Suggested NIC Interventions

Aspiration Precautions; Bottle Feeding; Breastfeeding Assistance; Enteral Tube Feeding; Fluid Monitoring; Kangaroo Care; Lactation Counseling; Nonnutritive Sucking; Swallowing Therapy; Teaching: Infant Safety; Tube Care: Umbilical Line



### Example NIC Activities—Bottle Feeding

Place nipple on top of tongue; Increase infant alertness by loosening clothing, rubbing hands/feet or talking to infant

## Nursing Interventions and Rationales

- Refer to care plans for **Disorganized Infant behavior** and **Risk for disorganized Infant behavior.**
- Interventions follow sequential pattern of implementation that can be adapted as appropriate.
- Provide developmentally supportive neonatal intensive care for preterm infants that facilitates self-regulation of the physiological/autonomic, motor, state organizational, attention-interaction systems). *Developmentally supportive care refers to the provision of social interactions and necessary nursing interventions in a fashion that supports the neurodevelopmental and physiological stability of the neonate (Als, 1982; Taquino, 1999). The goal of the disorganized feeder is to learn self-regulation and organization in the subsystems of functioning to be able to adequately nipple feed (VandenBerg, 1990).*
- Provide opportunities for skin-to-skin (kangaroo care) care. *Kangaroo care enhances earlier breastfeeding, physiological and behavioral organization, earlier parent-infant co-regulation, and becomes an important mode of communication between parents and infant, creating a sense of security and trust (Gale, 1998).*
- Discuss using "trophic" feedings for high-risk hospitalized infants as appropriate. **EB:** *This study indicates "trophic" feedings are small milk volumes given by oral or nasal gastric gavage feedings that nourish the gut and facilitate gastrointestinal development but do not contribute significantly to the infant's overall nutritional intake (Berseth, 1995). "Trophic" feedings provide minimum enteral nutrition and help the infant attain earlier full nutritional oral feedings and consequently are discharged home earlier (Anderson, 2002).*
- Implement gavage feedings (or another alternative feeding method) using breast milk whenever possible, before infant's readiness for feedings by mouth. *Even after a pre-*

*term infant develops the ability to suck and swallow, the infant may require too much energy to do so and gavage feedings may be necessary. Serious illness can interfere with a neonate's ability to suck, and calorie and nutrient needs are increased by the stress of illness (Lucas et al, 1997; Medoff-Cooper et al, 2000).*

- Provide naturalistic environment for tube feedings (naso-oral, gastric gavage, or other alternative tube feedings similar to oral feeding experience). Include pleasurable tactile experiences, hold in semiupright/flexed position, offer nonnutritive sucking (NNS), quiet environment, pace feeding, semidemand method contingent on infant behavior cues, rest breaks, burp, as appropriate. **EBN:** *Studies have demonstrated that sucking helps calm infants, thus raising the oxygen level; may aid digestion and inrease average daily weight gain; and may prepare infants for earlier nipple feedings and discharge (Pickler et al, 1996; Shiao, 1997). Study found gavage-fed, healthy, preterm infants 32 to <34 weeks postconceptional age transitioned faster to oral feeding using semidemand method without compromising their weight gain (McCain et al, 2001).*
- Assess infant's oral reflexes (i.e., root, gag, suck, and swallow). *Oral reflexes are necessary for successful oral feedings. Feeding by the nipple or breast should be encouraged to aid in the growth and maturity of the gastrointestinal tract and for comfort and oral gratification (Lau et al, 2000).*
- Prepare and structure the environment, minimizing unnecessary sensory stimuli. *Noxious stimuli must be kept to a minimum to decrease physiological stress on at-risk infants. The neonatal intensive care unit environment can interfere with normal development of the infant and breastfeeding success; therefore, this environment must be modified to enhance attachment and normal development (Baker & Rasmussen, 1997; Brown & Heermann, 1997).*
- Modify stimulation based on infant's physiological and behavioral state organization/disorganization. *Full-term infants are able to show appropriate and organized physiological and state behavior in response to internal and external stimuli whereas preterm infants' state behavior is less well organized and less well communicated to caregivers. Cardiorespiratory stability is necessary for nipple feedings (Shaio, 1997).*
- Feed infant in quiet alert state, the optimal state for feeding. *The infant must be able to find and grasp the nipple effectively and then be ready and eager to suck. The quiet alert state was found to be optimal for feeding preterm infants (Brandt, Andrews, & Kvale, 1998; McCain, 1997; Medoff-Cooper et al, 2000).*
- Position preterm infant in semiupright flexed feeding posture, head neutral alignment, slight chin tuck, back straight with shoulders/arms forward, hands midline keeping hips flexed 90 degrees. **EBN:** *Studies identified "total sucking pattern of the full-term newborn combines strong physiological flexion and high rib cage position to provide support for the tongue and jaw, which is essential for effective nippling" (Brandon, Holditch Davis, & Beylea, 1999; Brown & Heermann, 1997).*
- Before feeding, assess the infant's baseline parameters of vital signs, state, and activity level. *Disorganization in feeding is usually a temporary problem that nurses can help resolve with adequate understanding and educating parent how to effectively feed the disorganized feeder to facilitate self-regulation that will foster organized feeding behaviors. Assess oxygen requirement for infants with bronchipulmonary disease (BPD), respiratory distress syndrome (RDS), and chronic lung disease (CLD), these babies work hard at breathing,*

*gulp the feeding too quickly, and become exhausted, which increases the risk for aspiration (VandenBerg, 1990).*

- Provide 10 minutes of NNS prior to oral feeding. **EBN:** *This study demonstrated that 10 minutes of NNS was the most effective intervention promoting awake states and lower heart rates before feeding (McCain, 1995).*
- Determine the appropriate flow rate of nipple for preterm infants that facilitates 1:1:1 ratio of coordinated suck-swallow-breathe. *High-flow nipples often used to feed preterm infants may exacerbate the difficulties they have in coordinating suck-swallow and breathing (Matthews, 1994). For infants with disorganized feeding patterns, investigate using self-regulated oral feeding systems (liquid must be actively sucked before the liquid comes through the nipple hole versus a regular nipple that continually drips liquid in the infant's mouth). Some hospitals provide self-regulated feeding systems in their nurseries, whereas at other hospitals parents must purchase them at the time of hospital discharge.*
- Assess infant's ability to sustain coordinated suck-swallow-breathe pattern for 2 minutes. **EB:** *One of the variables of this study identified the inability to maintain a 2-minute suckle pattern is attributed to three underlying problems: fatigue, habituation, and respiratory (Palmer, 1993).*
- Assess infant's suck, swallow, and breathing coordination 1:1:1 ratio pattern during active sucking. *Disorganized sucking patterns occur when the infant does not stop to swallow and breathe after each suck, leading to respiratory difficulty that increases the risk of becoming apneic or bradycardic (VandenBerg, 1990). As infants mature they become more able to coordinate breathing with sucking and swallowing (Medoff-Cooper et al, 2000; Shiao, 1997).*
- Use techniques that support the infant's suck-swallow-breathe coordination and prevent development of abnormal compensatory patterns used to protect the airway. *If an infant is observed to continue sucking without pausing to breathe after each suck, intervene. Tip the infant and the bottle forward so no liquid collects in the nipple. This action will allow the infant to swallow the liquid in the oral-pharynx without expressing more liquid into the mouth; once the infant takes a breath, gently tip the infant and the bottle back to semiupright feeding position so the liquid returns in the nipple ready for the next suck. Repeat until the infant is able to coordinate suck-swallow-breathe (Matthews, 1994).*
- Provide oral support measures for preterm infants by giving jaw and/or cheek support as appropriate. **EBN:** *This study found oral support provided stability for the preterm infant's jaw and cheek and resulted in decreased frequency and length of pauses between bursts and did not interfere with cardiopulmonary functioning (Hill, 2000).*
- ▲ Collaborate with other health care providers (e.g., physician, neonatal nutritionist, physical and occupational therapists, lactation specialists) to develop a feeding plan. *Various health care providers contribute expertise to the care of an infant with special needs (Baker & Rasmussen, 1997; Caretto et al, 2000).*
- Allow appropriate time for nipple feeding to ensure infant's safety without exceeding calorie expenditure. **EBN:** *Nipple feeding can lead to nutritional deficits because of the increased metabolic demands placed on the at-risk infant by thermoregulation, work of respiration and feeding, and decreased ability to absorb nutrients (Hill, Kurkowski, & Garcia, 2000; Shaio, 1997).*
- Monitor the length of the feeding not to exceed 30 minutes. *Efficient feeders will con-*

*sume prescribed amounts within 15 minutes, and half of the amount within the first 5 minutes (Case-Smith et al, 1989).* **EBN:** *Studies correlate the length of the feeding with presence of stress indicators that interfere with feeding effectiveness (Glass & Wolf, 1994; McCain, 2003).*

- Encourage transitioning from standard-care scheduled feeding method to a semidemand feeding method contingent on infant behavior cues. **EBN:** *In this study gavage-fed infants that were provided NNS for 10 minutes every 3 hours, if awake (state 3 and higher), were offered oral nipple feedings. If they were not awake after NNS, they were allowed to sleep for an additional 30 minutes; if after the second assessment the infant was in a sleep state, the infant was gavage fed. Experimental infants, using the semidemand method, attained oral feedings sooner (McCain, 2001). This study found healthy preterm infants 32 to 33 weeks postconceptual age (PCA) who were given semidemand protocol that combined use of NNS to promote awake behavior for feeding were more often in a quiet-alert state, fed more efficiently, and were more often in a sleep state after feeding than their control counterparts (McCain, 2002).*

I

- Assess quality of parent-infant interactions. *The terms* approach/engagement *refer to the infant's attempt to attract the parent's attention, whereas* avoidance/disengagement *cues are the infant's attempt to interrupt or break away from the interaction or stimulation (Eriks, 1978) and their responses to either internal stimuli (hunger, pain, discomfort) or external stimuli (lights, noise, handling) in the environment (Blackburn, 1978). Feedings provide a window to assess the quality of parent-infant interactions. The ability of the parent(s) to read and respond in a contingent way to the infant's response is essential to support infants as they learn to interact with people and the environment. The most widely accepted definitions of infant cues are found in the Nursing Care Assessment Satellite Training literature and the Nursing Child Assessment Feeding Scales (NCAFS) (Barnard, 1978).*
- Assess for attachment behaviors that can positively or negatively affect a feeding. *Mothers who are warm, emotionally available, and sensitive in reading the infant cues and responding contingently to the infant's cues and communicated needs for comfort and nurturance are more likely to have infants securely attached to them (Ainsworth, 1978; Boris et al, 1999). Consequence of insecure attachment relationships may intensify feeding problems and may lead to more severe malnutrition (Chatoor et al, 1998).*
- Encourage family to participate in the feeding process. *Nurses can promote the psychosocial development of the at-risk infant and family by encouraging the caregiving ability of the parents (Moran et al, 1999).*

▲ Refer to a neonatal nutritionist, physical or occupational therapist, or lactation specialist as needed. *Collaborative practice with others who are specially trained to meet the needs of this vulnerable population will help ensure feeding and parenting success (Baker & Rasmussen, 1997; Caretto et al, 2000).*

## Home Care

- The above appropriate interventions may be adapted for home care use.
- Infants with risk factors and clinical indicators of feeding problems present prior to hospital discharge should be referred to appropriate community early-intervention service providers (e.g., community health nursing, Early-On, OT, speech pathologists, feeding specialists) to ensure effective feeding outcomes that facilitate adequate weight

gain for optimal growth and development. *Home visitation by maternal-child nurses, certified as lactation consultants, working collaboratively with the attending physician, midwife, or nurse practitioner is recommended for breastfeeding mothers whose infant is at risk for lactation failure that may lead to dehydration, weight loss, and hyperbilirubinemia (Locklin,1999). Reasons for rehospitalization of infants discharged from NICU during the first 2 weeks for non-life-threatening illness is for feeding difficulties and jaundice (Escobar, 1999).*

## Family Teaching

- Provide anticipatory guidance for infant's expected feeding course. *Knowing what to anticipate helps the family feel involved and enhances attachment (Caretto et al, 2000; Huckabay, 1999; Jaeger, Lawson, & Filteau, 1997).*
- Teach various effective feeding methods and strategies to parent(s). *Parents should be involved in the feeding process as soon as possible to enhance attachment through positive feedback about their ability to nurture a child (Bruschweiler, 1998; Huckabay, 1999). Feeding difficulties place the sick neonate at higher risk for failure to thrive and long-term hospitalization requiring parents to be an active partner of the NICU team, learning to care for and feed their babies well before hospital discharge (VandenBerg, 1990).*
- Teach parents how to read, interpret, and respond contingently to infant cues. *Parents' understanding of infant's cues may increase their involvement in caring for the infant by improving their perception of the infant's abilities (Brandt, Andrews, & Kvale, 1998; Medoff-Cooper et al, 2000).*
- Provide a family-focused caring environment that supports parents in their role as their infant's primary caregiver. Strengths are supported while vulnerabilities are partnered. **EB:** *A multisite study evaluated the effectiveness of family-focused, developmentally supportive care with low-birth-weight infants by emphasizing the importance of building nurturing relationships within the NICU environment among infants, parents, nurses, and staff where "strengths are emphasized while vulnerabilities are partnered" (Gilkerson, 1995).*
- Help parent(s) identify support systems, including immediate and extended family members and friends, prior to hospital discharge; if necessary, include these persons in family teaching sessions. *Recognize parents' lack of confidence and fears and encourage them to verbalize what they are. Be a compassionate and reflective listener and teacher.*
- Provide anticipatory guidance for the infant's discharge. *Parents need assistance in assuming responsibility for infant care as the day of discharge approaches (Baker & Rasmussen, 1997; Davis et al, 1996; Elliot & Reimer, 1998).*

## evolve WEBSITES FOR EDUCATION

See the EVOLVE website for World Wide Web resources for client education.

## REFERENCES

Ainsworth MDS, Blehar M, Waters E et al: *Patterns of attachment.* Hillsdale, NJ, 1978, Erlbaum.
Anderson DM, Loughead JL: Feeding the ill or preterm infant, *Neonatal Netw* 21(7):7, 2002.

Baker BJ, Rasmussen TW: Organizing and documenting lactation support of NICU families, *J Obstet Gynecol Neonatal Nurs* 26: 515, 1997.
Bernard KE: *Nursing Child Assessment Satellite Training (NCAST)*. Seattle, Nursing Child Assessment Feeding Scale (NCAFS), University of Washington.
Berseth CL: Minimal enteral feedings, *Clin Perinatol* 22(1):195,1995.
Boris NW, Aoki Y, Zeanah CH: The development of infant-parent attachment: considerations for assessment, *Infants Young Child* 11(4):1, 1999.
Brandon DH, Holditch-Davis D, Beylea M: Nursing care and the development of sleeping and waking behaviors in preterm infants, *Res Nurs Health* 22(3):217, 1999.
Brandt KA, Andrews CM, Kvale J: Mother-infant interaction and breast-feeding outcome 6 weeks after birth, *J Obstet Gynecol Neonatal Nurs* 27:169, 1998.
Brown LD, Heermann JA: The effect of developmental care on preterm infant outcome, *Appl Nurs Res* 10(4):190, 1997.
Bruschweiler SN: Early emotional care for mothers and infants, *Pediatrics* 102(5 suppl E):1278, 1998.
Caretto V, Topolski KF, Linkous CM et al: Current parent education on infant feeding in the neonatal intensive care unit: the role of the occupational therapist, *Am J Occup Ther* 54(1):59, 2000.
Case-Smith J, Cooper P, Scala V: Feeding efficiency of premature neonates, *Am J Occup Ther* 43(4):245, 1989.
Chatoor I, Ganiban J, Colin V et al: Attachment and feeding problems: a reexamination of nonorganic failure to thrive and attachment insecurity, *J Am Acad Child Adolesc Psychiatry* 37(11):1217, 1998.
Davis DW, Logsdon MC, Birkmer JC: Types of support expected and received by mothers after their infants' discharge from the NICU, *Issues Compr Pediatr Nurs* 19(4):263, 1996.
Elliott S, Reimer C: Postdischarge telephone follow-up program for breastfeeding preterm infants discharged from a special care nursery, *Neonatal Netw* 17(6):41, 1998.
Escobar GJ, Joffe S, Gardner MN et al: Rehospitalization in the first two weeks after discharge from the neonatal intensive care unit, *Pediatrics* 104(1):e2, 1999.
Gayle G, VandenBerg KA: Kangaroo care, *Neonatal Netw* 17(5):69, 1998.
Gilkerson L, Als H: Role of reflective process in the implementation of developmentally supportive care in the newborn intensive care nursery, *Infants Young Child* 7(4):20, 1995.
Glass RP, Wolf LS: A global perspective on feeding assessment in the neonatal intensive care unit, *Am J Occup Ther* 48(6):514, 1994.
Hill AS, Kurkowski TB, Garcia J: Oral support measures used in feeding the preterm infant, *Nurs Res* 49(1):2, 2000.
Huckabay LM: The effect on bonding behavior of giving a mother her premature baby's picture, *Sch Inq Nurs Pract* 13(4):349, 1999.
Jaeger MC, Lawson M, Filteau S: The impact of prematurity and neonatal illness on the decision to breast-feed, *J Adv Nurs* 25(4): 729, 1997.
Lau C, Alagugurusamy R, Schanler RJ et al: Characterization of the developmental stages of sucking in preterm infants during bottle feeding, *Acta Paediatr* 89(7):846, 2000.
Locklin MP, Jansson MJ: Home visits: strategies to protect the breastfeeding newborn at risk, *J Obstet Gynecol Neonatal Nurs* 28: (1):34, 1999.
Lucas A, Fewtrell MS, Davies PS et al: Breastfeeding and catch-up growth in infants born small for gestational age, *Acta Paediatr* 86:564, 1997.
Matthews GL: Supporting suck-swallow-breathe coordination during nipple feeding, *Am J Occup Ther* 48(6):561, 1994.
McCain GC: An evidence-based guideline for introducing oral feeding to healthy preterm infants, *Neonatal Netw* 22(5):45, 2003.
McCain GC, Gartside PS, Greenberg JM et al: A feeding protocol for healthy preterm infants that shortens time to oral feeding, *J Pediatr* 139(3):374, 2001.
McCain GC: Behavioral state activity during nipple feedings for preterm infants, *Neonatal Netw* 16(5):43, 1997.
McCain GC: Promotion of preterm infant nipple feeding with nonnutritive sucking, *J Pediatr Nurs* 10(1):3, 1995.
Medoff-Cooper B, McGrath JM, Bilker W: Nutritive sucking and neurobehavioral development in preterm infants from 34 weeks PCA to term, *MCN Am J Matern Child Nurs* 25(2):64, 2000.
Meier PP et al: Estimating milk intake of hospitalized preterm infants who breastfeed, *J Hum Lact* 12(1):21, 1996.
Meier PP, Brown LP, Hurst NM et al: Nipple shields for preterm infants: effect on milk transfer and duration of breastfeeding, *J Hum Lact* 16(2):106, 2000.
Moran M, Radzyminski SG, Higgins KR et al: Maternal kangaroo (skin-to-skin) care in the NICU beginning 4 hours postbirth, *MCN Am J Matern Child Nurs* 24(2):74, 1999.

Palmer MM, Crawley K, Blanco IA: Neonatal Oral-Motor Assessment Scale: a reliability study, *J Perinatol* 13(1):28, 1993.
Pickler RH, Frankel HB, Walsh KM et al: Effects of nonnutritive sucking on behavioral organization and feeding performance in pre-term infants, *Nurs Res* 45(3):132, 1996.
Shiao SY: Comparison of continuous versus intermittent sucking in very-low-birth-weight infants, *J Obstet Gynecol Neonatal Nurs* 26:313, 1997.
Taquino LT, Lockridge T: Caring for critically ill infants: strategies to promote physiological stability and improve developmental outcomes, *Crit Care Nurse* 19(6):64, 1999.
VandenBerg KA: Nippling management of the sick neonate in the NICU: the disorganized feeder, *Neonatal Netw* 9(1):9, 1990.

# Risk for Infection

evolve

*Gail B. Ladwig*

I

**NANDA**

## Definition

At increased risk for being invaded by pathogenic organisms

## Risk Factors

Invasive procedures; insufficient knowledge regarding avoidance of exposure to pathogens; trauma; tissue destruction and increased environmental exposure; rupture of amniotic membranes; pharmaceutical agents (e.g., immunosuppressants); malnutrition; increased environmental exposure to pathogens; immunosuppression; inadequate acquired immunity; inadequate secondary defenses (e.g., decreased hemoglobin, leukopenia, suppressed inflammatory response); inadequate primary defenses (e.g., broken skin, traumatized tissue, decrease in ciliary action, stasis of body fluids, change in pH secretions, altered peristalsis); chronic disease

## Related Factors (r/t)

See Risk Factors

**NOC**

## Outcomes (Nursing Outcomes Classification)

### Suggested NOC Outcomes

Immune Status; Knowledge: Infection Control; Risk Control; Risk Detection

**Example NOC Outcome with Indicators**

**Immune Status** as evidenced by the following indicators: Recurrent infections not present/Skin and mucosa integrity/Gastrointestinal (GI), Respiratory, Genitourinary (GU) function/Weight and body temperature in expected range (Rate each indicator of **Immune Status:** 1 = severely compromised, 2 = substantially compromised, 3 = moderately compromised, 4 = mildly compromised, 5 = not compromised [see Section I].)

## Client Outcomes

**Client Will (Specify Time Frame):**

- Remain free from symptoms of infection
- State symptoms of infection of which to be aware
- Demonstrate appropriate care of infection-prone site
- Maintain white blood cell count and differential within normal limits
- Demonstrate appropriate hygienic measures such as hand washing, oral care, and perineal care

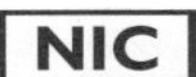

## Interventions (Nursing Interventions Classification)

### Suggested NIC Interventions

Immunization/Vaccination Administration, Infection Control, Infection Protection

**Example NIC Activities—Infection Control**

Wash hands before and after each patient care activity; ensure aseptic handling of all intravenous lines; ensure appropriate wound care technique; teach client and family members how to avoid infections

## Nursing Interventions and Rationales

- ▲ Observe and report signs of infection such as redness, warmth, discharge, and increased body temperature. **EB:** *Prospective surveillance study for nosocomial infection on hematology-oncology units should include fever of unknown origin as the single most common and clinically important entity (Engelhart et al, 2002).*
- ▲ Assess temperature of neutropenic clients every 4 hours; report a single temperature of greater than 38.5° C (100.4° F) or three temperatures of greater than 38° C (101.3° F) in 24 hours. *Neutropenic clients do not produce an adequate inflammatory response; therefore fever is usually the first and often the only sign of infection (Wujcik, 1993).*
- • Oral or tympanic thermometers may be used to assess temperature in adults and infants. **EBN:** *There was no significant difference between average tympanic and average oral temperatures in this study. The use of tympanic thermometers in addition to oral thermometers in obtaining temperatures is supported (Gilbert, Barton, & Counsell, 2002).* **EBN:** *Tympanic membrane temperature recordings in healthy preterm neonates are safe, accurate, easy, and comfortable for the baby and appropriate with this client group provided staff are trained in the technique (Bailey & Rose, 2001).*
- • Use oral thermometers for critically ill adults. **EBN:** *Oral thermometry is recommended as the best practice method for temperature evaluation in critical care patients when measurement of core temperature via a pulmonary artery catheter is not possible (Giuliano, 2000).*
- ▲ Note and report laboratory values (e.g., white blood cell count and differential, serum protein, serum albumin, and cultures). **EB:** *The white blood cell count and the automated absolute neutrophil count are better diagnostic tests for adults and most children (Cornbleet, 2002). Laboratory values are correlated with the client's history and physical examination to provide a global view of the client's immune function and nutritional status and to develop an appropriate plan of care for the diagnosis (Lehmann, 1991).*

- Remove the granulocytopenic client from areas exposed to construction dust so that the client will not inhale fungal spores. Remove all plants and flowers from the client's room. *Aspergillus, an organism that can cause fungal pneumonia, is commonly found in soil, water, and decomposing vegetation. This fungus can enter the hospital through an unfiltered air system, in dust stirred up during construction, or in food or ornamental plants (Calianno, 1999).*
- Assess skin for color, moisture, texture, and turgor (elasticity). Keep accurate, ongoing documentation of changes. Preventive skin assessment protocol, including documentation, assists in the prevention of skin breakdown. *Intact skin is nature's first line of defense against microorganisms entering the body (Kovach, 1995).*
- Carefully wash and pat dry skin, including skinfold areas. Use hydration and moisturization on all at-risk surfaces. *Maintaining supple, moist skin is the best method of keeping skin intact. Dry skin can lead to inflammation, excoriations, and possible infection episodes (Kovach, 1995).* Refer to care plan for **Risk for impaired Skin integrity. EBN:** *Atopic dermatitis is a common, chronic skin condition that is often seen in both children and adults. It can be managed in most patients by prescribing avoidance measures, good skin care, antihistamines, and conservative topical medications. Patients with more severe disease may require aggressive therapies such as phototherapy, balneo-phototherapy, or systemic agents (Mack, 2004).*
- Encourage a balanced diet, emphasizing proteins, fatty acids, and vitamins listed below. **EB:** *Nutrients that have been demonstrated to be required for the immune system to function efficiently include essential amino acids, the essential fatty acid linoleic acid, vitamin A, folic acid, vitamin $B_6$, vitamin $B_{12}$, vitamin C, vitamin E, Zn, Cu, Fe, and Se. Practically all forms of immunity may be affected by deficiencies in one or more of these nutrients (Calder & Kew, 2002).*
- Monitor weight loss, leaving 25% or more of food uneaten at most meals. **EBN:** *This study demonstrated the above criteria as significant predictors of protein calorie malnutrition (Crogan et al, 2002).*
- Use strategies to prevent nosocomial pneumonia (NP): assess lung sounds, sputum, and redness or drainage around stoma sites; use sterile water rather than tap water for mouth care of immunosuppressed clients; provide a clean manual resuscitation bag for each client; use sterile technique when suctioning; suction secretions above tracheal tube before suctioning; drain accumulated condensation in ventilator tubing into a fluid trap or other collection device before repositioning the client; assess patency and placement of nasogastric tubes; elevate the client's head to 30 degrees or higher to prevent gastric reflux of organisms in the lung; institute feeding as soon as possible; assess for signs of feeding intolerance—no bowel sounds, abdominal distention, increased residual, emesis. **EB:** *Hospital-acquired pneumonia is the second most common nosocomial infection but has the highest mortality (30%) and morbidity rates. The strategies listed are used to prevent NP (Tasota et al, 1998). Once treatment for pneumonia has begun, it must continue for 48 to 72 hours, the minimum time to evaluate a clinical response (Ruiz et al, 2000).* **EBN:** *NP is well documented as the second most common nosocomial infection. It is now more common in surgical patients than surgical-site or wound infection (Brooks, 2001).*
- Encourage fluid intake. *Fluid intake helps thin secretions and replace fluid lost during fever (Calianno, 1999).*

- Use appropriate "hand hygiene" (i.e., hand washing or use of alcohol-based hand rubs). *Improved adherence to hand hygiene has been shown to terminate outbreaks in health care facilities, to reduce transmission of antimicrobial resistant organisms (e.g., methicillin-resistant* Staphylococcus aureus*) and reduce overall infection rates (Centers for Disease Control and Prevention [CDC], 2002b).* **EBN:** *Meticulous infection control precautions are required to prevent health care–associated infection, with particular attention to hand hygiene and universal precautions. (Gould, 2004).*
- When using an alcohol-based hand rub, apply product to palm of one hand and rub hands together, covering all surfaces of hands and fingers, until hands are dry. Note that the volume needed to reduce the number of bacteria on hands varies by product. **EB:** *By introducing the use of hand rubbing with an alcoholic solution, there was significant improved hand-cleansing compliance (Girou & Oppein, 2001).* **EB:** *Alcohols exert the strongest and fastest activity against a wide spectrum of bacteria and fungi (but not bacterial spores), as well as enveloped (but less so against nonenveloped) viruses, being little influenced by interfering substances. They are of low toxicity and offer acceptable skin tolerability when made up with suitable emollients. The mode of their application is simple and three to four times more economical of time than wash procedures, features that help to increase the compliance with the rules of hand hygiene (Rotter, 2001).*
- Follow Standard Precautions and wear gloves during any contact with blood, mucous membranes, nonintact skin, or any body substance except sweat. Use goggles, gloves, and gowns when appropriate. *The first and most important tier of the new CDC guidelines is Standard Precautions. Because client examination and medical history cannot reliably identify every client with blood-borne pathogens, Standard Precautions apply to all clients. You must assume all clients are carrying blood-borne pathogens such as human immuno-deficiency virus (HIV) or hepatitis B or C virus (HBV or HCV). Standard Precautions exceed Universal Precautions. Transmission of blood-borne pathogens takes place via parenteral, mucous membrane, or nonintact skin exposure to blood and other body substances. You must take precautions whenever contact is likely with blood, mucous membranes, nonintact skin, or any body substance except sweat (CDC, 2002).* **EB:** *This study indicates that when risk for infection is high, powder-free gloves should be considered because powder may promote wound infection (Dave, Wilcox, & Kellett, 1999).*
- Follow Transmission-Based Precautions for airborne-, droplet-, and contact-transmitted microorganisms:
  - **Airborne:** Isolate the client in a room with monitored negative air pressure, with the room door closed, and the client remaining in the room. Always wear appropriate respiratory protection when you enter the room. For tuberculosis, you should wear an approved particulate respirator mask. Limit the movement and transport of the client from the room to essential purposes only. If at all possible, have the client wear a surgical mask during transport.
  - **Droplet:** Keep the client in a private room, if possible. If not possible, maintain a spatial separation of 3 feet from other beds or visitors. The door may remain open. You should wear a mask when you must come within 3 feet of the client. Some hospitals may choose to implement a mask requirement for droplet precautions for anyone entering the room. Limit transport to essential purposes and have the client wear a mask if possible.

- **Transmission:** Place the client in a private room if possible or with someone who has an active infection from the same microorganism. Wear clean, nonsterile gloves when entering the room. When providing care, change gloves after contact with any infective material such as wound drainage. Remove the gloves and wash your hands before leaving the room and take care not to touch any potentially infectious items or surfaces on the way out. Wear a gown if you anticipate your clothing may have substantial contact with the client or other potentially infectious items. Remove the gown before leaving the room. Limit transport of the client to essential purposes and take care that the client does not contact other environmental surfaces along the way. Dedicate the use of noncritical client care equipment to a single client. If use of common equipment is unavoidable, adequately clean and disinfect equipment before use with other clients.

*Standard Precautions are based on the likely routes of transmission of pathogens. The second tier of the new CDC guidelines is Transmission-Based Precautions. This replaces many old categories of isolation precautions and disease-specific precautions with three simpler sets of precautions. These three sets of precautions are designed to prevent airborne transmission, droplet transmission, and contact transmission (CDC, 2002).*

I

- • Sterile technique must be used when inserting urinary catheters. Catheters must be cared for at least every shift. **EB:** *The GU tract is the most common site of nosocomial infections in the acute care setting. Catheterization and instrumentation of the urinary tract are implicated as precipitating factors in approximately 80% of cases (Tasota et al, 1998).*
- • Use careful technique when changing and emptying urinary catheter bags; avoid cross-contamination. *Clients are most at risk for cross-infection during bag changing and emptying (Crow et al, 1993; Roe, 1993).*
- ▲ Use alternatives to indwelling catheters whenever possible (external catheters, incontinence pads, bladder control techniques). **EB:** *The GU tract is the most common site of nosocomial infections in the acute care setting. Catheterization and instrumentation of the urinary tract are implicated as precipitating factors in approximately 80% of cases (Tasota et al, 1998).*
- • Provide well-designed site care for all peripheral, central venous, and arterial catheters: standardize insertion technique; select catheters with as few lumens as necessary; avoid use of femoral catheters in clients with fecal or urinary incontinence; use aseptic technique for insertion and care; stabilize cannula and tubing; maintain a sterile occlusive dressing (change every 72 hours per hospital policy); label insertion sites and all tubing with date and time of insertion, inspect every 8 hours for signs of infection, record and report; replace peripheral catheters per hospital policy (usually every 48 to 72 hours); when fever of unknown origin develops, obtain culture. **EB:** *More than 40% of bloodstream infections in intensive care units (ICUs) are associated with short-term use of central venous catheters. Strict aseptic technique should be maintained. The risk of infection associated with use of triple-lumen catheters is as much as three times greater than the risk associated with single-lumen catheters. Clients with unexplained fever and signs of localized infection most likely have a catheter-related infection. The catheter should be removed and samples obtained for microbial culture (Tasota et al, 1998).* **EBN:** *Care in selection of site and catheter is important. The shortest catheter and smallest size should be used when possible. Accommodate the need to replace catheters before they occlude (Schmid, 2000).*

- Use careful sterile technique wherever there is a loss of skin integrity. **EB:** *Extensive literature search revealed that sterile gloves should be used gloves for postoperative wound dressing changes (St. Clair & Larrabee, 2002).*
- Ensure the client's appropriate hygienic care with hand washing; bathing; and hair, nail, and perineal care performed by either the nurse or the client. *Hygienic care is important to prevent infection in at-risk clients (Wujcik, 1993).*

▲ Recommend responsible use of antibiotics; use antibiotics sparingly. *Widespread use of certain antibiotics, particularly third-generation cephalosporins, has been shown to foster development of generalized beta-lactam resistance in previously susceptible bacterial populations. Reduction in the use of these agents, as well as imipenem and vancomycin, and concomitant increases in the use of extended-spectrum penicillins and combination therapy with aminoglycosides have been shown to restore bacterial susceptibility (Yates, 1999).* **EB:** *The reduction of endometritis by two thirds to three quarters and a decrease in wound infections justify a policy of recommending prophylactic antibiotics to women undergoing elective or nonelective cesarean section (Smaill & Hofmeyr, 2002).* **EB:** *Antibiotic prophylaxis is effective in the prevention of postoperative complications in appendectomized patients, whether the administration is given preoperatively, peroperatively, and postoperatively, and could be considered for routine in emergency appendectomies (Andersen et al, 2001).*

▲ Carefully screen and treat women with infertility who may have female genital tuberculosis. **EB:** *Female genital tuberculosis is a symptomless disease inadvertently uncovered during investigation for infertility. The condition is relatively rare and often arises secondary to a primary focus elsewhere. Symptomatic disease patient usually presents with infertility, pelvic pain, or menstrual irregularities. Diagnosis is daunting, even where grounds for suspicion exist. Molecular-based diagnostic methods are likely to play a prominent role in the future. Drug treatment is similar to that of pulmonary tuberculosis. Clinicians need to be aware of the existence of this important cause of infertility in women, in view of the continuing HIV epidemic and the current upsurge in tuberculosis worldwide, as well as the continuing migration of large numbers of women and their families out of areas where tuberculosis is endemic (Aliyu, Aliyu, & Salihu, 2004).*

### Pediatric

NOTE: Many of the above interventions are appropriate for the pediatric client.

- Follow meticulous hand hygiene when working with premature infants. **EB:** *In this study of* Serratia marcescens *in a neonatal intensive care unit (NICU) transmission was likely to occur through the hands of staff (Sarvikivi et al, 2004). Cross-transmission through transient hand carriage of a health care worker appeared to be the probable route of transmission in NICU (Milisavljevic et al, 2004).*
- Cluster nursing procedures to decrease number of contacts with infants allowing time for appropriate hand hygiene. **EBN:** *Enhancement of minimal handling and clustering of nursing procedures reduced the total patient contact episodes, which could help to overcome the major barrier of time constraints. A concurrent decrease in health care–associated infection rate and increase in hand hygiene compliance was observed in this study. (Lam, Lee, & Lau, 2004).*

- Assess child's temperature with a rectal thermometer after other vital signs have been obtained. **EBN:** *An inaccurate temperature can mean missed diagnoses.*
  - *Rectal temperature is the most accurate method.*
  - *Consider both reported and observed temperature readings when making treatment decisions.*
  - *Take temperature after other vital signs, since the procedure can affect heart and respiratory rates.*
  - *Fever in young children can be life-threatening, so assess for signs of septic shock or meningitis.*
  - *Have a high index of suspicion for serious bacterial infection in all neonates with fever.*
  - *Allow nurses to initiate the septic work-up for infants with fever.*
  - *A child's condition may deteriorate rapidly, so frequent reassessment is needed (Is your care, 2004).*

▲ Avoid the prophylactic use of topical cream in premature infants. **EB:** *Nosocomial sepsis is a frequent and serious complication of premature infants. The increased susceptibility of extremely low-birth-weight infants to infection has been attributed to less effective immune function compared to mature newborns and the invasive nature of necessary supportive care. Breakdown of the barrier function of the skin may be an additional risk factor for nosocomial sepsis. Prophylactic application of topical ointment increases the risk of coagulase negative staphylococcal infection and any nosocomial infection. A trend toward increased risk of any bacterial infection was noted in infants prophylactically treated. (Conner, Soll, & Edwards, 2004).*

I

## Geriatric

- Recognize that geriatric clients may be seriously infected but have less obvious symptoms. The immune system declines with aging. *The elderly may present with atypical manifestations of infections (Madhaven, 1994).*

▲ Suspect pneumonia when the client has symptoms of lethargy or confusion. **EB:** *Many elderly persons do not have the classic symptoms of community acquired pneumonia; instead, they may present with confusion, lethargy, tachypnea, anorexia, or abdominal pain. Prompt empiric treatment is essential. Recommended initial therapy choices include a beta-lactam agent with a macrolide, or an antipneumococcal fluoroquinolone (Patel & Criner, 2003).*

- Most clients develop NP by either aspirating contaminated substances or inhaling airborne particles. Refer to care plan for **Risk for Aspiration.**

▲ Carefully screen elderly women for salmonella with symptoms of urinary tract infections. **EB:** *Salmonellosis is a major cause of gastroenteritis in the United States and can lead to septicaemia, and other extraintestinal illness including urinary tract infections. National reporting of* Salmonella bacteriuria *increased in absolute incidence and as a proportion of all* Salmonella, *especially in elderly women, and may represent an increase in the incidence of* Salmonella *urinary tract infections (Sivapalasingam, 2004).*

▲ Foot care other than simple toenail cutting should be performed by a podiatrist.

▲ Observe and report if the client has a low-grade temperature or new onset of confusion. **EB:** *Residents of long-term care facilities who are suspected of having an infection and have one temperature reading of greater than 100° F (37.8° C), more than two readings of* *greater than 99° F (37.2° C), or an increase of 2° F (1.1° C) over baseline should be reported immediately to the on-site nurse, and appropriate testing should be done to determine site of infection (Bentley et al, 2002).* **EBN:** *Those caring for elderly patients must be alerted to the potential presence of infection when even low-grade temperature elevations appear for short periods. (Holtzclaw, 2003). In the majority of acute confusion in the elderly, the etiology was multifactorial infections and dehydration as the most common causes (Cacchione et al, 2003).*

- • During the peak of the influenza epidemic, limit visits by relatives and friends. *Hospital- and nursing home–acquired influenza A virus infection leads to high mortality in the elderly (Madhaven, 1994).*
- ▲ Recommend that the geriatric client receive an annual influenza immunization and one-time pneumococcal vaccine. **EB:** *Immunization against influenza is an effective intervention that reduces serologically confirmed cases by between 60% and 70% (Hull et al, 2002). Among the many infections to which the aged are susceptible, pneumonia and influenza combined are responsible for the greatest mortality (Madhaven, 1994). Oseltamivir prophylaxis was very effective in protecting nursing home residents from influenza-like illnesses and in halting an outbreak of influenza B. A comparable nursing home in this study that did not use this treatment had double the number of cases (Parker, Loewen, & Skowronski, 2001).*
- ▲ Recognize that chronically ill geriatric clients, particularly those with depression, have an increased susceptibility to infection; practice meticulous care of all invasive sites. *Depression has been noted as a risk factor for lethal infectious disease in disabled older adults, with reduced reactivity in humoral and cellular immunity (Shinkawa et al, 2002). A successful infection control program can provide the foundation for expanding performance improvement throughout the long-term care facility (Stevenson & Loeb, 2004).*
- ▲ Recognize that older adults are at risk for HIV/acquired immune deficiency syndrome (AIDS); institute Universal Precautions and appropriate instruction for all age groups. *Approximately 10% of AIDS cases occur in adults over age 50. Manifestations include* Pneumocystis carinii *pneumonia, herpes zoster, tuberculosis, cytomegalovirus, oral thrush,* Mycobacterium avium (M. intracellulare) *complex, and HIV dementia. Older women with HIV (compared with those without) are at higher risk for vaginal yeast infections, cervical dysplasia and carcinoma, condyloma, and pelvic inflammatory disease (Wooten-Bielski, 1999). Older adults are less likely to use a condom or to participate in routine HIV testing. Survival rates of elders with HIV are lower compared with younger patients (Chiao, Ries, & Sande, 1999) of all invasive sites.*

## Home Care

- • Some of the above interventions may be adapted for home care use. **EBN:** *Wound treatment in the community, when combined with comprehensive nursing assessment, can be effective while reducing costs (Carville, 2004).*
- ▲ Review standards for surveillance of infections in home care. *The Association for Professionals in Infection Control and Epidemiology has provided definitions for home care infection surveillance. Although the current material is a draft, it is in use and will be revised periodically (Anonymous, 2001).*
- • Maintain strong infection control policies. *Strong guidelines are important to avoid in-*

*fection in the home setting, especially addressing such issues as storage and use of irrigation solutions and supplies (Friedman, 2003).*

- • Assess home environment for general cleanliness, storage of food items, and appropriate waste disposal. Instruct as necessary in proper disposal and use of disinfecting agents. *Presence of waste and inappropriate storage of food items can contribute to the presence of pathogens.*
- ▲ Assess home care environment for appropriate disposal of used dressing materials. *Used dressing materials may contain or be a primary medium for growth of pathogens.*
- ▲ Role model all preventive behaviors in care of the client (e.g., Universal Precautions).
- • Do not visit the client when you are ill. *Demonstration is a more effective teaching strategy than verbalization.*
- • Maintain the cleanliness of all irrigation and cleansing solutions. Change solutions when cleanliness has not been maintained—do not wait to finish bottle. *Solutions exposed to contaminants provide a medium for growth of pathogens.*
- • Assess and teach clients about current medications and therapies that promote susceptibility to infection: corticosteroids, immunosuppressants, chemotherapeutic agents, and radiation therapy. *Knowledge of risk factors promotes vigilance in assessment, prompt reporting, and early treatment.*
- • Assess the client for knowledge of infections that have been drug resistant.
- ▲ Instruct the client to complete any course of prophylactic antibiotic therapy unless experiencing adverse side effects. *Prophylactic antibiotic therapy decreases the risk of infection.*
- • Monitor recurrent antibiotic use in infants. Instruct parents on appropriate indicators for medical visits, and on the influence of breastfeeding and day care at home for avoiding increased need for antibiotics. **EB:** *Families who sought frequent antibiotic therapy for infants with fever or cold had a low threshold for seeking medical help. Breastfeeding and care at home was found to decrease medical visits for antibiotics (Louhi-Pirkanniemi, 2004).*
- ▲ Monitor for the occurrence of infectious exacerbation of chronic obstructive pulmonary disease (COPD); refer to physician for treatment. *Nontypable* Haemophilus influenzae, Streptococcus pneumoniae, *and* Moraxella *can cause exacerbation of COPD (Sheikh & Sethi, 2001).*
- ▲ Refer for nutritional evaluation; implement dietary changes to support recovery and address antibiotic side effects. *Overgrowth of* Clostridium difficile *can cause abdominal pain, fever, and diarrhea. Inclusion of probiotics in the diet can counteract antibiotic-associated diarrhea (Vogelzang, 2001).*

## Client/Family Teaching

- ▲ Teach the client risk factors contributing to surgical wound infection, smoking, and higher body mass index. **EB:** *These are some of the factors associated with risk of surgical wound infection (Reilly, 2002).*
- ▲ Teach the client and family the symptoms of infection that should be promptly reported to a primary medical caregiver (e.g., redness; warmth; swelling; tenderness or pain; new onset of drainage or change in drainage from wound; increase in body temperature). **EB:** *Two thirds of wound infections occur after discharge (Reid et al, 2002).*

- ▲ Teach signs of HBV/AIDS symptoms: malaise, abdominal pain, vomiting or diarrhea, enlarged glands, rash; tuberculosis symptoms: cough, night sweats, dyspnea, changes in sputum, changes in breath sounds; insulin-dependent diabetes mellitus (IDDM) symptoms: sores or wounds that do not heal. *A high prevalence of HBV/AIDS, an increasing incidence of tuberculosis, and the general risk of diabetes are related to increased rate of infection.*
- ▲ Encourage high-risk persons, including health care workers, to have influenza vaccinations. *Vaccinations help to prevent viral NP (Calianno, 1999).*
- • Assess whether the client and family know how to read a thermometer; provide instructions if necessary. Chemical dot thermometers are easy to use and decrease risk of infection. Clients need to know that the instructions should be followed carefully and that electronic thermometers may be the best choice for accuracy. *Single-use clinical thermometers provide a safe alternative to the traditional mercury in glass thermometers for routine temperature taking (MacQueen, 2001).*
- • Instruct the client and family about the need for good nutrition, especially protein, and proper rest to prevent infection. *Optimal nutritional status contributes to health maintenance and the prevention of infection. The function of healthy cells is maintained by the provision of adequate nutrition (Felblinger, 2003).*
- • If the client has AIDS, discuss the continued need to practice safe sex, avoid nonsterile needle use, and maintain a healthy lifestyle to prevent infection.
- ▲ Refer the client and family to social services and community resources to obtain support in maintaining a lifestyle that increases immune function (e.g., adequate nutrition and rest, freedom from excessive stress).

## evolve WEBSITES FOR EDUCATION

See the EVOLVE website for World Wide Web resources for client education.

## REFERENCES


Aliyu MH, Aliyu SH, Salihu HM: Female genital tuberculosis: a global review, *Int J Fertil Womens Med* 49(3):123-136, 2004.

APIC Home Care Membership Section, Embry F, Chinnes LF: Draft definitions of surveillance of infection in home healthcare, *Home Healthc Nurse* 19(7):439-444, 2001.

Bentley DW, Bradley S, High Ket al: Practice guidelines for evaluation of fever and infection in long-term care facilities, *Clin Infect Dis* 31(3):640-653, 2000.

Brooks JA: Postoperative nosocomial pneumonia: nurse-sensitive interventions, *AACN Clin Issues* 12(2):305, 2001.

Cacchione PZ, Culp K, Laing J et al: Clinical profile of acute confusion in the long-term care setting, *Clin Nurs Res* 12(2):145-158, 2003.

Calder PC, Kew S: The immune system: a target for functional foods? *Br J Nutr* 88(Suppl 2):S165, 2002.

Calianno C: *Nosocomial pneumonia,* Springnet, Springhouse. Available at www.springnet.com/ce/ce965a.htm, accessed on March 29, 1999.

Carville K: A report on the effectiveness of comprehensive wound assessment and documentation in the community, *Prim Intent* 12(1):41, 2004.

Centers for Disease Control and Prevention, Hospital Infection Control Practices Advisory Committee: Recommendations for isolation precautions in hospitals, revised November 9, 2002a. Available at www.cdc.gov/ncidod/hip/isolat/isopart2.htm, accessed on March 16, 2003.

Centers for Disease Control and Prevention: Hand hygiene guidelines fact sheet, 2002b. Available at www.cdc.gov/od/oc/media/pressrel/fs021025.=htm, accessed on February 12, 2003.

Chiao EY, Ries KM, Sande MA: AIDS and the elderly, *Clin Infect Disease* 28:740, 1999.

Conner JM, Soll RF, Edwards WH: Topical ointment for preventing infection in preterm infants, *Cochrane Database Syst Rev* (1): CD001150, 2004.

Cornbleet PJ: Clinical utility of the band count, *Clin Lab Med* 22(1):101, 2002.

Crogan NL, Corbett CF, Short RA: The minimum data set: predicting malnutrition in newly admitted nursing home residents, *Clin Nurs Res* 11(3):341, 2002.

Crow R et al: *A study of patients with an indwelling urethral catheter and related nursing practice,* Guildford, Surrey, England, 1996, Nursing Practice Unit, University of Surrey.

Dave J, Wilcox MH, Kellett M: Glove powder: implications for infection control, *J Hosp Infect* 42(4):283, 1999.

Engelhart S, Glasmacher A, Exner M et al: Surveillance for nosocomial infections and fever of unknown origin among adult hematology-oncology patients, *Infect Control Hosp Epidemiol* 23(5):244, 2002.

Felblinger DM: Malnutrition, infection, and sepsis in acute and chronic illness, *Crit Care Nurs Clin North Am* 15(1):71, 2003.

Friedman MM: Infection control update for home care and hospice organizations, *Home Healthc Nurse* 21(11):753, 2003.

Gilbert M, Barton AJ, Counsell CM: Comparison of oral and tympanic temperatures in adult surgical patients, *Appl Nurs Res* 15(1):42, 2002.

Girou E, Oppein F: Handwashing compliance in a French university hospital: new perspective with the introduction of hand-rubbing with a waterless alcohol-based solution, *J Hosp Infect* 48(Suppl A):S55, 2001.

Giuliano KK, Giuliano AJ, Scott SS et al: Temperature measurement in critically ill adults: a comparison of tympanic and oral methods, *Am J Crit Care* 9(4):254, 2000.

Holtzclaw BJ: Use of thermoregulatory principles in patient care: fever management, *Online J Clin Innovat* 5(5):1-23, 2003.

Gould D: Systematic observation of hand decontamination, *Nurs Stand* 18(47):39-44, 2004.

Hull S, Hagdrup N, Hart B et al: Boosting uptake of influenza immunisation: a randomised controlled trial of telephone appointing in general practice, *Br J Gen Pract* 52(482):710, 2002.

Is your care of children with fever outdated? Don't miss warning signs: if you don't assume the worst, you may overlook sepsis or meningitis, *ED Nurs* 7(6):61-64, 2004.

Kovach T: The barrier defense: skin hydration as infection control, *J Pract Nurs* 45:13, 1995.

Lam BC, Lee J, Lau YL: Hand hygiene practices in a neonatal intensive care unit: a multimodal intervention and impact on nosocomial infection. *Pediatrics,* 2004 Nov; 114(5):e565-e571.

Lehmann S: Immune function and nutrition: the clinical role of the intravenous nurse, *J Intraven Nurs* 14:406, 1991.

Louhi-Pirkanniemi K: Recurrent antibiotic use in a small child and the effects on the family, *Scand J Prim Health Care* 22(1):16, 2004.

Mack 0053: Atopic dermatitis: an overview for the nurse practitioner, *J Am Acad Nurse Pract* 16(10):451-454, 2004.

Madhaven T: Infections in the elderly: current concepts in management, *Compr Ther* 20:465, 1994.

Mank A, van der Lelie H: Is there still an indication for nursing patients with prolonged neutropenia in protective isolation? An evidence-based nursing and medical study of 4 years experience for nursing patients with neutropenia without isolation, *Eur J Oncol Nurs* 7(1):17-23, 2003.

Milisavljevic V, Wu F, Larson E et al: Molecular epidemiology of Serratia marcescens outbreaks in two neonatal intensive care units, *Infect Control Hosp Epidemiol* 25(9):719-721, 2004.

Parker R, Loewen N, Skowronski D: Experience with oseltamivir in the control of a nursing home influenza B outbreak, *Can Commun Dis Rep* 27(5):37, 2001.

Patel N, Criner G: Community-acquired pneumonia in the elderly: update on treatment strategies, *Consultant* 43(6):689-690, 692, 695-7, 2003.

Pediatric corner. Don't get a sick child's temperature wrong: inaccurate readings can impact care, *ED Nursing* 7(6):64-65, 2004.

Reid R, Simcock JW, Chisholm L et al: Postdischarge clean wound infections: incidence underestimated and risk factors overemphasized, *ANZ J Surg* 72(5):339, 2002.

Reilly J: Evidence-based surgical wound care on surgical wound infection, *Br J Nurs* 11(Suppl 16):S4, 2002.

Roe B: Catheter-associated urinary tract infection: a review, *J Clin Nurs* 2:197, 1993.

Rotter ML: Arguments for alcoholic hand disinfection, *J Hosp Infect* 48(Suppl A):S4, 2001.

Ruiz M, Arosio C, Salman P et al: Diagnosis of pneumonia and monitoring of infection eradication, *Drugs* 60(6):1289, 2000.

Sarvikivi E, Lyytikinen O, Salmenlinna S et al: Clustering of Serratia marcescens infections in a neonatal intensive care unit, *Infect Control Hosp Epidemiol* 25(9):723-729, 2004.

I

Schmid MW: Risks and complications of peripherally and centrally inserted intravenous catheters, *Crit Care Nurs Clin North Am* 12(2):165, 2000.
Sheikh S, Sethi S: Management of infectious exacerbation of COPD, *Home Health Care Consult* 8(5):21, 2001.
Shinkawa M, Nakayama K, Hirai H et al: Depression and immunoreactivity in disabled older adults, *J Am Geriatr Soc* 50:198, 2002.
Sivapalasingam S, Hoekstra RM, McQuiston JR et al: Salmonella bacteriuria: an increasing entity in elderly women in the United States, *Epidemiol Infect* 132(5):897-902, 2004.
Stevenson KB, Loeb M: Topics in long-term care. Performance improvement in the long-term-care setting: building on the foundation of infection control, *Infect Control Hosp Epidemiol* 25(1):72-79, 2004.
St Clair K, Larrabee JH: Clean versus sterile gloves: which to use for postoperative dressing changes? *Outcomes Manag* 6(1):17, 2002.
Tasota FJ, Fisher EM, Coulson CF et al: Protecting ICU patients from nosocomial infections: practical measures for favorable outcomes, *Crit Care Nurse* 18(1):54, 1998.
Vogelzang JL: Nutrition in home care. Nonfunctional gut? Try a probiotic food, *Home Healthc Nurse* 19:467, 2001.
Wujcik D: Infection control in oncology patients, *Nurs Clin North Am* 28:639, 1993.
Yates RR: New intervention strategies for reducing antibiotic resistance, *Chest* 115(Suppl):24S, 1999.



# Risk for Injury

evolve

*Betty J. Ackley*

NANDA

## Definition

At risk of injury as a result of the interaction of environmental conditions interacting with the individual's adaptive and defensive resources

NOTE: This nursing diagnosis overlaps with other diagnoses such as **Risk for Falls, Risk for Trauma, Risk for Poisoning, Risk for Suffocation, Risk for Aspiration,** and if the client is at risk of bleeding, **Ineffective Protection.** Refer to care plans for these diagnoses if appropriate.

## Risk Factors

### External

Mode of transport or transportation; people or provider (e.g., nosocomial agents; staffing patterns; cognitive, affective, and psychomotor factors); physical (e.g., design, structure, and arrangement of community, building, and/or equipment); nutrients (e.g., vitamins, food types); biological (e.g., immunization level of community, microorganism); chemical (e.g., pollutants, poisons, drugs, pharmaceutical agents, alcohol, caffeine, nicotine, preservatives, cosmetics, dyes)

### Internal

Psychological (affective orientation); malnutrition; abnormal blood profile (e.g., leukocytosis/leukopenia); altered clotting factors; thrombocytopenia; sickle cell; thalassemia; decreased hemoglobin; immune-autoimmune dysfunction; biochemical, regulatory function (e.g., sensory dysfunction, integrative dysfunction, effector dysfunction, tissue hypoxia); developmental age (physiological, psychosocial); physical (e.g., broken skin, altered mobility)

## Related Factors (r/t)

See Risk Factors

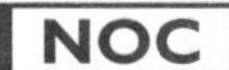

## Outcomes (Nursing Outcomes Classification)

### Suggested NOC Outcomes

Fall Prevention Behavior; Fetal Status: Intrapartum; Immune Status; Maternal Status: Intrapartum; Parenting: Psychosocial Safety; Personal Safety Behavior; Risk Control; Safe Home Environment

**Example NOC Outcome with Indicators**

**Risk Control** as evidenced by the following indicators: Monitors environmental risk factors/Develops effective risk control strategies/Follows selected risk control strategies (Rate each indicator of **Risk Control:** 1 = never demonstrated, 2 = rarely demonstrated, 3 = sometimes demonstrated, 4 = often demonstrated, 5 = consistently demonstrated [see Section I].)

## Client Outcomes

### Client Will (Specify Time Frame):

- Remain free of injuries
- Explain methods to prevent injury

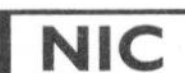

## Interventions (Nursing Interventions Classification)

### Suggested NIC Interventions

Behavior Modification; Health Education; Patient Contracting; Self-Modification Assistance

**Example NIC Activities—Health Education**

Identify internal or external factors that may enhance or reduce motivation for healthy behavior; determine current health knowledge and lifestyle behaviors of individual, family, or target group

## Nursing Interventions and Rationales

- Prevent iatrogenic harm to the hospitalized client by following these guidelines for giving care:
  - Use at least two methods to identify the client before administering medications or blood products, such as the client's name and medical record number or birth date.

- Prior to beginning any invasive or surgical procedure, have a final verification to confirm the correct client, the correct procedure, and the correct site for the procedure using active or passive communication techniques.
- When taking verbal or telephone orders, the orders should be written down, and then read back for verification to the individual giving the order.
- Standardize use of abbreviations and eliminate abbreviations that are prone to cause errors.
- Take high alert medications off the nursing unit, such as potassium chloride. Standardize concentrations of medications such as morphine in PCA pumps.
- Use only intravenous pumps that prevent free flow of intravenous solution when the tubing is taken out of the pump.
- Improve the effectiveness of alarm systems in the clinical area.
- Reduce the risk of infections by following CDC hand hygiene guidelines.
- Identify all of the client's current medications upon admission to a health care facility, and ensure that all health care staff have access to the information.
- Evaluate all clients for fall risk and take appropriate actions to prevent falls.

*These are the National Patient Safety Goals, and required actions to improve client safety in a hospital or health care facility from the Joint Commission of Hospital Accreditation (Chai, 2005).*

I

- • Thoroughly orient the client to environment.
- • Place call light within reach and show how to call for assistance; answer call light promptly.
- • Screen clients using a fall risk factor assessment tool to identify those at risk for falls. **EBN:** *This may reduce the incidence of client falls and provides an opportunity to offer health education to high-risk clients (Hsu et al, 2004).*
- ▲ Avoid use of restraints if at all possible. Obtain a physician's order if restraints are necessary. *The use of restraints has been associated with serious injuries, including rhabdomyolysis, brachial plexus injury, neuropathy, dysrhythmias, as well as strangulation, traumatic brain injuries, and all the consequences of immobility (Capezuti, 2004). Restraint-free extended care facilities were shown to have fewer residents with ADL deficiencies and fewer residents with bowel or bladder incontinence than facilities that use restraints (Castle & Fogel, 1998).* **EBN and EB:** *A study demonstrated that there was no increase in falls or injuries in a group of clients that were not restrained, versus a similar group that was restrained in a nursing home (Capezuti et al, 1999). Restrained elderly clients often experience an increased number of falls, possibly as a result of muscle deconditioning or loss of coordination (Tinetti, Liu, & Ginter, 1992).*
- • In place of restraints, use the following:
  - Well-staffed and educated nursing personnel with frequent client contact
  - Nursing units designed to care for clients with cognitive or functional impairments
  - Nonskid footwear
  - Alarm systems with ankle, above the knee, or wrist sensors
  - Bed or wheelchair alarms
  - Increased observation of the client
  - Locked doors to unit
  - Low or very low height beds

• = Independent; ▲ = Collaborative; EBN = Evidence-Based Nursing; EB = Evidence-Based

- ■ Border-defining pillow/mattress to remind the client to stay in bed
*These alternatives to restraints can be helpful to prevent falls (Capezuti et al, 1999; Capezuti, 2004; McCarter-Bayer, Bayer, & Hall, 2005).*

- • For an agitated client, consider providing individualized music of the client's choice. **EBN:** *One study demonstrated that hospitalized clients who previously were in restraints demonstrated more positive behaviors when listening to individualized music than did clients who were out of restraints but were not exposed to music (Janelli, Kanski, & Wu, 2002). Calming music was shown to be effective in decreasing agitation in persons with dementia (Remington, 2002).*
- • Review drug profile for potential side effects that may increase risk of injury. **EB:** *Benzodiazepines have a fivefold increase injury risk for drivers (Movig et al, 2004).*
- • Use one quarter– to one half–length side rails only, and maintain bed in a low position. Ensure that wheels are locked on bed and commode. Keep dim light in room at night. *Use of full side rails can result in the client climbing over the rails, leading with the head, and sustaining a head injury. Side rails with widely spaced vertical bars and side rails not situated flush with the mattress have been associated with asphyxiation deaths because of rail and in bed entrapment and should not be used (Capezuti, 2004; Hanger et al, 1999; Todd et al, 1997).*
- ▲ If the client has a new onset of confusion (delirium), recognize this is a medical emergency and refer for evaluation and treatment. Also provide reality orientation when interacting with him or her. Have family bring in familiar items, clocks, and watches from home to maintain orientation. If the client has chronic confusion with dementia, use validation therapy that reinforces feelings but does not confront reality. *Reality orientation can help prevent or decrease the confusion that increases risk of injury when the patient becomes agitated. Validation therapy is more effective for clients with dementia (Fine & Rouse-Bane, 1995).* (Refer to care plan for **Acute Confusion** if delirium or **Chronic Confusion** if dementia.)
- • Ask family to stay with the client to prevent the client from accidentally falling or pulling out tubes.
- • Remove all possible hazards in environment such as razors, medications, and matches.
- • Place an injury-prone client in a room that is near the nurses' station. *Such placement allows more frequent observation of the client.*
- • Help clients sit in a stable chair with armrests. Avoid use of wheelchairs and gerichairs except for transportation as needed. *Clients are likely to fall when left in a wheelchair or geri-chair because they may stand up without locking the wheels or removing the footrests. Wheelchairs do not increase mobility; people just sit in them the majority of the time (Lipson & Braun, 1993; Simmons et al, 1995).*
- ▲ Refer to physical therapy for strengthening exercises and gait training to increase mobility.
- ▲ For the agitated psychotic client, use nonphysical forms of behavior management, such as verbal intervention or show of force. If medication is required, use oral medications if at all possible. *Nonphysical behavior management is first-line strategy when dealing with the psychotic client; oral medications can be just as effective as intramuscular injections when used for agitation if the client will swallow them and avoid possible injury from intramuscular injections (Murphy, 2002).*

### Pediatric

- Teach parents the need for close supervision of all young children playing near water, including washing machines. **EB:** *Children can be harmed by washing machines by the wringer mechanism, also by hot water, and by drowning (Warner, Kenney, & Rice, 2003).*
- If child has epilepsy, recommend showers instead of tub baths, and no unsupervised swimming is ever allowed. *Most drowning accidents involving children are preventable if basic safety measures are taken (Bolte, 2000).*
- Assess the client's social economic status. **EB:** *Pediatric clients living in poverty are at higher risk for injury (Shenassa et al, 2004).*
- Never leave young children unsupervised around cooking areas. *Heat and fire from cooking are a hazard to young children.*
- Teach parents and children the need to maintain safety for the exercising child, including wearing helmets when biking, using breakaway bases for baseball, and having the needed conditioning for the activity. **EB:** *Wearing helmets while bicycling was shown to reduce the rate of head injury by 85% (Thompson, Rivara, & Thompson, 1989). Use of breakaway bases was shown to reduce the number of injuries in baseball and softball by 96% (Janda, Bir, & Kedroske, 2001).*
- Teach both parents and children the need for gun safety. *There are a number of programs available to teach gun safety, including Eddie the Eagle Gun Safe Program, Straight Talk about Risks (STAR), Steps to prevent Firearm Injury in the Home, and the Emergency Nurses Association Gun Safety Program (Howard, 2001).*

### Geriatric

- Encourage the client to wear glasses and hearing aids and to use walking aids when ambulating.
- If the client experiences dizziness because of orthostatic hypotension when getting up, teach methods to decrease dizziness, such as rising slowly, remaining seated several minutes before standing, flexing feet upward several times while sitting, sitting down immediately if feeling dizzy, and trying to have someone present when standing. *If orthostatic hypotension is present and there is minimal change in the heart rate, most likely the baroreceptors are not working to maintain blood pressure on arising. This is common in the elderly and can be from cardiovascular disease, neurological disease, or a medication effect (Sclater & Alagiakrishnan, 2004).*
- Discourage driving at night. *A decline in depth perception, slower recovery from glare, and night blindness are common in the elderly and make night driving a difficult and unsafe task (Beers & Berkow, 2000).*

### Multicultural

- Acknowledge racial/ethnic differences at the onset of care. **EBN:** *Acknowledgment of race/ethnicity issues will enhance communication, establish rapport, and promote treatment outcomes (D'Avanzo et al, 2001; Ludwick & Silva, 2000; Vontress & Epp, 1997). A recent study found that burns, guns, drowning, and being pierced/cut appeared to be particularly important mechanisms of injury for Hispanic children (Karr, Rivara, & Cummings, 2005).*

- Assess for the influence of cultural beliefs, norms, and values on the client's perceptions of risk for injury. **EBN:** *What the client considers risky behavior may be based on cultural perceptions (Cochran, 1998; Doswell & Erlen, 1998). Young, African-American, and Hispanic pregnant women are at higher risk for trauma in pregnancy and are most likely to benefit from primary trauma prevention efforts (Ikossi et al, 2005). African Americans, American Indians, and Alaska Natives were identified as high-risk groups who engaged in the following risky traffic-related behavior: not wearing seat belts, not using child safety seats, not wearing bicycle or motorcycle helmets, driving after drinking, driving while fatigued or distracted, speeding, running red lights, and aggressive driving (Schlundt, Warren, & Miller, 2004).*
- Assess whether exposure to community violence is contributing to risk for injury. **EBN:** *Exposure to community violence has been associated with increases in aggressive behavior and depression (Gorman-Smith & Tolan, 1998). Minority students, especially African-American and Hispanic students in lower grades, may participate in and may more often be victims of school violence (Hill & Drolet, 1999).*
- Use culturally relevant injury prevention programs whenever possible. **EBN:** *The Make It Safe program is a bilingual, culturally sensitive educational presentation for Hispanic families that focuses on living and working safely in a rural environment (National Rural Health Association, 1998).*
- Validate the client's feelings and concerns related to environmental risks. **EBN:** *Validation is therapeutic communication technique that lets the client know that the nurse has heard and understands what was said, and it promotes the nurse-client relationship (Heineken, 1998). A recent study found that ethnic minority families were less likely to engage in some safety practices and have less access to information regarding the availability and fitting of safety equipment (Mulvaney & Kendrick, 2004). Injuries were identified as the third leading cause of death among Hispanics and the leading cause for those Hispanic individuals 1 to 44 years of age (Mallonee, 2003).*

## Home Care

- Some of the above interventions may be adapted for home care use.
- Assess home environment for threats to safety: clutter, inappropriate storage of chemicals, slippery floors, scatter rugs, unsafe stairs and stairwells, blocked entries, dim lighting, extension cords across pathways, unsafe electrical or gas connections, unsafe heating devices, unsafe oxygen placement, high beds without rails, excessively hot water, pets, and pet excrement. **EB:** *Home hazard assessment and modification are personal safety measures to prevent falls (Gillespie et al, 2005). Identifying risks and implementing changes decreases risk of injury (National Center for Injury Prevention and Control, 2000). A Cochrane review found that there is insufficient evidence to determine the effects of interventions to modify environmental hazards in the home, more studies are needed (Lyons et al, 2003).*

▲ Instruct the client and family or caregivers in correcting identified hazards. Refer to occupational therapy services for assistance if needed. Notify landlord or code enforcement office of any structural building hazards.

- Provide assistive devices in bathrooms (e.g., hand rails, nonslip decals on the floor of the shower and bathtub). **EB:** *Home hazard assessment and modification are personal safety measures that are effective to prevent falls (Gillespie et al, 2005).*

- ▲ Refer to physical therapy services for the client and family education in safe transfers and ambulation and for strengthening exercises for ambulation and transfers.
- • Avoid extreme hot and cold around clients at risk for injury (e.g., heating pads, hot water for baths/showers). *Clients with decreased cognition or sensory deficits cannot discriminate extremes in temperature.*
- ▲ Monitor blood glucose patterns for indicators of need for client instruction or referral to physician for treatment changes. *Pattern management of glucose levels is essential to client care (Linekin, 2002). Intensive management of blood glucose is possible, using multiple daily injections or continuous subcutaneous insulin pumps, with reduction of diabetes complications by up to 60%. Continuous glucose sensor monitoring is also available (Unger, 2001). Tools for diabetes education for the visually impaired are available (Camporeale, 2001), as well as "talking" glucometers.*
- ▲ Provide a signaling device for clients who wander or are at risk for falls. If the client lives alone, provide a Lifeline or similar call device. *Orienting a vulnerable client to a safety net relieves anxiety of the client and caregiver and allows for rapid response to a crisis situation.*
- ▲ Provide medical identification bracelet for clients at risk for injury from dementia, seizures, or other medical disorders.



## Client/Family Teaching

- • Teach how to safely ambulate at home, including using safety measures such as handrails in bathroom.
- • Recommend client use a nightlight after dark. *A nightlight provides some light in the room to assist in orientation and improves visual acuity (Beers & Berkow, 2000).*
- • If the client has visual impairment, teach the client and caregiver to label with bright colors such as yellow or red significant places in environment that must be easily located (e.g., stair edges, stove controls, light switches). **EB:** *Color cues can improve the legibility of the environment and increase the ability to target objects quickly (Cooper, 1999).*
- • Encourage the use of proper car seats and safety belts. *The risk of fatal injury in motor vehicle accidents is decreased by 45% when a shoulder and lap safety belt is worn (SeguiGomez, 2000). Every state requires that children ride buckled up and use a car safety seat or belt correctly to prevent injuries to children (American Academy of Pediatrics, 2002).*
- • Instruct the client not to drive under the influence of alcohol or drugs. Assess for a substance abuse problem and refer to appropriate resources for drug and alcohol education. **EB:** *The use of alcohol or drugs (benzodiazepines, cocaine, or opiates) places increased risk for motor vehicle accidents. Alcohol and drug combinations were at the highest risk of experiencing injurious road accidents (Movig et al, 2004).*
- • Counsel the client not to use alcohol to protect from injury. **EB:** *People who drink are three times more likely to die from injury as are nondrinkers, or former drinkers of alcohol. The most common injury was drowning, but injury also was caused by motor vehicle accidents, falls, fire, poisoning, and an increased rate of suicide (Chen et al, 2005). A brief counseling session in the office setting was shown to be effective in decreasing injuries in problem drinkers (Dinh-Zarr et al, 2004).*

- Teach the client to avoid excessive noise at work or at home, wearing hearing protection when necessary. Any noise that hurts the ears or is above 90 decibels is excessive. *Hearing loss from excessive noise is common and preventable (Lusk, 2002).*

## evolve WEBSITES FOR EDUCATION

See the EVOLVE website for World Wide Web resources for client education.

## REFERENCES

American Academy of Pediatrics: Car safety seats, a guide for parents. Available at www.aap.org/family/carseatguide.htm, accessed on April 5, 2005.

Bolte R: Drowning: a preventable cause of death, *Patient Care* 34(7):129, 2000.

Camporeale J: Client challenge. Teaching an insulin-dependent blind patient about self-care, *Home Healthc Nurse* 19:247, 2001.

Capezuti E, Strumpf N, Evans L et al: Outcomes of nighttime physical restraint removal for severely impaired nursing home residents, *Am J Alzheimer's Dis Other Demen* 14(3):157, 1999.

Capezuti E: Minimizing the use of restrictive devices in dementia patients at risk for falling, *Nurs Clin North Am* 39:625, 2004.

Castle NG, Fogel B: Characteristics of nursing homes that are restraint free, *Gerontologist* 38(2):181, 1998.

Chai K: Patient safety goals and the impact on the JCAHO survey, *Cinahl Information Systems*, No 2005048933, 2005.

Chen LH, Baker SP Li G: Drinking history and risk of fatal injury: comparison among specific injury causes, *Accid Anal Prev* 37(2):245, 2005.

Cochran M: Tears have no color, *Am J Nurs* 98(6):53, 1998.

Cooper BA: The utility of functional colour cues: seniors' views, *Scand J Caring Sci* 13(3):186, 1999.

D'Avanzo CE et al: Developing culturally informed strategies for substance-related interventions. In Naegle MA, D'Avanzo CE, editors: *Addictions and substance abuse: strategies for advanced practice nursing,* St Louis, 2001, Mosby.

Dinh-Zarr T, Goss C, Heitman E et al: Interventions for preventing injuries in problem drinkers, *Cochrane Database Syst Rev* (3): CD001857, 2004.

Doswell W, Erlen J: Multicultural issues and ethical concerns in the delivery of revising care interventions, *Nurs Clin North Am* 33(2):353, 1998.

Evans L, Strumpf N: Myths about elder restraint, *Image J Nurs Sch* 22:124, 1990.

Fine JI, Rouse-Bane S: Using validating techniques to improve communication with cognitively impaired older adults, *J Gerontol Nurs* 21:39, 1995.

Gillespie LD et al: Interventions for preventing falls in elderly people, *Cochrane Database Syst Rev* (3):CD000340, 2005.

Gorman-Smith D, Tolan P: The role of exposure to community violence and developmental problems among inner city youth, *Dev Psychopathol* 10(1):101, 1998.

Hanger HC, Ball MC, Wood LA: An analysis of falls in the hospital: can we do without bedrails? *J Am Geriatr Soc* 47(5):529-31, 1999.

Heineken J: Patient silence is not necessarily client satisfaction: communication in home care nursing, *Home Healthc Nurse* 16(2): 115, 1998.

Howard PK: An overview of a few well-known national children's gun safety programs and ENA's newly developed program, *J Emerg Nurs* 27(5):485, 2001.

Heineken J: Patient silence is not necessarily client satisfaction: communication in home care nursing, *Home Healthc Nurse* 16(2): 115, 1998.

Hill SC, Drolet JC: School related violence among high school students in the United States 1993-1995, *J Sch Health* 69(7):264, 1999.

Hsu SS, Lee CL, Wang SJ et al: Fall risk factors assessment tool: enhancing effectiveness in falls screening, *J Nurs Res* 12(3):169, 2004.

Ikossi DG, Lazar AA, Morabito D et al: Profile of mothers at risk: an analysis of injury and pregnancy loss in 1,195 trauma patients, *J Am Col Surg* 200(1):49-56, 2005.

Janda DH, Bir C, Kedroske B: A comparison of standard versus breakaway bases: an analysis of a preventative intervention for softball and baseball foot and ankle injuries, *Foot Ankle Int* 22:810, 2001.

Janelli LM, Kanski GW, Wu YB. Individualized music—a different approach to the restraint issue, *Rehabil Nurs* 27(6):221, 2002.

Karr CJ, Rivara FP, Cummings P: Severe injury among Hispanic and non-Hispanic white children in Washington state, *Public Health Rep* 120(1):19-24, 2005.

Linekin PL: Diabetes pattern management, *Home Healthc Nurse* 20:168, 2002.

Lipson J, Braun S: *Toward a restraint-free environment: reducing the use of physical and chemical restraint in long-term care and acute settings,* Baltimore, 1993, Health Professions Press.

Ludwick R, Silva M: Nursing around the world: cultural values and ethical conflicts, *Online J Issues Nurs.* Available at www.nursingworld.org/ojin/ethcol/ethics_4.htm.

Lusk SL: Preventing noise-induced hearing loss, *Nurs Clin North Am* 37(2):257, 2002.

Lyons RA, Sander LV, Weightman AL et al: Modification of the home environment for the reduction of injuries, *Cochrane Database Syst Rev* (4):CD003600, 2003.

Mallonee S: Injuries among Hispanics in the United States: implications for research, *J Transcult Nurs* 14(3):217-226, 2003.

Movig KL, Mathijssen MP, Nagel PH et al: Psychoactive substance use and the risk of motor vehicle accidents, *Accid Anal Prev* 36(4):631, 2004.

Mulvaney C, Kendrick D: Engagement in safety practices to prevent home injuries in preschool children among white and non-white ethnic minority families, *Inj Prev* 10(6):375, 2004.

Murphy MC: The agitated psychotic patient: guidelines to ensure staff and patient safety, *J Am Psychiatr Nurses Assoc* 8(Suppl 4): S2, 2002.

National Rural Health Association: Make it safe: an injury prevention program for Hispanic farm workers and families at work and play, *Int Electronic J Health Ed* 1(4):219, 1998.

Remington R: Calming music and hand massage with agitated elderly, *Nurs Res* 51(5):317, 2002.

Sclater A, Alagiakrishnan K: Orthostatic hypotension. A primary care primer for assessment and treatment, *Geriatrics* 59(8):22, 2004.

Schlundt D, Warren R, Miller S: Reducing unintentional injuries on the nation's highways: a literature review, *J Health Care Poor Underserved* 15(1):76-98, 2004.

Shenassa ED, Stubbendick A, Brown MJ: Social disparities in housing and related pediatric injury: a multilevel study, *Am J Public Health* 94(4):633, 2004.

Simmons SF, Schnelle JF, MacRae PG et al: Wheelchairs as mobility restraints: predictors of wheelchair activity in nonambulatory nursing home residents, *J Am Geriatr Soc* 43:384, 1995.

Tinetti ME, Liu W-L, Ginter SF: Mechanical restraint use and fall-related injuries among residents of skilled nursing facilities, *Ann Intern Med* 116:369, 1992.

Todd JF, Ruhl CE, Gross TP: Injury and death associated with hospital bed side-rails: reports of the US Food and Drug Administration from 1985 to 1995, *Am J Public Health* 87(10):1675, 1997.

Unger J: Intensive management of type I diabetes, *Home Health Care Consult* 8(6):7, 2001.

Vontress CE, Epp LR: Historical hostility in the African American client: implications for counseling, *J Multicult Counseling Dev* 25:170, 1997.

Warner BL, Kenney BD, Rice M: Washing machine related injuries in children: a continuing threat, *Injury Prev* 9(4):357, 2003.

# Risk for perioperative positioning Injury

*Terri Foster*

**NANDA**

## Definition

At risk for injury as a result of the environmental conditions found in the perioperative setting

## Risk Factors

Disorientation; edema; emaciation; immobilization; muscle weakness; obesity; sensory/perceptual disturbances resulting from anesthesia (NANDA). High pressure for short periods of time and low pressure for extended periods of time are risk factors for tissue injury (AORN, 2004).

NOTE: The following systems are most frequently affected by surgical positioning: neurological, musculoskeletal, integumentary, respiratory, and cardiovascular. Risk factors contributing to the incidence of injury related to surgical positioning include but are not limited to the client's age; height; weight; nutritional status; skin condition; the presence of preexisting conditions such as diabetes, vascular, and/or respiratory disease; immunocompromise; impaired nerve function; physical mobility limitations such as arthritis, limited range of motion (ROM), presence of implants/prosthesis or malignancy; effects of anesthesia; staff's knowledge of the equipment; required position for the procedure; and the duration of the procedure (AORN, 2004). As a result of these factors, there is the potential for impaired tissue perfusion, impaired skin integrity, or neuromuscular or joint injury related to surgical positioning. The anesthetized client is at increased risk of injury due to positioning because anesthesia prevents the body's defense mechanism from warning the client of exaggerated stretching, twisting, or compression of his or her body (Power, 2002).

### Complications of Surgical Positioning

Complications of positioning include, but are not limited to, mechanical restriction of the rib cage, vasodilatation, hyper/hypotension, decreased cardiac output, inhibition of normal compensatory mechanisms, redistribution and congestion of the blood supply, and nerve and muscle trauma due to stretching and compression (AORN, 2004). **EBN:** *Studies have shown that procedures lasting more than 2.5 to 3 hours significantly increase the risk for pressure ulcer formation (AORN, 2004). Studies have also shown that a normal capillary interface pressure of 32 mm Hg or less should be maintained due to higher pressures causing occlusion and subsequent restriction/blockage of blood flow and ultimately tissue breakdown/ischemia (AORN, 2004). Research has shown that pressure ulcers will develop in 8.5% of all surgical patients whose procedure lasted more than 3 hours (Rothrock, 2003).*

Transient physiological reactions to surgical positioning include skin redness and/or bruising, lumbar backache, stiffness in the limbs and neck, numbness, and generalized muscle aches that usually resolve within 24 to 48 hours without treatment. Lumbar back pain, previously considered a transient physiological reaction to positioning, may be an indication of rhabdomyolysis (Anema, 2000).

More serious complications of surgical positioning include pressure ulcers, peripheral nerve injury, deep venous thrombosis, joint dislocation, compartment syndrome (impairment of microcirculation in soft tissue), rhabdomyolysis, and joint injury.

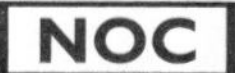


## Outcomes (Nursing Outcomes Classification)

### Suggested NOC Outcomes

Circulation Status; Neurological Status; Risk Control; Tissue Integrity: Skin and Mucous Membranes; Tissue Perfusion: Peripheral

**Example NOC Outcome with Indicators**

**Tissue Perfusion: Peripheral** as evidenced by the following indicators: Peripheral edema/Localized extremity pain/Skin integrity/Muscle function/Sensation/Peripheral pulses (Rate each indicator of **Tissue Perfusion: Peripheral:** 1 = severely compromised, 2 = substantially compromised, 3 = moderately compromised, 4 = mildly compromised, 5 = not compromised [see Section I].)

## Client Outcomes

### Client Will (Specify Time Frame):

- Demonstrate redness of the skin for less than 30 minutes at points of pressure; be free of injury related to positioning during the surgical procedure, including intact skin and free from pain or numbness associated with surgical positioning
- Demonstrate unchanged or improved physical mobility from preoperative status
- Demonstrate unchanged or improved cardiovascular status from preoperative status
- Demonstrate unchanged or improved peripheral sensory integrity from preoperative status
- Maintain sense of privacy and dignity

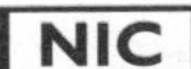

## Interventions (Nursing Interventions Classification)

### Suggested NIC Interventions

Positioning: Intraoperative; Pressure Ulcer Prevention; Risk Identification; Skin Surveillance

**Example NIC Activities—Positioning: Intraoperative**

Use an adequate number of personnel to transfer the client; maintain the client's proper body alignment

## Nursing Interventions and Rationales

### General Interventions for Any Surgical Patient

- The nurse must demonstrate knowledge of not only the equipment, but also anatomy and the application of physiological principles in order to properly position the client.
- A preoperative assessment should be completed prior to the surgical procedure to "identify physical alterations that may require additional precautions for procedure-specific positioning" (Beyea, 2002). *The preoperative assessment should include a chart review for information such as the patient's age, weight, preexisting medical conditions, presence of implanted devices or amputations, incontinence, laboratory test results, and determination of the client's range of motion/mobility. In addition, the type of anesthesia, length of the procedure, and position needed for the procedure should also be considered during the preoperative assessment (Armstrong et al, 2001). Preplanning ensures that the correct posi-*

*tioning devices and appropriate numbers of personnel are available to position the patient (AORN, 2004).*

- Clients with limited *range of motion/mobility* should be asked to position themselves under the nurse's guidance before induction of anesthesia so that the client can verify that a position of comfort has been obtained. **EB:** *Having the awake client assist in positioning is helpful for assessing range of comfort when the skeleton is distorted and for evaluating alternate positioning that will allow for maximum surgical site exposure (Martin, 2000).*
- Appropriate numbers of personnel should be present to assist in positioning the client. **EBN:** *Two people should assist an awake client to transfer from a cart/bed to the operating room (OR) table: one person on the stretcher side to assist the client onto the OR table and a second person on the far side of the OR table to prevent the client from falling off the table (Fortunato, 2000). A minimum of four persons are necessary when transferring/positioning an unconscious, obese, or weak client (Fortunato, 2000).*
- Monitor pressure being applied to the client intraoperatively by staff, equipment, and/or instruments. *Staff leaning on the client, or equipment and/or instruments resting on the client can cause redness and bruising and lead to pressure ulcers (Rothrock, 2003). An adequate clearance of 2 to 3 inches should be maintained in order to protect feet and protuberant parts from over bed tables, mayo stands, and frames (Fortunato, 2000). Injury due to retraction and manipulation of tissue has been observed during pelvic procedures (femoral nerve injuries) as well as during hip surgery (sciatic nerve injuries) (Fortunato, 2000). Head straps that are too tight or vigorous manual elevation of the mandible for airway maintenance can cause facial nerve injury (Fortunato, 2000).* **EB:** *A client undergoing cervical surgery sustained injury to her ulnar nerve due to pressure on the arm by a retractor bar, from the Thompson-Farley retractor system, during the procedure. As a result, continuous monitoring of somatosensory evoked potentials (SSEPs) is suggested with use of this retractor (Baumann, 2000).*
- Keep linens on the OR table free of wrinkles. *Folds and creases in linen can cause pressure indentations in the skin and lead to skin and tissue damage (Farley, 2002).*
- Equipment should be checked to verify it is in good working order and it should be used according to manufacturer's instructions. Verify that the equipment is clean, operating properly, free of sharp edges, able to maintain normal capillary interface pressure, and nonallergenic to the client (AORN, 2004; Rothrock, 2003). *Equipment that is working properly leads to client safety and aids in improved exposure of the surgical site (AORN, 2004). Many beds have a weight limit for safe use; therefore, it is necessary to check the equipment to ensure that it will tolerate the client's weight (Fortunato, 2000).*
- Reassess the client after positioning and periodically during the procedure for maintenance of proper alignment and skin integrity. *Changes in position can expose or injure body parts (e.g., shearing, friction, compression) that were protected previously (AORN, 2004). Once the client has been positioned, lifting him or her slightly for a moment may allow skin to realign with the skeleton and decrease potential for shearing, and so on (Rothrock, 2003).*
- Do not allow extremities to extend beyond/off the OR table. *Many beds have an extension that can be added to accommodate tall clients (Fortunato, 2000).*
- Avoid contact with metal when positioning the client.



I

- Avoid hyperextension of joints. *Extension of the head for long periods can result in a stiff neck, which causes more pain then the incision site (Fortunato, 2000). Hyperextension of joints can cause permanent injury to extremities (Fortunato, 2000).*
- Move and position clients slowly and smoothly. *Quick, jerky movements can cause musculoskeletal injury (Rothrock, 2003). Slow movement allows the body time to adjust to circulatory and respiratory changes, allows the abdominal contents to reposition, and allows the staff to have better control of the client's body (Fortunato, 2000).*
- Lock the OR table, cart, or bed and the stabilize the mattress before transfer/ positioning of the client (Fortunato, 2000). *An unlocked OR table, cart, or bed could lead to the client's sustaining a fall injury.*
- Pad the operating room table well. Use a static air overlay or full-length silicone gel pad to prevent pressure injuries. **EBN:** *Foam pads quickly compress under heavy body areas; therefore, they are not effective in reducing capillary interface pressure, whereas gel pads decrease pressure at a given point by redistributing the pressures across a larger surface area (AORN, 2004). Research shows that a static air overlay on the operating room table works best to reduce tissue interface pressure (Rothrock, 2003; Armstrong et al, 2001).*
- Prevent pooling of preparative solutions, blood, irrigation, urine, and feces. *Prior to initiating the skin prep, absorbent pads should be placed to collect any preoperative solutions that run off the area being prepped. Clean up as necessary. Pooling in areas of high pressure can increase the chances for the development of a more severe pressure sore and prolonged exposure to skin prep chemicals in pressure areas can lead to chemically induced contact dermatitis (Rothrock, 2003).*
- Ensure privacy and dignity for the client during positioning, by reducing unnecessary exposure (AORN, 2004).
- Implement measures to prevent inadvertent hypothermia (Beyea, 2002). **EBN:** *One study demonstrated that the use of warming blankets under clients was statistically significant in the increased development of pressure ulcers (Armstrong et al, 2001). Other research has shown that forced air warming over nonpressure areas can decrease the risk of pressure ulcers developing, by slowing the detrimental effects of hypothermia (Rothrock, 2003). Another study with results of clinical significance showed the incidence of pressure ulcers was reduced by almost half when intraoperative warming occurred (Rothrock, 2003).*
- If the client is positioned in Trendelenburg's/reverse Trendelenburg's or with the head of the bed raised/lowered every attempt should be made to lift the patient for several seconds, prior to prepping and draping, to allow the skin to realign itself. *When raising/lowering the head of the bed or placing the client in Trendelenburg's/reverse Trendelenburg's position gravity can cause the skeleton to be pulled, which in turn can lead to tearing, folding, and/or stretching of tissue (Rothrock, 2003).*
- Lift rather than pull or slide the client when positioning. *Sliding and pulling increase the incidence of skin injury (dermal abrasion or soft tissue injury) from shearing and friction (Fortunato, 2000).* **EBN:** *The use of technical aids and techniques when correctly positioning the client has been shown to decrease the intensity of pressure and shearing forces (Defloor et al, 2000).*
- Position the client's legs parallel and uncrossed. *Crossing of the client's ankles and legs*

*creates occlusive pressure on blood vessels and nerves that can lead to pressure necrosis (Fortunato, 2000).*

- Maintain alignment of head with cervical, thoracic, and lumbar spine. *Misalignment, flexion, and twisting may cause muscle and nerve damage, as well as airway interference. Proper alignment of the head and spine prevents neuromuscular strain.*
- Body supports and restraint straps (safety belt) should be loose and secured over waist or mid-thigh at least 2 inches above knees, avoiding bony prominences by placing a blanket between the strap and the client. *Adequate arterial circulation must be maintained to avoid changes in blood pressure, tissue perfusion (oxygenation), venous return, and thrombus formation. Occlusion and pressure on peripheral blood vessels should be avoided (Fortunato, 2000). The extremities and body should always be well supported so that prolonged pressure or stretching of peripheral nerves, which could result in sensory and/or motor loss, is avoided (Fortunato, 2000). Use of the safety belt during procedures performed in the lithotomy position can cause compression of abdominal structures and therefore should be used only when the client's legs are in the down position (Fortunato, 2000).*
- Recognize that the longer the surgery, the greater the chance of the client developing pressure ulcers. **EBN:** *The risk of developing an intraoperative pressure ulcer increases as the length of the surgical procedure increases, especially in procedures lasting longer than 3 hours (Rothrock, 2003; Armstrong, et al, 2001).*

## Supine Position (Dorsal Recumbent)

- Pad all bony prominences and positioning devices. *The occiput, scapulae, thoracic vertebrae, olecranon processes, sacrum/coccyx, calcanea, and knees are all pressure points in this position (AORN, 2004; Rothrock 2003). When tissue is compressed between a bony prominence and an inanimate surface, the high-pressure forces in the tissue surrounding the bone increase likelihood of pressure ulcer development around the bony prominence (Rothrock, 2003). Prolonged pressure to a localized area of the scalp can result in the development of alopecia in the area within the first few days to a week postoperatively (Rothrock, 2003). Skin overlying bony prominences supporting the weight of body parts can become relatively avascular with prolonged compression (Martin, 2000).*
- Place a safety strap 2 inches above the knees, with a sheet or blanket between the strap and the client's skin. *Safety straps should be snug enough to secure the client on the table, but loose enough to prohibit obstruction of circulation (Rothrock, 2003).*
- Support lumbar and popliteal areas. *Small pillows can be placed under the head, lumbar spine, and popliteal areas to relieve spine pressure. However, when placing a pillow under the knees, it should be placed proximal to the popliteal space and the snugness of the safety strap should be reassessed so as not to compress the popliteal artery, common peroneal nerve, and/or tibial nerve.*
- Use a pillow, padded footboard, or donut under the heels. *A support or footboard prevents prolonged plantar flexion and foot drop (Fortunato, 2000).*
- Arms positioned on padded armboards should be in the palms up position, with the armboards at less than a 90-degree angle (some sources recommend less than 60 degrees) to the body and the armboard pad level with the OR table pad. *Hyperabduction of the arm can cause stretching of the brachial plexus and compressed between the clavicle*

*and the first rib. This pressure/compression increases when the client's head is turned toward the opposite shoulder/arm. Another complication of hyperabduction of the arm is thrombosis. Injury to the brachial plexus, ulnar, and pudendal nerves, and axillary artery can occur when arms are placed at an angle 90 degrees or greater (AORN, 2004).*

- Arms positioned at the sides of the body should have the palms against the sides of the body and fingers extended along the length of the body. The sheet flaps should be brought down over the arms and tucked under the client's sides (Rothrock, 2003). *Lift sheets tucked under the side of the mattress can impair circulation or cause nerve torsion due to the combined weight of the mattress and the client's torso pressing on the arms (Fortunato, 2000).*
- When placing a pregnant client in the supine position, place a small roll under her right flank. *In the supine position, there is increased pressure to the inferior vena cava from the abdominal contents and the fetus, which can decrease the return of blood to the heart (Rothrock, 2003). Elevating the right buttocks has been shown to increase pressure to underlying structures of the left buttock and can result in sciatic neuropathy, so it is suggested that the client be kept in this position for as short a length of time as possible (Roy et al, 2002).*



## Prone Position (Modification: Kneeling, Jackknife, or Kraske Position)

- Provide an adequate number of personnel to accomplish "logroll" turning of the anesthetized client. **EBN:** *At least four persons are necessary to "logroll" a client in order to maintain proper body alignment (Rothrock, 2003).*
- Pad all bony prominences and positioning devices. The nose, forehead, chin, chest, breasts, genitalia, iliac crest, toes, patellas, and edges of the foot are at risk areas for pressure ulcer development in the prone position (Farley, 2002). **EBN:** *When tissue is compressed between a bony prominence and an inanimate surface, the high-pressure forces in the tissue surrounding the bone increase likelihood of pressure ulcer development around the bony prominence (Rothrock, 2003). Skin overlying bony prominences supporting the weight of body parts can become relatively avascular with prolonged compression (Martin, 2000).*
- Arms and heels should not be in contact with hard surfaces or hanging over the edge of the OR table. *When the arms hang over the edge of the bed, the potential exists for radial nerve compression due to the weight of the humerus against the bed rail.*
- Arms secured at the patient's sides should be in an elbow up position to decrease mattress pressure on the ulnar nerve. *The elbows should be padded to minimize risk of injury due to personnel leaning on the elbows (Rothrock, 2003).*
- When placing the client's arms on armboards, they should be brought down slowly and then forward with minimal abduction. Pad elbows and forearms to prevent injury to the ulnar nerve. Do not flex elbows beyond 90 degrees. **EB:** *Overabduction of the arms can result in shoulder dislocation and/or brachial plexus injury (Rothrock, 2003).*
- Place chest rolls from the acromioclavicular joint to the iliac crests. Chest rolls allow for the chest to be raised off the bed, thus allowing for easier movement of the diaphragm and easier lung expansion (Rothrock, 2003). **EB:** *The respiratory system is the system with the greatest vulnerability in the prone position due to compression of the abdominal wall and rib cage, restriction of normal anterior lateral movement, and inhibition of diaphragm movement (Rothrock, 2003). Note: Some surgeons prefer to use a laminectomy frame, but the same rationale applies.*

- Male genitalia and female breasts should be checked and positioned to eliminate pressure. Male genitalia should be allowed to hang loosely and without pressure. Female breasts should be angled toward the sternum to reduce compression on them. **EB:** *Misalignment of the patient's frame and limbs can lead to injury.*
- Place a bolster or pillow under the pelvis. **EB:** *Support of the pelvis decreases abdominal pressure on the inferior vena cava and male genitalia (Rothrock, 2003).*
- Place padding under the knees to prevent undo pressure on the patellas.
- Shoulders should be kept in a neutral position with the elbows bent at 90 degrees and the hands resting alongside the head (Goettler et al, 2002). **EB:** *The most common neurological injury due to positioning in the operating room is brachial plexus injury. Conditions that appear to cause brachial plexus injuries are abduction of the arms with external rotation and posterior shoulder displacement (Goettler et al, 2002).*
- Place the head, turned to one side, on a padded headrest, maintain neck in alignment with the spine, and protect the client's ears and eyes. Pad the head and eyeballs to avoid pressure from the operating table. *A padded headrest provides airway access (AORN, 2004).* **EB:** *A reported incident of unilateral blindness occurred in a client after prolonged compression of the eyeball during cervical spine surgery. As a result, it is suggested that Halo traction on a Mayfield support might be helpful to avoid continuous contact of the face with the operating table (Manfredini et al, 2000).*
- Care must be taken when positioning obese clients in the Kraske position (a modified form of the prone position). *Dangling skin folds can drop down into table crevasses. If they come in contact with metal, a grounding burn could occur during cautery use and when the table is repositioned horizontally, the skin folds could become trapped, incised, or even amputated (Martin, 2000).*
- Clients placed in the Kraske position should be observed for respiratory and circulatory changes. *The circulatory and respiratory positions are greatly affected when the client is placed in the Kraske position, due to restriction of anterior lateral chest movement and increased blood volume in the lungs and feet due to venous pooling (Rothrock, 2003).*

### Lateral Position (Lateral Chest or Kidney)

- Pad all bony prominences and positioning devices. The ears, shoulders, trochanters, medial portion of the knees, malleolus, edge of the feet, and elbows are all pressure points in this position (Farley, 2002). **EBN:** *When tissue is compressed between a bony prominence and an inanimate surface, the high-pressure forces in the tissue surrounding the bone increase likelihood of pressure ulcer development around the bony prominence (Rothrock, 2003). Skin overlying bony prominences supporting the weight of body parts can become relatively avascular with prolonged compression (Martin, 2000).* **EBN:** *Interface pressures are highest in the lateral position. In a study of five operating room table mattresses, all mattresses were fully compressed from the weight of the body when in the lateral position. The mattress showing the best pressure-reducing qualities in this position was the visco-elastic polyurethane and polyether mattress (Defloor et al, 2000).*
- Provide adequate personnel to properly position the client.
- Use a lift sheet to facilitate the turn. Lift sheets prevent skin injury resulting from shearing.
- Place a support under the head. *A pillow or support keeps the head properly aligned with*

*the cervical spine and thoracic vertebrae and lessens stretching of the brachial plexus (Rothrock, 2003).*

- Keep the top leg straight or slightly flexed and flex the bottom leg at the hip and knee. **EB:** *Flexing the bottom leg at the hip stabilizes the client on the table (Rothrock, 2003).*
- Place padded beanbags, sandbags, or bolsters against the back and abdomen. **EB:** *All of the tissue in contact with a rigid beanbag has increased interface pressure which can increase the risk of pressure ulcer formation (Rothrock, 2003).*
- Pad the lateral aspect of the bottom knee. **EB:** *Padding the lateral aspect of the bottom knee will help prevent pressure on the peroneal nerve (Rothrock, 2003).*
- Place a pillow between the client's legs lengthwise so that the pillow also supports the foot. *Pressing the bony prominences of one extremity against the other may cause injury to the peroneal and tibial nerves.*
- Pad the lower shoulder and bring it forward slightly; the lower arm is extended on a padded armboard. *Bringing the shoulder forward relieves pressure on the brachial plexus and improves chest expansion (Rothrock, 2003).*
- Place the upper arm on a padded raised armboard or over the lower arm with padding between the two arms. *Pressing the bony prominences of one extremity against the other may cause injury to the nerves.*
- Place an axillary roll at the apex of the scapula in the axillary space of the dependent arm. A bolster placed in this position will relieve pressure on the brachial plexus nerves and vessels and also facilitate chest expansion (Rothrock, 2003). **EBN:** *There is potential for injury when using bolsters, axillary rolls, and so on. These devices may induce compartment syndrome resulting in compression injury (Fritzlen et al, 2003).*
- When using positioning straps or tape to hold the client in the lateral position, place a towel or blanket between the client's skin and the strap/tape. **EB:** *Compression of the skin beneath the tape/strap can cause injury and should be avoided (Fortunato, 2000).*

### Lithotomy Position

- Pad all bony prominences and positioning devices. *The scapula, shoulders, occiput, sacrum, lateral knee, elbows, and ankles are all pressure points in this position (Farley, 2002). When tissue is compressed between a bony prominence and an inanimate surface, the high-pressure forces in the tissue surrounding the bone increase likelihood of pressure ulcer development around the bony prominence (Rothrock, 2003). Prolonged pressure to a localized area of the scalp can result in the development of alopecia in the area within the first few days to a week postoperatively (Rothrock, 2003). Skin overlying bony prominences supporting the weight of body parts can become relatively avascular with prolonged compression (Martin, 2000).*
- Check the stirrups to ensure they are fastened securely to the operating room table before placing the client in the lithotomy position. *If the stirrups slip, the patient could sustain a dislocated hip, muscle or nerve injury, or a fracture (Rothrock, 2003).*
- Position the client's arms loosely secured across the abdomen, extended on padded armboards, or at the client's sides. *Extreme care must be taken when positioning the client's arms at the sides in this position because the hand and fingers could get crushed or pinched in the operating room table when raising and lowering the lower third of the table for the procedure.*



I

- Pad the sacral area and provide a small lumbar roll. The client's buttocks should be even with the table edge once the lower portion of the operating room table has been lowered. A lumbar roll helps maintain normal lumbar concavity. **EB:** *When the buttocks extend beyond the edge of the table it causes strain on the lumbosacral muscles and ligaments, due to the client's body weight resting on the sacrum (Fortunato, 2000). The greatest amount of force is placed on the lower back muscles when the client is in the lithotomy position (Anema et al, 2000).*
- Stirrups should be positioned at equal height and adjusted according to the length of the client's legs and at the level of the client's upper thighs. *Positioning stirrups at equal height helps to prevent knee and hip injury.*
- Place the client's legs in the stirrups simultaneously, using one hand to hold the foot and the other to hold the calf at the knee. **EB:** *Raising the legs slowly and simultaneously reduces lumbar and sacral pressure and vascular congestion (AORN, 2004; Fortunato, 2000).*
- Lower the client's legs simultaneously and slowly, extending the legs fully. **EB:** *Lowering the legs slowly and simultaneously decreases lumbar and sacral pressure, and vascular congestion (AORN, 2004).*
- Minimize the height of the legs. **EB:** *Huge thighs can compress the outer abdomen and force abdominal contents midline, leading to increased pressure on the diaphragm (Martin, 2000).*
- Avoid hyperabduction of the thighs, and excessive external rotation and flexion of the hips. *Excess flexion of the hip and knee can cause venous obstruction (Anema et al, 2000, and can stretch the sciatic and obturator nerves and strain the hip joint and muscles (Irvin, et al, 2004; Rothrock, 2003).* **EB:** *Overflexion of the hip can lead to injury to the sciatic nerve due to overstretching. In a study involving 1170 clients placed in the lithotomy position, nerve injury occurred in 12 and the study showed that the age of the client, the type of operation, length of the operation (over 180 minutes), and improper positioning by staff all contributed to those who sustained injury (Gumus et al, 2002).*
- Select lithotomy leg holders with optimal body alignment and weight bearing in mind (e.g., combination knee-crutch-and-boot). *Product selection and evaluation should be based on identified needs and should promote client safety (AORN, 2004). Boot stirrups distribute weight evenly and allow controlled and limited abduction.*
- Pad all bony prominences and surfaces that may contact the leg support system. *When using candy cane stirrups, the ankle strap presses on the distal sural and plantar nerves, which could cause neuropathies of the foot. Knee crutch stirrups can put pressure on the posterior tibial, sural, and common peroneal nerves. Well-padded stirrups can still create some pressure on the back of the knees and lower extremities and could jeopardize the popliteal vessels and nerves (Fortunato, 2000).* **EBN:** *Research has shown that intramuscular pressures in the leg are increased, especially in the anterior and lateral compartments, with the leg in this position (Meyer et al, 2002).*

  NOTE: The hemilithotomy position (one leg in the lithotomy position) is often used when operating to repair a fractured hip or femur. Studies have shown that the uninjured leg in the lithotomy holder can develop compartment syndrome because of elevated intramuscular pressures, decreased perfusion, and the length of the procedure. Therefore, it has been suggested that the uninjured leg be supported at the heel rather than at the calf (Meyer et al, 2002).

- Arms should be positioned on armboards or loosely cradled over the lower abdomen and secured with the blanket. **EB:** *Arms should not rest on the chest due to possible impedance of respirations (Fortunato, 2000).*
- Assess the need for sequential compression stockings. *Sequential stockings aid in the prevention of thrombi/emboli.* **EB:** *Sequential compression stockings seem to closely resemble normal physiological conditions and could possibly decrease the risk of compartment syndrome (Anema et al, 2000). Deep vein thrombosis and pulmonary embolus are the most common complications of radical retropubic prostatectomy procedures, which are done in the lithotomy position (Michaels et al, 1998). Ace wraps or antiembolic stockings/devices are recommended if the client will be in the lithotomy position for longer then 2 hours (Rothrock, 2003).*
- Monitor the length of time the client remains in the lithotomy position. Clients who have been in the lithotomy position for 4 hours should be repositioned supine for 20 to 30 minutes in an attempt to avert peroneal nerve injury and/or development of compartment syndrome. **EB:** *The potential for complications is directly proportional to the length of time a client is in the lithotomy position (Anema et al, 2000). During a study of 991 clients who underwent surgery in the lithotomy position, it was found that increased duration in the lithotomy position was associated with increased risk of lower extremity neuropathy. These clients had no previous neuropathies and were well padded, thus leading to this conclusion. The study also found that the frequency of neuropathy increased markedly after 2 hours in the lithotomy position (Warner et al, 2000).* **EBN:** *A study involving 153 women undergoing gynecological procedures in the lithotomy position showed that 41% had pain in their lower extremities, unrelated to incisional site pain, postoperatively and women who were in the position longer than 60 minutes had significantly more pain than those who were in the position for under 60 minutes (Power, 2002). The results of this study were similar to those of Graling and Covin's study in 1992. Acute compartment syndrome has been reported in clients positioned in lithotomy position for prolonged surgical procedures (Meyer et al, 2002).*

  NOTE: If assessment reveals conditions that place the client at increased risk for injury in this position, attempting this position while the client is awake and can report any discomfort may help prevent positioning complications.
- To decrease the length of time the client is in the lithotomy position, evaluate the procedure to determine if any portion can be done in the supine position. **EB:** *During urethral reconstruction, research has shown that the risk of positioning injury is directly proportional to the length of time the client is in the high lithotomy position, with procedures that take less than 5 hours having minimal risk (Anema et al, 2000). To decrease the length of time the client is in the lithotomy position, these authors perform the penile flap dissection, during urethral reconstruction procedures, with the client in the supine position (Anema et al, 2000).*

## Trendelenberg's/Reverse Trendelenberg's Position

- Either of these positions can have adverse effects on both the circulatory system (i.e., increased blood pressure and intracranial pressure) and the respiratory system (i.e., diaphragm movement is impeded), which in most circumstances are monitored and controlled by anesthesia personnel.

- Modifications of both positions may be suggested and implemented by the nurse in collaboration with the surgeon and anesthesiologist.
- Padded shoulder braces may be used in the Trendelenburg position. They should be placed at an equal distance from the head of the table and lateral on the acromioclavicular joint, with a half inch of space allowed between the brace and the shoulder and without medial deviation towards the neck. **EB:** *Improperly placed shoulder braces can cause significant compression of the brachial plexus nerves (Philosophe, 2003).*
- Knees should be positioned at the break in the operating table. **EB:** *Positioning the knees at the break in the operating table prevent pressure on the peroneal nerves and leg veins (Fortunato, 2000).*
- Length of time in this position should be as short as possible. **EB:** *Lung volume is decreased, and the heart is compressed due to pressure of organs against the diaphragm in this position (Fortunato, 2000).*

## evolve WEBSITES FOR EDUCATION

See the EVOLVE website for World Wide Web resources for client education.

I

## REFERENCES


American Society of Anesthesiologists Task Force on Prevention of Perioperative Peripheral Neuropathies: Practice advisory for the prevention of perioperative peripheral neuropathies, *Anesthesiol* 92(4):1168, 2000.

Anema JG, Morey AF, McAninch JW et al: Complications related to the high lithotomy position during urethral reconstruction, *J Urol* 164(2):360, 2000.

AORN: Recommended practices for positioning the patient in the perioperative practice setting, *AORN Standards and Recommended Practices for Perioperative Nursing,* Denver, 341-346; 2004, The Association of Perioperative Registered Nurses.

Armstrong, D, Bortz, P: An integrative review of pressure relief in surgical patients, *AORN J* 73(3): 645-674, 2001.

Baumann S, Welch W, Bloom M: Intraoperative SSEP detection of ulnar nerve compression or ischemia in an obese patient: a unique complication associated with a specialized spinal retraction system, *Arch Phys Med Rehabil* 81(1):130, 2000.

Beyea, S. *Perioperative nursing data set: the perioperative nursing vocabulary,* ed 2, Denver, 2002, AORN, Inc.

Defloor T, DeSchuijmer J: Preventing pressure ulcers: an evaluation of four operating-table mattresses, *Appl Nurs Res* 13(3):134-141, 2000.

Farley M: Oh my, the pressure! *Can Operating Room Nurs J,* 9, 11-13, 20, June 2002.

Fortunato N: *Berry and Kohn's operating room technique, positioning the patient,* ed 9, St Louis, 2000, Mosby.

Fritzlen T, Kremer M, Biddle C: The AANA foundation closed malpractice claims study on nerve injuries during anesthesia care, *AANA J* 71(5):347-352, 2003.

Goettler CE, Pryor JP, Reilly PM: Brachial plexopathy after prone positioning, *Crit Care* 6:6, 2002.

Gumus E, Kendirci M, Horasanli K et al: Neurapraxic complications in operations performed in the lithotomy position, *World J Urol* 20(1):68, 2002.

Irvin W, Andersen W, Taylor P et al: Minimizing the risk of neurologic injury in gynecologic surgery, *Am Col Obstet Gynecol* 103(2):374-382, 2004.

Manfredini M, Ferrante R, Gildone A et al: Unilateral blindness as a complication of intraoperative positioning for cervical spinal surgery, *J Spinal Disord* 13(3):271, 2000.

Martin JT: Positioning aged patients, *Geriatr Anesth,* 18:1, 2000.

Mathias J: Pressure ulcers: sorting out the evidence, *OR Manager* 19(1):18-21, 2003.

Meyer RS, White KK, Smith JM et al: Intramuscular and blood pressure in legs positioned in the hemilithotomy position: clarification of risk factors for well-leg acute compartment syndrome, *J Bone Joint Surg Am* 84-A(10):1829-1835, 2002.

Michaels MJ, Lish MC, Mohler JL: Patient positioning for radical retropubic prostatectomy, *Urology* 51:5, 1998.

Philosophe R: Avoiding complications of laparoscopic surgery, *Fertil Steril* 80(Suppl 4):30-39, 2003.

Power H: Patient positioning outcomes for women undergoing gynaecological surgeries, *Can Oper Room Nurs J* 20(3):7-10, 27-30, 2002.

Rothrock J: *Alexander's care of the patient in surgery,* ed 12, St. Louis, 2003, Mosby.
Roy S, Levine AB, Herbison GJ et al: Intraoperative positioning during cesarean as a cause of sciatic neuropathy, *Obstet Gynecol* 99(4):652-3, 2002.
Mann W Jr: Complications of gynecological surgery. Available at www.uptodateonline.com, accessed March 5, 2005.
Warner MA, Warner DO, Harper CM et al: Lower extremity neuropathies associated with lithotomy positions, *Anesthesiology* 93(4):938-942, 2000.



# Decreased Intracranial adaptive capacity

*Pamela H. Mitchell*

**NANDA**

## Definition

Intracranial fluid dynamic mechanisms that normally compensate for increases in intracranial volumes are compromised, resulting in repeated disproportionate increases in intracranial pressure (ICP) in response to a variety of noxious and non-noxious stimuli

## Defining Characteristics

Repeated increases in ICP of greater than 10 mm Hg for more than 5 minutes following a variety of external stimuli; disproportionate increases in ICP following a single environmental or nursing maneuver stimulus; baseline ICP greater than 10 mm Hg; elevated P2 component of ICP waveform; wide-amplitude ICP waveform; volume-pressure response test variation (volume-pressure ratio of 2, pressure-volume index of less than 10) (Rauch, Mitchell, & Tyler, 1990; Kirkness et al, 2000.)

## Related Factors (r/t)

Decreased cerebral perfusion less than 50 to 60 mm Hg; sustained increase in ICP greater than 10 to 15 mm Hg; systemic hypotension with intracranial hypertension; brain injuries

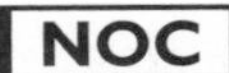

## Outcomes (Nursing Outcomes Classification)

### Suggested NOC Outcomes

Neurological Status; Neurological Status: Consciousness

**Example NOC Outcome with Indicators**

**Neurological Status** as evidenced by the following indicators: Consciousness/Intracranial pressure/Vital signs/Central motor control/Cranial sensory-motor function/Spinal sensory-motor function (Rate each indicator of **Neurological Status:** 1 = severely compromised, 2 = substantially compromised, 3 = moderately compromised, 4 = mildly compromised, 5 = not compromised [see Section I].)

## Client Outcomes

### Client Will (Specify Time Frame):

- Experience fewer than five episodes of disproportionate increases in intracranial pressure (DIICP) in 24 hours
- Have neurological status changes that are not triggered by episodes of DIICP
- Have cerebral perfusion pressure (CPP) remaining greater than 60 to 70 mm Hg in adults



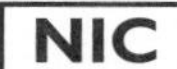

## Interventions (Nursing Interventions Classification)

### Suggested NIC Interventions

Cerebral Edema Management, Cerebral Perfusion Promotion, Intracranial Pressure (ICP) Monitoring, Neurological Monitoring

**Example NIC Activities—Cerebral Edema Management**

Monitor for confusion, changes in mentation, complaints of dizziness, syncope; allow ICP to return to baseline between nursing activities

## Nursing Interventions and Rationales

- For episodes of DIICP, do the following:
  - Reverse stimulus if readily apparent.
  - Evaluate position of the client. Head should be in midline without neck flexion to prevent intracranial trapping of jugular venous outflow. **EB and EBN:** *Positional changes of the head and neck are the most consistent triggers of sustained ICP elevations. Forward, lateral, and rotational neck flexion will result in increased ICP until the neck position is restored to a neutral position (Bader & Littlejohns, 1999; Simmons, 1997; Mavrocordatos, Bissonnette, & Ravussin, 2000).*
  - Return the client to original position if a position change has triggered DIICP. **EBN:** *No particular body position triggers DIICP unless combined with neck flexion; however, some individuals respond to passive turning to lateral or three-quarter prone positions. Routine physical therapy also does not trigger problematic increases in ICP (Brimioulle et al, 1997; Lee, 1989; Mitchell & Ackerman, 1992). Prone positioning may trigger significant increases in ICP and should be individually evaluated if used to improve lung functioning (Beuret et al, 2002).*

- Stop suctioning if routine suctioning is triggering DIICP. Follow preventive protocol if future suctioning is indicated. **EBN and EB:** *A standard series of three suctioning passes can result in stair-step elevation of ICP with each successive pass, even with full hyperoxygenation and hyperinflation before suctioning. Brief hyperventilation may be protective against these increases (Kerr et al, 1997). In well-sedated patients, endotracheal suctioning is not associated with cerebral ischemia even though ICP rises (Gemma et al, 2002; Kerr et al, 1999).*
- Have clients who can follow directions exhale through their mouth if they are doing a Valsalva maneuver. **EB:** *The Valsalva maneuver is accompanied by significant increase in ICP (Haykowsky et al, 2003). Open mouth breathing prevents the valsalva effect.* **EBN:** *If client's nonvolitional movements, such as posturing and unconscious straining, are causing a Valsalva maneuver, sedation or paralytics with sedation may be indicated (Kerr et al, 1998).*
- Reduce environmental noise and painful or unexpected touching of the client. **EBN and EB:** *All these factors have been shown to be potent noxious stimuli in individual adults and preterm infants but may not trigger DIICP in the majority of clients (Bellini et al 2003; Mitchell & Habermann, 1999).*

I

• Elevate head of bed if the client maintains CPP. **EBN and EB:** *Head elevation reduces the average ICP in groups of clients, but individuals may exhibit either no change or even increased ICP (Fan 2004; Winkelman, 2000). In addition, when cerebral autoregulation is impaired, even a small systemic blood pressure drop with head elevation may decrease the CPP to an unacceptable level (Chesnut, 1997; March et al, 1990; Fan 2004). Patients with large hemispheric stroke and subarachnoid hemorrhage may be particularly susceptible to reduced CPP and cerebral blood flow with head elevation (Schwarz et al, 2002; Wojner, El-Mitwalli, & Alexandrov, 2002). Optimal head position needs to be determined individually, depending on both ICP and CPP measurements (Simmons, 1997).*

▲ For DIICP, if baseline ICP rises above 15 mm Hg or CPP (mean arterial blood pressure minus mean ICP) is less than 60 mm Hg in adults for 5 minutes or more, do the following:

- Initiate protocols for lowering ICP according to a collaborative plan with attending physician if ICP remains elevated or CPP decreases outside parameters—usually ICP greater than 15 to 20 mm Hg or CPP less than 60 mm Hg for 10 or more minutes (less than 40 to 65 mm Hg in children). **EB:** *The Brain Trauma Foundation guidelines have been compiled by neurosurgical societies from systematic reviews of the research literature. Thereapeutic options for children have been compiled in the same manner by pediatric and trauma professional societies (Carney, Chesnut, & Kochanek, 2003). All recommendations are at the level of therapeutic options, rather than standards or guidelines, given the paucity of clinical research, particularly with children. Therapeutic option for adults to manage CPP has been updated to maintain pressure greater than 60 mm Hg based on observations that such a pressure level may be associated with better outcomes, without the risk of acute respiratory distress syndrome associated with aggressive attemts to maintain CPP greater than 70 mm Hg (Brain Trauma Foundation, 2000a, 2003). ICP and CPP thresholds in children are less clear, but the pediatric guidelines recommend an option to treat child ICP when it exceeds 20 mm Hg, and to maintain*

*CPP ranging from 40 to 65 mm Hg (Adelson et al, 2003). A small controlled study in adults with severe head injury demonstrated better control of both ICP and CPP variations with a standardized protocol consistent with the Severe Head Injury Guidelines (McKinley, Parmley, & Tonneson, 1999). A larger study showed significant decrease in length of hospital stay and a trend to better outcomes at 6 months with use of an adult guidelines-based protocol (Fakhry et al, 2004). The plan will vary by region and individual physician preference but is increasingly likely to include interventions consistent with Brain Trauma Foundation guidelines (Bulger et al, 2002; Huizenga et al, 2002).*

- Cerebrospinal fluid (CSF) drainage via ventriculostomy intermittently to maintain a given ICP level. **EB:** *CSF drainage will manage CPP by reducing ICP at least temporarily in both adults and children. It does not change adaptive capacity (intracranial compliance) (Adelson et al, 2003b).*
- Addition of sedation (e.g., morphine, midazolam, propofol) and analgesia with or without paralysis (e.g., atracurium, pancuronium [Pavulon]) if body movements or fighting respirator continuously stimulate a CPP decrease. **EBN and EB:** *The short-acting agents allow rapid reversal of both sedation and paralysis for short periods to provide periodic neurological examination (McClelland et al, 1995) and appear useful in reducing ICP/CPP variations during suctioning (Gemma et al, 2002; Kerr et al, 1998, 1999). However there is recent evidence that ICP/CPP overall values do not differ in those head-injured patients who receive sedation and paralysis compared with those who do not (Juul et al, 2000). There is insufficient evidence in children to recommend any common protocols (Adelson et al, 2003c).*
- Bolus administration of osmotic diuretic or other hyperosmotic agent (e.g., mannitol, mannitol plus furosemide) may be followed with continuous administration if CPP is not maintained with bolus administration. Note that it is essential to keep serum osmolality less than 320 mOsm/L to prevent hyperosmolality-related seizures. These agents primarily reduce vascular volume and not cerebral edema. The older practice of keeping clients volume depleted in an attempt to prevent cerebral edema is no longer advocated (Chesnut, 1995). **EB:** *Although mannitol produces dramatic changes in individual cases, the research base for on-going management is limited. The most recent Cochrane Review of use of mannitol for traumatic brain injury found few well-conducted studies and concluded that mannitol appears to be more beneficial than pentobarbital in reducing mortality and that treatment directed by ICP monitoring is more beneficial than that directed by observed neurological signs (Schierhout & Roberts, 2002). Hypertonic saline is an evidence-based alternative in children, with dosage for continuous infusion of 3% saline range between 0.1 and 1.0 mL/kg of body weight per hour, administered on a sliding scale to keep ICP below 20 mm Hg. The children's guidelines recommend cautious use of hypertonic saline, pending more extensive studies to document lack of toxicity and confirmation of effectiveness (Adelson et al, 2003d).*
- In adults, control hyperventilation, maintaining $P_{CO_2}$ of 30 to 35 mm Hg unless ICP continues to be refractory, in which case $P_{CO_2}$ may be briefly decreased below 30 mm Hg if ICP is responsive. Mild or prophylactic hyperventilation should be

avoided in children, unless ICP is refractory. **EB:** *Older standards of early hyperventilation of clients to levels as low as 25 mm Hg have been shown to have poorer outcomes than in similar clients not hyperventilated. Prophylactic use of hyperventilation may induce cerebral ischemia (Brain Trauma Foundation, 2000b). Although many clinicians continue to use extreme hyperventilation, major trauma centers recommend this only as a last resort in refractory intracranial hypertension (Chesnut, 1995). Adequate randomized controlled trials have not yet been done to definitely settle the question of benefit or harm from aggressive hyperventilation in either adults or children (Schierhout & Roberts, 2002; Adelson et al, 2003e).*

- • To prevent DIICP in clients at risk (clients with elevated P2 waveforms and ICP of less than 10 mm Hg; clients previously responsive to general stimuli), do the following:
  - Maintain 15- to 30-degree head elevation if CPP is maintained at greater than 70 mm Hg.
  - Maintain systemic blood pressure adequate to keep CPP greater than 70 mm Hg by body positioning and use of vasoactive protocols.
  - Maintain adequate respiratory status; suction if needed but not prophylactically. **EBN:** *If suctioning is required, may use aerosolized lidocaine or sedation to reduce associated coughing (Kerr et al, 1997, 1998, 1999). Preoxygenate, hyperventilate only very briefly, and limit number of catheter passes to one or two (Kerr et al, 1997).*
  - Use gentle touching and talking or family visitations. **EBN:** *These activities rarely stimulate DIICP (Schinner et al, 1995). Family voices and gentle touch may help stabilize ICP (Hepworth et al, 1994; Mitchell & Ackerman, 1992; Mitchell & Habermann, 1999; Treloar et al, 1991).*
  - Use mechanical turning beds if manual repositioning is a stimulus to DIICP. **EBN:** *These beds keep the head and neck in a neutral alignment and have been shown not to alter ICP overall (Tillett et al, 1993; Mitchell, 1993).*
  - Avoid 90-degree hip flexion and use of the knee gatch of the bed. **EBN:** *Hip flexion may trap venous blood in the intraabdominal space, increasing abdominal and intrathoracic pressure, which in turn reduces venous outflow from the head (Vos, 1993).*
  - Sequence nursing care to allow for recovery of baseline ICP between noxious activities, such as suctioning, and position changes that involve neck flexion. **EBN:** *Several studies have shown stair-step increases in ICP when a stimulus to DIICP is repeated several times within a short time (Kerr et al, 1993; Mitchell & Ackerman, 1992).*
- ▲ With regard to general ICP monitoring:
  - Monitor ICP and CPP continuously with alarm settings on. **EBN and EB:** *Secondary brain injury can result from even brief periods of hypoxia and hypotension. Data from the Traumatic Coma Data Bank and international studies have documented that even in well-attended intensive care units, periods of more than 5 minutes of systemic hypotension (systolic blood pressure of less than 90 mm Hg) or intracranial hypertension occur in 70% to 90% of clients (Jones et al, 1994; Miller, 1993) and that even a single recording of a hypotensive episode is generally associated with a doubling of mortality in clinical studies (Brain Trauma Foundation, 2000c).*
- ▲ Notify physician if nursing interventions and collaborative protocols do not maintain a

CPP of greater than 60 mm Hg and an ICP of less than 20 mm Hg for adults; 40 to 65 mm Hg for for infants and children.

- ■ Monitor neurological status and CPP, including level of arousal, ability to follow commands, response to painful stimuli if arousal is decreased, and brainstem signs (pupil response, respiratory pattern, symmetry of motor response, and vital signs).

▲ Notify physician of signs of neurological deterioration regardless of levels of ICP and CPP. *Brain shift and herniation will be manifested by these changes in neurological status and may occur at any level of ICP. If the client is sedated and paralyzed to control ICP, pupillary changes or changes in response to painful stimuli may be the only available sign of deterioration (Mitchell & Ackerman, 1992; Ross et al, 1989).*

## Home Care

NOTE: Clients experiencing potentially rapid changes in ICP are not candidates for home care. However, clients experiencing potentially gradual changes in ICP (i.e., clients with developmental delays resulting from genetic dysfunction), or clients post ICP changes secondary to brain trauma, may be served by home care with the following considerations:

I

- Some of the above interventions may be adapted for home care use.
- Identify baseline neurological data before discharge from institutional care. *Baseline data will help both to identify changes in status and to create an individualized care plan.*
- Evaluate neurological functioning at regular intervals. *Neurological function improvements require long-term intervention.*
- Instruct the caregiver about client-specific changes that will indicate increased ICP. Examples include changes in speech articulation and eye coordination, decreased ability to focus, increased seizure activity, and decreased coping ability. The nurse is cautioned that changes will be specific to the disability of the client. Early reporting of status changes allows for early intervention in neurologically impaired clients.
- Instruct the client/family in appropriate expectations of cognitive recovery following minor brain injury. **EBN:** *During the first 24 hours after minor brain injury, clients are likely to experience distractibility, impulsivity, irritability, and impaired executive function. The results of a study suggested that cognitive demands on clients should be reduced for at least 48 hours following injury and for 30 days or longer for clients who lost consciousness (Brewer, Metzger, & Therrien, 2002).*
- For clients with a history of traumatic brain injury, assess for mood, thought process, or personality disturbances and refer for appropriate mental health follow-up. *A 30-year follow-up study of individuals who suffered a traumatic brain injury found a substantial risk for depressive episodes, delusional disorder, or personality disturbances (Koponen et al, 2002).*
- Assist clients to identify resources/situations they can attend or in which they can participate to enhance a sense of valued fit. Identify and problem solve around issues of stress. **EBN:** *In a study of individuals living at home who had experienced traumatic brain injury, low sense of belonging (valued fit) and chronic stress were strong predictors of depression (Bay et al, 2002).*

- Institute case management of frail elderly to support continued independent living. *Neurological difficulties represent and can lead to increasing needs for assistance in using the health care system effectively. Case management combines nursing activities of the client and family assessment, planning and coordination of care among all health care providers, delivery of direct nursing care, and monitoring of care and outcomes. These activities are able to address continuity of care, mutual goal setting, behavior management, and prevention of worsening health problems (Guttman, 1999).*

## evolve WEBSITES FOR EDUCATION

See the EVOLVE website for World Wide Web resources for client education.

## REFERENCES

I

Adelson PD, Bratton SL, Carney NA et al: Guidelines for the acute medical management of severe traumatic brain injury in infants, children, and adolescents: cerebral perfusion pressure, *Pediatr Crit Care Med* 4(Suppl 3):S31, 2003a.

Adelson PD, Bratton SL, Carney NA et al: Guidelines for the acute medical management of severe traumatic brain injury in infants, children, and adolescents: the role of cerebrospinal fluid drainage in the treatment of severe pediatric traumatic brain injury. *Pediatr Crit Care Med* 4(Suppl 3):S38, 2003b.

Adelson PD, Bratton SL, Carney NA et al: Guidelines for the acute medical management of severe traumatic brain injury in infants, children, and adolescents: use of sedation and neuromuscular blockade in the treatment of severe pediatric traumatic brain injury, *Pediatr Crit Care Med* 4(Supl 3):S34, 2003c.

Adelson PD, Bratton SL, Carney NA et al: Guidelines for the acute medical management of severe traumatic brain injury in infants, children, and adolescents: use of hyperosmolar therapy in the management of severe pediatric traumatic brain injury, *Pediatr Crit Care Med* 4(Suppl 3):S40, 2003d.

Adelson PD, Bratton SL, Carney NA et al: Guidelines for the acute medical management of severe traumatic brain injury in infants, children, and adolescents: use of hyperventilation in the acute management of severe pediatric traumatic brain injury, *Pediatr Crit Care Med* 4(Suppl 3):S45, 2003e.

Bader M, Littlejohns L: Intracranial pressure monitoring. In Bulechek GM, McCloskey JC, editors: *Nursing interventions: effective nursing treatments,* Philadelphia, 1999, WB Saunders.

Bay E, Hagerty BM, Williams RA, et al: Chronic stress, sense of belonging, and depression among survivors of traumatic brain injury, *J Nurs Scholarship* 34(3):221, 2002.

Bellieni CV, Burroni A, Perrone S et al: Intracranial pressure during procedural pain, *Bio Neonate* 84(3):202, 2003.

Beuret P, Carton MJ, Nourdine K et al: Prone position as prevention of lung injury in comatose patients: a prospective, randomized, controlled study, *Intensive Care Med* 28(5):564, 2002.

Brain Trauma Foundation, American Association of Neurological Surgeons, Congress of Neurological Surgeons, Joint Section on Neurotrauma and Critical Care: Update to Guidelines for Management of Severe Traumatic Brain Injury: Cerebral Perfusion Pressure, Approved March 14, 2003. Available at www.2.braintrauma.org/guidelines/index.php, accessed on January 8, 2005.

Brain Trauma Foundation, American Association of Neurological Surgeons, Joint Section on Neurotrauma and Critical Care: Guidelines for cerebral perfusion pressure, *J Neurotrauma* 17(6-7):507, 2000a.

Brain Trauma Foundation, American Association of Neurological Surgeons, Joint Section on Neurotrauma and Critical Care: Hyperventilation, *J Neurotrauma* 17(6-7):513, 2000b.

Brain Trauma Foundation, American Association of Neurological Surgeons, Joint Section on Neurotrauma and Critical Care: Hypotension, *J Neurotrauma* 17(6-7):591, 2000c.

Brewer TL, Metzger BL, Therrien B: Trajectories of cognitive recovery following a minor brain injury, *Res Nurs Health* 25:269, 2002.

Brimioulle S, Moraine JJ, Norrenberg D et al: Effects of positioning and exercise on intracranial pressure in a neurosurgical intensive care unit, *Phys Ther* 77:1682, 1997.

Bulger EM, Nathens AB, Rivara FP et al: Management of severe head injury: institutional variations in care and effect on outcome, *Crit Care Med* 30(8):1870, 2002.

Carney NA, Chesnut R, Kochanek PM: Guidelines for the acute medical management of severe traumatic brain injury in infants, children, and adolescents, *Pediatr Crit Care Med*, 4(Suppl 3):S1, 2003.

Chesnut RM: Avoidance of hypotension: condition sine qua non of successful severe head-injury management, *J Trauma* 42(Suppl 5):S4, 1997.

Chesnut RM: Medical management of severe head injury: present and future, *New Horiz* 3:581, 1995.

Fakhry SM, Trask AL, Waller MA et al: Management of brain-injured patients by an evidence-based medicine protocol improves outcomes and decreases hospital charges, *J Trauma*, 56(3):492, 2004.

Fan JY: Effect of backrest position on intracranial pressure and cerebral perfusion pressure in individuals with brain injury: a systematic review, *J Neurosci Nurs* 36(5):278, 2004.

Gemma M, Tommasino C, Cerri M et al: Intracranial effects of endotracheal suctioning in the acute phase of head injury, *J Neurosurg Anesthesiol* 14(1):50, 2002.

Guttman R: Case management of the frail elderly in the community, *Clin Nurs Spec* 13(4):174, 1999.

Haykowsky MJ, Eves ND, Warburton DER: Resistance exercise, the Valsalva maneuver, and cerebrovascular transmural pressure, *Med Sci Sports Exerc* 35(1):65, 2003.

Hepworth JT, Hendrickson SG, Lopez J: Time series analysis of physiological response during ICU visitation, *West J Nurs Res* 16: 704, 1994.

Huizenga JE, Zink BJ, Maio RF et al: Guidelines for the management of severe head injury: are emergency physicians following them? *Acad Emerg Med* 9(8):806, 2002.

Jones PA, Andrews PJ, Midgley S et al: Measuring the burden of secondary insults in head-injured patients during intensive care, *J Neurosurg Anesthesiol* 6:4, 1994.

Juul N, Morris GF, Marshall SB et al: Neuromuscular blocking agents in neurointensive care, *Acta Neurochir Suppl* 76:467, 2000.

Kerr ME, Rudy EB, Brucia J et al: Head-injured adults: recommendations for endotracheal suctioning, *J Neurosci Nurs* 25:86, 1993.

Kerr ME, Rudy EB, Weber BB et al: Effect of short-duration hyperventilation during endotracheal suctioning in severe head-injured adults, *Nurs Res* 46:195, 1997.

Kerr ME, Weber BB, Sereika SM et al: Effect of endotracheal suctioning on cerebral oxygenation in traumatic brain-injured patients, *Crit Care Med* 27(12):2776, 1999.

Kirkness CJ, Mitchell PH, Burr RL et al: Intracranial pressure waveform analysis: clinical and research implications, *J Neurosci Nurs*, 32(5):271, 2000.

Koponen S, Taiminen T, Portin R et al: Axis I and II psychiatric disorders after traumatic brain injury: a 30-year follow-up study, *Am J Psychiatry* 159:1315, 2002.

Lee S: Intracranial pressure changes during positioning of patients with severe head injury, *Heart Lung* 18:411, 1989.

March K, Mitchell P, Grady S et al: Effects of backrest position on ICP and CPP, *J Neurosci Nurs* 22:375, 1990.

Mavrocordatos P, Bissonnette B, Ravussin P: Effects of neck position and head elevation on intracranial pressure in anaesthetized neurosurgical patients: preliminary results, *J Neurosurg Anesthesiol* 12(1):10, 2000.

McKinley BA, Parmley CL, Tonneson AS: Standardized management of intracranial pressure: a preliminary clinical trial, *J Trauma* 46:271, 1999.

Miller JD: Head injury, *J Neurol Neurosurg Psychiatry* 56:440, 1993.

Mitchell PH: Decreased adaptive capacity. In Kinney MR, Packa DR, Dunbar SB, editors: *AACN's clinical reference for critical care nursing*, ed 3, St Louis, 1993, Mosby.

Mitchell PH, Ackerman LL: Secondary brain injury reduction. In Bulechek GM, McCloskey JC, editors: *Nursing interventions*, ed 2, Philadelphia, 1992, WB Saunders.

Mitchell PH, Habermann B: Rethinking physiological stability: touch and intracranial pressure, *Biol Res Nurs* 1(1):12, 1999.

Rauch ME, Mitchell PH, Tyler ML: Validation of risk factors for the nursing diagnosis of decreased intracranial adaptive capacity, *J Neurosci Nurs* 22:173, 1990.

Ross DA, Olsen WL, Ross AM et al: Brain shift, level of consciousness and restoration of consciousness in patients with acute intracranial hematoma, *J Neurosurg* 71:498, 1989.

Schierhout G, Roberts I. Mannitol for acute traumatic brain injury, *Cochrane Database Syst Rev* 2, 2002.

Schinner KM, Chisholm AH, Grap MJ et al: Effects of auditory stimuli on intracranial pressure and cerebral perfusion pressure in traumatic brain injury, *J Neurosci* Nurs 27:348, 1995.

Schwarz S, Georgiadis D, Aschoff A et al: Effects of body position on intracranial pressure and cerebral perfusion in patients with large hemispheric stroke, *Stroke* 33(2):497, 2002.

Simmons BJ: Management of intracranial hemodynamics in the adult: a research analysis of head positioning and recommendations for clinical practice and future research, *J Neurosci Nurs* 29:44, 1997.

Tillett JM, Marmarou A, Agnew JP et al: Effect of continuous rotational therapy on intracranial pressure in the severely brain-injured patient, *Crit Care Med* 21(7):1005, 1993.



I

Treloar DM, Nalli BJ, Guin P et al: The effect of familiar and unfamiliar voice treatments on intracranial pressure in head-injured patients, *J Neurosci Nurs* 23(5):295, 1991.

Vos HR: Making headway with intracranial hypertension, *Am J Nurse* 93:28, 1993.

Williams A, Coyne SM: Effects of neck position on intracranial pressure, *Am J Crit Care* 2:68, 1993.

Winkelman C: Effect of backrest position on intracranial and cerebral perfusion pressures in traumatically brain-injured adults, *Am J Crit Care* 9(6):373, 2000.

Wojner AW, El-Mitwalli A, Alexandrov AV: Effect of head positioning on intracranial blood flow velocities in acute ischemic stroke: a pilot study, *Crit Care Nurs Q* 24(4):57, 2002.

# Deficient Knowledge (specify)

evolve

*Gail B. Ladwig*

**NANDA**

## Definition

Absence or deficiency of cognitive information related to a specific topic

## Defining Characteristics

Verbalization of the problem; inaccurate follow-through of instruction; inaccurate performance of test; inappropriate or exaggerated behaviors (e.g., hysterical, hostile, agitated, apathetic)

## Related Factors (r/t)

Lack of exposure, lack of recall, information misinterpretation, cognitive limitation, lack of interest in learning, unfamiliarity with information resources

**NOC**

## Outcomes (Nursing Outcomes Classification)

### Suggested NOC Outcomes

Knowledge: Diet, Disease Process, Energy Conservation, Health Behavior, Health Resources, Infection Control, Medication, Personal Safety, Prescribed Activity, Substance Use Control, Treatment Procedure(s), Treatment Regimen

**Example NOC Outcome with Indicators**

**Knowledge: Health Behavior** as evidenced by the following indicators: Description of: Healthy nutritional practices/Benefits of exercise/Safe use of prescription and nonprescription drugs (Rate each indicator of **Knowledge: Health Behavior:** 1 = none, 2 = limited, 3 = moderate, 4 = substantial, 5 = extensive [see Section I].)

## Client Outcomes

**Client Will (Specify Time Frame):**

- Explain disease state, recognize need for medications, and understand treatments
- Explain how to incorporate new health regimen into lifestyle
- State an ability to deal with health situation and remain in control of life
- Demonstrate how to perform health related procedure(s) satisfactorily
- List resources that can be used for more information or support after discharge

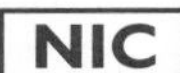


## Interventions (Nursing Interventions Classification)

### Suggested NIC Interventions

Teaching: Disease Process, Individual, Infant Safety

**Example NIC Activities—Teaching: Disease Process**

Discuss therapy/treatment options; describe rationale behind management/therapy/treatment recommendations

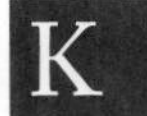


## Nursing Interventions and Rationales

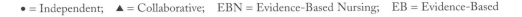

- Observe the client's ability and readiness to learn (e.g., mental acuity, ability to see or hear, no existing pain, emotional readiness, absence of language or cultural barriers) and previous knowledge. **EBN:** *Astute assessment is needed to determine the person's learning ability. A bowel management program for spinal cord–injured clients can be adjusted accordingly to either meet the needs of a self-directed learner or a dependent learner. Whichever the case, well-designed education materials will facilitate patient learning and the transfer of education from inpatient to community settings (Pryor& Jannings, 2004). Learning best occurs when learners are motivated and attend to the important aspects of what is to be learned (Forrest, 2004).*
- Assess barriers to learning (e.g., perceived change in lifestyle, financial concerns, cultural patterns, lack of acceptance by peers or coworkers). **EBN:** *The client brings to the learning situation a unique personality, established social interaction patterns, cultural norms and values, and environmental influences (Bohny, 1997).*
- Involve clients in writing specific outcomes for the teaching session, such as identifying what is most important to learn from their viewpoint and lifestyle. **EBN:** *This study indicated that clients were willing to take responsibility for playing their part in trying to optimize the outcome of their surgery (Edwards, 2002). In this study of women diagnosed with early breast cancer, the understanding of factors that are important to women when they are making decisions for medical treatment is a mandatory step in designing customized evidence-based decision support (Budden et al, 2003).*
- When teaching, build on the client's literacy skills. **EB:** *In clients with low literacy skills, materials should be short and have culturally sensitive illustrations (Mayeaux et al, 1996). The National Adult Literacy Survey reported that 44 million Americans could not read or write well enough to meet the needs of everyday living and working (Quirk, 2000).*
- Present material that is most significant to the client first, such as how to give injec-

tions or change dressings; present additional material once the client's most pressing educational needs have been met. *Information building begins with explaining simple concepts and moves on to explanations of complex application situations.*

- Use easy to understand language when giving information to clients. Encourage clients to ask the following questions: What is my main problem? What do I need to do? Why is it important for me to do this?" Have clients' repeat back information. **EB:** *An estimated 90 million Americans—nearly half of all adults in this country—cannot understand the complex language used in health care delivery. It is recommended to rewrite all hospital materials at a fifth-grade level, using graphics where appropriate. This includes informed consent and hospital information forms—everything a patient sees. "It cuts across the whole health system, not just patient education." Another initiative fosters patient "teach-backs" in which doctors or clinicians ask patients to repeat their care instructions back to them (Thrall, 2004).*
- ▲ Carefully evaluate information that is given to client regarding "disease state" focus on wellness. *In this study of clients with myocardial infarction, illness representation was predictive of the likelihood of experiencing a complication. Thus illness representation appears to be an important psychosocial factor in acute recovery from myocardial infarction (Cherrington et al, 2004).*

K

- Evaluate the readability of the material in pamphlets or written instructions. **EBN:** *Nonadherence of older adults to new medication regimens appears to be a function of decreased cognitive ability and comprehension of instruction, poor communication, and increased physical limitations (Hayes, 1998).*
- ▲ Use visual aids such as diagrams, pictures, videotapes, audiotapes, and interactive Internet websites. **EBN:** *Verbal reinforcement of personalized, written instructions appears to be the best-tested intervention. Computer-generated, personalized instructions improved adherence when compared with handwritten instructions (Hayes, 1998).* **EB:** *Leaflets are a useful resource for information provision (Kubba, 2000).* **EBN:** *An intervention of an educational video and written instructions designed to reduce prehospital delays in patients with chest pain showed a significant increase in the use of ambulances for the intervention group ($p = 0.03$) but not for the control group (Blank & Smithline, 2002).*
- ▲ Provide clients with appropriate preoperative information. **EBN:** *Research has shown the benefits of giving preoperative information to patients, which include decreased length of stay, less demand for analgesia postoperatively and increased patient satisfaction (Garretson et al, 2004).*
- ▲ Assess willingness of family to incorporate new information, immunizations, medical/dental care, and diet/behavior modifications in support of the client. **EBN:** *Attention needs to be directed at family adjustment factors. For example, women recovering from alcohol abuse are at risk for relapse if their spouse continues to drink alcohol (Murphy, 1993).* **EBN:** *Modification of eating patterns plus social and partnership support have had more success than modification alone (Keller et al, 1997).*
- ▲ Help the client identify community resources for continuing information and support. **EB:** *Community resources can offer financial and educational support. For example, role modeling and skill training have been used to monitor symptoms and solve asthma problems (Bartholomew et al, 2000).*

- ▲ Consider an experience-based group educational program for clients with type 2 diabetes. **EB:** *Findings in this study indicated that participating in the intervention program significantly decreased HbA1c by 0.4% at 24 months after baseline. The intervention group exercised more in order to lower blood-glucose levels and was also more able to predict current blood-glucose levels before measuring it (Sarkadi & Rosenqvist, 2004).* **EB:** *Group care per se was the major factor associated with improved knowledge, problem-solving ability, and quality of life in this study of clients with type 2 diabetes (Trento et al, 2004).*
- • Evaluate the client's learning through return demonstrations, verbalizations, or the application of skills to new situations. *Presenting information along with examples of how to apply the information has been found more successful than providing information alone in a home care setting (Duffy, 1997).*

## Pediatric

- ▲ Consider the developmental needs of teens when designing programs related to pregnancy. **EBN:** *Adolescent pregnancy remains a significant social, economic, and health issue in the United States. The unique developmental needs of the pregnant adolescent require attention when designing prenatal care services. The Centering Pregnancy model of group prenatal care provides education and support for young women in an active and developmentally appropriate environment. Evaluation data suggest that the model has encouraged excellent health care compliance, satisfaction with prenatal care, and low rates of preterm birth and low-birth-weight infants (Grady & Bloom, 2004).*
- ▲ Consider a pregnancy prevention intervention program for teens using Baby Think It Over infant simulator. **EBN:** *These findings suggest that simulated experiences can be a powerful strategy for effective learning about complex decisions regarding the risks of sexual activity and the realities of parenting (Didion & Gatzke, 2004).*

## Geriatric

- • Adapt the teaching process for the physical constraints of the aging process (e.g., speak clearly, use a variety of audio-visual-psychomotor methods, provide examples, and allow time for the client to repeat and review). **EBN:** *Adults are capable of learning at any age. Age modifies but does not inhibit learning (Dellasega et al, 1994). Older adults need practice to use new technology (Westerman & Davies, 2000).*
- • Ensure that the client uses necessary reading aids (e.g., eyeglasses, magnifying lenses, large-print text) or hearing aids. *Visual and hearing deficits require amplification or clarification of sensory input.*
- • Use printed material, videotapes, lists, diagrams, and Internet addresses that the client can refer to at another time. **EB:** *These methods provide a reference that can be used in a less stressful setting, decreasing barriers to learning. This study demonstrated the effectiveness of printed material and a Web-based format for education. The Web-based format demonstrated two additional benefits when compared with printed material: increased social support and decreased anxiety (Scherrer-Bannerman et al, 2000).*
- • Repeat and reinforce information during several brief sessions. *Understanding past information is essential to acquiring new knowledge. Brief sessions focus attention on essential information.*

K

- • Discuss healthy lifestyle changes that promote wellness for the older adult. **EBN:** *Greater efforts must be made both to improve preventive health care and enhance quality-of-life interventions of older people (Nolan, 2001).*
- • Evaluate readability of the material. **EBN:** *Nonadherence of older adults to new medication regimens appears to be a function of decreased cognitive ability, comprehension of instruction, poor communication, and increased physical limitations (Hayes, 1998).*
- ▲ Consider health education programs using television and newspapers. *There was a significant increase in stroke knowledge (52% more likely to know a risk factor and 35% know a symptom, $p = 0.032$) following this health education program as demonstrated through a telephone pretest and posttest (Becker et al, 2001).*

### Multicultural

- • Acknowledge racial/ethnic differences at the onset of care. **EBN:** *Acknowledgment of racial/ethnicity issues will enhance communication, establish rapport, and promote treatment outcomes (D'Avanzo et al, 2001; Ludwick & Silva, 2000; Vontress & Epp, 1997).*
- • Assess for the influence of cultural beliefs, norms, and values on the client's knowledge base. **EBN:** *The client's knowledge base may be influenced by cultural perceptions (Cochran, 1998; Doswell & Erlen, 1998; Leininger & McFarland, 2002).*
- • Use a neutral indirect style when addressing areas where improvement is needed when working with Native-American clients. **EBN:** *Using indirect statements such as "I had a client who tried 'X,' and it seemed to work very well" will help avoid resentment from the client (Seideman et al, 1996).*
- • Validate the client's feelings and concerns related to previous learning experiences. **EBN:** *Validation is therapeutic communication technique that lets the client know that the nurse has heard and understands what was said, and it promotes the nurse-client relationship (Heineken, 1998).*
- • Approach individuals of color with respect, warmth, and professional courtesy. **EBN:** *Instances of disrespect and lack of caring have special significance for individuals of color (D'Avanzo et al, 2001; Vontress & Epp, 1997).*
- • Provide health care information to mothers and grandmothers in African-American families. **EBN:** *Mothers and grandmothers are considered the gatekeepers of health care in the African-American community (Sterling & Peterson, 2003).*
- • Provide written health care information to patients with limited English proficiency in their native language. **EB:** *Patients with limited English proficiency were unable to understand routinely dispensed medication instructions written in English. Health care providers should not assume that limited English proficiency patients who are comfortable speaking English will understand a prescription label written in English (Leyva, Sharif, & Ozuah, 2005).*

### Home Care

NOTE: Because home care is an intermittent model of care having a goal of safety and optimal wellness of the client between visits, the importance of teaching (by the nurse) and learning (by the client) should not be understated. All of the previously mentioned interventions are applicable to the home setting.

- ▲ Select a space and time for teaching in which the client and/or caregiver can focus on information to be learned. *The home setting provides many distractions that may impair the ability of the client to learn.*

- ▲ Consider the complexity of material or behaviors to be learned. Adjust care plan and respective teaching and learning experiences accordingly to build client confidence in ability to learn (and change). *Confidence in ability to learn and change is part of readiness to learn.*
- • Assess the client for low or absent literacy. Use illustrations for instruction that are as closely equivalent as possible to written instructions. *Clients who are illiterate may assert their understanding of written instructions as a face-saving response. Clients with low literacy skills may demonstrate limitations in their understanding of written instructions.*
- • Assess the client/family learning needs and current level of knowledge. *Adult learners bring preexisting knowledge to a situation. Building on that knowledge is more effective than assuming total client/family ignorance. At the same time, inaccuracies in preexisting knowledge may need to be corrected.*
- • Assess for specific areas of learning that have the potential for strong emotional responses by the client or family/caregiver. Allow time for expression of feelings and encourage acceptance of need for learning. *An individual's perception of barriers and benefits has consistently been most predictive of subsequent behavior. Clinicians should develop interventions that increase benefits and decrease barriers (Fenn, 1998).*
- • Use visual aids and other available media that engage multiple senses to maximize learning. Leave visually oriented/written materials in home. **EB:** *The effectiveness of media-based interventions for educating patients about general process and risks of anesthesia were compared in this systematic review. The use of video and/or printed information can decrease patient anxiety and increase patient knowledge (Lee, Chui, & Gin, 2003).*
- • Document the client's and caregivers' responses to learning. *Clear documentation supports continuity in the learning experience.*
- • Explore resources for teaching relative to specific illnesses. **EBN:** *The Learning Needs Assessment Tool (LNAT) has been developed to assess family/environment, current knowledge, and learning style of clients with congestive heart failure (Lile, Buhmann, & Roders, 1999).*
- • Encourage self-care management of illness. Refer to care plan for **Powerlessness. EBN:** *Enhancing the client's perception of his or her ability to perform specific diabetes activities increased self-efficacy for diabetes management (Corbett, 1999).*
- ▲ Consider high-tech options for delivery of home-based instruction. **EBN:** *Televideo technology has been used effectively to improve self-management of diabetes (Bowles & Dansky, 2002). Interactive teleconferencing and on-site training for family caregivers positively influenced knowledge, self-perceived competence, and resourcefulness, with no significant difference between the program delivery types (Rosswurm et al, 2002).*

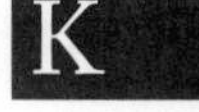

## evolve WEBSITES FOR EDUCATION

See the EVOLVE website for World Wide Web resources for client education.

## REFERENCES

Bartholomew LK, Gold RS, Parcel GS et al: Watch, discover, think, and act: evaluation of computer-assisted instruction to improve asthma self-management in inner-city children, *Patient Educ Couns* 39(2-3):269, 2000.

Becker K, Fruin M, Gooding T et al: Community-based education improves stroke knowledge, *Cerebrovasc Dis* 11(1):34, 2001.
Blank FS, Smithline HA: Evaluation of an educational video for cardiac patients, *Clin Nurs Res* 11(4):403, 2002.
Bohny B: A time for self-care: role of the home healthcare nurse, *Home Healthc Nurse* 15(4):281, 1997.
Bowles KH, Dansky KH: Teaching self-management of diabetes, *Home Healthc Nurse* 20(1):36, 2002.
Budden LM, Pierce PF, Hayes BA et al: Australian women's prediagnostic decision-making styles, relating to treatment choices for early breast cancer treatment, *Res Theory Nurs Pract* 17(2):117-136, 2003.
Cherrington CC, Moser DK. Lennie TA et al: Illness representation after acute myocardial infarction: impact on in-hospital recovery, *Am J Crit Care* 13(2):136-145, 2004.
Cochran M: Tears have no color, *Am J Nurs* 98(6):53, 1998.
Corbett CF: Research-based practice implications for patients with diabetes: part II: diabetes self-efficacy, *Home Healthc Nurse* 17: 587, 1999.
D'Avanzo CE et al: Developing culturally informed strategies for substance-related interventions. In Naegle MA, D'Avanzo CE, editors: *Addictions and substance abuse: strategies for advanced practice nursing,* St Louis, 2002, Mosby.
Dellasega C, Clark D, McCreary D et al: Nursing process: teaching elderly clients, *J Gerontol Nurs* 20(1):31-38, 1994.
Doswell W, Erlen J: Multicultural issues and ethical concerns in the delivery of revising care interventions, *Nurs Clin North Am* 33(2):353, 1998.
Duffy B: Using a creative teaching process with adult patients, *Home Healthc Nurse* 15(2):102, 1997.
Edwards C: A proposal that patients be considered honorary members of the healthcare team, *J Clin Nurs* 11(3):340, 2002.
Fenn M: Health promotion: theoretical perspectives and clinical applications, *Holist Nurs Pract* 12(2):1, 1998.
Forrest S: Learning and teaching: the reciprocal link, *J Contin Educ Nurs* 35(2):74-9, 2004.
Garretson S: Benefits of preoperative information programmes, *Nurs Stand* 18(47):33-7, 2004.
Grady MA, Bloom KC: Pregnancy outcomes of adolescents enrolled in a Centering Pregnancy program, *J Midwifery Womens Health* 49(5):412-420, 2004.
Hayes K: Randomized trial of geragogy-based medication instruction in the emergency department, *Nurs Res* 47(4):211, 1998.
Heineken J: Patient silence is not necessarily client satisfaction: communication in home care nursing, *Home Healthc Nurse* 16(2): 115, 1998.
Keller C, Oveland D, Hudson S: Strategies for weight control success in adults, *Nurse Pract* 22(3):37, 1997.
Kubba H: An evidence-based patient information leaflet about otitis media with effusion, *Clin Perform Qual Health Care* 8(2):93, 2000.
Leininger MM, McFarland MR: *Transcultural nursing: concepts, theories, research and practices,* ed 3, New York, 2002, McGraw-Hill.
Leyva M, Sharif I, Ozuah PO: Health literacy among Spanish-speaking Latino parents with limited English proficiency, *Ambul Pediatr* 5(1):56-59, 2005.
Lile JB, Buhmann J, Roders S: Development of a learning needs assessment tool for patients with congestive heart failure, *Home Healthcare Manag Pract* 11(6):11, 1999.
Ludwick R, Silva M: Nursing around the world: cultural values and ethical conflicts, *Online J Issues Nurs.* Available at www.nursingworld.org/ojin/ethcol/ethics_4.htm.
Mayeaux EJ Jr, Murphy PW, Arnold C et al: Improving patient education for patients with low literacy skills, *Am Physician* 53(1): 205, 1996.
Murphy SP: Coping strategies of abstainers from alcohol 3 years to post treatment, *Image J Nurs Sch* 25:32, 1993.
Nolan J: Improving the health of older people: what do we do? *Br J Nurs* 10(8):524, 2001.
Pryor J, Jannings W: Preparing patients to self-manage faecal continence following spinal cord injury, *JARNA* 7(2): 20-23, 2004.
Quirk PA: Screening for literacy and readability: implications for the advanced practice nurse, *Clin Nurse Spec*14(1):26, 2000.
Rosswurm MA, Larrabee JH, Zhang J: Training family caregivers of dependent elderly adults through on-site and telecommunications programs, *J Gerontol Nurs* 28(7):27, 2002.
Sarkadi A, Rosenqvist U: Experience-based group education in type 2 diabetes: a randomized controlled trial, *Patient Educ Couns* 53(3):291-298, 2004.
Scherrer-Bannerman A, Fofonoff D, Minshall D et al: Web-based education and support for patients on the cardiac surgery waiting list, *J Telemed Telecare* 6(Suppl 2):S72, 2000.
Seideman RY, Jacobson S, Primeaux M et al: Assessing American Indian families, *MCN Am J Matern Child Nurs* 21(6):274, 1996.
Sterling YM, Peterson JW: Characteristics of African American women caregivers of children with asthma, *MCN Am J Matern Child Nurs* 28(1):32, 2003.
Vontress CE, Epp LR: Historical hostility in the African American client: implications for counseling, *J Multicult Counsel Devel* 25:170, 1997.
Westerman SJ, Davies DR: Acquisition and application of new technology skills: the influence of age, *Occup Med* 50(7):478, 2000.

# Readiness for enhanced Knowledge (specify)

evolve

*Gail B. Ladwig*

**NANDA**

## Definition

The presence or acquisition of cognitive information related to a specific topic is sufficient for meeting health-related goals and can be strengthened

## Defining Characteristics

Expresses an interest in learning; explains knowledge of the topic; behaviors congruent with expressed knowledge; describes previous experiences pertaining to the topic

## Related Factors (r/t)

To be developed

K

**NOC**

## Outcomes (Nursing Outcomes Classification)

### Suggested NOC Outcome

Knowledge: Health Promotion

**Example NOC Outcome with Indicators**

**Knowledge: Health Promotion** as evidenced by the following indicator: Description of health behaviors that promote health/relevant health resources (Rate each indicator of **Knowledge: Health Promotion:** 1 = none, 2 = limited, 3 = moderate, 4 = substantial, 5 = extensive [see Section I].)

## Client Outcomes

**Client Will (Specify Time Frame):**

- Demonstrate knowledge of new information
- Meet personal health-related goals
- Explain how to incorporate new health regimen into lifestyle
- List sources to obtain information

**NIC**

## Interventions (Nursing Interventions Classification)

### Suggested NIC Interventions

Health Education, Learning Readiness Enhancement

**Example NIC Activities—Health Education**

Prioritize identified learner needs based on client preference, skills of nurse, resources available, and likelihood of successful goal attainment

## Nursing Interventions and Rationales

- Include clients as members of the health care team when providing education. **EBN:** *This study indicated that clients were willing to take responsibility for playing their part in trying to optimize the outcome of their surgery. Reconceptualization of clients as honorary members of the health care team may facilitate the development of a framework, within which the potential contribution of clients to their own care could be valued and supported more effectively (Edwards, 2002).* **EBN:** *Couples who had received a diagnosis of prostrate cancer in this study found that by engaging in the challenge of gathering a volume of facts and a variety of details, they felt could make informed decisions and regain a sense of control through the engagement in decision making related to treatment, surgeon, and hospital (Maliski, Heilemann, & McCorkle, 2002).*
- Use open-ended questions and encourage two-way communication. **EBN:** *Intervention strategies that use interpersonal communication, including the opportunity for mothers to ask questions, were most preferred. Strategies that involve one-way messages to mothers were least preferred (Gaffney & Altieri, 2001).*
- Provide appropriate individualized health education when clients visit health care providers. **EBN:** *The low rate of lifestyle advice reported in this study by clients implies that more preventive advice should be provided in primary care settings. More effective health promotion should be planned according to the needs of the practice population (Duaso & Cheung, 2002).* **EB:** *Having a regular doctor was found to have a greater impact than having a regular site on discretional preventive services, such as blood pressure and cholesterol level checkups (Xu & Tom, 2002).*
- Ensure that clients receive appropriate health-oriented education during hospitalization. **EBN:** *Hospitalized patients were shown to be in a "window of opportunity" for assisting the behavior change process of smoking cessation due to increased health motivation (Narsavage & Idemoto, 2003).*
- When developing written information, assess and provide information that is important to clients. **EBN:** *This randomized study of information compiled from focus group input led to major change in providing information and produced a leaflet that was more clear, more attractive, and more informative and that proved more satisfactory to clients (Chumbley et al, 2002).* **EBN:** *During child psychiatric hospitalization, parents in this study identified needing informational, emotional, and instrumental support (Scharer, 2002).*
- Carefully develop written materials to ensure that the client's literacy levels, including English as a second language, are addressed. *Functional illiteracy contributes to negative long-term health consequences for clients who must understand and adhere to complex health care instructions and therefore is of primary importance to community health nurses. This problem is compounded when English is the client's second language (Horner, Surratt, & Juliusson, 2000).* **EBN:** *Patients need and want comprehensible, written information (Semple & McGowan, 2002).*

- • Assist clients to find access to the Internet, libraries, and schools to find health information. **EB:** *Access, demographics, and, in particular, motivational factors all influence clients' interest in the Internet as a health resource (Mead et al, 2003).*
- • Assist clients with questions about health information to find quality sites on the Internet. **EB:** *More popular sites according to Google rank were more likely than less popular ones to contain information on ongoing clinical trials, results of trials, and opportunities for psychosocial adjustment. These characteristics were also associated with higher number of links as reported by Google and AltaVista. More popular sites by number of linking sites were also more likely to provide updates on breast cancer research, information on legislation and advocacy, and a message board service (Meric et al, 2002).* **EBN:** *Health care providers have important roles in helping their clients as well as the public locate, assess, and interpret health information (Houston & Ehrenberger, 2001).*
- ▲ Provide a previsit questionnaire to facilitate individualized proactive planning before the visit to health care provider. **EBN:** *More than 75% of all women in this study wanted information to help them make decisions on breast cancer prevention options, benefits, and risks. A previsit questionnaire facilitates individualized proactive planning before the visit (Stacey, DeGrasse, & Johnston, 2002).*
- ▲ Provide information about the prognosis, the alternatives of treatment, and the effects of treatment when the diagnosis is cancer. Consider providing informational leaflets. **EBN:** *The results of this study indicated that there is still much to do when it comes to informing cancer patients. Around half of the respondents had not received enough information about the prognosis, the alternatives of treatment, and the effects of cancer or treatment. Leaflets about cancer and related issues were the most popular source of additional information. Most respondents wanted information because it had a positive impact on their feelings and attitudes and it helped them to cope with their situation (Sainio & Eriksson, 2003).* **EB:** *In this study of clients with ovarian cancer, the three most important information needs, in all measurements, were information about the likelihood of a cure, the stage and spreading of the disease, and the different treatment options (Browall, Carlsson, & Horvath, 2004).*
- ▲ Provide appropriate health care information and screening for clients with physical disabilities. **EBN:** *In this study of 170 women with physical disabilities between the ages of 21 and 65 years, most (96%) had not had routine preventive gynecological cancer screening services in the past 5 years or information and treatment for complications (e.g., fatigue, spasticity, deconditioning, joint pain, depression), which are preventable. Preventive health care services should be provided to clients with disabilities (Coyle & Santiago, 2002). The Americans with Disabilities Act requires that diabetes educators provide reasonable accommodations to people with disabilities in response to their particular individual needs (Position Statement, 2002).*
- ▲ Before the initiation of a mood stabilizer, the potential benefits, risks, and adverse effects should be communicated to the patient. Provide information on potential severe and life-threatening adverse cutaneous drug reactions (ACDRs) to all clients on mood-stabilizing agents such as carbamazepine, lithium carbonate, valproic acid, topiramate, lamotrigine, gabapentin, and oxcarbazepine. Patients should be advised to seek medical attention if they suspect a drug-induced skin reaction. *Of all the psychotropic medications currently available, the mood-stabilizing agents have the highest incidence*

*of severe and life-threatening ACDRs. An exanthematous eruption in a patient treated with a mood-stabilizing agent should be viewed as possibly being the initial symptom of a severe and life-threatening ACDR, such as a hypersensitivity reaction, Stevens-Johnson syndrome, or toxic epidermal necrolysis (Warnock & Morris, 2003).*

- ▲ Refer to nurse practitioners for client education. Use the HOPE model (health-oriented patient education) instead of the DOPE model (disease-oriented health education). *The economics of prevention supports reimbursement of nurse practitioners for client education (Glanville, 2000).*
- • Refer to care plan for **Deficient Knowledge.**

## Pediatric

- ▲ Provide adolescents with cancer with developmentally appropriate information. **EBN:** *Research has shown that information on the cancer experience improves outcomes by decreasing uncertainty and increasing perceived support. Clients in this study rated the need for information as high (Decker et al, 2004)*

## Geriatric

- ▲ Consider using an interactive multimedia computer software program to disburse education. **EBN:** *Users of Personal Education Program (PEP) designed for the learning styles and psychomotor skills of older adults had greater knowledge of potential interactions of prescription medications with over-the-counter (OTC) drugs and alcohol than controls. Participants indicated a high degree of satisfaction with the PEP and reported their intent to make specific changes in self-medication behaviors (Neafsey et al, 2001).* **EB:** *A total of 42 patients age 51 to 92 years tested an interactive program on heart failure. They thought it was a better way of receiving information than reading a booklet or watching a video (Stromberg, Ahlen, & Fridlund, 2002).*

## Multicultural

- • Refer to **Deficient Knowledge** care plan.
- • Provide health care information to mothers and grandmothers in African-American families. **EBN:** *Mothers and grandmothers are considered the gatekeepers of health care in the African-American community (Sterling & Peterson, 2003).*

## Home Care

NOTE: Because home care is an intermittent model of care having a goal of safety and optimal wellness of the client between visits, the importance of teaching (by the nurse) and learning (by the client) should not be understated. All of the previously mentioned interventions are applicable to the home setting.

- ▲ Consider high-tech options for delivery of home-based instruction. **EBN:** *Televideo technology has been used effectively to improve self-management of diabetes (Bowles & Dansky, 2002). Interactive teleconferencing and on-site training for family caregivers positively influenced knowledge, self-perceived competence, and resourcefulness, with no significant difference between the program delivery types (Rosswurm, Larrabee, & Zhang, 2002).*

## evolve WEBSITES FOR EDUCATION

See the EVOLVE website for World Wide Web resources for client education.

## REFERENCES


Bowles KH, Dansky KH: Teaching self-management of diabetes, *Home Healthc Nurse* 20(1):36, 2002.

Browall M, Carlsson M, Horvath G: Information needs of women with recently diagnosed ovarian cancer, *Eur J Oncol Nurs* 8(3); 200-210, 2004.

Chumbley GM, Hall GM, Salmon P: Patient-controlled analgesia: what information does the patient want? *J Adv Nurs* 39(5):459, 2002.

Coyle CP, Santiago MC: Healthcare utilization among women with physical disabilities, *Medscape Womens Health* 7(4):2, 2002.

Decker C, Phillips CR, Haase JE: Information needs of adolescents with cancer, *J Pediatr Oncol Nurs* 21(6):327-334, 2004.

Didion J, Gatzke H: The Baby Think It Over experience to prevent teen pregnancy: a postintervention evaluation, *Public Health Nurs* 21(4):331-337, 2004.

Duaso MJ, Cheung P: Health promotion and lifestyle advice in a general practice: what do patients think? *J Adv Nurs* 39(5):472, 2002.

Edwards C: A proposal that patients be considered honorary members of the healthcare team, *J Clin Nurs* 11(3):340, 2002.

Gaffney KF, Altieri LB: Mothers' ranking of clinical intervention strategies used to promote infant health, *Pediatr Nurs* 27(5):510, 2001.

Glanville IK: Moving towards health-oriented patient education (HOPE), *Holist Nurs Pract* 14(2):57, 2000.

Horner SD, Surratt D, Juliusson S: Improving readability of patient education materials, *J Community Health Nurs 17(1):15, 2000.*

Houston TK, Ehrenberger HE: The potential of consumer health informatics, *Semin Oncol Nurs* 17(1):41, 2001.

Lee A, Chui PT, Gin T: Educating patients about anesthesia: a systematic review of randomized controlled trials of media-based interventions, *Anesth Analg* 96(5):1424-1431, 2003.

Maliski SL, Heilemann MV, McCorkle R: From "death sentence" to "good cancer": couples' transformation of a prostate cancer diagnosis, *Nurs Res* 51(6):391, 2002.

Mead N, Varnam R, Rogers A et al: What predicts patients' interest in the Internet as a health resource in primary care in England, *J Health Serv Res Policy* 8(1):33, 2003.

Meric F, Bernstam EV, Mirza NQ et al: Breast cancer on the world wide web: cross sectional survey of quality of information and popularity of websites, *BMJ* 324(7337):577, 2002.

Narsavage G, Idemoto BK: Smoking cessation interventions for hospitalized patients with cardio-pulmonary disorders, *Online J Issues Nurs*, 8(2):8, 2003.

Neafsey PJ, Strickler Z, Shellman J et al: Delivering health information about self-medication to older adults: use of touchscreen-equipped notebook computers, *J Gerontol Nurs* 27(11):19, 2001.

Position Statement: Diabetes education for people with disabilities, *Diabetes Educ* 28(6):916, 2002.

Rosswurm MA, Larrabee JH, Zhang J: Training family caregivers of dependent elderly adults through on-site and telecommunications programs, *J Gerontol Nurs* 28(7):27, 2002.

Sainio C, Eriksson E: Keeping cancer patients informed: a challenge for nursing, *Eur J Oncol Nurs*, Mar; 7(1):39-49, 2003.

Sarkadi A, Rosenqvist U: Experience-based group education in type 2 diabetes: a randomised controlled trial, *Patient Educ Couns* 53(3):291-298, 2004.

Scharer K: What parents of mentally ill children need and want from mental health professionals, *Issues Ment Health Nurs* 23(6): 617, 2002.

Semple CJ, McGowan B: Need for appropriate written information for patients, with particular reference to head and neck cancer, *J Clin Nurs* 11(5):585, 2002.

Stacey D, DeGrasse C, Johnston L: Addressing the support needs of women at high risk for breast cancer: evidence-based care by advanced practice nurses, *Oncol Nurs Forum* 29(6):e77, 2002.

Sterling YM, Peterson JW: Characteristics of African American women caregivers of children with asthma, *MCN Am J Matern Child Nurs* 28(1):32, 2003.

Stromberg A, Ahlen H, Fridlund B: Interactive education on CD-ROM: a new tool in the education of heart failure patients, *Patient Educ Couns* 46(1):75, 2002.

Taylor KL, Turner RO, Davis JL 3rd et al: Improving knowledge of the prostrate cancer-screening dilemma among African American men: an academic-community partnership in Washington, DC, *Public Health Rep* 116(6):590, 2001.

Thrall TH: Dump the MUMBO-JUMBO, *Hosp Health Netw* 78(10):70-74, 2004.
Trento M, Passera P, Borgo E et al: A 5-year randomized controlled study of learning, problem solving ability, and quality of life modifications in people with type 2 diabetes managed by group care, *Diabetes Care* 27(3):670-675, 2005.
Warnock JK, Morris DW: Adverse cutaneous reactions to mood stabilizers, *Am J Clin Dermatol* 4(1):21, 2003.
Xu KT: Access to care: usual source of care in preventive service use: a regular doctor versus a regular site, *Health Serv Res* 37(6): 1509, 2002.

# Sedentary Lifestyle

*Betty J. Ackley*

**NANDA**

## Definition

Reports a habit of life that is characterized by a low physical activity level

## Defining Characteristics

Chooses a daily routine lacking physical exercise, demonstrates physical deconditioning, verbalizes preference for activities low in physical activity

## Related Factors

Deficient knowledge of health benefits of physical exercise; lack of training for accomplishment of physical exercise; lack of resources (time, money, companionship, facilities); lack of motivation; lack of interest

**NOC**

## Outcomes (Nursing Outcomes Classification)

### Suggested NOC Outcome

Ambulation

**Example NOC Outcome with Indicators**

**Ambulation** as evidenced by the following indicators: Walks with effective gait/Walks at moderate pace/Walks up and down steps/Walks moderate distance (Rate each indicator of **Ambulation:** 1 = severely compromised, 2 = substantially compromised, 3 = moderately compromised, 4 = mildly compromised, 5 = not compromised [see Section I].)

## Client Outcomes

**Client Will (Specify Time Frame):**

- Increase physical activity to minimum of 10,000 steps per day
- Meet mutually defined goals of increased exercise
- Verbalize feeling of increased strength and ability to move

**NIC**

## Interventions (Nursing Interventions Classification)

### Suggested NIC Interventions

Exercise Therapy: Ambulation, Joint Mobility; Positioning

**Example NIC Activities—Exercise Therapy: Ambulation**

Assist the client to use footwear that facilitates walking and prevents injury; instruct in availability of assistive devices, if appropriate

## Nursing Interventions and Rationales

- Observe the client for cause of sedentary lifestyle. Determine whether cause is physical or psychological. *Some clients choose not to move because of psychological factors such as an inability to cope or depression.* See care plan for **Ineffective Coping** or **Hopelessness.**
- ▲ Assess for reasons why the client would be unable to participate in an exercise program; refer for evaluation by a primary care practitioner as needed.
- Use the Outcome Expectation for Exercise Scale to determine client's self-efficacy expectations and outcomes expectations toward exercise. **EBN:** *The client's self-efficacy expectations and outcome expectations for exercise will greatly influence his or her willingness to exercise. If the individual has a low outcome, interventions can be implemented to strengthen the expectations and hopefully improve exercise behavior (Resnick, Zimmerman, & Orwig, 2001).*
- Recommend the client enter an exercise program with a friend. **EBN:** *Findings from a study of exercise behavior found that friends have the strongest influence to keep on an exercise program, more than family members or experts (Resnick, Orwig, & Magaziner, 2002).*
- Recommend the client begin a walking program using the following criteria:
  - Purchase a pedometer
  - Determine common times when walking can be incorporated into usual lifestyle
  - Set goal of walking 10,000 steps per day, which equals 5 miles per day
  - If when comes home from work, does not have required number of steps, go for a walk until reach designated goal of 10,000 steps per day

  **EB:** *A study demonstrated that use of a pedometer resulted in two times the usual amount of activity and weight loss in overweight adults (VanWormer, 2004). Another study demonstrated that in middle-aged women, women who walked more had lower body mass index (BMI), and that women who walked 10,000 plus steps per day were in the normal range for BMI (Thompson et al, 2004).*

### Pediatric

- Encourage child to increase the amount of walking done per day; if child is willing, ask him or her to wear a pedometer to measure number of steps. **EB:** *A study demonstrated that the recommended number of steps per day to have a healthy body composition for the 6 to 12 year old is 12,000 for a girl and 15,000 for a boy (Tudor-Locke et al, 2004).*

• = Independent; ▲ = Collaborative; EBN = Evidence-Based Nursing; EB = Evidence-Based

- Encourage the adolescent to increase exercise to help themselves feel better. **EBN:** *Adolescents had positive feeling states once they began to exercise (Robbins, 2004).*

## Geriatric

- Assess ability to move using the Get Up and Go test. Ask the client to rise from a sitting position, walk 10 feet, turn, and return to the chair to sit. *Performance on this screening examination demonstrates the client's mobility and ability to leave the house safely (Robertson & Montagnini, 2004).*
- Recommend the client begin a regular exercise program, even if generally active. **EB:** *A research program demonstrated that people who exercise with a defined program had greater functional capacity or reserve than clients who had an active lifestyle, but no defined exercise program (Wellbery, 2005).*
- ▲ Refer the client to physical therapy for resistance exercise training as able including abdominal crunch, leg press, leg extension, leg curl, calf press, and more. **EB:** A *study demonstrated that 6 months of resistance exercise for the elderly greatly increased their aerobic capacity, possibly from increased skeletal muscle strength (Vincent et al, 2002). An additional study where clients in an extended care facility were put on a strength-, balance-, and endurance-training program, the client's balance and mobility improved significantly (Rydwik, Kerstin, & Akner, 2005). A Cochrane Review meta-analysis found that progressive resistance strength training for physical disability in older clients resulted in increased strength and positive improvements in some limitations (Latham et al, 2005).*

L

- Use the WALC Intervention (Walk; Address pain, fear, fatigue during exercise; Learn about exercise; Cue by self-modeling) to improve exercise adherence in the older adult. **EBN:** *The WALC Intervention resulted in more exercise and had greater self-efficacy expectations regarding exercise (Resnick, 2002).*
- Recommend the client begin a Tai Chi practice. **EB and EBN:** *Studies have demonstrated that tai chi improves balance in the elderly and may help prevent falls (Wolf et al, 2003; Taggart, 2002).*
- If client is frail, ensure good nutrition, appropriate medications, attention to vision and hearing deficits, and increase social support along with exercise. *Frailty in the elderly can be multifactorial and often can be ameliorated or reversed (Storey & Thomas, 2004).*
- If client is scheduled for an elective surgery that will result in admission into the intensive care unit (ICU) and immobility, or recovery from a knee replacement, initiate a prehabilitation program that includes a warm-up, aerobic strength, flexibility, and functional task work. **EBN and EB:** *By increasing the functional capacity of the individual prior to the stressor of inactivity, the predictable declines in physical activity can be prevented or alleviated (Topp et al, 2002). In a study clients who performed strength activities preoperatively walked significantly greater distances postoperatively after total hip replacement (Whitney & Parkman, 2002). Another study demonstrated that aerobic training along with strength and interval training was effective in fewer postoperative complications, shorter postoperative stays, and reduced functional disabilities (Carli & Zavorsky, 2005).*
- ▲ Evaluate the client for signs of depression (flat affect, insomnia, anorexia, frequent somatic complaints) or cognitive impairment (use Mini-Mental State Exam [MMSE]). Refer for treatment or counseling as needed. **EBN:** *Multiple studies have demon-*

*strated that depression and decreased cognition in the elderly correlate with decreased levels of functional ability (Resnick, 1998).*

### Home Care

- • Above interventions may be adapted for home care use.
- ▲ Assess home environment for factors that create barriers to mobility. Refer to occupational therapy services if needed to assist the client in restructuring home and daily living patterns.

## Client/Family Teaching

- • Work with the client using the Transtheoretical Model of behavior change and determine if the client is in the precontemplation, contemplation, preparation, action, or maintenance state of behavior change about exercise. Provide appropriate strategies to support change to exercising based on determined state of change. **EBN:** *The Transtheoretical Model of behavior change can be very useful for nurses to utilize to increase exercise behavior utilizing-stage appropriate interventions (Burbank, Reibe, & Padula, 2002). Use of the Transtheoretical Model of behavior change plus theory of self-efficacy suggests that both of these theories are helpful to increase exercise in the older adult (Resnick & Nigg, 2003).*
- • Develop a series of contracts with mutually agreed on goals of increased activity. Include measurable landmarks of progress, consequences for meeting or not meeting goals, and evaluation dates. Sign the contracts with the client. **EBN:** *Using a series of evolving contracts to modify behavior toward increasing activity helps the client learn skills to change behavior (Boehm, 1989; Steckel, 1974).*

L

## evolve WEBSITES FOR EDUCATION

See the EVOLVE website for World Wide Web resources for client education.

## REFERENCES

Boehm S: Patient contracting, *Annu Rev Nurs Res* 7:143, 1989.

Burbank PM, Reibe D, Padula CA: Exercise and older adults: changing behavior with the transtheoretical model, *Orthop Nurs* 21(4):51, 2002.

Carli F, Zavorsky GS: Optimizing functional exercise capacity in the elderly surgical population, *Curr Opin Clin Nutr Metab Care* 8(1):23, 2005.

Liepert J, Bauder H, Wolfgang HR: Treatment-induced cortical reorganization after stroke in humans, *Stroke* 31(6):1210, 2000.

Mills EM: The effect of low-intensity aerobic exercise on muscle strength, flexibility, and balance among sedentary elderly persons, *Nurs Res* 43:207, 1994.

Resnick B: Predictors of functional ability in geriatric rehabilitation patients, *Rehabil Nurs* 23(1):21, 1998.

Resnick B: Testing the effect of the WALC intervention on exercise adherence in older adults, *J Gerontol Nurs,* 28(6):40, 2002.

Resnick B, Nigg C: Testing a theoretical model of exercise behavior for older adults, *Nurs Res* 52(2):80, 2003.

Resnick B, Orwig D, Magaziner J: The effect of social support on exercise behavior in older adults, *Clin Nurs Res* 11(1):52, 2002.

Resnick B, Zimmerman S, Orwig D: Model testing for reliability and validity of the outcome expectations for exercise scale, *Nurs Res* 50(5):293, 2001.

Robbins LB, Pis MB, Pender NJ et al: Exercise self-efficacy, enjoyment, and feeling states among adolescents, *West J Nurs Res* 26(7):716, 2004.

Robertson RG, Montagnini M: Geriatric failure to thrive, *Am Fam Physician* 70(2):343, 2004.
Rydwik E, Kerstin F, Akner G: Physical training in institutionalized elderly people with multiple diagnoses—a controlled pilot study, *Arch Gerontol Geriatr* 40(1):29, 2005.
Steckel SB: The use of positive reinforcement in order to increase patient compliance, *AANNT J* 1:1:1974.
Story E, Thomas RL: Understanding and ameliorating frailty in the elderly, *Top Geriatr Rehabil* 20(1), 2004.
Taggart HM: Effects of tai chi exercise on balance, functional mobility, and fear of falling among older women, *Appl Nurs Res* 15(4):235, 2002.
Thompson DL, Rakow J, Perdue SM: Relationship between accumulated walking and body composition in middle-aged women, *Med Sci Sports Exerc* 36(5):911, 2004.
Topp R, Ditmyer M, King K et al: The effect of bed rest and potential of prehabilitation on patients in the intensive care unit. *AACN Clin Issues* 13(2):263, 2002.
Tudor-Locke C, Pangrazi RP, Corbin CB et al: BMI-referenced standards for recommended pedometer-determined steps/day in children, *Prev Med* 38(6):857, 2004.
VanWormer JJ: Pedometers and brief e-counseling: increasing physical activity for overweight adults *J Appl Behav Anal* 37(3):421, 2004.
Vincent KR, Braith RW, Feldman RA et al: Improved cardiorespiratory endurance following 6 months of resistance exercise in elderly men and women, *Arch Intern Med* 162:673, 2002.
Wellbery C: Physical function and levels of activity in the elderly, *Am Family Physician* 71(3):557, 2005.
Whitney JA, Parkman S: Preoperative physical activity, anesthesia, and analgesia: effects on early postoperative walking after total hip replacement, *Appl Nurs Res* 15(1):19, 2002.
Wolf SL, Sattin RW, Kutner M et al: Intense Tai Chi exercise training and fall occurrences in older, transitionally frail adults: a randomized, controlled trial. *J Am Geriatr Soc* 51(12):1693, 2003.

## Risk for Loneliness

*Gail B. Ladwig*

**NANDA**

### Definition

At risk for experiencing vague dysphoria

### Risk Factors

Affectional deprivation, social isolation, cathectic deprivation, physical isolation

### Related Factors (r/t)

See Risk Factors

**NOC**

### Outcomes (Nursing Outcomes Classification)

#### Suggested NOC Outcomes

Loneliness Severity, Social Interaction Skills, Social Involvement, Social Support

**Example NOC Outcome with Indicators**

**Loneliness Severity** as evidenced by the following indicator: Sense of social isolation/Difficulty in establishing contact with other people (Rate each indicator of **Loneliness Severity:** 1 = severe, 2 = substantial, 3 = moderate, 4 = mild, 5 = none [see Section I].)

## Client Outcomes

### Client Will (Specify Time Frame):

- Maintain one or more meaningful relationship (growth enhancing versus codependent or abusive in nature)—relationships allowing self-disclosure—and demonstrate a balance between emotional dependence and independence
- Participate in ongoing positive and relevant social activities and interactions that are personally meaningful
- Demonstrate positive use of time alone when socialization is not possible

NIC

## Interventions (Nursing Interventions Classification)

### Suggested NIC Interventions

Family Integrity Promotion, Socialization Enhancement, Visitation Facilitation

L

**Example NIC Activities—Socialization Enhancement**

Encourage enhanced involvement in already established relationships; use role playing to practice improved communication skills and techniques

## Nursing Interventions and Rationales

- Assess the client's perception of loneliness (Is the person alone by choice, or do others impose the aloneness?). **EBN:** *Among persons with severe mental illness, more than half identify problems with loneliness and social isolation (Perese et al, 2003).* Refer to care plan for **Social isolation.**
- Assess the client's ability and/or inability to meet physical, psychosocial, spiritual, and financial needs and how unmet needs further challenge the ability to be socially integrated (e.g., loss of job leading to inability to afford usual and familiar social interaction; fatigue; lack of energy necessary for social interaction and personal engagement; impaired skin integument and its relationship to real and/or perceived social isolation). NOTE: See care plan for **Disturbed Body image** if loneliness is associated with impaired skin integument. **EB:** *Existential loneliness is an issue that arises for women with human immunodeficiency virus (HIV) and needs to be given equal consideration alongside other forms of loneliness (Mayers & Svartberg, 2001).* **EBN:** *Patients' perception of general health, symptoms, and social support influences outcome (Lindsay et al, 2001).*
- Use active listening skills. Establish therapeutic relationship and spend time with the

client. **EBN:** *In this study, being truly present was listed as one behavior that demonstrated caring (Yonge & Molzahn, 2002).* **EBN:** *This study demonstrated the importance of presence and caring communication (Sundin et al, 2002).*

- Assist the client with identifying loneliness as a feeling and the causes related to loneliness. **EBN:** *Loneliness was the number one fear identified. Chi-square analysis showed that the homeless who did not stay in shelters were significantly longer-term residents ($p < 0.0001$) of the community and reported fear of loneliness significantly more frequently (Reichenbach et al, 1998).*
- Evaluate the client's desire for social interaction in relation to actual social interaction. **EB:** *The lonelier the student, the more dishonest, the more negative, and the less revealing was the quality of the self-disclosure in their ICQ ("I seek you") chat interaction (Leung, 2002).*
- Explore ways to increase the client's support system and participation in groups and organizations. **EB:** *Satisfaction with support networks was a potent predictor of self-esteem, emotional health, and loneliness in female survivors of violence and abuse (Fry & Barker, 2002).* **EBN:** *Encouragement by nurses is important in helping clients with mental illness to become part of support groups (Perese et al, 2003).* **EBN:** *The effects of a psychosocial group intervention on loneliness and social support in Japanese women with breast cancer demonstrated that the experimental group had significantly lower scores than the control group for loneliness and significantly higher scores for the number of confidants, satisfaction with confidants, and satisfaction with mutual aid (Fukui et al, 2003).*
- Encourage the client to be involved in meaningful social relationships that are characteristic of both giving and receiving support. **EBN:** *It is important to recognize that the positive relevance of social relationships is related to the content and quality of relationships (Gulick, 1994).*
- Encourage social support for patients with visual impairments. **EB:** *Results of a large, nationwide study, conducted in 1994 through 1999 at the University of Amsterdam, on the meaning of personal networks and social support for Dutch adolescents with visual impairments indicate that social support, especially the support of peers, is important to adolescents with visual impairments (Kef, 2002).*
- Encourage the client to develop closeness in at least one relationship. **EBN:** *Dependence and independence should be balanced in healthy relationships. Previous research has indicated that the development of a balanced level of emotional dependence and the ability to self-disclose are important factors in reducing the risk for loneliness (Mahon & Yarcheski, 1992).*

L

## Adolescents

- Assess the client's social support system. **EBN:** *Use a social support tool or validated assessment tool if possible (e.g., UCLA Loneliness Scale for adolescents [Mahon et al, 1995]). (See References for assessment tool.)*
- Evaluate the depth and level of character traits, shyness, and self-esteem, particularly of younger and middle adolescent clients.
- Evaluate the family stability of younger and middle adolescent clients and advocate and encourage healthy, growth-producing relationships with family and support sys-

tems. **EB:** *This study showed a fear of intimacy and loneliness among adolescents who were taught during childhood not to trust strangers (Terrell, Terrell, & Von Drashek, 2000).*

- For older adolescents, encourage close relationships with peers and involvement with groups and organizations. **EBN:** *Younger adolescents are at a higher risk for loneliness if they are shy or have low self-esteem. Younger adolescents rely more on parental relationships. An expanded set of relationships becomes increasingly important in alleviating loneliness as adolescents mature (Mahon & Yarcheski, 1992).*
- Consider use of pets to cope with loneliness. **EBN:** *In this study of homeless youths, participants identified pets as companions that provide unconditional love and decrease feelings of loneliness (Rew, 2000).* **EBN:** *Equine-facilitated psychotherapy, while not a new idea, is a little-known experiential intervention that offers the opportunity to achieve healing (Vidrine et al, 2002).*

## Geriatric

- Assess the client's adaptive sensory functions or any other health deviations that may limit or decrease his or her ability to interact with others. **EB:** *Greater loneliness was found to be associated with an increased probability of having a coronary condition, as were low levels of both emotional support and companionship (Sorkin et al, 2002).*
- ▲ Assess the client's potential or actual hearing loss or hearing impairment and make appropriate referrals if a problem is identified. *Because of the nature of this sensory deprivation, communication barriers are increased and human intimacy and self-esteem are negatively affected (Chen, 1994).* **EB:** *In addition, it is important to note that hearing impairments often go unnoticed and may not be obvious as are more visibly recognized handicaps (Chen, 1994).* **EB:** *This study demonstrated declines in speech understanding in noise and central auditory processing are common in the growing population of older women (Garstecki & Erler, 2001).*
- Assess caregivers for Alzheimer's disease clients for depression related to loneliness. **EBN:** *Loneliness was significantly related to depression in this secondary analysis of data from a sample of 242 husbands, wives, and daughters providing care for Alzheimer's disease family members (Beeson et al, 2000).*
- ▲ Identify community support systems specific to elderly populations. **EB:** *Aging is often accompanied by significant losses of family members and other social support systems, which may lead to loneliness and depression. A study of residents of a nursing facility showed that social relationships with other residents were a strong predictor of decreased depression and loneliness (Fessman & Lester, 2000).*
- Consider a retirement village. **EB:** *In this study of 323 residents in 25 retirement villages, participants reported that isolation and loneliness decreased when clients relocated to a retirement village (Buys, 2001).*
- Encourage support by friends and family when the decision to stop driving must be made. **EBN:** *In this study, increased loneliness and isolation affected the older driver, although an enhanced sense of responsibility was evident among friends and family. Findings suggest that the support offered by friends and family played a significant role in the decision to stop driving (Johnson, 1998).*

- Encourage physical activity such as aerobics or stretching and toning in a group. **EB:** *These activities decreased loneliness in former sedentary adults (N = 174, median age = 65.5 years) (McAuley et al, 2000).*
- Provide opportunities for indoor gardening. **EBN:** *This study examined the effects of indoor gardening on socialization, activities of daily living (ADLs), and perceptions of loneliness in elderly nursing home residents. There were significant pretest to posttest differences within groups on loneliness and guidance, reassurance of worth, and social integration (Brown et al, 2004).*
- Provide reading materials for clients who are able to read. *Older people who enjoyed reading for pleasure were rarely lonely (Rane-Szotak & Herth, 1994).*

## Multicultural

- Acknowledge racial/ethnic differences at the onset of care. *Acknowledgment of racial/ethnicity issues will enhance communication, establish rapport, and promote treatment outcomes (D'Avanzo et al, 2001).*
- Assess for the influence of cultural beliefs, norms, and values on the client's perception of social activity and relationships. *What the client considers normal social interaction may be based on cultural perceptions (Leininger, 1996).*
- Approach individuals of color with respect, warmth, and professional courtesy. *Instances of disrespect and lack of caring have special significance for individuals of color and may impede efforts to increase social outlets (D'Avanzo et al, 2001).*
- Assess the use of personal space needs, communication styles, acceptable body language, eye contact, perception of touch, and use of paraverbals when communicating with the client. *Nurses need to consider these when interpreting verbal and nonverbal messages (Siantz, 1991). Native Americans may consider avoidance of direct eye contact as a sign of respect and asking questions to be rude and intrusive (Seideman et al, 1996).*
- Use a family-centered approach when working with Latino, Asian-American, African-American, and Native-American clients. *Latinos may perceive family as source of support, solver of problems, and a source of pride. Asian Americans may regard the family as the primary decision maker and influence on individual family members (D'Avanzo et al, 2001).*
- Promote a sense of ethnic attachment. *Older Korean clients with strong ethnic attachments had lower levels of loneliness than those without strong attachments (Kim, 1999).*
- Validate the client's feelings regarding isolation and loneliness. *Validation lets the client know that the nurse has heard and understands what was said, and it promotes the nurse-client relationship (Giger & Davidhizar, 1995; Stuart & Laraia, 2001).*

## Home Care

- Above interventions may be adapted for home care use. Assess for depression with lonely elderly client and make appropriate referrals. **EBN:** *Findings have related loneliness in older adults to mental health problems especially depression (McInnis & White, 2001).*

▲ If the client is experiencing somatic complaints, evaluate client complaints to ensure physical needs are being met, and then identify relationship between somatic complaints and loneliness. **EBN:** *Three factors have been found to increase levels of loneliness among elderly individuals residing in a nursing home: lack of intimate relationships, increased dependency, and loss. Nurses in long-term care facilities are in a position to directly intervene with elderly resident (Hicks, 2000).*

- • Assist clients to identify resources/situations they can attend or in which they can participate to enhance a sense of valued fit. **EBN:** *In a study of individuals living at home who had experienced traumatic brain injury, low sense of belonging (valued fit) and chronic stress were strong predictors of depression (Bay et al, 2002).*
- ▲ Help the client to identify periods when loneliness is greatest (e.g., certain times of day, anniversaries of past special events). With the client's permission, refer for services of visiting volunteers. *The only agenda of visiting volunteers is to meet the social needs of the client. Long-term friendships sometimes develop from volunteer experiences.*
- • To keep older people independent, interventions to prevent loneliness should be explored. Consider using art as an intervention. *Study shows that extreme loneliness predicts admission to the nursing home (PSL Consulting Group, 1999).* **EBN:** *The findings of a qualitative study to investigate the plausibility of integrating masterworks of art with care of the chronically ill elderly demonstrated that masterworks of art can generate energy exchange between the elderly and caregivers, providing a plausible catalyst for meaningful interventions that transcend age and practice settings (Hodges, Keeley, & Grier, 2001).*
- • Identify alternatives to eating alone. *Clients are often susceptible to loneliness at mealtimes. Loneliness may contribute to nutritional deficiencies or excesses.*
- • Identify alternatives to being alone (e.g., telephone contact). **EBN:** *This research demonstrated social support can be provided to low-income pregnant women who may have little or no social support and feel alienated in a clinical setting by telephone (Bullock, Browning, & Geden, 2002).*
- • Consider using computers and the Internet to alleviate or reduce loneliness and social isolation. **EBN:** *This descriptive qualitative study used a Web page questionnaire and chat room interviews with online participants age 65 years and older who were living alone. Seven of the 10 participants used the computer to combat loneliness (Clark, 2002). In this study, Internet use was found to decrease loneliness and depression significantly, while perceived social support and self-esteem increased significantly (Shaw & Gant, 2002). This randomized controlled trial assessed the psychosocial impact of providing Internet access to older adults over a 5-month period. Among Internet users (N = 29) in the intervention group, there were trends toward less loneliness and less depression (White et al, 2002).*
- • Support religious beliefs. *Belief in a supreme being provides a feeling of ever-present help and prevents loneliness. If clients have regrets about their life, they may be separated from their usual source of religious comfort.*
- • Discuss the meaning of death and fears associated with dying alone. Explore the possibility of significant others being with the client at the time of death. *In later stages of life, individuals give significant thought to death and the meaning of their life. If they perceive their life as undesirable, they may fear death.*



L

## Client/Family Teaching

- Encourage positive use of solitude to prevent loneliness (e.g., reading, listening to music, enjoying nature and art). *A positive use of solitude plays a strong role in preventing or alleviating loneliness. The mentioned activities are flow activities—self-directed, independent activities that enhance well-being and decrease feelings of loneliness (Rane-Szotak & Herth, 1994).*
- Include the family in all client-teaching activities, and give them accurate information regarding the illness severity. **EBN:** *In this study of residents and family members in the first year in long-term care, by listening to residents and family members, nurses can improve life for residents and dignify them as individuals (Iwasiw et al, 2003).*
- Give family members something to do such as holding a hand, applying lotion, or assisting with feeding. **EB:** *Perceived family support was predictive of reduced loneliness in this study of women with HIV (Serovich et al, 2001).*
- Encourage family members to express caring by telling the client where they will be and sending messages when they cannot be present. *If people could spare a smile or a word for others who might be perceived as lonely, even if in doing so they selfishly think "There but for the grace of God go I," such a small gesture might just make the day of a lonely person a little less of an ordeal (Killeen, 1998). Everyone is lonely to some degree, no matter how much they pretend they are not: it is part of the human condition. Loneliness is such an innate part of the human psyche that it cannot be solved like a puzzle; it can only be alleviated and made less painful. This can only be achieved by increasing humankind's awareness of this distressing condition that all people to endure in some way, shape, or form, sometime during their lives, about which there is nothing to be embarrassed (Killeen, 1998).*

L

## evolve WEBSITES FOR EDUCATION

See the EVOLVE website for World Wide Web resources for client education.

## REFERENCES


Bay E, Hagerty BM, Williams RA et al: Chronic stress, sense of belonging, and depression among survivors of traumatic brain injury, *J Nurs Scholarship* 34(3):221, 2002.

Beeson R, Horton-Deutsch S, Farran C et al: Loneliness and depression in caregivers of persons with Alzheimer's disease or related disorders, *Issues Ment Health Nurs* 21(8):779, 2000.

Brown VM, Allen AC, Dwozan M et al: Indoor gardening and older adults: effects on socialization, activities of daily living, and loneliness, *J Gerontol Nurs* 30(10):34-42, 2004.

Bullock LF, Browning C, Geden E: Telephone social support for low-income pregnant women, *J Obstet Gynecol Neonatal Nurs* 31(6):658, 2002.

Buys LR: Life in a retirement village: implications for contact with community and village friends, *Gerontology* 47(1):55, 2001.

Chen H: Hearing in the elderly, relation of healing loss, loneliness, and self-esteem, *J Gerontol Nurs* 20:22, 1994.

Clark DJ: Older adults living through and with their computers, *Comput Inform Nurs* 20(3):117, 2002.

D'Avanzo CE et al: Developing culturally informed strategies for substance-related interventions. In Naegle MA, D'Avanzo CE, editors: *Addictions and substance abuse: strategies for advanced practice nursing,* St Louis, 2001, Mosby.

Fessman N, Lester D: Loneliness and depression among elderly nursing home patients, *Int J Aging Hum Dev* 51(2):137, 2000.

Fry PS, Barker LA: Quality of relationships and structural properties of social support networks of female survivors of abuse, *Genet Soc Gen Psychol Monogr* 128(2):139, 2002.

Fukui S, Koike M, Ooba A et al: The effect of a psychosocial group intervention on loneliness and social support for Japanese women with primary breast cancer, *Oncol Nurs Forum* 30(5):823-830, 2003.

Garstecki DC, Erler SF: Personal and social conditions potentially influencing women's hearing loss management, *Am J Audiol* 10:2, 2001.

Giger JN, Davidhizar RE: *Transcultural nursing,* ed 2, St Louis, 1995, Mosby.

Gulick E: Social support among persons with multiple sclerosis, *Res Nurs Health* 17:195, 1994.

Hicks TJ Jr: What is your life like now? Loneliness and elderly individuals residing in nursing homes, *J Gerontol Nurs* 26(8):15, 2000.

Hodges HF, Keeley AC, Grier EC: Masterworks of art and chronic illness experiences in the elderly, *J Adv Nurs* 36(3), 2001.

Iwasiw C, Goldenberg D, Bol N et al: Resident and family perspectives. The first year in a long-term care facility, *J Gerontol Nurs* 29(1):45-54, 2003.

Johnson J: Older rural adults and the decision to stop driving: the influence of family and friends, *J Community Health Nurs* 15(4): 205, 1998.

Kef S: Psychosocial adjustment and the meaning of social support for visually impaired adolescents, *J Visual Impairment Blindness* 96(1):22, 2002.

Killeen C: Loneliness: an epidemic in modern society, *J Adv Nurs* 28(4):762, 1998.

Kim O: Mediation effect of social support between ethnic attachment and loneliness in older Korean immigrants, *Res Nurs Health* 22(2):169, 1999.

Leininger MM: *Transcultural nursing: theories, research and practices,* ed 2, Hilliard, Ohio, 1996, McGraw-Hill.

Leung L: Loneliness, self-disclosure, and ICQ ("I seek you") use, *Cyberpsychol Behav* 5(3):241, 2002.

Lindsay GM, Smith LN, Hanlon P et al: The influence of general health status and social support on symptomatic outcome following coronary artery bypass grafting, *Heart* 85(1):80, 2001.

Mahon NE, Yarcheski A: Alternate explanations of loneliness in adolescents: a replication and extension study, *Nurs Res* 41:151, 1992.

Mahon NE, Yarcheski T, Yarcheski A: Validation of the revised UCLA loneliness scale for adolescents, *Res Nurs Health* 18:263, 1995.

Mayers AM; Svartberg M: Existential loneliness: a review of the concept, its psychosocial precipitants and psychotherapeutic implications for HIV-infected women, *Br J Med Psychol* 74(Pt 4):539, 2001.

McAuley E, Blissmer B, Marquez DX et al: Social relations, physical activity, and well-being in older adults, *Prev Med* 31(5):608, 2000.

McInnis GJ, White JH: A phenomenological exploration of loneliness in the older adult, *Arch Psychiatr Nurs* 15(3):128, 2001.

Perese EF, Getty C, Wooldridge P: Psychosocial club members' characteristics and their readiness to participate in a support group, *Issues Ment Health Nurs* 24(2):153, 2003.

PSL Consulting Group: Loneliness may foreshadow nursing home admission, doctor's guide. Available at www.pslgroup.com/dg/56afe.htm, accessed on March 31, 1999.

Rane-Szotak D, Herth K: A new perspective on loneliness in later life, *Issues Ment Health Nurs* 16:583, 1994.

Reichenbach E, McNamee M, Seibel L: The community health nursing implications of the self-reported health status of a local homeless population, *Public Health Nurs* 15(6):398, 1998.

Rew L: Friends and pets as companions: strategies for coping with loneliness among homeless youth, *J Child Adolesc Psychiatr Nurs* 13(3):125, 2000.

Seideman RY, Jacobson S, Primeaux M et al: Assessing American Indian families, *MCN Am J Matern Child Nurs* 21(6):274, 1996.

Serovich JM, Kimberly JA, Mosack KE et al: The role of family and friend social support in reducing emotional distress among HIV-positive women, *AIDS Care* 13(3):335, 2001.

Shaw LH, Gant LM: In defense of the Internet: the relationship between Internet communication and depression, loneliness, self-esteem, and perceived social support, *Cyberpsychol Behav* 5(2):157, 2002.

Siantz ML: How can we be more aware of culturally specific body language and use this awareness therapeutically? *J Psychosocial Nurs Ment Health Serv* 29(11):38, 1991.

Sorkin D, Rook KS, Lu JL: Loneliness, lack of emotional support, lack of companionship, and the likelihood of having a heart condition in an elderly sample, *Ann Behav Med* 24(4):290, 2002.

Stuart GW, Laraia MT: Therapeutic nurse-patient relationship. In Stuart GW, Laraia MT, editors: *Principles and practice of psychiatric nursing,* St Louis, 2001, Mosby.

Sundin K, Jansson L, Norberg A: Understanding between care providers and patients with stroke and aphasia: a phenomenological hermeneutic inquiry, *Nurs Inq* 9(2):93, 2002.

Terrell F, Terrell IS, Von Drashek SR: Loneliness and fear of intimacy among adolescents who were taught not to trust strangers during childhood, *Adolescence* 35(140):611, 2000.
Vidrine M, Owen-Smith P, Faulkner P: Equine-facilitated group psychotherapy: applications for therapeutic vaulting, *Issues Ment Health Nurs* 23(6):587, 2002.
White H, McConnell E, Clipp E et al: A randomized controlled trial of the psychosocial impact of providing Internet training and access to older adults, *Aging Ment Health* 6(3):213, 2002.
Yonge O, Molzahn A: Exceptional nontraditional caring practices of nurses, *Scand J Caring Sci* 16(4):399, 2002.

# Impaired Memory

evolve

*Graham J. McDougall Jr.*

M

**NANDA**

## Definition

Inability to remember or recall bits of information or behavioral skills, impaired memory may be attributed to pathophysiological or situational causes that are either temporary or permanent

## Defining Characteristics

Inability to recall factual information, inability to recall recent or past events, inability to learn or retain new skills or information, inability to determine whether a behavior was performed, observed or reported experiences of forgetting, inability to perform a previously learned skill, forgets to perform a behavior at a scheduled time

## Related Factors (r/t)

Fluid and electrolyte imbalance, neurological disturbances, excessive environmental disturbances, anemia, acute or chronic hypoxia, decreased cardiac output

**NOC**

## Outcomes (Nursing Outcomes Classification)

### Suggested NOC Outcomes

Cognitive Orientation; Memory; Neurological Status: Consciousness

**Example NOC Outcome with Indicators**

**Memory** as evidenced by the following indicators: Recalls immediate information accurately/Recalls recent information accurately/Recalls remote information accurately (Rate each indicator of **Memory:** 1 = severely compromised, 2 = somewhat compromised, 3 = moderately compromised, 4 = mildly compromised, 5 = not compromised [see Section I].)

## Client Outcomes

**Client Will (Specify Time Frame):**

- Demonstrate use of techniques to help with memory loss
- State has improved memory for everyday concerns

**NIC**

## Interventions (Nursing Interventions Classification)

### Suggested NIC Intervention

Memory Training, Realistic appraisal of memory

**Example NIC Activities—Memory Training**

Stimulate memory by repeating patient's last expressed thought, as appropriate; provide opportunity to use memory for recent events, such as questioning patient about a recent outing; give examples of external memory strategies (e.g., calendar)

## Nursing Interventions and Rationales

- Assess cognitive function and memory. The emphasis of the assessment is everyday memory, the day-to-day operations of memory in real-world ordinary situations (Cohen, 1989). Use an assessment tool such as the Mini-Mental State Examination (MMSE) and/or the Metamemory in Adulthood (MIA) questionnaire. *The MMSE can help determine whether the client has cognitive impairment and/or memory loss, delirium and needs to be referred for further evaluation and treatment (Agostinelli et al, 1994; Breitner & Welsh, 1995; McDougall, 1990). The MIA is reliable and nonthreatening assessment for nonimpaired individuals and has been validated to be effective (McDougall, 1990).*

▲ Determine whether onset of memory loss is gradual or sudden. If memory loss is sudden, refer the client to a physician or neuropsychologist for evaluation. *Acute onset of memory loss may be associated with neurological disease, medication effect, electrolyte disturbances, hypoxia, hypothyroidism, mental illness, or many other physiological factors (Breitner & Welsh, 1995; Elliott, 2000; Foreman et al, 2001).*

- Determine amount and pattern of alcohol intake. *Alcohol intake has been associated with blackouts; clients may function but not remember their actions. Long-term alcohol use causes Korsakoff's syndrome with associated memory loss; however, moderate consumption of alcohol may be health promoting (Britton et al, 2004; Perreira et al, 2002; Zimmerman et al, 2004). A study demonstrated that dementia and cognitive decline were positively associated with silent brain infarcts (Vermeer et al, 2003).*
- Note the client's current medications and intake of any mind-altering substances such as benzodiazepines, ecstasy, marijuana, cocaine, or glucocorticoids. *Benzodiazepines can produce memory loss for events that occur after taking the medication; information is not stored in long-term memory (Fluck et al, 1998; Mejo, 1992). Cocaine abuse has been shown to decrease memory (Butler & Frank, 2000). The ingestion of ecstasy has been associated with impaired memory, both short term and possibly long term (Gowing et al, 2002; Morgan et al, 2002).* **EB:** *Glucocorticoid therapy can cause a decrease in memory function that*

*is usually reversible once a person is off the medications (Wolkowitz et al, 1997). Clients receiving long-term prednisone performed significantly worse on memory tasks than matched control subjects (Keenan, 1996). Both infrequent and long-term use of marijuana is associated with impaired memory function (Curran et al, 2002; Solowij et al, 2002).*

- • Note the client's current level of stress. Ask if there has been a recent traumatic event. *Post-traumatic stress and anxiety-inducing general life factors may induce memory problems (Diamond et al, 2004; Jelicic et al, 2004). Elevated cortisol levels associated with stress have been shown to impair memory (Greendale et al, 2000; Lupien et al, 1994, 1997).*
- ▲ If stress is associated with memory loss, refer to a stress reduction clinic. If not available, suggest that the client meditate, receive massages, participate in moderate physical activity, all of which may promote stress reduction and reduce anxiety and depression *(Rees et al, 2004).* Encourage the client to develop an aerobic exercise program. **EB:** *A study demonstrated that aerobic exercise improved memory and executive function in depressed middle-age and older adults (Khatri et al, 2001).*
- • Determine the client's sleep patterns. If insufficient, refer to care plan for **Disturbed Sleep pattern. EB:** *Studies demonstrate that memory consolidation is enhanced by sleep (Gais et al, 2002; Peigneux et al, 2001).*
- ▲ Determine the client's blood sugar levels. If they are elevated, refer to physician for treatment and encourage healthy diet and exercise to improve memory. *Elevated blood sugar levels were associated with impaired memory (Convit, 2003).*
- ▲ If signs of depression such as weight loss, insomnia, or sad affect are evident, refer the client for psychotherapy. *Depression can result in source memory errors, in which case the client is not sure if he or she did something or just thought about doing it (Elias, 2001).*
- ▲ Perform a nutritional assessment. If nutritional status is marginal, confer with a dietitian and primary care practitioner to evaluate whether the client needs supplementation with foods or vitamins. Teach the client the need to eat a healthy diet with adequate intake of whole grains, fruits, and vegetables to decrease cerebrovascular infarcts. *Moderate, long-term deficiencies of nutrients may lead to loss of memory. This condition may be preventable or diminished through diet (Cataldo, DeBruyne, & Whitney, 1999). Adequate levels of vitamin E may help protect memory (Miller, 2000).* **EB:** *A large study demonstrated that people who ate mostly fruits and vegetables per day (9 or 10 servings) had decreased incidence of ischemic strokes (Joshipura et al, 1999).*
- ▲ Question the client about cholesterol level. If it is high, refer to physician or dietitian for help in lowering. Encourage the client to eat a healthy diet, avoiding saturated fats and *trans*-fatty acids. **EB:** *One study demonstrated that individuals who were prescribed statin medications that lowered cholesterol had a substantially lowered risk of developing dementia (Jick et al, 2000). A study demonstrated that high intake of saturated or* trans-*fatty acids may increase the risk of Alzheimer's disease (Morris et al, 2003).*
- • Suggest clients use cues, including alarm watches, electronic organizers, calendars, lists, or pocket computers, to trigger certain actions at designated times. *Cues and external cognitive strategies can help remind clients of certain actions (McDougall, 1999; Wilson & Moffat, 1992).*
- • Encourage the client to use external memory devices, such as a calendar for appointments, keep reminder lists, place a string around finger or rubber band around wrist as

M

reminders, or enlist someone else to remind him or her of important events. *Using reminders can serve as cues for memory-impaired clients.*

- Help the client set up a medication box that reminds the client to take medication at needed times; assist the client with refilling the box at intervals if necessary. *Medication boxes are effective because clients will know whether medication has been taken when corresponding compartments are empty.*
- If safety is an issue with certain activities (e.g., the client forgets to turn off stove after use or forgets emergency telephone numbers), suggest alternatives such as using a microwave or whistling teakettle for heating water and programming emergency numbers in telephone so that they are readily available.
- ▲ Refer the client to a memory clinic (if available), a neuropsychologist, or an occupational therapist. *Memory clinics can help the client learn ways to improve memory. Clinics may be more effective if work is done in groups because of increased support, reinforcement, and motivation (McDougall, 1999; Robinson, 1992).*
- For clients with memory impairments associated with dementia, refer to care plan for **Chronic Confusion.**

## Geriatric

- Assess for signs of depression. *Depression is the most important affective variable for memory loss in the older adult (McDougall, 1999).* **EB:** *Cognitive impairment is not an inevitable consequence of aging, even in very old age (Snowdon, 1997).*
- Evaluate all medications that the client is taking to determine whether they are causing the memory loss. *Many medications, prescription, over-the-counter, and herbals, may cause memory loss in the elderly, including anticholinergics, $H_2$-receptor antagonists, beta-blockers, digitalis, benzodiazepines, barbiturates, and even mild opiates (DeMaagd, 1995; Dergal et al, 2002; Sjogren et al, 2000).*
- Recommend that elderly clients maintain a positive attitude and active involvement with the world around them and that they maintain good nutrition. **EB:** *Findings from the Nun Study demonstrated that it is possible to maintain good cognitive function until extreme old age if elderly persons maintain active involvement with their environment and are able to avoid having vascular disease with infarction of brain tissue (Snowdon, 1997).*
- Encourage the elderly to believe in themselves and to work to improve their memory. *Negative attitudes and belief may decrease motivation and impair everyday memory function (McDougall, 1999).* **EB:** *Elderly clients may be able to improve their memory function up to 50% if they use appropriate strategies and invest the energy and time (Ball et al, 2002). New research has shown that there is formation of new neurons in the brain, a process called neurogenesis, throughout the life span, and stimulation of the brain is necessary for this formation (Eriksson et al, 1998).*
- ▲ Refer the client to a memory class that focuses on helping older adults learn memory strategies. **EBN and EB:** *Research has demonstrated that classes that focus on memory strategies could improve memory (McDougall, 2002). In memory impairment associated with strokes, there is insufficient evidence to determine if memory training is effective (Majid, Lincoln, & Weyman, 2002).*
- Help family develop a memory aid booklet or wallet that contains pictures and labels

M

from the client's life, or develop a video movie that includes familiar pictures with narration (Cohen, 2002). *Using memory aids helps clients with dementia make more factual statements and stay on topic and decreases the number of confused, erroneous, and repetitive statements made (Bourgeois, 1992).* **EB:** *Use of the memory book may also help decrease the number of depressive statements by the client (Bourgeois et al, 2001).*

- Help family label items such as the bathroom or sock drawer to increase recall. *A supportive environment that includes orientation can help increase the client's awareness (Green & Gildemeister, 1994).*

## Multiculturall

- Assess for the influence of cultural beliefs, norms, and values on the family or caregiver's understanding of impaired memory. If an African-American male is dealing with memory loss, encourage him to believe in his abilities. **EBN:** *What the family considers normal and abnormal health behavior may be based on cultural perceptions (Cochran, 1998).* **EBN:** *Nursing research demonstrated that there were no significant differences in the memories of African-American versus Caucasian men, but the African-American men had higher anxiety about memory function, used fewer memory strategies, and had a higher incidence of depression (McDougall & Holston, 2003).*
- Use bias-free instruments when assessing memory in the culturally diverse client. **EBN:** *Use of the MMSE without modification for ethnic bias resulted in younger Hispanics being categorized as more severely impaired than others (Mulgrew et al, 1999).*

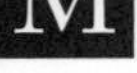

- Inform the client's family or caregiver of meaning of and reasons for common behavior observed in the client with impaired memory. *An understanding of impaired memory behavior will enable the client family/caregiver to provide the client with a safe environment.*
- Validate family members' feelings regarding the impact of the client's behavior on family lifestyle. **EBN:** *Even though validation therapy for dementia is a communication technique that lets the client know that the nurse has heard and understands what was said, and it promotes the nurse-client relationship, there is insufficient evidence from randomized trials to make any conclusion about its efficacy for people with dementia or cognitive impairment (Neal & Briggs, 2003; Heineken, 1998).*

## Home Care

- Above interventions may be adapted for home care use.
- Arrange cues for medication taking that are focused around daily events (e.g., meals and bedtimes). **EBN:** *Older adults report the use of internal memory strategies to compensate for age-related memory loss; specifically they prefer event-based prescription medication instructions (Branin, 2001).*
- Assess the client's need for outside assistance with recall of treatment, medications, and willingness/ability of family to provide needed support. *During initial phase of home care, increased frequency of visits may be necessary to compensate for the client's inability to recall treatment, medications. Counting of medications may be needed to determine if the client is following medication regimen. Telephone calls from family/friends may help to remind the client of treatment schedule.*

- Identify a checking-in support system (e.g., Lifeline or significant others). *Checking in ensures the client's safety.*
- Keep furniture placement and household patterns consistent. *Change increases risk of impaired memory and decreased functioning.*
- ▲ In the presence of a medical disorder, institute case management of frail elderly to support continued independent living. *Memory difficulties often represent and can lead to increasing needs for assistance in using the health care system effectively. Case management combines nursing activities of the client and family assessment, planning and coordination of care among all health care providers, delivery of direct nursing care, and monitoring of care and outcomes. These activities are able to address continuity of care, mutual goal setting, behavior management, and prevention of worsening health problems (Guttman, 1999).*

### Client/Family Teaching

- When teaching the client, determine what the client knows about memory techniques and then build on that knowledge. *New material is organized in terms of what knowledge already exists, and efficient teaching should attempt to take advantage of what is already known in order to graft on new material (McDougall, 1999; Wilson & Moffat, 1992).*
- When teaching a skill to the client, set up a series of practice attempts. Begin with simple tasks so that the client can be positively reinforced and progress to more difficult concepts. *Distributed practice with correct recall attempts can be a very effective teaching strategy. Widely distribute practice over time if possible (Camp et al, 1993, 2002).*
- Teach clients to use memory techniques such as repeating information they want to remember, making mental associations to remember information, and placing items in strategic places so that they will not be forgotten. These methods increase recall of information the client thinks is important. *The internal methods of increasing memory can be effective, especially if used along with external methods such as calendars, lists, and other methods (McDougall, 1999).*

M

## evolve WEBSITES FOR EDUCATION

See the EVOLVE website for World Wide Web resources for client education.

## REFERENCES

Agostinelli B, Demers K, Garrigan D et al: Targeted interventions. Use of the Mini-Mental State Exam, *J Gerontol Nurs* 20(8):15, 1994.

Ball K, Berch DB, Helmers KF et al: Advanced cognitive training for independent and vital elderly study group, *JAMA* 288(18): 2271-2281, 2002.

Bourgeois MS: *Conversing with memory-impaired individuals using memory aids: a memory aid workbook,* Gaylord, Mich, 1992, Northern Speech Services.

Bourgeois MS, Dijkstra K, Burgio L et al: Memory aids as an augmentative and alternative communication strategy for nursing home residents with dementia, *AAC Augment Altern Commun* 17(3):196, 2001.

Branin JJ: The role of memory strategies in medication adherence among the elderly, *Home Health Care Serv Q* 20(2):1, 2001.

Breitner JC, Welsh KA: Diagnosis and management of memory loss and cognitive disorders among elderly persons, *Psychiatr Serv* 46:29, 1995.

Neal M, Briggs M: Validation therapy for dementia, *Cochrane Database Syst Rev* (3):CD001394, 2003.
Britton A, Singh-Manoux A, Marmot M: Alcohol consumption and cognitive function in the Whitehall II Study, *Am J Epidemiol* 160(3):240, 2004.
Butler LF, Frank EM: Neurolinguistic function and cocaine abuse, *J Med Speech Lang Pathol* 8(3):199, 2000.
Camp CJ, Foss JW, Stevens AB et al: Memory training in normal and demented elderly populations: the E-I-E-I-O model, *Exp Aging Res* 19(3):277-290, 1993.
Camp CJ, Cohen-Mansfield J, Capezuti EA: Use of nonpharmacologic interventions among nursing home residents with dementia, *Psychiatr Serv* 53(11):1397-1401, 2002.
Cataldo CB, DeBruyne LK, Whitney EN: *Nutrition and diet therapy: principles and practice,* ed 5, Belmont, Calif, 1999, Wadsworth.
Cochran M: Tears have no color, *Am J Nurs* 98(6):53, 1998.
Cohen G: Everyday memory. In Cohen G, editor: *Memory in the real world,* Hillsdale, NJ 1989, Lawrence Erlbaum.
Cohen GD: Creative interventions for Alzheimer's disease: familiar activities, videos can help patients copy with memory loss, *Geriatrics* 57(3):62, 2002.
Convit A, Wolf OT, Tarshish C et al: Reduced glucose tolerance is associated with poor memory performance and hippocampal atrophy among normal elderly, *Proc Natl Acad Sci U S A* 100(4):2019, 2003.
Curran HV, Brignell C, Fletcher S et al: Cognitive and subjective dose-response effects of acute oral delta 9-tetrahydrocannabinol (THC) in infrequent cannabis users, *Psychopharmacology (Berl)* 164(1):61, 2002.
DeMaagd G: High-risk drugs in the elderly population, *Geriatr Nurs* 16:198, 1995.
Dergal JM, Gold JL, Laxer DA et al: Potential interactions between herbal medicines and conventional drug therapies used by older adults attending a memory clinic, *Drugs Aging* 19(11):879-886, 2002.
Diamond DM, Park CR, Woodson JC: Stress generates emotional memories and retrograde amnesia by inducing an endogenous form of hippocampal LTP, *Hippocampus* 14(3):281-291, 2004.
Elias J: Why caregiver depression and self-care abilities should be part of the PPS case mix methodology, *Home Healthc Nurse* 19(1):23, 2001.
Elliott B: Case report. Diagnosing and treating hypothyroidism, *Nurs Pract* 25(3):92, 2000.
Eriksson PS, Perfilieva E, Bjork-Eriksson T et al: Neurogenesis in the adult human hippocampus, *Nat Med* 4(11):1313, 1998.
Fluck E, File SE, Springett J et al: Does the sedation resulting from sleep deprivation and lorazepam cause similar cognitive deficits? *Pharmacol Biochem Behav* 59(4):909, 1998.
Foreman MD, Wakefield B, Culp K et al: Delirium in elderly patients: an overview of the state of the science. *J Gerontol Nurs* 27(4):12, 2001.
Gais S, Molle M, Helms K et al: Learning-dependent increases in sleep spindle density, *J Neurosci* 22(15):6830, 2002.
Gowing LR, Henry-Edwards SM, Irvine RJ et al: The health effects of ecstasy: a literature review, *Drug Alcohol Rev* 21(1):53, 2002.
Green PM, Gildemeister JE: Memory aging research and memory support in the elderly, *J Neurosci Nurs* 26:241, 1994.
Greendale GA, Kritz-Silverstein D, Seeman T et al: Higher basal cortisol predicts verbal memory loss in postmenopausal women: Rancho Bernardo Study, *J Am Geriatr Soc* 48(12):1655, 2000.
Guttman R: Case management of the frail elderly in the community, *Clin Nurs Spec* 13(4):174, 1999.
Heineken J: Patient silence is not necessarily client satisfaction: communication in home care nursing, *Home Healthc Nurse* 16(2): 115, 1998.
Jelicic M, Merckelbach H: Traumatic stress, brain changes, and memory deficits: a critical note, *J Nerv Ment Dis* 192(8):548-53, 2004.
Jick H, Zornberg GL, Jick SS et al: Statins and risk of dementia, *Lancet* 356(9242):1627, 2000.
Joshipura KJ, Ascherio A, Manson JE et al: Fruit and vegetable intake in relation to ischemic stroke, *JAMA* 282(13):1233, 1999.
Keenan PA: Chronic prednisone use causes memory loss, *Neurology* 47:1396, 1996.
Khatri P, Babyak M, Croughwell ND et al: Effects of exercise training on cognitive functioning among depressed older men and women, *J Aging Phys Activity* 9(1):43, 2001.
Lupien S, Lecours AR, Lussier I et al: Basal cortisol levels and cognitive deficits in human aging, *J Neurosci* (5 Pt 1):2893, 1994.
Lupien SJ, Gaudreau S, Tchiteya BM et al: Stress-induced declarative memory impairment in healthy elderly subjects: relationship to cortisol reactivity, *J Clin Endocrinol Metab* 82(7):2070-2075, 1997.
Majid MJ, Lincoln NB, Weyman N: Cognitive rehabilitation for memory deficits following stroke, *Cochrane Database Syst Rev* (3):CD002293, 2002.
McDougall GJ: Older adults' metamemory: coping, depression, and self-efficacy, *Appl Nurs Res* 6:28, 1993.
McDougall GJ: Cognitive interventions among older adults, *Annu Rev Nurs Res* 17:219, 1999.

McDougall GJ. Memory improvement in octogenarians, *Appl Nurs Res* 15(1):2, 2002.
McDougall GJ: A review of screening instruments for assessing cognition and mental status in older adults, *Nurs Pract* 15(11):18, 1990.
McDougall GJ, Holston EC: Black and white men at risk for memory impairment, *Nurs Res* 52(1):42, 2003.
Mejo SL: Anterograde amnesia linked to benzodiazepines, *Nurse Pract* 17:44, 1992.
Miller JW: Vitamin E and memory: is it vascular protection? *Nutr Rev* 58(4):109-111, 2000.
Morgan MJ, McFie L, Fleetwood HJ et al: Ecstasy (MDMA): are the psychological problems associated with its use reversed by prolonged abstinence? *Psychopharmacology (Berl)* 159(3), 294-303, 2002.
Mulgrew CL, Morgenstern N, Shetterly SM et al: Cognitive functioning and impairment among rural elderly Hispanics and non-Hispanic whites as assessed by the Mini-Mental State Examination, *J Gerontol B Psychol Sci Soc Sci* 54(4):P223-230, 1999.
Peigneux P, Laureys S, Delbeuck X et al: Sleeping brain, learning brain. The role of sleep for memory systems, *Neuroreport* 12(18): A111, 2001.
Perreira KM, Sloan FA: Excess alcohol consumption and health outcomes: a 6-year follow-up of men over age 50 from the health and retirement study. *Addiction* 97(3):301, 2002.
Rees K, Bennett P, West R et al: Psychological interventions for coronary heart disease, *Cochrane Database Syst Rev* (2): CD002902, 2004.
Robinson S: Occupational therapy in a memory clinic, *Br J Occup Ther* 55:394, 1992.
Schwartz RH, Gruenewald PJ, Klitzner M et al: Short-term memory impairment in cannabis-dependent adolescents, *Am J Dis Child* 143(8):1214, 1989.
Sjogren P, Thomsen AB, Olsen AK: Impaired neuropsychological performance in chronic nonmalignant pain patients receiving long-term oral opioid therapy, *J Pain Symptom Manage* 19(2):100, 2000.
Snowdon DA: Aging and Alzheimer's disease: lessons from the Nun Study, *Gerontologist* 37(2):150, 1997.
Solowij N, Stephens RS, Roffman RA et al: Cognitive functioning of long-term heavy cannabis users seeking treatment, *JAMA* 287(9):1123, 2002.
Vermeer SE, Prins ND, den Heijer T et al: Silent brain infarcts and the risk of dementia and cognitive decline, *N Engl J Med* 348(13):1215, 2003.
Wilson BA, Moffat N: *Clinical management of memory problems,* San Diego, 1992, Singular.
Wolkowitz OM, Reus VI, Canick J et al: Glucocorticoid medication, memory and steroid psychosis in medical illness, *Ann N Y Acad Sci* 823:81, 1997.
Zimmerman T, McDougall GJ Jr, Becker H: Older women's cognitive and affective response to moderate drinking, *Int J Geriatr Psychiatry*, 19(11):1095-1102, 2004.

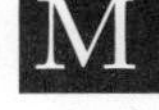


# Impaired bed Mobility

*Brenda Emick-Herring*

**NANDA**

## Definition

Limitation of independent movement from one bed position to another

## Defining Characteristics

Impaired ability to turn from side to side; impaired ability to move from supine to sitting or sitting to supine; impaired ability to "scoot" or reposition self in bed, impaired ability to move from supine to prone or prone to supine, impaired ability to move from supine to long sitting or long sitting to supine

## Related Factors (r/t)

Intolerance to activity, decreased strength and endurance, pain or discomfort, perceptual or cognitive impairment, neuromuscular impairment, musculoskeletal impairment, depression, severe anxiety

Suggested functional level classifications include the following:
0—Completely independent
1—Requires use of equipment or device
2—Requires help from another person
3—Requires help from another person and equipment device
4—Dependent (does not participate in activity)

**NOC**

## Outcomes (Nursing Outcomes Classification)

### Suggested NOC Outcomes

Mobility; Self-Care: Activities of Daily Living (ADLs)

**Example NOC Outcome with Indicators**

**Mobility** as evidenced by the following indicator: Body positioning performance/Gait/Joint movement (Rate each indicator of **Mobility:** 1 = severely compromised, 2 = substantially compromised, 3 = moderately compromised, 4 = mildly compromised, 5 = not compromised [see Section I].)

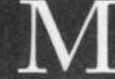


## Client Outcomes

**Client Will (Specify Time Frame):**

- Demonstrate optimal independence in positioning, exercising, and performing functional activities in bed
- Demonstrate ability to direct others on how to do bed positioning, exercising, and functional activities

**NIC**

## Interventions (Nursing Interventions Classification)

### Suggested NIC Intervention

Bed Rest Care

**Example NIC Activities—Bed Rest Care**

Position in proper alignment; teach bed exercises as appropriate

## Nursing Interventions and Rationales

- Perform physical assessment to determine the client's risk for intracranial pressure (ICP), respiratory, and cardiovascular abnormalities, increased muscle tone, aspiration, pressure ulcer, and pain. *These conditions warrant certain bed positions to prevent compli-*

*cations (Palmer & Wyness, 1988; Sullivan, 2000; Wound, Ostomy, and Continence Nurses Society,* 2003). **EBN:** *Authors suggested use of the semirecumbent position to reduce risk of aspiration in enteral tube fed client even though a lit search indicated lack of quality research to prove it (Williams & Leslie, 2004). Head of bed elevation of 30 degrees reduced ICP (Fan, 2004). A retrospective study showed staff improvement of identifying clients at high risk for pressure ulcer and repositioning of bed-bound patients, after a new model for prevention was used in 17 hospitals (Lyder et al, 2004).*

- Use critical thinking and priority setting to decide most therapeutic bed positions and frequency of turns; base this on clients history, risk profile, and preventative needs. *Positioning for one condition may negatively affect another. For example, elevation of head of bed is therapeutic for persons with increased ICP and tube feedings, but may be contraindicated with acute ischemic stroke and high risk for pressure ulcers (Fan, 2004; Sullivan, 2000; Williams & Leslie, 2004).* **EBN:** *Therapeutic bed positions are recommended from the author's assimilation of multisystem (neurological, cardiovascular, pulmonary status) study results (Sullivan, 2000). Results indicated a flat to 15 degree head of bed elevation may increase blood flow to ischemic tissue in acute stroke survivors (Wojner et al, 2002). Evidence-based guidelines recommend clients be turned at least every 2 to 4 hours if on a pressure-reducing mattress and at least every 2 hours if on a standard foam mattress (Wound, Ostomy, and Continence Nurses Society, 2003).*
- Raise the head of the to 30 degrees if the client has increased intracranial pressure (ICP). Refer to care plan for **Decreased Intracranial adaptive capacity.** *Head of bed elevation decreases ICP (Fan, 204; Sullivan, 2000).*
- Assist client to sit upright during and after feedings or ingestion of pills if dysphagia presents. Refer to care plan for **Impaired Swallowing.** *Helps prevent aspiration of food, liquids, and pills (Flannery & Pugh, 2004).*
- Periodically position the client in an upright sitting position as tolerated. If vital signs and oxygen saturation levels are stable, dangle patient if applicable. *Being vertical reduces the work of the heart and abnormal posturing; it changes intravascular pressure and stimulates neural reflexes; it improves lung ventilation, aeration, symmetrical body alignment, and awareness of the surroundings (Metzler & Harr, 1996; Palmer & Wyness, 1988).* **EB:** *A review of studies demonstrated there are few indications for bed rest; it may even delay recovery or cause harm (Allen, Glasziou, & Del Mar, 1999). A randomized trial found that assisting patients with community-acquired pneumonia to sit up out of bed for 20 minutes the first day of hospitalization, with progressive mobilization thereafter, shortened length of stay by a day (Mundy et al, 2003).*
- Maintain the head of the bed at the lowest degree of elevation possible, depending on medical condition to prevent pressure ulcer. *If unable to tolerate a low head of bed, then check the sacrum often for signs of pressure. Sacral shearing risk is high when the head of the bed is above 30 degrees because skin may stick to linen if clients slide down, causing skin to pull away from underlying muscle tissue and bone (Wound, Ostomy, and Continence Nurses Society, 2003).*
- Position the bed flat at intervals, unless contraindicated for a medical reason. *Helps maintain body alignment and normalize tone; is the start position for bed mobility tasks; and is the position of most clients' beds at home (Kumagai, 1998).*

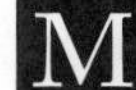

- Tilt patients 30 degrees or less while side lying. *A full side-lying position places high pressure on the trochanter (Defloor, 2000; Hoeman, 2002).*
- Place a pillow under heels of immobile, supine-lying patients unless contraindicated, e.g., postoperatively after total knee replacement. *A pillow lengthwise under the calves lowers heel interface pressure (Wound, Ostomy, and Continence Nurses Society, 2003).*
- Prevent complications of immobility. *The inability to be upright disturbs many body systems (Metzler & Harr, 1996; Murphy, 1997; Olson, 1967).*
- If high risk for pressure ulcer development, place the client on a static or dynamic surface in bed. Routinely place palm of hand under the overlay and susceptible bony areas to check for "bottoming out" (body sinks into mattress thus the recommended one inch between the surface and client is absent). Refer to care plan for **Risk for impaired Skin integrity.** *Pressure-relieving devices such as these help prevent or treat pressure ulcers (Wound, Ostomy, and Continence Nurses Society, 2003; Gutierrez, 2002; Johnson & Nolde-Lopez, 2002).*

▲ Place the client with stage III or IV pressure ulcer on low-air-loss surface or air-fluidized bed. Consult enterostomal therapy nurse to determine appropriate surface for complex clients (Wound, Ostomy, and Continence Nurses Society, 2003).

- Encourage the client to take deep breaths, cough, reposition self, drink adequate fluids, and use incentive spirometer. *This prevents atelectasis and possible pneumonia.*
- Ensure the client receives adequate fiber, fluid, and a stool softener and/or bulking agent to prevent constipation. Refer to care plan for **Constipation.** *Immobility leads to constipation because peristalsis slows, and abdominal muscles weaken, this plus loss of gravity during defecation makes it hard to pass stool (Folden, 2002, Fried & Fried, 2001).*
- Recognize clients at risk for venous thromboembolism (VTE) and implement prophylactic measures such as antiembolic stockings, elastic wraps, sequential compression devices; joint range-of-motion (ROM) and leg exercises; adequate fluid intake and anticoagulant medications. Refer to care plan for **Ineffective Tissue perfusion.** *Prolonged immobility, major surgery, multiple trauma, previous deep vein thrombosis (DVT) or pulmonary embolism (PE), hip fracture, cancer, spinal cord injury, cardiac or pulmonary failure, and older age are high-risk factors (Anderson & Spencer, 2003; Proctor & Greenfield, 2001).* **EBN:** *A quantitative study concluded that changing the needle after withdrawing heparin from a vial did not reduce the size of ecchymoses at the injection site of subjects (Klingman, 2000).*
- Encourage fluid intake of 2000 to 3000 mL/day as tolerated by medical condition. *Increased fluids help flush mobilized calcium and bacteria from the body to prevent kidney stones and urinary infection (Maas & Specht, 2001; Mahoney, 2001).*
- Take scrupulous care of indwelling Foley catheter; detect and report signs of urinary tract infection as early as possible. *Loss of weight bearing on bones and presence of an indwelling catheter can lead to increased urinary calculi and infection (McConnell, 1984; Murphy, 1997; Rubin, 1988).*
- Implement the following interventions during bed mobility activities:
  - Place positioning devices such as pillows or foam wedges between bony prominences.
  - Use lifting or lateral transferring devices such as trapeze, bed linen, mechanical lateral transfer aid, ceiling mounted lift or transfer chair, and bed scale to move (rather than drag) for dependent or obese individuals (Jenkins & Egersett, 2004; Wound,

Ostomy, and Continence Nurses Society, 2003). *Devices protect against mechanical forces, e.g., pressure, friction, and shear (Wound, Ostomy, and Continence Nurses Society, 2003). NOTE: A trapeze may be contraindicated in persons with cardiac disease and stroke because of the isotonic effect. Trapeze use is also discouraged with hemiplegcs because gripping with the sound hand elicits hypertonicity and flexion in the hemiplegic side (Bobath, 1978; Hoeman, 2002).* **EBN:** *Manual lifting often causes overexertion back stress and injuries to staff and may be uncomfortable to clients (Owen, Welden, & Kane, 1999).*

- Use large beds and special equipment to reposition the bariatric (very obese) client, such as air mattress overlay with rotation function, trapeze, and stirrup and pulley attached to an overhead traction system (to place one leg in thus raising it during pericare). Logroll and tilt dependent bariatric client (avoid full side-lying position) until familiar with his or her ability to help turn in bed. *The air mattress overlay reduces skin shear and frictional burn plus decreases resistance for staff to overcome when moving heavy clients in bed. If the client starts to slide out of bed in the side-lying position, it is difficult for staff to stop the motion (Dionne, 2002).*
- Apply elbow pads to comatose clients, to those with arm restraints, and to clients who use their elbows to prop or scoot themselves up in bed. Apply nocturnal elbow splint to promote extension if an ulnar nerve palsy exists or if there is pain at the elbow and paresthesia in the ulnar side of the fourth and fifth fingers. *Prolonged compression or repetitive flexion producing pressure on the ulnar nerve can lead to neuropathy and nerve damage (Congress of Neurological Surgeons, 2002). An enclosure bed for agitated and confused clients may alleviate wrist and chest restraints, thus prevent elbow abrasions.*

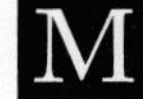

- Teach proper range of motion (ROM) and self-care activities, and apply extremity splints/boots on a rotating schedule to prevent joint contracture and disuse syndrome. *Immobility, chronic spasticity, and muscle weakness/atrophy from connective tissue changes contribute to joint contractures (Fried & Fried, 2001).*
- Explain the importance of exhaling when pulling self up or rolling in bed and during any activity that precipitates breath holding or straining. *This prevents the Valsalva maneuver and increased intraabdominal, and intrathoracic pressure, which elevate blood pressure and impair myocardial and cerebral perfusion (Rodriguez, 1998).*
- If movement intensifies pain level, then preventatively administer analgesics before bed repositioning, exercising, or self-cares. *Nurses must accept clients' definition and self-rating of pain, and need for analgesics (McCaffery & Pasero, 1999). Robinson and Shannon (2002) summarized medications to specifically relieve neuropathic pain, which may occur with peripheral nerve injury and secondarily to disuse.* **EBN:** *A phenomenological study demonstrated nurses took action to intervene for postoperative patients pain, thus affecting quality of care (Soderhamn & Idwall, 2003).*
- Assist clients to splint an incision, wound, or other painful abdominal area with a pillow as they change positions, cough, or perform functional activities.

▲ Administer oral antispasmodic medications as prescribed to control muscle spasms that interfere with movement. *A therapeutic level is one that prevents spasms but does not produce muscle weakness (Finocchiaro & Herzfeld, 1998).*

▲ Apply ice as ordered by physician to sites after nerve and motor point blocks and assess for side effects of pain, sensory deficits, or vascular problems. *Injections with phenol, ethanol, or botulinum toxin may be given locally (to the ankle, foot, knee, fingers) to prevent contractures and reduce spasticity that interferes with hygiene, ROM, positioning, standing, pressure prevention, and comfort (Gormley, 1999; Gracies et al, 1997; McKinley et al, 2002).*

▲ Recognize that intractable chronic spasticity and pain can interrupt function, bed/chair positioning, hygiene, and quality of life. If conservative treatment fails, some clients benefit from continuous intrathecal baclofen infusion (CITB) through an implanted pump in the spinal canal. **EBN:** *Follow-up with 18 clients receiving CITB treatment indicated the majority had a significant decrease in tone and nursing care and increased function (Rawicki, 1999).* **EB:** *Spasticity decreased in 25 subjects as measured by the Ashworth score. Subjects' answers to two open-ended questions relating to quality of life were positive (Gianino et al, 1998).*

▲ Refer clients to a dietitian, or provide dietary information to promote normal body weight. *Excessive weight places extra work and stress on body parts during bed mobility activities and may prevent tolerance to prone positioning.*

## Exercising

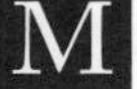


- Perform passive ROM at least twice a day to immobile body parts. Support limb above and below the joint being ranged (e.g., hold the forearm and hand while ranging the wrist). *ROM maintains joint and muscle movement and prevents contracture. Muscles can only get stronger by working. Adequate support of the joint allows for staff to detect ease or resistance to movement (Hoeman, 2002).*
- Range hemiplegic client's affected upper extremity with the shoulder in slight external rotation. *Spasticity pulls hemiplegic shoulders into retraction, which prevents normal gliding movement. External rotation prevents soft tissue from becoming pinched between the bones thus reducing pain (Borgman & Passarella, 1991).*
- Perform ROM slowly and rhythmically. Do not range beyond the point of pain in those with sensation; range only to the point of resistance in those with poor sensation and mental awareness. *Fast, jerky ROM creates pain and increases tone. Slow, rhythmical movements relax and lengthen spastic muscles so they can be ranged further. Slow joint movement with gentle stretch may also elicit muscle relaxation.* NOTE: *This is not the case for those with rigidity, as in Parkinson's disease (Palmer & Wyness, 1988).*
- Reinforce clients' self-initiated practice of exercise programs, developed by therapists including muscle setting, active strengthening, contraction of muscles against resistance, and weight lifting. *Allowing clients to initiate exercise programs early on encourages self-responsibility. Active exercise and weight lifting helps maintain muscle tone and strength. Muscle setting shortens muscle fibers without moving limbs or joints. Progressive resistive exercises cause muscles to work against gentle force and gravity, which stimulates muscle lengthening (Hoeman, 2002, Finocchiaro & Herzfeld, 1998).*
- Intervene for misalignment, flaccidity and spasticity, inability to shift weight, reduced sensation, and excessive effort while moving. *Therapeutic bed positioning and moving can counteract such problems, enhance sensation, and restore more normal tone and posture (Bobath, 1978; Gee & Passarella, 1985; Kumagai, 1998; Palmer & Wyness, 1988).*
- Use manual guidance and verbal cueing during bed mobility to facilitate more normal tone, posture, and movement. Allow clients to do as much of the activity as they can.

*Clients need the opportunity to feel more normal tone and posture so they do not relearn abnormal patterns (Ossman & Campbell, 1990; Passarella & Lewis, 1987).*

## Positioning

- Incorporate the following measures to promote normal tone and prevent complications. Refer to Ossman and Campbell (1990), and Kumagai (1998), and Gee and Passarella (1985) for detailed instructions.
  - Position head and neck in midline. *Head, neck, and trunk alignment normalizes muscle tone in the extremities thus decreases spasticity (Bobath, 1978).*
  - Use a flat pillow when clients are supine if neck flexion occurs. Use a small pillow behind the head and/or between the shoulder blades if extension occurs. *This prevents flexor or extensor tone and contractures of the head and neck (Bobath, 1978; Palmer & Wyness, 1988).*
  - If lateral head flexion occurs, lace a sandbag under the pillow along one or both sides of the head when the client is supine, and place one or two pillows under the head in the side-lying position. *Lateral head flexion and rotation may occlude the internal jugular vein, thus preventing cerebral ventricular outflow, which can increase ICP (Palmer & Wyness, 1988).*
  - Change the position of clients' shoulders and arms frequently. Abduct the shoulders of persons with high paraplegia or quadriplegia horizontally to 90 degrees briefly twice a day. *Positioning their arms in the horizontal plane provides full range of motion (Pires 1989).*
  - Do not position hemiplegics shoulders in abduction. *Too much abduction increases spasticity around the scapula, inhibits normal gliding movements, and thus pinches soft tissue (Borgman & Passarella, 1991).*
  - Apply resting forearm, wrist, and hand splints as ordered. Routinely check underlying skin for pressure and poor circulation. Strictly adhere to on/off orders. *Splints maintain hands and wrists in neutral position, and immobilize inflamed joints as a means of controlling pain.*
  - Use hard cone or splint in hands as ordered to help prevent hand contractures. **EBN:** *Soft rolls may elicit flexor patterns in the wrists and hands. Instead, a hard cone is suggested because it likely inhibit the long flexors of the hand (Jamieson & Dayhoff, 1980).*
  - Elevate the affected arm of persons with hemiplegia and apply an isotoner glove. *Paralysis allows lymph fluid to collect in the dependent hand; therefore venous insufficiency occurs, which further limits motion (Borgman & Passarella, 1991).*
  - Place a thin pillow under the weak pelvic girdle, hip, and upper thigh of persons with hemiplegia. Place a trochanter roll along the outside of the legs of persons with hemiplegia or leg paralysis. *These actions maintain hip and leg alignment (Bobath, 1978).*
  - Strictly maintain leg abduction in persons with a surgical hip pinning or hip replacement by placing an abductor splint or pillow between the legs. *Abduction stabilizes the new prosthesis in the joint (Hoeman, 2002).*
  - Apply foot splints, boots, or high-top tennis shoes as recommended by the physical therapist. Routinely assess underlying skin for signs of pressure. *This intervention helps prevent foot drop while in bed. Footboards are undesirable because pressure on the*

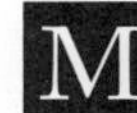


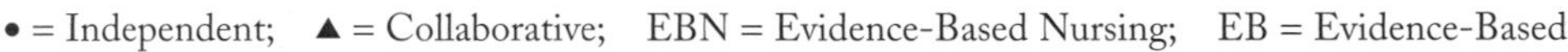

*ball of the foot stimulates plantar flexion and spasticity (Bobath, 1978; Hoeman, 2002; Palmer & Wyness, 1988).*

- Assist clients to lie prone or semiprone routinely (may be contraindicated in those with cardiopulmonary disturbances or increased intracranial pressure). *Promotes drainage and mobilizes secretions from dependent lobes of the lung. It also enhances hip and trunk extension, so is therapeutic for persons with leg amputations, paralysis, and brain injury (Kumagai, 1998; Palmer & Wyness, 1988).*
- Position hemiplegics on the unaffected and affected sides. Position the affected shoulder slightly forward by moving the shoulder, not the arm. *Weight bearing and protraction of the shoulder reduces tone. Moving the affected shoulder versus the arm prevents shoulder pain (Bobath, 1978; Borgman & Passarella, 1991).*

• Components of normal bed mobility include rolling, bridging, scooting, long sitting, and sitting upright. Most movements start with the client supine, flat in bed. *Normal movements are bilateral, segmental, well-timed, and effortless. They involve set positions, weight bearing and shifting, trunk centering, and stabilization against gravity (Borgman & Passarella, 1991; Gee & Passarella, 1985; Kumagai, 1998).*

### Bed Mobility—Rolling

• Assist the client into the set position for rolling. For hemiplegics, this includes the following:
  - Moving the shoulder and arm on the side to which the client will turn outward with palm facing up
  - Flexing the knees with the feet flat on the bed

• For persons with bilateral leg paralysis, this includes the following:
  - Crossing the outside leg over the other leg or manually flexing the outside leg
  - Placing the arms in front of the chest with the hands clasped together

  *Set positions are those normal postures assumed to prepare the body for purposeful movements (Gee & Passarella, 1985; Kumagai, 1998).*

• Instruct and guide the client to roll over segmentally (e.g., start by turning the head toward the direction of the turn, then move the shoulders/arms/trunk, as the hips and flexed knees follow). *Staff should be prepared to assist the affected side of hemiplegics, and the legs of paraplegics and quadriplegics (Bobath, 1978; Kumagai, 1998).*

Note: For safety, always logroll a client with spinal cord injury and persons with severe back pain or recent back surgery. Refer to Kumagai (1998) for detailed information on turning paralyzed persons.

### Bed Mobility—Bridging

• Teach clients to use bridging (lifting hips off the bed) during functional activities such as using the bedpan or pulling up pants. *Bridging is a bilateral activity that prepares the legs and feet for weight bearing while the hips are extended (Gee & Passarella, 1985).*

• Reinforce the set position (e.g., knees flexed and feet flat on the bed close to the buttocks. Assist by preventing external rotation of the legs). *The closer the feet are to the buttocks, the higher the hips can lift up; pain, limited ROM, a fracture, and arthritis may limit knee flexion though (Gee & Passarella, 1985).*

- Have the client rest his or her arms and hands on the bed alongside the trunk.
- Instruct the client to push down on the bed with the feet thus lifting his/her buttocks. Assistance may be needed to lift the pelvis upward or to hold a weak foot down.

### Bed Mobility—Scooting Laterally

- Communicate which direction the client is to move toward and help the client bridge.
- Support the client's pelvis to the extent needed as he or she pushes down on the bed with the feet, and lifts the hips up and over onto the side of the bed. *The lower body is moved first in lateral scooting.*
- Instruct the client then lift head and shoulders up off the bed and move them and the trunk sideways. If the client has hemiplegia, support the affected shoulder from the scapula and help move the trunk as needed.

### Bed Mobility—Side-Lying to Sitting Upright

- Assess whether the client is over to one side of the bed far enough; if not, help the client to move over. *This will reduce the risk of sliding off the edge of the bed while sitting up.*
- Assist or cue the client turn on his/her side (to the affected side if hemiplegic if possible. *Weight bearing on the hemiplegic decreases tone, promotes bilateral activity, and provides sensory stimulation (Bobath, 1978).*
- Instruct the client to lower the legs slowly over the edge of the bed with knees flexed and close to chest unless the client has recently had back or neck surgery, or has back pain. If so, the legs should be lowered slowly off the bed by staff at the same time the client lifts his/her head and pushes up with the arms, keeping the spine straight. *Lowering legs over the edge of the bed reduces the amount of weight to be shifted and managed while sitting up. However, in cases of back surgery or pain, legs are moved in unison with the body because the weight of freely hanging legs could aggravate back pain and surgical stability.*
- Ask the client to lift his or her head off the bed.
- Ensure that the bottom shoulder is positioned slightly forward before sitting up (move it forward from the shoulder). *This allows the elbow to take weight as the body moves upright (Bobath, 1978; Ossman & Campbell, 1990).*
- Instruct the client to bear weight on the bottom arm and elbow while at the same time pushing against the mattress with the palm of other hand to sit up (Kumagai, 1998).
- Help the client sit up by placing one of your hands under the bottom shoulder blade to keep it well forward and pushing down on the opposite with your other hand. Shift the client's weight; do not lift it. Encourage the client to complete as much of the movement as possible. *Protraction of the shoulder helps prevent abnormal tone and pain. The shoulder and pelvis are key points of control for guiding the movements (Gee & Passarella, 1985; Ossman & Campbell, 1990). The nurse's weight shifts from the front foot to back foot so leverage, not strength is used (Gee & Passarella, 1985).*
- Assist clients to sit on the edge of the bed with weight on both buttocks. Hips and knees should flex to 90 degrees, and if possible, feet should be flat on the floor (Bobath, 1978).

### Bed Mobility—Long Sitting (for Clients with Paretic or Immobile Legs)

- Assess the client's ability for 100-degree straight leg raises; if absent, avoid this position. *Straight leg raises test hamstring tone. If hamstrings are too tight and long sitting is attempted, the back extensor muscles will be overstretched and the person will lose passive stability of the trunk (Kumagai, 1998).*
- Cue the client to start from the flat and supine position and to grasp the side rails.
- Instruct client to pull self up to a sitting position. If hand function is poor, teach the client to raise the head/trunk and then push against the mattress with flexed forearms, until sitting upright. The legs remain in extension as the client sits up.

### Geriatric

- Discriminately raise the side rails. Try alternatives such as body pillows, height-adjustable beds, bed alarms, and antislip floor mats next to the bed instead. *Falls and entrapment related to bed rails can cause injury and death (Todd et al, 1997).* **EBN:** *BedSafe, an interdisciplinary quality improvement project, demonstrated that assessment of which residents to try to stop bedrail use with, education, trials of alternative measures, and evaluation decreased use of bedrails and falls (Hoffman et al, 2003).*
- Develop strategies for bed positioning and mobility based on the client's multiple chronic and disabling conditions. *Comorbid conditions are high in the elderly.*
- Assess caregivers' strength, health history, and cognitive status to predict ability and risk for helping clients with bed mobility at home. Explore alternative options if risk is too high. *Caregivers are often themselves frail elders with chronic health problems who cannot physically help the client (McAnaw, 2001).*
- Assess the client's stamina and energy level during bed mobility activities; rest breaks may be needed. *Aging clients may have poor energy reserves and may fatigue due to respiratory and circulatory impairments (McAnaw, 2001).*
- Spread out bed activities and exercise programs rather than clumping them together. *Anticipate that day-to-day energy thus abilities may fluctuate.*
- Incorporate memory aids and strategies (e.g., written schedules, directions, sketches, or notes), timers, and so on so that clients with cognitive decline can function as independently as possible.

### Home Care

▲ Utilize nurse case managers, care coordinators, or social workers to assess support systems and identify need for assistive technology devices and community or home health services. *Professional advocates can help clients understand and locate assistive technology and services along with funding sources in their communities (Berry & Ignash, 2003).*

- Encourage use of the client's regular bed in the home unless contraindicated for medical reasons. Foam wedges or blocks can raise the head of bed if necessary. Place indented or grooved-out areas in wood pieces under each leg of the bed and set bed against the walls in a corner of the room. *Emotionally, persons may benefit from sleeping in their own bed, with their partner. Use of blocks and the wall will help secure the bed in place.*
- Suggest rearranging furniture at home to make it accessible and to meet sleeping, toileting, and living needs. *Converting a main level room into a suite for living and sleeping*

M

*purposes and decorating it cozily yet functionally may be emotionally soothing and prevent an institutional look (Yearns, 1995).*

- Discuss the psychological and physical benefits of allowing clients to be as self-sufficient as possible with bed mobility even though it may be time consuming. *Caregivers may try to help or save time by "doing for" their loved one; with discussion about prevention of helplessness and disuse syndromes and how to promote self-esteem, caregivers may willing alter their care approach.*
- Prepare family members for potential regression in clients' self-care during the transition from hospital to home. *Relocation anxiety may interfere with independence. The confidence building, coaching, and teaching strategies listed below may be needed to help client cope (Theuerkauf, 1996).*
- Offer emotional support and suggest community social supports to help with adjustment and independence issues. *The home environment may trigger the reality of loss and changing abilities (Hoeman, 1996).*
- Provide information about options for durable medical equipment and assistive technology and help families creatively discover ways to access funding sources to pay for such devices (Berry & Ignash, 2003).

▲ In the presence of medical disorder, institute case management of the frail elderly to support continued independent living. *Case management combines client and family assessment, planning and coordination of care among all health providers, and monitoring of care and outcomes. They address continuity of care, mutual goal setting, behavior management, and prevention of worsening health problems (Guttman, 1999).*

- Refer to the Home Care interventions of the care plan for **Impaired physical Mobility.**

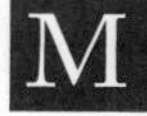

## Client/Family Teaching

- Use various sensory modalities to teach the client, family, and caregivers correct techniques for ROM, exercising, repositioning, and bed mobility activities.
- Give visual information (e.g., demonstrations, sketches, instructional videos, written instructions) (Allen, 2002).
- Give tactile stimulation (e.g., manual guidance, hand-on-hand technique, return demonstrations, note taking).
- Give auditory information (e.g., verbal instructions, instructional audiotapes, verbal repetition of instructions, self-talk during a motor activity, reading aloud written instructions). *Repeated practice and sensory stimulation helps motor learning and memory retention (Allen, 2002; Bobath, 1978).*
- Schedule time with family and caregivers for education and practice. Suggest that family members come prepared with questions and wear comfortable and safe clothing and shoes for practice. *Practice provides opportunity for hands-on learning.*
- Teach caregivers proper body mechanics and use of assistive devices (if applicable) while assisting clients with bed mobility activities. *This prevents injury and discomfort.*

## evolve WEBSITES FOR EDUCATION

See the EVOLVE website for World Wide Web resources for client education.

## REFERENCES


Allen C, Glasziou P, Del Mar C: Bed rest: a potentially harmful treatment needing more careful evaluation, *Lancet* 354(9186): 1229, 1999.

Allen, JC: Outcome-directed client and family education. In Hoeman SP, editor: *Rehabilitation nursing: process, application, and outcomes,* ed 3, St. Louis, 2002, Mosby.

Anderson FA, Spencer FA: Risk factors for venous thromboembolism, *Circulation* 107(23 Suppl 1):I9, 2003.

Berry BE, Ignash S: Assistive technology: providing independence for individuals with disabilities, *Rehabil Nurs* 28(1):6, 2003.

Bobath B: *Adult hemiplegia: evaluation and treatment,* London, 1978, William Heinemann Medical Books.

Borgman MF, Passarella PM: Nursing care of the stroke patient using Bobath principles: an approach to altered movement, *Nurs Clin North Am* 26(4):1019, 1991.

Congress of Neurological Surgeons: Medical student curriculum in neurosurgery. Available at www.neurosurgery.org/cns/meetings/curriculum/d1.html, 2002.

Defloor T: The effect of position and mattress on interface pressure, *Appl Nurs Res* 13(1):2, 2000.

Dionne M: 10 tips for safe mobility in the bariatric population, *Rehabil Manag* 15(8):28, 2002.

Fan JY: Effect of backrest position on intracranial pressure and cerebral perfusion pressure in individuals with brain injury: A systematic review, *J Neurosci Nurs* 36(5):278, 2004.

Finocchiaro D, Herzfeld S: Neurological deficits associated with spinal cord injury. In Chin PA, Finocchiaro D, Rosebrough A: *Rehabilitation nursing practice,* New York, 1998, McGraw-Hill.

Flannery J, Pugh SB: Stroke rehabilitation. In Flannery J: *Rehabilitation nursing secrets,* St Louis, 2004, Mosby.

Folden S: Practice guidelines for the management of constipation in adults, *Rehabil Nurs* 27(5):169, 2002.

Fried KM and Fried GW: Immobility. In Derstine J, Hargrave SD, editors: *Comprehensive rehabilitation nursing*, Philadelphia, 2001, WB Saunders.

Gee ZL, Passarella PM: *Nursing care of the stroke patient: therapeutic approach,* Pittsburgh, 1985, AREN.

Gianino JM, York MM, Paice JA et al: Quality of life: effect of reduced spasticity from intrathecal baclofen, *J Neurosci Nurs* 30(1): 47, 1998.

Gormley MH: Management of spasticity in children: part 1: chemical denervation, *J Head Trauma Rehabil* 14(1):97, 1999.

Gracies JM et al: Traditional pharmacological treatments for spasticity, part I: local treatments, *Muscle Nerve Suppl* 6:S61, 1997.

Gutierrez A: Pressure lessons, *Rehabil Manag* 15(9):44, 2002.

Guttman R: Case management of the frail elderly in the community, *Clin Nurs Spec* 13(4):174, 1999.

Hoeman SP: Coping with chronic, disabling, or developmental disorders. In Hoeman SP, editor: *Rehabilitation nursing: process and application,* ed 2, St Louis, 1996, Mosby.

Hoeman SP: Movement, functional mobility, and activities of daily living. In Hoeman SP, editor: *Rehabilitation nursing: process, application, and outcomes,* ed 3, St. Louis, 2002, Mosby.

Hoffman SB et al: BedSafe: a bed safety project for frail older adults, *J Gerontol Nurs* 29(11):34, 2003.

Jamieson S, Dayhoff NE: A hard hand-positioning device to decrease wrist and finger hypertonicity: a sensorimotor approach for the patient with nonprogressive brain damage, *Nurs Res* 29:285, 1980.

Jenkins L, Egersett, M: Better lifts and transfers, *Rehabil Manag* 17(9):24, 2004.

Johnson KMM, Nolde-Lopez G: Skin integrity. In Hoeman SP, editor: *Rehabilitation nursing: process, application, and outcomes,* ed 3, St Louis, 2002, Mosby.

Klingman L: Effects of changing needles prior to administering heparin subcutaneously, *Heart Lung* 29(1):70, 2000.

Kumagai KAS: Physical management of the neurologically involved client: techniques for bed mobility and transfers. In Chin PA, Finocchiaro D, Rosebrough A, editors: *Rehabilitation nursing practice,* New York, 1998, McGraw-Hill.

Lyder CH et al: Preventing pressure ulcers in Connecticut hospitals by using the plan—study-act model of quality improvement, *Jt Comm J Qual Saf* 30(4):205, 2004.

Maas ML, Specht JP: Impaired physical mobility. In Maas ML et al, editors: *Nursing care of older adults: diagnoses, outcomes, and interventions,* St Louis, 2001, Mosby.

Mahoney D: Nursing management of the patient with spinal cord injury. In Derstine JB, Hargrave SD, editors: *Comprehensive rehabilitation nursing*, Philadelphia, 2001, WB Saunders.

McAnaw MB: Normal changes with aging. In Maas ML et al, editors: *Nursing care of older adults: diagnoses, outcomes and interventions,* St Louis, 2001, Mosby.

McCaffery M, Pasero C: *Pain: clinical manual,* ed 2, St Louis, 1999, Mosby.

McConnell J: Preventing urinary tract infections, *Geriatr Nurs* 5(8):361, 1984.

McKinley WO, Gittler MS, Kirshblum SC et al: Spinal cord injury medicine. 2. Medical complications after spinal cord injury: identification and management, *Arch Phys Med Rehabil* 83(Suppl 1):S58, 2002.

Metzler DJ, Harr J: Positioning your patient properly, *Am J Nurs* 96(3):33, 1996.
Mundy LM et al: Early mobilization of patients hospitalized with community-acquired pneumonia, *Chest* 124(3):883, 2003.
Murphy JB: Dysmobility and immobility. In Ham RJ, Sloane PD, editors: *Primary care geriatrics: a case-based approach,* ed 3, St Louis, 1997, Mosby.
Olson EV: The hazards of immobility, *Am J Nurs* 67:781, 1967.
Ossman NJ, Campbell M: *Therapist guide: adult positions, transitions, and transfers—reproducible instruction cards for caregivers,* Tucson, 1990, Communication Skill Builders.
Owen BD, Welden N, Kane J: What are we teaching about lifting and transferring patients? *J Res Nurs Health* 22(1):3, 1999.
Palmer M, Wyness MA: Positioning and handling: important considerations in the care of the severely head-injured patient, *J Neurosurg Nurs* 20(1):42, 1988.
Passarella PM, Lewis N: Nursing application of Bobath principles in stroke care, *J Neurosurg Nurs* 19(2):106, 1987.
Pires M: Spinal cord injuries: coping with devastating damage. In Ursevich PR, editor: *Coping with neurologic problems proficiently,* ed 2, Nursing '84 Skillbook series, Springhouse, Penn, 1984, Springhouse.
Proctor MC, Greenfield LJ: Thromboprophylaxis in an academic medical center, *Cardiovasc Surg* 9(5):426, 2001.
Rawicki B: Treatment of cerebral origin spasticity with continuous intrathecal baclofen delivered via an implantable pump: long-term follow-up review of 18 patients, *J Neurosurg* 91(5):733, 1999.
Robinson MD, Shannon S: Rehabilitation of peripheral nerve injuries, *Phys Med and Rehabil Clin North Am* 13(1):109, 2002.
Rodriguez L: Medical-surgical complications in the rehabilitation client. In Chin PA, Finocchiaro D, Rosebrough A, editors: *Rehabilitation nursing practice,* New York, 1998, McGraw-Hill.
Rubin M: The physiology of bedrest, *Am J Nurs* 88:50, 1988.
Theuerkauf A: Self-care and activities of daily living. In Hoeman SP, editor: *Rehabilitation nursing: process and application,* ed 2, St Louis, 1996, Mosby.
Soderhamn O, Idvall E: Nurses' influence on quality of care in postoperative pain management: a phenomenological study, *Int J Nurs Prac,* 9:26, 2003.
Sullivan J: Positioning of patients with severe traumatic brain injury: research-based practice, *J Neurosci Nurs* 32(4):204, 2000.
Todd JF, Rhul CE, Gross TP: Injury and death associated with hospital bed side-rails: reports to the US Food and Drug Administration from 1985-1995, *Pub Health Briefs* 87(10):1675, 1997.
Williams TA, Leslie, GD: A review of the nursing care of enteral feeding tubes in critically ill adults: Part I, *Intensive Crit Care Nurs* 20(6):330, 2004.
Wojner AW, El-Mitwalli A, Alexandrov AV: Effect of head positioning on intracranial blood flow velocities in acute ischemic stroke: a pilot study, *Crit Care Nurs Q* 24(4):57, 2002.
Wound, Ostomy, and Continence Nurses Society (WOCN): *Guideline for prevention and management of pressure ulcers* (WOCN clinical practice guideline, no 2), Glenview, Ill, 2003, The Society.
Yearns MH: Modest home makeovers to improve farmhouse accessibility: how our AgrAgbility team used this fast, affordable alternative to remodeling with the Miller family, *Technol Disabil* 4:49, 1995.



## Impaired physical Mobility

evolve

*Betty J. Ackley and Teepa Snow*

**NANDA**

### Definition

A limitation in independent, purposeful physical movement of the body or of one or more extremities

### Defining Characteristics

Postural instability during performance of routine ADLs; limited ability to perform gross motor skills; limited ability to perform fine motor skills; uncoordinated or jerky movements; limited range of motion (ROM); difficulty turning; decreased reaction time; movement-induced shortness of breath; gait changes (e.g., decreased walking speed, difficulty initiating gait, small steps, shuffles feet, exaggerated lateral postural sway); engages in substitutions for movement (e.g., increased attention to other's activity, controlling behavior, focus on preillness/predisability); slowed movement; movement-induced tremor

## Related Factors

Medications; prescribed movement restrictions; discomfort; lack of knowledge regarding value of physical activity; body mass index greater than 30; sensoriperceptual impairments; neuromuscular impairment; pain; musculoskeletal impairment; intolerance to activity/decreased strength and endurance; depressive mood state or anxiety; cognitive impairment; decreased muscle strength, control, and/or mass; reluctance to initiate movement; sedentary lifestyle or disuse or deconditioning; selective or generalized malnutrition; loss of integrity of bone structures; developmental delay; joint stiffness or contractures; limited cardiovascular endurance; altered cellular metabolism; lack of physical or social environmental supports; cultural beliefs regarding age-appropriate activity

Suggested functional level classifications include the following:

0—Completely independent
1—Requires use of equipment or device
2—Requires help from another person for assistance, supervision, or teaching
3—Requires help from another person and equipment device
4—Dependent (does not participate in activity)



**NOC**

## Outcomes (Nursing Outcomes Classification)

### Suggested NOC Outcomes

Ambulation; Ambulation: Wheelchair; Mobility; Self-Care: Activities of Daily Living (ADLs); Transfer Performance

**Example NOC Outcome with Indicators**

**Ambulation** as evidenced by the following indicators: Walks with effective gait/Walks at moderate pace/ Walks up and down steps/Walks moderate distance (Rate each indicator of **Ambulation:** 1 = severely compromised, 2 = substantially compromised, 3 = moderately compromised, 4 = mildly compromised, 5 = not compromised [see Section I].)

## Client Outcomes

### Client Will (Specify Time Frame):

- Increase physical activity
- Meet mutually defined goals of increased mobility
- Verbalize feeling of increased strength and ability to move

- Demonstrate use of adaptive equipment (e.g., wheelchairs, walkers) to increase mobility

NIC

## Interventions (Nursing Interventions Classification)

### Suggested NIC Interventions

Exercise Therapy: Ambulation, Joint Mobility; Positioning

**Example NIC Activities—Exercise Therapy: Ambulation**

Assist the client to use footwear that facilitates walking and prevents injury; instruct in availability of assistive devices, if appropriate

## Nursing Interventions and Rationales

- • Screen for mobility skills in the following order: (1) bed mobility; (2) supported and unsupported sitting; (3) transition movements such as sit to stand, sitting down, and transfers; and (4) standing and walking activities. Use a tool such as the Assessment Tool for Safe Patient Handling and Movement. *The abilities of the client should be assessed to determine how best to facilitate movement and protect the nurse from harm (Nelson et al, 2003).*
- • Observe the client for cause of impaired mobility. Determine whether cause is physical or psychological. *Some clients choose not to move because of psychological factors such as an inability to cope or depression.* Refer to care plan for **Ineffective Coping** or **Hopelessness.**
- • Monitor and record the client's ability to tolerate activity and use all four extremities; note pulse rate, blood pressure, dyspnea, and skin color before and after activity. Refer to the care plan for **Activity intolerance.**
- ▲ Before activity, observe for and, if possible, treat pain. Ensure that the client is not oversedated. *Pain limits mobility and is often exacerbated by movement.*
- ▲ Consult with physical therapist for further evaluation, strength training, gait training, and development of a mobility plan. *Techniques such as gait training, strength training, and exercise to improve balance and coordination can be very helpful for rehabilitating clients (Tempkin et al, 1997).*
- ▲ Obtain any assistive devices needed for activity, such as gait belt, walker, cane, crutches, or wheelchair, before the activity begins. *Assistive devices can help increase mobility (Nelson et al, 2004).*
- • If the client is immobile, perform passive ROM exercises at least twice a day unless contraindicated; repeat each maneuver three times. *Inactivity rapidly contributes to muscle shortening and changes in periarticular and cartilaginous joint structure. The formation of contractures starts after 8 hours of immobility (Fletcher, 2005; Fried & Fried, 2001).*
- ▲ If the client is immobile, consult with physician for a safety evaluation before beginning an exercise program; if program is approved, begin with the following exercises:
  - ■ Active ROM exercises using both upper and lower extremities (e.g., flexing and extending at ankles, knees, hips)

M

- Chin-ups and pull-ups using a trapeze in bed (may be contraindicated in clients with cardiac conditions)
- Strengthening exercises such as gluteal or quadriceps sitting exercises

*These exercises help reverse weakening and atrophy of muscles (Kasper et al, 2005).*

- If client is immobile, consider use of a transfer chair, a chair that becomes a stretcher. *Utilizing a transfer chair where the client is pulled onto a flat surface and then seated upright in the chair can help previously immobile clients get out of bed (Nelson et al, 2003).*
- Help the client achieve mobility and start walking as soon as possible if not contraindicated. **EB:** *A study has shown that bed rest for primary treatment of medical conditions or after health care procedures is associated with worse outcomes than early mobilization (Allen, Glasziou, & Del Mar, 1999). A meta-analysis of research demonstrated that early mobilization for acute limb injuries generally resulted in improved function, less pain, and earlier return to work and sports (Ebell, 2005).*
- Use a gait-walking belt when ambulating the client. *Gait belts help improve the care givers grasp, reducing the incidence of injuries (Nelson, 2003).*
- Apply any ordered brace before mobilizing the client. Braces support and stabilize a body part, allowing increased mobility.
- Initiate a "No Lift" policy where appropriate assistive devices are utilized for manual lifting. *A study in six Veterans Administration (VA) hospitals demonstrate that workman's comp costs decreased significantly after initiation of a "No Lift" program, and it was predicted that $5 million would be saved within 9 years (Nelson et al, 2003).*
- Increase independence in ADLs, encouraging self-efficacy and discouraging helplessness as the client gets stronger. *Providing unnecessary assistance with transfers and bathing activities may promote dependence and a loss of mobility.*
- If client has had a cerebrovascular accident (CVA) with hemiparesis, consider use of constraint-induced movement therapy (CIMT), where the functional extremity is purposely constrained and the client is forced to use the involved extremity. *Constraint therapy is estimated to benefit about half of the total CVA population (Barker, 2005).* **EB:** *The plasticity of the brain allows the brain to rewire and reroute neural connections to take up the work of the injured area of the brain (National Institute of Neurological Disorders and Stroke, 2004; Liepert et al, 2000).*
- If the client does not feed or groom self, sit side-by-side with the client, put your hand over the client's hand, support the client's elbow with your other hand, and help the client feed self; use the same technique to help the client comb hair. *This feeding technique increases client mobility, range of motion, and independence, and clients often eat more food (Pedretti, 1996).*

M

## Geriatric

- Assess ability to move using the "Get Up and Go" test. Ask the client to rise from a sitting position, walk 10 feet, turn, and return to the chair to sit. *Performance on this screening exam demonstrates the client's mobility and ability to leave the house safely (Robertson & Montagnini, 2004).*
- Help the mostly immobile client achieve mobility as soon as possible, depending on physical condition. *In the elderly, mobility impairment can predict increased mortality and*

*dependence; however, this can be prevented by physical exercise (Fletcher, 2005; Hirvensalo, Rantanen, & Heikkinen, 2000).*

- If client is frail, ensure good nutrition, appropriate medications, attention to vision and hearing deficits, and increase social support along with exercise. *Frailty in the elderly can be multifactorial and often can be ameliorated or reversed (Storey & Thomas, 2004).*
- Use the Outcome Expectation for Exercise Scale to determine client's self-efficacy expectations and outcomes expectations toward exercise. **EBN:** *The client's self-efficacy expectations and outcome expectations for exercise will greatly influence his or her willingness to exercise. If the individual has a low outcome, interventions can be implemented to strengthen the expectations and hopefully improve exercise behavior (Resnick, Zimmerman, & Orwig, 2001).*
- For a client who is mostly immobile, minimize cardiovascular deconditioning by positioning the client in the upright position several times daily. *The hazards of bed rest in the elderly are multiple, serious, quick to develop, and slow to reverse. Deconditioning of the cardiovascular system occurs within days and involves fluid shifts, fluid loss, decreased cardiac output, decreased peak oxygen uptake, and increased resting heart rate (Fletcher, 2005; Kasper et al, 2005; Resnick & Daly, 1998).*
- If the client is mostly immobile, encourage him or her to attend a low-intensity aerobic chair exercise class that includes stretching and strengthening chair exercises. **EBN:** *A study of sedentary elderly subjects demonstrated that chair exercises have been shown to increase flexibility and balance (Mills, 1994).*
- Initiate a walking program in which the client walks with or without help every day as part of daily routine. **EBN:** *Walking programs in extended care facilities have been shown to be effective in improving ambulatory status and decreasing disability and the number of falls in the elderly (Koroknay et al, 1995).*

▲ Refer the client to physical therapy for resistance exercise training as able, including abdominal crunch, leg press, leg extension, leg curl, calf press, and more. **EB:** A *study demonstrated that 6 months of resistance exercise for the elderly greatly increased their aerobic capacity, possibly from increased skeletal muscle strength (Vincent et al, 2002). An additional study where clients in an extended care facility were put on a strength, balance, and endurance training program, the client's balance and mobility improved significantly (Rydwik, Kerstin, & Akner, 2005).*

- Use the WALC Intervention (Walk; Address pain, fear, fatigue during exercise; Learn about exercise; Cue by self-modeling) to improve exercise adherence in the older adult. **EBN:** *The WALC Intervention resulted in more exercise and had greater self-efficacy expectations regarding exercise (Resnick, 2002).*
- If client is scheduled for an elective surgery that will result in admission into ICU and immobility, or recovery from a knee replacement, initiate a prehabilitation program that includes a warm-up, aerobic strength, flexibility, and functional task work. **EBN and EB:** *By increasing the functional capacity of the individual prior to the stressor of inactivity, the predictable declines in physical activity can be prevented or alleviated (Topp et al, 2002). In a study clients who performed strength activities preoperatively walked significantly greater distances postoperatively after total hip replacement (Whitney & Parkman, 2002). Another study demonstrated that aerobic training along with strength and*

M

*interval training was effective in fewer postoperative complications, shorter postoperative stays and reduced functional disabilities (Carli & Zavorsky, 2005).*

▲ Evaluate the client for signs of depression (flat affect, insomnia, anorexia, frequent somatic complaints) or cognitive impairment (use Mini-Mental State Exam [MMSE]). Refer for treatment or counseling as needed. **EBN:** *Multiple studies have demonstrated that depression and decreased cognition in the elderly correlate with decreased levels of functional ability (Fletcher, 2005; Resnick, 1998).*

• Watch for orthostatic hypotension when mobilizing elderly clients. Have the client dangle at the side of the bed with legs hanging over the edge of the bed, flex and extend feet several times after sitting up, then stand up slowly with someone holding the client. If client becomes light headed or dizzy, return them to bed immediately. *Orthostatic hypotension as a result of cardiovascular system changes, chronic diseases, and medication effects is common in the elderly (Dingle, 2003).*

• Be very careful when getting a mostly immobile client up. Be sure to lock the bed and wheelchair and have sufficient personnel to protect the client from falls. *Elderly clients most commonly sustain the most serious injuries when they fall.* **EB:** *The most important preventative measure to reduce the risk of injurious falls for nonambulatory residents involves increasing safety measures while transferring, including careful locking of equipment such as wheelchairs and beds before moves (Thapa et al, 1996).*

• Do not routinely assist with transfers or bathing activities unless necessary. *The nursing staff may contribute to impaired mobility by helping too much. Encourage client independence (Kasper et al, 2005).*

• Use gestures and nonverbal cues when helping clients move if they are anxious or have difficulty understanding and following verbal instructions. *Nonverbal gestures are part of a universal language that can be understood when the client is having difficulty with communication.*

• Recognize that wheelchairs are not a good mobility device and often serve as a mobility restraint. **EB:** *Wheelchairs can be very effective restraints. In one study, only 4% of residents in wheelchairs were observed to propel them independently; only 45% could propel them, even with cues and prompts; no residents could unlock them without help; the wheelchairs were not fitted to residents; and residents were not trained in propulsion (Simmons et al, 1995).*

• Ensure that chairs fit clients. Chair seat should be 3 inches above the height of the knee. Provide a raised toilet seat if needed. *Raising the height of a chair can dramatically improve the ability of many older clients to stand up. Low, deep, soft seats with armrests that are far apart reduce a person's ability to get up and down without help.*

• If the client is mainly immobile, provide opportunities for socialization and sensory stimulation (e.g., television and visits). Refer to the care plan for **Deficient Diversional activity.** *Immobility and a lack of social support and sensory input may result in confusion or depression in the elderly (Fletcher, 2005).* Refer to nursing interventions for **Acute Confusion** or **Hopelessness** as appropriate.

## Home Care

• Above interventions may be adapted for home care use.

▲ Begin discharge planning as soon as possible with case manager or social worker to assess need for home support systems, assistive devices, and community or home health services.

- ▲ Assess home environment for factors that create barriers to physical mobility. Refer to occupational therapy services if needed to assist the client in restructuring home and daily living patterns.
- ▲ Refer to home health aide services to support the client and family through changing levels of mobility. Reinforce need to promote independence in mobility as tolerated. *Providing unnecessary assistance with transfers and bathing activities may promote dependence and a loss of mobility (Fletcher, 2005).*
- ▲ Refer to physical therapy for gait training, strengthening, and balance training. *Physical therapists can provide direct interventions as well as assess need for assistive devices (e.g., cane, walker).*
- • Assess skin condition at every visit. Establish a skin care program that enhances circulation and maximizes position changes. *Impaired mobility decreases circulation to dependent areas. Decreased circulation and shearing place the client at risk for skin breakdown.*
- • Once the client is able to walk independently, and needs an exercise program, suggest the client enter an exercise program with a friend. **EBN:** *Findings from a study of exercise behavior found that friends have the strongest influence to keep on an exercise program, more than family members or experts (Resnick, Orwig, & Magaziner, 2002).*
- • Provide support to the client and family/caregivers during long-term impaired mobility. *Long-term impaired mobility may necessitate role changes within the family and precipitate caregiver stress.* Refer to the care plan for **Caregiver role strain**.
- ▲ Institute case management of frail elderly to support continued independent living. *Impaired mobility can lead to increasing needs for assistance in using the health care system effectively. Case management combines nursing activities of the client and family assessment, planning and coordination of care among all health care providers, delivery of direct nursing care, and monitoring of care and outcomes. These activities are able to address continuity of care, mutual goal setting, behavior management, and prevention of worsening health problems (Guttman, 1999).*

## Client/Family Teaching

- • Teach the client to get out of bed slowly when transferring from the bed to the chair.
- • Teach the client relaxation techniques to use during activity.
- • Teach the client to use assistive devices such as a cane, a walker, or crutches to increase mobility.
- • Teach family members and caregivers to work with clients during self-care activities such as eating, bathing, grooming, dressing, and transferring rather than having the client be a passive recipient of care. *Maintaining as much independence as possible helps maintain mobility skills (Lipson & Braun, 1993).*
- • Work with the client using the Transtheoretical Model of behavior change and determine if the client is in the precontemplation, contemplation, preparation, action, or maintenance state of behavior change about exercise. Provide appropriate strategies to support change to exercising based on determined state of change. **EBN:** *The Transtheoretical Model of behavior change can be very useful for nurses to increase exercise behavior utilizing stage-appropriate interventions (Burbank, Reibe, & Padula, 2002). Use of the*

*Transtheoretical Model of behavior change plus theory of self-efficacy suggests that both of these theories are helpful in increasing exercise in the older adult (Resnick & Nigg, 2003).*

- Develop a series of contracts with mutually agreed on goals of increased activity. Include measurable landmarks of progress, consequences for meeting or not meeting goals, and evaluation dates. Sign the contracts with the client. **EBN:** *Using a series of evolving contracts to modify behavior toward increasing activity helps the client learn skills to change behavior (Boehm, 1989; Steckel, 1974).*

## evolve WEBSITES FOR EDUCATION

See the EVOLVE website for World Wide Web resources for client education.

## REFERENCES


Allen C, Glasziou P, Del Mar C: Bed rest: a potentially harmful treatment needing more careful evaluation, *Lancet* 354(9186): 1229, 1999.

Barker E: New hope for stroke patients, *RN* 68(2):38, 2005.

Boehm S: Patient contracting, *Annu Rev Nurs Res* 7:143, 1989.

Burbank PM, Reibe D, Padula CA: Exercise and older adults: changing behavior with the transtheoretical model, *Orthop Nurs* 21:4, 2002.

Carli F, Zavorsky GS: Optimizing functional exercise capacity in the elderly surgical population, *Curr Opin Clin Nutr Metab Care* 8(1):23, 2005.

Dingle M: Role of dangling when moving from supine to standing position, *Br J Nurs* 12(6):346, 2003.

Ebell M: Early mobilization better for acute limb injuries, *Am Family Physician* 71(4), 2005.

Fletcher K: Immobility: geriatric self-learning module, *Medsurg Nurs* 14(1):35, 2005.

Fried KM, Fried GW: Immobility. In Derstine JB, Hargrove SD: *Comprehensive rehabilitation nursing,* Philadelphia, 2001, WB Saunders.

Guttman R: Case management of the frail elderly in the community, *Clin Nurs Spec* 13(4):174, 1999.

Halfmann PL, Keller C, Allison M: Pragmatic assessment of physical activity, *Nurse Pract Forum* 8(4):160, 1997.

Hirvensalo M, Rantanen T, Heikkinen E: Mobility difficulties and physical activity as predictors of mortality and loss of independence in the community-living older population, *J Am Geriatr Soc* 48(5):493, 2000.

Koroknay VJ, Werner P, Cohen-Mansfield J et al: Maintaining ambulation in the frail nursing home resident: a nursing administered walking program, *J Gerontol Nurs* 21:18, 1995.

Liepert J, Bauder H, Wolfgang HR et al: Treatment-induced cortical reorganization after stroke in humans, *Stroke* 31(6):1210, 2000.

Lipson J, Braun S: *Toward a restraint-free environment: reducing the use of physical and chemical restraint in long-term care and acute settings,* Baltimore, 1993, Health Professions Press.

Mills EM: The effect of low-intensity aerobic exercise on muscle strength, flexibility, and balance among sedentary elderly persons, *Nurs Res* 43:207, 1994.

National Institute of Neurological Disorders and Stroke: Stroke: hope through research. Available at www.ninds.nih.gov/disorders/stgroke/detail_stroke.htm, accessed March 5, 2005.

Nelson A, Owen B, Lloyd JD et al: Safe patient handling movement, *AJN* 103(3):32, 2003.

Nelson A, Powell-Cope G, Gavin-Dreschnack D et al: Technology to promote safe mobility in the elderly, *Nurs Clin North Am* 39:649, 2004.

Pedretti LW: *Occupational therapy: practice skills for physical dysfunction*, ed 4, St Louis, 1996, Mosby.

Resnick B: Predictors of functional ability in geriatric rehabilitation patients, *Rehabil Nurs* 23(1):21, 1998.

Resnick B: Testing the effect of the WALC intervention on exercise adherence in older adults, *J Gerontol Nurs,* 28(6):40, 2002.

Resnick B, Daly MP: Predictors of functional ability in geriatric rehabilitation patients, *Rehabil Nurs* 23(1):21, 1998.

Resnick B, Nigg C: Testing a theoretical model of exercise behavior for older adults, *Nurs Res* 52(2):80, 2003.


M

Resnick B, Orwig D, Magaziner J: The effect of social support on exercise behavior in older adults, *Clin Nurs Res* 11(1):52, 2002.

Resnick B, Zimmerman S, Orwig D: Model testing for reliability and validity of the outcome expectations for exercise scale, *Nurs Res* 50:5, 2001.

Robertson RG, Montagnini M: Geriatric failure to thrive, *Am Family Physician*, 70(2):343, 2004.

Rydwik E, Kerstin F, Akner G: Physical training in institutionalized elderly people with multiple diagnoses—a controlled pilot study, *Arch Gerontol Geriatr* 40(1):29, 2005.

Simmons SF, Schnelle JF, MacRae PG et al: Wheelchairs as mobility restraints: predictors of wheelchair activity in nonambulatory nursing home residents, *J Am Geriatr Soc* 43:384, 1995.

Steckel SB: The use of positive reinforcement in order to increase patient compliance, *AANNT J* 1:1:1974.

Story E, Thomas RL: Understanding and ameliorating fraility in the elderly, *Top Geriatr Rehabil* 20(1):4, 2004.

Tempkin T, Tempkin A, Goodman H: Geriatric rehabilitation, *Nurs Pract Forum* 8(2):59, 1997.

Thapa PB, Brockman KG, Gideon P et al: Injurious falls in nonambulatory nursing home residents: a comparative study of circumstances, incidence, and risk factors, *J Am Geriatr Soc* 44:273, 1996.

Topp R, Ditmyer M, King K et al: The effect of bed rest and potential of prehabilitation on patients in the intensive care unit. *AACN Clin Issues* 13:2, 2002.

Vincent KR, Braith RW, Feldman RA et al: Improved cardiorespiratory endurance following 6 months of resistance exercise in elderly men and women, *Arch Intern Med* 162:673, 2002.

Whitney JA, Parkman S: Preoperative physical activity, anesthesia, and analgesia: effects on early postoperative walking after total hip replacement, *Appl Nurs Res* 15:1, 2002.

# Impaired wheelchair Mobility

*Brenda Emick-Herring*

M

**NANDA**

## Definition

Limitation of independent operation of wheelchair within environment

## Defining Characteristics

Impaired ability to operate a manual or power wheelchair on even or uneven surface; impaired ability to operate manual or power wheelchair on an incline or decline; impaired ability to operate wheelchair on curbs

## Related Factors (r/t)

Intolerance to activity; decreased strength and endurance; pain or discomfort; perceptual or cognitive impairment; neuromuscular impairment; musculoskeletal impairment; depression; severe anxiety

Suggested functional level classifications include the following:
0—Completely independent
1—Requires use of equipment or device
2—Requires help from another person for assistance, supervision, or teaching
3—Requires help from another person and equipment or device
4—Dependent—does not participate in activity

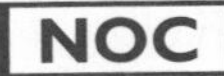

## Outcomes (Nursing Outcomes Classification)

### Suggested NOC Outcome

Ambulation: Wheelchair

**Example NOC Outcome with Indicators**

**Ambulation: Wheelchair** as evidenced by the following indicators: Propels wheelchair safely/Transfers to and from wheelchair/Maneuvers curbs, doorways, ramps (Rate each indicator of **Ambulation: Wheelchair:** 1 = severely compromised, 2 = substantially compromised, 3 = moderately compromised, 4 = mildly compromised, 5 = not compromised [see Section I].)

## Client Outcomes

**Client Will (Specify Time Frame):**

- Demonstrate optimal independence in operating and moving a wheelchair or other device equipped with wheels
- Demonstrate the ability to direct others in operating and moving a wheelchair or other device equipped with wheels
- Demonstrate therapeutic positioning, pressure relief, and safety principles while operating and moving wheelchair or other device equipped with wheels

**NIC**

## Interventions (Nursing Interventions Classification)

### Suggested NIC Interventions

Exercise Therapy: Muscle Control; Positioning: Wheelchair

**Example NIC Activities—Positioning: Wheelchair**

Select the appropriate wheelchair for the patient; monitor for patient's inability to maintain correct posture in wheelchair

## Nursing Interventions and Rationales

- • Assist client to put on and take off equipment (e.g., braces, corsets, orthoses, immobilizers, and abdominal binders) in bed. *Provide stabilization and alignment of body parts; the abdominal binder prevents postural hypotension, supports abdominal contents, and increases vital capacity. For hemodynamic stability, the binder must be put on and taken off in bed.*
- ▲ Obtain referrals for physical therapy (PT), occupational therapy (OT), or a wheelchair seating clinic (Gavin-Dreschnack, 2004). *The wheelchair seating system fits the build, abilities, postural support needs, comfort, and pressure ulcer prevention of the client.*
- • Realize the seating system allows the client to propel the chair, safely and ably use the hands, reach the foot rests and floor with the feet, stand up from the chair without

falling, and in the disabled is part of their identity (Cox 2004; Cooper et al, 2000; Minkel, 2001). *Wheelchair seating and cushion systems are the basis of postural support for clients and allow functional activities. Poor posture (slouching, side leaning, and sliding down) can cause deformities, discomfort, high skin pressure, overuse of physical restraints, and trunk compression.*

- Keep the right cushion and wheelchair with the right patient (Gavin-Dreschnack, 2004). *Individualized chair and seating systems promote functional independence and prevent medical complications. Proper cushions lessen shock impact, pressure, and repetitive vibration, which may lead to fatigue, pain, and improper body mechanics (Cooper et al 2000; Paleg 2002; Saur 1999).*
- Use of contoured surfaces/cushions/cutouts/supports, strict continence management, adequate nutrition and hydration, and repositioning are key strategies to prevent sitting-acquired pressure ulcers. Never use doughnut-type cushions or sheepskin (Cooper et al 2000; Paleg, 2002; Saur, 1999; Wound, Ostomy, and Continence Nurses Society, 2003). *Such options allow immobile clients to remain seated longer, and they distribute body mass to lower peak pressures over the bony ischial tuberosities. Doughnuts place high pressure on surrounding tissue, and sheepskin offers no pressure relief.* **EBN:** *Four cushions tested had varying pressure-reducing abilities. Healthy subjects had maximum pressure at the buttock-seat interface on a pressure-reducing cushion when they slid down or slouched in a chair. The least pressure occurred when the chair was tilted back with legs (not heels) resting on a stool. In straight sitting there was less pressure with feet on the floor versus a stool (Defloor & Grypdonck, 1999).*

▲ Obtain a PT, OT, or wheelchair seating clinic referral for cushion reevaluation if signs of pressure exist after chair sitting. *Professionals perform pressure mapping to evaluate cushion stiffness (ability to prevent bottoming out), dampening (ability to soften impact during activity), and envelopment (ability to contain the buttock); it ultimately assesses pressure distribution at the seat-cushion interface (e.g., where the seat-buttock make contact (Swaine, 2003).* **EB:** *A pilot study indicated high buttock-cushion interface pressure was associated with pressure ulcer development (Brienza et al, 2001).*

- Emphasize importance of weight shifts every 15 minutes with safety belts in place, including lateral leans (leaning toward one side of chair); forward leans (leaning forward as arms lie alongside thighs); and pushups if balance and trunk control are present (pushing up with hands on armrests to lift buttocks off the seat). *Such intermittent relief helps prevent pressure ulcers related to capillary occlusion from great force on small bony areas (McCourt, 1993; Minkel, 2000).*
- Manually tilt the wheelchair backward 45 to 65 degrees for 3 to 5 minutes, hourly. Client may also sit with the back of the wheelchair reclined (150 degrees) with legs on leg/foot rests (Minke, 2000; Pellow 1999). *This lowers tissue pressure and is used to prolong sitting time in immobile persons.* **EBN:** *When wheelchairs of two quadriplegics were tilted to 45 degrees or more or reclined to at least 150 degrees, pressure at their ischial tuberosities decreased significantly (Pellow, 1999).*
- Activate passive standing position in wheel chair if applicable, or if client has partial weight bearing, stand him/her briefly (Wound, Ostomy, and Continence Nurses Society, 2003). *Removes tissue pressure over bony prominences.*
- Inspect skin under orthoses, braces, and so on once removed and check bony promi-

nences after client returns to bed. *Early detection of pressure allows for early pressure relief strategy implementation (Wound, Ostomy, and Continence Nurses Society, 2003).*

- Place feet level with both feet on foot rests or on the floor when passively sitting in the wheelchair. *There is less pressure on sacral and buttock tissue sitting upright with feet on the floor than with feet on foot rests (Rader et al, 1999).*
- Routinely assess the clients sitting posture and help reposition him/her into sound alignment as needed. **EBN:** *Nurses only spent 6% of their time deliberately repositioning stroke patients with poor posture and asymmetry; they indirectly improved posture while helping clients with tasks such as getting ready to eat (Dowswell et al, 2000).*
- Place clients feet securely on foot rests and fasten seat belts across the top of the thighs before propelling the wheelchair. *Securing feet on foot plates prevents foot injuries and seat belts help stabilize and hold the pelvis in place (Rader et al, 1999).*
- Remove leg and foot rests from wheelchairs of clients who can "walk" it by taking short steps with their legs while seated to move the chair. *Foot rests may cause skin tears, bruising, or postural alignment problems.*
- Implement precautionary measures including use of friction-coated projection hand rims and leather gloves as clients propel manual wheelchairs. *Friction-coated projection rims are less invasive and slippery than aluminum rims. Persons without finger flexor function use palm action against the projection rims to propel a wheelchair; leather gloves help protect against palm sores and calluses.*
- Guide clients' hands onto wheelchair rims and explain how to push forward on both wheel rims to move ahead, to push the right rim to turn left and vice versa, and to pull backward on both wheel rims to back up (Wilson & Kerr, 1988).
- Use a wheelchair low enough so both feet touch flat on the floor.
- Guide and instruct clients with unilateral arm and leg function to propel the wheelchair by (1) raising that foot plate then putting foot flat on the floor, (2) placing sound hand on the wheel rim, (3) pushing forward with the sound hand while (4) "walking" the chair forward by extending the knee, putting the heel then the entire foot on the floor, flexing the knee and pulling the chair forward. NOTE: A hemi, one-arm drive wheelchair is recommended for persons with hemiplegia (Wilson & Kerr, 1988).
- Recommend clients back their wheelchairs (wheeled devices) into an elevator. If entering face first, instruct them to turn chair around to face the elevator doors. *This allows clients to see the control panel, floor monitor display, and doors opening and they can exit by wheeling forward (Minor & Minor, 1999).*
- Reinforce principle of descending a curb backward ("popping a wheelie") if balance, trunk control, strength, and timing are adequate. Client needs to lean slightly forward and guide both wheels off curb at the same time. *Backward descent carries less risk of clients losing control and falling forward out of the wheelchair. If someone helps the client, backing down the curb places less stress on the helper.*
- Recommend ascending curbs in a forward position by popping a wheelie or having an assistant tilt the chair back, place the front wheels over the curb, and roll the back wheels up it. If surface is soft (muddy, sandy) go up curb backward via a wheelie. *The front casters will not roll on soft surfaces. A backward approach will require less energy and prevent getting stuck or injured from falling forward (Younker Rehabilitation Center, 1990).*

- During assisted wheelies, the helper must hold the wheelchair until all four wheels are back on the ground and the client has balance and control of the wheelchair. *Releasing the grip too soon may alter the client's balance and cause injury (Younker Rehabilitation Center, 1990).*
- When client has unilateral neglect, agnosia, or proprioception deficits, nurses should reinforce the team's compensatory strategies as clients propel the wheelchair, enter doorways, and detect and avoid obstacles. Strategies may include visual scanning, self-talk, self-questioning about what could be wrong, and manual guiding. *Too often nurses physically move the wheelchair or obstacle when clients run into doorways, furniture, etc., instead of cueing clients to detect and solve the problem.*
- Use an individualized wheelchair with clients sitting as upright as possible versus a geri-chair when feeding dysphagic elders. *Prolonged use of geri-chairs promote a fetal-type posture. If they are reclined a lot, their heads are forced into an extensor pattern. When fed in this position, there is high risk for aspiration (Gavin-Dreschnack, 2004).*

▲ Implement and teach the following measures (Berry & Ignash, 2004; Cooper et al, 2004; Minkel, 2000; Nylund et al, 2000), which prevent upper extremity pain and joint degeneration from overuse and repetitive strain related to manual wheelchair propulsion, push-ups, and transfers, especially if clients are overweight:
  - ▲ Consult therapists for ROM, exercises, strengthening, and gentle stretching, and for wheelchair setup, seat height and "pushing" evaluations.
  - ■ Encourage doing more leans and chair tilts versus push-ups as weight shifts.
  - ■ Ensure transfer surfaces are as even in height as possible.
  - ▲ Advocate for ultralightweight manual; or pushrim-activated power assisted or electric powered wheelchairs (therapists and physicians will need to document evaluations and write letters of necessity to justify/request funding from payors).
  - ■ Stress that clients maintain normal versus extra body weight.
  - ■ Reinforce these principles as clients propel their wheelchairs, "Use long and smooth strokes that limit high forces and rate of loading on the pushrim," and "Allow the hand to naturally drift down when letting go of the pushrim; make an effort to keep the hand below the pushrim when not in contact with the pushrim" (Koontz & Boninger, 2004, p. 21). **EB:** *Individualized forward adjustment of the axle position on ultralightweight manual wheelchairs, combined with personal wheelchair fitting, improved propulsion biomechanics and likely lessens the risk of upper extremity nerve injury (Boninger et al, 2000). Persons with tetraplegia had more frequent and intense shoulder pain than those with paraplegia. Functional tasks creating the greatest pain in both groups included pushing up an incline and wheeling longer than 10 minutes. Pain was also intense while sleeping (Curtis et al, 1999).*
  - ■ Remind clients to avoid putting pressure on their elbows and remind them to distribute pressure the length of the arm during repositioning and weight shifts. Splints (especially nocturnal), elbow pads, assistance with transfers, and temporary use of an electric wheelchair may relieve tendonitis. *Arms are overworked during propulsion, transfers, repositioning, upper dressing, and thus they are at risk for painful syndromes (Congress of Neurological Surgeons, 2002; Minkel, 2000).*
  - ■ Recognize the value systems of clients and nurses regarding use of a wheelchair may

M

create tension. *Need for a wheelchair may symbolize weakness and loss of autonomy to clients; it may symbolize increased independence and functioning to professionals (Minkel, 2000).* **EBN:** *This phenomenological study found wheelchair users had frustration with barriers, accessibility, independence issues, societal attitudes toward people with disability, and lack of understanding by others (Pierce, 1998).*

▲ Offer support and referrals to help clients cope with issues related to physical disability and loss of independence (Minkel, 2000). *Clients may experience depression and anxiety with physical loss and inability to walk.*

• Suggest and help clients transition from a manual to a powered wheelchair if progressive physical disability occurs (Minkel, 2000). *An electric wheelchair helps protect shoulder and arm joints; reduces pain, energy and time demands; and helps maintains independence.* **EB:** *Eight interviewees, 6 to 24 months after switching to a powered mobility device, responded that the change positively affected their roles, occupational performance, interests, independence, and self-esteem (Buning, Angelo, & Schmeler, 2001).*

• Request and receive clients' permission before moving their unoccupied wheelchair within the room or out to the hall or another room (Cox, 2004; Gavin-Dreschnack, 2004). *Chronic wheelchair users may view the chair as part of their identity and independence; they may become stressed if it is not readily available.*

## Geriatric

• Alternate wheelchair mobility with rest periods. *Increased resting heart rate and blood pressure, and decreased maximal oxygen uptake, vital capacity, and strength in the elderly indicate activity intolerance (Radwanski, 2002).*

▲ Avoid using restraints on elderly, fidgeting clients because they slide down in a wheelchair or try to reposition themselves. Rather, assess for deformities, spinal curvatures, abnormal tone, discomfort, and limited joint range. If present, obtain a consult for a proper wheelchair seating system. *Standard wheelchair seats and backs sag and are uncomfortable whereas more solid seats and backrests, specialized supports, and cushions give postural stability, pressure relief, and comfort (Defloor & Grypdonck, 1999; Minkel, 2001; Rader et al, 1999; Taylor 2003). Elderly clients may move to get comfortable or to do a task, which may inadvertently result in poor posture and sliding down in the chair thus nurses may unnecessarily restrain them (Rader et al, 1999).*

• Ensure proper lower-extremity positioning when clients are sitting up. Do not use elevating leg rests to prevent them from sliding down in the wheelchair, instead use custom foot rests. Place both feet either on foot rests or on the floor when the wheelchair is stationary. *Tight hamstrings and a posterior pelvic tilt are common in the elderly, these may pull the pelvis toward the front of the chair. Special leg/foot rests help accommodate for this. An unequal foot level accentuates tight hamstrings and posterior tilt, thus contributing to discomfort and malalignment (Gee & Passarella, 1985; Rader et al, 1999).*

▲ Assess for side effects of medications and potential need for dosage readjustments to increase wheelchair mobility tolerance. *Antidepressants, diuretics, and benzodiazepines can cause postural hypotension and dizziness, and antihypertensive and cardiac medications often create hypotension and dizziness, and may alter cardiac output (Halm, 2001; Skidmore-Roth, 2001).*

- Allow the client to propel the wheelchair independently at his or her own speed. Avoid rushing client. *Elders often move slowly because of diminished ROM and strength, stiff joints, cardiopulmonary compromise, and discomfort.*

## Home Care

- Assess the home environment for barriers to wheelchair accessibility and for a support system for emergency and contingency care (e.g., Lifeline). *Impaired mobility and wheelchair use may pose a life threat during crises such as falls or orthostatic hypotension.* **EB:** *In two connected studies, 37% of respondents living at home had fallen from their wheelchairs, 46% of the fallers had sustained injury, and 36% had not made common home modifications (Berg et al, 2002).*
- Arrange traffic patterns so they are wide enough for a wheelchair or wheeled device to get around in. *Adequate space prevents damage to skin (especially on knuckles of hands), wheelchair, walls, woodwork, and furniture and increases independence (Yearns & Huntoon, 1997).*
- Explain a 5-foot turning space is necessary to maneuver wheelchairs, in e.g., in a bathroom, doorways need to be 32 to 36 inches wide, entrance ramps or paths should slope 1 inch per foot, and one outside entrance should have space enough to open the door and accommodate the wheelchair or wheeled device in (Yearns & Huntoon, 1997).
- Suggest simple and economical changes such as replacing door hardware with fold-back hinges, removing doorway encasements if doorways are too narrow, and removing or replacing thresholds if existing ones are too high. *Universal design literature recommends ways to modify (and build) homes and appliances to make them more accessible.*
- Suggest rearranging room functions, furniture, and storage so that toileting, sleeping, bathing, and preparing and eating meals can safely take place on one level of the home. *The ability to perform these activities is critical for staying in one's own home (Yearns & Huntoon, 1997).*

▲ Request a PT and OT referrals to evaluate wheelchair skills and safety; teach clients how to improve endurance, propel wheelchair on carpet and irregular surfaces, how to get back into wheelchair if he or she falls (or intentionally moves) onto the floor; and to make home modifications for safety (Berg et al, 2002). **EB:** *A cohort study concluded the Wheelchair Skills Test (WST) is a short, reliable test that professionals can use to assess clients manual wheelchair skills. Further test refinement is underway (Kirby et al, 2004).*

- Reinforce clients or caregiver assess for skin breakdown daily and establish programs to enhance circulation and decrease risk of sitting-acquired pressure ulcers. *Impaired mobility decreases circulation and applies pressure to dependent areas.*

▲ Supply home health aide services as appropriate for assistance with ADLs, bathing, and skin care. *Mobility impairments may serve as a barrier to self-care.*

▲ Provide support to clients and make referrals to medical social services or mental health/support group services. *Loss of independence may create anger and frustration. Counseling and support groups allow for validation of feelings and alternative methods of problem solving.*

▲ Provide client with information about advocacy, accessibility, assistive technology, po-

M

tential funding, and issues under the Americans with Disabilities Act. *Information, assistive devices, and funding create the potential for greater independence (Berry & Ignash, 2003; Minor & Minor, 1999).*

▲ Investigate community resources and written information for locating wheelchair parts and services for repair and tune up if the client is unable to do it (an annual tune-up is wise).

## Client/Family Teaching

- Suggest that the client test-drive wheelchairs and try out cushions and postural supports before purchasing them. *Equipment is very expensive, and different makes and models have different advantages and disadvantages (Minkel, 2000).*
- Discuss advantages, disadvantages, and long-term care involved with various cushions that distribute pressure. (1) Air cushions evenly distribute pressure, can be changed to optimize flotation, wash easily in case of incontinence, and are lightweight, but they leak air and need reinflation. As flotation increases, a lightweight client's sense of stability may decrease. (2) Gel cushions are durable and give support because they contour to the buttock; however, they may be hot, heavy, and create a moist environment. The gel must be pushed back in place to provide pressure relief. (3) Foam cushions are light, inexpensive, and can be cut to fit client contour but they compress and break down. They may need to be replaced and are not waterproof (Kurfuerst & Chew, 2003; Paleg, 2002). **EB:** *Individual seating interventions focused on support for spinal and pelvic posture, pressure distribution, and wheelchair functionality. Most subjects experienced pain relief with ergonomic seating interventions (Samuelsson et al, 2001). Researchers found most wheelchair uses had significant pain and rated comfort and mobility as key features of a wheelchair. Seating prototype testing found seat adjustability and low-back support improved comfort (Crane & Hobson, 2003).*
- Instruct and have the client return demonstrate reinflation of pneumatic tires; encourage the client to monitor tire pressure every 2 to 3 weeks. *Low tire pressure impacts the repetitive strain to the shoulder and wrist that occurs with manual wheelchair use.* **EB:** *Tire pressure that is at or below 50% of what the manufacturer recommends increases wheeling/rolling resistance and energy expenditure (Sawatzky et al, 2002).*
- Instruct clients and family to remove as many wheelchair parts as possible when lifting wheelchair into the car. Check that armrests and all parts of chair are fastened securely before picking them or the chair up. Check temperature of wheelchair or wheeled device before sitting in it. *Removing parts reduces the weight that needs to be lifted, locking parts into place prevents dropping them, and checking temperature of chair and parts prevents skin from being burned or chilled (Younker Rehabilitation Center, 1990).*

▲ Teach or secure social service referrals to educate clients on financial coverage/regulations of third-party payors and HCFA for durable medical equipment. Realize that light and ultralight wheelchairs are easier to propel and are more comfortable and adjustable than heavier models. They are expensive, but over time cost less to operate than heavier chairs. *It is important to recognize the advantages, cost, and durability of different wheelchair models before deciding on a purchase (Cooper et al, 2000).*

- Teach the client the importance of using seatbelts or chair tie-downs when riding in motor vehicles. If unavailable, clients in wheelchairs should be transported in large, heavy vehicles. *Clients need restraint protection in case of abrupt vehicle maneuvers (Shaw, 2000).*

## evolve WEBSITES FOR EDUCATION

See the EVOLVE website for World Wide Web resources for client education.

## REFERENCES


Berg K, Hines M, Allen S: Wheelchair users at home: few modifications and many injurious falls, *Am J Pub Health* 92(1):48, 2002.

Berry BE, Ignash S: Assistive technology: providing independence for individuals with disabilities, *Rehabil Nurs* 28(1):6, 2003.

Boninger ML, Baldwin M, Cooper RA et al: Manual wheelchair pushrim biomechanics and axle position, *Arch Phys Med Rehabil* 81:608, 2000.

Brienza DM, Karg PE, Geyer MJ et al: The relationship between pressure ulcer incidence and buttock-seat cushion interface pressure in at-risk elderly wheelchair users, *Arch Phys Med Rehabil* 82(4):529, 2001.

Buning ME, Angelo JA, Schmeler MR: Occupational performance and the transition to powered mobility: a pilot study, *Am J Occup Ther* 55(3): 339, 2001.

Cooper RA, Schmeler MR, Cooper R et al: Long-term rehab: advanced seating systems, parts I and II, *Rehab Manag* 13(2-3):58, 2000.

Cooper RA, Cooper R, Boninger ML: Push for power, *Rehab Manag* 17(2):32, 2004.

Congress of Neurological Surgeons: Medical student curriculum in neurosurgery: diagnosis and management of peripheral nerve injury and entrapment. Available at www.neurosurgery.org/cns/meetings/curriculum/dl.html.

Cox, DI: Not your parent's wheelchair, *Rehab Manag* 17(7):26, 2004.

Crane B, Hobson D: Room for discussion, *Rehab Manag* 16(1):30, 2003.

Curtis KA, Drysdale GA, Lanza RD et al: Shoulder pain in wheelchair users with tetraplegia and paraplegia, *Arch Phys Med Rehabil* 80(4):453, 1999.

Defloor T, Grypdonck MH: Sitting posture and prevention of pressure ulcers, *Appl Nurs Res* 12(3):136, 1999.

Dowswell G, Dowswell T, Young J: Adjusting stroke patients' poor position: an observational study, *J Adv Nurs* 32(2):286, 2000.

Gavin-Dreschnack, D: Effects of wheelchair posture on patient safety, *Rehabil Nurs*, 29(6):221, 2004.

Gee ZL, Passarella PM: *Nursing care of the stroke patient: therapeutic approach*, Pittsburgh, 1985, America Rehabilitation Educational Network.

Halm M: Altered tissue perfusion. In Maas ML et al, editors: *Nursing care of older adults: diagnoses, outcomes, and interventions,* St Louis, 2001, Mosby.

Kirby RL, Dupuis DJ, Macphee AH et al: The wheelchair skills test (version 2.4): measurement properties, *Arch Phys Med Rehabil* 85(5):794, 2004.

Koontz AM, Bonninger M: Proper propulsion, *Rehab Manag* 16(6):18, 2003.

Kurfuerst S, Chew F: Cushion conclusions, *Rehab Manag* 16(7):52, 2003.

McCourt A: *The specialty practice of rehabilitation nursing: a core curriculum,* ed 3, Skokie, Ill, 1993, Rehabilitation Nursing Foundation.

Minkel JL: Seating and mobility considerations for people with spinal cord injury, *Phys Ther* 80(7):701, 2000.

Minkel JL: Sitting outside of the box, *Rehab Manag* 14(8):50, 2001.

Minor MAD, Minor SD: *Patient care skills,* ed 4, Stamford, Conn, 1999, Appleton and Lange.

Nyland J, Quigley P, Huang C et al: Preserving transfer independence among individuals with spinal cord injury, *Spinal Cord* 38: 649, 2000.

Paleg G: The prevention struggle, *Rehab Manag* 15(8):40, 2002.

Pellow TR: A comparison of interface pressure readings to wheelchair cushions and positioning: a pilot study, *Can J Occup Ther* 66(3):140, 1999.

Pierce LL: Barriers to access: frustrations of people who use a wheelchair for full-time mobility, *Rehabil Nurs* 23(3):120, 1998.

Rader J, Jones D, Miller LL: Individualized wheelchair seating: reducing restraints and improving comfort and function, *Top Geriatr Rehabil* 15(2):34, 1999.

Radwanski MB: Gerontological rehabilitation nursing. In Hoeman SP, editor: *Rehabilitation nursing: process, application, and outcomes,* ed 3, St Louis, 2002, Mosby.




M

Samuelsson K, Larsson H, Thyberg M et al: Wheelchair seating intervention. Results from a client-centered approach, *Disabil Rehabil* 23(15):677, 2001.

Saur T: Long-term rehab: seating and positioning in the newly injured, *Rehab Manag* 12(6):70, 1999.

Sawatzky BJ, Denison I, Kim W: Rolling, rolling, rolling, *Rehab Manag* 15(6):36, 2002.

Shaw G: Wheelchair rider risk in motor vehicles: a technical note, *J Rehabil Res Dev* 37(1):89, 2000.

Skidmore-Roth L: *Mosby's nursing drug reference,* St Louis, 2001, Mosby.

Swaine JM: Seeing the difference, *Rehab Manag* 16(9):26, 2003.

Taylor SJ: An overview of evaluation for wheelchair seating for people who have had strokes, *Top Stroke Rehabil* 10(1):95, 2003.

Wilson G, Kerr VL: Wheelchairs: selection, uses, adaptation, and maintenance. In Sine RD et al, editors: *Basic rehabilitation techniques: a self-instructional guide,* ed 3, Gaithersburg, Md, 1988, Aspen.

Yearns MH, Huntoon R: *A home for all ages: convenient, comfortable, and attractive,* handout for 47th Annual Conference of the National Council on the Aging, HDFS-H-294, March 1997.

Wound, Ostomy, and Continence Nurses Society (WOCN): *Guideline for prevention and management of pressure ulcers* (WOCN clinical practice guideline, no 2), Glenview, Ill, 2003, The Society.

Younker Rehabilitation Center: *Wheelchair mobility class: do's and don'ts,* Physical Therapy Patient Teaching Sheet, no 105, 1990. (Available from Younker Rehabilitation Center, Iowa Health System, 1200 Pleasant, Des Moines, IA 50309.)


# Nausea

evolve

*Betty J. Ackley and Gail B. Ladwig*

**NANDA**

## Definition

N

A subjective unpleasant wavelike sensation in the back of the throat, epigastrium, or throughout the abdomen that may lead to the urge or need to vomit

## Defining Characteristics

Usually precedes vomiting, but may be experienced after vomiting or when vomiting does not occur; accompanied by pallor, cold and clammy skin, increased salivation, tachycardia, gastric stasis, and diarrhea; accompanied by swallowing movements affected by skeletal muscles; reports "nausea" or "sick to stomach"

## Related Factors (r/t)

### Treatment related

Gastric irritation: pharmaceuticals (e.g., aspirin, nonsteroidal anti-inflammatory drugs [NSAIDS], steroids, antibiotics), alcohol, iron, and blood, gastric distention: delayed gastric emptying caused by pharmacological interventions (e.g., narcotics administration, anesthesia agents), pharmaceuticals (e.g., analgesics, antiviral for human immunodeficiency virus [HIV], aspirin, opioids, chemotherapeutic agents), toxins (e.g., radiotherapy)

### Biophysical

Biochemical disorders (e.g., uremia, diabetic ketoacidosis, pregnancy), cardiac pain, cancer of stomach or intraabdominal tumors (e.g., pelvic or colorectal cancers), esophageal or pancreatic disease, gastric distention due to delayed gastric emptying, pyloric intestinal obstruction, genitourinary and biliary distention, upper bowel stasis, compression of the stomach (liver, spleen, or other organ enlargement that slows the stomach functioning (squashed stomach syndrome), excess food intake, gastric irritation due to pharyngeal and/or peritoneal inflammation, liver or splenetic capsule stretch, local tumors (e.g., acoustic neuroma, primary or secondary brain tumors, bone metastases at base of skull), motion sickness, Menière's disease, or labyrinthitis

### Physical factors

Examples included increased intracranial pressure, meningitis, and toxins (e.g., tumor-produced peptides, abnormal metabolites due to cancer)

### Situational

Psychological factors (e.g., pain, fear, anxiety, noxious odors, taste, unpleasant visual stimulation)

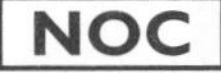

## Outcomes (Nursing Outcomes Classification)

### Suggested NOC Outcomes

Comfort Level; Hydration; Nausea and Vomiting Severity; Nutritional Status: Food and Fluid Intake, Nutrient Intake

**Example NOC Outcome with Indicators**

**Nausea and Vomiting Severity** as evidenced by the following indicators: Frequency of nausea/Intensity of nausea/Distress of nausea (Rate each indicator of **Nausea and Vomiting Severity:** 1 = severe, 2 = substantial, 3 = moderate, 4 = mild, 5 = none [see Section I].)

N

## Client Outcomes

### Client Will (Specify Time Frame):

- State relief of nausea
- Explain methods they can use to decrease nausea and vomiting (N&V)

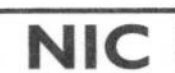

## Interventions (Nursing Interventions Classification)

### Suggested NIC Interventions

Distraction, Medication Administration, Progressive Muscle Relaxation, Simple Guided Imagery, Therapeutic Touch

**Example NIC Activities—Distraction**

Encourage the client to choose the distraction technique(s) desired, such as music, engaging in conversation or telling a detailed account of event or story, guided imagery, or humor; advise the client to practice the distraction technique before it is needed, if possible

## Nursing Interventions and Rationales

- Determine cause of N&V (e.g., medication effects, viral illness, food poisoning, extreme anxiety, anesthetic agents, pregnancy). *Since most episodes of N&V are now preventable, it is important for the cause to be determined (Garrett et al, 2003).*
- Provide distraction from sensation of nausea using soft music, television, and videos per the client preference. *Distraction can help direct attention away from the sensation of nausea (Garrett et al, 2003).* **EBN:** *Music therapy has been shown to decrease N&V in chemotherapy clients (Ezzone et al, 1998).*
- Apply a cold washcloth to the forehead of a nauseated client. *This is a distraction technique to help the client deal with nausea.*
- ▲ Apply supplemental oxygen if ordered. **EB:** *The use of supplemental oxygen has been shown to decrease nausea and vomiting in trauma clients during ambulance transport (Kober et al, 2002) and also postoperative clients (Greif et al, 1999).*
- Maintain a quiet, well-ventilated environment free of strong odors from food, perfume or cleaning solutions. *Odors can cause or exacerbate N & V (Garrett et al, 2003).*
- Avoid sudden movement of the client; allow the client to lie still. *Movement can trigger further N&V (Garrett et al, 2003).*
- If nausea is associated with frequent vomiting, assess client for fluid and electrolyte imbalances. *Protracted vomiting can cause hyponatremia, hypokalemia, or dehydration (Garrett et al, 2003).*
- Keep a clean emesis basin and tissues within the client's reach.
- Provide oral care after the client vomits. *Oral care helps remove the taste and smell of vomitus, thus reducing the stimulus for further vomiting.*

- Stay with the client to give support, place hand on shoulder, and hold the emesis basin. *Human support can be helpful and comforting to an uncomfortable client.* **EBN:** *A study demonstrated that clients with nausea that received purposeful touch as an intervention, had decreased nausea (Dune, 2002).*
- After vomiting is controlled and nausea abates, begin offering the client small amounts of clear fluids such as clear soda or preferably ginger ale, and then bland foods such as crackers or dry toast; progress to a soft diet. *Ginger root (found in some ginger ales) has been shown to be more effective than a placebo for treatment of postoperative N&V (Thompson, 1999).*
- Remove cover of food tray before bringing it into the client's room. *The sudden, concentrated food odors that come when the cover is removed in front of the client can trigger nausea (Quinton, 1998).*
- ▲ Refer clients with HIV for management of antiretroviral-related nausea. **EBN:** *A nursing study demonstrated that nausea associated with combination antiretroviral therapy was quite common and may adversely affect medication adherence (Reynolds & Neidig, 2002).*

### Nausea in Pregnancy

- Recommend that the woman eat dry crackers or dry toast in bed before arising and then get up slowly. Also advise to chew gum or suck hard candies, eat small frequent meals, avoid foods with offensive odors, and avoid preparing food or shopping when nauseated. *These are traditional strategies for alleviating nausea (Grodner, Long, & DeYoung, 2004).*

▲ Discuss with the primary care practitioner the possibility of using transcutaneous electrical stimulation in the form of Relief Band Device (Woodside Biomedical) to help relieve nausea. **EB:** *The results of a systematic review of the studies showed that the results of using P6 acupressure in pregnancy are equivocal (Jewell & Young, 2005).*

▲ Consider the use of continuous acupressure at P6 applied by Sea-Bands with acupressure buttons to both wrists or P6 acupressure. **EBN:** *Sea-Bands with acupressure buttons were demonstrated to be a noninvasive, inexpensive, safe, and effective treatment for the N&V of pregnancy (Steele et al, 2001).*

▲ Refer for acupuncture. **EB:** *Acupuncture is an effective treatment for women who experience nausea and dry retching in early pregnancy (Smith, Crowther, & Beilby, 2002).*

## Nausea Following Surgery

• Medicate the client for nausea as ordered. **EB:** *Antiemetic medications can reduce the incidence of postoperative nausea and vomiting (PONV), and use of more than one medication may be needed (Apfel et al, 2004).*

▲ Alleviate postoperative pain using ordered analgesic agents (refer to care plan for **Acute Pain**). *Pain sensation is known to be a factor in the development of postoperative N&V (Thompson, 1999).*

• Ensure that the nauseated client is not hypotensive. Check blood pressure and note signs of postural hypotension. *Postural hypotension can be caused by deficient fluid volume following surgery and can result in nausea (Garrett et al, 2003; Thompson, 1999).*

• Consider use of a recliner chair postoperatively if not contraindicated. **EBN:** *A study demonstrated that clients who used a recliner-chair postoperatively had fewer adverse symptoms such as nausea, severe pain, and delayed voiding (Agodoa et al, 2002).*

• Recommend that client sit down when experiencing nausea. **EB:** *Women undergoing gynecological surgery presenting with orthostatic dysregulation and arterial hypotension in their history exhibit an increased risk of PONV (Pusch et al, 2002).*

▲ Refer for possible use of isopropyl alcohol (IPA) inhalation for treatment of postoperative N&V for patients who have general anesthesia for a surgical procedure. **EBN:** *The results of this show IPA to be effective for postoperative N&V and that there was no significant difference between the standard treatment protocol or antiemetics and treatment with IPA. Treatment with IPA was significantly more cost effective than standard drug treatment (Merritt, Okyere, & Jasinski, 2002).*

▲ Consult with primary care practitioner for use of nonpharmacological techniques such as acupuncture, electroacupuncture, acupoint stimulation, or transcutaneous electrical nerve stimulation as an adjunct for controlling postoperative N&V. **EB:** *Nonpharmacological techniques demonstrated that they were equivalent to commonly used antiemetic drugs in preventing vomiting following surgery, especially within 6 hours of surgery in adults (Lee & Done, 1999). A study of the use of acupuncture for postoperative nausea and vomiting demonstrated a significant reduction in vomiting in postoperative gynecological surgery (Streitberger et al, 2004). P6 acupoint stimulation seems to reduce the risk of nausea in postoperative surgical patients (Lee & Done, 2005).*

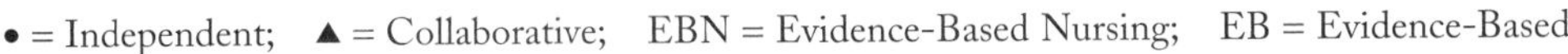
• = Independent; ▲ = Collaborative; EBN = Evidence-Based Nursing; EB = Evidence-Based

- ▲ Teach the use of acupressure on two acupressure points on the wrist. **EBN:** *This study confirmed the effectiveness of acupressure in preventing postoperative N&V (Ming et al, 2002).*
- • Use relaxation, imagery and distraction techniques for nausea: encourage the client to take slow, deep breaths. *Deep breaths can serve as a distraction technique and can help rid the body of the anesthetic agent (Thompson, 1999).*

### Nausea Following Chemotherapy

- ▲ Consult with physician regarding need for antiemetic medications either prophylactic or when N&V occurs. *N&V is among the most distressing side effects of chemotherapy (Bender et al, 2002). Preventing N&V is important; one serious bout can result in anticipatory nausea for the remainder of the client's treatments (Garrett et al, 2003).*
- ▲ Use antiemetics and a nursing intervention program of increased access to support and increased information. **EBN:** *In comparative antiemetic trials of 162 women with ovarian cancer receiving cisplatin-based chemotherapy, the group receiving antiemetics and the nursing intervention above reported less nausea (Borjeson et al, 2002).*
- ▲ If nausea is associated with the use of opioids, consult with primary care practitioner for possible use of alternative pain medication and consider the possible use of olanzapine as an antiemetic for advanced cancer patients. *Opiods can stimulate the vomiting center (Garrett et al, 2003).* **EB:** *This study suggests an antiemetic effect of olanzapine, an atypical antipsychotic, in patients with advanced cancer requiring opioid analgesics for pain (Passik et al, 2002).*
- ▲ Consult with primary care provider on the use of transcutaneous electrical nerve stimulation as an adjunct for controlling chemotherapy-induced N&V. *Antiemetic medications may stop vomiting, but not nausea (Roscoe et al, 2000). Transcutaneous electric nerve stimulation, using the ReliefBand, was shown to be an effective adjunct to medications for controlling nausea in gynecological oncology clients (Pearl et al, 1999).*
- • Help the client learn how to use acupressure for nausea, applying pressure bilaterally at P6 and ST36 acupressure points on the back of the wrist and by the knee. **EBN:** *Finger acupressure may be effective to relieve chemotherapy-induced nausea (Dibble et al, 2000). Research supports the use of acupressure along with antiemetic drugs, this is supported by a National Institutes of Health (NIH) consensus statement (Collins & Thomas, 2004).*
- ▲ For clients who continue to experience nausea after antiemetic drugs or other treatments, consult with the primary care practitioner regarding the possibility of using acupuncture or transcutaneous nerve stimulation wristband to control N&V. *Acupuncture has been shown to effectively control chemotherapy-induced N&V in adults (Collins & Thomas, 2004; Acupuncture, 2000). Nerve stimulation for this patient receiving methotrexate demonstrated it as a valid alternative to other first-line antiemetic therapies (Wilson, 2002).*
- • Offer the nauseated client a 10-minute foot massage. **EBN:** *Foot massage was shown to be an effective way to decrease nausea, pain, and anxiety in a group of oncology clients (Grealish, Lomasney, & Whiteman, 2000).*
- • If client has anticipatory nausea, utilize interventions such as education, relaxation therapy, imagery to help client decrease nausea associated with event. **EBN:** *Nurses are*

*in a position to identify clients at highest risk for developing anticipatory nausea and to implement strategies to prevent/minimize it (Eckert, 2001).*

### Geriatrics

- ▲ Administer antiemetic drugs carefully; watch for side effects. *Elderly clients have increased risk of side effects such as extrapyramidal effects or sedation from antiemetic drugs (Johnson et al, 1997).*
- ▲ Evaluate NSAIDs as a possible cause of nausea. *NSAIDs are commonly taken for arthritis pain in elderly clients and can cause nausea, as well as abdominal pain and ulcers (Peura, 2003).*

### Home Care

- • Above interventions may be adapted for home care use.
- ▲ Assess for causes of nausea in the hospice care client such as constipation, bowel obstruction, adverse effects of medications and onset of increased intracranial pressure, refer to primary care practitioner if needed. *There can be multiple causes of nausea in the client with advanced cancer (Haughney, 2004).*
- • Assist the client and family with identifying and avoiding irritants in the home setting that exacerbates nausea (e.g., strong odors from food, plants, perfume, and room deodorizers).

## Client/Family Teaching

- • Teach the client techniques to use when uncomfortable, including relaxation techniques, guided imagery, hypnosis, and music therapy (Garrett et al, 2003). **EBN:** *Eight Chinese breast cancer patients receiving doxorubicin and cyclophosphamide demonstrated that progressive muscle relaxation treatment is an effective adjuvant method to decrease N&V in chemotherapy recipients (Molassiotis, 2000). Guided imagery has been shown to effectively decrease nausea associated with chemotherapy (Troesch, 1993). Music therapy has been shown to be helpful for decreasing N&V in clients receiving high-dose chemotherapy (Ezzone et al, 1998).*

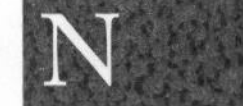

## evolve WEBSITES FOR EDUCATION

See the EVOLVE website for World Wide Web resources for client education.

## REFERENCES


Acupuncture: National Institutes of Health consensus development conference statement, *Dermatol Nurs* 12(2):126, 2000.

Agodoa SE, Holder MA, Fowler SM: Effects of recliner-chair versus traditional hospital bed on postsurgical diagnostic laparoscopic recovery time, *J Perianesth Nurs* 17(5):318, 2002.

Apfel CC, Korttila K, Abdalla M et al: A factorial trial of six interventions for the prevention of postoperative nausea and vomiting, *N Eng J Med* 350(24), 2441, 2004.

Bender CM, McDaniel RW, Murphy-Ende K et al: Chemotherapy-induced nausea and vomiting, *Clin J Oncol Nurs* 6(2):94, 2002.

Borjeson S, Hursti TJ, Tishelman C et al: Treatment of nausea and emesis during cancer chemotherapy. Discrepancies between antiemetic effect and well-being, *J Pain Sympt Manag* 24(3):345, 2002.

Collins KB, Thomas DJ: Acupuncture and acupressure for the management of chemotherapy-induced nausea and vomiting, *J Am Acad Nurse Pract* 16(2):76, 2004.
Dibble SL, Chapman J, Mack KA et al: Acupressure for nausea: results of a pilot study, *Oncol Nurs Forum* 27(1):41, 2000.
Dodd MJ: Side effects of cancer chemotherapy, *Annu Rev Nurs Res* 11:77, 1993.
Dune LS: Nausea relief and purposeful touch: decreasing distress by altering the perceptual field, Texas Woman's University PhD, Order No AA13046305, 2002.
Eckert RM: Understanding anticipatory nausea, *Oncol Nurs Forum* 28(10):1553, 2001.
Ezzone S, Baker C, Rosselet R et al: Music as an adjunct to antiemetic therapy, *Oncol Nurs Forum* 25(9):1551, 1998.
Garrett K, Tsuruta K, Walker S et al: Managing nausea and vomiting. Current strategies, *Crit Care Nurse* 23(1):31-50, 2003.
Grealish L, Lomasney A, Whiteman B: Foot massage: a nursing intervention to modify the distressing symptoms of pain and nausea in patients hospitalized with cancer, *Cancer Nurs* 23(3):237, 2000.
Greif R, Laciny S, Rapf B et al: Supplemental oxygen reduces the incidence of postoperative nausea and vomiting, *Anesthesiology* 91(5):1246, 1999.
Grodner M, Long S, DeYoung S: *Foundations and clinical applications of nutrition: a nursing approach*, ed 3, St Louis, 2004, Mosby.
Haughney A: Nausea and vomiting in end-stage cancer, *Am J Nurs* 104(11):40-48, 2004.
Jewell D, Young G: Interventions for nausea and vomiting in early pregnancy, *Cochrane Database Syst Rev* (4):CD000145, 2005.
Johnson MH, Moroney CE, Gay CF: Relieving nausea and vomiting in patients with cancer: a treatment algorithm, *Oncol Nurs Forum* 24(1):51, 1997.
Kober A, Fleischackl R, Scheck T et al: A randomized controlled trial of oxygen for reducing nausea and vomiting during emergency transport of patients older than 60 years with minor trauma, *Mayo Clinic Proceedings* 77(1):35, 2002.
Lee A, Done ML: Stimulation of the wrist acupuncture point P6 for preventing postoperative nausea and vomiting, *Cochrane Database Syst Rev* (3):CD003281, 2005.
Lee A, Done ML: The use of nonpharmacologic techniques to prevent postoperative nausea and vomiting: a meta-analysis, *Anesth Analg* 88(6):1362, 1999.
Merritt BA, Okyere CP, Jasinski DM: Isopropyl alcohol inhalation: alternative treatment of postoperative nausea and vomiting, *Nurs Res* 51(2):125, 2002.
Ming JL, Kuo BI, Lin JG et al: The efficacy of acupressure to prevent nausea and vomiting in post-operative patients, *J Adv Nurs* 39(4):343, 2002.

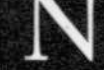

Molassiotis A: A pilot study of the use of progressive muscle relaxation training in the management of post-chemotherapy nausea and vomiting, *Eur J Cancer Care (Engl)* 9(4):230, 2000.
Morse JM, Bottorff JL, Hutchinson S: The phenomenology of comfort, *J Adv Nurs* 20:189, 1994.
Passik SD, Lundberg J, Kirsh KL et al: A pilot exploration of the antiemetic activity of olanzapine for the relief of nausea in patients with advanced cancer and pain, *J Pain Sympt Manag* 23(6):526, 2002.
Pearl ML, Fischer M, McCauley DL et al: Transcutaneous electrical nerve stimulation as an adjunct for controlling chemotherapy-induced nausea and vomiting in gynecologic oncology patients, *Cancer Nurs* 22(4):307, 1999.
Peura DA: Evaluating the approaches to safe and effective analgesia for older patients with arthiritis, *Adv Stud Med* 3(3):128, 2003.
Pusch F, Berger A, Wildling E et al: Preoperative orthostatic dysfunction is associated with an increased incidence of postoperative nausea and vomiting, *Anesthesiology* 96(6):1381, 2002.
Quinton D: Anticipatory nausea and vomiting in chemotherapy, *Prof Nurse* 13(10):663, 1998.
Reynolds NR, Neidig JL: Characteristics of nausea reported by HIV-infected patients initiating combination antiretroviral regimens, *Clin Nurs Res* 11(1):71, 2002.
Roscoe JA, Morrow GR, Hickok JT et al: Nausea and vomiting remain a significant clinical problem: trends over time in controlling chemotherapy-induced nausea and vomiting in 1413 patients treated in community clinical practices, *J Pain Sympt Manag* 20(2):113, 2000.
Smith C, Crowther C, Beilby J: Acupuncture to treat nausea and vomiting in early pregnancy: a randomized controlled trial, *Birth* 29(1):1, 2002.
Steele NM, French J, Gatherer-Boyles J et al: Effect of acupressure by Sea-Bands on nausea and vomiting of pregnancy, *J Obstet Gynecol Neonatal Nurs* 30(1):61, 2001.
Streitberger K, Diefenbacher M, Bauer A et al: Acupuncture compared to placebo-acupuncture for postoperative nausea and vomiting prophylaxis: a randomized placebo-controlled patient and observer blind trial, *Anaesthesia* 59(2):142, 2004.
Thompson HJ: The management of post-operative nausea and vomiting, *J Adv Nurs* 29(5):1130, 1999.

Troesch LM, Rodehaver CB, Delaney EA et al: The influence of guided imagery on chemotherapy-related nausea and vomiting, *Oncol Nurs Forum* 20:1179, 1993.
Wilson JK, Phelps KC, Feldman SR: Use of transcutaneous nerve stimulation wristband to treat methotrexate-induced nausea, *J Cutan Med Surg* 6(6):551, 2002.

# Unilateral Neglect

*Betty J. Ackley*

**NANDA**

## Definition

Lack of awareness and attention to one side of the body

## Defining Characteristics

Consistent inattention to stimuli on an affected side, does not look toward affected side, inadequate positioning and/or safety precautions with regard to the affected side, inadequate self-care, leaves food on plate on the affected side

## Related Factors (r/t)

Effects of disturbed perceptual abilities (e.g., hemianopsia [one-sided blindness]), neurological illnesses, trauma

NOTE: Because the right hemisphere is dominant in directing attention, unilateral neglect is more common if neurological pathology occurs in the right hemisphere of the brain, which results in left-sided neglect (Katz et al, 2000). Also, unilateral neglect often occurs with damage to the right parietal lobe, the right frontal lobe, the thalamus, and basal ganglia (Pierce & Buxbaum, 2002).

**NOC**

## Outcomes (Nursing Outcomes Classification)

### Suggested NOC Outcomes

Body Image; Body Positioning: Self-Initiated; Mobility; Self-Care: Activities of Daily Living (ADLs)

**Example NOC Outcome with Indicators**

**Mobility** as evidenced by the following indicators: Balance/Coordination/Gait/Muscle movement (Rate each indicator of **Mobility:** 1 = severely compromised, 2 = substantially compromised, 3 = moderately compromised, 4 = mildly compromised, 5 = not compromised [see Section I].)

## Client Outcomes

**Client Will (Specify Time Frame):**

- Demonstrate techniques that can be used to minimize unilateral neglect
- Care for both sides of the body appropriately and keep affected side free from harm
- Return to the highest functioning level possible based on personal goals and abilities

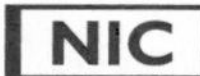

## Interventions (Nursing Interventions Classification)

### Suggested NIC Intervention

Unilateral Neglect Management

**Example NIC Activities—Unilateral Neglect Management**

Provide realistic feedback about patient's perceptual deficit; touch unaffected shoulder when initiating conversation

## Nursing Interventions and Rationales



- Monitor the client for signs of unilateral neglect (e.g., not washing, shaving, or dressing one side of the body; sitting or lying inappropriately on affected arm or leg; failing to respond to stimuli on the contralateral side of lesion; eating food on only one side of plate; or failing to look to one side of the body). *Looking, listening, touching, and searching deficits occur on the affected side of the body and may or may not be associated with a loss of vision, sensation, or motion on the affected side (Plummer, Morris, & Dunai, 2003).*
- If available, use the "star cancellation test" to evaluate presence of unilateral neglect. **EB:** *The star cancellation test consists of a series of big and little stars and words scattered on a page. When directed to cross out all the little stars, clients with unilateral neglect will miss stars on one side of the paper (Halligan et al, 1989; Taylor et al, 1994).*
- Use the Draw-A-Man test as a means of verifying the presence of unilateral neglect. **EB:** *The Draw-A-Man test is a valid and reliable method of determining clients who have unilateral neglect (Chen-Sea, 2000).*
- Use the wheelchair collision test for screening for behavior assessment of unilateral neglect; set up four round chairs in two rows and ask the client in a wheelchair to propel the wheelchair around the chairs. **EB:** *The wheelchair collision test is a simple screening test with reliability and validity to evaluate behavior unilateral neglect (Qiang et al, 2005).*
  *NOTE: Of the 62 assessment tools for evaluation of the presence of unilateral neglect, 28 of them are standardized (Jmenon & Korner-Bitensky, 2004.)*
- Provide a safe, well-lighted, and clutter-free environment. Place call light on unaffected side. Cue the client to environmental hazards when mobile. *Cognitive impairment may accompany neglect; safety is of paramount importance.*

- Nursing interventions for clients with unilateral neglect should be implemented in the following stages as the client progresses:
  - **Stage I:** Focus attention mainly on nonneglected side.
    - ❑ Set up environment so that most activity is on unaffected side.
    - ❑ Keep the client's personal items within view and on unaffected side.
    - ❑ Position the client's bed so that activity is on unaffected side.

  *The initial priority is client safety.*
  - **Stage II:** Help the client develop an awareness of neglected side.
    - ❑ Gradually focus the client's attention on affected side.
    - ❑ Gradually move personal items and activity to affected side.
    - ❑ Stand on the client's affected side when assisting with ambulation or ADLs.

  *The goal now is for the client to develop an awareness of the neglected side.*
  - **Stage III:** Help the client develop ability to compensate for neglect.
    - ❑ Encourage the client to bathe and groom affected side first.
    - ❑ Focus touch and talking on affected side; use a positive approach (e.g., "Mary, turn your head to the left and you'll see your daughter").
    - ❑ Use constant and positive reminders to keep the client scanning the entire environment.
    - ❑ Use bright yellow or red stickers on outer margins in reading or writing exercises. Have the client look for the sticker before reading or writing.
    - ❑ Help the client do ordinary tasks, compensating for their neglect situation. Use cues and anchors to promote attention to the neglected side and help the client develop compensatory mechanisms to deal with the neglect syndrome (Kalbach, 1991).

  *Care of clients with unilateral neglect includes providing stimuli on the affected side of the body, especially task-oriented activities which encourage the client to look towards the affected side (Carr & Sheperd, 2002).* **EB:** *A study demonstrated that clients discovered and gradually compensated for their unilateral neglect during meaningful occupational or life situations (Tham, Borell, & Gustavsson, 2000).*
- Recognize that unilateral neglect can improve following a stroke, and it is practical to postpone evaluation until 2 weeks after a stroke. **EB:** *A study demonstrated that neglect diminished within 6 months, but only 13% of the subjects studied had complete recovery (Appelros et al, 2004).*

▲ Refer to a rehabilitation team including a nurse rehabilitation specialist, a neuropsychologist, an occupational therapist, and physical therapist for continued help in dealing with unilateral neglect. *A number of different treatments for unilateral neglect are effective; others show limited evidence of lasting improvement (Pierce & Buxbaum, 2002; Gottlieb & Miesner, 2004). Both the occupational therapist and the neuropsychologist can help ameliorate symptoms of unilateral neglect (Freeman, 2001).* **EB:** *Research has shown that there is some evidence that cognitive rehabilitation for unilateral spatial neglect improves performance, but its effect on disability is not clear. Further studies are needed (Bowen, Lincoln, & Dewey, 2002).*

▲ Refer client to an opthmologist who specializes in low vision rehabilitation. By use of specialized glasses with built in prisms, more normal vision may be restored. *The specialized glasses work to increase vision to allow the client to be more independent (Gottlieb & Miesner, 2004).*

### Home Care

- Many of the listed interventions may be adapted for use in the home care setting.
- Position bed at home so that client gets out of bed on unaffected side. *Positioning the bed so that the client gets out on the unaffected side can increase safety.*

### Client/Family Teaching

- Explain pathology and symptoms of unilateral neglect to both the client and family.
- Teach the client how to scan regularly to check the position of body parts and to regularly turn head from side to side for safety when ambulating, using a wheelchair, or doing other tasks. Recommend the client think of self like a horizon-illuminating lighthouse. **EB:** *The use of the visual image of being a lighthouse was shown to improve function in a neglect client when walking, using a wheelchair, or engaging in problem-solving activities (Niemeier, Cifu, & Kishore, 2001).*
- Teach caregivers positive cueing (reminders to help the client remember to interact with entire environment).

## evolve WEBSITES FOR EDUCATION

See the EVOLVE website for World Wide Web resources for client education.

## REFERENCES


Appelros P et al: Recovery from unilateral neglect after right-hemisphere stroke, *Disabil Rehabil* 26(8):471, 2004.

Bowen A, Lincoln NB, Dewey M: Cognitive rehabilitation for spatial neglect following stroke, *Cochrane Database Syst Rev* (2):CD003586, 2002.

Carr JH, Shepherd RB: *Stroke rehabilitation—guidelines for exercise and training to optimize motor skill*, Boston, 2002, Butterworth-Heinemann.

Chen-Sea M: Unilateral neglect and functional significance among patients with stroke, *OTJR* 21(4):223, 2001.

Freeman E: Unilateral spatial neglect: new treatment approaches with potential application to occupational therapy, *Am J Occup Ther* 55:401, 2001.

Gottlieb DD, Miesner N: Innovative concepts in hemianopsia and complex visual loss-low vision rehabilitation for our older population, *Top Geriatr Rehabil* 20(3):212, 2004.

Halligan PW, Marshall JC, Wade DT: Visuospatial neglect: underlying factors and test sensitivity, *Lancet* 2(8668):908, 1989.

Kalbach LR: Unilateral neglect: mechanisms and nursing care, *J Neurosci Nurs* 23:125, 1991.

Katz N et al: Relationships of cognitive performance and daily function of clients following right hemisphere stroke: predictive and ecological validity of the LOTCA Battery, *Occup Ther J Res* 20(1):3, 2000.

Jmenon A, Korner-Bitensky N: Evaluating unilateral spatial neglect post stroke: working your way through the maze of assessment choices, *Top Stroke Rehabil* 11(3):41, 2004.

Niemeier JP, Cifu DX, Kishore R: The lighthouse strategy: improving the functional status of patients with unilateral neglect after stroke and brain injury using a visual imagery intervention, *Top Stroke Rehabil* 8(2):10, 2001.

Pierce SM, Buxbaum LJ: Treatments of unilateral neglect: a review, *Arch Phys Med Rehabil* 83:256, 2002.

Plummer P, Morris ME, Dunai J: Assessment of unilateral neglect, *Phys Ther* 83(8):732, 2003.

Qiang W, Sonoda S, Suzuki M et al: Reliability and validity of a wheelchair collision test for screening behavior assessment of unilateral neglect after stroke, *Am J Phys Med Rehabil* 84(3):161, 2005.

Riddoch MF, Humphreys GW: The effect of cueing on unilateral neglect, *Neuropsychologist* 21:589, 1983.

Taylor D, Ashburn A, Ward CD: Asymmetrical trunk posture, unilateral neglect and motor performance following stroke, *Clin Rehabil* 8:48, 1994.

Tham K, Borell L, Gustavsson A: The discovery of disability: a phenomenological study of unilateral neglect, *Am J Occup Ther* 54, 398-406, 2000.

# Noncompliance

*Betty J. Ackley and Gail B. Ladwig*

**NANDA**

## Definition

Behavior of person and/or caregiver that fails to coincide with a health-promoting or therapeutic plan agreed on by the person (and/or family and/or community) and health care professional; in the presence of an agreed-on, health-promoting, or therapeutic plan, person's or caregiver's behavior is fully or partially nonadherent and may lead to clinically ineffective or partially ineffective outcomes

## Defining Characteristics

Behavior indicative of failure to adhere (directly observed or verbalized by patient or significant others) (critical); objective tests (e.g., physiological measures, detection of physiological markers); evidence of development of complications; evidence of exacerbation of symptoms; failure to keep appointments; failure to progress

## Related Factors (r/t)

### Health Care Plan

Duration, significant others, cost, intensity, complexity

### Individual Factors

Personal and developmental abilities; health beliefs, cultural influences, spiritual values; individual's value system; knowledge and skill relevant to the regimen behavior; motivational forces

### Health System

Satisfaction with care, credibility of provider, access and convenience of care, financial flexibility of plan, client-provider relationships, provider reimbursement of teaching and follow-up, provider continuity and regular follow-up, individual health coverage, communication and teaching skills of the provider

### Network

Involvement of members in health plan; social value regarding plan; perceived beliefs of significant others

NOTE: The nursing diagnosis **Noncompliance** is judgmental and places blame on the client (Ward-Collins, 1998). The authors recommend use of the diagnosis **Ineffective Therapeutic regimen management** in place of the diagnosis **Noncompliance.** The diagnosis **Ineffective Therapeutic regimen management** has interventions that are developed by both the health care providers and the client. It is a more respectful and efficacious nursing diagnosis than **Noncompliance.**

NOC

## Outcomes (Nursing Outcomes Classification)

### Suggested NOC Outcomes

Adherence Behavior, Compliance Behavior, Pain Level, Symptom Control, Treatment Behavior: Illness or Injury

**Example NOC Outcome with Indicators**

**Adherence Behavior** as evidenced by the following indicators: Uses strategies to maximize health/Uses strategies to eliminate unhealthy behavior/Provides rationale for adopting a health regimen/Uses strategies to eliminate unhealthy behavior (Rate each indicator of **Adherence Behavior:** 1 = never demonstrated, 2 = rarely demonstrated, 3 = sometimes demonstrated, 4 = often demonstrated, 5 = consistently demonstrated [see Section I].)

## Client Outcomes

**Client Will (Specify Time Frame):**

- Describe consequence of continued noncompliance with treatment regimen
- State goals for health and the means by which to obtain them
- Communicate an understanding of disease and treatment
- List treatment regimens and expectations and agree to follow through
- List alternative ways to meet goals
- Describe the importance of family participation to help achieve goals

N

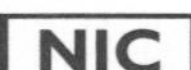

## Interventions (Nursing Interventions Classification)

### Suggested NIC Interventions

Health System Guidance; Self-Modification Assistance

**Example NIC Activities—Health System Guidance**

Inform the client of appropriate community resources and contact persons; inform the client how to access emergency services by telephone and vehicle, as appropriate

## Nursing Interventions and Rationales

- Ask the client why he or she has not complied with the prescribed treatment. Have the client "tell his or her story." Listen nonjudgmentally. *Compliance assessment should begin with a nonthreatening discussion with the client.*
- Make the client an active partner in his or her own health care management. Recognize that the client has absolute control over whether he or she follows the health care regimen. Always treat the client with respect, and develop mutual outcomes for treatment. *If the client feels respected and is involved in decision making, compliance will increase. Many clients report that how they are treated by health professionals has a great im-*

*pact on whether they follow advice (Lannon, 1997). The traditional paternalistic approach to health care results in many clients failing to follow the prescribed treatment (Tsoneva & Shaw, 2004).*

- • Work with the client to problem solve how to handle the illness and need for medications or prescribed care. **EBN:** *In clinical trials, it was shown that self-efficacy was enhanced when people solved problems that they themselves identified (Bodenheimer et al, 2002).*
- • If the client is in denial: provide information, communicate unconditional positive regard, avoid distancing yourself, and look for opportunities for authentic contact with your client, being present psychologically and physically. *The most important thing you can do for someone who appears to be in denial is to take the time to genuinely connect (Robinson, 1999).* **EBN:** *The relationship between the client and provider is very important in increasing adherence behavior (Russell, Krantz, & Neville, 2004).*
- • Observe for cause of noncompliance (see Related Factors). Recognize that noncompliance is very common. **EBN:** *Adherence to treatment among persons with chronic disorders constitutes a significant problem; half of clients have difficulty following their regimen (Dunbar-Jacob et al, 2000).*
- • Recognize that behavioral change comes slowly, and often in stages (Prochaska, 1994):
  - ■ Precontemplation—change is not contemplated; unaware of problem or risk
  - ■ Contemplation—aware that problem exists; no specific plans or commitment to change
  - ■ Preparation—plan to take action within the next 30 days
  - ■ Action—now taking action to improve health; often behavior not consistently carried out
  - ■ Maintenance—consistently engages in healthful behavior for more than 6 months

  *Individuals tend to cycle through the stages of change, often not in a linear progression, and may go through the cycle several times. The most important thing is unconditional acceptance of the person, understanding of the behavior, and subtle encouragement when asked. Make information available, but do not preach or force information on clients (Samuelson, 1998).*
- • Determine the client's and family's knowledge of illness and treatment. Teach them about the illness and purpose of the treatment regimen if necessary. *Knowledge is power, and with it comes increased control; the more control clients have, the more likely they are to comply with the prescribed regimen.*
- • Observe whether locus of control is internal or external for the client. Recognize that people with external locus of control are more likely to be noncompliant because they do not believe they can help themselves. They believe that it is a matter of luck or destiny that they are ill. *Clients with an internal locus of control are more compliant (Muscari, 1998).*
- ▲ Monitor the client for signs of depression that may cause noncompliance. Refer for treatment if appropriate. **EBN:** *Depression can cause increased incidence of "source memory errors," resulting in the client being unable to remember if he or she did something or just thought about doing it, which can be very serious when it involves taking needed medications (Elias, 2001). Depression can also cause apathy, in which case the client does not care whether he or she takes needed actions for health.*

N

- Monitor the client's ability to follow directions, solve problems, concentrate, and read. **EB:** *A national survey found that almost half of the adult population has deficiencies in reading or computation skills. Literacy is defined as the basic ability to read and speak English, whereas functional health literacy is the ability to read, understand, and act on health information. Up to 48% of English-speaking patients do not have adequate functional health literacy (Andrus & Roth, 2002).* **EB:** *More than 90 million Americans have limited literacy skills. Almost 2 million U.S. residents cannot speak English, and millions more speak it poorly (Dreger & Tremback, 2001).*
- Avoid using threats, pressure, and inappropriate fear arousal to increase compliance. *These measures are unethical and generally ineffective. If clients are "browbeaten" and attempts are made to shame, induce guilt, or embarrass the client, the noncompliant client will only dig deeper in his or her resolve not to change (Samuelson, 1998).*
- Determine whether the client's support system helps or hinders therapy. Bring family members and significant others into the educational process as desired by the client. **EB:** *Schizophrenic clients who have little family support are more likely to be noncompliant than are those with family support, especially if there is a history of substance abuse and difficulty recognizing own symptoms (Olfson et al, 2000).*
- Listen to the client's descriptions of abilities; encourage the client to use these abilities in self-care. When dealing with complex health care regimens, start the client with small behavioral changes (e.g., have chemotherapy client rinse mouth with a saliva substitute twice daily). When one step has been accomplished, add another step. *The client is often overwhelmed by what is expected and needs help with managing behavioral changes (Boehm, 1992).*
- Work with the client to develop cues that trigger-needed health care behaviors (e.g., checking blood sugar level before putting on makeup each morning), including weekends, holidays, and vacations. *Associating cues with desired behaviors increases the frequency of these behaviors. Compliance often decreases when the client no longer has a usual routine.*
- Work with the client to develop an instruction and reminder sheet that fits medications and treatments into the client's lifestyle. *Visual reminders help increase compliance (Schlenk, Dunbar-Jacob, & Engberg, 2004).*
- Observe the noncompliant client for possibility of secondary gain such as increased attention if the client continues to be ill and noncompliant. *Adolescent clients may use noncompliance as a passive form of manipulation to control their relationships with others to avoid school, work, or the legal system. Also, sometimes the illness has become part of the client's self-concept and identity and therefore meets needs (Muscari, 1998).*

▲ Consider allowing the client to take his or her own medications while in the hospital if appropriate. *Clients who learned to take medications successfully in the hospital were less likely to be readmitted in a group of mental health clients (DeProspero & Riffle, 1997).*

- Develop a mutually agreed-on written contract with the client regarding needed health care behaviors; give reinforcement as the client meets defined goals. *A client contract that helps the client analyze behaviors and choose behavioral strategies can be very effective in changing health care behaviors (Boehm, 1992).* **EBN:** *The nursing intervention of*

N

*patient contracting provides a concrete means of keeping track of actions to meet health-related goals.*

▲ Consult with primary care practitioner regarding the possibility of simplifying the health care regimen so that it more easily fits into the client's lifestyle (e.g., taking medications one time per day versus four times per day). *Complex regimens and inconvenient dose scheduling decrease compliance (Crane, Kirby, & Kooperman, 1996).*

▲ Refer for compliance therapy (motivational interviewing and cognitive behavioral therapy) for medication management for clients with schizophrenia. **EBN:** *Failure to keep up their antipsychotic medication is a major cause of relapse in people with psychosis. Compliance therapy is effective in enhancing concordance and reducing the risk of relapse (Gray, Robson, & Bressington, 2002).* **EBN:** *Compliance therapy, based on cognitive-behavioral techniques, appears to be effective in enhancing compliance and preventing relapse in people with schizophrenia on antipsychotic medication (Gray, Wykes, & Gournay, 2002; White, 2004).*

## Geriatric

• Make the client an explicit medication instruction using bulleted lists and simple icons. **EB:** *Several studies have demonstrated that use of a medication schedule increased compliance (Esposito, 1995; Raynor, Booth, & Blenkinsopp, 1993).*

▲ If the client has sensory and coordination deficits, use a medication organizer and have the home health nurse or family place the client's medications in daily compartments. *Careful labeling, self-administration of medicine programs, simplification of drug regimens, and the use of medication compliance devices can help promote patient adherence in older patients (McGraw & Drennan, 2001).*

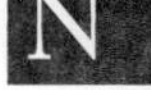

• Help the client feel like a partner in managing health care condition; use caring, encouragement, written goals, and a "power with" relationship with nurse. **EBN:** *These methods have been shown to increase self-efficacy and empower elderly clients to manage their condition (Muscari, 1998; Resnick, 1996).*

▲ Ask clients if they can afford medications. Refer for financial help from social worker or case manager if needed. **EB:** *A small but growing proportion of Americans are unable to afford prescribed medications (Kennedy, Coyne, & Sclar, 2004).*

▲ Monitor the client for signs of depression associated with noncompliance (e.g., refusing to eat or take medications). Refer the client for treatment of depression as needed. *Noncompliance in the elderly may be a form of indirect self-destructive behavior that is associated with depression and leads to suicide (Meisekothen, 1993).* **EBN:** *One study demonstrated that depressed clients were three times more likely than nondepressed clients to be noncompliant (DiMatteo, Lepper, & Croghan, 2000).*

• Use repetition, verbal cues, and memory aids such as pictures, schedule, or reminder sheet when teaching the health care regimen. Use events such as meals, bedtime, and so on, as reminders when to take medications. **EBN:** *There may be age-related memory deficits that necessitate an increased use of measures that cue the client to perform needed health care behaviors (Dunbar-Jacob et al, 2000). This research demonstrated that older adults reported greater use of internal memory strategies and a preference for event-based over time-based prescription medication instructions (Branin, 2001).*

- Consider assistive medication technology: talking reminders, pill dispensers, and so on. *Elderly clients are relying on technology to help them adhere to increasingly complex medication regimens (Logue, 2002; Schlenk, Dunbar-Jacob, & Engberg, 2004).*

## Multicultural

- Assess for the influence of cultural beliefs, norms, and values on the client's ability to modify health behavior. **EBN:** *What the client considers normal and abnormal health behavior may be based on cultural perceptions (Cochran, 1998; Doswell & Erlen, 1998; Leininger & McFarland, 2002). Adherence to medical treatment is influenced by the person's health beliefs, health practices, specific disease, treatment time frame, medication regimen, and cognitive-affective status, worldview, and language (Barron et al, 2004). Minority patients expressed concerns and barriers to adherence that included cost, difficulty of obtaining medication, daily life hassles, and a general distrust of the medical establishment (Bender & Bender, 2005).*
- Discuss with the client those aspects of their health behavior/lifestyle that will remain unchanged by their health status. **EBN:** *Aspects of the client's life that are meaningful and valuable to him or her should be understood and preserved without change (Leininger & McFarland, 2002).*
- Negotiate with the client regarding the aspects of health behavior that will need to be modified. **EBN:** *Give and take with the client will lead to culturally congruent care (Leininger & McFarland, 2002).*
- Assess the role of fatalism on the client's ability to modify health behavior. **EBN:** *Fatalistic perspectives, which involve the belief that you cannot control your own fate, may influence health behaviors in some African-American and Latino populations (Chen, 2001; Harmon et al, 1996; Phillips et al, 1999).*
- Validate the client's feelings regarding the impact of health status on current lifestyle. **EBN:** *Validation is therapeutic communication technique that lets the client know that the nurse has heard and understands what was said, and it promotes the nurse-client relationship (Heineken, 1998). Latinas' cognitions about medications were directly related to inadequate adherence (Arcia, Fernandez, & Jaquez, 2004).*
- Use mechanical reminders to cue patients as a means to improve adherence. **EBN:** *African-American and Hispanic women who used an electronic monitoring bottle for 6 months showed significant increases in adherence (Robbins et al, 2004).*

## Home Care

NOTE: Because the home care nurse enters the client's home as a guest, the ability of the nurse to establish a supportive, therapeutic relationship is especially important. A paradigm shift in nurses' view of noncompliance has been proposed, to include the recognition of clients as experts on their own lives, and the assessment of client social context to determine possible rationales for not following professional advice (Russell et al, 2003).

- Above interventions may be adapted for home care use.
- Before providing any care, review the Home Health Care Bill of Rights with the client, including the right to refuse treatment. *Identifying the rights of the client demonstrates respect of the health care system and its representatives for client wishes.*

- If included in agency policies and procedures, also review patient responsibilities with the client, which is often part of a printed Bill of Rights. *Reviewing responsibilities helps the client define roles of mutual respect and partnership with the health care provider.*
- When the client is noncompliant, redefine personal and health priorities (contract for services) with the client to determine alternative motivational strategies or health actions to meet health goals. *For clients to carry out desired health actions, they must perceive actions as beneficial to self and the cost of the health action as not being greater than the benefit (Rosenstock, 1974).*
- Institute self-care management to maximize client responsibility for own care. Refer to care plan for **Powerlessness. EB:** *Client participation in care has been increased by using multiple components of self-regulation in interventions for asthma, anxiety, and smoking (Clark, Gong, & Kaciroti, 2001; Clark & Nothwehr, 1997; Clark & Starr-Schneidkraut, 1994).*
- Elicit and answer questions respectfully regarding illness and treatment, correcting any misconceptions and highlighting the importance of assisting the client to incorporate treatment plan into daily lifestyle. Do not use medical jargon in explanations. *Living situations that may interfere with adherence include inability to afford medications and lack of available transportation. Factors important to compliance with prescribed medications have been identified as the client's perceptions of his or her disease and treatment, physician's perceptions, manner assumed by physician, language used to communicate with the client, the client's living situation, regular medication review, and continuity of health care provision (Claesson et al, 1999).*
- Explore barriers to medical regimen adherence. Review medications and treatment regularly for needed modifications. Take complaints of side effects seriously and serve as the client advocate to address changes as indicated. *The presence of uncomfortable side effects frequently motivates clients to deviate from the medication regimen. A discussion of treatment regimen with coronary heart disease noted that physicians do not always adhere to guideline recommendations; adherence to guidelines and long-term strategies would prompt use of the most effective agents with the lowest incidence of side effects, aiding client adherence (Erhardt, 1999). Older adults do not always take their antidepressant medications. They may not consider the medications helpful and may experience uncomfortable side effects. Their experience with the medications should be solicited (Prabhakaran & Butler, 2002).*

▲ If noncompliance compromises the client's health status, refer for psychiatric home health care services to assess the client's motivation and implement therapeutic regimen. **EBN:** *Psychiatric home care nurses can address issues relating to the client's nonadherence to treatment and inability to adjust to changes in health status. Behavioral interventions in the home can assist the client to participate more effectively in treatment plan (Patusky, Rodning, & Martinez-Kratz, 1996).*

▲ If noncompliant behavior continues and the client chooses not to cooperate with medical regimen, the home health care agency cannot continue to provide services. *Reimbursement guidelines and agency policies do not support the continued use of health care resources when the client makes an informed decision to not follow the prescribed regimen.*

- If care is to be terminated, identify all possible alternatives for the client, and assist with making an informed choice about future health actions. *Some regulatory guidelines require health care providers to give written notice of discontinuance of care using established time frames. Noncompliance and a plan for termination of care notwithstanding, it remains the goal and ethical responsibility of home health care providers to promote optimal wellness, independence, and safety.*
- Respect the wishes of terminally ill clients to refuse selected aspects of medical regimen. With terminally ill clients, do not terminate care. Provide those aspects of care that the client and family or caregivers will accept. *The goal of hospice care is to provide comfort and dignity in the dying process.*

## Client/Family Teaching

▲ Teach clients about medication side effects (e.g., mental changes, sexual dysfunction) so that they understand them and feel comfortable discussing them. *Many medications can cause side effects such as changes in mental function and impotence, which can lead to noncompliance.*

- Teach clients to control their "self-talk" by giving themselves positive messages that will be used to promote desired behaviors, such as taking medications and controlling food intake. **EBN:** *Self-talk has been shown to be a common motivating method for behavior changes (McSweeney, 1993).*

## evolve WEBSITES FOR EDUCATION



See the EVOLVE website for World Wide Web resources for client education.

## REFERENCES


Andrus MR, Roth MT: Health literacy: a review, *Pharmacotherapy* 22(3):282, 2002.

Arcia E, Fernandez MC, Jaquez M: Latina mothers' stances on stimulant medication: complexity, conflict, and compromise, *J Dev Behav Pediatr* 25(5):311-317, 2004.

Barron F, Hunter A, Mayo R et al: Acculturation and adherence: issues for health care providers working with clients of Mexican origin, *J Transcult Nurs* 15(4):331-337, 2004.

Bender BG, Bender SE: Patient-identified barriers to asthma treatment adherence: responses to interviews, focus groups, and questionnaires, *Immunol Allergy Clin North Am* 25(1):7-30, 2005.

Bodenheimer T, Lorig K, Holman H et al: Patient self-management of chronic disease in primary care, *JAMA* 288(19):2469, 2002.

Boehm S: Patient contracting. In Bulechek GM, McCloskey JC, editors: *Nursing interventions: essential nursing treatments,* Philadelphia, 1992, WB Saunders.

Branin JJ: The role of memory strategies in medication adherence among the elderly, *Home Healthcare Serv Q* 20(2):1, 2001.

Chen YC: Chinese values, health and nursing, *J Adv Nurs* 36(2):270, 2001.

Claesson S, Morrison A, Wertheimer AI et al: Compliance with prescribed drugs: challenges for the elderly population, *Pharm World Sci* 21(6):256, 1999.

Clark NM, Gong M, Kaciroti N: A model of self-regulation for control of chronic diseases, *Health Educ Behav* 28:769, 2001.

Clark NM, Nothwehr F: Self-management of asthma by adult patients, *Patient Educ Couns* 32:S5, 1997.

Clark NM, Starr-Schneidkraut NJ: Management of asthma by patients and families, *Am J Respir Crit Care Med* 149:S54, 1994.

Cochran M: Tears have no color, *Am J Nurs* 98(6):53, 1998.

Crane K, Kirby B, Kooperman D: Patient compliance for psychotropic medications, *J Psychosoc Nurs* 34(1):8, 1996.

DeProspero T, Riffle WA: Improving patients' drug compliance, *Psychiatr Serv* 48(11):1468, 1997.


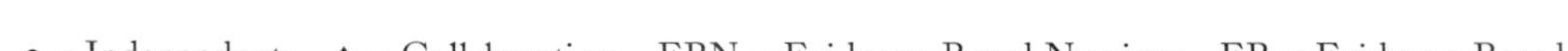

DiMatteo MR, Lepper HS, Croghan TW: Depression is a risk factor for noncompliance with medical treatment: meta-analysis of the effects of anxiety and depression on patient adherence, *J Psychosoc Nurs Ment Health Serv* 38(5):37, 2000.
Doswell W, Erlen J: Multicultural issues and ethical concerns in the delivery of revising care interventions, *Nurs Clin North Am* 33(2):353, 1998.
Dreger V, Tremback T: Optimize patient health by treating literacy and language barriers, *AORN J* 75(2):280, 2002.
Dunbar-Jacob J, Erlen JA, Schlenk EA et al: Adherence in chronic disease, *Annu Rev Nurs Res* 18:48, 2000.
Elias JW: Why caregiver depression and self-care abilities should be part of the PPS case mix methodology, *Home Healthc Nurse* 19(1):23, 2001.
Erhardt ER: The essence of effective treatment and compliance is simplicity, *Am J Hypertens* 12(10 Pt 2):105S, 1999.
Esposito L: The effects of medication education on adherence to medication regimens in an elderly population, *J Adv Nurs* 21:935, 1995.
Gray R, Robson D, Bressington D: Medication management for people with a diagnosis of schizophrenia, *Nurs Times* 98(47):38, 2002.
Gray R, Wykes T, Gournay K: From compliance to concordance: a review of the literature on interventions to enhance compliance with antipsychotic medication, *J Psychiatr Ment Health Nurs* 9(3):277, 2002.
Harmon MP, Castro FG, Coe K: Acculturation and cervical cancer: knowledge, beliefs, and behaviors of Hispanic women, *Women Health* 24(3):37, 1996.
Heineken J: Patient silence is not necessarily client satisfaction: communication in home care nursing, *Home Healthc Nurse* 16(2): 115, 1998.
Kennedy J, Coyne J, Sclar D: Drug affordability and prescription noncompliance in the United States: 1997-2002, *Clin Ther* 26(4):607, 2004.
Lannon SL: Using a health promotion model to enhance medication compliance, *J Neurosci Nurs* 29(3):170, 1997.
Leininger MM, McFarland MR: *Transcultural nursing: concepts, theories, research and practices,* ed 3, New York, 2002, McGraw-Hill.
Logue RM: Self-medication and the elderly: how technology can help, *Am J Nurs* 102(7):51, 2002.
McGraw C, Drennan V: Self-administration of medicine and older people, *Nurs Stand* 15(18):33, 2001.
McSweeney JC: Making behavior changes after a myocardial infarction, *West J Nurs Res* 15(4):441, 1993.
Meisekothen LM: Noncompliance in the elderly: a pathway to suicide, *J Am Acad Nurs Pract* 5(2):67, 1993.
Muscari ME: Rebels with a cause, *Am J Nurs* 98(12):26, 1998.
Olfson M, Mechanic D, Hansell S et al: Predicting medication noncompliance after hospital discharge among patients with schizophrenia, *Psychiatr Serv* 51(2):216, 2000.
Patusky KL, Rodning C, Martinez-Kratz M: Clinical lessons in psychiatric home care: a case study approach, *J Home Healthc Manag* 9:18, 1996.
Phillips JM, Cohen MZ, Moses G: Breast cancer screening and African American women: fear, fatalism, and silence, *Oncol Nurs Forum* 26(3):561, 1999.
Prabhakaran P, Butler R: What are older peoples' experiences of taking antidepressants? *J Affect Disord* 70:319, 2002.
Prochaska JO et al: *Changing for good: a revolutionary six stage program for overcoming bad habits and moving your life positively forward,* New York, 1994, Avon Books.
Raynor OK, Booth TG, Blenkinsopp A: Effects of computer generated reminder charts on patients' compliance with drug regimens, *BMJ* 306:1158, 1993.
Resnick B: Motivation in geriatric rehabilitation, *Image* 28(1):41, 1996.
Robinson AW: Getting to the heart of denial, *Am J Nurs* 99(5):38, 1999.
Robbins B, Rausch KJ, Garcia RI et al: Multicultural medication adherence: a comparative study, *J Gerontol Nurs* 30(7):25-32, 2004.
Rosenstock I: Health belief model and preventive behavior. In Becker M, editor: *The health belief model and personal health behavior,* Thorofare, NJ, 1974, CB Slack.
Russell J, Krantz S, Neville S: The patient-provider relationship and adherence to highly active antiretroviral therapy, *J Assoc Nurses AIDS Care* 15(5):40, 2004.
Russell S, Daly J, Hughes E et al: Nurses and 'difficult' patients: negotiating noncompliance, *J Adv Nurs* 43(3):281, 2003.
Samuelson M: Stages of change: from theory to practice, *Art Health Promotion* 2(5):1, 1998.
Schlenk EA, Dunbar-Jacob J, Engberg S: Medication non-adherence among older adults: a review of strategies and interventions for improvement, *J Gerontol Nursing* 30(7):33, 2004.

Tsoneva J, Shaw J: Understanding patients' beliefs and goals in medicine-taking, *Prof Nurse* 19(8):466-468, 2004.
Ward-Collins D: "Noncompliant": isn't there a better way to say it?, *AJN* 98(5):27-31, 1998.
White RB: Adherence to the dialysis prescription: partnering with patients for improved outcomes, *Nephrol Nurs J* 31(4):432, 2004.

# Readiness for enhanced Nutrition

*Betty J. Ackley*

**NANDA**

## Definition

A pattern of nutrient intake that is sufficient for meeting metabolic needs and can be strengthened

## Defining Characteristics

Expresses willingness to enhance nutrition; eats regularly; consumes adequate food and fluid; expresses knowledge of healthy food and fluid choices; follows an appropriate standard for intake (e.g., the food pyramid, U.S. Dietary Guidelines or America Diabetic Association guidelines); safe preparation and storage for food and fluids; attitude toward eating and drinking is congruent with health goals

N

## Related Factors (r/t)

Motivation to improve health through diet

**NOC**

## Outcomes (Nursing Outcomes Classification)

### Suggested NOC Outcomes

Nutritional Status; Nutritional Status: Food and Fluid Intake, Nutrient Intake; Weight Control

**Example NOC Outcome with Indicators**

**Nutritional Status** as evidenced by the following indicators: Food and fluid intake/Body mass index/Weight/height ratio/Hematocrit (Rate each indicator of **Nutritional Status:** 1 = severe deviation from normal range, 2 = substantial deviation from normal range, 3 = moderate deviation from normal range, 4 = mild deviation from normal range, 5 = no deviation from normal range [see Section I].)

## Client Outcomes

### Client Will (Specify Time Frame):

- Explain how to eat according to the U.S. Dietary Guidelines

- Design dietary modifications to meet individual long-term goal of health, using principles of variety, balance, and moderation
- Weigh within normal range for height and age

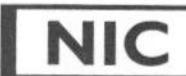

## Interventions (Nursing Interventions Classification)

### Suggested NIC Interventions

Nutrition Management, Nutritional Counseling, Weight Reduction Assistance

**Example NIC Activities—Nutrition Management**

Determine the client's motivation for changing eating habits; develop with the client a method to keep a daily record of intake

## Nursing Interventions and Rationales

- Ask the client to keep a one day to three day food diary where everything eaten or drank is recorded. Analyze the quality, quantity, and pattern of food intake. *Use of a food diary will be helpful for both the client and the nurse, to examine usual foods eaten and patterns of eating.* **EBN and EB:** *Self-monitoring helps the client assess adherence to self-determined performance criteria and progress toward desired goals. Self-monitoring serves an important role in the maintenance of internal standards of behavior (Fleury, 1991). Development of self-monitoring tools that meet the needs of clients increase dietary reporting and promote self-efficacy (Mossavar-Rahmani et al, 2004).*
- Advise the client to measure food periodically. Help the client learn usual portion sizes. *Measuring food alerts the client to normal portion sizes. Estimating amounts can be extremely inaccurate.* **EB:** *A study where women were served either larger portions, or more calorie dense foods in the same portion size demonstrated that extra calories were eaten, and the women subjects did not realize it and decrease their calories for dinner (Kral et al, 2004).*
- Help the client determine their body mass index (BMI). Use a chart or one of the formulas below:
  - Weight in kilograms divided by height (in meters) squared ($kg/m^2$)
  - Weight in pounds multiplied by 705, divided by height in inches, divided again by height in inches.

  *A normal BMI is 20 to 25, 26 to 29 is overweight, and a BMI of greater than 30 is obese (Nix, 2005). If BMI is greater than 25, refer to* **Imbalanced Nutrition: more than body requirements.**
- Recommend the client use the interactive Food Pyramid site at/www.MyPyramid.gov to determine the number of calories to eat and gain more information on how to eat in a healthy fashion.
- Recommend the client follow the Dietary Guidelines for Americans which can be found at www.healthierus.gov/dietaryguidelines. Use the Food Guide Pyramid to analyze the quality of the diet. *Dietary Guidelines are written by national experts and based on research in nutrition.*
- Recommend the client eat a healthy breakfast every morning. **EB:** *A study demonstrated*

*that people who skip breakfast are more likely to overeat in the evening (deCastro, 2004). Another study demonstrated that people who skipped breakfast were 450 times more likely to be obese (Ma et al, 2003).*

- Recommend the client avoid eating in fast food restaurants. **EB:** *A 15-year study demonstrated that people who frequently eat fast foods gain an average of 10 pounds more than those who eat fast food less often, and were two times more likely to develop insulin resistance which can lead to diabetes (Periera, 2005).*
- Review the client's current exercise level. With the client and primary health care provider, design a long-term exercise program. Encourage the client to adopt an exercise program that involves 45 minutes of exercise five times/week. *Exercise is important for increased energy expenditure, for maintenance of lean body mass, and as part of a total change in lifestyle, but a health risk appraisal should be performed on all previously sedentary individuals beginning a program of exercise (Lutz & Przytulski, 2001). Moderately intense physical activity for 30 to 45 minutes 5 to 7 days/week can expend the 1500 to 2000 calories/week that appear to be necessary to maintain weight loss. Cross-sectional and longitudinal studies illustrate that persons who increase their physical activity also increase their resting metabolic rate (Rippe & Hess, 1998).* Refer to care plan **Sedentary Lifestyle** for more interventions on increasing activity.
- Demonstrate the use of food labels to make healthful choices. Alert the client/family to focus on serving size, total fat, and simple carbohydrate. *The standardized food label in bold type simplifies the search for information. Fats and sugars contribute the least to a healthful diet and the most to excessive calorie intake. Generally clients should eat foods that are no more than 30% fat.*
- Determine the client's knowledge of the need for supplements. Discourage the client from taking excessive amounts of vitamins unless prescribed by a physician. *If the client eats a healthy diet, there is generally no need for supplementation. If the client is over age 50 years, one multivitamin per day is generally recommended.* **EB:** *A review of clinical trials concluded that antioxidant supplements are unlikely to reduce the risk of heart disease, and high doses of individual supplements can have adverse effects (Kris-Etherton et al, 2004). Another review of 14 randomized trial demonstrated that intake of antioxidant supplementation did not prevent gastrointestinal (GI) cancers, and intake seemed to increase mortality (Bjelakovic et al, 2004).*

N

## Carbohydrates

- Encourage the client to *decrease* intake of sugars including intake of soft drinks, desserts, and candy. Limit sugar intake to 12 teaspoons of added sugar daily. *Sugar predisposes to dental caries, and also is a source of calories that is empty of other nutrients (Cataldo, DeBruyne, & Whitney, 2003). A 20-ounce cola drink contains 17 teaspoons of sugar (Tufts University, 2004).* **EB:** *Consuming excessive amounts of fructose, which is used to sweeten soft drinks, and insufficient high-fiber grains is associated with development of type 2 diabetes (Wu et al, 2004).*
- Recommend the client eat whole grains whenever possible, and explain how to find whole grains using the food label. **EB:** *Intake of whole grains (3 servings per day) has been shown to decrease the incidence of type 2 diabetes in men and women (McKeown et al, 2002; Meyer et al, 2000). It has also been shown to decrease heart disease (Liu et al,*

*1999). Intake of refined grains in women was associated with an increased risk of hemorrhagic strokes (Oh, 2005).*

- Evaluate the client's usual intake of fiber. In general, high-fiber foods take longer to eat and contain fewer calories than most other foods. **EB:** *Increased dietary fiber was associated with lower body weight and waist-to-hip ratios, as well as predicted weight gain more strongly than did fat consumption (Ludwig et al, 1999; Slavin, 2005).*
- Recommend the client eat five to nine fruits and vegetables per day, with a minimum of two servings of fruit and three servings of vegetables. Encourage client to eat a rainbow of fruits and vegetables because bright colors are associated with increased nutrients. *Both fruits and vegetables are excellent sources of vitamins and also phytochemicals that help protect from disease.* **EB:** *An epidemiological study demonstrated a decreased incidence of cardiovascular disease deaths and overall mortality with an increased intake of fruits and vegetables (Bazzano et al, 2002). Intake of fruits and vegetables can help prevent heart disease, stroke, hypertension, high cholesterol, some types of cancer, diverticulitis and guard against cataract and macular degeneration (Hung, Joshipura, & Jiang, 2004).*

## Fats

- Recommend the client limit intake of saturated fats and *trans*-fatty acids; instead increase intake of vegetable oils such as canola oil, and olive oil. Limit fat intake to around 30% of total calories per day. *Intake of both saturated fat and trans-fatty acids raise the low-density lipoprotein (LDL) level, which predisposes to atherosclerosis. Trans-fatty acids also lower the high-density lipoproteins (HDL), which are thought to be protective against heart disease (Cataldo, DeBruyne, & Whitney, 2003).*
- Recommend client use low-fat choices when selecting and cooking meat, also when selecting diary products.
- Recommend that the client eat cold-water fish such as salmon, tuna, or mackerel at least two times per week to ensure adequate intake of omega-3 fatty acids. If unwilling to eat fish, suggest sources such as flaxseed, soy, or walnuts. NOTE: Fish oil capsules should be taken cautiously; some brands can be contaminated with mercury or pesticides. Intake of excessive omega-3 fatty acids can result in bleeding. **EB:** *Multiple studies have demonstrated that intake of omega-3 fatty acids by fish intake or fish oil capsules results in decreased incidence of sudden cardiac death (Albert et al, 2002a; Jones, 2002; Marchioli et al, 2002). A study demonstrated that consumption of fish was associated with a significantly reduced progression of coronary artery atherosclerosis in postmenopausal women with coronary artery disease (Erkkil et al, 2004). In addition, increasing intake of omega-3 fatty acids may be helpful in risk reduction for autoimmune disorders, some kinds of cancer, diabetes, and arthritis (Connor, 2000).*

## Protein

- Recommend the client decrease intake of red meat and processed meats, instead eat more poultry, fish, and dairy sources of protein. *Women who eat more red and processed meats, along with processed grains and increased sweets consumption, have higher rates of cerebrovascular accidents (CVAs) (Fung, 2004).*
- Recommend the client eat meatless meals at intervals and try alternative sources of protein, including nuts, especially almonds (one handful), and nut butters. **EB:** *Fre-*

*quent nut consumption was associated with a reduced risk of coronary heart disease in a study of registered nurses (Hu et al, 1998). Consumption of nuts and peanut butter was shown to probably decrease the incidence of type 2 diabetes in women (Jiang et al, 2002). In a study conducted on physicians, nut consumption demonstrated that those whose diet included the most nuts had the lowest risk of dying from heart disease (Albert et al, 2002b). An additional study demonstrated that intake of almonds to a regular diet resulted in decreased risk factors for cardiovascular disease and other chronic diseases (Jaceldo-Siegel et al, 2004).*

- Recommend the client eat beans and especially soy as an alternative to animal proteins at intervals. Introduce the client to soy products such as flavored soy milk. *Eating soy as a substitute for animal products reduces the incidence of coronary artery disease by reducing blood lipids, oxidized LDL, homocysteine, and blood pressure (Jenkins et al, 2002). NOTE: Women with diagnosed estrogen-dependent cancer of the breast should generally avoid eating soy foods.*

## Fluid and Electrolytes

- Recommend the client choose and prepare foods with less salt, aiming for a maximum of 2300 mg per day, which is approximately 1 teaspoon (Dietary Guidelines for Americans, 2005).
- If the client drinks alcohol, encourage him or her to drink in moderation—no more than one drink per day for women and two drinks per day for men. *Consuming more than a moderate amount of alcohol is one of the main causes of hypertension in both men and women (Krousel-Wood, 2004).*
- Recommend client increase intake of water, to at least 2000 mL or 2 quarts per day. A guideline is 1 to 1.5 mL of fluid per each calorie needed, so an average intake would be between 2000 and 3000 mL/day, or at least 8 cups of fluid (Grodner, Long, & DeYoung, 2004). *The adequate intake recommendation is 3 L for the 19- to 30-year-old male and 2.2 L for the 19- to 30-year-old female. Water balance studies suggest that adult men require 2.5 L per day (Institute of Medicine, 2004).*

N

## Geriatric

- Assess changes in lifestyle and eating patterns. *Energy needs decrease an estimated 5% per decade after age 40 years, but often, eating patterns remain unchanged from youth (Lutz & Przytulski, 2001).*
- ▲ Recommend the client discuss the need for a low-dose balanced multiple vitamin and mineral supplement with physician. *It is generally recommended that anyone over age 50 should take a multivitamin every day to ensure that adequate amounts of vitamins and minerals are obtained.* **EB:** *Some studies have demonstrated increased immunity and decreased rate of infections in older people who take a vitamin supplement (Chandra, 1997; Johnson & Porter, 1997).*
- Assess fluid intake. Recommend routine drinks of water regardless of whether thirsty. *The elderly are predisposed to deficient fluid volume because of decreased fluid in body, decreased thirst sensation, and decreased ability to concentrate urine (Bennett, 2000; Suhayda & Walton, 2002).*
- Observe for socioeconomic factors that influence food choices (e.g., funds, cooking fa-

cilities). *Even those on restricted budgets and with limited facilities can be assisted to choose food sources of a balanced diet.*

- Suggest a variety of seasonings. *The ability to taste sweet, bitter, sour, and salty declines in most, but not all, older persons (Morley, 1997).*

## Multicultural

- Assess for dietary intake of essential nutrients. **EBN:** *Studies have shown that African-American women have calcium intakes of less than 75% of the recommended daily allowance (RDA) (Zablah et al, 1999). Hispanics with type 2 diabetes also often have inadequate protein nutritional status (Castenada et al, 2000). Mexican-American women have a higher prevalence of iron-deficiency anemia than non-Hispanic white females (Frith-Terhune et al, 2000). Rural African-American men had low caloric intakes coupled with high fat intakes but nutrient deficiencies (Vitolins et al, 2000). African-American adolescents have some of the highest levels of vitamin D deficiency (Gordon et al, 2004).*
- Assess for the influence of cultural beliefs, norms, and values on the client's nutritional knowledge. *What the client considers normal dietary practices may be based on cultural perceptions (Cochran, 1998; Doswell & Erlen, 1998; Leininger & McFarland, 2002). Among African-Americans, there was a general perception that "eating healthfully" meant giving up part of their cultural heritage, trying to conform to the dominant culture, and the sense that friends and relatives usually were not supportive of dietary changes (James, 2004).*
- Discuss with the client those aspects of their diet that will remain unchanged. *Aspects of the client's life that are meaningful and valuable to them should be understood and preserved without change (Leininger & McFarland, 2002).*
- Determine the motivational factors operating within the client at the present time. **EBN:** *African-American women were motivated to increase their physical activity by personal and familial histories of heart disease and related risk factors (Banks-Wallace, 2000).*
- Negotiate with the client regarding the aspects of his or her diet that will need to be modified. *Give and take with the client will lead to culturally congruent care (Leininger & McFarland, 2002).*
- Explore strategies that appeal to the client. **EBN:** *Group interventions that include spiritual and community building may be especially effective for promoting physical activity among African-American woman (Banks-Wallace, 2000). African-American women tried more commercial diet products and ceased their weight loss efforts sooner than did European-American women (Tyler, Allan, & Alcozer, 1997). A recent study using the Parent as Teachers site to deliver a dietary change program via personal visits, newsletters, and group meetings was successful in reducing the percentage of calories from fat and increasing fruit and vegetable consumption among participating parents (Haire-Joshu et al, 2003).*
- Validate the client's feelings regarding the impact of current lifestyle, finances, and transportation on ability to obtain nutritious food. **EBN:** *Validation is therapeutic communication technique that lets the client know that the nurse has heard and understands what was said, and it promotes the nurse-client relationship (Heineken, 1998).*
- Encourage family meals. **EB:** *Frequency of family meals was positively associated with intake of fruits, vegetables, grains, and calcium-rich foods and negatively associated with soft drink consumption (Neumark-Sztainer et al, 2003).*

N

## Client/Family Teaching

- The majority of interventions above involve teaching.
- Work with the family members regarding information on how to improve nutritional status. *If the client and family select the nutritional plan, they are more likely to comply with it, particularly if the client does not do the marketing and cooking.*
- Teach the importance of exercise in a weight control program. *A physically conditioned person uses more fat for energy at rest and with exercise than a sedentary person does. The majority of patients will benefit from establishing walking as a cornerstone of their physical activity program (Rippe, Crossley, & Ringer, 1998).*

## evolve WEBSITES FOR EDUCATION

See the EVOLVE website for World Wide Web resources for client education.

## REFERENCES


Albert CM et al: Blood levels of long-chain n-3 fatty acids and the risk of sudden death, *N Engl J Med* 346(15):1113, 2002a.

Albert CM et al: Nut consumption and decreased risk of sudden cardiac death in the Physicians' Health Study, *Arch Intern Med* 162(2):1382, 2002b.

Banks-Wallace J: Staggering under the weight of responsibility: the impact of culture on physical activity among African American women, *Multicult Nurs Health* 6:24, 2000.

Bazzano LA et al: Fruit and vegetable intake and risk of cardiovascular disease in U.S. adults: the first National Health and Nutrition Examination Survey epidemiologic follow-up study, *Am J Clin Nutr* 76:1, 2002.

Bennett JA: Dehydration: hazards and benefits, *Geriatr Nurs* 21(2):84, 2000.

Bjelakovic G et al: Antioxidant supplements for prevention of gastrointestinal cancers: a systematic review and meta-analysis, *Lancet* 364(9441):1219, 2004.

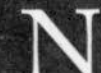

Castenada C, Bermudez OI, Tucker KL: Protein nutritional status and functions are associated with type II diabetes in Hispanic elders, *Am J Clin Nutr* 72(1):89, 2000.

Cataldo CB, DeBruyne LK, Whitney EN: *Nutrition and diet therapy,* Belmont, Calif, 2003, Thomason Wadsworth.

Chandra RD: Graying of the immune system: can nutrient supplements improve immunity in the elderly? *JAMA* 277:1398, 1997.

Cochran M: Tears have no color, *Am J Nurs* 98(6):53, 1998.

Connor WE: Importance of n-3 fatty acids in health and disease, *Am J Clin Nutr* 71(1 suppl):171S, 2000.

DeCastro JM: The time of day of food intake influences overall intake in humans, *J Nutr* 134(1), 2004.

Dietary Guidelines for Americans 2005. Available at www.healthierus.gov/dietary guidelines, accessed April 19, 2005.

Doswell W, Erlen J: Multicultural issues and ethical concerns in the delivery of revising care interventions, *Nurs Clin North Am* 33(2):353, 1998.

Erkkil AT et al: Fish intake is associated with a reduced progression of coronary artery atherosclerosis in postmenopausal women with coronary artery disease, *Am J Clin Nutr* 80(3):626, 2004.

Fleury J: Empowering potential: a story of wellness motivation, *Nurs Res* 40:288, 1991.

Frith-Terhune AL et al: Iron deficiency anemia: higher prevalence in Mexican American than in non-Hispanic white females in the third National Health and Nutrition Examination Survey, 1988-1994, *Am J Clin Nutr* 72(4):963, 2000.

Fung TT et al: Prospective study of major dietary paterns and stroke risk in women, *Stroke* 35(9):2014, 2004.

Gordon CM, DePeter KC, Feldman HA et al: Prevalence of vitamin D deficiency among healthy adolescents, *Arch Ped Ad Med* 158(6):531-537, 2004.

Haire-Joshu D, Brownson RC, Nanney MS et al: Improving dietary behavior in African Americans: the Parents As Teachers High 5, Low Fat Program, *Prev Med* 36(6):684-691, 2003.

Heineken J: Patient silence is not necessarily client satisfaction: communication in home care nursing, *Home Healthcare Nurse* 16(2):115, 1998.

Hu FB et al: Frequent nut consumption and risk of coronary heart disease in women: prospective cohort study, *BMJ* 317(7169): 1341, 1998.

Hung HC, Joshipura KJ, Jiang R: Fruit and vegetable intake and risk of major chronic disease, *J Natl Cancer Inst* 96:1577, 2004.

Institute of Medicine: Applications of dietary reference intakes for electrolytes and water, *National Academy of Sciences*, National Academies Press, 2004.

Jaceldo-Siegel K et al: Almond supplementation without advice on food replacement induces favourable nutrient modifications to the habitual diets of free-living individuals, *Br J Nutr* 92(3):533, 2004.

James DC: Factors influencing food choices, dietary intake, and nutrition-related attitudes among African Americans: application of a culturally sensitive model, *Ethn Health* 9(4):349-367, 2004.

Jenkins DJ et al: Effects of high-and low-isoflavone soyfoods on blood lipids, oxidized LDL, homocysteine, and blood pressure in hyperlipidemic men and women, *Am J Clin Nutr* 76(2):365, 2002.

Jiang R et al: Nut and peanut butter consumption and risk of type 2 diabetes in women, *JAMA* 288(20):2554, 2002.

Johnson MA, Porter KH: Micronutrient supplementation and infection in institutionalized elders, *Nutr Rev* 55:400, 1997.

Jones PJ: Effect of n-3 polyunsaturated fatty acids on risk reduction of sudden death, *Nutr Rev* 60:12, 2002.

Kral TV et al: Combined effects of energy density and portion size on energy intake in women, *Am J Clin Nutr* 79(6), 2004.

Kris-Etherton PM et al: Antioxidant vitamin supplements and cardiovascular disease, *Circulation* 110(5), 2004.

Krousel-Wood MA et al: Primary prevention of essential hypertension, *Med Clin North Am* 88(1):223, 2004.

Leininger MM, McFarland MR: *Transcultural nursing: concepts, theories, research and practices,* ed 3, New York, 2002, McGraw-Hill.

Liu S et al: Whole grain consumption and risk of coronary heart disease: results from the Nurses' Health Study, *Am J Clin Nutr* 70(3):412, 1999.

Ludwig DS et al: Dietary fiber, weight gain, and cardiovascular disease risk factors in young adults, *JAMA* 282:1539, 1999.

Lutz CA, Przytulski KR: *Nutrition and diet therapy,* ed 3, Philadelphia, 2001, FA Davis.

Ma Y et al: Association between eating patterns and obesity in a free-living U.S. adult population, *Am J Epidiomol,* 158(1):85, 2003.

Marchioli R et al: Early protection against sudden death by n-3 polyunsaturated fatty acids after myocardial infarction, *Circulation* 105(16):1987, 2002.

McKeown NM, Meigs JB, Liu S: Whole-grain intake is favorably associated with metabolic risk factors for type 2 diabetes and cardiovascular disease in the Framingham Offspring Study, *Am J Clin Nutr* 76:2, 2002.

Meyer KA et al: Carbohydrates, dietary fiber, and incident type 2 diabetes in older women, *Am J Clin Nutr* 71(4):921, 2000.

Morley JE: Anorexia of aging: physiologic and pathologic, *Am J Clin Nutr* 66:760, 1997.

Mossavar-Rahmani Y et al: Additional self-monitoring tools in the dietary modification component of the women's health initiative, *J Am Diet Assoc* 104(1):76, 2004.

Nonas CA: A model for chronic care of obesity through dietary treatment, *J Am Diet Assoc* 98(suppl 2):S16, 1998.

Neumark-Sztainer D et al: Family meal patterns: associations with sociodemographic characteristics and improved dietary intake among adolescents, *J Am Diet Assoc,* 103(3):317-322, 2003.

Oh K et al: Carbohydrate intake, glycemic index, glycemic load, and dietary fiber in relation to risk of stroke in women, *Am J Epidemiol* 161(2):161, 2005.

Pereira MA et al: Dietary fiber and risk of coronary heart disease: a pooled analysis of cohort studies, *Arch Intern Med* 164(4), 2004.

Pereira MA, Kartashov AI, Ebbeling CB et al: Fast-food habits, weight gain, and insulin resistance (the CARDIA study): 15-year prospective analysis, *Lancet* 365(9453):36, 2005.

Rippe JM, Crossley S, Ringer R: Obesity as a chronic disease: modern medical and lifestyle management, *Jam Diet Assoc* 98(suppl 2):S9, 1998.

Rippe JM, Hess S: The role of physical activity in the prevention and management of obesity, *J Am Diet Assoc* 98(Suppl 2): S31, 1998.

Slavin JL: Dietary fiber and body weight, *Nutrition* 21(3):411, 2005.

Suhayda R, Walton JC: Preventing and managing dehydration, *Medsurg Nurs* 11(6):267, 2002.

Tufts University: How much sugar is right? *Health and Nutrition Letter* 22(4), 2004.

Tyler DO, Allan JD, Alcozer FR: Weight loss methods used by African American and Euro American women, *Res Nurs Health* 20:413, 1997.

Vitolins MZ et al: Ethnic and gender variation in the dietary intake of rural elders, *J Nutr Elderly* 19(3):15, 2000.

Wu T et al: Fructose, glycemic load, and quantity and quality of carbohydrate in relation to plasma C-peptide concentrations in US women, *Am J Clin Nutr* 80(4), 2004.

Zablah EM et al: Barriers to calcium intake in African American women, *J Hum Nutr* 12(2):123, 1999.

N

# Imbalanced Nutrition: less than body requirements evolve

*Betty Ackley and Carroll A. Lutz*

## NANDA

### Definition

Intake of nutrients insufficient to meet metabolic needs

### Defining Characteristics

Body weight less than 20% under ideal weight; pale conjunctival and mucous membranes; weakness of muscles required for swallowing or mastication; sore, inflamed buccal cavity; satiety immediately after ingesting food; reported or evidence of lack of food; reported inadequate food intake less than RDA; reported altered taste sensation; perceived inability to ingest food; misconceptions; loss of weight with adequate food intake; aversion to eating; abdominal cramping; poor muscle tone; abdominal pain with or without pathology; lack of interest in food; capillary fragility; diarrhea and/or steatorrhea; excessive loss of hair; hyperactive bowel sounds; lack of information; misinformation

### Related Factors (r/t)

Inability to ingest or digest food or absorb nutrients because of biological, psychological, or economic factors

N

## NOC

### Outcomes (Nursing Outcomes Classification)

#### Suggested NOC Outcomes

Nutritional Status; Nutritional Status: Food and Fluid Intake, Nutrient Intake; Weight Control

#### Example NOC Outcome with Indicators

**Nutritional Status** as evidenced by the following indicators: Food and fluid intake/Body mass index/Weight/height ratio/Hematocrit (Rate each indicator of **Nutritional Status:** 1 = severe deviation from normal range, 2 = substantial deviation from normal range, 3 = moderate deviation from normal range, 4 = mild deviation from normal range, 5 = no deviation from normal range [see Section I].)

### Client Outcomes

**Client Will (Specify Time Frame):**

- Progressively gain weight toward desired goal
- Weigh within normal range for height and age
- Recognize factors contributing to underweight

- Identify nutritional requirements
- Consume adequate nourishment
- Be free of signs of malnutrition

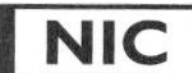

## Interventions (Nursing Interventions Classification)

### Suggested NIC Interventions

Eating Disorders Management; Electrolyte Management: Hypophosphatemia; Enteral Tube Feeding; Feeding; Nutrition Management; Nutrition Therapy; Nutritional Counseling; Nutritional Monitoring; Swallowing Therapy; Weight Gain Assistance; Weight Management

**Example NIC Activities—Nutrition Management**

Ascertain the client's food preferences; provide the client with high-protein, high-calorie, nutritious finger foods and drinks that can be readily consumed, as appropriate

## Nursing Interventions and Rationales

- • Monitor for signs of malnutrition including: brittle hair that is easily plucked, bruises, dry skin, pale skin and conjunctiva, muscle wasting, smooth red tongue, cheilosis, "flaky paint" rash over lower extremities, and disorientation (Kasper et al, 2005).
- • Note laboratory test results as available: serum albumin, serum total protein, serum ferritin, transferrin, hemoglobin, hematocrit, and electrolytes. *A serum albumin level of less than 3.5 is considered an indicator of risk of poor nutritional status (DiMaria-Ghaliili & Amella, 2005).*
- • Weigh the client daily in acute care, weekly in extended care under same conditions.
- ▲ Determine healthy body weight for age and height. Refer to dietitian for complete nutrition assessment if 10% under healthy body weight or if rapidly losing weight. *In the developed world, protein-calorie malnutrition (PCM) most often accompanies a disease process.*
- ▲ Monitor food intake; record percentages of served food that is eaten (25%, 50%); consult with dietitian for actual calorie count if needed.
- • Observe the client's relationship to food. Attempt to separate physical from psychological causes for eating difficulty. *It may be difficult to tell if the problem is physical or psychological. Refusing to eat may be the only way the client can express some control, and it may also be a symptom of depression.*
- • Compare usual food intake with the Food Guide Pyramid, noting slighted or omitted food groups. *Milk consumption has decreased among children while intake of fruit juices and carbonated beverages has increased.* **EB:** *A higher incidence of bone fractures in teenage girls has been associated with a greater consumption of carbonated beverages (Wyshak, 2000); possibly also related is the substitution of soda for milk. Omission of entire food groups increases risk of deficiencies.*

• = Independent; ▲ = Collaborative; EBN = Evidence-Based Nursing; EB = Evidence-Based

- If the client is a vegetarian, evaluate vitamin $B_{12}$ and iron intake. *Strict vegetarians may be at particular risk for vitamin $B_{12}$ and iron deficiencies. Special care should be taken when implementing vegetarian diets for pregnant women, infants, children, and the elderly. A dietitian can usually furnish a balanced vegetarian diet (with adequate substitutes for omitted foods) for inpatients and can provide instruction for outpatients.*
- Observe the client's ability to eat (time involved, motor skills, visual acuity, and ability to swallow various textures). *Clients in institutions are susceptible to protein-calorie malnutrition (PCM) or protein-energy malnutrition when they are unable to feed themselves.* **EB:** *Poor vision was associated with lower protein and energy (calorie) intakes in home care clients independent of other medical conditions (Payette et al, 1995).*

NOTE: If the client is unable to feed self, refer to Nursing Interventions and Rationales for **Feeding Self-care deficit.** If the client has difficulty swallowing, refer to Nursing Interventions and Rationales for **Impaired Swallowing.**

- ▲ If the client is recovering from a GI disorder such as gastroenteritis, surgery, previous obstruction and is malnourished, consult with dietitian regarding use of a clear liquid product that contains increased amounts of protein and calories such as citrotein, Boost Breeze, or Resource Fruit Beverage.
- For the client with anorexia, who will not eat foods, consider offering 30 mL of a nutritional supplement in a medication cup every hour. **EB:** *A Cochrane Review found that use of oral nutritional supplements was more effective than dietary advice from a dietitian, further studies are needed (Baldwin, Parsons, & Logan, 2001). An additional Cochrane Review demonstrated that there was a small but consistent weight gain along with a positive effect on mortality and a shorter length of hospital stay in elderly clients who received a nutritional supplement (Milne, Potter, & Avenell, 2005).*
- For the client who is malnourished, and can eat, offer small quantifies of food, served in an appetizing fashion, at frequent intervals. *Small, frequent feedings are often effective in getting food into clients who otherwise would not eat.*
- If the client lacks endurance, schedule rest periods before meals and open packages and cut up food for the client. *Nursing assistance with ADLs will conserve the client's energy for activities that the client values.*
- When the client is malnourished, watch carefully for signs of infection and maintain every action possible to protect the client from infection. *Protein-energy malnutrition is associated with a significant impairment of cell-mediated immunity (Chandra, 2002). Infection may result in confusion, anorexia, and negative nitrogen balance, all of which contribute to protein-energy malnutrition (Kamel et al, 1998).*
- Assess for recent changes in physiological status that may interfere with nutrition. *The consequences of malnutrition can lead to a further decline in the patient's condition that then becomes self-perpetuating if not recognized and treated. Extreme cases of malnutrition can lead to septicemia, organ failure, and death (Arrowsmith, 1997).*
- If the client is pregnant, ensure that she is receiving adequate amounts of folic acid by eating a balanced diet and taking prenatal vitamins as ordered. *All women of childbearing potential are urged to consume 400 mcg of synthetic folic acid from fortified foods or supplements in addition to food folate from a varied diet (National Academy of Sciences, 1998).*

- • Provide companionship at mealtime to encourage nutritional intake. *Mealtime usually is a time for social interaction; often clients will eat more food if other people are present at mealtimes.* **EB:** *Compared with married subjects, mean weight loss and the prevalence of weight loss were significantly higher among widowed subjects who ate more solitary meals, more commercial meals per week, and fewer snacks and homemade meals (Shahar et al, 2001).*
- • Monitor state of oral cavity (gums, tongue, mucosa, teeth). Provide good oral hygiene before and after meals. *Good oral hygiene enhances appetite; the condition of the oral mucosa is critical to the ability to eat. The oral mucosa must be moist, with adequate saliva production to facilitate and aid in the digestion of food.*
- • If a client has anorexia and dry mouth from medication side effects, offer sips of fluids throughout the day, along with sugarless hard candy and chewing gum to stimulate saliva formation (DiMaria-Ghalili & Amella, 2005).
- • Determine relationship of eating and other events to onset of nausea, vomiting, diarrhea, or abdominal pain.
- • Determine time of day when the client's appetite is the greatest. Offer highest calorie meal at that time. *Clients with liver disease often have their greatest appetite at breakfast time.*
- ▲ Administer antiemetics and pain medications as ordered and needed before meals. *Antiemetics are more effective when given before nausea occurs. The presence of pain decreases the appetite.*
- • Prepare the client for meals. Clear unsightly supplies and excretions. Avoid invasive procedures before meals. *A pleasant environment helps promote intake.*
- • If client is nauseated, remove cover of food tray before bringing it into the client's room. *The sudden, concentrated food odors that come when the cover is removed in front of the client can trigger nausea (Quinton, 1998).*
- • If vomiting is a problem, discourage consumption of favorite foods. *If favorite foods are consumed and then vomited, the client may later reject them.*
- • Work with the client to develop a plan for increased activity. *Immobility leads to negative nitrogen balance that fosters anorexia.*
- • If the client is anemic, offer foods rich in iron and vitamins $B_{12}$, C, and folic acid. *Heme iron in meat, fish, and poultry is absorbed more readily than nonheme iron in plants. Vitamin C increases the solubility of iron. Vitamin $B_{12}$ and folic acid are necessary for erythropoiesis (Lutz & Przytulski, 2001).*
- • For the agitated client, offer finger foods (sandwiches, fresh fruit) and fluids. *If a client cannot be still, food can be consumed while pacing.*
- ▲ If client has been malnourished for a significant length of time, consult with dietitian and refeed carefully after correcting electrolyte balance. Watch for heart and respiratory failure. *Be aware of clients at risk for refeeding syndrome: those with frank starvation, with anorexia nervosa, and those with chronic illness and malnutrition. Refeeding syndrome, a potentially fatal condition, occurs in some malnourished clients when nutrients are given (orally, by tube feeding, or parenterally) in excess of the client's ability to metabolize them. Clients at risk of refeeding syndrome must be monitored carefully for electrolyte imbalances, congestive heart failure, and respiratory failure (Lutz & Przytulski, 2001).*

N

## Geriatric

- Assess for protein-energy malnutrition in elderly clients regardless of setting. Use a screening tool such as the Mini Nutritional Assessment. *It is imperative to assess elderly clients for malnutrition because it is so common in the elderly population (DiMaria-Ghalili & Amella, 2005).* **EB:** *Twenty percent of hospitalized elderly veterans consumed less than 50% of their energy requirements and had higher rates of in-hospital and 90-day mortality (Sullivan et al, 1999). Protein-energy undernutrition at hospital discharge was a strong independent risk factor for mortality in outpatients followed for 4.5 years (Sullivan and Walls, 1998).* **EBN:** *When followed for 6 months in a long-care hospital, 84% of patients had an intake below estimated energy expenditure and 30% had intakes below their estimated basal metabolic rates (Elmstahl et al, 1997).*
- Assess for factors contributing to a current acute illness. **EBN:** *The strongest contributing factor to acute confusion in nursing home residents was inadequate fluid intake followed by dementia and a fall within 30 days (Mentes et al, 1999).*
- Implement strategies to ensure good nutrition to prevent recurrence of illness. **EB:** *Individuals with any amount of weight loss and no improvement in serum albumin levels during the first month following hospitalization for medical or surgical services were at a much higher risk of readmission than those who maintained or increased their discharge weight and repleted their serum albumin concentrations (Friedmann et al, 1997). Interpret laboratory findings cautiously. Compromised kidney function makes reliance on urine samples for nutrient analyses less reliable in the elderly than in younger persons.* **EBN:** *Because it is correlated to urine specific gravity and urine osmolality, observing urine color is a low-cost method of monitoring dehydration (Wakefield et al, 2002).*
- Offer high protein supplements based on individual needs and capabilities. *Patients with decreased kidney function may not be able to excrete the waste products from protein metabolism.*
- Give the client a choice of supplements to increase personal control. If the client is unwilling to drink a glass of liquid supplement, offer 30 mL/hr in a medication cup. **EB:** *Alternatively, offer 3 oz of supplement with each medication pass (Lewis & Boyle, 1998). Often the elderly will take medications when they will not take food. The supplement is then served as a medicine.*
- Offer liquid energy supplements. *When given liquid preloads 60 minutes before the next meal, older persons consistently ate a greater total energy load (Morley, 1997).* **EB:** *Elderly nursing home residents gained an average of 3.3 lb in 60 days when consuming an average of 400 kilocalories (kcal) per day of oral supplements (Lauque et al, 2000). A Cochrane Review demonstrated that there was a small but consistent weight gain along with a positive effect on mortality and a shorter length of hospital stay in elderly clients who received a nutritional supplement (Milne, Potter, & Avenell, 2005).*
- Unless medically contraindicated, permit self-selected seasonings and foods.
- Serve food in a restaurant style manner if possible. *Older persons rate flavor as the most important determinant of their food choice but ability to taste declines in most but not all aging clients, most often affecting salt receptors and least often sweet receptors. Blindfolded older subjects have about one half the ability of younger subjects to recognize blended foods,*

*which predominantly results from a decline in olfactory sense (Morley, 1997).* **EB:** *Elderly people generally eat more when they go out to eat (Castro, 2002).*

- Play relaxing dinner music during mealtime. **EBN:** *On a nursing home ward for patients with dementia, the patients ate more calmly and spent more time with dinner when music was played (Ragneskog et al, 1996). Musical selections with a slow tempo, at or below the human heart rate, have usually been used to dampen environmental noises that might otherwise startle clients. Fewer incidents of agitated behaviors occurred during the weeks that music was played compared with weeks without music (Denney, 1997).*
- Assess components of bone health: calcium intake, the elderly adult needs 1200 mg and adequate amount of vitamin D.
- Consider social factors that may interfere with nutrition (e.g., lack of transportation, inadequate income, lack of social support). *Nutritional deficiencies are seen in at least one third of the elderly in industrialized countries (Chandra, 1997). In most surveys, poverty was found to be the major social cause of food insecurity and weight loss, but friendship networks play an important role in maintaining adequate food intake (Morley, 1997).* **EB:** *One study demonstrated that increasing the number of people present at meals was effective in increasing food intake in free-living elderly (Castro, 2002).*
- Assess for psychological and mental factors that impact nutrition. Watch for signs of depression. *Malnutrition is commonly found with depression in the elderly (Stewart, 2004).* **EB:** *Nutritional risk independently increased the likelihood of death in cognitively impaired older adults (Keller & Ostbye, 2000). In persons with depression, 90% of the elderly lose weight, compared with 60% of younger persons (Morley, 1997). Emotions affect food intake, a study demonstrated that the presence of anxiety and anger decreased food intake in the elderly (Paquet et al, 2003).*

▲ Consider the effects of medications on food intake. Appetite-stimulating drugs may have a role in some cases. *The side effects of drugs are a major cause of weight loss in older persons (Morley, 1997). Medications linked to protein-energy malnutrition in nursing home residents include digoxin, theophylline, nonsteroidal anti-inflammatory drugs, iron supplements, and psychoactive drugs (Kamel et al, 1998).* **EB:** *Compared with a placebo, megestrol acetate improved appetite and promoted weight gain in geriatric patients (Yeh et al, 2000).*

▲ Provide appropriate food textures for chewing ease. Insert dentures (if needed) before meals. Assess fit of dentures. Refer for dental consultation if needed. *The bony structure of jaws changes over time, requiring adjustment of dentures. The most common feeding difficulties among geriatric rehabilitation clients involved dentures (lack of or ill fitting) and oral infections (Keller, 1997).*

NOTE: If the client is unable to feed self, refer to Nursing Interventions and Rationales for **Feeding Self-care deficit.** If client has impaired physical function, malnutrition, depression and cognitive impairment, please refer to care plan on **Adult Failure to Thrive.**

## Multicultural

- Assess for dietary intake of essential nutrients. **EB:** *Studies have shown that African-American women have calcium intakes of less than 75% of the RDA (Zablah et al, 1999).*



N

*Hispanics with type 2 diabetes also often have inadequate protein nutritional status (Castaneda et al, 2000). Mexican-American women have a higher prevalence of iron-deficiency anemia than non-Hispanic white females (Frith-Terhune et al, 2000). Rural African-American men had low caloric intakes coupled with high fat intakes but nutrient deficiencies (Vitolins et al, 2000). African-American adolescents have some of the highest levels of vitamin D deficiency (Gordon et al, 2004).*

- Assess for the influence of cultural beliefs, norms, and values on the client's nutritional knowledge. *What the client considers normal dietary practices may be based on cultural perceptions (Cochran, 1998; Doswell & Erlen, 1998; Leininger & McFarland, 2002). Among African Americans, there was a general perception that "eating healthfully" meant giving up part of their cultural heritage, trying to conform to the dominant culture, and the sense that friends and relatives usually were not supportive of dietary changes (James, 2004).*
- Discuss with the client those aspects of their diet that will remain unchanged. *Aspects of the client's life that are meaningful and valuable to them should be understood and preserved without change (Leininger & McFarland, 2002).*
- Negotiate with the client regarding the aspects of his or her diet that will need to be modified. *Give and take with the client will lead to culturally congruent care (Leininger and McFarland, 2002).*
- Validate the client's feelings regarding the impact of current lifestyle, finances, and transportation on ability to obtain nutritious food. *Validation is a therapeutic communication technique that lets the client know that the nurse has heard and understands what was said, and it promotes the nurse-client relationship (Heineken, 1998).*
- Encourage family meals. **EB:** *Frequency of family meals was positively associated with intake of fruits, vegetables, grains, and calcium-rich foods and negatively associated with soft drink consumption (Neumark-Sztainer et al, 2003).*



## Home Care

- Above interventions may be adapted for home care use.
- Monitor food intake. Instruct the client in intake of small frequent meals and liquid supplements (e.g., Ensure, Instant Breakfast). *Until definitive causes can be isolated for intervention, it is important for clients to maintain intake as much as possible. Reducing meal size and eating more often may help. Multiple causes of anorexia and weight loss in older adults have been suggested, from social isolation to GI dysfunction. Altered neurochemistry has been implicated (Blanton et al, 1999).*
- Assess clients' willingness to eat; fashion interventions accordingly. **EBN:** *Older adults reported that their willingness to eat influenced appetite, and factors influencing appetite included mood, personal values (independence and integrity), wholesomeness (being in good health), food (preparation, consistency, and freshness), eating environment (pleasantness), and meal companionship (Wikby & Fagerskiold, 2004).*

▲ Assess the client for depression. Refer for mental health services as indicated. *Decreased appetite with weight loss is part of the syndrome of depression. Return of appetite is unlikely unless the underlying depression is treated.*

- Recognize that older women may continue their younger preoccupation with weight and recurrent dieting, despite being at normal weight. Assess source of low weight or weight loss with this in mind. *Reports suggest that elderly women continue to be preoc-*

*cupied with being thin. Increased awareness of eating habits and weight preoccupation in elderly women is recommended (Fallaz et al, 1999).*

- ▲ Monitor the effect of total parenteral nutrition (TPN) as ordered by physician. *TPN requires monitoring for potential complications and client/caregiver education (Gorski, 2001).*
- ▲ In the presence of depression diagnosis, refer for psychiatric home health care services for client reassurance and implementation of therapeutic regimen. *Poor appetite and weight loss are symptoms of depression.* **EBN:** *Psychiatric home care nurses can address issues relating to assessment and treatment of the client's depression. Behavioral interventions in the home can assist the client to participate more effectively in a treatment plan (Patusky, Rodning, & Martinez-Kratz, 1996).*

## Client/Family Teaching

- Help the client/family identify the area to change that will make the greatest contribution to improved nutrition. *Change is difficult. Multiple changes may be overwhelming.*
- Build on the strengths in the client's/family's food habits. Adapt changes to their current practices. *Accepting the client's/family's preferences shows respect for their culture.*
- Select appropriate teaching aids for the client's/family's background.
- Implement instructional follow-up to answer the client's/family's questions.
- Suggest community resources as suitable (food sources, counseling, Meals on Wheels, senior centers).
- Teach the client and family how to manage tube feedings or parenteral therapy at home.

## evolve WEBSITES FOR EDUCATION

See the EVOLVE website for World Wide Web resources for client education.

N

## REFERENCES


Arrowsmith H: Malnutrition in hospital: detection and consequences, *Br J Nurs* 6:1131, 1997.

Baldwin C, Parsons T, Logan S: Dietary advice for illness-related malnutrition in adults, *Cochrane Database Syst Rev* (2): CD002008, 2001.

Blanton et al: Neurochemical alterations during age-related anorexia, *Proc Soc Exp Biol Med* 221(3): 153, 1999.

Castaneda C, Bermudez OI, Tucker KL: Protein nutritional status and functions are associated with type II diabetes in Hispanic elders, *Am J Clin Nutr* 72(1):89, 2000.

Castro JM: Age-related changes in the social, psychological, and temporal influences on food intake in free-living, healthy, adult humans, *J Gerontology* 57A(6), 2002.

Chandra RK: Nutrition and the immune system: an introduction, *Am J Clin Nutr* 66:S460, 1997.

Chandra RK: Nutrition and the immune system from birth to old age, *Eur J Clin Nutr* 56 (Suppl 3):S73, 2002.

Cochran M: Tears have no color, *Am J Nurs* 98(6):53, 1998.

Denney A: Quiet music: an intervention for mealtime agitation? *J Gerontol Nurs* 23:16, 1997.

DiMaria-Ghalili RA, Amella E: Nutrition in older adults, *Am J Nurs* 105(3):40, 2005.

Doswell W, Erlen J: Multicultural issues and ethical concerns in the delivery of revising care interventions, *Nurs Clin North Am* 33(2):353, 1998.

Elmstahl S et al: Malnutrition in geriatric patients: a neglected problem? *J Adv Nurs* 26:851, 1997.

Fallaz et al: Weight loss preoccupation in aging women, *J Nutr Health Aging* 3(3):177, 1999.

Friedmann JM et al: Predicting early nonelective hospital readmission in nutritionally compromised older adults, *Am J Clin Nutr* 65:1714, 1997.

Frith-Terhune AL et al: Iron deficiency anemia: higher prevalence in Mexican American than in non-Hispanic white females in the third National Health and Nutrition Examination Survey, 1988-1994, *Am J Clin Nutr* 72(4):963, 2000.

Gordon CM et al: Prevalence of vitamin D deficiency among healthy adolescents, *Arch Pediatr Adolesc Med* 158(6):531-537, 2004.
Gorski LA: TPN update: making each visit count, *Home Healthc Nurse* 19(1):15, 2001.
Heineken J: Patient silence is not necessarily client satisfaction: communication in home care nursing, *Home Healthc Nurse* 16(2): 115, 1998.
James DC: Factors influencing food choices, dietary intake, and nutrition-related attitudes among African Americans: application of a culturally sensitive model, *Ethn Health* 9(4): 349-367, 2004.
Kamel HK, Thomas DR, Morley JE: National deficiencies in long-term care: part II. Management of protein-energy malnutrition and dehydration, *Ann Long Term Care* 6:250, 1998.
Kasper DL: *Harrison's principles of internal medicine*, ed 16, New York, 2005, McGraw-Hill.
Keller HH: Nutrition problems and their association with patient outcomes in a geriatric rehabilitation setting, *J Nutr Elderly* 17(2):1, 1997.
Keller HH, Ostbye T: Do nutrition indicators predict death in elderly Canadians with cognitive impairment? *Can J Public Health* 91:220, 2000.
Kreiter SR et al: Nutritional rickets in African American breast-fed infants, *J Pediatr* 137:153, 2000.
Lauque S et al: Protein-energy oral supplementation in malnourished nursing-home residents. A controlled trial, *Age Ageing* 29: 51, 2000.
Leininger MM, McFarland MR: *Transcultural nursing: concepts, theories, research and practices,* ed 3, New York, 2002, McGraw-Hill.
Lewis DA, Boyle KD: Nutritional supplement use during medication administration: selected case studies, *J Nutr Elderly* 17:53, 1998.
Lutz CA, Przytulski KR: *Nutrition and diet therapy,* ed 3, Philadelphia, 2001, FA Davis.
Mentes J et al: Acute confusion indicators: risk factors and prevalence using MDS data, *Res Nurs Health* 22:95, 1999.
Milne AC, Potter J, Avenell A: Protein and energy supplementation in elderly people at risk from malnutrition, *Cochrane Database Syst Rev* (2):CD003288, 2005.
Morley JE: Anorexia of aging: physiologic and pathologic, *Am J Clin Nutr* 66:760, 1997.
Morley JE, Thomas DR, Kamel H: Nutritional deficiencies in long-term care: part I, *Ann Long Term Care* 6(5):183, 1998.
National Academy of Sciences: *Dietary reference intakes,* Washington, DC, 1998, National Academy Press.
Nelson ME et al: Effects of high-intensity strength training on multiple risk factors for osteoporotic fractures, *JAMA* 272(24): 1909, 1994.

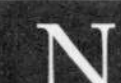

Neumark-Sztainer D et al: Family meal patterns: associations with sociodemographic characteristics and improved dietary intake among adolescents, *J Am Diet Assoc* 103(3):317-322, 2003.
Paquet C et al: Direct and indirect effects of everyday emotions on food intake of elderly patients in institutions, *J Gerentol* 58A(2), 2003.
Patusky KL, Rodning C, Martinez-Kratz M: Clinical lessons in psychiatric home care: a case study approach, *J Home Healthc Manag* 9:18, 1996.
Payette H et al: Predictors of dietary intake in a functionally dependent elderly population in the community, *Am J Public Health* 85:677, 1995.
Quinton D: Anticipatory nausea and vomiting in chemotherapy, *Prof Nurse* 13(10): 663, 1998.
Ragneskog H et al: Dinner music for demented patients: analysis of video-recorded observations, *Clin Nurs Res* 5:262, 1996.
Shahar DR et al: The effect of widowhood on weight change, dietary intake, and eating behavior in the elderly population, *J Aging Health* 13:189, 2001.
Stewart JT: Why don't physicians consider depression in the elderly? *Postgrad Med* 115(6):57, 2004.
Sullivan DH, Sun S, Walls RC: Protein-energy undernutrition among elderly hospitalized patients: a prospective study, *JAMA* 281:2013, 1999.
Sullivan DH, Walls RC: Protein-energy undernutrition and the risk of mortality within six years of hospital discharge, *J Am Coll Nutr* 17:571, 1998.
Vitolins MZ et al: Ethnic and gender variation in the dietary intake of rural elders, *J Nutr Elderly* 19(3):15, 2000.
Wakefield B et al: Monitoring hydration status in elderly veterans, *West J Nurs Res* 24:132, 2002.
Wikby K, Fagerskiold A: The willingness to eat: an investigation of appetite among elderly people, *Scand J Caring Sci* 18:120, 2004.
Wyshak G: Teenaged girls, carbonated beverage consumption, and bone fractures, *Arch Pediatr Adolesc Med* 154:610, 2000.
Yeh S et al: Improvement in quality-of-life measures and stimulation of weight gain after treatment with megesterol acetate oral suspension in geriatric cachexia: results of a double-blind, placebo-controlled study, *J Am Geriatr Soc* 48:485, 2000.

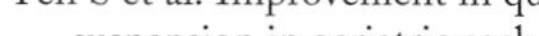

Zablah EM et al: Barriers to calcium intake in African American women, *J Hum Nutr* 12(2):123, 1999.

# Imbalanced Nutrition: more than body requirements evolve

*Betty Ackley and Carroll A. Lutz*

NANDA

## Definition

Intake of nutrients that exceeds metabolic needs

## Defining Characteristics

Triceps skin fold of more than 25 mm in women; triceps skin fold of more than 15 mm in men; body weight more than 20% over ideal for height and frame; eating in response to external cues (e.g., time of day, social situation); eating in response to internal cues other than hunger (e.g., anxiety); reported or observed dysfunctional eating pattern (pairing food with other activities); sedentary activity level; concentration of food intake at the end of the day

## Related Factors (r/t)

Excessive intake in relation to metabolic need; deficient knowledge related to desirability of nutritional supplements

NOC

## Outcomes (Nursing Outcomes Classification)

### Suggested NOC Outcomes

Nutritional Status: Food and Fluid Intake, Nutrient Intake; Weight Control

**Example NOC Outcome with Indicators**

**Weight Control** as evidenced by the following indicators: Demonstrates progress toward target weight/ Balances exercise with caloric intake/Maintains recommended eating pattern/Controls preoccupation with food (Rate each indicator of **Weight Control:** 1 = never demonstrated, 2 = rarely demonstrated, 3 = sometimes demonstrated, 4 = often demonstrated, 5 = consistently demonstrated [see Section I].)

## Client Outcomes

### Client Will (Specify Time Frame):

- State pertinent factors contributing to weight gain
- Identify behaviors that remain under client's control
- Claim ownership for current eating patterns
- Design dietary modifications to meet individual long-term goal of weight control, using principles of variety, balance, and moderation
- Accomplish desired weight loss in a reasonable period (1 to 2 lb per week)
- Incorporate appropriate activities requiring energy expenditure into daily life



N

## NIC

## Interventions (Nursing Interventions Classification)

### Suggested NIC Interventions

Eating Disorders Management, Nutrition Management, Nutritional Counseling, Weight Management, Weight Reduction Assistance

**Example NIC Activities—Weight Management**

Determine client's motivation for changing eating habits; develop with client a method to keep daily record of intake

## Nursing Interventions and Rationales

- Ask the client to keep a one day to three day food diary where everything eaten or drank is recorded. *Use of a food diary will be helpful for both the client and the nurse, to examine usual foods eaten and patterns of eating.* **EBN and EB:** *Self-monitoring helps the client assess adherence to self-determined performance criteria and progress toward desired goals. Self-monitoring serves an important role in the maintenance of internal standards of behavior (Fleury, 1991). Development of self-monitoring tools that meet the needs of clients increase dietary reporting and promote self-efficacy (Mossavar-Rahmani et al, 2004).*
- Advise the client to measure food periodically. Help the client learn usual portion sizes. *Measuring food alerts the client to normal portion sizes. Estimating amounts can be extremely inaccurate.* **EB:** *A study where women were served either larger portions, or more calorie dense foods in the same portion size demonstrated that extra calories were eaten, and the women subjects did not realize it and decrease their calories for dinner (Kral et al, 2004).*
- Help the client determine their body mass index (BMI). Use a chart or one of the formulas below:
  - Weight in kilograms divided by height (in meters) squared (kg/m$^2$)
  - Weight in pounds multiplied by 705, divided by height in inches, divided again by height in inches

  *A normal BMI is 20 to 25, 26 to 29 is overweight, and a BMI of greater than 30 is obese (Nix, 2005).*
- Recommend the client follow the U.S. Dietary Guidelines, which can be found at www.healthierus.gov/dietaryguidelines. *Dietary Guidelines are written by national experts and based on research in nutrition.*
- Recommend the client use the interactive Food Guide Pyramid site at www.MyPyramid.gov to determine the number of calories to eat, and gain more information on how to eat in a healthy fashion.
- Establish a reasonable goal for the client's body weight and for weight loss (e.g., 1 to 2 lb per week). **EB:** *Because subjects in one study achieved comparable weight loss on liquid formula diets of 420, 600, or 800 calories/day, choosing the higher-energy diets may minimize adverse side effects (Foster et al, 1992).*
- Recommend that client lose weight slowly, based on a healthy eating pattern and increased exercise. The number of calories consumed should be at least 1600 for men, and 1300 for women. *Slower weight loss is generally more likely to be lasting weight*

*loss. It is important that increased activity is included to help burn more calories (Ruser, Federman, & Kashaf, 2005).*

- Demonstrate the use of food labels to make healthful choices. Alert the client/family to focus on serving size, total fat, and simple carbohydrate. *The standardized food label in bold type simplifies the search for information. Fats and sugars contribute the least to a healthful diet and the most to excessive calorie intake. Generally clients should eat foods that are no more than 30% fat.*
- Initiate a client contract that involves rewarding and reinforcing progressive goal attainment. *Client contracts can help clients learn to analyze their behavior and to choose effective behavioral strategies as well as provide a progress report to reinforce the behaviors.*
- Weigh the client twice a week under the same conditions. *It is important to most clients and contributes to their progress to have the tangible reward that the scale shows. Monitoring twice a week gives frequent feedback to encourage the client to continue with the program.*
- Watch the client for signs of depression: flat affect, poor sleeping habits, lack of interesting in life. *Depression is found in at least one third of all obese persons (Ruser, Federman, & Kashaf, 2005).*
- Determine the client's knowledge of the need for supplements. Discourage the client from taking excessive amounts of vitamins unless prescribed by a physician. *If the client eats a healthy diet, there is generally no need for supplementation. If the client is over 50, one multiple vitamin per day is generally recommended.* **EB:** *A review of clinical trials concluded that antioxidant supplements are unlikely to reduce the risk of heart disease, and high doses of individual supplements can have adverse effects (Kris-Etherton et al, 2004). Another review of 14 randomized trial demonstrated that intake of antioxidant supplementation did not prevent GI cancers, and intake seemed to increase mortality (Bjelakovic et al, 2004).*

N

### Pattern of Dietary Intake

- Recommend the client eat a healthy breakfast every morning. **EB:** *A study demonstrated that people who skip breakfast are more likely to overeat in the evening (deCastro, 2004). Another study demonstrated that people who skipped breakfast were 450 times more likely to be obese (Ma et al, 2003).*
- Recommend the client avoid eating in fast food restaurants. **EB:** *A 15-year study demonstrated that people who often eat fat foods gain an average of 10 lb more than those who eat fast food less often, and were two times more likely to develop insulin resistance which can lead to diabetes (Pereira et al, 2005).*

▲ Obtain a thorough history. Refer to a dietitian if the client has a medical condition. *The most appropriate clients for the nursing intervention of weight management are adults with no other major health problems requiring medical nutritional therapy.*

### Recommended Foods/Fluids

- Encourage the client to increase intake of vegetables and fruits to at least five servings per day, preferably 9 servings per day. **EB:** *A study demonstrated that women who increased their fruit and vegetable intake to 4 servings per day had a 24% lower risk of obesity than those who ate only 2 servings per day (He et al, 2004).*

- Encourage the client to eat at least 3 whole grain servings per day, preferably more. **EB:** *A study demonstrated that men who ate more whole grains had decreased weight gain (Koh-Banerjee et al, 2004).*
- Evaluate the client's usual intake of fiber. *In general, high-fiber foods take longer to eat and contain fewer calories than most other foods.* **EB:** *High dietary fiber intake was associated with lower body weight and waist-to-hip ratio and predicted weight loss more strongly than did level of fat consumption (Ludwig et al, 1999).*
- Encourage the client to *decrease* intake of sugars including intake of soft drinks, desserts, and candy. S*ugar predisposes to dental caries, and also is a source of calories that is empty of other nutrients (Nix, 2005). Consuming excessive amounts of fructose, which is used to sweeten soft drinks, other foods with a high glycemic index, and insufficient high-fiber grains may result in development of type 2 diabetes (Wu et al, 2004).*
- Recommend client increase intake of water, to at least 2000 mL or 2 quarts per day. A guideline is 1 to 1.5 ml of fluid per each calorie needed, so an average intake would be between 2000 and 3000 mL/day, or at least 8 cups of fluid (Grodner, Long, & DeYoung, 2004). *The Adequate Intake recommendation is 3 L for the 19- to 30-year-old male and 2.2 L for the 19- to 30-year-old female. Water balance studies suggest that adult men require 2.5 liters per day (Institute of Medicine, 2004).*
- For more information on healthy eating, refer to Nursing Interventions for **Readiness for enhanced Nutrition.**

### Behavioral Methods for Weight Loss

N

- Familiarize the client with the following behavior modification techniques (Lutz & Przytulski, 2001):
  - Self-monitoring of food intake, including keeping a food and exercise diary
  - Graphing weight weekly
  - Controlling stimuli that causes overeating, such as watching television with frequent food-related commercials
  - Limiting food intake to one site in the home
  - Sitting down at the table to eat
  - Planning food intake for each day
  - Rearranging the schedule to avoid inappropriate eating
  - Saving or rescheduling everyday activities for times when one is hungry
  - Avoiding boredom; keeping a list of activities on the refrigerator
  - For a party, eating before arriving, sitting away from the snack foods, and substituting lower-calorie beverages for alcoholic ones
  - Deciding beforehand what to order in a restaurant
  - Bringing only healthy foods into the house to decrease temptation
  - Slowing mealtime by swallowing food before putting more food on the utensil, pausing for a minute during the meal and attempting to increase the number of pauses, and trying to be the last one to finish eating
  - Drinking a glass of water before each meal; taking sips of water between bites of food

- Charting one's progress
- Making an agreement with oneself or a significant other for a meaningful reward and not rewarding oneself with food
- Changing one's mindset, as in control of eating behavior
- Viewing exercise as a means of controlling hunger
- Practicing relaxation techniques
- Imagining oneself ordering a side salad, diet dressing, low-fat milk, and a small hamburger at a fast-food restaurant
- Visualizing oneself enjoying a fresh apple in preference to apple pie

*There are multiple behavior methods to change the style of eating and help the client deal with the reality of decreasing food intake.*

## Physical Activity

- Assess for reasons why the client would be unable to participate in an exercise program; refer for evaluation by a primary care practitioner as needed. Encourage activity to help with weight loss. **EB:** *Diet plus exercise produced greater and better-sustained weight loss than either diet or exercise alone (Miller, 1997).*
- Use the Outcome Expectation for Exercise Scale to determine client's self-efficacy expectations and outcomes expectations toward exercise. **EBN:** *The client's self-efficacy expectations and outcome expectations for exercise will greatly influence his or her willingness to exercise. If the individual has a low outcome, interventions can be implemented to strengthen the expectations and hopefully improve exercise behavior (Resnick, Zimmerman, & Orwig, 2001).*
- Recommend the client enter an exercise program with a friend. **EBN:** *Findings from a study of exercise behavior found that friends have the strongest influence to keep on an exercise program, more than family members or experts (Resnick, Orwig, & Magaziner, 2002).*
- Recommend the client begin a walking program using the following guidelines:
  - Buy a pedometer
  - Determine times when walking can be incorporated into usual lifestyle
  - Set a goal of walking 10,000 steps per day, or 5 miles per day.
  - If when comes home from work, does not have required number of steps, go for a walk until reach designated goal of 10,000 steps per day.

  **EB:** *A study demonstrated that use of a pedometer resulted in two times the usual amount of activity and weight loss in overweight adults (VanWormer, 2004). Another study demonstrated that in middle-age women, women who walked more had lower BMIs, and that women who walked 10,000 or more steps per day were in the normal range for BMI (Thompson et al, 2004).*

## Pediatric

- Work with parents of the overweight child by encouraging the following behaviors:
  - Emphasize providing good food, not depriving children of food. *Trying to get children to eat less or move more for weight control generally backfires and makes the child preoccupied with food and unwilling to move unless forced.*

N

- Accept the child's natural size and shape, the child needs the parents unconditional love.
- Make family meals a priority.
- Involve the child in helping plan menus, doing cooking and preparation as appropriate for the child's age.
- Be active with children.
- Encourage children to love their bodies

*These methods can help children who are overweight without causing harm to the child (Satter, 2005).*

- Determine the child's BMI after the child is age 3 years (Fowler-Brown, Kahwati, 2004). *The Centers for Disease Control and Prevention's (CDC) BMI chart for children and teens is available at www.cdc.gov/nccdphp/dnpa/bmi/bmi-for-age.htm.* **EB:** *Research has demonstrated that kids who are overweight or obese have a higher risk for being overweight or obese as adults and even children in the high normal weight range have an elevated risk of becoming overweight or obese (Field et al, 2005).*
- Work with the child and parent to develop an appropriate weight maintenance plan, including behavior methods of weight loss, as well as increased activity. *The goal with a child is often to maintain existing weight as the body grows taller (Fowler-Brown, Kahwati, 2004).* **EB:** *A Cochrane Review showed that there is insufficient data to determine the effectiveness of obesity prevention programs, although reduction in sedentary behaviors and increased activity are probably appropriate (Campbell et al, 2002).*
- Encourage child to increase the amount of walking done per day, if the child is willing, ask them to wear a pedometer to measure number of steps. **EB:** *A study demonstrated that the recommended number of steps per day to have a healthy body composition for the 6 to 12 year old is 12,000 for the girl and 15,000 for the boy (Tudor-Locke et al, 2004).*
- Do not use food as a reward for good behavior, especially not foods that are concentrated sources of sugar or fat. *Rewarding the child with "treats" can give the child a life-long craving for high sugar and fat foods.*
- Recommend the child decrease television viewing, watching movies, and playing video games. Ask parents to limit television to 1 to 2 hours per day maximum (Calamaro & Faith, 2004). **EB:** *Children receiving a 6-month classroom curriculum to reduce television, videotape, and video game use showed significant decreases in BMI and triceps skin folds compared with controls (Robinson, 1999). A study demonstrated that children who watch television 5 hours or more per day were 4.6 times more likely to be overweight versus children who watched television 0 to 2 hours per day (Gortmaker et al, 1996).*

## Geriatric

- Assess changes in lifestyle and eating patterns. Energy needs decrease an estimated 5% per decade after the age of 40 years, but often eating patterns remain unchanged from youth.

N

- Assess fluid intake. Recommend routine drinks of water regardless of thirst. *Thirst sensation becomes dulled in the elderly.*
- Observe for socioeconomic factors that influence food choices (e.g., inadequate funds or cooking facilities). *Even those on restricted budgets and with limited facilities can be helped to choose food sources for a balanced diet.*
- Suggest a variety of seasonings. *The ability to taste sweet, bitter, sour, and salty declines in most, but not all, older persons (Miller, 2004).*

## Multicultural

- Assess for the influence of cultural beliefs, norms, acculturation and values on the client's nutritional knowledge and practices. *What the client considers normal dietary practices may be based on cultural perceptions (Cochran, 1998; Doswell & Erlen, 1998; Leininger & McFarland, 2002). Among African-Americans, there was a general perception that "eating healthfully" meant giving up part of their cultural heritage, trying to conform to the dominant culture, and the sense that friends and relatives usually were not supportive of dietary changes (James, 2004). A higher risk for obesity among Latino immigrants was associated with length of residence in the United States and may be due to acculturation processes such as the adoption of the unhealthy dietary practices (i.e., a diet high in fat and low in fruits and vegetables) and sedentary lifestyles of the host country (Kaplan et al, 2004). Another study suggests that acculturation to the United States is a risk factor for obesity-related behaviors among Asian-American and Hispanic adolescents (Unger et al, 2004). One Mexican-American pediatrician reported that the primary complaint of his Mexican-American parents is that their children do not eat enough despite being obviously overweight (Garcia, 2004). Research findings suggest that nutrition education efforts targeting Latina mothers of young children can be culturally reframed to identify positive eating behaviors rather than focusing on a child's weight (Crawford et al, 2004).*
- Encourage parental efforts at increasing physical activity and decreasing dietary fat for their children. **EB:** *Physical activity and dietary fat consumption were inversely related among African-American girls (Thompson et al, 2004). Interventions to increase physical activity among preadolescent African-American girls may benefit from a parental component to encourage support and self-efficacy for daughters' physical activity (Adkins et al, 2004).*
- Assess for the influence of cultural beliefs, norms, and values on the client's ideal of acceptable body weight and body size. *Ideal body weight and size may be based on cultural perceptions (Leininger & McFarland, 2002).* **EB:** *African-American women report more satisfaction with body size than other women (Miller et al, 2000). Overweight Hispanic women with high levels of binge eating and depression preferred a slim body ideal (Fitzgibbon et al, 1998).*
- Discuss with the client those aspects of his or her diet that will remain unchanged, and work with the client to adapt cultural core foods. *Aspects of the client's life that are meaningful and valuable to the client should be understood and preserved without change (Leininger & McFarland, 2002). Core foods are those foods that are universal, staple, important, and consistently used in the culture (Sanjur, 1995).* **EB:** *Dramatic weight loss was achieved in Hawaii using a culturally appropriate methodology (Shintani et al, 1991).*

N

- Negotiate with the client regarding the aspects of his or her diet that will need to be modified. *Give and take with the client will lead to culturally congruent care (Leininger & McFarland, 2002).*
- Validate the client's feelings regarding the impact of current lifestyle, finances, and transportation on the ability to obtain and prepare nutritious food. *Validation is a therapeutic communication technique that lets the client know that the nurse has heard and understood what was said, and it promotes the nurse-client relationship (Heineken, 1998).*
- Limit television viewing and consumption of soft drinks. **EB:** *Longer hours of child television viewing and higher soft drink intake was associated with the occurrence of overweight for Hispanic children (Ariza et al, 2004; Giammattei et al, 2003).*
- Encourage family meals. **EB:** *Frequency of family meals was positively associated with intake of fruits, vegetables, grains, and calcium-rich foods and negatively associated with soft drink consumption (Neumark-Sztainer et al, 2003).*

## Client/Family Teaching

- Provide the client and family with information regarding the treatment plan options. *If the client and family select the treatment plan, they are more likely to comply with it, particularly if the client does not do the marketing and cooking.*
- Inform the client about the health risks associated with obesity, which include cancer, diabetes, heart disease, strokes, hypertension, gastroesophageal reflux, gallstones, osteoarthritis, and venous thrombosis (Nutrition Action, 2004). **EB:** *The risk of death from all causes—cardiovascular disease, cancer, and other diseases—increases throughout the range of moderate and severe overweight for both men and women in all age groups (Calle et al, 1999).*
- Inform the client and family of the disadvantages of trying to lose weight by dieting alone. *Resting metabolic rate is decreased as much as 45% with extreme calorie restriction. The decrease persists after the diet period has ended, which leads to the "yo-yo effect." With a reduced-calorie diet alone, as much as 25% of the weight lost can be lean body mass rather than fat. Resting energy expenditure is positively related to lean body mass.*
- Teach the importance of exercise in a weight control program. *A physically conditioned person uses more fat for energy at rest and with exercise than a sedentary person does. The majority of clients will benefit from establishing walking as a cornerstone of their physical activity program (Rippe, Crossley, & Ringer, 1998).*
- Recommend the client receive adequate amounts of sleep. **EB:** *Sleep deprivation, less than 7 hours per night, is associated with an increased risk of obesity (Tufts University, 2005). Another study demonstrated an association between short sleep duration and obesity in young adults (Hasler et al, 2004). Sleep curtailment in young healthy men resulted in increased hunger and appetite (Spiegel et al, 2004).*
- Teach stress reduction techniques as alternatives to eating. *The client should have available a variety of healthy behaviors to substitute for unhealthy ones.*

## evolve WEBSITES FOR EDUCATION

See the EVOLVE website for World Wide Web resources for client education.

## REFERENCES


Adkins S, Sherwood NE, Story M et al: Physical activity among African-American girls: the role of parents and the home environment, *Obes Res* 12(Suppl):S38-S45, 2004.

Allan JD: A biomedical and feminist perspective on women's experiences with weight management, *West J Nurs Res* 16:524, 1994.

Ariza AJ, Chen EH, Binns HJ et al: Risk factors for overweight in five-to six-year-old Hispanic-American children: a pilot study, *J Urban Health* 81(1):150-161, 2004.

Banks-Wallace J: Staggering under the weight of responsibility: the impact of culture on physical activity among African American women, *Multicult Nurs Health* 6:24, 2000.

Bjelakovic G, Nikolova D, Simonetti RG et al: Antioxidant supplements for prevention of gastrointestinal cancers: a systematic review and meta-analysis, *Lancet*, 364(9441):1219, 2004.

Calamaro CJ, Faith MS: Preventing childhood overweight, *Nutr Today* 39(5):194, 2004.

Calle EE: Body-mass index and mortality in a prospective cohort of US adults, *N Engl J Med* 34:1097, 1999.

Campbell K, Waters E, O'Meara S et al: Interventions for preventing obesity in children, *Cochrane Database Syst Rev* (2): CD001871, 2002.

Cochran M: Tears have no color, *Am J Nurs* 98(6):53, 1998.

de Castro JM: The time of day of food intake influences overall intake in humans, *J Nutr* 134(1):104, 2004.

Doswell W, Erlen J: Multicultural issues and ethical concerns in the delivery of nursing care interventions, *Nurs Clin North Am* 33(2):353, 1998.

Field AE, Cook NR, Gillman MW: Weight status in childhood as a predictor of becoming overweight or hypertensive in early adulthood, *Obes Res J* 13(1):163, 2005.

Fitzgibbon ML, Spring B, Avellone ME et al: Correlates of binge eating in Hispanic, black and white women, *Int J Eat Disord* 24(1):43, 1998.

Fleury J: Empowering potential: a theory of wellness motivation, *Nurs Res* 40:288, 1991.

Foster GD, Wadden TA, Peterson FJ et al: A controlled comparison of three very-low-calorie diets: effects on weight, body composition and symptoms, *Am J Clin Nutr* 55:811, 1992.

Fowler-Brown A, Kahwati LC: Prevention and treatment of overweight in children and adolescents, *Am Family Physician* 69(11): 2591, 2004.

Garcia RS: No come nada, *Health Aff* 23(2):215-219, 2004.

Giammattei J, Blix G, Marshak HH et al: Television watching and soft drink consumption: associations with obesity in 11-to 13-year-old schoolchildren, *Arch Pediatr Adolesc Med* 157(9):882-886, 2003.

Gortmaker SL, Must A, Sobol AM et al: Television viewing as a cause of increasing obesity among children in the United States, 1986-1990, *Arch Pediatr Adolesc Med* 150:356, 1996.

Grodner M, Long S, DeYoung S: *Foundations and clinical applications of nutrition*, St. Louis, 2004, Mosby.

Hasler G, Buysse DJ, Klaghofer R et al: The association between short sleep duration and obesity in young adults: a 13-year prospective study, *Sleep* 27(4):661, 2004.

He K, Hu FB, Colditz GA et al: Changes in intake of fruits and vegetables in relation to risk of obesity and weight gain among middle-aged women, *Int J Obes Relat Metab Disord* 28(12):1569, 2004.

Heineken J: Patient silence is not necessarily client satisfaction: communication in home care nursing, *Home Healthc Nurse* 16(2): 115, 1998.

Institute of Medicine: Applications of dietary reference intakes for electrolytes and water, *National Academy of Sciences*, 2004, National Academies Press.

James DC: Factors influencing food choices, dietary intake, and nutrition-related attitudes among African Americans: application of a culturally sensitive model, *Ethn Health* 9(4):349-367, 2004.

Kaplan MS, Huguet N, Newsom JT et al: The association between length of residence and obesity among Hispanic immigrants, *Am J Prev Med* 27(4):323-326, 2004.

Koh-Banerjee P, Franz M, Sampson L et al: Changes in whole-grain, bran, and cereal fiber consumption in relation to 3 year weight gain among men, *Am J Clin Nutr* 80(5):1237, 2004.

Kral TV, Roe LS, Rolls BJ: Combined effects of energy density and portion size on energy intake in women, *Am J Clin Nutr* 79(6):962, 2004.

Kris-Etherton PM, Lichtenstein AH, Howard BV et al: Antioxidant vitamin supplements and cardiovascular disease, *Circulation* 110(5):637, 2004.

Leininger MM, McFarland MR: *Transcultural nursing: concepts, theories, research and practices,* ed 3, New York, 2002, McGraw-Hill.
Ludwig DS, Pereira MA, Kroenke CH et al: Dietary fiber, weight gain, and cardiovascular disease risk factors in young adults, *JAMA* 282(16):1539, 1999.
Lutz CA, Przytulski KR: *Nutrition and diet therapy,* ed 3, Philadelphia, 2001, FA Davis.
Ma Y, Bertone ER, Stanek EJ, III et al: Association between eating patterns and obesity in a free-living US adult population, *Am J Epidiomol* 158(1):85, 2003.
Miller KJ, Gleaves DH, Hirsch TG et al: Comparisons of body image by race/ethnicity and gender in a university population, *Int J Eat Disord* 27(3):310, 2000.
Miller WC: A meta-analysis of the past 25 years of weight loss research using diet, exercise or diet plus exercise intervention, *Int J Obes Relat Metab Disord* 21:941, 1997.
Miller CA: *Nursing for wellness in older adults,* ed 4, Philadelphia, 2004, JB Lippincott.
Morley JE: Anorexia of aging: physiologic and pathologic, *Am J Clin Nutr* 66:760, 1997.
Mossavar-Rahmani Y, Henry H, Rodabough R et al: Additional self-monitoring tools in the dietary modification component of the women's health initiative, *J Am Diet Assoc* 104(1):76, 2004.
Neumark-Sztainer D, Hannan PJ, Story M et al: Family meal patterns: associations with sociodemographic characteristics and improved dietary intake among adolescents, *J Am Diet Assoc* 103(3):317-322, 2003.
Nix S: *Williams' basic nutrition and diet therapy*, St. Louis, 2005, Mosby.
Nutrition Action: Ten myths that won't quit, *Nutrition Action Health Letter* 32(10), 2004.
Pereira MA, Kartashov AI, Ebbeling CB: Fast-food habits, weight gain, and insulin resistance (the CARDIA study): 15-year prospective analysis, *Lancet* 365(9453):36, 2005.
Resnick B, Orwig D, Magaziner J: The effect of social support on exercise behavior in older adults, *Clin Nurs Res* 11(1):52, 2002.
Resnick B, Zimmerman S, Orwig D: Model testing for reliability and validity of the outcome expectations for exercise scale, *Nurs Res* 50:5, 2001.
Rippe JM, Crossley S, Ringer R: Obesity as a chronic disease: modern medical and lifestyle management, *J Am Diet Assoc* 98(Suppl 2):S9, 1998.
Rippe JM, Hess S: The role of physical activity in the prevention and management of obesity, *J Am Diet Assoc* 98(Suppl 2):S31, 1998.



Robinson TN: Reducing children's television viewing to prevent obesity: a randomized controlled trial, *JAMA* 282:1561, 1999.
Ruser CB, Federman DG, Kashaf SS: Whittling away at obesity and overweight, *Postgrad Med* 117(1):31, 2005.
Sanjur D: *Hispanic foodways, nutrition, and health,* Needham Heights, Mass, 1995, Allyn and Bacon.
Satter E: *Your child's weight, helping without harming*. Madison, Wis, 2005, Kelcy Press.
Shintani TT, Hughes CK, Beckham S et al: Obesity and cardiovascular risk intervention through the ad libitum feeding of traditional Hawaiian diet, *Am J Clin Nutr* 53(6 Suppl):1647S, 1991.
Spiegel K, Tasali E, Penev P et al: Brief communication: sleep curtailment in healthy young men is associated with decreased leptin levels, elevated ghrelin levels, and increased hunger and appetite, *Ann Intern Med* 141(11):846, 2004.
Thompson D, Jago R, Baranowski T et al: Covariability in diet and physical activity in African-American girls, *Obes Res* 12(Suppl):S46-S54, 2004.
Thompson DL, Rakow J, Perdue SM: Relationship between accumulated walking and body composition in middle-aged women, *Med Sci Sports Exerc* 36(5):911, 2004.
Tudor-Locke C, Pangrazi RP, Corbin CB et al: BMI-referenced standards for recommended pedometer-determined steps/day in children, *Prev Med* 38(6):857, 2004.
Tufts University: Getting enough sleep helps you stay slim, *Health Nutr Let* 22(11):2, 2005.
Tyler DO, Allan JD, Alcozer FR: Weight loss methods used by African American and Euro-American women, *Res Nurs Health* 20:413, 1997.
Unger JB, Reynolds K, Shakib S et al: A. Acculturation, physical activity, and fast-food consumption among Asian-American and Hispanic adolescents, *J Community Health* 29(6):467-481, 2004.
VanWormer JJ: Pedometers and brief e-counseling: increasing physical activity for overweight adults *J Appl Behav Anal* 37(3):421, 2004.
Wu T, Giovannucci E, Pischon T et al: Fructose, glycemic load, and quantity and quality of carbohydrate in relation to plasma C-peptide concentrations in U.S. women, *Am J Clin Nutr* 80(4):1043, 2004.

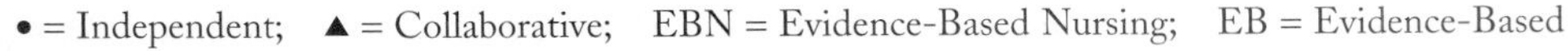

# Risk for imbalanced Nutrition: more than body requirements

*Betty Ackley*

**NANDA**

## Definition

At risk for intake of nutrients that exceeds metabolic needs

## Risk Factors

Reported use of solid food as major food source before 5 months of age; concentration of food intake at end of day; reported or observed obesity in one or both parents; reported or observed higher baseline weight at beginning of each pregnancy; rapid transition across growth percentiles in infants or children; pairing of food with other activities; observed use of food as reward or comfort measure; eating in response to internal cues other than hunger (e.g., anxiety); eating in response to external cues (e.g., time of day, social situation); dysfunctional eating patterns

**NOC**

## Outcomes (Nursing Outcomes Classification)

### Suggested NOC Outcomes

Nutritional Status: Food and Fluid Intake, Nutrient Intake; Weight Control

N

**Example NOC Outcome with Indicators**

**Weight Control** as evidenced by the following indicators: Demonstrates progress toward target weight/Balances exercise with caloric intake/Maintains recommended eating pattern/Controls preoccupation with food (Rate each indicator of **Weight Control:** 1 = never demonstrated, 2 = rarely demonstrated, 3 = sometimes demonstrated, 4 = often demonstrated, 5 = consistently demonstrated [see Section I].)

## Client Outcomes

**Client Will (Specify Time Frame):**

- Explain concept of a balanced diet
- Compare current eating pattern with recommended healthy one
- Design dietary modifications to meet individual long-term goal of weight control, using principles of variety, balance, and moderation
- Identify role of exercise in weight control

**NIC**

## Interventions (Nursing Interventions Classification)

### Suggested NIC Interventions

Nutrition Management; Nutritional Counseling; Weight Management

**Example NIC Activities—Weight Management**

Determine client's motivation for changing eating habits; develop with client a method to keep daily record of intake

### Nursing Interventions and Rationales

Refer to care plan for **Imbalanced Nutrition: more than body requirements**

## Impaired Oral mucous membrane

evolve

*Betty J. Ackley*

**NANDA**

### Definition

Disruptions of lips and soft tissues of oral cavity

### Defining Characteristics

Purulent drainage or exudates; gingival recession, pockets deeper than 4 mm; tonsils enlarged beyond what is developmentally appropriate; smooth, atrophic, sensitive tongue; geographic tongue; mucosal denudation; presence of pathogens; difficulty in speech; self-report of bad taste; gingival or mucosal pallor; oral pain/discomfort; xerostomia (dry mouth); vesicles, nodules, or papules; white patches/plaques, spongy patches, or white curdlike exudate; oral lesions or ulcers; halitosis; edema; hyperemia; desquamation; coated tongue; stomatitis; self-report of difficult eating or swallowing; self-report of diminished or absent taste; bleeding; macroplasia; gingival hyperplasia; fissures; cheilitis; red or bluish masses (e.g., hemangiomas)

### Related Factors (r/t)

Chemotherapy; chemical exposure (e.g., alcohol, tobacco, acidic foods, regular use of inhalers); depression; immunosuppression; aging-related loss of connective, adipose, or bone tissue; barriers to professional care; cleft lip or palate; medication side effects; lack of or decreased salivation; chemical trauma (e.g., acidic foods, drugs, noxious agents, alcohol); pathological conditions—oral cavity (radiation to head or neck); nothing-by-mouth status for more than 24 hours; mouth breathing; malnutrition or vitamin deficiency; dehydration; infection; ineffective oral hygiene; mechanical factors (e.g., ill-fitting dentures, braces, tubes [endotracheal/nasogastric], surgery in oral cavity); decreased platelet count; immunocompromise; radiation therapy; barriers to oral self-care; diminished hormone levels (women); stress; loss of supportive structures

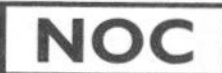

## Outcomes (Nursing Outcomes Classification)

### Suggested NOC Outcomes

Oral Hygiene; Tissue Integrity: Skin and Mucous Membranes

**Example NOC Outcome with Indicators**

**Oral Hygiene** as evidenced by the following indicators: Cleanliness of mouth/Moisture of oral mucosa and tongue/Color of mucous membranes/Oral mucosa integrity (Rate each indicator of **Oral Hygiene:** 1 = severely compromised, 2 = substantially compromised, 3 = moderately compromised, 4 = mildly compromised, 5 = not compromised [see Section I].)

## Client Outcomes

### Client Will (Specify Time Frame):

- Maintain intact, moist oral mucous membranes that are free of ulceration and debris
- Demonstrate measures to regain or maintain intact oral mucous membranes

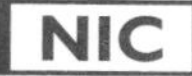

## Interventions (Nursing Interventions Classification)

### Suggested NIC Intervention

Oral Health Restoration

**Example NIC Activities—Oral Health Restoration**

Use soft toothbrush for removal of dental debris; instruct client to avoid commercial mouthwashes

O

## Nursing Interventions and Rationales

- ▲ Inspect the oral cavity at least once daily and note any discoloration, lesions, edema, bleeding, exudate, or dryness. Refer to a physician or specialist as appropriate. *Oral inspection can reveal signs of oral disease, symptoms of systemic disease, drug side effects, or trauma of the oral cavity (White, 2000).*
- Assess for mechanical agents such as ill-fitting dentures and chemical agents such as frequent exposure to tobacco that could cause or increase trauma to oral mucous membranes. **EB:** *Denture wearing and being edentulous can be related to a decreased quality of life and risk for undiagnosed oral disease (Weyant et al, 2004).*
- Monitor the client's nutritional and fluid status to determine if it is adequate. Refer to the care plan for **Deficient Fluid volume** or **Imbalanced Nutrition: less than body requirements** if applicable. *Dehydration and malnutrition predispose clients to impaired oral mucous membranes.*
- Encourage fluid intake of up to 3000 mL/day if not contraindicated by the client's medical condition. *Fluids help increase moisture in the mouth, which protects the mucous membranes from damage and helps the healing process (Roberts, 2000).*

- Determine the client's mental status. If the client is unable to care for him- or herself, oral hygiene must be provided by nursing personnel. The nursing diagnosis **Bathing/hygiene Self-care deficit** is then also applicable.
- Determine the client's usual method of oral care and address any concerns regarding oral hygiene. *Whenever possible, build on the client's existing knowledge base and current practices to develop an individualized plan of care.*
- If the client does not have a bleeding disorder and is able to swallow, encourage the client to brush the teeth with a soft toothbrush using fluoride-containing toothpaste at least twice per day. **EBN and EB:** *The toothbrush is the most important tool for oral care. Brushing the teeth is the most effective method for reducing plaque and controlling periodontal disease (American Dental Association [ADA], 2004; Pearson & Hutton, 2002; Stiefel, 2000; DeWalt, 1975).*
- Encourage the client to brush the tongue with the toothbrush, or use a tongue scraper twice a day. **EB:** *The tongue scraper was shown to be more effective than brushing in removing volatile sulfur compounds which are associated with halitosis (Pedrazzi et al, 2004). Another study demonstrated that tongue brushing or scraping resulted in improved taste sensation and reduced the coating on the tongue (Quirynen et al, 2004).*
- If the client does not have a bleeding disorder, encourage the client to floss once per day or use an interdental cleaner. **EB:** *Floss is useful to remove plaque buildup between the teeth (Brown & Yoder, 2002; ADA, 2004).*

## Client Receiving Chemotherapy/Radiation

- Ensure that the client receives a comprehensive oral examination before initiation of chemotherapy or radiation, with aggressive preventative dental care given as needed (National Institutes of Health [NIH], 1990; Sonis & Kunz, 1988).
- Provide instructions about the need for and method of providing frequent oral care to the patient one week before radiotherapy. **EBN:** *In one study, Shieh et al demonstrated that instructions on oral care given 1 week prior to radiation resulted in reduced mucositis as opposed to instructions given 1 day before, or no instructions (Shieh et al, 1997).*
- For measurement of presence or severity of mucositis, use the Oral Mucositis Assessment Scale (OMAS). **EB:** *This is an instrument that has two components; clinician's assessment of presence and severity of mucositis, and patient report about pain, difficulty swallowing, and ability to eat (Sonis et al, 1999). For more information about measurement of oral mucositis, please refer to Eilers and Epstein (2004).*
- For the client receiving bolus fluorouracil, use cryotherapy with ice chips dissolving in client's mouth for 5 minutes before and 25 minutes after bolus administration of fluorouracil to reduce the severity of mucositis (Cascinu et al, 1994; Mahood et al, 1991; Rocke et al, 1993).
- Give the client frequent sips of water, and ask client to rinse the mouth with water regularly. **EBN:** *The use of water to moisten the mouth has been shown to be as effective as many other agents (Joanna Briggs Institute, 2004).*
- Provide ice chips frequently to keep the mouth moist. **EB:** *There is some evidence that ice chips help prevent mucositis (Clarkson, Worthington, & Eden, 2003).*

▲ If radiation induced mucositis, request an order for benzydamine hydrochloride as a mouthwash for prevention or treatment of radiation induced mucositis. **EB:** *Ben-*

O

*zydamine is effective in relieving mouth pain and severity of mucositis (Epstein et al, 2001; Epstein et al, 1989; Lever, Dupuis, & Chan, 1987).*

- • Help client use a mouth rinse of salt and soda every 1 to 2 hours for prevention and treatment of stomatitis. **EBN:** *A study demonstrated that there was no difference in the rate of cessation of symptoms of stomatitis when three different mouthwashes were used: chlorhexidine, lidocaine, Benadryl and Maalox, and salt and soda (Dodd et al, 2000).*
- ▲ If the mouth is severely inflamed and it is painful to swallow, contact the physician for a topical anesthetic or analgesic order. Modification of oral intake (e.g., soft or liquid diet) may also be necessary to prevent friction trauma. The nursing diagnosis **Imbalanced Nutrition: less than body requirements** may apply.
- • If the client's platelet count is lower than 50,000/mm$^3$ or the client has a bleeding disorder, use a specially made toothbrush designed for sensitive or diseased tissue, or a toothette that is not soaked in glycerin or flavorings; if the client cannot tolerate a toothbrush or a toothettte, a piece of gauze wrapped around a finger can be used to remove plaque and debris (Brown & Yoder, 2002).
- • Use tap water or normal saline to provide oral care; do not use commercial mouthwashes containing alcohol or hydrogen peroxide. Also, do not use lemon-glycerin swabs. *Alcohol dries the oral mucous membranes (Rogers, 2001).* **EBN:** *Hydrogen peroxide can cause mucosal damage and is extremely foul-tasting to clients (Tombes & Gallucci, 1993). Use of lemon-glycerin swabs can result in decreased salivary amylase and oral moisture, as well as erosion of tooth enamel (Foss-Durant & McAffee, 1997; Poland, 1987).*
- • Use foam sticks to moisten the oral mucous membranes, clean out debris, and swab out the mouth of the edentulous client. Do not use foam sticks to clean the teeth unless the platelet count is very low and the client is prone to bleeding gums. *Foam sticks are useful for cleansing the oral cavity of a client who is edentulous (Curzio & McCowan, 2000).* **EBN:** *Foam sticks are not effective for removing plaque; the toothbrush is much more effective (DeWalt, 1975; Pearson & Hutton, 2002).*
- • Keep the lips well lubricated using a lip balm that is water or aloe-based. *This is a comfort measure (Joanna Briggs Institute, 2004; Sadler, 2003).*

O

## Client on a Ventilator

- • Use a pediatric-size toothbrush to brush teeth, use suction to remove secretions. **EBN:** *Brushing the teeth is effective in removing dental plaque (Pearson, 1996; Stiefel et al, 2000). Further research is needed because brushing may increase tranlocation of bacteria from the oral cavity to the trachea or bloodstream if the contamination is not sufficiently removed from the oral cavity. A study is now being conducted combining mechanical cleaning plus an antibacterial application (Munro & Grap, 2004).*
- • Use water as a rinsing agent and mouthwash. **EBN:** *The use of water to moisten the mouth has been shown to be as effective as many other agents (Joanna Briggs Institute, 2004).*
- ▲ Apply chlorhexidine gluconate in the oral cavity by swab or spray early after intubation if ordered. **EBN:** *A study demonstrated that the use of chlorohexidine gluconate administered early after intubation decreased positive cultures of bacteria and may decrease VAP (Grap et al, 2004). More studies are needed before this technique can be recommended for practice.*

- Provide scrupulous oral care to a critically ill client. *Cultures of the teeth of critically ill clients have yielded significant bacterial colonization, which can lead to nosocomial pneumonia (Scannapieco, Stewart, & Mylotte, 1992).*
- ▲ If whitish plaques are present in the mouth or on the tongue and can be rubbed off readily with gauze, leaving a red base that bleeds, suspect a fungal infection and contact the physician for follow-up. *Oral candidiasis (moniliasis) is extremely common secondary to antibiotic therapy, steroid therapy, human immunodeficiency virus (HIV) infection, diabetes, or treatment with immunosuppressive drugs, and should be treated with oral or systemic antifungal agents (Epstein & Chow, 1999).*
- Refer to the care plan for **Impaired Dentition** if the client has problems with the teeth.

## Geriatric

- Determine the functional ability of the client to provide his or her own oral care. Refer to **Bathing/hygiene Self-care deficit.** *Interventions must be directed toward both treatment of the functional loss and care of oral health (Avlund, Holm-Pedersen, & Schroll, 2001).*
- Provide appropriate oral care to the elderly with a self care deficit, brushing the teeth after every meal. **EB:** *Several studies have shown that the rate of pneumonia was decreased by providing oral care after every meal (Watando et al, 2004; Yoneyama et al, 2002).*
- Carefully observe the oral cavity and lips for abnormal lesions such as white or red patches, masses, ulcerations with an indurated margin, or a raised granular lesion. *Malignant lesions are more common in elderly persons than in younger persons, especially if there is a history of smoking or alcohol use, and many elderly persons rarely visit a dentist (Aubertin, 1997).*
- Ensure that dentures are removed and scrubbed at least once daily, removed and rinsed thoroughly after every meal, and removed and kept in an appropriate solution at night. *This is an evidence-based protocol for denture care (Curzio & McCowan, 2000). Denture plaque containing* Candida *organisms can cause denture-induced stomatitis, which is more common in clients with unhealthy lifestyles and poor oral hygiene than in others (Nikawa, Hamada, & Yamamoto, 1998; Sakki et al, 1997).*
- If the client has xerostomia, evaluate medications to see if they could be the cause, provide synthetic saliva products to moisten the oral cavity, and offer frequent sips of water and sugarless gum or candy to provide lubrication. *Xerostomia is common in the elderly for many reasons, including medication use and aging. The goal is to keep the mouth moist to prevent stomatitis (Walton, Miller, & Tordecilla, 2001).*



## Home Care

- The interventions described previously may be adapted for home care use.
- ▲ If dryness is a side effect of the client's medication(s), instruct the client in the use of artificial saliva. Monitor sodium intake in hypertensive clients. Use alternatives to sodium chloride rinses. *Frequent rinsing with sodium chloride places the client at risk for exacerbation of hypertension or heart failure.*

- Instruct the client to avoid alcohol-based or hydrogen peroxide–based commercial products for mouth care and to avoid other irritants to the oral cavity (e.g., tobacco, spicy foods). *Oral irritants can further damage the oral mucosa and increase the client's discomfort.*
- Instruct the client in ways to soothe the oral cavity (e.g., cool beverages, Popsicles, viscous lidocaine).
- If the client often breathes by mouth, add humidity to the room unless contraindicated.

▲ If necessary, refer for home health aide services to support the family in oral care and observation of the oral cavity.

## Client/Family Teaching

- Teach the client how to inspect the oral cavity and monitor for signs and symptoms of infection or complications, and when to call the health care practitioner (Rogers, 2001).
- Teach the client and family if necessary how to perform appropriate mouth care.

## evolve WEBSITES FOR EDUCATION

See the EVOLVE website for World Wide Web resources for client education.

## REFERENCES


American Dental Association: Cleaning your teeth and gums. Available at www.ada.org/public/topics/cleaning_faq.asp, accessed April 5, 2005.

Aubertin MA: Oral cancer screening in the elderly: the home healthcare nurse's role, *Home Healthc Nurse* 15(9):594, 1997.

Avlund K, Holm-Pedersen P, Schroll M: Functional ability and oral health among older people: a longitudinal study from age 75 to 80, *J Am Geriatr Soc* 49:7, 2001.

Brown CG, Yoder LH: Stomatitis: an overview, *Am J Nurs* 102(Suppl 4):20, 2002.

Cascinu S et al: Oral cooling (cryotherapy), an effective treatment for the prevention of 5-fluorouracil-induced stomatitis, *Eur J Cancer B Oral Oncol* 30B(4):234-236, 1994.

Clarkson JE, Worthington HV, Eden OB: Interventions for preventing oral mucositis or oral candidiasis for patients with cancer receiving chemotherapy, *Cochrane Database Syst Rev* (3):CD000978, 2003.

Curzio J, McCowan M: Getting research into practice: developing oral hygiene standards, *Br J Nurs* 9(7):434, 2000.

DeWalt EM: Effect of timed hygienic measures on oral mucosa in a group of elderly subjects, *Nurs Res* 24:104, 1975.

Dodd MJ, Dibble SL, Miaskowski C et al: Randomized clinical trial of the effectiveness of three commonly used mouthwashes to treat chemotherapy-induced mucositis, *Oral Surg Oral Med Oral Pathol Oral Radiol Endod* 90(1):39, 2000.

Eilers J, Epstein JB: Assessment and measurement of oral mucositis, *Semin Oncol Nurs* 20(1):22, 2004.

Epstein JB, Chow AW: Oral complications associated with immunosuppression and cancer therapies, *Infect Dis Clin North Am* 13(4):901, 1999.

Epstein JB, Silverman S Jr, Paggiarino DA et al: Benzydamine HCl for prophylaxis of radiation-induced oral mucositis: results from a multi-center, randomized, double-blind, placebo-controlled clinical trial, *Cancer* 92(4):875, 2001.

Epstein JB, Stevenson-Moore P, Jackson S et al: Prevention of oral mucositis in radiation therapy: a controlled study with benzydamine hydrochloride rinse, *Int J Radiat Oncol Biol Phys* 16(6):1571, 1989.

Foss-Durant AM, McAffee A: A comparison of three oral care products commonly used in practice, *Clin Nurs Res* 6:1, 1997.

Grap MJ, Munro CL, Elswick RK Jr et al: Duration of action of a single, early oral application of chlorhexidine on oral microbial flora in mechanically ventilated patients: a pilot study, *Heart Lung* 33(2):83, 2004.

Joanna Briggs Institute: Prevention and treatment of oral mucosistis in cancer patients: Best Practice Information Sheet. Available at www.joannabriggs.edu.au/best_practice/bp5.php, accessed April 5, 2005.

Lever SA , Dupuis LL, Chan SL: Comparative evaluation of benzydamine oral rinse in children with antineoplastic-induced stomatitis, *Drug Intell Clin Pharm* 21:359, 1987.


O

Mahood DJ, Dose AM, Loprinzi CL et al: Inhibition of fluorouracil-induced stomatitis by oral cryotherapy, *J Clin Oncol* 9(3):449, 1991.
Munro CL, Grap MJ: Oral health and care in the intensive care unit: state of the science, *Am J Crit Care* 13(1):25-33, 2004.
National Instututes of Health Consensus Development Panel: NIH Consensus statement: oral complications of cancer therapies, *NCI Monogr* 3, 1990.
Nikawa H, Hamada T, Yamamoto T: Denture plaque—past and recent concerns, *J Dent* 26(4):299, 1998.
Pearson LS: A comparison of the ability of foam swabs and toothbrushes to remove dental plaque: implications for nursing practice, *J Adv Nurs* 23:62, 1996.
Pearson LS, Hutton JL: A controlled trial to compare the ability of foam swabs and toothbrushes to remove dental plaque, *J Adv Nurs* 39:5, 2002.
Pedrazzi V, Sato S, de Mattos Mda G et al: Tongue-cleaning methods: a comparative clinical trial emplying a toothbrush and a tongue scraper, *J Periodontol* 75(7):1009, 2004.
Poland JM: Comparing Moi-Stir to lemon-glycerin swabs, *Am J Nurs* 87(4):422, 1987.
Quirynen M, Avontroodt P, Soers C et al: Impact of tongue cleaners on microbial load and taste, *J Clin Periodontol* 31(7):5-6, 2004.
Roberts J: Developing an oral assessment and intervention tool for older people: 2, *Br J Nurs* 9(18):2033, 2000.
Rocke LK, Loprinzi CL, Lee JK et al: A randomized clinical trial of two different durations of oral cryotherapy for prevention of 5-fluorouracil-related stomatitis, *Cancer* 72:2234, 1993.
Rogers BB: Mucositis in the oncology patient, *Nurs Clin North Am* 36:4, 2001.
Sadler GR, Stoudt A, Fullerton JT et al: Managing the oral sequelae of cancer therapy, *Medsurg Nurs* 12(1):28, 2003.
Sakki TK, Knuuttila ML, Laara E et al: The association of yeasts and denture stomatitis with behavioral and biologic factors, *Oral Surg Oral Med Oral Pathol Oral Radiol Endod* 84(6):624, 1997.
Scannapieco FA, Stewart EM, Mylotte JM: Colonization of dental plaque by respiratory pathogens in medical intensive care patients, *Crit Care Med* 20(6):740, 1992.
Shieh SH et al: Mouth care for nasopharyngeal cancer patients undergoing radiotherapy, *Oral Oncol* 33(1), 1997.
Sonis S, Kunz A: Impact of improved dental services on the frequency of oral complications of cancer therapy for patients with non-head-and-neck malignancies, *Oral Surg Oral Med Oral Pathol* 65, 1988.
Sonis ST, Eilers JP, Epstein JB et al: Validation of a new scoring system for the assessment of clinical trial research of oral mucositis induced by radiation or chemotherapy, Mucositis Study Group, *Cancer* 85(10):2103-2113, 1999.
Stiefel KA, Damron S, Sowers NJ et al: Improving oral hygiene for the seriously ill patient: implementing research-based practice, *Medsurg Nurs* 9(1):40, 2000.
Tombes MB, Gallucci B: The effects of hydrogen peroxide rinses on the normal oral mucosa, *Nurs Res* 42(6):332, 1993.
Walton JC, Miller J, Tordecilla L: Elder oral assessment and care, *Medsurg Nurs* 10:1, 2001.
Watando A, Ebihara S, Ebihara T et al: Daily oral care and cough reflex sensitivity in elderly nursing home patients, *Chest* 126(4):1066, 2004.
Weyant RJ, Pandav RS, Plowman JL et al: Medical and cognitive correlates of denture wearing in older community-dwelling adults, *J Am Geriatr Soc* 52(4):596, 2004.
White R: Nurse assessment of oral health: a review of practice and education, *Br J Nurs* 9(5):260, 2000.
Yoneyama T, Yoshida M, Ohrui T et al: Oral care reduces pneumonia in older patients in nursing homes, *J Am Geriatr Soc* 50(3):340, 2002.

P

# Pain: Assessment Guide and Equianalgesic Chart

*Chris Pasero and Margo McCaffery*

## ASSESSMENT: USE OF PAIN RATING SCALES

### Nursing Assessment/Diagnosis of Pain Sensation

Ask the client about the current level of pain if at all possible. The client's self-report of pain is the single most reliable indicator of how much pain the client is experiencing. The pain intensity rating given by the client is always what is recorded in the patient's record.

• = Independent; ▲ = Collaborative; EBN = Evidence-Based Nursing; EB = Evidence-Based

## Basic Measures of Pain

The hierarchy of importance of basic measures of pain is as follows:

- Client's self-report
- Report of parent, family, or others close to client
- Behaviors (e.g., facial expressions, body movements, crying)
- Physiological measures which are not sensitive or specific indicators of pain (American Pain Society, 2004) Use opioids with caution in the older client. **EBN:** *Elders are more sensitive to the analgesic effects of opioid drugs because they experience a higher peak effect and a longer duration of pain relief (Giuffre et al, 1991). Reduce the initial recommended adult starting opioid dosage by 25% to 50%, especially if the client is frail and debilitated; then increase the dosage by 25% on an individual basis if needed (Ardery et al, 2003).* (See **Acute Pain.**)

## Client/Family Teaching—Use of Pain Rating Scale

NOTE: When it is obvious that pain is severe (e.g., following trauma or major surgery), a pain rating scale need not be used initially. Give an analgesic and wait until the client is better able to understand and use the pain rating scale.

- Explain the primary purposes of a pain rating scale. Show the client and family the scale. This step allows quick, consistent communication between client and caregiver/nurse/physician. Emphasize that the client must volunteer information because the caregivers may not know when the client has pain. *This step also helps establish a pain relief goal that is satisfactory to the client.*
- Explain the specific pain rating scale (e.g., 0 to 10; 0 = no pain and 10 = worst possible pain). When a numerical scale is used, verify that the client can count to the number used. If the client does not understand whatever scale is standard in that clinical setting, use another scale.
- Discuss the word *pain.* Explain that pain is discomfort that may occur anywhere in the body; may have various characteristics such as aching, hurting, pulling, tightness, burning, or pricking; and may be mild to severe. If the client prefers some other term such as hurt, use that word. To verify that the client understands how the word pain (or other word preferred by client) is used, ask client to give two examples of pain he or she has now or has experienced.
- Ask client to practice using the pain rating scale by rating the current pain or past painful experiences.
- Establish a comfort-function goal. Ask the client what pain rating would be acceptable or satisfactory while at rest and active. *This helps set a realistic initial goal. Zero pain is not always possible.*
- Once the initial goal is achieved, the possibility of better pain relief can be considered. Emphasize to the client that satisfactory pain relief is a level of pain that is noticeable but not distressing and enables the client to sleep, eat, and perform other required or desired physical activities. Pain rated at higher than 3 on a 0 to 10 pain rating scale interferes significantly with daily function. *Perceived quality of life appears to be comparable across cultures, with pain ratings of higher than 5 interfering markedly with a person's ability to enjoy life (Pasero & McCaffery, 2004b).* (See **Acute Pain.**)



P

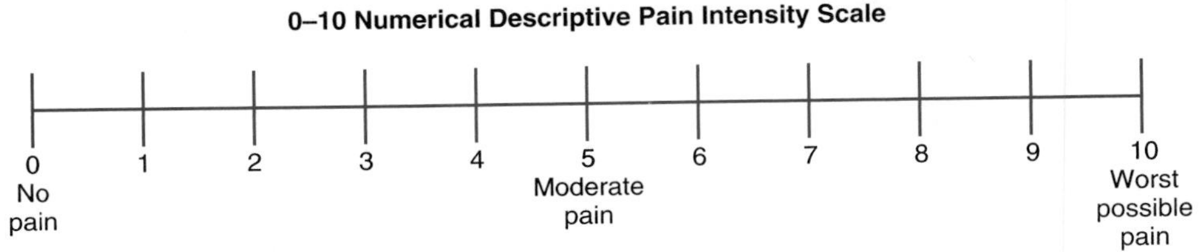


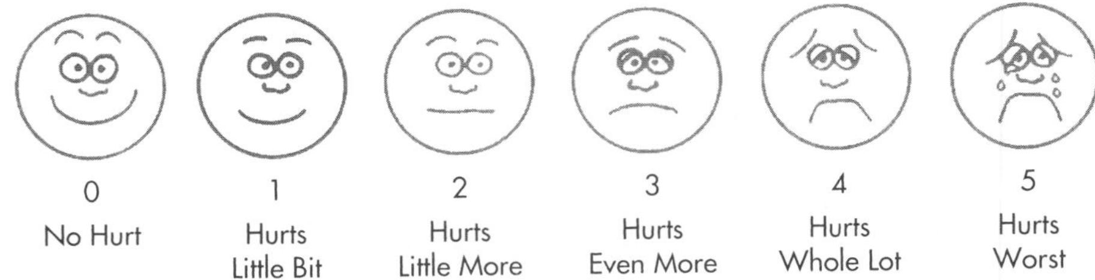


From Wong DL, Hockenberry-Eaton M, Wilson D, Winkelstein ML: *Wong's Essentials of Pediatric Nursing*, ed 6, St Louis, 2001, Mosby. Reprinted with permission.

## HOW TO USE THE WONG-BAKER FACES PAIN SCALE

**Original instructions:** Explain to the person that each face is for a person who feels happy because he has no pain (hurt) or sad because he has some or a lot of pain. **Face 0** is very happy because he doesn't hurt at all. **Face 1** hurts just a little bit. **Face 2** hurts a little more. **Face 3** hurts even more. **Face 4** hurts a whole lot. **Face 5** hurts as much as you can imagine, although you don't have to be crying to feel this bad. Ask the person to choose the face that best desribes how he is feeling.

A rating scale is recommended for persons age 3 years and older.

**Brief word instructions:** Point to each face using the words to describe the pain intensity. Ask the child to choose face that best describes own pain and record the appropriate number.

## HOW TO USE THE FACES PAIN SCALE – REVISED (FPS-R)

"These faces show how much something can hurt. This face (point to the left-most face) shows no pain (or hurt). The faces show more and more pain (point to each face from left to right) up to this one (point to the right-most face)—it shows very much pain. Point to the face that shows how much you hurt (right now)." NOTE: Numbers are not shown to children. **EB:** *The Faces Pain Scale was shown to be valid using 4 to 12 year olds postoperatively. It was further validated with 600 children ages 4-to 5 years receiving immunizations (Wood et al, 2003; Hicks et al, 2001).*

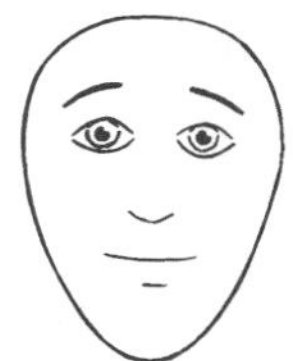 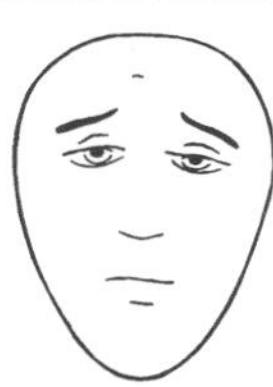 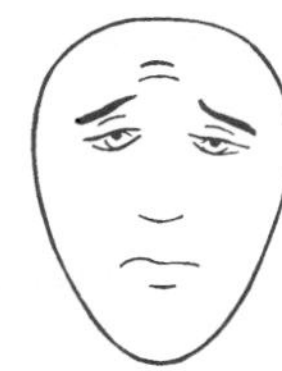 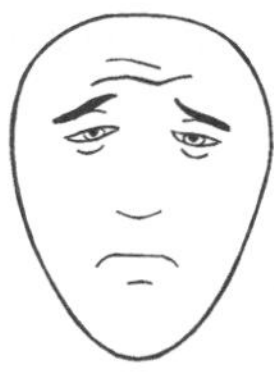 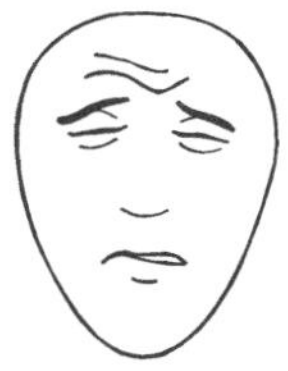 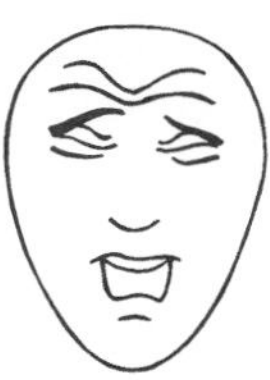

From the *Pediatric Pain Sourcebook.* Original copyright © 2001. Used with permission of the International Association for the Study of Pain and the Pain Research Unit, Sydney Children's Hospital, Randwick NSW 2031, Australia.

## REFERENCES


American Pain Society (APS): Pain: current understanding of assessment, management and treatment. Available at www.ampainsoc.org, accessed November 2004.

American Pain Society: The assessment and management of acute pain in infants, children, and adolescents: a position statement from the American Academy of Pediatrics Committee on psychosocial aspects of child and family health and American Pain Society Task Force on pain in infants, children and adolescents. Available at www.ampainsoc.org, accessed November 2004.

Hicks CL et al: The Faces Pain Scale–Revised: toward a common metric in pediatric pain measurement, *Pain* 93:2, 2001.

Lawlor P et al: Dose ratio between morphine and hydromorphone in patients with cancer pain: a retrospective study, *Pain* 72(1): 79-85, 1997.

Mandfredi PL et al: Intravenous methadone for cancer pain unrelieved by morphine and hydromorphone: clinical observations, *Pain* 70:99, 1997.

Portenoy RK: Opioid analgesics. In Portenoy RK, Kanner RM, editors: *Pain management: theory and practice,* Philadelphia, 1996, FA Davis.

Spagrud LJ, Hon BA, Piira T et al, Pain control: children's self-report of pain intensity, *Am J Nurs* 103:12, 2003.

Wood, C et al: Self-assessment by the Faces Pain Scale: revised of immediate post-vaccination pain following administration of Priorix versus MMRII as a second dose in 4 to 6 year old children, Poster, Sixth International Symposium on Pediatric Pain. Special Interest Group on Pain in Childhood. International Association for the Study of Pain, Sydney, 2003.




## A GUIDE TO USING EQUIANALGESIC CHARTS

- Equianalgesic means approximately the same pain relief.
- The equianalgesic chart is a guideline. Doses and intervals between doses are titrated according to the individual's response.
- The equianalgesic chart is helpful when switching from one drug to another, or switching from one route of administration to another.
- Dosages in the equianalgesic chart for moderate to severe pain are not necessarily starting doses. The doses suggest a ratio for comparing the analgesia of one drug to another.
- For elders, initially reduce the recommended adult opioid dose for moderate to severe pain by 25% to 50%.
- The longer the patient has been receiving opioids, the more conservative the starting doses of a *new* opioid.

## Equianalgesic Chart: Approximate Equivalent Doses of Opioids for Moderate to Severe Pain

| Analgesic | Parenteral (IM, SC, IV) route*†(mg) | PO route* (mg) | Comments |
|---|---|---|---|
| **μ-Opiod Agonists** | | | |
| Morphine | 10 | 30 | Standard for comparison<br>Multiple routes of administration<br>Available in immediate-release and controlled-release formulations<br>Active metabolic M6G can accumulate with repeated dosing in renal failure |
| Codeine | 130 | 200<br>NR | IM has unpredictable absorption and high side effect profile<br>Used PO for mild to moderate pain<br>Usually compounded with nonopioid (e.g., Tylenol #3). |
| Fentanyl | 100 mcg/hr parenterally and transdermally ≅ 4 mg/hr morphine parenterally; 1 mcg/hr transdermally ≅ 2 mg/24 hr morphine PO | — | Short half-life, but at a steady state, slow elimination from tissues can lead to a prolonged half-life (up to 12 hr)<br>Start opioid-naïve patients on no more than 25 mcg/h transdermally<br>Transdermal fentanyl NR for acute pain management<br>Available by oral transmucosal route |
| Hydrocodone (as in Vicodin, Lortab) | | 30?<br>(NR) | Equianlagesic information lacking |
| Hydromorphone (Dilaudid) | 1.5 | 7.5 | Useful alternative to morphine<br>No evidence that metabolites are clinically relevant; shorter duration than morphine<br>Available in high-potency parenteral formulation (10 mg/mL) useful for SC infusion; 3 mg rectal ≅ 650 mg aspirin PO. With repeated dosing (e.g., PCA), it is more likely that 2 to 3 mg parenteral hydromorphone = 10 mg parenteral morphine. |
| Levorphanol (Levo-Dromoran) | 2 | 4 | Longer acting than morphine when given repeatedly<br>Long half-life can lead to accumulation within 2 to 3 days of repeated dosing |
| Meperidine | 75 | 300<br>NR | No longer preferred as a first-line opioid for the management of acute or chronic pain due to potential toxicity from accumulation of metabolite, normeperidine<br>Normeperidine has 15-to 20 hr half-life and is not reversed by naloxone |

## Equianalgesic Chart: Approximate Equivalent Doses of Opioids for Moderate to Severe Pain—cont'd

| Analgesic | Parenteral (IM, SC, IV) route*†(mg) | PO route* (mg) | Comments |
|---|---|---|---|
| **μ-Opiod Agonists—cont'd** | | | |
| Meperidine—cont'd | | | NR in elderly or patients with impaired renal function<br>NR by continuous IV infusion |
| Methadone (Dolophine) | 10 | 29 | Longer acting than morphine when given repeatedly<br>Long half-life can lead to delayed toxicity from accumulation within 3 to 5 days<br>Start PO dosing on PRN schedule<br>In opioid-tolerant patients converted to methadone, start with 10% to 25% of equianalgesic dose |
| Oxycodone | — | 20 | Used for moderate pain when combined with a nonopioid (e.g., Percocet, Tylox)<br>Available as a single entity in immediate-release and controlled-release formulations (e.g., OxyContin)<br>Can be used like PO morphine for severe pain |
| Oxymorphone (Numorphan) | 1 | 10 rectal | Used for moderate to severe pain<br>No PO formulation |
| **Agonist-Antagonist Opioids** | | | |
| Not recommended for severe, escalating pain. If used in combination with μ-agonists, may reverse analgesia and precipitate withdrawal in opioid-dependent patients | | | |
| Buprenorphine (Buprenex) | 0.4 | — | Not readily reversed by naloxone<br>NR for laboring patients |
| Butorphanol (Stadol) | 2 | — | Available in nasal spray |
| Dezocine (Dalgan) | 10 | — | |
| Nalbuphine (Nubain) | 10 | — | |
| Pentazocine (Talwin) | 60 | 180 | |

From McCaffery M, Pasero C: *Pain: clinical manual*, St. Louis, 1999, Mosby.

*IM,* intramuscular; *SC,* subcutaneous; *IV,* intravenous; *PO,* by mouth; *FDA,* Food and Drug Administration; *NR,* not recommended; "≅," roughly equal to.

*Duration of analgesia is dose-dependant; the higher the dose, usually the longer the duration.

†IV boluses may be used to produce analgesia that lasts approximately as long as IM or SC doses. However, of all routes of administration, IV produces the highest peak concentration of the drug, and the peak concentration is associated with the highest level of toxicity, e.g., sedation. To decrease the peak effect and lower the level of toxicity, IV boluses may be administered more slowly (e.g., 10 mg of morphine over a 15 minute period) or smaller doses may be administered more often (e.g., 5 mg of morphine every 1 to 1.5 hours).



P

# Acute Pain

evolve

*Chris Pasero and Margo McCaffery*

## NANDA

### Definition

Pain is whatever the experiencing person says it is, existing whenever the person says it does (McCaffery, 1968); unpleasant sensory and emotional experience arising from actual or potential tissue damage or described in terms of such damage (International Association for the Study of Pain); sudden or slow onset of pain of any intensity from mild to severe with anticipated or predictable end and a duration of less than six months (North American Nursing Diagnosis Association International [NANDA-I])

### Defining Characteristics

#### Subjective

Pain is always subjective and cannot be proved or disproved. A client's report of pain is the most reliable indicator of pain (American Pain Society, 2004). A client with cognitive ability who can speak or point should use a pain rating scale (e.g., 0 to 10) to identify the current level of pain intensity (self-report) and determine a comfort-function goal (Pasero & McCaffery, 2004b; McCaffery & Pasero, 1999). Establishment of a comfort-function goal involves helping the client to select a pain rating level that will allow the client to easily perform identified functional goals (e.g., a pain rating of 3 on a scale of 0 to 10 to cough, deep breathe, and ambulate).

P

#### Objective

Expressions of pain are extremely variable and cannot be used in lieu of self-report. Neither behavior nor vital signs can substitute for the client's self-report (McCaffery & Pasero, 1999, 2001). However, observable responses to pain may be helpful in assessing clients who cannot or will not use a self-report pain rating scale. Observable responses may be loss of appetite and inability to deep breathe, ambulate, sleep, or perform ADLs. Clients may show guarding, self-protective behavior, self-focusing or narrowed focus, distraction behavior ranging from crying to laughing, and muscle tension or rigidity. In sudden and severe pain, autonomic responses such as diaphoresis, blood pressure and pulse changes, pupillary dilation, or increases or decreases in respiratory rate and depth may be present.

### Related Factors (r/t)

Actual or potential tissue damage (mechanical [e.g., incision or tumor growth], thermal [e.g., burn], or chemical [e.g., toxic substance])

**NOC**

## Outcomes (Nursing Outcomes Classification)

### Suggested NOC Outcomes

Comfort Level, Pain Control, Pain Level

**Example NOC Outcome—Pain Level**

Reported **Pain Level.** (Rate pain intensity: 0 = no pain, 1 to 3 = mild pain, 4 to 6 = moderate pain, 7 to 9 = severe pain, 10 = worst possible pain.) In cognitively impaired clients, demonstrates reduction in pain behaviors or improved function.

## Client Outcomes

**Client Will (Specify Time Frame):**

- Use pain rating scale to identify current pain intensity and determine comfort/function goal (if client has cognitive abilities)
- Describe how unrelieved pain will be managed
- Report that pain management regimen relieves pain to satisfactory level with acceptable and manageable side effects
- Perform activities of recovery with reported acceptable level of pain (if pain is above comfort-function goal, take action that decreases pain or notify a member of health care team)
- If cognitively impaired, demonstrate a reduction in pain behaviors, have manageable and tolerable side effects, and perform recovery activities satisfactorily
- State ability to obtain sufficient amounts of rest and sleep
- Describe nonpharmacological method that can be used to help control pain

P

**NIC**

## Interventions (Nursing Interventions Classification)

### Suggested NIC Interventions

Analgesic Administration, Pain Management, Patient-Controlled Analgesia (PCA) Assistance

**Example NIC Activities—Pain Management**

Ensure that client receives attentive analgesic care; perform a comprehensive assessment of pain, including location, characteristics, onset/duration, frequency, quality, intensity or severity, and precipitating factors

## Nursing Interventions and Rationales

▲ Determine whether the client is experiencing pain at the time of the initial interview. If so, intervene at that time to provide pain relief. Assess and document the intensity, character, onset, duration, and aggravating and relieving factors of pain during the initial evaluation of the client. *The initial assessment and documentation provides direction for the pain treatment plan. A comprehensive pain assessment includes all characteristics of the pain that the client can provide. The client's report of the pain is considered the single most reliable data (American Pain Society, 2004; Joint Commission on Accreditation of Healthcare Organizations [JCAHO], 2000).*

- Assess pain in a client using a self-report 0 to 10 numerical pain rating scale or the Faces Pain Scale. **EB:** *Single-item ratings of pain intensity are valid and reliable as measures of pain intensity (Jensen, 2003).*
- Question the client regarding pain at frequent intervals, often at the same time as doing vital signs. *Pain assessment is as important as taking vital signs and the American Pain Society suggests applying the concept of pain assessment as the "fifth vital sign" (American Pain Society, 2004).*
- Ask the client to describe past experiences with pain and the effectiveness of methods used to manage pain, including experiences with side effects, typical coping responses, and the way the client expresses pain. **EBN:** *A study involving 270 people with cancer pain revealed that those surveyed had a number of concerns (barriers) that affected their willingness to report pain and use analgesics (Ward et al, 1993). Many harbored fears and misconceptions regarding the use of analgesics, management of side effects, and risk of addiction.*
- Question the client regarding the level of pain that they think is appropriate to achieve a state of comfort and appropriate function. Attempt to keep below that level, preferably much lower. *The pain rating that allows the client to have comfort and appropriate function should be determined as this allows a tangible way to measure outcomes of pain management (Griffie, 2003).*
- Describe the adverse effects of unrelieved pain. **EBN and EB:** *Numerous pathophysiological and psychological morbidity factors may be associated with pain. One study demonstrated that persistent unrelieved pain suppressed immune function, which can lead to infection and other complications (Page & Ben-Eliyahu, 1997). Analgesics, such as opioids and local anesthetics, have been shown to block immunosuppression (Page & Ben-Eliyahu, 1997). Another study showed that critically ill clients with severe pain had a significantly higher incidence of atelectasis than those with less pain (Puntillo & Weiss, 1994).*
- Assess and document the intensity of the pain and discomfort after any known pain-producing procedure, with each new report of pain, and at regular intervals. *Systematic ongoing assessment and documentation provide direction for the pain treatment plan; adjustments are based on the client's responses. The client's report of pain is the single most reliable indicator of pain (American Pain Society, 2004; JCAHO, 2000).*
- If the client is cognitively impaired and unable to report pain and use a pain rating scale, assess and document behaviors that might be indicative of pain (e.g., change in activity, loss of appetite, guarding, grimacing, moaning) (Herr, 2002). *The absence of behaviors thought to be indicative of pain does not necessarily mean that pain is absent (Pasero, 2003a, b; McCaffery & Pasero, 1999).* **EBN:** *Certain behaviors have been shown to be indicative of pain and can be used to assess pain in clients who cannot use a self-report pain rating tool (e.g., in the cognitively impaired client). The clinician should be aware that*



P

*pain expression is highly individual and what may be a pain behavior in one client may not be in another. Pain assessment must be individualized (Herr, 2002).*

- • Assume that pain is present and treat accordingly in a client who has a pathological condition or who is undergoing a procedure thought to be painful. *Pain is associated with certain pathological conditions (e.g., fractures) and procedures (e.g., surgery). In the absence of the client's report of pain (e.g., anesthetized, critically ill, or cognitively impaired client), the clinician should assume pain is present and treat accordingly (Pasero, 2003b; Herr, 2002; McCaffery & Pasero, 1999).*
- • Prevent pain when possible during procedures such as venipuncture. Use a topical local anesthetic such as EMLA cream, or LMX-4. *Venipuncture pain is often not minor pain to the child or adult experiencing the pain. Nurses are obligated to minimize all kinds of pain (Wong, 2003).*
- • Determine the client's current medication use. *Obtain a complete history of medications the client is taking or has taken to help prevent drug-drug interactions and toxicity problems that can occur when incompatible drugs are combined or when allergies are present. The history will also provide the clinician with an understanding of what medications have been tried and were or were not effective in treating the client's pain (American Pain Society, 2004; McCaffery & Pasero, 1999).*
- ▲ Explore the need for both opioid (narcotic) and nonopioid analgesics. *Pharmacological interventions are the cornerstone of management of moderate to severe pain (American Pain Society, 2004; Pasero 2003a; McCaffery & Pasero, 1999). All analgesic options are considered. Unless contraindicated, all clients with acute pain should receive a nonopioid agent around the clock (ATC). The analgesic regimen should include a nonopioid even if pain is severe enough to require the addition of an opioid (Pasero, 2003a; McCaffery & Pasero 1999). Combining analgesics can result in acceptable pain relief with lower dosages of each analgesic than would be possible with one analgesic alone. Lower dosages can result in fewer or less severe side effects (American Pain Society, 2004; Pasero, 2003a; McCaffery & Pasero, 1999).*
- ▲ Obtain a prescription to administer a nonopioid, such as acetaminophen, a nonselective nonsteroidal anti-inflammatory drug (NSAID), or a cyclooxygenase-2 (COX-2) selective NSAID ATC, unless contraindicated. *Unless contraindicated, all clients with acute pain should receive a nonopioid ATC. The analgesic regimen should include a nonopioid, even if pain is severe enough to require the addition of an opioid (American Pain Society, 2004; Pasero, 2003a; McCaffery & Pasero, 1999).* **EB:** *Oral celecoxib is an effective oral analgesic for acute postoperative pain (Barden et al, 2003).*
- ▲ Obtain a prescription to administer an opioid analgesic if indicated, especially for severe pain. *Opioid analgesics are indicated for the treatment of moderate to severe pain (American Pain Society, 2004; McCaffery & Pasero, 1999; Pasero, 2003a).*
- ▲ Administer opioids orally or intravenously (IV), not intramuscularly (IM). Use a preventive approach to keep pain at or below an acceptable level. Provide PCA and intraspinal routes of administration when appropriate and available. *The least invasive route of administration capable of providing adequate pain control is recommended. The IM route is avoided because of unreliable absorption, pain, and inconvenience. The IV route is preferred for rapid control of severe pain. For ongoing pain, give analgesia ATC. For inter-*

*mittent pain, prn dosing is appropriate (American Pain Society, 2004; Pasero, 2003a; McCaffery & Pasero, 1999).* **EBN:** *One study demonstrated that patient-controlled-analgesia was more effective in controlling pain than on demand IM injections (Chang, Ip, Cheung, 2004).*

- Explain to the client the pain management approach that has been ordered, including therapies, medication administration, side effects, and complications. *One of the most important steps toward improved control of pain is a better client understanding of the nature of pain, its treatment, and the role the client needs to play in pain control (American Pain Society, 2004; McCaffery & Pasero, 1999).*
- Discuss the client's fears of under treated pain, overdose, and addiction. *Because of the many misconceptions regarding pain and its treatment, education about the ability to control pain effectively and correction of myths about the use of opioids should be included as part of the treatment plan. Addiction is unlikely when clients use opioids for pain management (American Pain Society, 2004; McCaffery & Pasero, 1999; McCaffery, Pasero, & Portenoy, 2004).* **EBN:** *A survey of 270 people with cancer pain revealed that many harbored fears and misconceptions regarding the use of analgesics, management of side effects, and risk of addiction (Ward et al, 1993).*

▲ When opioids are administered, assess pain intensity, sedation, and respiratory status at regular intervals. Assess sedation and respiratory status at least every 2 hours in opioid-naïve clients (those who have not been taking regular daily doses of opioids) during the first 24 hours of opioid therapy. Decrease the opioid dose if the client is excessively sedated. *Opioids may cause respiratory depression because they reduce the responsiveness of carbon dioxide chemoreceptors located in the respiratory centers of the brain. Because even more opioid is required to produce respiratory depression than is required to produce sedation, clients with clinically significant respiratory depression are usually also sedated. Respiratory depression can be prevented by assessing sedation and decreasing the opioid dose when the client is arousable but has difficulty staying awake (McCaffery & Pasero, 1999; Pasero & McCaffery, 2002).*



▲ Review the client's flow sheet and medication records to determine overall degree of pain relief, side effects, and analgesic requirements during the previous 24 hours. **EBN:** *One study showed that systematic tracking of pain was an important factor in improving pain management (Faries et al, 1991).*

▲ Administer supplemental opioid doses as needed to keep pain ratings at or below the comfort-function goal. *An order for prn supplementary opioid doses between regular doses is an essential backup (American Pain Society, 2004; McCaffery & Pasero, 2003; McCaffery & Pasero, 1999).*

▲ Obtain prescriptions to increase or decrease opioid doses as needed; base prescriptions on the client's report of pain severity and response to the previous dose in terms of relief, side effects, and ability to perform the activities of recovery. Increase or decrease the dosage of opioid based on assessment of the client's response. *Clients' responses, and therefore their analgesic requirements, vary widely, so it is less important to focus on the amount given than on the response (McCaffery & Pasero, 1999). It is important that nurses knowledgeable in pain management have an "as needed" range of opioid doses available to provide appropriate pain relief (American Pain Society, 2004b).*

▲ When the client is able to tolerate oral analgesics, obtain a prescription to change to the oral route; use an equianalgesic chart to determine initial dose. (Refer to the Equianalgesic Chart before this care plan.) *The oral route is preferred because it is the most convenient and cost effective (American Pain Society, 2004). Use of equianalgesic doses when switching from one opioid or route of administration to another will help to prevent loss of pain control from underdosing and side effects from overdosing (McCaffery, 2003; McCaffery & Pasero, 2003).*

• In addition to administering analgesics, support the client's use of nonpharmacological methods to help control pain, such as distraction, imagery, relaxation, and application of heat and cold. *Cognitive-behavioral strategies can restore the client's sense of self-control, personal efficacy, and active participation in his or her own care (American Pain Society, 2004).*

• Teach and implement nonpharmacological interventions when pain is relatively well-controlled with pharmacological interventions. *Nonpharmacological interventions should be used to supplement, not replace, pharmacological interventions (American Pain Society, 2004).*

• Plan care activities around periods of greatest comfort whenever possible. *Pain diminishes the client's activity. Performing care actions at times when the client is rested and pain is well controlled will make it easier for the client to achieve recovery or rehabilitation milestones (McCaffery & Pasero, 1999).*

▲ Ask the client to describe appetite, bowel elimination, and ability to rest and sleep. Administer medications and treatments to improve these functions. Obtain a prescription for a peristaltic stimulant to prevent opioid-induced constipation. *Because there is great individual variation in the development of opioid-induced side effects, these side effects should be monitored and, if their development is inevitable (e.g., constipation), prophylactically treated. Opioids cause constipation by decreasing bowel peristalsis (Plaisance & Ellis, 2002; McCaffery & Pasero, 1999).*

P

### Pediatric

• For the neonate, use oral sucrose for pain of short duration such as heel stick or venipuncture. *Neonates are as sensitive to pain as adults, and premature infants are thought to be highly sensitive. Oral sucrose briefly produces analgesia in neonates up to age 6 months of age (Pasero, 2004).*

• Use a topical local anesthetic such as EMLA cream, or LMX-4. before performing venipuncture in an infant or child. *Venipuncture pain is often not minor pain to the child experiencing the pain. Nurses are obligated to minimize all kinds of pain (Wong, 2003).*

• For the neonate experiencing moderate to severe pain, utilize opioid analgesics and anesthetics in appropriate dosages. *Neonates experiencing endotracheal intubation and chest tube placement or other procedures causing pain should receive adequate pain medication (Pasero, 2004).*

• For the young child (age 1 to 4 years) use a Faces Pain Scale to determine the level of pain present. **EB:** *The Faces Pain Scale was shown to be valid using 4 to 12 year olds postoperatively. It was further validated with 600 children age 4 to 5 years receiving immunizations (Wood et al, 2003; Hicks et al, 2001).*

## Geriatric

- ▲ Always take the older client's reports of pain seriously and ensure that the pain is relieved. *In spite of what many professionals and clients believe, pain is not an expected part of normal aging (American Geriatric Society Panel on Persistent Pain in Older Persons, 2002; Herr, 2002; McCaffery & Pasero, 1999).*
- • When assessing pain, speak clearly, slowly, and loudly enough for the client to hear, and if the client uses a hearing aid, be sure it is in place; repeat information as needed. Be sure the client can see well enough to read the pain scale (use an enlarged scale) and written materials. *Elders often have difficulty hearing and seeing. Comprehension is improved when instructions are given slowly and clearly and when the client can see visual aids (Herr, 2002).*
- • Handle the client's body gently. Allow the client to move at his or her own speed. *Elders are particularly susceptible to injury during care activities. Caregivers must be patient and expect that the older client will move more slowly than younger clients; they may also perform better and experience less pain during care activities when they are allowed to move themselves (McCaffery & Pasero, 1999).*
- ▲ Use acetaminophen and NSAIDs with low gastrointestinal side-effect profiles, such as the selective COX-2 NSAIDs (celecoxib) and watch for side effects, such as gastrointestinal disturbances and renal dysfunction. *Elders are at increased risk for gastric and renal toxicity from NSAIDs (Fine, 2004; Hutchinson, 2004; American Geriatric Society Panel on Persistent Pain in Older Persons, 2002).*
- ▲ Avoid or use with caution drugs with a long half-life, such as the NSAID piroxicam (Feldene), and the opioids methadone (Dolophine) and levorphanol (LevoDromoran). *The higher prevalence of renal insufficiency in elders compared with younger persons can result in toxicity from drug accumulation (Fick et al, 2003; American Geriatric Society Panel on Persistent Pain in Older Persons, 2002; McCaffery & Pasero, 1999).*
- ▲ Use opioids with caution in the older client. **EBN:** *Elders are more sensitive to the analgesic effects of opioid drugs because they experience a higher peak effect and a longer duration of pain relief (Giuffre et al, 1991). Reduce the initial recommended adult starting opioid dosage by 25% to 50%, especially if the client is frail and debilitated; then increase the dosage by 25% on an individual basis if needed (Ardery et al, 2003).*
- ▲ Avoid the use of opioids with toxic metabolites, such as meperidine (Demerol) and propoxyphene (Darvon, Darvocet), in older clients. *Meperidine's metabolite, normeperidine, can produce central nervous system (CNS) irritability, seizures, and even death; propoxyphene's metabolite, norpropoxyphene, can produce CNS toxicity. Both of these metabolites are eliminated by the kidneys, which makes meperidine and propoxyphene particularly poor choices for older clients, many of whom have at least some degree of renal insufficiency (Ardery et al, 2003; Fick et al, 2003; American Geriatrics Society, 2002; McCaffery & Pasero, 1999).*

## Multicultural

- • Assess for the influence of cultural beliefs, norms, and values on the client's perception and experience of pain. **EB:** *One study showed that the Native-American patients may think that asking for pain medication is disrespectful because it implies that health care pro-*

*viders don't know what they are doing (Brant et al, 2001). A recent study with African-American elders found the use of prayer or faith for pain management, care, and prevention was very common (Ibrahim et al, 2004). A representational approach first developed at the University of Wisconsin-Madison School of Nursing offers a flexible framework for nurses to get cancer patients to delve deeply into their own belief systems about health, disease, pain, and so on, and to add sound concepts that will work for their pain management. The program is called Representational Intervention to Decrease Cancer Pain (RIDcancer-Pain) and has the following 6 steps:*

1. Representational assessment—the patient describes beliefs about cancer pain along five dimensions: identity, cause, timeline, consequences and cure/control
2. Exploring misconceptions, with emphasis on their origins
3. Creating conditions for conceptual change by discussing the limitations of holding beliefs that are misconceptions (i.e., what one loses by maintaining those beliefs)
4. Introducing replacement information
5. Summarizing and discussing benefits of adopting beliefs that are credible replacements
6. Developing a plan and strategies. (Ward, Donovan & Gunnarsdottir, in press)

- Assess for the effect of fatalism on the client's beliefs regarding the current state of comfort. **EBN:** *Fatalistic perspectives, which involve the belief that one cannot control one's own fate, may influence health behaviors in some African-American and Latino populations (Phillips, Cohen, & Moses, 1999; Harmon, Castro, & Coe, 1996).*
- Assess for pain disparities among racial and ethnic minorities. **EB:** *Racial and ethnic minorities tend to be undertreated for pain when compared with non-Hispanic whites (Green et al, 2003).*
- Incorporate safe and effective folk health care practices and beliefs into care whenever possible. It is the responsibility of the caregiver to ensure that safe and effective pain management is provided. Although support of an individual's health care beliefs is recommended, when research does not support the safety or effectiveness of a method or when research does not exist, this should be explained fully to the client (McCaffery & Pasero, 1999). **EBN:** *Incorporating folk health care beliefs and practices into pain management care increased compliance with the treatment plan (Juarez, Ferrell, & Borneman, 1998).*
- Use a family-centered approach to care. **EBN:** *Involving the family in pain management care increased compliance with the treatment regimen (Juarez, Ferrell, & Borneman, 1998).*
- Teach information about pain medications and their side effects, how to work with health care providers to manage pain, and encouragement to use religious faith to cope with pain. **EB:** *Socioeconomically disadvantaged African-American and Hispanic patients benefit from educational interventions on pain that dispel myths about opioids and teach patients to communicate assertively about their pain with their physicians and nurses (Anderson et al, 2002).*
- Use culturally relevant pain scales (e.g., the Oucher Scale), if available, to assess pain in the client. **EBN:** *Clients from minority cultures may express pain differently than clients from the majority culture. The Oucher Scale is available in African-American and Hispanic versions and is used to assess pain in children (Beyer, Denyes, & Villarruel, 1992).*
- Ensure that directions for medication use are available in the client's language of

P

choice and are understood by the client and caregiver. **EB:** *Use of bilingual instructions for medication administration increased compliance with the pain management plan (Juarez, Ferrell, & Borneman, 1998). Using specific phrases in Spanish to assess acute pain in non–English-speaking Hispanic patients helps provide timely pain assessment and management (Collins, Gullette, & Schnepf, 2004).*

## Home Care

- Develop the treatment plan with the client and caregivers. *Client input into the plan of care improves the likelihood of successful management.*
- ▲ Develop a full medication profile, including medications prescribed by all physicians and all over-the-counter medications. Assess for drug interactions. Instruct the client to refrain from mixing medications without physician approval. *Pain medications may significantly affect or be affected by other medications and may cause severe side effects. Some combinations of drugs are specifically contraindicated (American Pain Society, 2004; Pasero, 2003a).*
- Assess the client's and family's knowledge of side effects and safety precautions associated with pain medications (e.g., use caution in operating machinery when opioids are first taken or dosage has been increased significantly). *The cognitive effects of opioids usually subside within a week of initial dosing or dosage increases (McCaffery & Pasero, in press). The use of long-term opioid treatment does not appear to affect neuropsychological performance.* **EB:** *Pain itself may reduce performance on neuropsychological tests more than oral opioid treatment (Sjogren et al, 2000).*
- If medication is administered using highly technological methods, assess the home for the necessary resources (e.g., electricity) and ensure that there will be responsible caregivers available to assist the client with administration. *Some routes of medication administration require special conditions and procedures to be safe and accurate (McCaffery & Pasero, 1999).*
- ▲ Assess the knowledge base of the client and family with regard to highly technological medication administration. Teach as necessary. Be sure the client knows when, how, and whom to contact if analgesia is unsatisfactory. *Appropriate instruction in the home increases the accuracy and safety of medication administration (McCaffery & Pasero, 1999).*



## Client/Family Teaching

NOTE: To avoid the negative connotations associated with the words *drugs* and *narcotics,* use the term *pain medicine* when teaching clients.

- Provide written materials on pain control such as *Understanding Your Pain: Using a Pain Rating Scale* (McCaffery, Pasero, & Portenoy, 2001) (see instructions on the use of pain rating scales) and *Taking Oral Opioid Analgesics* (McCaffery, Pasero, & Portenoy, 2004). *Written materials are provided in addition to verbal instructions so that the client will have a reference during treatment (McCaffery & Pasero, 1999).*
- Discuss the various discomforts encompassed by the word *pain* and ask the client to give examples of previously experienced pain. Explain the pain assessment process and the purpose of the pain rating scale. *It is often difficult for clients to understand the con-*

*cept of pain and describe their pain experience. Using alternative words and providing a complete description of the assessment process, including the use of scales, will ensure that an accurate treatment plan is developed (McCaffery & Pasero, 1999, 2001).*

- ▲ Teach the client to use the pain rating scale to rate the intensity of past or current pain. Ask the client to set a comfort-function goal by selecting a pain level on the rating scale that makes it easy to perform recovery activities (e.g., turn, cough, deep breathe). If pain is above this level, the client should take action that decreases pain or notify a member of the health care team. (See information on teaching clients to use the pain rating scale.) *The use of comfort-function goals provides direction for the treatment plan. Changes are made according to the client's response and achievement of the goals of recovery or rehabilitation (Pasero & McCaffery, 2004).*
- ▲ Demonstrate medication administration and the use of supplies and equipment. If PCA is ordered, determine the client's ability to press the appropriate button. Remind the client and staff that the PCA button is for client use only. *Appropriate instruction increases the accuracy and safety of medication administration (McCaffery & Pasero, 1999).*
- • Reinforce the importance of taking pain medications to keep pain under control. *Teaching clients to stay on top of their pain and prevent it from getting out of control will improve the ability to accomplish the goals of recovery (Pasero & McCaffery, 2004).*
- • Reinforce that taking opioids for pain relief is not addiction and that addiction is very unlikely to occur. *The development of addiction when opioids are taken for pain relief is rare (American Pain Society, 2004).*
- • Demonstrate the use of appropriate nonpharmacological approaches in addition to pharmacological approaches for helping to control pain, such as application of heat and/or cold, distraction techniques, relaxation breathing, visualization, rocking, stroking, music listening, and television watching. *Nonpharmacological interventions are used to complement, not replace, pharmacological interventions (American Pain Society, 2004; McCaffery & Pasero, 1999).*

P

## evolve WEBSITES FOR EDUCATION

See the EVOLVE website for World Wide Web resources for client education.

## REFERENCES


American Geriatric Society Panel on Persistent Pain in Older Persons: The management of persistent pain in older persons, *J Am Geriatr Soc* 50(S205):1-20, 2002.

The American Pain Society: Pain: current understanding of assessment, management and treatments. Available at www.ampainsoc.org/ce/npc, accessed on September 6, 2004.

Anderson KO, Richman SP, Hurley J et al.: Cancer pain management among underserved minority outpatients: perceived needs and barriers to optimal control, *Cancer* 94(8):2295-2304, 2002.

Ardery G, Herr KA, Titler MG et al: Assessing and managing acute pain in older adults: a research base to guide practice, *Medsurg Nurs* 12(1):7, 2003.

Barden J, Edwards J, McQuay HJ et al: Single dose oral celecoxib for postoperative pain, *Cochrane Database Syst Rev* (2): CD004233, 2003.

Beyer J, Denyes M, Villarruel A: The creation, validation, and continuing development of the Oucher: a measure of pain intensity in children, *J Pediatr Nurs* 7(5):335, 1992.

Brant, JM. Cultural implications of pain education, a Native American example, presented at Cancer Pain and Education for Patients and the Public conference, City of Hope National Medical Center, Duarte, Calif, October 18, 2001.
Chang AM, Ip WY, Cheung TH: Patient-controlled analgesia versus conventional intramuscular injection: a cost effectiveness analysis, *J Adv Nurs* 46(5):531, 2004.
Collins AS, Gullette D, Schnepf M: Break through language barriers, *Nurs Manag* 35(8):34-36, 2004.
Faries JE, Mills DS, Goldsmith KW et al: Systematic pain records and their impact on pain control, *Cancer Nurs* 14(6):306, 1991.
Fick DM, Cooper JW, Wade WE et al: Updating the Beers criteria for potentially inappropriate mediation use in older adults, *Arch Int Med* 163:2716-2724, 2003.
Fine P: Pharmacological management of persistent pain in older patients, *Clin J Pain* 20(4):220-226, 2004.
Giuffre M, Asci J, Arnstein P et al: Postoperative joint replacement pain: description and opioid requirement, *J Post Anesth Nurs* 6(4):239, 1991.
Green CR, Anderson KO, Baker TA et al: The unequal burden of pain: confronting racial and ethnic disparities in pain, *Pain Med* 4(3):277-294, 2003.
Griffie J: Pain control: addressing inadequate pain relief, *Am J Nurs* 103(8):61-63, 2003.
Harmon MP, Castro FG, Coe K: Acculturation and cervical cancer: knowledge, beliefs, and behaviors of Hispanic women, *Women Health* 24(3):37, 1996.
Herr K: Pain assessment in cognitively impaired older adults, *Am J Nurs* 102(12):65, 2002.
Humphrey C: *Home care nursing handbook,* ed 2, Gaithersburg, Maryland, 1994, Aspen.
Ibrahim SA, Zhang A, Mercer MB et al: Inner city African-American elderly patients' perceptions and preferences for the care of chronic knee and hip pain: findings from focus groups, *J Gerontol Series A Biol Sci Med Sci* 59(12):1318-1322, 2004.
Joint Commission on Accreditation of Healthcare Organizations: *2000 Hospital accreditation standards,* Oakbrook Terrace, Ill, 2000, The Commission.
Jensen MP: The validity and reliability of pain measures in adults with cancer, *J Pain* 4(1):2, 2003.
Juarez G, Ferrell BR, Borneman T: Influence of culture on cancer pain management in Hispanic clients, *Cancer Pract* 6(5):262, 1998.
Leininger MM: *Transcultural nursing: theories, research and practices,* ed 2, Hilliard, Ohio, 1996, McGraw-Hill.
McCaffery M: *Nursing practice theories related to cognition, bodily pain and man-environment interactions,* Los Angeles, 1968, University of California at Los Angeles Students' Store.
McCaffery M: Culturally sensitive pain assessment, *Am J Nurs* 99(8):18, 1999.
McCaffery M: What is the role of nondrug methods in the nursing care of patients with acute pain? *Pain Manage Nurs* 3(3):77-80, 2002.
McCaffery M: Switching from IV to PO, *Am J Nurs* 103(5):62-63, 2003.
McCaffery M, Pasero C: *Pain: clinical manual,* ed 2, St. Louis, 1999, Mosby.
McCaffery M, Pasero C, Portenoy RK: *Understanding your pain: using a pain rating scale,* Chadds Ford, Pa, 2001, Endo Pharmaceuticals.
McCaffery M, Pasero C, Portenoy RK: *Understanding your pain: taking oral opioid analgesics,* Chadds Ford, Pa, 2004, Endo Pharmaceuticals.
McCaffery M, Pasero C: Pain control: breakthrough pain, *Am J Nurs* 103(4):83, 2003.
Page GG, Ben-Eliyahu S: The immune-suppressive nature of pain, *Semin Oncol Nurs* 13(1):10, 1997.
Pasero C: Multimodal analgesia in the PACU, *J Perianesth Nurs* 18(4):265-268, 2003a.
Pasero C: Pain in the critically ill, *J Perianesth Nurs* 18(6):422-425, 2003b.
Pasero C: Pain control: pain relief for neonates, *Am J Nurs* 104(5):44, 2004.
Pasero C, McCaffery M: Pain control: patient's report of pain, *Am J Nurs* 101(12):73, 2001.
Pasero C, McCaffery M: Monitoring opioid-induced sedation, *Am J Nurs* 102(2):67-68, 2002.
Pasero C, McCaffery M: Pain control: controlled-release oxycodone, *Am J Nurs* 104(1):30, 2004a.
Pasero C, McCaffery M: Pain control: comfort-function goals, *Am J Nurs* 104(9):77, 2004b.
Phillips JM, Cohen MZ, Moses G: Breast cancer screening and African American women: fear, fatalism, and silence, *Oncol Nurs Forum* 26(3):561, 1999.
Plaisance L, Ellis JA: Opioid-induced constipation, *Am J Nurs* 102(3):72-73, 2002.
Puntillo K, Weiss SJ: Pain: its mediators and associated morbidity in critically ill cardiovascular surgical clients, *Nurs Res* 43(3):1, 1994.
Sjogren P, Olsen AK, Thomsen AB et al: Neuropsychological performance in cancer clients: the role of oral opioids, pain and performance status, *Pain* 86(3):237, 2000.

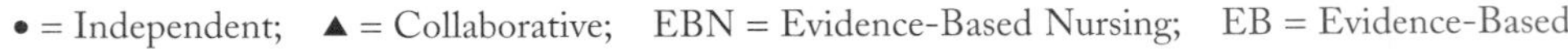

Ward S, Donovan H, Gunnarsdottir S et al: A representational intervention to decrease cancer pain (RIDcancerPain), in press.
Ward SE, Goldberg N, Miller-McCauley V et al: Client-related barriers to management of cancer pain, *Pain* 52(3):319, 1993.
Wong D: Pain control; topical local anesthetics, *Am J Nurs* 103(6):42-45, 2003.
Wood C et al: Self-assessment by the Faces Pain Scale: revised of immediate post-vaccination pain following administration of Priorix versus MMRII as a second dose in 4 to 6 year old children, Poster, Sixth International Symposium on Pediatric Pain, Sydney, 2003, Special Interest Group on Pain in Childhood, International Association for the Study of Pain.

# Chronic Pain

evolve

*Chris Pasero and Margo McCaffery*

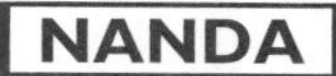

## Definition

Pain is whatever the experiencing person says it is, existing whenever the person says it does (McCaffery, 1968); unpleasant sensory and emotional experience arising from actual or potential tissue damage or described in terms of such damage (International Association for the Study of Pain); sudden or slow onset of pain of any intensity from mild to severe, constant or recurring, without anticipated or predictable end and a duration of greater than six months (NANDA-I); state in which the individual experiences pain that persists for a period beyond the usual course of acute illness or a reasonable duration for the injury to heal, is associated with a chronic pathological process, or recurs at intervals for months or years (Bonica, 1990)

## Defining Characteristics

### Subjective

Pain is always subjective and cannot be proved or disproved. The client's report of pain is the most reliable indicator of pain (American Pain Society, 2004). Clients with cognitive abilities who can speak or point should use a pain rating scale (e.g., 0 to 10) to identify their current level of pain intensity (self-report) and determine a comfort-function goal (Pasero & McCaffery, 2004). Establishment of a comfort-function goal involves assisting clients in selecting a pain rating that will allow them to easily perform identified functional goals (e.g., a pain rating of 3 on a scale of 0 to 10 to work or walk the dog).

### Objective

Expressions of pain are extremely variable and cannot be used in lieu of self-report. Neither behavior nor vital signs can substitute for the client's self-report (American Pain Society, 2004; McCaffery & Pasero, 1999). However, observable responses to pain may be helpful in pain assessment, especially in clients who cannot or will not use a self-report pain rating scale. Observable responses may be loss of appetite or the inability to ambulate, perform ADLs, work, or sleep. Clients may show guarding, self-protective be-



P

havior, self-focusing or narrowed focus, distraction behavior ranging from crying to laughing, and muscle tension or rigidity. In sudden severe pain, autonomic responses such as diaphoresis, blood pressure and pulse changes, pupillary dilation, and increase or decrease in respiratory rate and depth may be present but are usually not seen with chronic pain that is relatively stable. Clients with chronic or persistent cancer or nonmalignant pain may experience threats to self-image; a perceived lack of options for coping; and worsening helplessness, anxiety, and depression. Chronic pain may affect almost every aspect of the client's daily life, including concentration, work, and relationships.

## Related Factors (r/t)

Actual or potential tissue damage; tumor progression and related pathology; diagnostic and therapeutic procedures; central or peripheral nerve injury (neuropathic pain)

NOTE: The cause of chronic nonmalignant pain may not be known because pain study is a new science and an area encompassing diverse types of problems.

**NOC**

## Outcomes (Nursing Outcomes Classification)

### Suggested NOC Outcomes

Comfort Level; Pain Control; Pain: Disruptive Effects; Pain Level

**Example NOC Outcome—Pain Level**

**Reported Pain Level.** (Rate **Pain Level:** 0 = no pain, 1 to 3 = mild pain, 4 to 6 = moderate pain, 7 to 9 = severe pain, 10 = worst possible pain.) In cognitively impaired clients, demonstrates a reduction in pain behaviors or improved function.

P

## Client Outcomes

**Client Will (Specify Time Frame):**

- Use pain rating scale to identify current level of pain intensity, determine comfort/function goal, and maintain a pain diary (if client has cognitive abilities)
- Describe total plan for pharmacological and nonpharmacological pain relief, including how to safely and effectively take medicines and integrate nondrug therapies
- Demonstrate ability to pace self, taking rest breaks before they are needed
- Function on acceptable ability level with minimal interference from pain and medication side effects (if pain is above comfort-function goal, take action that decreases pain or notify a member of health care team)
- If cognitively impaired, demonstrate a reduction in pain behaviors, have manageable and tolerable side effects, and perform ADLs satisfactorily

**NIC**

## Interventions (Nursing Interventions Classification)

### Suggested NIC Interventions

Analgesic Administration; Pain Management

**Example NIC Activities—Pain Management**

Ensure that client receives attentive analgesic care; perform comprehensive assessment of pain, including location, characteristics, onset and duration, frequency, quality, intensity or severity, and precipitating factors

## Nursing Interventions and Rationales

- ▲ Determine whether the client is experiencing pain at the time of the initial interview. If so, intervene at that time to provide pain relief. Assess and document the intensity, character, onset, duration, and aggravating and relieving factors of pain during the initial evaluation of the client. *The initial assessment and documentation provide direction for the pain treatment plan. A comprehensive pain assessment includes all characteristics of the pain that the client can provide. The client's report of the pain is considered the single most reliable datum (American Pain Society, 2004; Joint Commission on Accreditation of Healthcare Organizations [JCAHO], 2000).*
- • Assess pain in a client using a self-report 0 to 10 numerical pain rating scale or a faces pain rating scale. **EB:** *Single-item ratings of pain intensity are valid and reliable as measures of pain intensity (Jensen, 2003).*
- • Question the client regarding pain at frequent intervals, often at the same time as doing vital signs. *Pain assessment is as important as taking vital signs and the American Pain Society suggests applying the concept of pain assessment as the "fifth vital sign" (American Pain Society, 2004).*
- • Tell the client to report pain location, intensity, and quality when experiencing pain. Assess and document the intensity of pain and discomfort after any known pain-producing procedure, with each new report of pain, and at regular intervals. *Systematic ongoing assessment and documentation provide direction for the pain treatment plan; adjustments are based on the client's response. The client's report of pain is the single most reliable indicator of pain (American Pain Society, 2004).*
- • Question the client regarding the level of pain that they think is appropriate to achieve a state of comfort and appropriate function. Attempt to keep pain level no higher than that level, preferably much lower. *The pain rating that allows the client to have comfort and appropriate function should be determined and this allows a tangible way to measure outcomes of pain management (Pasero & McCaffery, 2004; Griffie, 2003).*
- • Ask the client to describe past and current experiences with pain and the effectiveness of the methods used to manage the pain, including experiences with side effects, typical coping responses, and the way the client expresses pain. **EBN:** *A study of 270 people with cancer pain revealed that those surveyed had a number of concerns (barriers) that affected their willingness to report pain and use analgesics (Ward et al, 1993). Many harbored fears and misconceptions regarding the use of analgesics, management of side effects, and risk of addiction.*
- • Describe the adverse effects of unrelieved pain. **EBN and EB:** *Numerous athophysiological and psychological morbidity factors may be associated with pain. One study demonstrated that persistent unrelieved pain suppressed immune function, which can lead to infection, increased tumor growth, and other complications (Page & Ben-Eliyahu, 1997). Analgesics such as opioids and local anesthetics have been shown to block immunosuppression (Page & Ben-Eliyahu, 1997).*

P

- Ask the client to maintain a diary of pain ratings, timing, precipitating events, medications, treatments, and steps that work best to relieve pain. **EBN:** *Studies have shown that systematic tracking of pain was an important factor in improving pain management (Schumacher, Koresawa, & West et al, 2002; Faries et al, 1991).*
- If the client is cognitively impaired and unable to report pain and use a pain rating scale, assess and document behaviors that might be indicative of pain (e.g., change in activity, loss of appetite, guarding, grimacing, moaning). *The absence of behaviors thought to be indicative of pain does not necessarily mean that pain is absent (Pasero, 2003b; Herr, 2002; McCaffery & Pasero, 1999).* **EBN:** *Certain behaviors have been shown to be indicative of pain and can be used to assess pain in clients who cannot use a self-report pain rating tool (e.g., in the cognitively impaired client). The clinician should be aware that pain expression is highly individual, and what may be a pain behavior in one client may not be in another. Pain assessment must be individualized (Herr, 2002).*

▲ Assume that pain is present and treat accordingly in clients who have a pathological condition or are undergoing a procedure thought to be painful. *Pain is associated with certain pathological conditions (e.g., arthritis) and procedures (e.g., surgery). In the absence of the client's report of pain (e.g., in critically ill or cognitively impaired clients), the clinician should assume that pain is present and treat accordingly (Pasero, 2003b).*

- Determine the client's current medication use. To aid in planning pain treatment, obtain a medication history. *Obtaining a complete history of medications the client is taking or has taken can help to prevent drug-drug interactions and toxicity problems that can occur when incompatible drugs are combined or when allergies are present. The history will also provide the clinician with an understanding of what medications have been tried and were or were not effective in treating the client's pain (American Pain Society, 2004; McCaffery and Pasero, 1999).*

▲ Explore the need for medications from the three classes of analgesic: opioids (narcotics), nonopioids (acetaminophen, nonselective nonsteroidal anti-inflammatory drugs [NSAIDs], and COX-2 [cyclo-oxygenase-2] selective NSAIDs), and adjuvant medications. For chronic neuropathic pain, consider adjuvant medications that are analgesic, such as anticonvulsants and antidepressants. *The analgesic regimen should include a nonopioid drug around the clock (ATC), even if pain is severe enough to require the addition of an opioid (American Pain Society, 2004). Some types of pain respond to nonopioid drugs alone. If the pain is not responding, however, consider increasing the dosage or adding an opioid. At any level of pain, analgesic adjuvants may be useful (American Pain Society, 2004). Analgesic combinations may enhance pain relief. Combining analgesics can result in acceptable pain relief with lower dosages of each analgesic than would be possible with one analgesic alone. Lower dosages can result in fewer or less severe side effects (Pasero, 2003a; McCaffery & Pasero, 1999).*

▲ For persistent cancer pain, obtain a prescription to administer opioid analgesics. When pain persists or increases, an opioid such as oxycodone should be added to the nonopioid. If this is not effective, switch to morphine or other single-entity opioids (Pasero & McCaffery, 2004). **EB:** *Research has demonstrated that controlled-release oxycodone is comparable to controlled-release morphine with less side-effects such as vomiting, itching, and hallucinations (Mucci-LoRusso et al, 1998; Heiskanen & Kalso, 1997).*

▲ For persistent chronic nonmalignant pain, discuss the use of opioid analgesics with the

P

health care team and obtain a prescription to administer if appropriate. *The use of opioid analgesics for chronic nonmalignant pain is both legal and clinically important. These agents should be used for clients with chronic nonmalignant pain (e.g., osteoarthritis, rheumatoid arthritis) when other medications and nonpharmacological interventions produce inadequate pain relief and the client's quality of life is affected by the pain (American Pain Society, 2004).*

▲ The oral route for pain medication administration is preferred. If the client is receiving parenteral analgesia, use an equianalgesic chart to convert to a controlled release, long-acting oral medication as soon as possible (McCaffery, 2003). (Refer to the Equianalgesic Chart at the start of this section.) *The least invasive route of administration capable of providing adequate pain control is recommended. The oral route is preferred because it is the most convenient and cost effective (McCaffery, 2003). Avoid the intramuscular (IM) route because of unreliable absorption, pain, and inconvenience. Repeated IM injections can produce sterile abscesses.*

▲ Establish ATC dosing and administer supplemental opioid doses for breakthrough pain as needed to keep pain ratings at or below the comfort-function goal. *An order for PRN breakthrough dose, which is 1/6 to 1/10 of the total daily opioid dose and is an essential backup because breakthrough pain is common in clients with chronic pain (McCaffery & Pasero, 2003).*

▲ Ask the client to describe appetite, bowel elimination, and ability to rest and sleep. Administer medications and treatments to improve these functions. Always obtain a prescription for a stool softener and a peristaltic stimulant daily to prevent opioid-induced constipation in clients taking regular daily doses of opioids. *Because there is great individual variation in the development of opioid-induced side effects, they should be monitored and, if their development is inevitable (e.g., constipation), prophylactically treated. Opioids cause constipation by decreasing bowel peristalsis (Plaisance & Ellis, 2002; McCaffery & Pasero, 1999).*

• Explain to the client the pain management approach that has been ordered, including therapies, medication administration, side effects, and complications. *One of the most important steps toward improved control of pain is a better client understanding of the nature of pain, its treatment, and the role the client needs to play in pain control (American Pain Society, 2004).*

• Discuss the client's fears of undertreated pain, addiction, and overdose. *Because of the many misconceptions regarding pain and its treatment, education about the ability to control pain effectively and correction of myths about the use of opioids should be included as part of the treatment plan (McCaffery & Pasero, 1999; McCaffery, Pasero, & Portenoy, 2004). Opioid tolerance and physical dependence are expected with long-term opioid treatment and should not be confused with addiction (American Pain Society, 2004). Addiction is unlikely after clients use opioids for pain relief (McCaffery, Pasero, & Portenoy, 2004; Pasero & McCaffery, 2004).* **EBN:** *A survey of 270 people with cancer pain revealed that many harbor fears and misconceptions regarding the use of analgesics, management of side effects, and risk of addiction (Ward et al, 1993).*

▲ Review the client's pain diary, flow sheet, and medication records to determine the overall degree of pain relief, side effects, and analgesic requirements for an appropriate period (e.g., 1 week). **EBN:** *Systematic tracking of pain was found to be an important factor in improving pain management (Faries et al, 1991; Schumacher, Koresawa, West et al, 2002).*

- ▲ Obtain prescriptions to increase or decrease analgesic doses when indicated. Base prescriptions on the client's report of pain severity and the comfort-function goal and response to previous dose in terms of relief, side effects, and ability to perform ADLs and comply with the prescribed therapeutic regimen. *Analgesic dosages should be adjusted to achieve pain relief with manageable and tolerable adverse effects (Pasero, 2003a; McCaffery & Pasero, 1999).*
- ▲ If opioid dose is increased, monitor sedation and respiratory status for a brief time. *Clients receiving long-term opioid therapy generally develop tolerance to the respiratory depressant effects of these agents (Pasero & McCaffery, 2002).*
- ▲ In addition to the use of analgesics, support the client's use of nonpharmacological methods to help control pain, such as physical therapy, group therapy, distraction, imagery, relaxation, massage, and application of heat and cold. *Cognitive-behavioral strategies can restore the client's sense of self-control, personal efficacy, and active participation in his or her own care (American Pain Society, 2004).*
- • Teach and implement nonpharmacological interventions when pain is relatively well controlled with pharmacological means. *Nonpharmacological interventions should be used to supplement, not replace, pharmacological interventions (American Pain Society, 2004).*
- • Encourage the client to plan activities around periods of greatest comfort whenever possible. Pain diminishes activity. *Clients will find it easier to perform their ADLs and enjoy social activities when they are rested and pain is under control (Pasero & McCaffery, 2004).*
- • Explore appropriate resources for management of pain on a long-term basis (e.g., hospice, pain care center). *Most clients with cancer or chronic nonmalignant pain are treated for pain in outpatient and home care settings. Plans should be made to ensure ongoing assessment of the pain and the effectiveness of treatments in these settings (American Pain Society, 2004).*
- • If the client has progressive cancer pain, assist the client and family with handling issues related to death and dying. *Peer support groups and pastoral counseling may increase the client's and family's coping skills and provide needed support (American Pain Society, 2004).*
- • Assist the client and family in minimizing the effects of pain on interpersonal relationships and daily activities such as work and recreation. **EBN:** *Pain can reduce clients' options to exercise control, diminish psychological well-being, and make them feel helpless and vulnerable. Therefore clinicians should encourage active client involvement in effective and practical methods to manage pain (Hitchcock, Ferrell, & McCaffery, 1994).*

P

## Pediatric

- • For the young child (1 to 4 years of age) use a Faces Pain Scale to determine the level of pain present. **EB:** *The Faces Pain Scale was shown to be valid using 4 to 12 year olds postoperatively. It was further validated with 600 children age 4 to 5 years receiving immunizations (Wood et al, 2003; Hicks et al, 2001).*
- • Help children and adolescents learn and utilize techniques such as relaxation and cognitive behavioral techniques to handle pain. **EBN:** *Studies have shown that the use of psychological interventions can reduce the frequency and severity of pain in children and adolescents (Eccleston, Morley, & Williams et al, 2002).*

## Geriatric

- ▲ Always take an older client's reports of pain seriously and ensure that the pain is relieved. *In spite of what many professionals and clients believe, pain is not an expected part of normal aging (American Geriatric Society Panel on Persistent Pain in Older Persons, 2002; Herr, 2002; McCaffery & Pasero, 1999). Unrelieved pain can cause decreased cognition, depression, mood disorders and reduced ADLs (Davis & Srivastava, 2003; Pasero & McCaffery, 2004).*
- • When assessing pain, speak clearly, slowly, and loudly enough for the client to hear, and if the client uses a hearing aid, be sure it is in place; repeat information as needed. Be sure the client can see well enough to read the pain scale (use an enlarged scale) and written materials. **EBN:** *Older clients often have difficulty hearing and seeing. Comprehension is improved when instructions are given slowly and clearly and when clients can see visual aids (Herr, 2002).*
- • *In the absence of the client's report of pain (e.g., anesthetized, critically ill, or cognitively impaired client), the clinician should assume pain is present and treat accordingly (Herr, 2002; McCaffery & Pasero, 1999; Pasero, 2003b).*
- • Handle the client's body gently. Allow the client to move at his or her own speed. *Elders are particularly susceptible to injury during care activities. Caregivers must be patient and expect that older clients will move more slowly than younger clients; they may also perform better and experience less pain when they are allowed to move themselves (McCaffery & Pasero, 1999).*
- ▲ Use acetaminophen and NSAIDs with low gastrointestinal side-effect profiles, such as a COX-2 selective NSAID, choline and magnesium salicylates (Trilisate), and diflunisal (Dolobid), and watch for side effects, such as gastrointestinal disturbances and bleeding problems. *Elders are at increased risk for gastric and renal toxicity from NSAIDs (Davis and Srivastava, 2003; American Geriatric Society Panel on Persistent Pain in Older Persons, 2002). Opioids ATC are preferable to long-term administration of nonselective NSAIDs in the older client because of an increased risk for NSAID adverse effects (Fine, 2004; American Geriatric Society Panel on Persistent Pain in Older Persons, 2002).*
- ▲ Avoid or use with caution drugs with a long half-life, such as the NSAID piroxicam (Feldene), and the opioids methadone (Dolophine) and levorphanol (LevoDromoran). *The higher prevalence of renal insufficiency in elders compared with younger persons can result in toxicity from drug accumulation (American Geriatric Society Panel on Persistent Pain in Older Persons, 2002; American Pain Society, 2004; Fick et al, 2003; McCaffery & Pasero, 1999).*
- ▲ Use opioids cautiously in the older client with moderate to severe pain unrelieved by NSAIDs. Reduce initial doses by 25% to 50%. After titrating to comfort with a short-acting opioid, switch to an extended-release opioid. **EBN:** *Older clients are more sensitive to the analgesic effects of opioid drugs because they experience a higher peak effect and a longer duration of pain relief (Giuffre et al, 1991). Reduce the initial recommended adult starting opioid dosage by 25% to 50%, especially if the client is frail and debilitated; then increase the dosage by 25% on an individual basis if needed (Ardery et al, 2003).*
- ▲ Avoid the use of opioids with toxic metabolites, such as meperidine (Demerol) and

propoxyphene (Darvon, Darvocet), in older clients. *Meperidine's metabolite, normeperidine, can produce central nervous system (CNS) irritability, seizures, and even death; propoxyphene's metabolite, norpropoxyphene, can produce CNS toxicity. Both of these metabolites are eliminated by the kidneys, which makes meperidine and propoxyphene particularly poor choices for older clients, many of whom have at least some degree of renal insufficiency (Ardery et al, 2003; Fick et al, 2003; McCaffery & Pasero, 1999).*

▲ Monitor for signs of depression in the elders, refer for treatment if needed. **EB:** *A study demonstrated that treatment of depression in elders with arthritis, also helped decrease pain and improve functional abilities (Lin, Katon, & Von Korff, 2003).*

## Multicultural

- Assess for the influence of cultural beliefs, norms, and values on the client's perception and experience of pain. **EB:** *One study showed that the Native-American patients may think that asking for pain medication is disrespectful because it implies that health care providers don't know what they are doing (Brant, 2001). A recent study with African-American elders found the use of prayer or faith for pain management, care, and prevention very common (Ibrahim et al, 2004). A "representational approach" first developed at the University of Wisconsin-Madison School of Nursing offers a flexible framework for nurses to get cancer patients to delve deeply into their own belief systems about health, disease, pain, and so on, and to add sound concepts that will work for their pain management. The program is called Representational Intervention to Decrease Cancer Pain (RIDcancerPain) and has the following 6 steps:*
  1. Representational assessment—the patient describes beliefs about cancer pain along five dimensions (identity, cause, timeline, consequences and cure/control)
  2. Exploring misconceptions, with emphasis on their origins
  3. Creating conditions for conceptual change by discussing the limitations of holding beliefs that are misconceptions (i.e., what one loses by maintaining those beliefs
  4. Introducing replacement information
  5. Summarizing and discussing benefits of adopting beliefs that are credible replacements
  6. Developing a plan and strategies (Ward, Donovan, & Gunnarsdottir, in press)
- Assess for the effect of fatalism on the client's beliefs regarding the current state of comfort. **EBN:** *Fatalistic perspectives, which involve the belief that one cannot control one's own fate, may influence health behaviors in some African-American and Latino populations (Harmon, Castro, & Coe, 1996; Phillips, Cohen, & Moses, 1999).*
- Assess for pain disparities among racial and ethnic minorities. **EB:** *Racial and ethnic minorities tend to be undertreated for pain when compared with non-Hispanic whites (Green et al, 2003).*
- Incorporate safe and effective folk health care practices and beliefs into care whenever possible. It is the responsibility of the caregiver to ensure that safe and effective pain management is provided. Although support of an individual's health care beliefs is recommended, when research does not support the safety or effectiveness of a method or when research does not exist, this should be explained fully to the client (McCaffery & Pasero, 1999). **EBN:** *Incorporating folk health care beliefs and practices into pain*

P

*management care increased compliance with the treatment plan (Juarez, Ferrell, & Borneman, 1998).*

- Use a family-centered approach to care. **EBN:** *Involving the family in pain management care increased compliance with the treatment regimen (Juarez, Ferrell, & Borneman, 1998).*
- Teach information about pain medications and their side effects, how to work with health care providers to manage pain, and encouragement to use religious faith to cope with pain. **EB:** *Socioeconomically disadvantaged African-American and Hispanic patients benefit from educational interventions on pain that dispel myths about opioids and teach patients to communicate assertively about their pain with their physicians and nurses (Anderson et al, 2002).*
- Use culturally relevant pain scales (e.g., the Oucher Scale), if available, to assess pain in the client. **EBN:** *Clients from minority cultures may express pain differently than clients from the majority culture. The Oucher Scale is available in African American and Hispanic versions and is used to assess pain in children (Beyer, Denyes, & Villarruel, 1992).*
- Ensure that directions for medication use are available in the client's language of choice and are understood by the client and caregiver. **EB:** *Use of bilingual instructions for medication administration increased compliance with the pain management plan (Juarez, Ferrell, & Borneman, 1998). Using specific phrases in Spanish to assess acute pain in non–English-speaking Hispanic patients helps provide timely pain assessment and management (Collins, Gullette, & Schnepf, 2004).*

## Home Care

- Develop the treatment plan with the client and caregivers. *Clients and caregivers will be more likely to follow the treatment plan when their input is considered (McCaffery & Pasero, 1999).*

▲ Develop a full medication profile, including medications prescribed by all physicians and all over-the-counter medications. Assess for drug interactions. Instruct the client to refrain from mixing medications without physician approval. *Pain medications may significantly affect or be affected by other medications and may cause severe side effects. Some combinations of drugs are specifically contraindicated.*

- Assess the client's and family's knowledge of side effects and safety precautions associated with pain medications (e.g., use caution if operating machinery when opioids are first taken or dosage has been increased significantly). *The cognitive effects of opioids usually subside within a week of initial dosing or dose increases (McCaffery & Pasero, 1999). The use of long-term opioid treatment does not appear to affect neuropsychological performance.* **EB:** *Pain itself may reduce performance on neuropsychological tests more than oral opioid treatment (Sjogren et al, 2000).*

▲ Collaborate with the health care team (including the client and family) on an ongoing basis to determine an optimal pain control profile. Identify the most effective interventions and the medication administration routes most acceptable to the client and family. **EBN:** *Success in pain control is partially dependent on the acceptability of the suggested intervention. Acceptability promotes compliance. Dosages vary among routes and will need to be adjusted accordingly to avoid breakthrough or transitional pain (Bohnet, 1995).*

P

- ▲ If medication is administered using highly technological methods, assess the home for necessary resources (e.g., electricity) and ensure that responsible caregivers will be available to assist the client with administration. *Some routes of medication administration require special conditions and procedures to be safe and accurate (McCaffery & Pasero, 1999).*
- ▲ Assess the knowledge base of the client and family for highly technological medication administration. Teach as necessary. Be sure the client knows when, how, and whom to contact if analgesia is unsatisfactory. *Appropriate instruction in the home increases the accuracy and safety of medication administration (McCaffery & Pasero, 1999).*
- • Support the client and family in the use of opioid analgesics. *Well-intentioned friends and family may create added stress by expressing judgment or fears regarding the use of opioid analgesics (McCaffery & Pasero, 1999).*

## Client/Family Teaching

NOTE: To avoid the negative connotations associated with the words *drugs* and *narcotics,* use the term *pain medicine* when teaching clients.

- • Provide written materials on pain control such as *Understanding Your Pain: Using a Pain Rating Scale* (McCaffery, Pasero, & Portenoy, 2001) (see instructions on the use of a pain rating scale) and *Taking Oral Opioid Analgesics* (McCaffery, Pasero, & Portenoy, 2004). *Written materials are provided in addition to verbal instructions so that the client will have a reference during treatment (McCaffery & Pasero, in press).*
- • Discuss the various discomforts encompassed by the word pain and ask the client to give examples of previously experienced pain. Explain the pain assessment process and the purpose of the pain rating scale. *It is often difficult for clients to understand the concept of pain and describe their pain experience. Using alternative words and providing a complete description of the assessment process, including the use of scales, will ensure that an accurate treatment plan is developed (McCaffery & Pasero, 1999, 2001). Teach clients to use the pain rating scale to rate the intensity of past or current pain.*
- ▲ Ask the client to set a comfort-function goal by selecting a pain level on the rating scale that takes it easy to perform recovery activities (e.g., turn, cough, deep breathe). If pain is above this level, the client should take action that decreases pain or notify a member of the health care team. (See information on teaching clients to use the pain rating scale.) *The use of comfort-function goals provides direction for the treatment plan. Changes are made according to the client's response and achievement of the goals of recovery or rehabilitation (McCaffery & Pasero, 1999).*
- ▲ Discuss the total plan for pharmacological and nonpharmacological treatment, including the medication plan for ATC administration and supplemental doses, the maintenance of a pain diary, and the use of supplies and equipment. *Appropriate instruction increases the accuracy and safety of medication administration (McCaffery & Pasero, 1999).*
- • Reinforce the importance of taking pain medications to keep pain under control. *Teaching clients to stay on top of their pain and prevent it from getting out of control will improve their ability to perform ADLs and accomplish goals (Pasero & McCaffery, 2004).*
- • Reinforce that taking opioids for pain relief is not addiction and that addiction is very unlikely to occur. *The development of addiction when opioids are taken for pain relief is*

*rare (American Pain Society, 2004; McCaffery, Pasero, & Portenoy, 2004; McCaffery & Pasero, 1999).*

- Explain to a client with chronic neuropathic pain the process of taking adjuvant analgesics (e.g., tricyclic antidepressants). *A low dose of adjuvant analgesic is used initially and the dose is increased gradually. Pain relief is delayed, and the adjuvant analgesics must be taken daily. Teaching clients that, although the medicine is an antidepressant, it is used for analgesia and not depression will increase understanding of the drug. Comparable teaching should take place when an anticonvulsant is prescribed for analgesia (McCaffery & Pasero, 1999).*
- Suggest the client with cancer try having a massage, with aromatherapy if desired. **EB:** *Both massage and aromatherapy massage have short term benefits on psychological well-being for the client with cancer (Fellowes, Barnes, & Wilkinson, 2004).*
- Emphasize to the client the importance of pacing himself or herself and taking rest breaks before they are needed. *Clients will find they are able to perform their ADLs and achieve goals better when they are rested (Pasero & McCaffery, 2004).*
- ▲ Demonstrate the use of appropriate nonpharmacological approaches in addition to pharmacological approaches for helping to control pain (e.g., physical therapy, group therapy, distraction, imagery, and application of heat and cold).
- Teach and implement nonpharmacological interventions when pain is relatively well controlled with pharmacological means. *Nonpharmacological interventions are used to supplement, not replace, pharmacological interventions (American Pain Society, 2004; McCaffery & Pasero, 1999).*

## evolve WEBSITES FOR EDUCATION

See the EVOLVE website for World Wide Web resources for client education.

## REFERENCES

American Geriatric Society Panel on Persistent Pain in Older Persons: The management of persistent pain in older persons, *J Am Geriatr Soc* 50:S205, 1-20, 2002.

The American Pain Society, Pain: Current understanding of assessment, management and treatments, Available at www.ampainsoc.org/ce/npc, accessed on September 6, 2004.

Anderson KO et al: Cancer pain management among underserved minority outpatients: perceived needs and barriers to optimal control, *Cancer* 94(8):2295-2304, 2002.

Ardery G, Herr KA, Titler MG et al: Assessing and managing acute pain in older adults: a research base to guide practice, *Med-Surg Nurs* 12:1, 2003.

Beyer J, Denyes M, Villarruel A: The creation, validation, and continuing development of the Oucher: a measure of pain intensity in children, *J Pediatr Nurs* 7(5):335, 1992.

Bohnet N: Chronic pain management in the home care setting, *J Wound Ostomy Continence Nurs* 22:135, 1995.

Bonica JJ: Definitions and taxonomy of pain. In Bonica JJ, editor: *The management of pain,* Philadelphia, 1990, Lea and Febiger.

Brant JM: Cultural implications of pain education, presented at Cancer Pain and Education for Patients and the Public Conference, City of Hope National Medical Center, Duarte, Calif, October 18, 2001.

Collins AS, Gullette D, Schnepf M: Break through language barriers, *Nurs Manage* 35(8):34-36, 38, 2004.

Davis MP, Srivastava M: Demographics, assessment and management of pain in the elderly, *Drugs Aging* 20(1):23, 2003.

Eccleston C, Morley S, Williams A et al: Systematic review of randomized controlled trials of psychological therapy for chronic pain in children and adolescents with a subset meta-analysis of pain relief, *Pain* 99, 2002.

Faries JE et al: Systematic pain records and their impact on pain control, *Cancer Nurs* 14:306, 1991.



P

Fellowes D, Barnes K, Wilkinson S: Aromatherapy and massage for symptom relief in patients with cancer, *The Cochrane Librar,* CD002287, 2004.

Fick DM, Cooper JW, Wade WE et al: Updating the Beers criteria for potentially inappropriate mediation use in older adults, *Arch Int Med* 163:2716-2724, 2003.

Fine P: Pharmacological management of persistent pain in older patients, *Clin J Pain* 20(4):220-226, 2004.

Giuffre M, Asci J, Arnstein P et al: Postoperative join replacement pain: description and opioid requirement, *J Post Anesthesia Nursing* 6:4, 1991.

Green CR: et al: The unequal burden of pain: confronting racial and ethnic disparities in pain, *Pain Med* 4(3):277-294, 2003.

Griffie J: Pain control: addressing inadequate pain relief, *AJN* 8, 62-63, 103, 2003.

Griffin ME et al: Nonsteroidal anti-inflammatory drug use and increased risk for peptic ulcer disease in elderly persons, *Ann Intern Med* 11:257, 1991.

Harmon MP, Castro FG, Coe K: Acculturation and cervical cancer: knowledge, beliefs, and behaviors of Hispanic women, *Women Health* 24(3):37, 1996.

Heiskanen T, Kalso E: Controlled-release oxycodone and morphine in cancer related pain, *Pain* 73(1):37 1997.

Herr K: Pain assessment in cognitively impaired older adults, *Am J Nurs* 102(12):65, 66, 68, 2002.

Hicks CL et al: The Faces Pain Scale—Revised: toward a common metric in pediatric pain measurement, *Pain* 93(2):173, 2001.

Hitchcock LS, Ferrell BR, McCaffery M: The experience of chronic nonmalignant pain, *J Pain Symptom Manage* 9:312, 1994.

Hutchison R: Cox-2-selective NSAIDS, *AJN* 104(3), 2004.

Jensen MP: The validity and reliability of pain measures in adults with cancer, *J Pain* 4(1):52-55, 2003.

Joint Commission on Accreditation of Healthcare Organizations (JCAHO): *Hospital Accreditation Standards*, Oakbrook Terrace, Ill, 2000, The Commission.

Juarez G, Ferrell B, Borneman T: Influence of culture on cancer pain management in Hispanic clients, *Cancer Pract* 6(5):262, 1998.

Leininger MM, McFarland M: *Transcultural nursing: concepts, theories, research and practices,* Hilliard, Ohio, 2002, McGraw-Hill.

Lin EHB, Katon W, Von Korff M et al: Effect of improving depression care on pain and functional outcomes among older adults with arthritis, *JAMA* 290(18):2428, 2003.

McCaffery M: *Nursing practice theories related to cognition, bodily pain, and man-environment interactions,* Los Angeles, 1968, University of California at Los Angeles Students' Store.

McCaffery M: Ferrell BR: How would you respond to these clients in pain? *Nursing* 21(6):34, 1991.

McCaffery M: Culturally sensitive pain assessment, *Am J Nurs* 99(8):18, 1999.

McCaffery M: What is the role of nondrug methods in the nursing care of patients with acute pain? *Pain Management Nursing* 3(3):77-80, 2002.

McCaffery M, Pain control: switching from IV to PO, *Am J Nurs* 103(5):62-63, 2003.

McCaffery M, Pasero C: *Pain: clinical manual,* ed 2, St Louis, Mosby, 1999.

McCaffery M, Pasero C: Pain control: breakthrough pain, *Am J Nurs* 103(4):83, 84, 86, 2003.

McCaffery M, Pasero C, Portenoy RK: *Understanding your pain: using a pain rating scale,* Chadds Ford, Pa, 2001, Endo Pharmaceuticals.

McCaffery M, Pasero C, Portenoy RK: *Understanding your pain: taking oral opioid analgesics,* Chadds Ford, Pa, 2004, Endo Pharmaceuticals.

Mucci-LoRuso P et al: Controlled release oxycodone compared with controlled-release morphine in the treatment of cancer pain: randomized, double-blind, parallel-group study, *Eur J Pain* 2(2):239, 1998.

Page GG, Ben-Eliyahu S: The immune-suppressive nature of pain, *Semin Oncol Nurs* 13(1):10, 1997.

Pasero C: Multimodal analgesia in the PACU, *J PeriAnesthesia Nursing* 18(4):265-268, 2003a.

Pasero C: Pain in the critically ill, *J PeriAnesthesia Nursing* 18(6):422-425, 2003b.

Pasero, C, McCaffery M: Pain control: patient's report of pain, *Am J Nurs* 101(12):73-74, 2001.

Pasero C, McCaffery M: Monitoring opioid-induced sedation, *Am J Nurs* 102(2):67-68, 2002.

Pasero C, McCaffery M: Pain control: controlled-release oxycodone, *Am J Nurs* 104(1):30-32, 2004a.

Pasero, C, McCaffery M: Pain control: comfort-function goals, *Am J Nurs* 104(9):77-78, 81, 2004b.

Phillips JM, Cohen MZ, Moses G: Breast cancer screening and African American women: fear, fatalism, and silence, *Oncol Nurs Forum* 26(3):561, 1999.

Plaisance L, Ellis JA: Opioid-induced constipation. *Am J Nurs* 102(3):72-73, 2002.
Schumacher KL, Koresawa S, West C et al: The usefulness of a daily pain management diary for outpatients with cancer-related Pain, *Oncol Nurs Forum* 29(9):1304, 2002.
Sjogren P et al: Neuropsychological performance in cancer clients: the role of oral opioids, pain and performance statu, *Pain* 86: 237, 2000.
Ward S et al: Client-related barriers to management of cancer pain, *Pain* 52:319, 1993.
Ward S, Donovan H, Gunnarsdottir S et al: A representational intervention to decrease cancer pain (RIDcancerPain), in press.
Wood C et al: Self-assessment by the Faces Pain Scale: revised of immediate post-vaccination pain following administration of Priorix versus MMRII as a second dose in 4 to 6 year old children, Poster, Sixth International Symposium on Pediatric Pain, Sydney, 2003, Special Interest Group on Pain in Childhood, International Association for the Study of Pain.

# Readiness for enhanced Parenting

*T. Heather Herdman*

**NANDA**

## Definition

Pattern of providing an environment for children or other dependent person(s) that is sufficient to nurture growth and development and can be strengthened

## Defining Characteristics

Expresses willingness to enhance parenting, children or other dependent person(s) express satisfaction with home environment, emotional and tacit support of children or dependent person(s) is evident, bonding or attachment is evident, physical and emotional needs of children or other dependent person(s) are met, realistic expectations of children or other dependent person(s) are exhibited

**NOC**

## Outcomes (Nursing Outcomes Classification)

### Suggested NOC Outcomes

Child Development: 1 Month, 2 Months, 4 Months, 6 Months, 12 Months, Preschool, Middle Childhood, Adolescence; Growth; Health-Promoting Behavior; Health-Seeking Behavior; Immunization Behavior; Knowledge: Breastfeeding, Child Physical Safety, Diet, Health Behavior, Health Resources, Infection Control, Medication, Personal Safety; Leisure Participation; Nutritional Status; Parent-Infant Attachment; Parenting Performance; Parenting: Psychosocial Safety; Risk Control; Risk Detection; Role Performance; Safe Home Environment; Self-Esteem

### Example NOC Outcome with Indicators

**Parenting Performance** as evidenced by the following indicators: Provides regular preventive and episodic health care/Stimulates cognitive and social development/Stimulates emotional and spiritual growth/Interacts positively with child/Empathizes with child/Expresses satisfaction with parental role/Expresses positive self-esteem (Rate each indicator of **Parenting Performance:** 1 = never demonstrated, 2 = rarely demonstrated, 3 = sometimes demonstrated, 4 = often demonstrated, 5 = consistently demonstrated [see Section I].)

## Client Outcomes

### Client/Family Will (Specify Time Frame):

- Affirm desire to improve parenting skills to further support growth and development of children
- Demonstrate loving relationship with children
- Provide a safe, nurturing environment
- Assess risks in home/environment and takes steps to prevent possibility of harm to children
- Meet physical, psychosocial, and spiritual needs or seek appropriate assistance

NIC

## Interventions (Nursing Interventions Classification)

### Suggested NIC Interventions

Anticipatory Guidance; Attachment Promotion; Developmental Enhancement: Adolescent, Child; Family Integrity Promotion: Childbearing Family; Infant Care; Newborn Care; Parent Education: Adolescent, Childrearing Family, Infant; Parenting Promotion; Teaching: Infant Stimulation

P

### Example NIC Activities—Parenting Promotion

Assist parents to have realistic expectations appropriate to developmental and ability level of child; assist parents with role transition and expectations of parenthood

## Nursing Interventions and Rationales

- Use family-centered care and role modeling for holistic care of families. **EBN:** *Specific techniques of role modeling and reflective practice are suggested as effective approaches to teach the family sensitive care in clinical settings in which families are part of the care environment (Tomlinson et al, 2002).*
- Assess parents' feelings when dealing with a child who has a chronic illness. **EBN:** *Knowing how parents feel about a child's asthma is the first step in helping them manage this common chronic disease (Clark & Chalmers, 2003).*
- Encourage positive parenting: respect for children, understanding of normal development, and use of creative and loving approaches to meet parenting challenges. **EBN:** *Understanding normal development is a first step so that parents can distinguish common be-*

*haviors for a given stage of development from "problems." Central to positive parenting is developing approaches that can be used in place of anger, manipulation, punishment, and rewards (Ahmann, 2002).*

- Promote low-tech interventions, such as massage and multisensory interventions (maternal voice, eye-to-eye contact, and rocking) to reduce maternal and infant stress and improve mother-infant relationship. **EBN:** *Giving birth to infants in adverse situations (war, natural disasters, and so on) can affect infant growth and development long-term. One article explores neurohormonal aspects of stress and social bonding and offers strategies aimed at reducing maternal and infant stress and improving the mother-infant relationship (White-Traut, 2004). Another pilot study suggests a model of incorporating infant massage into a planned parenting enhancement program may promote effective parenting through a special focus on infant stimulation through massage (Porter & Porter, 2004).*
- Provide opportunities for mother-infant skin-to-skin contact (kangaroo care [KC]) for preterm infants. **EB:** *One study showed that the neurodevelopmental profile was more mature for infants receiving KC. Results underscore the role of early KC in the maturation of the autonomic and circadian systems in preterm infants (Feldman & Eidelman, 2003).*
- Provide the parent with the opportunity to assist in the newborn's first bath, allowing a flexible bath time. **EBN:** *A flexible bathing time is recommended depending on the characteristics and stability of the newborn and family desires. Axillary temperatures as measured at four different times did not differ significantly between infants bathed within 1 hour of birth and those bathed 4 to 6 hours after birth (Behring, Vezeau, & Fink, 2003).*
- When the person who is ill is the parent, use family-centered assessment skills to determine the impact of an adult's illness on the child and then guide the parent through those topics that are most likely to be of concern, including (a) the name of the illness, (b) the cause of the illness, (c) the potential contagion or spread of the illness, and (d) the ultimate impact of the illness on the life of the child. **EBN:** *The pediatric nurse, by embracing core principles of openness and honesty and by providing concrete developmental information, can empower parents to support their own children (McCue & Bonn, 2003).*
- ▲ Have family members participate in client conferences that involve all members of the health care team. *Conferences allow for distribution of information, input by all members at one time, and a decrease in anxiety levels of family members.*
- ▲ Help parents develop realistic expectations of their child's development. **EBN:** *This study demonstrated the potential of parent training and support to alter the style of interactions between parents and their children (Letourneau et al, 2001).*
- Provide practical and psychological assistance for parents of patients with psychiatric diagnoses, such as schizophrenia. **EBN:** *Parents of patients with schizophrenia show levels of burden that are closely connected with the illness curve of their children; forty percent of parents may experience constantly high levels of burden. Parents may be overloaded with their long-term caring tasks, and provision of practical and psychological assistance can be of benefit (Jungbauer et al, 2003).*

## Multicultural

- Assess for the influence of cultural beliefs, norms, and values on the client's perception

P

of parenting. **EBN:** *What the client considers normal parenting may be based on cultural perceptions (Leininger & McFarland, 2002; Cochran, 1998; Doswell & Erlen, 1998).*

- Acknowledge racial/ethnic differences at the onset of care. **EB:** *Acknowledgment of racial/ethnicity issues will enhance communication, establish rapport, and promote treatment outcomes (D'Avanzo et al, 2001).*
- Acknowledge that value conflicts from acculturation stresses may contribute to increased anxiety and significant conflict with children. **EBN:** *Challenges to traditional beliefs and values are anxiety provoking. Less acculturated parents may experience conflict with their more acculturated children as the children demand greater independence and freedom (True, 1995). Immigrant mothers scored significantly lower on the evaluation of parenting knowledge than U.S.-born mothers (Bornstein & Cote, 2004). Chinese immigrant mothers identified that a larger perceived acculturation gap was associated with more parenting difficulties (Buki, Ma, & Strom, 2003).*
- Acknowledge and praise parenting strengths noted. **EBN:** *Such acknowledgment will increase trust and foster a working relationship with the parent (Seideman et al, 1996). Clinicians could explore and support the positive qualities of authoritative parenting in Mexican descent families (Varela et al, 2004).*

## Home Care

- The nursing interventions described previously should be used in the home environment with adaptations as necessary.
- ▲ Refer to a parenting program to facilitate learning of parenting skills. **EBN:** *At the end of an 8-week parenting program, parents demonstrated statistically significant reduced levels of clinical anxiety and depression. Parents showed an increase in more positive ratings of personality states, such as not shouting at their children and being more calm and energetic, at the end of the program (Long et al, 2001).*

P

## Client/Family Teaching

- Refer to Client/Family Teaching for **Impaired Parenting** and **Risk for impaired Parenting** for suggestions that may be used with minor adaptations.
- Teach parents home safety: reduction of hot water temperature, proper poison storage, use of smoke alarms, and installation of safety gates for stairs. **EB:** *Counseling coupled with convenient access to reduced-cost products appears to be an effective strategy for promoting children's home safety (Gielen, McDonald, & Wilson, 2002).*
- Teach parents and young teens conflict resolution using a hypothetical conflict solution with and without a structured conflict resolution guide. **EBN:** *Parents and young teens do not use a systematic method of solving disagreements, but with structured guidance, the parents and teens are able to resolve conflicts (Riesch et al, 2003).*
- ▲ Refer mothers of children with type 1 diabetes for community support in babysitting, child care, or respite. **EBN:** *A study of mothers raising young children older than age 4 years with type 1 diabetes highlights the importance of identifying family and/or community resources that could reduce some of the tremendous stress and burden of responsibility experienced after a child is diagnosed with diabetes (Sullivan-Bolyai et al, 2003).*
- Support empowerment of parents of children with asthma. **EBN:** *Asthma is the most common chronic illness in children and has a significant impact on children and their fami-*

*lies. Empowering parents by facilitating their sense of control resulted in increased knowledge and ability to make decisions regarding their child's care (McCarthy et al, 2002).*

- Teach families the importance of monitoring television viewing and limiting exposure to violence. **EBN:** *Media violence can be hazardous to children's health, and studies point overwhelmingly to a causal connection between media violence and aggressive attitudes, values, and behaviors in some children. Nurses can teach children and parents about the effects of media violence and advise them on how to avoid exposure (Muscari, 2002).*
- Consider individual and/or group based parenting programs for teenage mothers. **EB:** *This systematic review indicated that results favored those engaged in individual and/or group parenting programs in the areas of mother-infant interaction, language development, parental attitudes, parental knowledge, maternal mealtime communication, maternal self-confidence and maternal identity (Coren & Barlow, 2004).*
- Consider group based parenting programs for parents for children under the age of three years with emotional and behavioral problems. **EB:** *This meta-analysis indicated that results favored those engaged in parenting programs in terms of improving the emotional and behavioral adjustment of children under age 3 (Barlow & Parsons, 2003).*
- Consider group-based parenting programs for parents with anxiety, depression and/or low self-esteem. **EB:** *This meta-analysis indicated that parenting programs can make a significant contribution to the short-term psychosocial health of mothers, and that they therefore have a potential role to play in the promotion of mental health (Barlow & Coren, 2004).*

▲ Refer adolescent parents for comprehensive psychoeducational parenting classes. **EBN:** *This study indicated that a comprehensive pyschoeducational parenting group can be effective in changing parenting attitudes and beliefs (Thomas et al, 2004).*

## evolve WEBSITES FOR EDUCATION

See the EVOLVE website for World Wide Web resources for client education.

P

## REFERENCES


Ahmann E: Promoting positive parenting: an annotated bibliography, *Pediatr Nurs* 28(4):382, 2002.

Barlow J, Coren E: Parent-training programmes for improving maternal psychosocial health, *Cochrane Database Syst Rev,* CD002020, 2004.

Barlow J, Parsons J: Group-based parent-training programmes for improving emotional and behavioral adjustment in 0-3 year old children, *Cochrane Database Syst Rev,* (3)CD003680, 2003.

Behring A, Vezeau TM, Fink R: Timing of the newborn first bath: a replication, *Neonatal Netw* 22(1):39, 2003.

Bornstein MH, Cote LR: "Who is sitting across from me?" Immigrant mothers' knowledge of parenting and children's development, *Pediatrics* 114(5):e557-564, 2004.

Buki LP, Ma TC, Strom RD et al: Chinese immigrant mothers of adolescents: self-perceptions of acculturation effects on parenting, *Cultur Divers Ethnic Minor Psychol* 9(2):127-140, 2003.

Clark BA, Chalmers KL: Helping parents cope, *Can Nurse* 99(2):19, 2003.

Cochran M: Tears have no color, *Am J Nurs* 98(6):53, 1998.

Coren E, Barlow J: Individual and group-based parenting programmes for improving psychosocial outcomes for teenage parents and their children, *Cochrane Database Syst Rev,* CD002964, 2004.

D'Avanzo CE et al: Developing culturally informed strategies for substance-related interventions. In Naegle MA, D'Avanzo CE, editors: *Addictions and substance abuse: strategies for advanced practice nursing,* St Louis, 2001, Mosby.

Doswell W, Erlen J: Multicultural issues and ethical concerns in the delivery of nursing care interventions, *Nurs Clin North Am* 33(2):353, 1998.

Feldman R, Eidelman A: Skin-to-skin contact (kangaroo care) accelerates autonomic and neurobehavioural maturation in preterm infants, *Dev Med Child Neurol* 45(4):274, 2003.

Gielen AC, McDonald EM, Wilson ME: Effects of improved access to safety counseling, products, and home visits on parents' safety practices: results of a randomized trial, *Arch Pediatr Adolesc Med* 156(1):33, 2002.

Jungbauer J, Wittmund B, Dietrich S et al: Subjective burden over 12 months in parents of patients with schizophrenia, *Arch Psychiatr Nurs* 17(3):126-134, 2003.

Leininger MM, McFarland MR: *Transcultural nursing: concepts, theories, research and practices,* ed 3, New York, 2002, McGraw-Hill.

Long A, McCarney S, Smyth G et al: The effectiveness of parenting programmes facilitated by health visitors, *J Adv Nurs* 34(5): 611, 2001.

McCarthy MJ, Herbert R, Brimacombe M et al: Empowering parents through asthma education, *Pediatr Nurs* 28(5):465, 2002.

McCue K, Bonn R: Helping children through an adult's serious illness, *Pediatr Nurs* 29(1):47, 2003.

Muscari M: Media violence: advice for parents, *Pediatr Nurs* 28(6):585, 2002.

Porter LS, Porter BO: A blended infant massage-parenting enhancement program for recovering substance-abusing mothers, *Pediatr Nur* 30(5):363-372, 389-390, 401, 2004.

Riesch SK, Gray J, Hoeffs M et al: Conflict and conflict resolution: parent and young teen perceptions, *J Pediatr Health Care* 17(1):22, 2003.

Schiffman RF, Omar MA, McKelvey LM: Mother-infant interaction in low-income families. *MCN Am J Matern Child Nurs* 28(4):246-251.

Seideman RY, Jacobson S, Primeaux M et al: Assessing American Indian families, *MCN Am J Matern Child Nurs* 21(6):274, 1996.

Sullivan-Bolyai S, Deatrick J, Gruppuso P et al: Constant vigilance: mothers' work parenting young children with type 1 diabetes, *J Pediatr Nurs* 18(1):21, 2003.

Thomas DV, Looney SW: Effectiveness of a comprehensive psychoeducational intervention with pregnant and parenting adolescents: a pilot study, *J Child Adolesc Psychiatr Nurs* 17(2):66-77, 2004.

Tomlinson PS, Thomlinson E, Peden-McAlpine C et al: Clinical innovation for promoting family care in paediatric intensive care: demonstration, role modelling and reflective practice, *J Adv Nurs* 38(2):161, 2002.

True RH: Mental health issues of Asian/Pacific island women. In Adams DL, editor: *Health issues for women of color: a cultural diversity perspective,* Thousand Oaks, Calif, 1995, Sage.

Varela RE, Vernberg EM, Sanchez-Sosa JJ et al: Parenting style of Mexican, Mexican American, and Caucasian-non-Hispanic families: social context and cultural influences, *J Fam Psychol* 18(4):651-657, 2004.

White-Traut R.: Providing a nurturing environment for infants in adverse situations: multisensory strategies for newborn care, *J Midwifery Womens Health* 49(4 Suppl 1):36, 2004.



# Impaired Parenting

evolve

*T. Heather Herdman*

**NANDA**

## Definition

Inability of primary caretaker to create, maintain, or regain an environment that promotes optimum growth and development of the child

## Defining Characteristics

### Infant/child

Poor academic performance, frequent illness, running away, physical and psychological trauma or abuse, frequent accidents, lack of attachment, failure to thrive, behavioral disorders, poor social competence, lack of separation anxiety, poor cognitive development

### Parental

Inappropriate child care arrangements, rejection of or hostility toward child, statements of inability to meet child's needs, inflexibility in meeting needs of child or situation, poor or inappropriate caretaking skills, regular punitive behavior, inconsistent care, child abuse, inadequate child health maintenance, unsafe home environment, verbalization of inability to control child, negative statements about child, verbalization of role inadequacy or frustration, inappropriate visual, tactile, or auditory stimulation of child, abandonment, insecure attachment or lack of attachment to infant, inconsistent behavior management, child neglect, little cuddling, maternal-child interaction deficit, poor parent-child interaction

## Related Factors (r/t)

### Social

Lack of access to resources; social isolation; lack of resources; poor home environment; lack of family cohesiveness; inadequate child care arrangements; lack of transportation; unemployment or job problems; role strain or overload; marital conflict, declining satisfaction; lack of value of parenthood; change in family unit; low socioeconomic class; unplanned or unwanted pregnancy; presence of stress (e.g., financial or legal difficulties, recent crisis, cultural move); lack of or poor parental role model; single parenthood; lack of social support network; lack of involvement of father of child; history of being abusive; history of being abused; financial difficulties; maladaptive coping strategies; poverty; poor problem-solving skills; inability to put child's needs before own; low self-esteem; relocation; legal difficulties

### Knowledge

Lack of knowledge about child health maintenance; lack of knowledge about parenting skills; unrealistic expectations for self, infant, partner; limited cognitive functioning; lack of knowledge about child development; inability to recognize and act on infant cues; low educational level or attainment; poor communication skills; lack of cognitive readiness for parenthood; preference for physical punishment



### Physiological

Physical illness

### Infant/child

Premature birth; illness; prolonged separation from parent; not desired gender; attention deficit hyperactivity disorder; difficult temperament; separation from parent at birth; lack of goodness of fit (temperament) with parental expectations; unplanned or unwanted child; handicapping condition or developmental delay; multiple births; altered perceptual abilities

### Psychological

History of substance abuse or dependencies, disability, depression, difficult labor and/or delivery, young age, especially adolescence, history of mental illness, high number of or closely spaced pregnancies, sleep derivation or disruption, lack of or late prenatal care, separation from infant/child

NOTE: It is important to reaffirm that adjustment to parenting in general is a normal maturational process that elicits nursing behaviors to prevent potential problems and to promote health.

NOC

## Outcomes (Nursing Outcomes Classification)

### Suggested NOC Outcomes

Abuse Cessation; Abuse Protection; Abuse Recovery: Emotional; Abusive Behavior Self-Restraint; Child Development: 2 Months, 4 Months, 6 Months, 2 Years, 3 Years, 4 Years, Preschool, Middle Childhood, Adolescence; Coping; Knowledge: Child Physical Safety; Neglect Recovery; Parent-Infant Attachment; Parenting Performance; Parenting: Psychosocial Safety; Role Performance; Safe Home Environment; Social Support

**Example NOC Outcome with Indicators**

**Abuse Recovery: Emotional** as evidenced by the following indicators: Demonstration of confidence/Demonstration of impulse control/Self-advocacy/Expressions of feeling empowered/Demonstration of positive interpersonal relationships/Demonstration of provision of safety for child (Rate each indicator of **Abuse Recovery: Emotional:** 1 = none, 2 = limited, 3 = moderate, 4 = substantial, 5 = extensive [see Section I].)

P

## Client Outcomes

### Client Will (Specify Time Frame):

- Affirm desire to develop constructive parenting skills to support infant/child growth and development
- Initiate appropriate measures to develop a safe, nurturing environment
- Acquire and display attentive, supportive parenting behaviors
- Identify strategies to protect child from harm and/or neglect and initiate action when indicated

NIC

## Interventions (Nursing Interventions Classification)

### Suggested NIC Interventions

Abuse Protection Support: Child; Attachment Promotion; Caregiver Support; Developmental Enhancement: Adolescent, Child; Environmental Management: Attachment Process; Family Integrity Promotion; Family Support; Family Therapy; Infant Care; Parent Education: Adolescent, Childrearing Family, Infant

**Example NIC Activities—Abuse Protection Support: Child**

Identify whether adult at risk has close friends or family available to help with children when needed; monitor for signs of neglect in high-risk families

## Nursing Interventions and Rationales

- • Use the Parenting Risk Scale to assess parenting. **EB:** *One study demonstrated that the Parenting Risk Scale is a reliable and valid measure for the systemic assessment of five key dimensions of parenting (Mrazek, Mrazek, & Klinnert, 1995).*
- • Examine the characteristics of parenting style and behaviors, including the following:
  - ■ Emotional climate at home
  - ■ Attribution of negative traits to the child
  - ■ Failure to support the child's increases in autonomy
  - ■ Type of interaction with the infant/child
  - ■ Competition with the child for attention of spouse/significant other
  - ■ Lack of knowledge/concern about health maintenance or behavioral problems
  - ■ Other behaviors or concerns

  **EB:** *Children are at risk for neglect, abuse, and other negative psychosocial outcomes in families with dysfunctions (Mrazek, Mrazek, & Klinnert, 1995).*
- ▲ Institute abuse/neglect protection measures if there is evidence of an inability to cope with family stressors or crisis, signs of parental substance abuse are observed, or a significant level of social isolation is apparent. *The risk of abuse/neglect is higher in families with high levels of stress, substance abuse, or lack of social support systems (Devlin & Reynolds, 1994).* **EBN:** *Maternal difficult life circumstances, psychiatric-mental health symptoms, educational level, maternal experience in the family of origin, and parenting stress explained 74% of the variance in maternal sensitivity and responsiveness of mothers with their toddlers in the laboratory setting (LeCuyer-Maus, 2003).*
- ▲ For a mother with a toddler, assess maternal depression, perceptions of difficult temperament in the toddler, and low maternal self-efficacy. Make appropriate referral. **EBN:** *Self-efficacy is defined as one's judgment of how effectively one can execute a task or manage a situation that may contain novel, unpredictable, and stressful elements. A cyclic relationship among depression, perceived difficult temperament, and self-efficacy has been identified. Negative feelings about oneself and one's child are likely to negatively influence the parent-child relationship (Gross et al, 1994).*
- • Appraise the parent's resources and the availability of social support systems. Determine the single mother's particular sources of support, especially the availability of her own mother and partner. Encourage the use of healthy, strong support systems. *Before adequate interventions and education can be initiated, the current support system and concerns must be understood. The mother's partner and her mother are often important sources of support (Zacharia, 1994).*
- • Provide education to at-risk parents on behavioral management techniques such as looking ahead, giving good instructions, providing positive reinforcement, redirecting, planned ignoring, and instituting time-outs. **EB:** *These behavioral management tech-*

P

*niques are effective approaches for dealing with ineffective parent-child interactions and improving family relationships (Nicholson et al, 2002).*

- Support parents' competence in appraising their infant's behavior and responses. **EBN:** *Parents must be supported and welcomed as active collaborators in their infant's care (Lawhon, 2002).*
- Promote low-tech interventions, such as massage and multisensory interventions (maternal voice, eye-to-eye contact, and rocking) to reduce maternal and infant stress and improve mother-infant relationship. **EBN:** *Giving birth to infants in adverse situations (war, natural disasters, and so on) can affect infant growth and long-term development. One article explores neurohormonal aspects of stress and social bonding and offers strategies aimed at reducing maternal and infant stress and improving the mother-infant relationship (White-Traut, 2004). Another pilot study suggests a model of incorporating infant massage into a planned parenting enhancement program may promote effective parenting through a special focus on infant stimulation through massage (Porter & Porter, 2004).*
- Encourage kangaroo care (KC) by parents of preterm infants. **EB:** *Parents have been found to be more sensitive and to show more positive affect, touch, and adaptation to infant cues when participating in KC (Feldman et al, 2002).*
- Model age-appropriate and cognitively appropriate caregiver skills by doing the following:
  - Communicating with the child at an appropriate cognitive level of development
  - Giving the child tasks and responsibilities appropriate to age or functional age/level
  - Instituting safety considerations such as the use of assistive equipment
  - Encouraging the child to perform activities of daily living as appropriate

  *These activities illustrate parenting and childrearing skills and behaviors for parents and family (McCloskey & Bulechek, 1992).*
- Encourage mothers to understand and capitalize on their infants' capacity to interact, particularly in the very early months of life. **EBN:** *This study suggested that nurses should routinely assess parent-child interactions in all high-risk, disadvantaged families with very young children (Schiffman, Omar, & McKelvey, 2003).*
- Provide practical and psychological assistance for parents of patients with psychiatric diagnoses, such as schizophrenia. *Parents of patients with schizophrenia show levels of burden that are closely connected with the illness curve of their children; 40% of parents may experience constantly high levels of burden. Parents may be overloaded with their long-term caring tasks, and provision of practical and psychological assistance can be of benefit (Jungbauer et al, 2003).*

▲ Provide programs for homeless mothers with severe mental illness who have lost physical custody of their children. **EBN:** *One study suggests that programs for homeless mothers with severe mental illness can effect changes that promote family reunification. Changes in housing, psychosis, substance use, and therapeutic relationships predicated reunification (Hoffman & Rosenheck, 2001).*

▲ Provide a recovery program that includes instruction in parenting skills and child development for mothers who are addicted to cocaine. **EBN:** *Women addicted to cocaine who are parenting children need strong encouragement from the health care system to* *begin a recovery program and also to gain parenting skills. Lack of parenting knowledge may be a major barrier for them (Coyer, 2003).*

## Multicultural

- Assess for the influence of cultural beliefs, norms, and values on the client's perception of parenting. **EBN:** *What the client considers normal parenting may be based on cultural perceptions (Cochran, 1998; Doswell & Erlen, 1998; Leininger & McFarland, 2002).*
- Acknowledge racial/ethnic differences at the onset of care. **EBN:** *Acknowledgment of racial/ethnicity issues will enhance communication, establish rapport, and promote treatment outcomes (D'Avanzo et al, 2001; Ludwick & Silva, 2000; Vontress & Epp, 1997).*
- Approach individuals of color with respect, warmth, and professional courtesy. **EBN:** *Instances of disrespect have special significance for individuals of color (D'Avanzo et al, 2001; Vontress & Epp, 1997).*
- Give a rationale when assessing African-American individuals about sensitive issues. **EBN:** *African Americans may expect white caregivers to hold negative and preconceived ideas about them. Giving a rationale for questions will help reduce this perception (D'Avanzo et al, 2001; Vontress & Epp, 1997).*
- Acknowledge that value conflicts from acculturation stresses may contribute to increased anxiety and significant conflict with children. **EBN:** *Challenges to traditional beliefs and values are anxiety provoking. Less acculturated parents may experience conflict with their more acculturated children as the children demand greater independence and freedom (True, 1995). Immigrant mothers scored significantly lower on the evaluation of parenting knowledge than U.S.-born mothers (Bornstein & Cote, 2004). Chinese immigrant mothers identified that a larger perceived acculturation gap was associated with more parenting difficulties (Buki, Ma, & Strom, 2003).*
- Use a neutral, indirect style when addressing areas in which improvement is needed, such as a need for verbal stimulation, when working with Native-American clients. **EBN:** *Using indirect statements such as "Other mothers have tried . . ." or "I had a client who tried 'X,' and it seemed to work very well" will help to avoid resentment from the parent (Seideman et al, 1996).*
- Provide support for Chinese families caring for children with disabilities. **EBN:** *The care of children with handicaps strains and violates the Chinese culturally expected order of parental obligations. The following themes emerged: disruptions to natural order, public opinions on what constitutes personhood and ordered bodies, and the establishment of moral reputations linked to shame and blame and the gendered division of parenting (Holroyd, 2003).*
- Acknowledge and praise parenting strengths noted. **EBN:** *Such acknowledgment will increase trust and foster a working relationship with the parent (Seideman et al, 1996). Clinicians could explore and support the positive qualities of authoritative parenting in Mexican descent families (Varela et al, 2004).*
- Validate the client's feelings regarding parenting. **EBN:** *Validation is a therapeutic communication technique that lets the client know that the nurse has heard and understood what was said, and it promotes the nurse-client relationship (Heineken, 1998).*
- Facilitate modeling and role playing to help the family improve parenting skills. **EBN:**

*It is helpful for the family and the client to practice parenting skills in a safe environment before trying them in real-life situations (Rivera-Andino & Lopez, 2000).*

## Home Care

- The interventions described previously may be adapted for home care use.
- Assess parenting stress at each home visit to provide appropriate support and anticipatory guidance to families of children with chronic disease. **EB:** *A study of parents of infants with congenital cardiac abnormalities ages 2 to 12, showed that parents found it difficult to set limits or discipline children with heart disease; older age of the child was associated with higher parenting stress scores (Uzark et al, 2003).*
- ▲ Assess the single mother's history regarding childhood and partner abuse, and current status regarding depressive symptoms, abusive parenting attitudes (lack of empathy, favorable opinion of corporal punishment, parent-child role-reversal, inappropriate expectations). Refer for mental health services as indicated. **EBN:** *In a study of low-income single mothers, findings indicated high levels of abuse, depressive symptoms, and abusive parenting attitudes, with little history of previous mental health treatment. Past history of partner and child abuse predicted higher daily stress leading to lower self-esteem. The presence of more depressive symptoms and daily stressors was associated with greater anger. Greater anger was associated with lower parental empathy. Partner abuse predicted higher levels of abusive parenting attitudes (Lutenbacher, 2002).*
- ▲ Implement behavioral parent training (BPT), including enhancement of skills in child-directed play, effective use of commands, use of discipline measures such as imposing time-outs and providing immediate and natural consequences, problem solving, and communication strategies. **EBN:** *Initial work (Gross, Fogg, & Tucker, 1995) and follow-up at 1 year (Tucker et al, 1998) of a behavioral training program for parents showed improvements in maternal self-efficacy and stress reduction, and in the quality of maternal-infant interaction. A higher amount of BPT was associated with fewer maternal critical statements and negative physical behaviors.*

P

## Client/Family Teaching

- Consider individual and/or group based parenting programs for teenage mothers. **EB:** *This systematic review indicated that results favored those engaged in individual and/or group parenting programs in the areas of mother-infant interaction, language development, parental attitudes, parental knowledge, maternal mealtime communication, maternal self-confidence and maternal identity (Coren & Barlow, 2004).*
- Consider group based parenting programs for parents for children under the age of three years with emotional and behavioral problems. **EB:** *This meta-analysis indicated that results favored those engaged (Barlow & Parsons, 2003).*
- Consider group-based parenting programs for parents with anxiety, depression, and/or low self-esteem. **EB:** *This meta-analysis indicated that parenting programs can make a significant contribution to the short-term psychosocial health of mothers, and that they therefore have a potential role to play in the promotion of mental health (Barlow & Coren, 2004).*
- ▲ Refer adolescent parents for comprehensive psychoeducational parenting classes. **EBN:** *This study indicated that a comprehensive pyschoeducational parenting group can be effective in changing parenting attitudes and beliefs (Thomas et al, 2004).*

- Explain individual differences in children's temperaments and compare and contrast with the parents' expectations. Help parents determine and understand the implications of their child's temperament. **EBN:** *Promoting parental understanding of temperament facilitates development of more realistic expectations (Melvin, 1995; McClowry, 1992).*
- Discuss sound disciplinary techniques, which include catching children being good, listening actively, conveying positive regard, ignoring minor transgressions, giving good directions, using praise, and imposing time-outs. *A variety of opinions exist about disciplinary methods. Proper discipline provides children with security, and clearly enforced rules help them learn self-control and social standards. Parenting classes can be beneficial when the parent has had little formal or informal preparation (Herman-Staab, 1994).*
- Encourage positive parenting: respect for children, understanding of normal development, and creative and loving approaches to meet parenting challenges. **EBN:** *Understanding normal development is a first step so parents can distinguish common behaviors for a given stage of development from "problems." Central to positive parenting is developing approaches that can be used in place of anger, manipulation, punishment, and rewards (Ahmann, 2002).*
- Plan parental education directed toward the following age-related parental concerns:
  - Birth to 2 years—transition, sleep, aggression
  - 3 to 5 years—transition, parent-child relationship, sleep
  - 6 to 10 years—school, parent-child relationship, divorce
  - 11 to 18 years—parent-child relationship, divorce, school

  *Parents with children of any age may seek basic information about a variety of concerns, which can be anticipated and addressed by providing ongoing information and support (Jones, Maestri, & McCoy, 1993).*
- ▲ Initiate referrals to community agencies, parent education programs, stress management training, and social support groups. *The parent needs support to manage angry or inappropriate behaviors. Use of support systems and social services can provide an opportunity to decrease feelings of inadequacy (Baker, 1994; Campbell, 1992).*
- ▲ Provide information regarding available telephone counseling services. *Telephone counseling services can provide confidential advice and support to families who might not otherwise have access to help in dealing with behavioral problems and parenting concerns (Jones, Maestri, and McCoy, 1993).*
- Refer to the care plan for **Delayed Growth and development** for additional teaching interventions.

## evolve WEBSITES FOR EDUCATION

See the EVOLVE website for World Wide Web resources for client education.

## REFERENCES

Ahmann E: Promoting positive parenting: an annotated bibliography, *Pediatr Nurs* 28(4):382, 2002.

Baker NA: Avoid collisions with challenging families, *MCN Am J Matern Child Nurs* 19:97, 1994.

Barlow J, Coren E: Parent-training programmes for improving maternal psychosocial health, *Cochrane Database Syst Rev* (1): CD002020, 2004.

Barlow J, Parsons J: Group-based parent-training programmes for improving emotional and behavioral adjustment in 0-3 year old children, *Cochrane Database Syst Rev* (1):CD003680, 2003.
Bornstein MH, Cote LR: "Who is sitting across from me?" Immigrant mothers' knowledge of parenting and children's development, *Pediatrics* 114(5):e557-564, 2004.
Buki LP, Ma TC, Strom RD et al: Chinese immigrant mothers of adolescents: self-perceptions of acculturation effects on parenting, *Cult Divers Ethnic Minor Psychol* 9(2):127-140, 2003.
Campbell JM: Parenting classes: focus on discipline, *J Community Health Nurs* 9:197, 1992.
Cochran M: Tears have no color, *Am J Nurs* 98(6):53, 1998.
Coren E, Barlow J: Individual and group-based parenting programmes for improving psychosocial outcomes for teenage parents and their children, *Cochrane Database Syst Rev* (3):2CD002964, 2004.
Coyer SM: Women in recovery discuss parenting while addicted to cocaine, *MCN Am J Matern Child Nurs* 28(1):45, 2003.
D'Avanzo CE et al: Developing culturally informed strategies for substance-related interventions. In Naegle MA, D'Avanzo CE, editors: *Addictions and substance abuse: strategies for advanced practice nursing,* St Louis, 2001, Mosby.
Devlin BK, Reynolds E: Child abuse: how to recognize it, how to intervene, *Am J Nurs* 94:26, 1994.
Doswell W, Erlen J: Multicultural issues and ethical concerns in the delivery of nursing care interventions, *Nurs Clin North Am* 33(2):353, 1998.
Feldman R, Eidelman AI, Sirota L et al: Comparison of skin-to-skin (kangaroo) and traditional care: parenting outcomes and preterm infant behavior, *Pediatrics* 110(1):16, 2002.
Gross D, Fogg L, Tucker S: The efficacy of parent training for promoting positive parent-toddler relationships, *Res Nurs Health* 18:489, 1995.
Gross D, Conrad B, Fogg L et al: A longitudinal model of maternal self-efficacy, depression, and difficult temperament during toddlerhood, *Res Nurs Health* 17:207, 1994.
Heineken J: Patient silence is not necessarily client satisfaction: communication in home care nursing, *Home Healthc Nurse* 16(2): 115, 1998.
Herman-Staab B: Screening, management and appropriate referral for pediatric behavior problems, *Nurs Pract* 19:40, 1994.
Hoffman D, Rosenheck R: Homeless mothers with severe mental illnesses and their children: predictors of family reunification, *Psychiatr Rehabil J* 25(2):163, 2001.
Holroyd EE: Chinese cultural influences on parental caregiving obligations toward children with disabilities, *Qual Health Res* 13(1):4, 2003.
Jones LC, Maestri BO, McCoy K: Why parents use the warm line, *MCN Am J Matern Child Nurs* 18:258, 1993.
Jungbauer J, Wittmund B, Dietrich S et al: subjective burden over 12 months in parents of patients with schizophrenia, *Arch Psychiatr Nurs* 17(3):126-134, 2003.
Lawhon G: Facilitation of parenting the premature infant within the newborn intensive care unit, *J Perinat Neonatal Nurs* 16(1): 71, 2002.
LeCuyer-Maus E: Stress and coping in high-risk mothers: difficult life circumstances, psychiatric-mental health symptoms, education, and experiences in their families of origin, *Public Health Nurs* 20(2):132, 2003.
Leininger MM, McFarland MR: *Transcultural nursing: concepts, theories, research and practices,* ed 3, New York, 2002, McGraw-Hill.
Ludwick R, Silva M: Nursing around the world: cultural values and ethical conflicts, *Online J Issues Nurs,* August 14, 2000. Available at www.nursingworld.org/ojin/ethcol/ethics_4.htm, accessed June 19, 2003.
Lutenbacher M: Relationships between psychosocial factors and abusive parenting attitudes in low-income single mothers, *Nurs Res* 51:158, 2002.
McCloskey JC, Bulechek GM, editors: *Nursing interventions classification (NIC),* St Louis, 1992, Mosby.
McClowry SG: Temperament theory and research, *Image* 24:319, 1992.
Melvin N: Children's temperament: intervention for parents, *J Pediatr Nurs* 10:152, 1995.
Mrazek DA, Mrazek P, Klinnert M: Clinical assessment of parenting, *J Am Acad Child Adolesc Psychiatry* 34: 272, 1995.
Nicholson B, Anderson M, Fox R et al: One family at a time: a prevention program for at-risk parents, *J Couns Dev* 80(3):362, 2002.
Porter LS, Porter BO: A blended infant massage-parenting enhancement program for recovering substance-abusing mothers, *Pediatric Nursing* 30(5):363-372, 389-390, 401, 2004.
Rivera-Andino J, Lopez L: When culture complicates care, *RN* 63(7):47, 2000.
Schiffman RF, Omar MA, McKelvey LM: Mother-infant interaction in low-income families. *MCN Am J Matern Child Nurs* 28(4):246-251, 2003.
Seideman RY et al: Assessing American Indian families, *MCN Am J Matern Child Nurs* 21(6):274, 1996.

Thomas DV, Looney SW: Effectiveness of a comprehensive psychoeducational intervention with pregnant and parenting adolescents: a pilot study, *J Child Adolesc Psychiatr Nurs* 17(2):66-77, 2004.
True RH: Mental health issues of Asian/Pacific island women. In Adams DL, editor: *Health issues for women of color: a cultural diversity perspective,* Thousand Oaks, Calif, 1995, Sage.
Tucker S, Gross D, Fogg L et al: The long-term efficacy of a behavioral parent training intervention for families with 2-year-olds, *Res Nurs Health* 21:199, 1998.
Uzark K, Jones K: Parenting stress and children with heart disease, *J Pediatr Health Care* 17(4):163-168, 2003.
Varela RE, Vernberg EM, Sanchez-Sosa JJ et al: Parenting style of Mexican, Mexican American, and Caucasian-non-Hispanic families: social context and cultural influences, *J Fam Psychol* 18(4):651-657, 2004.
Vontress CE, Epp LR: Historical hostility in the African American client: implications for counseling, *J Multicult Counseling Dev* 25:170, 1997.
White-Traut, R.: Providing a nurturing environment for infants in adverse situations: multisensory strategies for newborn care, *J Midwifery Womens Health* 49(4):36-41, 2004.
Zacharia R: Perceived social support and social network of low-income mothers of infants and preschoolers: pre-and postparenting program, *J Community Health Nurs* 11:11, 1994.

# Risk for impaired Parenting

*T. Heather Herdman*

**NANDA**

## Definition

Risk for inability of the primary caretaker to create, maintain, or regain an environment that promotes the optimum growth and development of the child

## Risk Factors

### Social

Marital conflict, declining satisfaction, history of being abused, poor problem-solving skills, role strain/overload, social isolation, legal difficulties, lack of access to resources, lack of value of parenthood, relocation, poverty, poor home environment, lack of family cohesiveness, lack of or poor parental role model, lack of involvement of father of child, history of being abusive, financial difficulties, low self-esteem, lack of resources, unplanned or unwanted pregnancy, inadequate child care arrangements, maladaptive coping strategies, low socioeconomic class, lack of transportation, change in family unit, unemployment or job problems, single parenthood, lack of social support network, inability to put child's needs before own, stress

### Knowledge

Low educational level or attainment, unrealistic expectations of child, lack of knowledge about parenting skills, poor communication skills, preference for physical punishment, in ability to recognize and act on infant cues, low cognitive functioning, lack of knowledge about child health maintenance, lack of knowledge about child development, lack of cognitive readiness for parenthood

### Physiological

Physical illness

### Infant/child

Multiple births; handicapping condition or developmental delay; illness; altered perceptual abilities; lack of goodness of fit (temperament) with parental expectations; unplanned or unwanted child; premature birth; not desired gender; difficult temperament; attention deficit/hyperactivity disorder; prolonged separation from parent; separation from parent at birth

### Psychological

Separation from infant/child; large number of closely spaced children; disability; sleep deprivation or disruption; difficult labor and/or delivery; young age (especially adolescence); depression; history of mental illness; lack of or late prenatal care; history of substance abuse or dependence

NOTE: It is important to reaffirm that adjustment to parenting in general is a normal maturational process that elicits nursing behaviors to prevent potential problems and to promote health.

NOC

## Outcomes (Nursing Outcomes Classification)

### Suggested NOC Outcomes

Abuse Recovery: Emotional, Physical, Sexual; Abusive Behavior Self-Restraint; Caregiver Emotional Health; Caregiver Stressors; Coping; Parent-Infant Attachment; Parenting Performance; Risk Control: Unintended Pregnancy; Social Interaction Skills

P

**Example NOC Outcome with Indicators**

**Parenting Performance** as evidenced by the following indicators: Provides for child's needs/Interacts positively with child/Expresses realistic expectations of parental role/Exhibits a loving relationship with child/Expresses satisfaction with parental role (Rate each indicator of **Parenting Performance:** 1 = never demonstrated, 2 = rarely demonstrated, 3 = sometimes demonstrated, 4 = often demonstrated, 5 = consistently demonstrated [see Section I].)

## Client Outcomes

### Client Will (Specify Time Frame):

- Successfully establish a nurturing parenting role
- Affirm desire to acquire and maintain constructive parenting skills to support infant/child growth and development
- Maintain appropriate measures to develop a safe, nurturing environment
- Display attentive, supportive parenting behaviors
- Have knowledge of strategies to protect child from harm and/or neglect

## NIC

## Interventions (Nursing Interventions Classification)

### Suggested NIC Interventions

Abuse Protection Support: Child; Attachment Promotion; Caregiver Support; Developmental Enhancement: Adolescent, Child; Environmental Management: Attachment Process; Family Integrity Promotion; Family Support; Family Therapy; Infant Care; Kangaroo Care; Parent Education: Adolescent, Childrearing Family, Infant; Risk Identification: Childbearing Family; Role Enhancement

**Example NIC Activities—Kangaroo Care**

Determine and monitor parent's level of confidence in caring for infant; encourage parent to initiate infant care

## Nursing Interventions and Rationales

Note: Management of a risk diagnosis necessitates approaches using primary and secondary prevention. Primary prevention interventions include activities such as safety instruction and focus on forestalling the development of a disease or condition. Early detection through screening, monitoring, and surveillance is secondary prevention (Shortridge & Valanis, 1992).

- Conduct risk identification, noting the presence of a history of abuse, parental/family stressors, strength and adequacy of social support systems, established coping styles, and other related factors (see Related Factors). *Identification of a family at risk signals special teaching and referral needs (McCloskey & Bulechek, 1992).*
- Screen for maternal psychiatric-mental health symptoms and negative experiences in the mother's family of origin. **EBN:** *Early detection can provide opportunities for intervention with these mothers (LeCuyer-Maus, 2003). One study partially explains the relationship between maternal abuse history and mental health status, and parenting attitudes. The findings underscore the need for health care providers to consider the mental health status and abuse histories of low-income single mothers (Lutenbacher, 2002).*
- Support parents' competence in appraising their infant's behavior and responses. **EBN:** *Parents must be supported and welcomed as active collaborators in their infant's care.*
- Promote low-tech interventions, such as massage and multisensory interventions (maternal voice, eye-to-eye contact, and rocking) to reduce maternal and infant stress and improve mother-infant relationship. **EBN:** *Giving birth to infants in adverse situations (war, natural disasters, and so on) can affect infant growth and development long-term. One article explores neurohormonal aspects of stress and social bonding and offers strategies aimed at reducing maternal and infant stress and improving the mother-infant relationship (White-Traut, 2004). Another pilot study suggests a model of incorporating infant massage into a planned parenting enhancement program may promote effective parenting through a special focus on infant stimulation through massage (Porter & Porter, 2004).*
- Encourage kangaroo care (KC) by parents of preterm infants. **EB:** *Parents have been found to be more sensitive and to show more positive affect, touch, and adaptation to infant cues when participating in KC (Feldman et al, 2002).*



P

- Provide education to at-risk parents on behavioral management techniques such as looking ahead, giving good instructions, providing positive reinforcement, redirecting, planned ignoring, and using time-outs. **EB:** *These behavioral management techniques are effective approaches for dealing with ineffective parent-child interactions and improving family relationships (Nicholson et al, 2002).*
- Monitor parent-infant interactions that may signal interrupted or inadequate attachment or other parenting issues. *Early detection can lead to early intervention, which can prevent or limit problems (McCloskey & Bulechek, 1992).*
- Encourage mothers to understand and capitalize on their infants' capacity to interact, particularly in the very early months of life. **EBN:** *This study suggested that nurses should routinely assess parent-child interactions in all high-risk, disadvantaged families with very young children (Schiffman, Omar, & McKelvey, 2003).*
- Provide practical and psychological assistance for parents of patients with psychiatric diagnoses, such as schizophrenia. *Parents of patients with schizophrenia show levels of burden that are closely connected with the illness curve of their children; forty percent of parents may experience constantly high levels of burden. Parents may be overloaded with their long-term caring tasks, and provision of practical and psychological assistance can be of benefit (Jungbauer et al, 2003).*
- Refer to the care plan for **Impaired Parenting** for other interventions as appropriate to the situation.

## Multicultural

- Assess for the influence of cultural beliefs, norms, and values on the client's perception of parenting. **EBN:** *What the client considers normal parenting may be based on cultural perceptions (Cochran, 1998; Doswell & Erlen, 1998; Leininger & McFarland, 2002).*
- Acknowledge racial/ethnic differences at the onset of care. **EBN:** *Acknowledgment of racial/ethnicity issues will enhance communication, establish rapport, and promote treatment outcomes (D'Avanzo et al, 2001; Ludwick & Silva, 2000; Vontress & Epp, 1997).*
- Approach individuals of color with respect, warmth, and professional courtesy. **EBN:** *Instances of disrespect have special significance for individuals of color (D'Avanzo et al, 2001; Vontress & Epp, 1997).*
- Give a rationale when assessing African-American individuals about sensitive issues. **EBN:** *Many African-Americans expect Caucasian caregivers to hold negative and preconceived ideas about them. Giving a rationale for questions will help reduce this perception (D'Avanzo et al, 2001; Vontress & Epp, 1997).*
- Acknowledge that value conflicts from acculturation stresses may contribute to increased anxiety and significant conflict with children. **EBN:** *Challenges to traditional beliefs and values are anxiety provoking. Less acculturated parents may experience conflict with their more acculturated children as the children demand greater independence and freedom (True, 1995). Immigrant mothers scored significantly lower on the evaluation of parenting knowledge than U.S.-born mothers (Bornstein & Cote, 2004). Chinese immigrant mothers identified that a larger perceived acculturation gap was associated with more parenting difficulties (Buki et al, 2003).*
- Use a neutral, indirect style when addressing areas in which improvement is needed

P

(such as a need for verbal stimulation) when working with Native American clients. **EBN:** *Using indirect statements such as "Other mothers have tried . . ." or "I had a client who tried 'X,' and it seemed to work very well" will assist in avoiding resentment from the parent (Seideman et al, 1996).*

- Acknowledge and praise parenting strengths noted. **EBN:** *Such acknowledgment will increase trust and foster a working relationship with the parent (Seideman et al, 1996). Clinicians could explore and support the positive qualities of authoritative parenting in Mexican descent families (Varela et al, 2004).*
- Validate the client's feelings regarding parenting. **EBN:** *Validation is a therapeutic communication technique that lets the client know that the nurse has heard and understood what was said, and it promotes the nurse-client relationship (Heineken, 1998).*
- Facilitate modeling and role playing to help the family improve parenting skills. **EBN:** *It is helpful for the family and the client to practice parenting skills in a safe environment before trying them in real-life situations (Rivera-Andino & Lopez, 2000).*

### Home Care

- The interventions described previously may be adapted for home care use.
- Assess parenting stress at each home visit to provide appropriate support and anticipatory guidance to families of children with chronic disease. **EB:** *A study of parents of infants with congenital cardiac abnormalities ages 2 to 12, showed that parents found it difficult to set limits or discipline children with heart disease; older age of the child was associated with higher parenting stress scores (Uzark et al, 2003).*

## Client/Family Teaching

- Consider individual and/or group based parenting programs for teenage mothers. **EB:** *This systematic review indicated that results favored those engaged in individual and/or group parenting programs in the areas of mother-infant interaction, language development, parental attitudes, parental knowledge, maternal mealtime communication, maternal self-confidence, and maternal identity (Coren & Barlow, 2004).*
- Consider group based parenting programs for parents for children under the age of three years with emotional and behavioral problems. **EB:** *This meta-analysis indicated that results favored those engaged in parenting programs in terms of improving the emotional and behavioral adjustment of children under age 3 (Barlow & Parsons, 2003).*
- Consider group-based parenting programs for parents with anxiety, depression, and/or low self-esteem. **EB:** *This meta-analysis indicated that parenting programs can make a significant contribution to the short-term psychosocial health of mothers, and that they therefore have a potential role to play in the promotion of mental health (Barlow & Coren, 2004).*

▲ Refer adolescent parents for comprehensive psychoeducational parenting classes. **EBN:** *This study indicated that a comprehensive pyschoeducational parenting group can be effective in changing parenting attitudes and beliefs (Thomas et al, 2004).*

▲ Initiate referrals to an appropriate community agency for early follow-up if an actual problem is identified.

- Refer to the care plan for **Impaired Parenting** for additional teaching interventions.

## evolve WEBSITES FOR EDUCATION

See the EVOLVE website for World Wide Web resources for client education.

## REFERENCES


Barlow J, Coren E: Parent-training programmes for improving maternal psychosocial health. *Cochrane Database Syst Rev* (1):CD002020, 2004.

Barlow J, Parsons J: Group-based parent-training programmes for improving emotional and behavioral adjustment in 0-3 year old children, *Cochrane Database Syst Rev* (1):CD003680, 2003.

Bornstein MH, Cote LR: "Who is sitting across from me?" Immigrant mothers' knowledge of parenting and children's development, *Pediatrics* 114(5):e557-564, 2004.

Buki LP, Ma TC, Strom RD et al: Chinese immigrant mothers of adolescents: self-perceptions of acculturation effects on parenting, *Cult Divers Ethnic Minor Psychol* 9(2):127-140, 2003.

Cochran M: Tears have no color, *Am J Nurs* 98(6):53, 1998.

Coren E, Barlow J: Individual and group-based parenting programmes for improving psychosocial outcomes for teenage parents and their children, *Cochrane Database Syst Rev* (3):CD002964, 2004.

D'Avanzo CE et al: Developing culturally informed strategies for substance-related interventions. In Naegle MA, D'Avanzo CE, editors: *Addictions and substance abuse: strategies for advanced practice nursing,* St Louis, 2001, Mosby.

Doswell W, Erlen J: Multicultural issues and ethical concerns in the delivery of nursing care interventions, *Nurs Clin North Am* 33(2):353, 1998.

Feldman R, Eidelman AI, Sirota L et al: Comparison of skin-to-skin (kangaroo) and traditional care: parenting outcomes and preterm infant behavior, *Pediatrics* 110(1):16, 2002.

Heineken J: Patient silence is not necessarily client satisfaction: communication in home care nursing, *Home Healthc Nurse* 16(2): 115, 1998.

Jungbauer J, Wittmund B, Dietrich S et al: Subjective burden over 12 months in parents of patients with schizophrenia, *Arch Psychiatr Nurs* 17(3):126-134, 2003.

Lawhon G: Facilitation of parenting the premature infant within the newborn intensive care unit, *J Perinat Neonatal Nurs* 16(1): 71, 2002.

LeCuyer-Maus E: Stress and coping in high-risk mothers: difficult life circumstances, psychiatric-mental health symptoms, education, and experiences in their families of origin, *Public Health Nurs* 20(2):132, 2003.

Leininger MM, McFarland MR: *Transcultural nursing: concepts, theories, research and practices,* ed 3, New York, 2002, McGraw-Hill.

Ludwick R, Silva M: Nursing around the world: cultural values and ethical conflicts, *Online J Issues Nurs,* August 14, 2000. Available at www.nursingworld.org/ojin/ethcol/ethics_4.htm, accessed June 19, 2003.

Lutenbacher M: Relationships between psychosocial factors and abusive parenting attitudes in low-income single mothers, *Nurs Res* 51(3):158, 2002.

McCloskey JC, Bulechek GM, editors: *Nursing interventions classification (NIC),* St Louis, 1992, Mosby.

Nicholson B, Anderson M, Fox R et al: One family at a time: a prevention program for at-risk parents, *J Couns Dev* 80(3):362, 2002.

Porter LS, Porter BO: A blended infant massage-parenting enhancement program for recovering substance-abusing mothers, *Pediatric Nursing, 30*(5): 363-372, 389-390, 401, 2004.

Rivera-Andino J, Lopez L: When culture complicates care, *RN* 63(7):47, 2000.

Schiffman RF, Omar MA, McKelvey LM: Mother-infant interaction in low-income families. *MCN Am J Matern Child Nurs* 28(4):246-251, 2003.

Seideman RY et al: Assessing American Indian families, *MCN Am J Matern Child Nurs* 21(6):274, 1996.

Shortridge L, Valanis B: The epidemiological model applied in community health nursing. In Stanhope M, Lancaster J, editors: *Community health nursing: process and practice for promoting health,* ed 3, St Louis, 1992, Mosby.

Thomas DV, Looney SW: Effectiveness of a comprehensive psychoeducational intervention with pregnant and parenting adolescents: a pilot study, *J Child Adolesc Psychiatr Nurs* 17(2):66-77, 2004.

True RH: Mental health issues of Asian/Pacific island women. In Adams DL, editor: *Health issues for women of color: a cultural diversity perspective,* Thousand Oaks, Calif, 1995, Sage.

Uzark K, Jones K: Parenting stress and children with heart disease. *J Pediatr Health Care* 17(4):163-168, 2003.

Varela RE, Vernberg EM, Sanchez-Sosa JJ et al: Parenting style of Mexican, Mexican American, and Caucasian-non-Hispanic families: social context and cultural influences, *J Fam Psychol* 18(4):651-657, 2004.




P

Vontress CE, Epp LR: Historical hostility in the African American client: implications for counseling, *J Multicult Counseling Dev* 25:170, 1997.

White-Traut, R.: Providing a nurturing environment for infants in adverse situations: multisensory strategies for newborn care, *J Midwifery Womens Health* 49(4):36-41, 2004.

# Risk for Peripheral neurovascular dysfunction

evolve

*Betty J. Ackley*

**NANDA**

## Definition

At risk for disruption in circulation, sensation, or motion of an extremity

## Risk Factors

Trauma; fractures; mechanical compression (e.g., tourniquet, cane, cast, brace, dressing, restraints); orthopedic surgery; immobilization; burns; vascular obstruction

**NOC**

## Outcomes (Nursing Outcomes Classification)

### Suggested NOC Outcomes

Circulation Status; Joint Movement: Passive; Neurological Status: Spinal Sensory/Motor Function; Risk Detection; Tissue Perfusion: Peripheral

**Example NOC Outcome with Indicators**

**Tissue Perfusion: Peripheral** will be intact as evidenced by the following indicators: Distal peripheral pulses/Sensation/Skin color/Muscle function/Skin integrity/Peripheral edema/Localized extremity pain (Rate each indicator of **Tissue Perfusion: Peripheral:** 1 = severely compromised, 2 = substantially compromised, 3 = moderately compromised, 4 = mildly compromised, 5 = not compromised [see Section I].)

## Client Outcomes

### Client Will (Specify Time Frame):

- Maintain circulation, sensation, and movement of an extremity within client's own normal limits
- Explain signs of neurovascular compromise and ways to prevent venous stasis



P

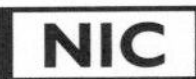

## Interventions (Nursing Interventions Classification)

### Suggested NIC Interventions

Exercise Therapy: Joint Mobility; Peripheral Sensation Management

**Example NIC Activities—Peripheral Sensation Management**

Monitor for paresthesia: numbness, tingling, hyperesthesia, and hypoesthesia; monitor for thrombophlebitis and deep vein thrombosis (DVT)

## Nursing Interventions and Rationales

- Perform neurovascular assessment every 1 to 4 hours or every 15 minutes as ordered.
- Use the six **P**'s of assessment:
  - **Pain**—Assess severity (on a scale of 1 to 10), quality, radiation, and relief by medications. *Diffuse pain that is aggravated by passive movement and is unrelieved by medication can be an early symptom of compartment syndrome or a symptom of limb ischemia (Kasirajan & Ouriel, 2002; Walls, 2002).*
  - **Pulses**—Check the pulses distal to the injury. Check the uninjured side first to establish a baseline for a bilateral comparison. *An intact pulse generally indicates a good blood supply to the extremity, although compartment syndrome may be present even if the pulse is intact (Walls, 2002).*
  - **Pallor/Poikilothermia**—Check color and temperature changes below the injury site. Check capillary refill. If pallor is present, record the level of coldness carefully. *A cold, pale, or bluish extremity indicates arterial insufficiency or arterial damage, and a physician should be notified (Kasirajan & Ouriel, 2002). A reddened, warm extremity may indicate infection (Kasper, 2005). Normal capillary refill time is 3 seconds or less (McConnell, 2002).*



  - **Paresthesia** (change in sensation)—Check by lightly touching the skin proximal and distal to the injury. Ask if the client has any unusual sensations such as hypersensitivity, tingling, prickling, decreased feeling, or numbness. *Changes in sensation are indicative of nerve compression and damage and can also indicate compartment syndrome (Kasirajan & Ouriel, 2002; Walls, 2002).*
  - **Paralysis**—Ask the client to perform appropriate range-of-motion exercises in the unaffected and then the affected extremity. *Paralysis is a late and ominous symptom of compartment syndrome or limb ischemia (Kasirajan & Ouriel, 2002; Walls, 2002).*
  - **Pressure**—Check by feeling the extremity; note new onset of firmness of the extremity. *With compartment syndrome, the affected area becomes taut and feels firm when touched (Walls, 2002).*
- Monitor the client for symptoms of compartment syndrome evidenced by pain greater than expected, pain with passive movement, decreased sensation, weakness, loss of movement, absence of pulse, and tension in the skin that surrounds the muscle compartment. These symptoms are not always present and can be difficult to assess. *Compartment syndrome is characterized by increased pressure within the muscle compartment, which compromises circulation, viability, and function of tissues (Edwards, 2004; Walls, 2002).*

- • Monitor appropriate application and function of corrective device (e.g., cast, splint, traction) every 1 to 4 hours as needed. *An improperly applied device can cause nerve damage, circulatory impairment, or pressure ulcers.*
- • Position the extremity in correct alignment with each position change; check every hour to ensure appropriate alignment.
- ▲ Get the client out of bed and mobilize the client as soon as possible, after consultation with the physician. *Immobility is a risk factor for deep vein thrombosis (DVT); early ambulation can help prevent clot formation (Roman, 2005).*
- ▲ Monitor for signs of DVT, especially in high-risk populations, including persons older than 40 years of age; persons with immobility or obesity; persons taking estrogen or oral contraceptives; persons with a history of trauma, surgery, or previous DVT; and persons with a cerebrovascular accident, varicose veins, malignancy, or cardiovascular disease. **EBN:** *These are identified risk factors that increase the incidence of DVT and have been validated using a DVT risk scale (Autar, 1996, 2003).*
- ▲ Apply graduated compression stockings if ordered; measure carefully to ensure proper fit, removing at least daily to assess circulation and skin condition. **EBN and EB:** *A meta-analysis of 11 studies demonstrated that graduated compression stockings reduced the incidence of DVT in a high-risk orthopedic surgical population and that additional antithrombotic measures, along with stocking use, decreased the incidence even further (Joanna Briggs Institute, 2001). The use of graduated compression stockings, alone or in conjunction with other prevention modalities, prevents DVT in hospitalized clients (Amarigiri & Lees, 2005).*
- ▲ Watch for and report signs of DVT as evidenced by pain, deep tenderness, swelling in the calf and thigh, and redness in the involved extremity. Take serial leg measurements of the thigh and leg circumferences. In some clients, a tender venous cord can be felt in the popliteal fossa. Do not rely on Homans' sign. *Thrombosis with clot formation is usually first detected as edema of the involved leg and then as pain. Homans' sign is not reliable (Kasper, 2005).*
- ▲ Help the client perform prescribed exercises every 4 hours as ordered.
- • Provide a nutritious diet and adequate fluid replacement. *Good nutrition and sufficient fluids are needed to promote healing and prevent complications.*

## Geriatric

- • Use heat and cold therapies cautiously. *Elderly clients often have decreased sensation and circulation.*

## Home Care

- • Assess the knowledge base of the client and family following any institutional care.
- • Teach about the disease process and care as necessary. *The length of time of institutional care and teaching may have been very short and insufficient for learning.*
- • If risk is related to fractures and cast care, teach the family to complete a neurovascular assessment; it may be performed as often as every 4 hours but is more commonly done two to three times per day. *A risk requiring monitoring more often than every 4 hours for longer than 24 hours indicates a need for institutionally based care.*



P

- If the fracture is peripheral, position the limb for comfort and change position frequently, avoiding dependent positions for extended periods. *Changes in position enhance circulation.*
- ▲ Refer to physical therapy services as necessary to establish an exercise program and safety in transfers or mobility within limitations of physical status.
- Establish an emergency plan. *Having a predetermined plan will save valuable time in the event of emergency.*

### Client/Family Teaching

- Teach the client and family to recognize signs of neurovascular dysfunction and report signs immediately to the appropriate person.
- Emphasize proper nutrition to promote healing.
- ▲ If necessary, refer the client to a rehabilitation facility for instruction in proper use of assistive devices and measures to improve mobility without compromising neurovascular function.

## evolve WEBSITES FOR EDUCATION

See the EVOLVE website for World Wide Web resources for client education.

## REFERENCES

Amarigiri SV, Lees TA: Elastic compression stockings for prevention of deep vein thrombosis, *Cochrane Database Syst Rev* (3): CD001484, 2005.

Autar R: Nursing assessment of clients at risk of deep vein thrombosis (DVT): the Autar DVT scale, *J Adv Nurs* 23:763, 1996.

Autar R: The management of deep vein thrombosis: the Autar DVT risk assessment scale re-visited, *J Orthop Nurs* 7(3):114, 2003.

Edwards S: Acute compartment syndrome, *Emerg Nurse* 12(3):32, 2004.

Feldman CB: Caring for feet: patients and nurse practitioners working together, *Nurse Pract Forum* 9(2):87, 1998.

Joanna Briggs Institute: Best practice: graduated compression stockings for the prevention of post-operative venous thromboembolism, *EB Pract Inform Sheets Health Profes* 5:2, 2001.

Kasirajan K, Ouriel K: Current options in the diagnosis and management of acute limb ischemia, *Prog Cardiovasc Nurs* 17:1, 2002.

Kasper DL et al: *Harrison's principles of internal medicine,* ed 16, New York, 2005, McGraw-Hill.

McConnell EA: Assessing neurovascular status in a casted limb, *Nursing* 32(9):20, 2002.

Roman M: Deep vein thrombosis: an overview, *Med-Surg Matters* 14(1), 2005.

Tumbarello C: Acute extremity compartment syndrome, *J Trauma Nurs* 7(2):30, 2000.

Walls M: Orthopedic trauma, *RN* 65:7, 2002.

P

# Risk for Poisoning

*Betty J. Ackley*

**NANDA**

### Definition

Accentuated risk of accidental exposure to, or ingestion of, drugs or dangerous products in doses sufficient to cause poisoning

## Risk Factors

### External

Unprotected contact with heavy metals or chemicals; storage of medicines in unlocked cabinets accessible to children or confused persons; presence of poisonous vegetation; presence of atmospheric pollutants, paint, lacquer, and so on, in poorly ventilated areas or without effective protection; flaking, peeling paint or plaster in presence of young children; chemical contamination of food and water; availability of illicit drugs potentially contaminated by poisonous additives; presence of large supplies of drugs in home; placement or storage of dangerous products within reach of children or confused persons

### Internal

Verbalization that occupational setting is without adequate safeguards, reduced vision, lack of safety or drug education, lack of proper precautions, insufficient finances, cognitive or emotional difficulties

## Related Factors (r/t)

See Risk Factors.

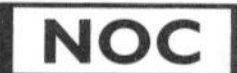

## Outcomes (Nursing Outcomes Classification)

### Suggested NOC Outcomes

Knowledge: Child Physical Safety, Medication, Personal Safety; Parenting Performance; Risk Control; Risk Control: Alcohol Use, Drug Use; Risk Detection; Safe Home Environment

**Example NOC Outcome with Indicators**

**Risk Control** as evidenced by the following indicators: Monitors environmental risk factors/Develops effective risk control strategies (Rate each indicator of **Risk Control:** 1 = never demonstrated, 2 = rarely demonstrated, 3 = sometimes demonstrated, 4 = often demonstrated, 5 = consistently demonstrated [see Section I].)

P

## Client Outcomes

**Client Will (Specify Time Frame):**

- Prevent inadvertent ingestion of or exposure to toxins or poisonous substances
- Explain and undertake appropriate safety measures to prevent ingestion of or exposure to toxins or poisonous substances

NIC

## Interventions (Nursing Interventions Classification)

### Suggested NIC Interventions

Environmental Management: Safety; First Aid; Health Education; Medication Management; Surveillance; Surveillance: Safety

**Example NIC Activities—Environmental Management: Safety**

Identify safety hazards in the environment (i.e., physical, biological, and chemical); remove hazards from the environment when possible

## Nursing Interventions and Rationales

- • When a client comes to the hospital with possible poisoning, begin care following the "ABCs," and administer oxygen if needed. *Poisoning is an emergency and should be treated as such (Broderick, 2004).*
- • Obtain a thorough history of what was ingested, how much, and when, and ask to look at the container. Note the client's age, weight, medications, and any medical conditions. *A thorough history is critical to success of treatment (Broderick, 2004).*
- • Inspect carefully for signs of ingestion of poisons, including an odor on the breath, a trace of the substance on the clothing, burns or redness around the mouth and lips, as well as signs of confusion, vomiting, or dyspnea. **EB:** *It is important to look for signs of ingestion of poison before initiating treatment because up to 40% of children who present with poisoning have not actually been exposed to the suspected toxin (Hwang, 2003).*
- • Note results of toxicology screens, arterial blood gasses, blood glucose levels, and any other ordered laboratory tests. *If there is incomplete or inaccurate information about what was ingested, laboratory tests may be needed to determine treatment (Broderick, 2004).*
- ▲ Initiate any ordered treatment for poisoning quickly. *The goal is to prevent further absorption of the agent; charcoal is most effective if administered in the first hour after ingestion of the poison (Bryant & Singer, 2003).*
- • Prevent iatrogenic harm to the hospitalized client by following these guidelines for administering medications:
  - ▪ Use at least two methods to identify the client before administering medications or blood products, such as the client's name and medical record number or birth date.
  - ▪ When taking verbal or telephone orders, the orders should be written down, and then read back for verification to the individual giving the order.
  - ▪ Standardize use of abbreviations and eliminate those that are prone to cause errors.
  - ▪ Take high alert medications off the nursing unit, such as potassium chloride. Standardize concentrations of medications such as morphine in PCA pumps.
  - ▪ Use only intravenous (IV) pumps that prevent free flow of IV solution when the tubing is taken out of the pump.
  - ▪ Identify all of the client's current medications on admission to a health care facility, and ensure that all health care staff have access to the information.

  *These are the National Patient Safety Goals and are required actions to improve client safety in a hospital or health care facility from the Joint Commission of Hospital Accreditation (Chai, 2005).*
- • Detect possible interactions and cumulative or other adverse effects among prescribed medications, self-administered over-the-counter (OTC) products, culturally based home treatments, herbal remedies and foods. *Serious consequences may occur if interactions are not identified, herbal preparations can be toxic.*

P

## Pediatrics

- ▲ Evaluate lead exposure risk and consult the health care provider regarding lead screening measures as indicated (public/ambulatory health). *Lead poisoning is one of the most common and preventable types of childhood poisoning today. Assessment of exposure risk and blood level testing are important preventive measures (Dennis, Staley, & Curtis, 2002).*
- • Supply "Mr.Yuk" labels for families with children. *Implementing poisoning prevention program strategies benefits the client and family (Dart & Ramack, 2003). Information on how to obtain "Mr Yuk" labels is available at www.chp.edu/mryuk/05a_mryuk.php.*
- • Provide guidance for parents/caregivers regarding age-related safety measures, including the following:
  - Store potentially harmful substances in the original containers with safety closures intact.
  - Recognize that no container is completely "childproof."
  - Avoid storage of medications or toxic substances in food containers.
  - Place poisonous houseplants out of the reach of infants and children; preferably remove them from the home. Teach children not to put leaves or berries into their mouths.
  - Keep cleaning agents, disinfectants, and other hazardous materials out of sight and out of children's reach; keep them locked up.
  - Do not take medications in front of children; children mimic parents' behaviors.
  - Do not suggest that medications such as aspirin and children's vitamins are candy.
  - If interrupted when using a harmful product, take it with you; children can get into it within seconds.
  - Use extreme caution with pesticides and gardening materials close to children's play areas.
  - Keep perfume and makeup out of reach of children.

  *Infants have a high level of hand-to-mouth behavior and will ingest anything. Young children may inadvertently ingest poisonous materials, particularly if those materials are thought to be food or beverage (Broderick, 2004; Dart & Rumack, 2003).* **EB:** *A study of poisoning incidences in children where the child was brought to the emergency department demonstrated that 73% of the parents received no instructions on how to prevent another incidence of poisoning (Demorest et al, 2004).*
- • Teach the family to keep the home safe for children by keeping harmful cleaning products and all liquids containing hydrocarbons away from children and using child-resistant packaging as available. *Liquid products that contain more than 10% hydrocarbons (e.g., cosmetics such as hair oils, automotive chemicals, cleaning solvents, or water repellents) are now required to be in child-resistant packaging. When these products enter the lungs inadvertently, they can cause chemical pneumonia and death in children (Barone, 2002).*
- • Advise families that syrup of ipecac is generally no longer recommended to be kept and used in the home. *Syrup of ipecac is not considered very effective and can delay or hamper administration of charcoal admixture that may be more effective (Rudolph et al, 2003).*

*There is a high aspiration potential with these clients. Giving ipecac may delay the administration or reduce the effectiveness of activated charcoal, oral antidotes, and whole bowel irrigation (Ressel, 2004).*

## Geriatric

- Caution the client and family to avoid storing medications with similar appearances close to one another (e.g., nitroglycerin ointment near toothpaste or denture creams). *Confusion and visual impairment can place the older person at risk of incorrectly identifying of the contents.*
- Place medications in a medication box that indicates when medications are to be taken. *Failing eyesight, the use of multiple drugs, and difficulty in remembering whether a medication was taken are among the causes of accidental poisoning in older persons.* **EB:** *A study that reviewed causes of calls to poison information centers by adults over age 50 demonstrated that most of the calls related to errors in taking drugs, and then adverse drug reactions (Skarupski, Mrvos, & Krenzelok, 2004).*
- Remind the older client to store medications out of reach when young children come to visit. *Children are inquisitive and may ingest medicines in containers without safety caps.*

## Home Care

- The interventions described previously may be adapted for home care use.
- Provide the client and/or family with a poison control diagram to be kept on the refrigerator or a bulletin board. Ensure that the telephone number for local poison control information is readily available.
- Prepour medications for a client who is at risk of ingesting too much of a given medication because of mistakes in preparation. Delegate this task to the family or caregivers if possible. *Elderly clients who live alone are at greatest risk of poisoning.*
- Identify poisonous substances in the immediate surroundings of the home, such as a garage or barn, including paints and thinners, fertilizers, rodent and bug control substances, animal medications, gasoline, and oil. Label with the name, a poison warning sign, and a poison control center number. Lock out of the reach of children. *Dangerous poisonous substances can be found in areas other than the internal home setting. Curious children are at risk for ingestion when exploring.*
- Identify the risk of toxicity from environmental activities such as spraying trees or roadside shrubs. Contact local departments of agriculture or transportation to obtain material substance data sheets or to prevent the activity in desired areas. *Very young children, women who are of childbearing age or who are pregnant, and the elderly are at greatest risk.*
- Avoid carbon monoxide poisoning. Instruct the client and family in the importance of using a carbon monoxide detector in the home, having the chimney professionally cleaned each year, having the furnace professionally inspected each year, ensuring that all combustion equipment is properly vented, and installing a chimney screen and cap to prevent small animals from moving into the chimney. *Many deaths each year are attributed to carbon monoxide poisoning. Take these precautions to protect the child and family (Jordan, 2002).*

### Multicultural

- Assess housing for pathways of lead poisoning. **EB:** *Minority individuals are more likely to reside in older and substandard housing. About 74% of privately owned, occupied housing units in the United States built before 1980 contain lead-based paint (Centers for Disease Control and Prevention, 2001).*
- Prompt caregivers to take action to prevent lead poisoning. **EB:** *A lead poisoning awareness campaign targeted at ethnic minority parents of preschool-age children respondents reported an increase in steps to prevent lead poisoning after exposure to the campaign (McLaughlin et al, 2004).*
- Inform minority parents of children who present for treatment of a poisoning episode of poisoning prevention education as part of the medical encounter. **EB:** *Research suggests that young children experiencing a first poisoning episode will have a second occurrence and that poisoning prevention education may prevent repeat poisoning occurrence (Demorest, Posner, Osterhoudt, & Henretig, 2004).*
- Poison control centers (PCC's) should offer information in bilingual and bicultural manner. **EB:** *Research suggests that PCCs are underused by low-income minority and Spanish-speaking parents because of lack of knowledge and misconception. A videotape intervention was highly effective in changing knowledge, attitudes, behaviors, and behavioral intentions concerning the PCC within this population (Kelly, Huffman, Mendoza, & Robinson, 2003; Shepherd, Larkin, Velez, & Huddleston, 2004).*

## Client/Family Teaching

- Counsel the client and family members regarding medication safety:
  - Avoid sharing prescriptions.
  - Read and follow labeling instructions on all products; adjust dosage for age.
  - Avoid excessive amounts and/or frequency of doses. ("If a little does some good, a lot should do more.")

  *Each year, thousands of adverse drug-related events occur, including poisoning. Poisoning is a major cause of morbidity and mortality.*
- Advise the family to post first aid charts and poison center instructions in an accessible location. Poison control center telephone numbers should be posted close to each telephone, and the number programmed into cell phones. *A poison control center should always be called immediately before initiating any first aid measures. The national toll-free number is (800) 222-1222; the agency will connect the caller to the closest poison control center (Broderick, 2004).*
- Advise family when calling the poison control center to:
  - Give as much information as possible, including your name, location, and telephone number, so that the poison control operator can call back in case you are disconnected or summon help if needed.
  - Give the name of the potential poison ingested and, if possible, the amount and time of ingestion. If the bottle or package is available, give the trade name and ingredients if they are listed.
  - Be prepared to tell the person the child's height and weight.

P

- Describe the state of the poisoning victim. Is the victim conscious? Are there any symptoms? What is the person's general appearance, skin color, respiration, breathing difficulties, mental status (alert, sleepy, unusual behavior)? Is the person vomiting? Having convulsions?

*Rapid initiation of proper treatment reduces mortality and morbidity and decreases emergency department visits and inpatient admissions. Consultation with a poison control center is necessary to assess and treat poisoned clients (Broderick, 2004; Ressel, 2004).*

- • Encourage the client and family to take first aid and other types of safety-related programs. *These programs raise participants' level of emergency preparation.*
- ▲ Initiate referrals to peer group interventions, peer counseling, and other types of substance abuse prevention/rehabilitation programs when substance abuse is identified as a risk factor. **EBN:** *Clients with substance abuse problems are at risk for contact with tainted substances or for overdose. The peer pressure factor is extremely strong for adolescents; rehabilitation programs providing nonpunitive and skill-focused approaches are most effective (Anderson, 1996).*

## evolve WEBSITES FOR EDUCATION

See the EVOLVE website for World Wide Web resources for client education.

## REFERENCES


Anderson NLR: Decisions about substance abuse among adolescents in juvenile detention, *Image J Nurs Sch* 28:65, 1996.

Barone S: Child-resistant packaging, *Consumer Product Safety Review* 6(3):3, 2002.

Broderick M: Pediatric poisoning! *RN* 67(9):37-38, 40-42, 2004.

Bryant S, Singer J: Management of toxic exposure in children, *Emerg Med Clin North Am* 21(1):101, 2003.

Centers for Disease Control and Prevention: Sources and pathways of lead exposure. In *Preventing lead poisoning in young children,* Atlanta, 2001, The Center.

Chai K: Patient safety goals and the impact on the JCAHO survey, *Cinahl Information Systems*, No 2005048933, 2005.

Dart RC, Rumack BA: Poisoning. In Hay WW et al, editors: *Current pediatrics: diagnosis and treatment*, ed 16, New York, 2003, McGraw-Hill.

Demorest RA, Posner JC, Osterhoudt KC et al: Poisoning prevention education during emergency department visits for childhood poisoning, *Pediatr Emerg Care* 20(5):281, 2004.

Hwang CF, Foot CL, Eddie G: The utility of the history and clinical signs of poisoning in childhood: a prospective study, *Ther Drug Monit* 25(6):728, 2003.

Jordan RA: Preventing CO poisoning: carbon monoxide, *Consumer Product Safety Review* 6(3):4, 2002.

Kelly NR, Huffman LC, Mendoza FS et al: Effects of a videotape to increase use of poison control centers by low-income and Spanish-speaking families: a randomized, controlled trial, *Pediatrics* 111(1):21-26, 2003.

Kim DY, Staley F, Curtis G: Relation between housing age, housing value and childhood blood levels in children in Jefferson County, Ky, *Am J Public Health* 92(5):769, 2002.

McLaughlin TJ, Humphries O Jr, Nguyen T et al: "Getting the lead out" in Hartford, Connecticut: a multifaceted lead-poisoning awareness campaign, *Environ Health Perspect* 112(1):1-5, 2004.

Ressel GW: AAP releases policy statement on poison treatment in the home, *Am Family Physician* 69(3):741, 2004.

Rudolph CD et al: *Rudolph's pediatrics*, ed 21, New York, 2003, McGraw-Hill.

Shepherd G, Larkin GL, Velez LI et al: Language preferences among callers to a regional Poison Center, *Vet Hum Toxicol* 46(2): 100-101, 2004.

Skarupski KA, Mrvos R, Krenzelok EP: A profile of calls to a poison information center regarding older adults, *J Aging Health* 16(2):228, 2004.

# Post-trauma syndrome

*Michele Walters*

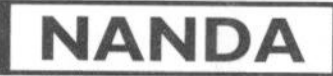


## Definition

Sustained maladaptive response to a traumatic, overwhelming event

### Defining Characteristics

Avoidance; repression; difficulty in concentrating; grief; intrusive thoughts; neurosensory irritability; palpitations; enuresis (in children); anger and/or rage; intrusive dreams; nightmares; aggression; hypervigilance; exaggerated startle response; hopelessness; altered mood state; shame; panic attack; alienation; denial; horror; substance abuse; depression; anxiety; guilt; fear; gastric irritability; detachment; psychogenic amnesia; irritability; numbing; compulsive behavior; flashbacks; headaches

### Related Factors (r/t)

Events outside range of usual human experience; physical and psychosocial abuse; tragic occurrence involving multiple deaths; epidemic; sudden destruction of one's home or community; confinement as prisoner of war or criminal victimization (torture); war; rape; natural and/or manmade disaster; serious accident; witnessing of mutilation, violent death, or other horror; serious threat or injury to self or loved ones; industrial or motor vehicle accident; military combat

**NOC**

## Outcomes (Nursing Outcomes Classification)

### Suggested NOC Outcomes

Abuse Cessation; Abuse Protection; Abuse Recovery: Emotional, Sexual; Coping; Impulse Self-Control; Self-Mutilation Restraint

#### Example NOC Outcome with Indicators

**Abuse Recovery: Emotional** as evidenced by the following indicator: Trauma-induced psychoneurotic behaviors, conduct disorders, and learning difficulties (Rate indicator of **Abuse Recovery: Emotional:** 1 = extensive, 2 = substantial, 3 = moderate, 4 = limited, 5 = none [see Section I].)

### Client Outcomes

**Client Will (Specify Time Frame):**

- Return to pretrauma level of functioning as quickly as possible
- Acknowledge traumatic event and begin to work with the trauma by talking about the experience and expressing feelings of fear, anger, anxiety, guilt, and helplessness

- Identify support systems and available resources and be able to connect with them
- Return to and strengthen coping mechanisms used in previous traumatic event
- Acknowledge event and perceive it without distortions
- Assimilate event and move forward to set and pursue life goals

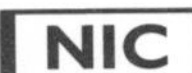

## Interventions (Nursing Interventions Classification)

### Suggested NIC Interventions

Counseling, Support System Enhancement

**Example NIC Activities—Counseling**

Encourage expression of feelings; assist client in identifying strengths and reinforcing these

## Nursing Interventions and Rationales

- Observe for a reaction to a traumatic event in all clients regardless of age. **EB:** *In a survey of 5877 persons, 1703 reported experiencing a traumatic event, and combat was reported as the worst trauma. Men who have faced combat are more likely to have lifetime post-traumatic stress disorder (PTSD), delayed onset of PTSD symptoms, and unresolved symptoms. They are also more likely to be unemployed, fired, and divorced, and to be physically abusive spouses (Prigerson, Maciejewski, & Rosenheck, 2001).*
- Provide a safe and therapeutic environment. *This will assist the client in regaining control (Townsend, 2003).*
- Remain with the client and provide support during periods of overwhelming emotions. *Presence of a trusted individual may calm fears for personal safety.* **EBN:** *The importance of trust was found to be a key element in a nurse-client relationship (Lowenberg, 2003).*
- Assist the individual to try to comprehend the trauma if possible. **EB:** *A stronger sense of coherence as the ability to perceive a stressor as comprehensible, manageable, and meaningful render the client somewhat resilient to symptoms of PTSD (Engelhan et al, 2003).*
- Use touch with the client's permission (e.g., a hand on the shoulder, holding a hand). **EBN:** *A meta-analysis of therapeutic touch indicated that therapeutic touch has a positive, medium effect on physiological and psychological variables (Peters, 1999).*
- Explore and enhance available support systems. **EB:** *Support systems decrease isolation and encourage communication, which may reduce negative affect and enhance the understanding and assimilation of the event (Engelhan et al, 2003).*
- Assist the client in regaining previous sleeping and eating habits. **EBN:** *Associated behavioral symptoms after a traumatic event may include substance abuse, eating disorders, high-risk sexual behavior, suicidality, and revictimization (Seng et al, 2004).*

▲ Provide the client with pain medication if they are experiencing physical pain. **EB:** *Pain may act as a proprioceptive trigger, stimulating post-tramatic reactions (Martz, 2004).*

▲ Consider the use of medication. **EB:** *Medications can be effective for treating PTSD. The* *largest trials showing efficacy have been with selective serotonin reuptake inhibitors (SSRIs) (Stein et al, 2000).*

- Help the client use positive cognitive restructuring to reestablish feelings of self-worth. **EB:** *In two studies of 159 and 138 motor vehicle accidents survivors, cognitive strategies to control intrusive negative thoughts played a major role in reducing post-traumatic stress in accident victims (Steil & Ehlers, 2000).* **EB:** *Results from one study showed that cognitive-behavioral interventions were more effective than other interventions for reducing occupational stress (van der Klink et al, 2001).*
- Provide the means for the client to express feelings through therapeutic drawing. **EBN:** *Expressive techniques such as therapeutic drawing can be used to facilitate the emotional work of coping with chronic trauma or life-threatening events and facilitate a better understanding of the experience to health care professionals (Locsin et al, 2003).*
- Encourage the client to return to the normal routine as quickly as possible. *Nurses can help traumatized children and adolescents relearn flexible responses in order to begin processing traumatic memories.*
- Talk to and assess the client's social support after a traumatic event. *The International Critical Incident Stress Foundation (2001) suggests telling children the facts that are appropriate to their age group. Listen to what they have to say. Provide reassurance of safety by touch and holding. Allow children to grieve and mourn and validate the normalcy of their reactions.* **EB:** *Higher social support is found to be associated with a significantly reduced risk of poor perceived mental health (Coker et al, 2002).*

## Geriatric

- Use environmental assessment skills to identify elderly clients who are traumatized by disaster, loss, or both. *The elderly who live alone are at greatest risk. Early intervention can minimize the response.*
- Observe the client for concurrent losses that may affect coping skills. *As the elderly grow older, losses are multiplied and compounded.*
- Allow the client more time to establish trust and express anger, guilt, and shame about the trauma. Review past coping skills and give the client positive reinforcement for successfully dealing with other life crises. *Clients who have adjusted positively to aging and can put events into proper perspective may adjust to loss more positively.*

▲ Monitor the client for clinical signs of depression and anxiety; refer to a physician for medication if appropriate. *Depression in the elderly is underestimated in this country.*

- Instill hope. *The energy generated by hope can help the elderly cope, overcome obstacles, and maintain normal functioning.*

## Multicultural

- Assess for the influence of cultural beliefs, norms, and values on the client's ability to cope with a traumatic experience. **EBN:** *What the client views as healthy coping may be based on cultural perceptions (Cochran, 1998; Doswell & Erlen, 1998; Leininger & McFarland, 2002).*
- Acknowledge racial/ethnic differences at the onset of care. **EBN:** *Acknowledgment of race/ethnicity issues will enhance communication, establish rapport, and promote posi-*

*tive treatment outcomes (D'Avanzo et al, 2001, Ludwick & Silva, 2000; Vontress & Epp, 1997). Black veterans' rate of service connection for PTSD was 43% compared with 56% for other respondents (P = 0.003) even after adjusting for differences in PTSD severity and functional status (Murdoch et al, 2003). Race has been identified as a factor in who receives treatment for trauma (Koenen, 2003).*

- Use a family-centered approach when working with Latino, Asian, African-American, and Native-American clients. **EBN:** *Latinos may perceive the family as a source of support, solver of problems, and source of pride. Asian Americans may regard the family as the primary decision maker and influence on individual family members (D'Avanzo et al, 2001). A school-based program using a family approach to treat traumatized immigrant children showed modest decline in trauma-related mental health problems (Kataoka et al, 2003).*
- When working with Asian-American clients, provide opportunities by which the family can save face. **EBN:** *Asian-American families may avoid situations and discussion of issues that they perceive will bring shame on the family unit (D'Avanzo et al, 2001).*
- Validate the client's feelings regarding the trauma. **EBN:** *Validation is a therapeutic communication technique that lets the client know that the nurse has heard and understood what was said, and it promotes the nurse-client relationship (Heineken, 1998).*
- Incorporate cultural traditions as appropriate. **EB:** *Activities such as tundra walks and time with elders were supported in treatment of trauma for the Yup'ik and Cup'ik Eskimo of Southwest Alaska (Mills, 2003).*

### Home Care

- ▲ Assess family support and the response to the client's coping mechanisms. Refer the family for medical social services or other counseling as necessary. *Persons who have not shared the client's traumatic experience may have unrealistic expectations about recovery and recovery time. Support may be denied if the client's response to the trauma does not stay within support system expectations.*
- • Provide a stable routine of day-to-day activities consistent with pretrauma experience. Do not force a new routine on the client. *Resuming a pretrauma routine can be reassuring to the client and can help place the trauma in perspective. Imposing an undesired routine can further isolate the client.*
- ▲ If the client is receiving medications, assess the client's self-medicating ability. Assign a responsible person to administer medications if necessary. *Crisis creates a feeling of helplessness. The client may be unable to make the simplest decisions (Spradley, 1990).*
- ▲ Assess the impact of the trauma on significant others (e.g., a father may have to take over his partner's parenting responsibility after she has been raped and injured). Provide empathy and caring to significant others. Refer for additional services as necessary. *Traumatic events can pose a crisis for both significant others and the involved client.*

## Client/Family Teaching

- Explain to the client and family what to expect the first few days after the traumatic event and in the future. *Knowing what to expect can minimize much of the anxiety that accompanies a traumatic response.*

- Teach positive coping skills and avoidance of negative coping skills. **EBN:** *Taking a direct action to resolve the problem itself is associated with higher levels of coping efficacy, while wishful thinking coping is associated with lower levels of coping efficacy (Tsay et al, 2001). Depressive coping is found to have a high correlation with PTSD (Schnyder et al, 2000).*
- Teach stress reduction methods such as deep breathing, visualization, meditation, and physical exercise. Encourage their use especially when intrusive thoughts or flashbacks occur. **EB:** *After a traumatic event, it is tempting for clients to maladaptively cope with their overwhelming emotions, which can establish unhealthy patterns for the future (Lang et al, 2003).*
- Encourage other healthy living habits of proper diet, adequate sleep, regular exercise, family activities, and spiritual pursuits. *A wide range of preventive, educational, and supportive interventions for trauma survivors are used. Despite this, there is a lack of research to prove their effectiveness (Schnurr & Green, 2004).*

▲ Refer the client to peer support groups. **EB:** *Peer support decreases the sense of social isolation and enhances knowledge, which may reduce the negative effects and enhance the understanding and assimilation of the event (Engelhan et al, 2003).*

- Instruct the family in ways to be helpful to and supportive of the traumatized person. Emphasize the importance of listening and being there. Also emphasize that there are no magic phrases capable of easing the person's emotional suffering.

▲ Consider the use of complementary and alternative therapies. **EB:** *Suggest the use of humanistic treatments (complementary and alternative medicine) for clients who have catastrophic illness or injuries (Halstead, 2001).*

## evolve WEBSITES FOR EDUCATION

See the EVOLVE website for World Wide Web resources for client education.

P

## REFERENCES


Cochran M: Tears have no color, *Am J Nurs* 98(6):53, 1998.

Coker A, Smith P, Thompson M et al: Social support protects against the negative effects of partner violence on mental health, *J Womens Health Gend Based Med* 11:465-476, 2002.

D'Avanzo CE et al: Developing culturally informed strategies for substance-related interventions. In Naegle MA, D'Avanzo CE, editors: *Addictions and substance abuse: strategies for advanced practice nursing,* St Louis, 2001, Mosby.

Doswell W, Erlen J: Multicultural issues and ethical concerns in the delivery of nursing care interventions, *Nurs Clin North Am* 33(2):353, 1998.

Engelhan I, van den Hout M, Vheyen J: The sense of coherende in early pregnancy and crisis support and posttraumatic stress after pregnancy loss: a prospective study, *Behav Med* 29:80-84, 2003.

Halstead LS: The John Stanley Coulter lecture: the power of compassion and caring in rehabilitation healing, *Arch Phys Med Rehabil* 82(2):149, 2001.

Heineken J: Patient silence is not necessarily client satisfaction: communication in home care nursing, *Home Healthc Nurse* 16(2): 115, 1998.

International Critical Incident Stress Foundation: Children's reactions and needs after disaster, 2001. Available at www.icisf.org/article.html, accessed January 5, 2005.

Irwin HJ: Proneness to dissociation and traumatic childhood events, *J Nerv Ment Dis* 182(8):456, 1994.

Kataoka SH, Stein BD, Jaycox LH et al: A school-based mental health program for traumatized Latino immigrant children, *J Am Acad Child Adolesc Psychiatry* 42(3):311-318, 2003.

Koenen KC, Goodwin R, Struening E et al: Posttraumatic stress disorder and treatment seeking in a national screening sample, *J Trauma Stress* 16(1):5-16, 2003.
Lang A, Rodgers C, Laffaye C et al: Sexual trauma, posttraumantic stress disorder, and health behavior, *Behav Med* 28:150-158, 2003.
Leininger MM, McFarland MR: *Transcultural nursing: concepts, theories, research and practices,* ed 3, New York, 2002, McGraw-Hill.
Locsin R, Barnard A, Matua A et al: Surviving ebola: understanding experience through artistic expression, *Int Nurs Rev* 50:156-166, 2003.
Lowenberg J: The nurse-client relationship in a stress management clinic, *Holist Nurs Pract* 17(2):99-109, 2003.
Ludwick R, Silva M: Nursing around the world: cultural values and ethical conflicts, *Online J Issues Nurs* August 14, 2000. Available at www.nursingworld.org/ojin/ethcol/ethics_4.htm, accessed June 19, 2003.
Martz E: Death anxiety as a predictor of posttraumatic stress levels among individuals with spinal cord injuries, *Death Stud* 28:1-17, 2004.
Mills PA: Incorporating Yup'ik and Cup'ik Eskimo traditions into behavioral health treatment, *J Psychoactive Drugs* 35(1):85-88, 2003.
Mollica RF, Lavelle J: Southeast Asian refugees. In Comas-Diaz L, Griffith EEH, editors: *Clinical guidelines in cross-cultural mental health,* New York, 1988, John Wiley and Sons.
Murdoch M, Hodges J, Cowper D et al: Racial disparities in VA service connection for posttraumatic stress disorder disability, *Med Care* 41(4):536-549, 2003.
Peters R: The effectiveness of therapeutic touch: a meta-analytic review, *Nurs Sci Q* 12(1):52, 1999.
Prigerson HG, Maciejewski PK, Rosenheck RA: Combat trauma: trauma with highest risk of delayed onset and unresolved post-traumatic stress disorder symptoms, unemployment, and abuse among men, *J Nerv Ment Dis* 189(2):99, 2001.
Seng J, Low L, Sparbel K et al: Abuse-related post-traumatic stress during the childbearing year, *J Adv Nurs* 46(6):604-613, 2004.
Schnurr PP, Green BL: Understanding relationships among trauma, post-traumatic stress disorder, and health outcomes, *Adv Mind Body Med* 20(1):18-29, 2004.
Schnyder U, Morgeli H, Nigg C et al: Early psychological reactions to life-threatening injuries, *Crit Care Med* 28(1):86, 2000.
Spradley B: *Community health nursing, concepts and practice,* ed 3, Glenview, Ill, 1990, Scott, Foresman/Little, Brown.
Steil R, Ehlers A: Dysfunctional meaning of posttraumatic intrusions in chronic PTSD, *Behav Res Ther* 38(6):537, 2000.
Townsend M: *Psychiatric mental health nursing: concepts of care,* ed 4, Philadelphia, 2003, FA Davis.
Tsay S-L, Tuls Halstead M, McCrone S et al: Predictors of coping efficacy, negative moods and post-traumatic stress syndrome following major trauma, *Int J Nurs Pract* 7:74, 2001.
van der Klink JJ, Blonk RW, Schene AH et al: The benefits of interventions for work-related stress, *Am J Public Health* 91(2):270, 2001.
Vontress CE, Epp LR: Historical hostility in the African American client: implications for counseling, *J Multicult Couns Devel* 25: 170, 1997.
Zungu-Dirwayi N, van Der Linden GJ et al: Pharmacotherapy for posttraumatic stress disorder, *Cochrane Database Syst Rev* (4): CD002795, 2000.



## Risk for Post-trauma syndrome

*Michele Walters*

**NANDA**

### Definition

At risk for sustained maladaptive response to a traumatic, overwhelming event

### Risk Factors

Exaggerated sense of responsibility; perception of event; survivor's role in the event; occupation (e.g., police, fire, rescue, corrections, emergency department, mental health worker); displacement from home; inadequate social support; nonsupportive environment; diminished ego strength; duration of event

NOC

## Outcomes (Nursing Outcomes Classification)

### Suggested NOC Outcomes

Abuse Cessation; Abuse Protection; Abuse Recovery: Emotional; Aggression Self-Control; Anxiety Self-Control; Coping; Grief Resolution; Sleep

**Example NOC Outcome with Indicators**

**Abuse Recovery: Emotional** as evidenced by the following indicator: Trauma-induced psychoneurotic behaviors, conduct disorders, and learning difficulties (Rate indicator of **Abuse Recovery: Emotional:** 1 = extensive, 2 = substantial, 3 = moderate, 4 = limited, 5 = none [see Section I].)

## Client Outcomes

**Client Will (Specify Time Frame):**

- Identify symptoms associated with post-traumatic stress disorder (PTSD) and seek help
- Identify the event in realistic, cognitive terms
- State that he or she is not to blame for the event

NIC

## Interventions (Nursing Interventions Classification)

### Suggested NIC Interventions

Counseling; Support System Enhancement

**Example NIC Activities—Counseling**

Encourage expression of feelings; assist client in identifying strengths and reinforcing these

## Nursing Interventions and Rationales

- Assess for PTSD in a client who has chronic illness, anxiety, or personality disorder; was a witness to serious injury or death; or experienced sexual molestation. **EB:** *PTSD has emerged as the most common anxiety disorder in women. There are also high rates of PTSD in chronically ill and psychiatric clients (Yen et al, 2002; McFarlane, 2000; Stein et al, 2000).*
- Consider the use of the Stanford Acute Stress Reaction Questionnaire to evaluate anxiety and dissociation symptoms after traumatic events. *This test was developed to assess dissociative and anxiety symptoms that research suggests trauma victims experience after the traumatic event (Cardena et al, 2000).*

- Assess for ongoing symptoms of dissociation, avoidant behavior, hypervigilance and re-experiencing. **EB:** *A study of acute stress disorder as a predictor of PTSD identified these symptoms as being 79% predictable of subsequent PTSD cases (Brink, 2004).*
- Assess for past experiences with traumatic events. **EB:** *As individuals become accustomed to traumatic situations, they can develop stress inoculation and acquire coping skills. This is supported by previous research suggesting that prolonged exposure results in habituation (Ronen et al, 2004).*
- Consider screening for PTSD in a client who is a high user of medical care. **EB:** *Traumatized clients who are at risk for PTSD are found to be high users of medical care (Stein et al, 2000).*
- Provide peer support to contact co-workers experiencing trauma to remind them that others in the organization are concerned about their welfare; provide an opportunity to discuss the traumatic incident and assess for the need for further post-trauma services. *The purpose of peer support in a post-trauma program is to ensure that each person involved in potentially traumatic incidents will receive the support and services necessary to make a successful recovery. Without the availability of peers, some individuals will certainly be overlooked. Peer supporters are not counselors. Their tasks include contacting co-workers to remind them that others in the organization are concerned about their welfare, providing the opportunity to discuss the incident, and assessing for the need for further post-trauma services (Post Trauma Resources, 2001).*
- Provide post-trauma debriefings. Effective post-trauma coping skills are taught, and each participant creates a plan for his or her recovery. During the debriefing, the facilitators assess participants to determine their needs for further services in the form of post-trauma counseling. For maximum effectiveness, the debriefing should occur within 2 to 5 days of the incident. *A debriefing is a specially designed group meeting that provides the opportunity to discuss the traumatic incident experiences and post-trauma consequences (Post Trauma Resources, 2001).*
- Provide post-trauma counseling. Counseling sessions are extensions of debriefings and include continued discussion of the traumatic event and post-trauma consequences, and the further development of coping skills. *Immediate post-trauma responses cannot be prevented. Long-term problems can develop if post-trauma consequences are not managed. With immediate and effective responses to duty-related trauma, most of these long-term problems can be prevented (Post Trauma Resources, 2001).*
- Instruct the client to use the following critical incident stress management techniques:



**Things to Try: Critical Incident Stress Debriefing (CISD)**

- Within the first 24 to 48 hours, engaging in periods of appropriate physical exercise alternated with relaxation will alleviate some of the physical reactions.
- Structure your time—keep busy.
- You're normal and are having normal reactions—don't label yourself as crazy.
- Talk to people—talk is the most healing medicine.
- Be aware of numbing the pain with overuse of drugs or alcohol; you don't need to complicate the stress with a substance abuse problem.
- Reach out—people do care.

- Maintain as normal a schedule as possible.
- Spend time with others.
- Help your co-workers as much as possible by sharing feelings and checking out how they are doing.
- Give yourself permission to feel rotten and share your feelings with others.
- Keep a journal—write your way through those sleepless hours.
- Do things that feel good to you.
- Realize that those around you are under stress.
- Don't make any big life changes.
- Do make as many daily decisions as possible to give you a feeling of control over your life (i.e., if someone asks you what you want to eat, answer them even if you're not sure).
- Get plenty of rest.
- Reoccurring thoughts, dreams, or flashbacks are normal—don't try to fight them; they'll decrease over time and become less painful.
- Eat well-balanced and regular meals (even if you don't feel like it).

*The CISD process is specifically designed to prevent or mitigate the development of PTSD among emergency services professions. CISD represents an integrated "system" of interventions that is designed to prevent and/or alleviate the adverse psychological reactions that are so often experienced by those engaged in emergency services, public safety, and disaster response functions. CISD interventions are especially directed toward the mitigation of post-traumatic stress reactions (International Critical Incident Stress Foundation, 2004).*

- • Assess for a history of life-threatening illness such as cancer and provide appropriate counseling. *People with histories of cancer can now be considered to be at risk for PTSD. The physical and psychological impact of having a life-threatening disease, of undergoing cancer treatment, and of living with recurring threats to physical integrity and autonomy constitute traumatic experiences for many cancer clients (National Cancer Institute, 2004).*

P

## Pediatric

- • Children with cancer should continue to be assessed for PTSD into adulthood. **EBN:** *In children surviving childhood cancer, PTSD symptoms may continue to emerge into young adulthood (Hobbie et al, 2000; Meeske et al, 2001).*
- • Provide protection for a child who has witnessed violence or who has had traumatic injuries. Help the child to acknowledge the event and to express grief over the event. **EB:** *Children who witness violent events that threaten the family's integrity are at highest risk for development of PTSD (Silva et al, 2000). One study supported the need for psychological evaluation and treatment for children who have had disfiguring traumatic injuries (Rusch et al, 2000).*
- • Consider implementation of a school-based program for children to decrease PTSD after catastrophic events. **EBN:** *The Catastrophic Stress Intervention was implemented following Hurricane Hugo to decrease mental stress by increasing the children's understanding of stress, enhancing their self-efficacy and social support, and thus decreasing the symptoms of PTSD (Hardin et al, 2002).*

## Multicultural

- Assess for the influence of cultural beliefs, norms, and values on the client's ability to cope with a traumatic experience. **EBN:** *What the client views as healthy coping may be based on cultural perceptions (Cochran, 1998; Doswell & Erlen, 1998; Leininger & McFarland, 2002).*
- Use a family-centered approach when working with Latino, Asian, African-American, and Native-American clients. **EBN:** *Latinos may perceive the family as a source of support, solver of problems, and source of pride. Asian Americans may regard the family as the primary decision maker and influence on individual family members (D'Avanzo et al, 2001). A school-based program using a family approach to treat traumatized immigrant children showed modest decline in trauma-related mental health problems (Kataoka et al, 2003).*
- Acknowledge racial/ethnic differences at the onset of care. **EBN:** *Acknowledgment of race/ethnicity issues will enhance communication, establish rapport, and promote positive treatment outcomes (D'Avanzo et al, 2001; Ludwick & Silva, 2000). African-American veterans' rate of service connection for PTSD was 43% compared with 56% for other respondents (P = 0.003) even after adjusting for differences in PTSD severity and functional status (Murdoch et al, 2003). Race has been identified as a factor in who receives treatment for trauma (Koenen, 2003).*
- Assure the client of confidentiality. **EBN:** *Many Indo-Chinese women will not discuss traumatic events like rape if they think that other staff members or their families, husbands, or community members may find out (Mollica & Lavelle, 1988).*
- Validate the client's feelings regarding the trauma and allow the client to tell the trauma story. **EBN:** *Validation is a therapeutic communication technique that lets the client know that the nurse has heard and understood what was said, and it promotes the nurse-client relationship (Heineken, 1998). Through the trauma story, the clinician can bridge the disrupted social connection that exists between the client, his or her family, and the community (Mollica & Lavelle, 1988).*
- Incorporate cultural traditions as appropriate. **EB:** *Activities such as tundra walks and time with elders were supported in treatment of trauma for the Yup'ik and Cup'ik Eskimo of Southwest Alaska (Mills, 2003).*

P

## Home Care

▲ Assess the client's ability to meet primary needs of shelter, nourishment, and safety. Refer to medical social services, state departments of human services, or other organizations as appropriate. *Clients in need of primary life requirements are unable to master a higher level of coping.*

- Identify other losses or stressors that may affect coping ability (e.g., role or relationship changes, deaths). *The presence of other stressors can compound the risk of post-trauma stress response and ineffective coping.*

▲ Assess the family's response to the client's risk. Refer the family to medical social services or mental health services or support groups as necessary. Provide nursing support. *Individuals in the client's support systems may not understand or be able to cope with the risk involved in selected occupations or the response to selected traumatic events in the cli-*

*ent's experience. This is a barrier to the provision of immediate and ongoing support to the client.*

- ▲ If the client is on medication, assess its effectiveness and the client's compliance with the regimen. Identify who administers the medication. *Clients with diminished ego strength may have difficulty adhering to a medication regimen.*
- • Assist the client in the home in identifying and establishing daily patterns that have meaning for the client. *Daily patterns provide the client and support system with structure, stability, and a point of reference for perspective development.*
- • For a client who is displaced from the home, identify internal values that can be maintained while the client is displaced, such as respite, contact with specific persons, and honesty. *Maintaining internal values reinforces ego strength, supports dignity, and promotes hope. NOTE: Hope should not be misconstrued to mean that a client displaced from the home can return home if this is not possible.*
- ▲ Encourage the client to verbalize feelings of risk and trauma to therapeutic staff or other supportive persons. Refer to medical social services or mental health/support group services as appropriate. *Expressing feelings validates client feelings, fears, and needs. Professional support systems may be a necessary substitute for inadequate personal support systems on a temporary basis.*
- ▲ Evaluate the client's response to a traumatic or critical event. If screening warrants, refer to a therapist for counseling/treatment. *Critical incident debriefing has become a controversial intervention. A review of psychological debriefing has concluded that little evidence exists to support its use. Early intervention recommendations are to assess the need for sustained treatment, provide psychological first aid, and provide education about trauma and information about treatment resources. Recommendations for secondary prevention of PTSD include education, anxiety management, cognitive restructuring, exposure, and relapse prevention (Litz et al, 2002).*
- • Refer to the care plan for **Post-trauma syndrome**.

P

## Client/Family Teaching

- • Instruct family and friends to use the following critical incident stress management techniques (International Critical Incident Stress Foundation, 2004):
  - ■ Listen carefully.
  - ■ Spend time with the traumatized person.
  - ■ Offer your assistance and a listening ear, even if the person has not asked for help.
  - ■ Help the person with everyday tasks like cleaning, cooking, caring for the family, and minding children.
  - ■ Give the person some private time.
  - ■ Don't take the individual's anger or other feelings personally.
  - ■ Don't tell the person that he or she is "lucky it wasn't worse"; such statements do not console traumatized people. Instead, tell the person that you are sorry such an event has occurred and you want to understand and assist him or her.
- • Teach the client and family to recognize symptoms of PTSD and to seek treatment when the client does the following (McDermott & Cvitanovich, 2000):
  - ■ Relives the traumatic event by thinking or dreaming about it often

- Is unsettled or distressed in other areas of his or her life such as in school, at work, or in personal relationships
- Avoids any situation that might cause him or her to relive the trauma
- Demonstrates a certain amount of generalized emotional numbness
- Shows a heightened sense of being on guard

- Instruct the parents to monitor a child who sustained minor injuries for symptoms of PTSD. **EB:** *The child's perception of threat and fear of death at the time of or immediately after the accident is significantly more related to development of the symptoms of PTSD than is the severity of the injuries sustained (McDermott & Cvitanovich, 2000).*
- Provide education to explain that acute stress disorder symptoms are normal reactions that are likely to resolve. Instruct to seek help if the symptoms persist. **EB:** *This will assist in identifying the client that is in need of a referral for treatment of post-traumatic stress disorder (Winston et al, 2002).*

## evolve WEBSITES FOR EDUCATION

See the EVOLVE website for World Wide Web resources for client education.

## REFERENCES

Brink E: Acute stress disorder as a predictor of post-traumatic stress disorder in physical assault victims, *J Interpers Violence* 19(6): 709-726, 2004.

Cardena E, Koopman C, Classen C et al: Psychometric properties of the Stanford Acute Stress Reaction Questionnaire (SASRQ): a valid and reliable measure of acute stress, *J Trauma Stress* 13(4):719, 2000.

Cochran M: Tears have no color, *Am J Nurs* 98(6):53, 1998.

D'Avanzo CE et al: Developing culturally informed strategies for substance-related interventions. In Naegle MA, D'Avanzo CE, editors: *Addictions and substance abuse: strategies for advanced practice nursing,* St Louis, 2001, Mosby.

Doswell W, Erlen J: Multicultural issues and ethical concerns in the delivery of nursing care interventions, *Nurs Clin North Am* 33(2):353, 1998.

Hardin SB, Weinrich S, Weinrich M et al: Effects of a long-term psychosocial nursing intervention on adolescents exposed to catastrophic stress, *Issues Ment Health Nurs* 23(6):537, 2002.

Heineken J: Patient silence is not necessarily client satisfaction: communication in home care nursing, *Home Healthc Nurse* 16(2): 115, 1998.

Hobbie WL, Stuber M, Meeske K et al: Symptoms of posttraumatic stress in young adult survivors of childhood cancer, *J Clin Oncol* 18(24):4060, 2000.

International Critical Incident Stress Foundation: Critical incident stress information, signs and symptoms. Available at www.icisf.org/CIS.html, accessed on December 18, 2004.

Kataoka SH, Stein BD, Jaycox LH et al: A school-based mental health program for traumatized Latino immigrant children, *J Am Acad Child Adolesc Psychiatry* 42(3):311-318, 2003.

Koenen KC, Goodwin R, Struening E et al: Posttraumatic stress disorder and treatment seeking in a national screening sample, *J Trauma Stress* 16(1):5-16, 2003.

Leininger MM, McFarland MR: *Transcultural nursing: concepts, theories, research and practices,* ed 3, New York, 2002, McGraw-Hill.

Litz BT, Gray MJ, Bryant RA et al: Early intervention for trauma: current status and future direction, *Clin Psychol Sci Pract* 9:112, 2002.

Ludwick R, Silva M: Nursing around the world: cultural values and ethical conflicts, *Online J Issues Nurs* August 14, 2000. Available at www.nursingworld.org/ojin/ethicol/ethics_4.htm, accessed on June 9, 2005.

McDermott BM, Cvitanovich A: Posttraumatic stress disorder and emotional problems in children following motor vehicle accidents: an extended case series, *Aust N Z J Psychiatry* 34:446, 2000.

McFarlane AC: Traumatic stress in the 21st century, *Aust N Z J Psychiatry* 34(6):919, 2000.

Meeske KA, Ruccione K, Globe DR et al: Posttraumatic stress, quality of life, and psychological distress in young adult survivors of childhood cancer, *Oncol Nurs Forum* 28(3):481, 2001.
Mills PA: Incorporating Yup'ik and Cup'ik Eskimo traditions into behavioral health treatment, *J Psychoactive Drugs* 35(1):85-88, 2003.
Mollica RF, Lavelle J: Southeast Asian refugees. In Comas-Diaz L, Griffith EEH, editors: *Clinical guidelines in cross-cultural mental health,* New York, 1988, John Wiley and Sons.
National Cancer Institute: Posttraumatic stress disorder. Available at www.cancer.gov/cancerinfo/pdq/supportivecare/post-traumatic-stress/HealthProfessional, accessed on November 22, 2004.
Post Trauma Resources: Tools for an unsafe world, 2001. Available at www.posttrauma.com/tools.htm, accessed on June 20, 2003.
Ronen T, Gahav G, Appel N: Adolescent stress responses to a single acute stress and to continuous external stress: terrorist attacks, *J Loss Trauma* 8:261-282, 2004.
Rusch MD, Grunert BK, Sanger JR et al: Psychological adjustment in children after traumatic disfiguring injuries: a 12 month follow-up, *Plast Reconstr Surg* 106(7):1451, 2000.
Silva RR, Alpert M, Munoz DM et al: Stress and vulnerability to posttraumatic stress disorder in children and adolescents, *Am J Psychiatry* 157(8):1229, 2000.
Stein MB, McQuaid JR, Pedrelli P et al: Posttraumatic stress disorder in the primary care medical setting, *Gen Hosp Psychiatry* 22(4):261, 2000.
Winston F, Kassam-Adams N, Vivarelli-O'Neill C et al: Acute stress disorder in children and their parents after pediatric traffic injury, *Pediatrics* 109(6):e90, 2002.
Yen S, Shea MT, Battle CL et al: Traumatic exposure and posttraumatic stress disorder in borderline, schizotypal, avoidant, and obsessive-compulsive personality disorders: findings from the collaborative longitudinal personality disorders study, *J Nerv Ment Dis* 190(8):510, 2002.

# Powerlessness

evolve

*Kathleen L. Patusky*

P

**NANDA**

## Definition

Perception that one's own actions will not significantly affect an outcome; perceived lack of control over current situation or immediate happening

## Defining Characteristics

### Low

Expressions of uncertainty about fluctuating energy levels; passivity

### Moderate

Nonparticipation in care or decision making when opportunities are provided; resentment, anger, and guilt; reluctance to express true feelings; passivity; dependence on others that may result in irritability; fearing alienation from caregivers; expressions of dissatisfaction and frustration because of inability to perform previous tasks/activities; expression of doubt regarding role performance; does not monitor progress; does not defend self-care practices when challenged; inability to seek information regarding care

### Severe

Verbal expressions of having no control over self-care, or influence over situation, or influence over outcome; apathy; depression regarding physical deterioration that occurs despite client's compliance with regimens

## Related Factors (r/t)

Health care environment; interpersonal interactions; lifestyle of helplessness; illness-related regimen

**NOC**

## Outcomes (Nursing Outcomes Classification)

### Suggested NOC Outcomes

Depression Self-Control; Health Beliefs; Health Beliefs: Perceived Ability to Perform, Perceived Control, Perceived Resources; Participation in Health Care Decisions

**Example NOC Outcome with Indicators**

**Health Beliefs: Perceived Control** as evidenced by the following indicators: Perceived responsibility for health decisions/Beliefs that own decisions and actions control health outcomes (Rate each indicator of **Health Beliefs: Perceived Control:** 1 = very weak belief, 2 = weak belief, 3 = moderately strong belief, 4 = strong belief, 5 = very strong belief [see Section I].)



## Client Outcomes

### Client Will (Specify Time Frame):

- State feelings of powerlessness and other feelings related to powerlessness (e.g., anger, sadness, hopelessness)
- Identify factors that are uncontrollable
- Participate in planning and implementing care; make decisions regarding care and treatment when possible
- Ask questions about care and treatment
- Verbalize hope for the future and sense of participation in planning and implementing care

**NIC**

## Interventions (Nursing Interventions Classification)

### Suggested NIC Interventions

Cognitive Restructuring, Complex Relationship Building, Mutual Goal Setting, Self-Esteem Enhancement, Self-Responsibility Facilitation

**Example NIC Activities—Self-Responsibility Facilitation**

Encourage independence but assist client when unable to perform; assist client to identify areas in which client could readily assume more responsibility

## Nursing Interventions and Rationales

NOTE: Before implementation of interventions in the face of client powerlessness, nurses should examine their own philosophies of care to ensure that control issues or lack of faith in client capabilities will not bias the ability to intervene sincerely and effectively. *Professional self-reflection has been identified as an important element in the maintenance of an empowerment philosophy. Such reflection helps the nurse come to terms with the cognitive dissonance of trying to empower clients within organizations that are inherently disempowering (Clark & Krupa, 2002). One perspective holds that power is not an individual attribute but rather a relational attribute, in that power relations exist between persons and are embedded in nested circles of power within levels of society (McCubbin, 2001). Thus the nurse must consider his or her power relations with clients, as well as the best means to negotiate the client's power relations within the social structure (e.g., healthcare system).*

- Observe for factors contributing to powerlessness (e.g., immobility, hospitalization, unfavorable prognosis, lack of support system, misinformation about situation, inflexible routine, chronic illness). *Correctly identifying the actual or perceived problem is essential to providing appropriate support measures.* **EBN:** *A phenomenological study identified the essence of ill health as powerlessness, involving the self image of worthlessness (fostered by an inability to meet societal norms), the sense of being imprisoned by circumstances (due to limited choices and abilities), and emotional suffering (with apathy and negative feelings threatening autonomy) (Strandmark, 2004). Complaints of powerlessness by people with chronic complaints such as fatigue or low back pain, are often dismissed (Dzurec et al, 2002; Lane, 2000). In a study of clients' perceptions of their health care, clients who expressed powerlessness at not being believed by staff (e.g., regarding their level of pain) (Nordgren & Fridlund, 2001).*
- Be alert to client behaviors that attempt to assert power, even if they seem confrontational. Assist clients to channel their behaviors in an effective manner. **EBN:** *Strategies women have used to regain control over uncertain illness trajectories included exiting (changing health care providers when dissatisfied), noncompliance (when medical advice did not seem to make sense), confrontation (especially when clients' perspectives were questioned or ignored), persuasion/insistence, making demands, and demonstrative distancing (refusing to participate in discussion) (Asbring & Narvanen, 2004).*
- Assess for **ineffective Therapeutic regimen management** or **Noncompliance. EBN:** *Ineffective adherence to the therapeutic regimen or noncompliance can be an assertion of the need for control (Gibson & Kenrick, 1998).*
- Assess the client's locus of control related to his or her health. **EBN:** *An external locus of control can lead a client to believe that he or she has no power over a situation (Gibson & Kenrick, 1998).*
- Assess for signs/symptoms of hopelessness depression and pay particular attention to the availability of social support. Hopelessness depression is characterized by a nega-



P

tive cognitive style (i.e., a tendency to perceive negative events as stable and global). *When negative life events occur, depression based on hopelessness can result, especially when social support is low or absent (Johnson et al, 2001; Joiner et al, 2001). In a study of individuals living at home who had experienced traumatic brain injury, low sense of belonging (valued fit) and chronic stress were strong predictors of depression. In this participant group, level of social support did not predict depression (Bay, Hagerty, Williams et al, 2002).* **EB:** *Lack of social support for men with HIV has been shown to increase hopelessness and thereby increase the risk for onset of depressive symptoms (Johnson et al, 2001).*

- Establish a therapeutic relationship with the client by spending one-on-one time with him or her, assigning the same caregiver, keeping commitments (e.g., saying, "I will be back to answer your questions in the next hour"), providing encouragement, and being empathetic. **EBN:** *In mothers undergoing the loss of a newborn, empowerment was experienced when the mothers felt a sense of nearness, encouragement, and empathy. Powerlessness was experienced when there was a sense of distance, violation, or disconnection (Lundqvist, Nilstun, & Dykes, 2002).*
- Allow the client to express hope, which may range from "I hope my coffee will be hot" to "I hope I will die with my significant other here." Listen to the client's priorities and incorporate those priorities in the therapeutic regimen wherever possible. *Hope is a way of coping with a stressful situation and motivates the client to continue living. Motivation is necessary in the change process. Listening to priorities without addressing them leads to frustration for the client.*
- Allow the client to share feelings. Evaluate the influence those feelings could have on the client's decision making and actions. Help the client focus on objective elements of his or her situation, rather than on the emotionally threatening aspects of the experience. *The experience of feeling overwhelmed by a medical situation can increase feelings of powerlessness.* **EBN:** *Sharing feelings often leads to the realization that similar feelings are experienced by others, and this realization can lead to a feeling of solidarity and reduce powerlessness (de Schepper, Francke, & Abu-Saad, 1997). Emotional responses to illness influence client behavior, coping efforts, and motivation for change; focusing on emotional rather than objective features of a threatening situation can increase negative emotional responses (Johnson, 1999).*
- Support clients' efforts to regain control of their lives by learning everything they can about their illnesses. **EBN:** *Women with chronic fatigue syndrome or fibromyalgia reported strategies to regain control, including acquiring knowledge about their illnesses (Asbring & Narvanen, 2004). Individuals on ventilators in a critical care unit identified seeking control over treatments, questioning and interpreting the environment as methods of reclaiming the world (Johnson, 2004).*
- Encourage the client to participate in self-regulation and self-care management of the client's illness. Have the client assist in planning care whenever possible (e.g., determining what time to bathe, taking pain medication before uncomfortable procedures, expressing food and fluid preferences). Document specifics in the care plan. *Self-regulation is a component of self-care management in which the client learns to monitor his or her own symptoms, make judgments about the meaning and seriousness of the symptoms, select strategies to manage the illness, try out the strategies, and evaluate whether they*

P

*were successful (Allen & Hagerty, 2003). Self-regulation and self-care management promote feelings of self-efficacy; confidence about managing chronic illness increases (Lorig et al, 2001). The more that clients participate in their own care, the less powerless they feel.* **EBN:** *In a study of clients' perceptions of their health care, clients expressed powerlessness because they were not part of decision-making (Nordgren & Fridlund, 2001).*

- Encourage the client to share his or her beliefs, thoughts, and expectations about his or her illness. *Self-regulation theory assumes that clients use perceptions, interpretations, and expectations about the illness experience to regulate their responses and behaviors (Johnson, 1999).*
- Make the time to learn the client's needs and be sure that nurse and client are operating with mutual understanding. **EBN:** *In a study of clients' perceptions of their health care, clients who expressed powerlessness believed that the staff's time constraints prevented them from being responsive to client needs (Nordgren & Fridlund, 2001).*
- Assist the client in specifying the health goals he or she would like to achieve, prioritizing those goals with regard to immediate concerns, and identifying actions that will achieve the goals. Offer feedback and education to ensure that goals and the expected time frame for meeting them are realistic. Goals may need to be small to be attainable (e.g., dangle legs at bedside for 2 days, then sit in chair 10 minutes for 2 days, then walk to window). *Self-regulation theory assumes that people develop a hierarchy of goals and that the discrepancy between what these goals are and what exists motivates action to reduce the discrepancy (Johnson, 1999). Goals must be realistic and achievable; otherwise, the inability to perceive progress will increase hopelessness and powerlessness.*
- Help the client identify factors not under his or her control. *Identifying factors within the client's control encourages the client to take some control of the situation. Acknowledging those factors not under the client's control provides the opportunity to address irritations and frustrations, while providing information crucial to insuring realistic goal setting.*
- Assist the client in identifying a repertoire of strategies to implement in managing his or her symptoms. **EBN:** *Clients who have multiple strategies to choose from in addressing situations have more success in managing symptoms than clients who use only one behavior (Taylor, 1999).*
- Encourage the client in goal-directed activities that promote a sense of accomplishment, especially regular exercise. *Goal direction enhances self-efficacy, an important antecedent of empowerment (Finfgeld, 2004; Fitzsimons & Fuller, 2002).* **EBN:** *In a study of menopausal women, it was found that regular exercise promoted a sense of self-fulfillment and an increasing sense of power (Jeng, Yang, Chang et al, 2004).*
- Discuss with the client areas in which he or she feels the need to protect himself or herself or others, and the strategies used. Support appropriate protective measures while assisting the client in identifying more effective and stress-reducing measures. *The ability to protect the self is an important part of retaining a sense of power or control over one's life.* **EBN:** *In a study of individuals living with a catastrophic illness or injury, participants felt the need to protect themselves from insensitive statements by others, including health care providers. A need to protect significant others was felt because of the additional physical and emotional burdens on caregivers. Protective strategies used included hiding the extent of the problem, concealing distress, trying to do things themselves, and trad-*

P

*ing what assistance they could provide to friends in exchange for physical care. The strategies were directed at maintaining social support but were themselves stressful (Dewar, 2001).*

- Recognize the client's need to experience a sense of reciprocity in dealing with others. Negotiate actions that the client can contribute to the caregiving partnership with both family and nurse (e.g., have the client prepare a cup of tea for the nurse during visits if the client is able). *A sense of control is promoted when the client feels he or she is able to exchange something of equitable value.* **EBN:** *Ill or injured individuals made attempts to exchange what skills they could for physical care in attempts to gain a feeling of equity (Dewar, 2001). For older adults, a lack of reciprocity (equitable exchange) was associated with depression, although older adults receiving home care services seemed to have adjusted to the lack of reciprocity (Patusky, 2000).*
- Help the client to identify and persist with self-care strategies that are effective; extinguish strategies that are ineffective. *Evaluation of strategies used is an important part of self-care management.*
- Allow time for questions (15 to 20 minutes each shift); have the client write down questions; encourage the client to record a summary of answers received if desired or practicable, or provide written material that reinforces answers. *Encouraging the client to write down questions and answers emphasizes the importance of client input and nurses' willingness to attend to that input; facilitates memory of questions and answers when the client may be distracted by health or other concerns; and provides the client with material that can be reviewed to refresh memory of the answers and offer reassurance in the absence of the nurse.* **EB:** *In a study of women during a hospital stay, 10% to 40% of the women reported the experiences of not being listened to, loss of privacy and dignity, and loss of day-to-day control—in short, powerlessness (Polimeni & Moore, 2002).* **EBN:** *Particularly for clients experiencing a first-time hospitalization, powerlessness was found to result from lack of staff support (in the form of not being listened to) and lack of information about their illness or medical treatment (Blockley, 2003).*
- Keep items the client uses and needs, such as a urinal, tissues, telephone, and television controls, within reach. *Well-being can be affected much more by choices related to activities of daily living (ADLs) like eating, sleeping, and grooming than by those related to larger, occasional events (Tolley, 1997). The client is able to participate in his or her own care if care devices are accessible. Participation in care provides a sense of control.*
- Give realistic and sincere praise for accomplishments. *Giving realistic praise assists the client in developing positive feelings and enhances self-concept (Meddaugh & Peterson, 1997).* **EBN:** *Sincerity promotes a sense of connectedness with the nurse. Clients with chronic obstructive pulmonary disease (COPD) reported that they value a sense of effectiveness and connectedness in their attempts to maintain personal integrity (Leidy & Haase, 1999).*
- Keep interactions with the client focused on the client, not on the family or physician. Actively listen to the client. *For a teen, this will support the developing ego. Directly focusing on the client also aids the client in practicing decision-making skills and increases the client's investment in adapting behavior (Hennessy-Harstad, 1999). It is important to convey the message that the client is unique and valued. Letting the client know that the schedule is tailored to meet his or her needs instead of tailored to the institution helps the client maintain a sense of self (Tolley, 1997). The client can expend a lot of energy holding*

*in unacceptable or frightening feelings. Listening to the client and encouraging these feelings to be expressed allows the energy to be released and used in other ways (Clark, 1993).*

- Acknowledge subjective concerns or fears. *All feelings are personal and have meaning for the client.*
- Encourage the client to take control of as many ADLs as possible; keep the client informed of all care that will be given. *Clients are more amenable to therapy if they know what to expect and can perform some tasks independently.* **EBN:** *Particularly for clients experiencing a first-time hospitalization, powerlessness was found to result from lack of information about their illness or medical treatment (Blockley, 2003).*
- Develop a contract with the client that states the client's and nurse's responsibilities and privileges. *Contracting can encourage the client to assume responsibility and increase motivation (Kubsch & Wichowski, 1997). A contract helps give a situation structure and clarifies what may or may not happen and who has responsibility for the client's care.*
- In evaluating outcomes implemented to address powerlessness, look to changes in the client, changes in relationships with others, and changes in behavior. **EBN:** *In response to interventions, clients achieve increased self-confidence and self-esteem; improved relationships with families and friends, as well as with health care providers; and the ability to make healthier choices for themselves (Falk-Rafael, 2001).*
- Refer to the care plans for **Hopelessness** and **Spiritual distress.**

## Geriatric

▲ Initiate focused assessment questioning and education regarding syndromes common in the elderly. **EBN:** *Older adults may not recognize the need for treatment when they misjudge symptoms and may initiate ineffective self-care treatment or seek no treatment at all (Edwardson & Dean, 1999).*

- Explore feelings of powerlessness—the feeling that the client's behavior will not affect outcomes. *Powerlessness can be exhibited as apathy, depression, expressions of no control, nonparticipation, indecisiveness, and passivity (Meddaugh & Peterson, 1997).* **EBN:** *Older adults who engaged in effective strategies to control their health problems experienced fewer depressive symptoms, particularly in the presence of acute physical symptoms (Wrosch, Schulz, & Heckhausen, 2002). Older adults who reported restricted activity due to arthritis and low levels of perceived control used more health services, had more physician visits, required more laboratory tests, and had longer hospital stays over a 1-year period than did study participants who expressed perceived high control (Chipperfield & Greenslade, 1999).*
- Explore personality resources and inner strengths that the client has used in the past. Incorporate these into the treatment plan. **EBN:** *While resources and strengths cultivated by older adults over the years often go unrecognized, they contribute to the older adult's sense of coherence (perception that life is meaningful, comprehensible, and manageable) and have been shown to optimize quality of life in older women with chronic health problems (Nesbitt & Heidrich, 2000).*
- Establish therapeutic relationships by listening; participate with the client in generating choices and incorporate his or her statement of limitations. **EBN:** *An individualized approach to health promotion, providing education that will support the individual client's needs, creates a partnership relationship that permits the nurse to enhance self-*

P

*care practices of the older adult and thereby promote self-care ability and activity (Leenerts, Teel, & Pendleton, 2002; Resnick, 2001).*

- Emphasize client control in all possible ADLs. *A study of older adults in nursing homes demonstrated that exposing older hospitalized adults to uncontrollable, disempowering circumstances could lead to the development of dependence based on learned helplessness. The dependence could be alleviated by fostering an expectation of control over activities, which lead to the development of a sense of mastery (Faulkner, 2001).*
- Encourage the positive use of solitude—reading, listening to music, enjoying nature—to prevent loneliness. Encourage socialization with others when possible; advocate for the client regarding family visitation if relationships are viewed positively by the client. **EBN:** *Loneliness, helplessness, and boredom can occur in older adults in nursing homes who lack companionship, have no opportunity to care for others, and find little variety in their lives (Slama & Bergman-Evans, 2000).*

▲ Monitor the use of alternative therapies but do not intervene unless the therapy interacts negatively with the existing therapeutic regimen. Ensure that all health care providers involved with the client are aware of the alternative therapies being used. *Older women in particular may use alternative therapies learned in their roles as mothers, midwives, and shamans. Familiarity with these alternatives to a patriarchal medical model can increase control over health and enhance prevention and self-care (Gaylord, 1999).*

## Multicultural

- Assess for the influence of cultural beliefs, norms, and values on the client's feelings of powerlessness. *The client's expressions of powerlessness may be based on cultural perceptions or expectations (Leininger, 1996).* **EBN:** *Older Chinese adults who had fallen reported powerlessness, fear, and care seeking. Powerlessness was expressed as lack of control, self-comforting, and lack of emotion. Falls were perceived as unpredictable and not preventable, which provoked fear that the older adult might become dependent and a care burden on others (Kong et al, 2002). Elderly Taiwanese men with heart trouble identified powerlessness as arising from lacking choice in living arrangements, having no control over discomfort, being unable to obtain care and companionship from families and friends, failing to get medical information about their disease and treatment options, or expecting deteriorating health and receiving no assistance (Shih et al, 2000).*
- Assess the effect of fatalism on the client's expression of powerlessness. *Fatalistic perspectives, which involve the belief that one cannot control one's own fate, may influence health behaviors in some African-American, Latino, and Native-American populations (Green et al, 2004; Harmon, Castro, & Coe, 1996; Phillips, Cohen, & Moses, 1999; Ramirez et al, 2002).*
- Encourage spirituality as a source of support to decrease powerlessness. *African Americans and Latinos may identify spirituality, religiousness, prayer, and church-based approaches as coping resources (Samuel-Hodge et al, 2000; Bourjolly, 1998; Mapp & Hudson, 1997).*
- Validate the client's feelings regarding the impact of health status on current lifestyle. **EBN:** *Validation lets the client know that the nurse has heard and understood what was said, and it promotes the nurse-client relationship (Heineken, 1998). In focus groups convened to determine the elements clients wanted to be addressed in diabetes education, power-*

P

*lessness was reported as a concern of African-American clients. Previous diabetes education programs had not addressed this element, but its inclusion in future programming was recommended (Blanchard et al, 1999).*

- For inner-city clients, help the client to redefine behaviors as ways of coping with a hostile environment and to reconnect with community supports. **EBN:** *Powerlessness among inner-city African Americans can arise in reaction to inner-city environments, poverty, and racism. Strategies that involve redefining behavior and reconnecting to the community promote empowerment (Dancy et al, 2001).*
- Use an empowerment approach when working with African-American women. **EB:** *Three strategies of empowerment for working with African-American women caregivers were identified as (1) raising critical group consciousness through storytelling; (2) teaching concrete problem-solving skills; and (3) teaching advocacy skills and mobilizing resources (Chadiha et al, 2004).*

## Home Care

▲ Include an initial and ongoing assessment and evaluation of potential abuse and neglect. Photograph evidence of abuse or neglect when possible. *A common dynamic of abusive situations is powerlessness. Victims of abuse perceive themselves to be powerless to change the situation. Indeed, the abuser fosters this perception and may threaten violence or death if the victim attempts to leave. Chronic abuse and neglect of the elderly by the spouse or other family member is often hidden until home care personnel are actively involved.*

▲ If neglect or abuse is suspected, identify an emergency plan that addresses the problem immediately, ensures client safety, and includes a report to the appropriate authorities. *Client safety is a nursing priority. An emergency plan should address either immediate removal to a safe environment or identification of appropriate steps to take in the event of abuse, and the securing of resources for anticipated action (e.g., telephone is accessible, bag is packed, alternative living arrangements are available). Reporting abuse is a legal requirement of health care workers.*

- Develop a therapeutic relationship in the home setting that respects the client's domain. **EBN:** *Effective home care involves negotiation between the nurse and the client within the context of territoriality, shared perception of situations, an amicable working relationship, role synchronization, knowledge, and taboo topics. The process empowers and makes vulnerable both nurse and client (Spiers, 2002).*
- Develop a written contract with the client that designates what care will be given and who has responsibility for care elements. Focus should be on care that is controlled by the client. Enable the client to develop his or her own resources actively. *A written contract reassures the client that the designation of control of care will be honored.*

▲ Empower the client by encouraging the client to guide specifics of care such as wound care procedures and dressing and grooming details. Confirm the client's knowledge and document in the chart that the client is able to guide procedures. Document in the home and in the chart the preferred approach to procedures. Orient the family and caregivers to the client's role. *Accurate documentation of the client's knowledge and abilities supports teamwork with the health care team and avoids conflict.* **EBN:** *Negotiation, reciprocity, shared decision making, creation of opportunities, and effective information and support are key elements of empowerment in the home. Empowerment is not a transfer of power* *from one person to another; it involves recognizing the power that each person has and assisting the client in identifying and using his or her own power (Houston and Cowley, 2002).*

- Identify the client's concerns and implement interventions to address the consequences of disability in clients with medical illness. **EB:** *In a study of cancer clients being cared for at home, primary factors influencing vulnerability to depression and suicide were identified as real or feared loss of autonomy and independence, concerns about being a burden on others, hopelessness about their condition, and fear of suffering (Filiberti et al, 2001).*
- Enhance self-efficacy by creating an environment that supports physical activities; provide support in the form of encouragement, anticipatory guidance, sharing of how others perform, and realistic assessment of the client's abilities. **EBN:** *Increasing self-efficacy in clients with heart failure can decrease symptomatology and improve quality of life (Borsody et al, 1999).*
- Respect the client's choices regarding desired assistance. Identify knowledge deficits and provide education to address them to ensure that the client's choice is accurately informed. **EBN:** *The client may identify a problem but choose not to receive help at this time. Assessment is an opportunity to discuss health needs, not a condition for treatment (Houston & Cowley, 2002).*
- Assess the affective climate within the family and family support system, including other caregivers. Instruct the family in appropriate expectations of the client and in the specifics of the client's illness. Encourage the family and client in efforts toward educating friends and co-workers regarding appropriate expectations for the client. Serve as the client's advocate. *Negative affective climate may interfere with the client's ability to adhere to the treatment plan, as well as with adjustment to health changes.* **EBN:** *Recognize that clients with an illness requiring extensive physical assistance may become caught in a dilemma: they may be dependent on others for assistance but that very dependence may hamper their ability to respond naturally within the relationship or to require that caregivers meet certain standards. Abuse is also a possibility (Curry, Hassouneh-Phillips, & Johnston-Silverberg, 2001).* Refer to care plan for **Risk for other-directed Violence.** *Clients experiencing a catastrophic illness or injury felt distressed by family members' or friends' comments that indicated a lack of understanding of the illness experience (Dewar, 2001).*
- Evaluate the powerlessness of caregivers, to ensure they continue their ability to care for the client. Provide assistance using interventions from this care plan. **EB:** *In a study of next of kin of cancer patients receiving palliative home care, powerlessness and helplessness was reported regarding patient's suffering, fading away, and next of kin's feeling of inadequacy. Multiple physical and psychological symptoms resulted in the next of kin, including loss of appetite, anxiety, and depression, along with anger, guilt, and loneliness (Milberg, Strang, & Jakobsson, 2004).*
- Be aware of and assist clients with potential needs for help in negotiating the health care system. **EB:** *Among individuals with disabilities, powerlessness may arise as a response to failures of the system to provide needed services (Helgoy, Ravneberg, & Solvang, 2003).*

▲ Refer for homemaker or psychiatric home health care services for respite, client reassurance, and implementation of a therapeutic regimen. *Responsibility for a person who perceives him- or herself to be powerless can promote high caregiver stress. Respite care decreases caregiver stress. The presence of caring individuals is reassuring to both the client and caregivers, especially during periods of client anxiety or depression. For a client with*

P

*powerlessness, especially if accompanied by depression, the interventions described earlier can be used, modified for the home setting.*

- ▲ Explain all relevant symptoms, procedures, treatments, and expected outcomes. *By increasing knowledge and adapting new behaviors, clients learn that they have some control over their health (Hennessy-Harstad, 1999). With knowledge comes power; the health care professional must ensure that clients have a sound knowledge base from which to make informed decisions (Meddaugh & Peterson, 1997). Clients are more amenable to therapy and better able to initiate appropriate self-care if they know what to expect.* **EBN:** *In a study of clients' perceptions of their healthcare, clients who expressed powerlessness described a lack of knowledge and information about treatment strategies (Nordgren & Fridlund, 2001).*
- ▲ Provide written instructions for treatments and procedures for which the client will be responsible. *A written record provides a concrete reference so that the client and family can clarify any verbal information that was given. People tend to forget half of what they hear within a few minutes, so it is important for nurses to supplement oral instructions with written material (Wong, 1992).*
- ▲ Continually assess the client for signs of inappropriate exercise of self-care. Confront such applications of self-care; instruct the client in the dangers that inappropriate care may present and in alternatives for care that would be more effective. *Although inappropriate self-care may represent an attempt to exercise personal power, clients who elect this action without sufficient knowledge of illness syndromes or treatment alternatives may deny themselves necessary and effective treatment.* **EBN:** *Clients often attempt to implement treatment on their own (e.g., through the use of previous prescribed medications, home remedies, or OTC medication) and may not be aware that they are misjudging a need for professional services or selecting less than optimal treatment options (Edwardson & Dean, 1999).*
- • Teach stress reduction, relaxation, and imagery. Many cassette tapes are available on relaxation and meditation. Assist the client with relaxation based on the client's preference indicated in the initial assessment. *These techniques can restore power in the client by allowing the client to learn how to control the autonomic nervous system and other physiological mechanisms (Johnson, Dahlen, & Roberts, 1997). Relaxation techniques, desensitization, and guided imagery can help clients to cope, increase their control, and allay anxiety (Narsavage, 1997).*
- • Teach cognitive-behavioral activities, such as active problem solving, reframing (reappraising the situation from a different perspective), or thought stopping (in response to a negative thought, picturing a large stop sign and replacing the image with a prearranged positive alternative). Teach the client to confront his or her own negative thought patterns (or cognitive distortions), such as catastrophizing (expecting the very worst), dichotomous thinking (perceiving events as belonging in only one of two opposite categories), or magnification (placing distorted emphasis on a single event). *Cognitive-behavioral activities address clients' assumptions, beliefs, and attitudes about their situations, fostering modification of these elements to be as realistic and optimistic as possible. Persons with negative cognitive styles tend to perceive situations as overwhelming, resistant to improvement, and all-encompassing. Through cognitive-behavioral interventions, clients become more aware of their cognitive choices in adopting and maintaining their belief*

P

*systems, thereby exercising greater control over their own reactions (Hagerty and Patusky, 2003; Sinclair et al, 1998).*

- Help the client practice assertive communication techniques. **EBN:** *Clients with conditions such as quadriplegia need to be assertive so that they can direct their care and be as independent as possible (Bach & McDaniel, 1993).*
- Role play (e.g., say, "Tell me what you are going to ask your doctor."). *Role playing is the most commonly used technique in assertiveness training. It deconditions the anxiety that arises from interpersonal encounters by allowing the client to practice how he or she might respond in a given situation. Anxiety levels tend to be higher in situations that are unfamiliar.*
- Identify the strengths of the caregiver and efforts to gain control of unpredictable situations. Help the caregiver to stay connected with a client who may be behaving differently than usual, to make life as routine as possible, to help the client set goals and sustain hope, and to allow the client space to experience progress. **EBN:** *Identifying positive caregiver responses to the client's illness will assist the caregiver in tolerating his or her own feelings of powerlessness. Family members of persons with severe mental illness have found it helpful to work at staying connected to the person with mental illness, finding a role that they can feel comfortable with, and helping the relative move forward (Rose, 1998).*

▲ Refer the client to support groups, pastoral care, or social services. *There is an assignment of power in the imparting of advice (Bonhote, Romano-Egan, & Cornwell, 1999). These services help decrease levels of stress, increase levels of self-esteem, and reassure clients that they are not alone.*

## evolve WEBSITES FOR EDUCATION

See the EVOLVE website for World Wide Web resources for client education.



## REFERENCES


Allen KS, Hagerty BM: Depression in primary care: empowering depressed patients to monitor their recurrent depression, in press, 2003.

Asbring P, Narvanen A: Patient power and control: a study of women with uncertain illness trajectories, *Qual Health Res* 14(2): 226, 2004.

Bach C, McDaniel R: Quality of life in quadriplegic adults: a focus group study, *Rehabil Nurs* 18:364, 1993.

Bay E, Hagerty BM, Williams RA et al: Chronic stress, sense of belonging, and depression among survivors of traumatic brain injury, *J Nurs Scholarship* 34(3):221, 2002.

Blanchard MA, Rose LE, Taylor J et al: Using a focus group to design a diabetes education program for an African American population, *Diabetes Educ* 25(6):917, 1999.

Blockley C: Experiences of first time hospitalisation for acute illness, *Nurs Prax N Z* 19(2):19, 2003.

Bonhote K, Romano-Egan J, Cornwell C: Altruism and creative expressions in a long-term older adult psychotherapy group, *Issues Ment Health Nurs* 20(6):603, 1999.

Borsody JM, Courtney M, Taylor K et al: Using self-efficacy to increase physical activity in patients with heart failure, *Home Healthcare Nurs* 17:113, 1999.

Bourjolly JN: Differences in religiousness among black and white women with breast cancer, *Soc Work Health Care* 28(1):21, 1998.

Chadiha LA, Adams P, Biegel DE et al: Empowering African American women informal caregivers: a literature synthesis and practice strategies, *Soc Work* 49(1):97-108, 2004.

Chipperfield JG, Greenslade L: Perceived control as a buffer in the use of health care services, *J Gerontol B Psychol Sci Soc Sci* 54B: 146, 1999.
Clark CC, Krupa T: Reflections on empowerment in community mental health: giving shape to an elusive idea, *Psychiatric Rehab J* 25(4):341, 2002.
Clark S: Challenges in critical care nursing: helping patients and families cope, *Crit Care Nurs* 13(4 Suppl):1, 1993.
Curry MA, Hassouneh-Phillips D, Johnston-Silverberg A: Abuse of women with disabilities: an ecological model and review, *Viol Against Women* 7(1):60, 2001.
Dancy BL, McCreary L, Daye M et al: Empowerment: a view of two low-income African-American communities, *J Natl Black Nurses Assoc* 12(2):49, 2001.
de Schepper AM, Francke AL, Abu-Saad HH: Feelings of powerlessness in relation to pain: ascribed causes and reported strategies, *Cancer Nurs* 20(6):422, 1997.
Dewar A: Protecting strategies used by sufferers of catastrophic illness and injuries, *J Clin Nurs* 19:600, 2001.
Dzurec LC, Hoover PM, Fields J: Acknowledging unexplained fatigue of tired women, *J Nurs Scholarsh* 34:41, 2002.
Edwardson SR, Dean, KJ: Appropriateness of self-care responses to symptoms among elders: identifying pathways of influence, *Res Nurs Health* 22:329, 1999.
Falk-Rafael AR: Empowerment as a process of evolving consciousness: a model of empowered caring, *Adv Nurs Sci* 24(1):1, 2001.
Faulkner M: The onset and alleviation of learned helplessness in older hospitalized people, *Aging Ment Health* 5:379, 2001.
Filiberti A, Ripamonti C, Totis A et al: Characteristics of terminal cancer patients who committed suicide during a home palliative care program, *J Pain Symptom Manage* 22:544, 2001.
Finfgeld DL: Empowerment of individuals with enduring mental health problems: results from concept analyses and qualitative investigations, *Adv Nurs Sci* 27(1):44, 2004.
Fitzsimons S, Fuller R: Empowerment and its implications for clinical practice in mental health: a review, *J Ment Health* 11(5): 481, 2002.
Gaylord S: Alternative therapies and empowerment of older women, *J Women Aging* 11(2-3):29, 1999.
Gibson JM, Kenrick M: Pain and powerlessness: the experience of living with peripheral vascular disease, *J Adv Nurs* 27(4):737, 1998.
Green BL, Lewis RK, Wang MQ et al: Powerlessness, destiny, and control: the influence on health behaviors of African Americans, *J Community Health* 29(1):15-27, 2004.
Hagerty B, Patusky K: Mood disorders: depression and mania. In Fortinash KM, Holoday-Worret PA, editors: *Psychiatric mental health nursing,* ed 3, St Louis, 2003, Mosby.
Harmon MP, Castro FG, Coe K: Acculturation and cervical cancer: knowledge, beliefs, and behaviors of Hispanic women, *Women Health* 24(3):37, 1996.
Heineken J: Patient silence is not necessarily client satisfaction: communication in home care nursing, *Home Healthc Nurse* 16(2): 115, 1998.
Helgoy I, Ravneberg B, Solvang P: Service provision for an independent life, *Disability Soc* 18(4):471, 2003.
Hennessy-Harstad EB: Empowering adolescents with asthma to take control through adaptation, *J Pediatr Health Care* 13:273, 1999.
Houston AM, Cowley S: An empowerment approach to needs assessment in health visiting practice, *J Clin Nurs* 11:640, 2002.
Jeng C, Yang S, Chang P: Menopausal women: perceiving continuous power through the experience of regular exercise, *J Clin Nurs* 13:447, 2004.
Johnson JE: Self-regulation theory and coping with physical illness, *Res Nurs Health* 22:435, 1999.
Johnson JG, Alloy LB, Panzarella C et al: Hopelessness as a mediator of the association between social support and depressive symptoms: findings of a study of men with HIV, *J Consult Clin Psychol* 69:1056, 2001.
Johnson LH, Dahlen R, Roberts SL: Supporting hope in congestive heart failure patients, *Dimens Crit Care Nurs* 16(2):65, 1997.
Johnson P: Reclaiming the everyday world: how long-term ventilated patients in critical care seek to gain aspects of power and control over their environment, *Intensive Crit Care Nurs* 20:190, 2004.
Joiner TE Jr, Steer RA, Abramson LY et al: Hopelessness depression as a distinct dimension of depressive symptoms among clinical and non-clinical samples, *Behav Res Ther* 39:523, 2001.
Kong KS, Lee Fk FK, Mackenzie AE et al: Psychosocial consequences of falling: the perspective of older Hong Kong Chinese who had experienced recent falls, *J Adv Nurs* 37:234, 2002.
Kubsch S, Wichowski HC: Restoring power through nursing intervention, *Nurs Diagn* 8(1):7, 1997.
Lane P: Adults with chronic low back pain feel frustrated, unsupported, and powerless with healthcare, social, and legal systems, *Evid Based Nurs* 3(1):29, 2000.

P

Leenerts MH, Teel CS, Pendleton MK: Building a model of self-care for health promotion in aging, *J Nurs Scholarsh* 34:355, 2002.
Leidy NK, Haase JE: Functional status from the patient's perspective: the challenge of preserving personal integrity, *Res Nurs Health* 22:67, 1999.
Leininger MM: *Transcultural nursing: theories, research and practices,* ed 2, Hilliard, Ohio, 1996, McGraw-Hill.
Lorig KR, Ritter P, Stewart AL et al: Chronic disease self-management program: 2-year health status and health care utilization outcomes, *Med Care* 39:1217, 2001.
Lundqvist A, Nilstun T, Dykes A: Both empowered and powerless: mothers' experiences of professional care when their newborn dies, *Birth* 29(3):192, 2002.
Mapp I, Hudson R: Stress and coping among African American and Hispanic parents of deaf children, *Am Ann Deaf* 142(1):48, 1997.
McCubbin M: Pathways to health, illness and well-being: from the perspective of power and control, *J Community Appl Soc Psychol* 11:75, 2001.
Meddaugh D, Peterson B: Removing powerlessness from the nursing home, *Nurs Homes* 46(8):32, 1997.
Milberg A, Strang P, Jakobsson M: Next of kin's experience of powerlessness and helplessness in palliative home care, *Support Care Cancer* 12:120, 2004.
Narsavage GL: Promoting function in clients with chronic lung disease by increasing their perception of control, *Holist Nurs Pract* 12(1):17, 1997.
Nesbitt BJ, Heidrich SM: Sense of coherence and illness appraisal in older women's quality of life, *Res Nurs Health* 23:25, 2000.
Nordgren S, Fridlund B: Patients' perceptions of self-determination as expressed in the context of care, *J Adv Nurs* 35(1):117, 2001.
Patusky KL: *Event-generated dependence and its psychological sequelae in older adults,* doctoral dissertation, Ann Arbor, Mich, 2000, University of Michigan.
Phillips JM, Cohen MZ, Moses G: Breast cancer screening and African American women: fear, fatalism, and silence, *Oncol Nurs Forum* 26(3):561, 1999.
Polimeni A, Moore S: Insights into women's experiences of hospital stays: perceived control, powerlessness and satisfaction, *Behav Change* 19(1):52, 2002.
Ramirez JR, Crano WD, Quist R et al: Effects of fatalism and family communication on HIV/AIDS awareness variations in American and Anglo parents and children, *AIDS Educ Prev* 14(1):29, 2002.
Resnick B: Motivating older adults to engage in self-care, *Pat Care Nurs Pract* 4:13, 2001.
Rose LE: Gaining control: family members relate to persons with severe mental illness, *Res Nurs Health* 21:363, 1998.

Samuel-Hodge CD, Headen SW, Skelly AH et al: Influences on day-to-day self-management of type 2 diabetes among African American women: spirituality, the multi-caregiver role, and other social context factors, *Diabetes Care* 23(7): 928, 2000.
Shih SN, Shih FJ, Chen CH et al: The forgotten faces: the lonely journey of powerlessness experienced by elderly single Chinese men with heart disease in Taiwan, *Geriatr Nurs* 21:254, 2000.
Sinclair VG, Wallston KA, Dwyer KA et al: Effects of a cognitive-behavioral intervention for women with rheumatoid arthritis, *Res Nurs Health* 21:315, 1998.
Slama CA, Bergman-Evans B: A troubling triangle: an exploration of loneliness, helplessness, and boredom of residents of a veterans home, *J Psychosoc Nurs Ment Health* Serv 38(12):36, 2000.
Spiers JA: The interpersonal contexts of negotiating care in home care nurse-patient interactions, *Qual Health Res* 12:1033, 2002.
Strandmark M: Ill heath is powerlessness: a phenomenological study about worthlessness, limitations and suffering, *Scand J Caring Sci* 18:135, 2004.
Taylor D: Effectiveness of professional peer group treatment: symptom management for women with PMS, *Res Nurs Health* 22: 496, 1999.
Tolley M: Power to the patient, *J Gerontol Nurs* 23(10):7, 1997.
Wong M: Self-care instructions: do patients understand educational materials? *Focus Crit Care* 19:47, 1992.
Wrosch C, Schulz R, Heckhausen J: Health stresses and depressive symptomatology in the elderly: the importance of health engagement control strategies, *Health Psychol* 21:340, 2002.

# Risk for Powerlessness

*Kathleen L. Patusky*

**NANDA**

## Definition

At risk for perceived lack of control over a situation and/or one's ability to significantly affect an outcome

## Related Factors (r/t)

### Physiological

Chronic or acute illness (e.g., hospitalization, intubation, ventilator use, suctioning); acute injury or progressive debilitating disease process (e.g., multiple sclerosis); aging (e.g., decreased physical strength, decreased mobility); dying

### Psychosocial

Lack of knowledge of illness or health care system; lifestyle of dependency with inadequate coping patterns; absence of integrality (e.g., essence of power); decreased self-esteem; low or unstable body image

**NOC**

## Outcomes (Nursing Outcomes Classification)

### Suggested NOC Outcomes

Depression Self-Control; Health Beliefs; Health Beliefs: Perceived Ability to Perform, Perceived Control, Perceived Resources; Participation in Health Care Decisions

**Example NOC Outcome with Indicators**

**Health Beliefs: Perceived Control** as evidenced by the following indicators: Perceived responsibility for health decisions/Belief that own decisions and actions control health outcomes (Rate each indicator of **Health Beliefs: Perceived Control:** 1 = very weak, 2 = weak, 3 = moderate, 4 = strong, 5 = very strong [see Section I].)

## Client Outcomes

### Client Will (Specify Time Frame):

- State feelings of powerlessness and other feelings related to powerlessness (e.g., anger, sadness, hopelessness)
- Identify factors that are uncontrollable



P

- Participate in planning and implementing care; make decisions regarding care and treatment when possible
- Ask questions about care and treatment
- Verbalize hope for the future and sense of participation in planning and implementing care

**NIC**

## Interventions (Nursing Interventions Classification)

### Suggested NIC Interventions

Cognitive Restructuring; Complex Relationship Building; Mutual Goal Setting; Self-Esteem Enhancement; Self-Responsibility Facilitation

**Example NIC Activities—Self-Responsibility Facilitation**

Encourage independence but assist client when unable to perform; assist client in identifying areas in which he or she could readily assume more responsibility

## Nursing Interventions and Rationales, Client/Family Teaching

See the care plan for **Powerlessness.**

# Ineffective Protection

*Gail B. Ladwig*

P

**NANDA**

## Definition

Decrease in ability to guard self from internal or external threats such as illness or injury

## Defining Characteristics

Maladaptive stress response, neurosensory alteration, impaired healing, deficient immunity, altered clotting, dyspnea, insomnia, weakness, restlessness, pressure ulcers, perspiring, itching, immobility, chilling, fatigue, disorientation, cough, anorexia

## Related Factors (r/t)

Abnormal blood profiles (e.g., leukopenia, thrombocytopenia, anemia, coagulation); extremes of age; inadequate nutrition; alcohol abuse; drug therapies (e.g., antineoplastic, corticosteroid, immune, anticoagulant, thrombolytic); treatments (e.g., surgery, radiation); diseases such as cancer and immune disorders

**NOC**

## Outcomes (Nursing Outcomes Classification)

### Suggested NOC Outcomes

Health Promoting Behavior, Blood Coagulation, Endurance, Immune Status

**Example NOC Outcome with Indicators**

**Immune Status** as evidenced by the following indicators: Recurrent infections not present/Tumors not present/Gastrointestinal function/Respiratory function/Weight loss/Body temperature/Absolute WBC count (Rate each indicator of **Immune Status:** 1 = severely compromised, 2 = substantially compromised, 3 = moderately compromised, 4 = mildly compromised, 5 = not compromised [see Section I].)

WBC, white blood cell

## Client Outcomes

### Client Will (Specify Time Frame):

- Remain free of infection
- Remain free of any evidence of new bleeding
- Explain precautions to take to prevent infection
- Explain precautions to take to prevent bleeding

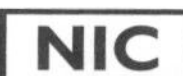

## Interventions (Nursing Interventions Classification)

### Suggested NIC Interventions

Bleeding Precautions, Infection Control, Infection Protection



**Example NIC Activities—Infection Control**

Monitor for systemic and localized signs and symptoms of infection; inspect skin and mucous membranes for redness, extreme warmth, or drainage

## Nursing Interventions and Rationales

- Take temperature, pulse, and blood pressure (e.g., every 1 to 4 hours). *Prospective surveillance study for nosocomial infection on hematology-oncology units should include fever of unknown origin as the single most common and clinically important entity (Engelhart et al, 2002). Changes in vital signs can indicate the onset of bleeding or infection.*
- ▲ Observe nutritional status (e.g., weight, serum protein and albumin levels, muscle mass, usual food intake). Work with the dietitian to improve nutritional status if needed. All clients diagnosed with HIV should have a dietary consult. *Early assessment of nutrition, good management of nutrition, and psychological support are essential for meeting the needs of the neutropenic client (Rust, Simpson, & Lister, 2000).* **EB:** *Nutrient status is an important factor contributing to immune competence: undernutrition impairs the*

*immune system (Calder & Kew, 2002).* **EBN:** *Nutrition complications of HIV infection, including wasting syndrome, nutrient deficiencies, and metabolic complications, have been well-documented over the last 25 years (Coyne-Meyers & Trombley, 2004).*
- Observe the client's sleep pattern; if altered, see Nursing Interventions and Rationales for **Disturbed Sleep patterns.**
- Determine the amount of stress in the client's life. If stress is uncontrollable, see Nursing Interventions and Rationales for **Ineffective Coping.** *Uncontrolled stress depresses immune system function (Carter, 1993).*

## Prevention of Infection

- ▲ Monitor for and report any signs of infection (e.g., fever, chills, flushed skin, drainage, edema, redness, abnormal laboratory values, and pain) and notify the physician promptly. *The immune system is stimulated with the onset of infection, which results in classic signs of infection. In the neutropenic client, antibiotics must be given promptly because a delay increases morbidity and mortality (Quadri & Brown, 2000).* **EBN:** *In many cases, changes in hematological parameters may be the initial sign of an occult infectious or inflammatory disorder (Szymanski, 2001).*
- Use appropriate "hand hygiene" (i.e., hand washing or use of alcohol-based hand rubs). *Improved adherence to hand hygiene has been shown to terminate outbreaks of infection in health care facilities, to reduce transmission of antimicrobial-resistant organisms (e.g., methicillin-resistant* Staphylococcus aureus*) and to reduce overall infection rates (U.S. Department of Health and Human Services, 2002).*
- When using an alcohol-based hand rub, apply product to palm of one hand and rub hands together, covering all surfaces of hands and fingers, until hands are dry. Note that the volume needed to reduce the number of bacteria on hands varies by product. **EB:** *Introducing the use of hand rubbing with an alcoholic solution resulted in significantly improved hand-cleansing compliance (Girou & Oppein, 2001). Alcohols exert the strongest and fastest activity against a wide spectrum of bacteria and fungi (but not bacterial spores), as well as enveloped viruses (but less so against nonenveloped viruses) and are little influenced by interfering substances. They are of low toxicity and offer acceptable skin tolerability when formulated with suitable emollients. The mode of their application is simple and they are three to four times more economical of time than wash procedures, features that help to increase compliance with the rules of hand hygiene (Rotter, 2001).*
- Consider warming the client before elective surgery. **EBN:** *In clients undergoing elective hernia repair, varicose vein surgery, or breast surgery, preoperative warming using a local device or a warm air blanket reduced the incidence of wound infection after surgery (Borbasi & Brougham, 2002).*
- ▲ If the client's immune system is depressed, notify the physician of elevated temperature, even in the absence of other symptoms of infection. *Clients with depressed immune function are unable to mount the usual immune responses to the onset of infection; fever may be the only sign of infection. A neutropenic client with fever represents an absolute medical emergency (Burney, 2000; Quadri & Brown, 2000).*
- If WBC count is severely decreased (i.e., absolute neutrophil count of <1000/$mm^3$), initiate the following precautions:
  - Take vital signs every 4 hours.



P

- ■ Complete a head-to-toe assessment twice daily, including inspection of oral mucosa, invasive sites, wounds, urine, and stool; monitor for onset of new complaints of pain.
- ■ Avoid any invasive procedures, including catheterization, injections, or rectal or vaginal procedures. *Infectious agents can invade when a treatment damages the skin or mucous membranes, which are natural barriers against infection (Flyge, 1993).*

▲ Administer granulocyte growth factor therapy as ordered. *Myeloid growth factors for granulocytes are more useful for preventing than for treating neutropenic infections in cancer clients (Glaspy, 2000). Clinical trials suggest that granulocyte-macrophage colony-stimulating factor (sargramostim [Leukine], Immunex Corporation, Seattle) has clinical benefits beyond enhancing neutrophil recovery, including shortening the duration of mucositis and diarrhea, stimulating dendritic cells, preventing infection, acting as an adjuvant vaccine agent, and facilitating antitumor activity (Buchsel et al, 2002).*

• Take meticulous care of all invasive sites; use chlorhexidine gluconate for cleansing. **EBN:** *Use of chlorhexidine gluconate for vascular catheter site care reduced catheter-related bloodstream infections and catheter colonization more than use of povidone iodine (Chaiyakunapruk et al, 2002).*

• Provide frequent oral care. *The effects of chemotherapy or radiation leave the mouth inflamed; combined with immunosuppression, this can result in stomatitis. Good oral care can help prevent this complication (Dose, 1995).*

▲ Refer for prophylactic medication to prevent oral candidiasis. **EB:** *There is strong evidence from randomized controlled trials that drugs absorbed or partially absorbed from the gastrointestinal (GI) tract prevent oral candidiasis in the client receiving treatment for cancer. There is also evidence that these drugs are significantly better at preventing oral candidiasis than drugs not absorbed from the GI tract (Worthington, Clarkson, & Eden, 2003).*

▲ Refer for appropriate prophylactic antifungal treatment and avoid pathogen exposure (through air filtration, regular hand hygiene, avoidance of plants and flowers). Practical measures can be taken to avoid exposing the client to fungi (Maertens, Vrebos, & Boogaerts, 2001). **EB:** *IV amphotericin B is the only antifungal agent for which there is evidence suggesting that its use might reduce mortality. It should therefore be preferred when prophylactic or empirical antifungal therapy is indicated in cancer clients with neutropenia (Gotzsche & Johansen, 2002).*

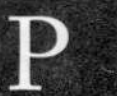


• Have the client wear a mask when leaving the room. **EB:** *To prevent nosocomial pulmonary aspergillosis during hospital construction, neutropenic clients with hematological malignancy were required to wear high-efficiency filtering masks when leaving their rooms. The rate of nosocomial aspergillosis decreased from 0.73 per 1000 hospital client-days during fiscal years 1993 to 1996 to 0.24 per 1000 hospital client-days during fiscal years 1996 to 1999 (Raad et al, 2002).*

• Limit and screen visitors to minimize exposure to contagion.

• Help the client bathe daily.

• Serve the client well-cooked food only; avoid all raw foods, including salads. Avoid serving processed meats, cheeses, yogurt, and beer or wine. Have the client drink sterile or boiled water only, and make ice cubes out of sterile water (Fenelon, 1998; Rust, Simpson, & Lister, 2000). *Data are lacking to confirm that consumption of neutropenic diets diminishes the rate of infection. Most centers use guidelines that recommend specific di-*

*etary restrictions during a period of immunosuppression (Rust, Simpson, & Lister, 2000; Smith and Besser, 2000).*

- Ensure that the client is well nourished. Provide food with protein and consider vitamin supplements. If appetite is suppressed, institute a dietary referral. Keep track of serum albumin levels, as well as transferrin and prealbumin levels. **EB:** *It is essential that the nurse ensure adequate nutrition for the neutropenic client. If the client cannot eat and the GI system is temporarily damaged, it may be necessary for the client to receive total parenteral nutrition. Levels of the visceral proteins (albumin, transferrin, and prealbumin) are an indirect measure of nutritional status (Rust, Simpson, & Lister, 2000). Nutrients that have been demonstrated (in either animal or human studies) to be required for the immune system to function efficiently include essential amino acids, the essential fatty acid linoleic acid, vitamin A, folic acid, vitamin $B_6$, vitamin $B_{12}$, vitamin C, vitamin E, zinc, copper, iron, and selenium. Practically all forms of immunity may be affected by deficiencies in one or more of these nutrients (Calder & Kew, 2002).* **EBN:** *For clients with HIV some experts recommend protein requirements of 1.0 to 1.4 g/kg for maintenance and 1.5 to 2.0 g/kg for anabolism. There is a general consensus that all individuals with HIV benefit from a daily multivitamin and mineral supplement at levels of 100% of the U.S. recommended daily intake (RDI). Nutrition therapy for HIV wasting is similar to that for other chronic diseases and begins with nutrition counseling. For persistent weight loss, standard oral supplements may be useful (Coyne-Meyers & Trombley, 2004).*
- Help the client to cough and practice deep breathing regularly. Maintain an appropriate activity level.
- Obtain a private room for the client. Take ordered precautions, including the use of a protective isolation or laminar airflow room, a Shinki bioclean room (SBCR), and/or high-energy particulate air (HEPA) filters if available and appropriate. Recognize that cotton cover gowns may not be effective in decreasing infection. *A private room is always necessary for neutropenic clients. There is no standardization of infection prevention practices nationwide for bone marrow transplant clients (Poe et al, 1994). A client with an absolute neutrophil count of less than 1000/mm$^3$ is severely neutropenic, has an impaired immune function, and is extremely prone to infection. Precautions should be taken to limit exposure to pathogens (Wujcik, 1993).* **EBN:** *A pilot study investigating the routine use of cotton cover gowns in the care of neutropenic clients found that the rates of infection were no different than when cover gowns were not used (Kenny & Lawson, 2000).* **EB:** *In a retrospective cohort study, the use of HEPA filters provided protection for highly immunocompromised clients with hematological malignancies and demonstrated effectiveness in controlling outbreaks of infection due to air contamination with* Aspergillus conidia *(Hahn et al, 2002).* **EBN:** *The SBCR is equal or superior to the laminar airflow room in preventing infection during neutropenia. Other advantages for the SBCR are a low level of noise (40 dB), easy control of temperature and humidity, and efficient removal of odor (Shinjo et al, 2002).* **EBN:** *Abandoning protective isolation combined with increased hygienic measures in nursing of patients with severe neutropenia does not increase the risk of infections, but improves the quality of care and patient satisfaction and reduces costs (Mank & van der Lelie, 2003).*

P

▲ Watch for signs of sepsis, including change in mental status, fever, shaking, chills, and hypotension. If present, notify the physician promptly. *Change in mental status, fever, shaking, chills, and hypotension are indicators of sepsis (Flyge, 1993).*

## Pediatric

▲ Suggest kangaroo care (KC), frequent and exclusive or nearly exclusive breastfeeding, and early discharge from hospital for low-birth-weight infants. **EBN:** *Although KC appears to reduce severe infant morbidity without any serious deleterious effect reported, there is still insufficient evidence to recommend its routine use in low-birth-weight infants. Well-designed, randomized, controlled trials of this intervention are needed (Conde-Agudelo, Diaz-Rossello, & Belizan, 2003).*

- For hand hygiene with low-birth-weight infants, use alcohol hand rub and gloves. **EBN:** *The introduction of the alcohol hand rub and glove protocol was associated with a 2.8-fold reduction in the incidence of late onset systemic infection, and also a significant decrease in the incidence of MRSA septicemia and NEC in very-low-birth-weight infants. This decrease in infection rate was maintained throughout the second 36-month period (Ng et al, 2004).*
- Avoid prophylactic application of topical ointment in preterm infants. **EBN:** *Prophylactic application of topical ointment increases the risk of coagulase negative staphylococcal infection and any nosocomial infection. A trend toward increased risk of any bacterial infection was noted in infants prophylactically treated. Topical ointment should not be used routinely in preterm infants (Conner, Soll, & Edwards, 2004).*

## Geriatric

- If not contraindicated, promote exercise to strengthen the immune system in the elderly. **EB:** *The results of a study of adults age 62 years and older suggest that lifestyle factors, including exercise, may influence immune response to influenza immunization. The practice of regular, vigorous exercise was associated with enhanced immune response following influenza vaccination in older adults (Kohut et al, 2002).*
- Give elderly clients with imbalanced nutrition a nutritional supplement to enhance immune function. **EB:** *Nineteen subjects age 65 years and older with a body mass index (BMI) of 25 or less received either a complete liquid nutritional supplement containing energy, vitamins, and minerals, including enhanced levels of antioxidants, or a noncaloric placebo drink for 7 months. The study indicated that consumption of this complete liquid nutritional supplement may have a beneficial effect on antibody response to influenza vaccination in the elderly population (Wouters-Wesseling et al, 2002).*
- Refer to the care plan for **Risk for Infection** for more interventions related to the prevention of infection.

## Prevention of Bleeding

- Monitor the client's risk for bleeding; evaluate results of clotting studies and platelet counts. *Laboratory studies give a good indication of the seriousness of the bleeding disorder.*
- Watch for hematuria, melena, hematemesis, hemoptysis, epistaxis, bleeding from mucosa, petechiae, and ecchymoses. *These types of bleeding can be detected in a bleeding disorder (Ellenberger, Hass, & Cundiff, 1993; Paschall, 1993).*

- ▲ Give medications orally or intravenously only; avoid giving them intramuscularly, subcutaneously, or rectally (Shuey, 1996). Apply pressure for a longer time than usual to invasive sites such as venipuncture or injection sites. *Additional pressure is needed to stop bleeding of invasive sites in clients with bleeding disorders.*
- • Take vital signs often; watch for changes associated with fluid volume loss. *Excessive bleeding causes decreased blood pressure and increased pulse and respiratory rates.*
- • Monitor menstrual flow, if relevant; have the client use pads instead of tampons. *Menstruation can be excessive in clients with bleeding disorders. Use of tampons can increase trauma to the vagina.*
- • Have the client use a moistened toothette or a very soft child's toothbrush instead of a toothbrush. Have the client use alcohol-free dental products and avoid flossing. *These actions help prevent trauma to the oral mucosa, which could result in bleeding (Shuey, 1996).*
- • Ask the client either not to shave or to use an electric razor only. *This helps prevent any unnecessary trauma that could result in bleeding (Shuey, 1996).*
- • To decrease risk of bleeding, avoid administering salicylates or nonsteroidal anti-inflammatory drugs (NSAIDs) if possible. *Salicylates and NSAIDs can cause GI bleeding; salicylates interfere with platelet function and can increase bleeding.*

### Home Care

- • Some of the interventions described previously may be adapted for home care use.
- • Consider institution of a nurse-administered mobile care unit for monitoring anticoagulant therapy. **EBN:** *Establishment of anticoagulation therapy management (ATM) clinics led to improvements in quality of care, in terms of improved control of international normalized ratio (INR) and reduced complications. From the year before to the year after implementation of an ATM program, the percentage of in-range INRs increased from 40.7% to 58.5%. The percentage in the modified target range also increased from 50.0% to 62.9% (Gill & Landis, 2002).*
- ▲ For terminally ill clients, teach and institute all of the aforementioned noninvasive precautions that will maintain quality of life. Discuss with the client, family, and physician the consequences of contracting infection. Determine which precautions do not maintain quality of life and should not be used (e.g., physical assessment twice daily, multiple vital sign assessments). *Multiple assessments and other invasive procedures are recovery-based, cure-focused activities. The client and physician must agree on an approach to care for the client's remaining life.*

## Client/Family Teaching

### Depressed Immune Function

- • Teach precautions to take to decrease the chance of infection (e.g., avoiding uncooked fruits or vegetables, using appropriate self-care, ensuring a safe environment).
- • Teach the client and family how to take a temperature. Encourage the family to take the client's temperature between 3 PM and 7 PM at least once daily. *For most people,*



P

*the difference between high and low values throughout the day is about 2.0° F (1.1° C) (97° to 99° F [36.1° to 37.2° C]) with the lowest value typically occurring in the early morning hours (2 AM to 5 AM) and the highest values commonly occurring in the evening 7 PM to 10 PM) (Round-the-Clock Systems, 2003).*

- ▲ Teach the client and family to notify the physician of elevated temperature, even in the absence of other symptoms of infection. *Clients with depressed immune function are unable to mount the usual immune response to the onset of infection; fever may be the only sign of infection present (Wujcik, 1993).*
- • Teach the client to avoid crowds and contact with persons who have infections. *Teach the need for good nutrition, avoidance of stress, and adequate rest to maintain immune system function. Client education to increase nutrition, manage stress, and perform self-care can reduce the risk of neutropenic infection (Carter, 1993).*

### Bleeding Disorder

- ▲ Teach the client to wear a medical alert bracelet and notify all health care personnel of the bleeding disorder. *Emergency identification schemes such as medical alert bracelets use emblems that alert health care professionals to potential problems and can ensure appropriate and prompt treatment (Morton et al, 2002).*
- • Teach the client and family the signs of bleeding, precautions to take to prevent bleeding, and action to take if bleeding begins. Caution the client to avoid taking OTC medications without the permission of the physician. *Medications containing salicylates can increase bleeding.*
- • Teach the client to wear loose-fitting clothes and avoid physical activity that might cause trauma.

## evolve WEBSITES FOR EDUCATION

See the EVOLVE website for World Wide Web resources for client education.

P

## REFERENCES


Borbasi S, Brougham L: Warming patients before clean surgery reduced the incidence of postoperative wound infection, *Evid Based Nurs* 5(2):48, 2002.

Buchsel PC, Forgey A, Grape FB et al: Granulocyte macrophage colony-stimulating factor: current practice and novel approaches, *Clin J Oncol Nurs* 6(4):198, 2002.

Burney KY: Tips for timely management of febrile neutropenia, *Oncol Nurs Forum* 27(4):617, 2000.

Calder PC, Kew S: The immune system: a target for functional foods? *Br J Nutr* 88(Suppl 2):S165, 2002.

Carter LW: Influences of nutrition and stress on people at risk for neutropenia: nursing implications, *Oncol Nurs Forum* 20(8):1241, 1993.

Chaiyakunapruk N, Veenstra DL, Lipsky BA et al: Chlorhexidine compared with povidone-iodine solution for vascular catheter-site care: a meta-analysis, *Ann Intern Med* 136(11):792, 2002.

Conde-Agudelo A, Diaz-Rossello JL, Belizan JM: Kangaroo mother care to reduce morbidity and mortality in low birthweight infants, *Cochrane Database Syst Rev* (2):CD002771, 2003.

Conner JM, Soll RF, Edwards WH: Topical ointment for preventing infection in preterm infants, *Cochrane Database Syst Rev* (1): CD001150, 2004.

Coyne-Meyers K, Trombley LE: A review of nutrition in human immunodeficiency virus infection in the era of highly active antiretroviral therapy, *Nutr Clin Pract* 19(4):340-355, 2004.

Dose AM: The symptom experience of mucositis, stomatitis, and xerostomia, *Semin Oncol Nurs* 11:248, 1995.

Ellenberger BJ, Hass L, Cundiff L: Thrombotic thrombocytopenia purpura: nursing during the acute phase, *Dimens Crit Care Nurs* 12:58, 1993.

Engelhart S, Glasmacher A, Exner M et al: Surveillance for nosocomial infections and fever of unknown origin among adult hematologyoncology patients, *Infect Control Hosp Epidemiol* 23(5):244, 2002.

Fenelon L: Strategies for prevention of infection in short-duration neutropenia, *Infect Control Hosp Epidemiol* 19(8):590, 1998.

Flyge HA: Meeting the challenge of neutropenia, *Nursing* 23(7):60, 1993.

Gill JM, Landis MK: Benefits of a mobile, point-of-care anticoagulation therapy management program, *Joint Comm J Qual Improv* 28(11):625, 2002.

Girou E, Oppein F: Handwashing compliance in a French university hospital: new perspective with the introduction of hand-rubbing with a waterless alcohol-based solution, *J Hosp Infect* 48(Suppl A):S55, 2001.

Glaspy JA: Hematologic supportive care of the critically ill cancer patient, *Semin Oncol* 27(3):375, 2000.

Gotzsche PC, Johansen HK: Routine versus selective antifungal administration for control of fungal infections in patients with cancer, *Cochrane Database Syst Rev,* CD000026, 2002.

Hahn T, Cummings KM, Michalek AM et al: Efficacy of high-efficiency particulate air filtration in preventing aspergillosis in immunocompromised patients with hematologic malignancies, *Infect Control Hosp Epidemiol* 23(9):525, 2002.

Kenny H, Lawson E: The efficacy of cotton cover gowns in reducing infection in nursing neutropenic patients: an evidence-based study, *Int J Nurs Pract* 6(3):135, 2000.

Kohut ML, Cooper MM, Nickolaus MS et al: Exercise and psychosocial factors modulate immunity to influenza vaccine in elderly individuals, *J Gerontol A Biol Sci Med Sci* 57(9):M557, 2002.

Maertens J, Vrebos M, Boogaerts M: Assessing risk factors for systemic fungal infections, *Eur J Cancer Care (Engl)* 10(1):56, 2001.

Morton L et al: Importance of emergency identification schemes, *Emerg Med J* 19(6):584, 2002.

Ng PC, Wong HL, Lyon DJ et al: Combined use of alcohol hand rub and gloves reduces the incidence of late onset infection in very low birthweight infants, *Arch Dis Child Fetal Neonatal Ed* 89(4):F336-340, 2004.

Paschall FE: Thrombotic thrombocytopenic purpura: the challenges of a complex disease process, *AACN Clin Issues* 4:655, 1993.

Poe SS, Larson E, McGuire D et al: A national survey of infection prevention practices on bone marrow transplant units, *Oncol Nurs Forum* 21(10):1687, 1994.

Quadri TL, Brown AE: Infectious complications in the critically ill patient with cancer, *Semin Oncol* 27(3):335, 2000.

Raad I, Hanna H, Osting C et al: Masking of neutropenic patients on transport from hospital rooms is associated with a decrease in nosocomial aspergillosis during construction, *Infect Control Hosp Epidemiol* 23(1):41, 2002.

Rotter ML: Arguments for alcoholic hand disinfection, *J Hosp Infect* 48(Suppl A):S4, 2001.

Round-the-Clock Systems: Circadian rhythms. Available at www.matrices.com/Workplace/Learning/sw.circadian.html, accessed on April 5, 2005.

Rust DM, Simpson JK, Lister J: Nutritional issues in patients with severe neutropenia, *Semin Oncol Nurs* 16(2):152, 2000.

Shinjo K, Takeshita A, Yanagi M et al: Efficacy of the Shinki bioclean room for preventing infection in neutropenic patients, *J Adv Nurs* 37(3):227, 2002.

Shuey KM: Platelet-associated bleeding disorders, *Semin Oncol Nurs* 12(1):15, 1996.

Smith LH, Besser SG: Dietary restrictions for patients with neutropenia: a survey of institutional practices, *Oncol Nurs Forum* 27(3):515, 2000.

Szymanski N: Infection and inflammation in dialysis patients: impact on laboratory parameters and anemia. Case study of the anemic patient, *Nephrol Nurse J* 28(3):337, 2001.

U.S. Department of Health and Human Services, Centers for Disease Control and Prevention: Hand hygiene guidelines fact sheet, 2002. Available at www.cdc.gov/od/oc/media/pressrel/fs021025.htm, accessed on April 5, 2005.

Worthington HV, Clarkson JE, Eden OB: Interventions for preventing oral candidiasis for patients with cancer receiving treatment, *Cochrane Database Syst Rev,* CD003807, 2003.

Wouters-Wesseling W, Rozendaal M, Snijder M et al: Effect of a complete nutritional supplement on antibody response to influenza vaccine in elderly people, *J Gerontol A Biol Sci Med Sci* 57(9):M563, 2002.

Wujcik D: Infection control in oncology patients, *Nurs Clin North Am* 28:639, 1993.

P

# Rape-trauma syndrome

*Linda Hutson*

## NANDA

### Definition

Sustained maladaptive response to forced, violent sexual act (penetration may not actually occur) (Ohio Revised Code) against victim's will and consent

### Defining Characteristics

Fear; disorganization; change in relationships; confusion; physical trauma (e.g., bruising, tissue irritation, injuries identified by use of new technology); suicide attempt(s); denial; guilt; paranoia; humiliation; embarrassment; aggression; muscle tension and/or spasms; mood swings; dependence; powerlessness; nightmares and sleep disturbances; sexual dysfunction; desire for revenge; phobias; loss of self-esteem; inability to make decisions; dissociative disorders; self-blame; hyperalertness; vulnerability; substance abuse; depression; helplessness; anger; anxiety; agitation; shame; shock

### Related Factors (r/t)

Rape, sexual assault, abuse

## NOC

### Outcomes (Nursing Outcomes Classification)

#### Suggested NOC Outcomes

Abuse Cessation; Abuse Protection; Abuse Recovery: Emotional, Sexual; Coping; Impulse Self-Control; Self-Mutilation Restraint

**Example NOC Outcome with Indicators**

**Abuse Recovery: Sexual** as evidenced by the following indicators: Acknowledgment of right to disclose abusive situation/Expression of right to have been protected from abuse (Rate each indicator of **Abuse Recovery: Sexual:** 1 = none, 2 = limited, 3 = moderate, 4 = substantial, 5 = extensive [see Section I].)

R

### Client Outcomes

**Client Will (Specify Time Frame):**

- Share feelings, concerns, and fears
- Recognize that the rape or attempt was not client's own fault
- State that, no matter what the situation, no one has the right to assault another
- Describe medical/legal treatment procedures and reasons for treatment
- Report absence of physical complications or pain

- Identify support people and be able to ask them for help in dealing with this trauma
- Function at same level as before crisis, including sexual functioning
- Recognize that it is normal for full recovery to take a minimum of 1 year

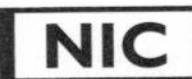

## Interventions (Nursing Interventions Classification)

### Suggested NIC Interventions

Counseling, Rape-Trauma Treatment

**Example NIC Activities—Counseling**

Explain rape protocol and obtain consent to proceed through protocol; encourage expression of feelings

## Nursing Interventions and Rationales

- • Observe the client's responses, including anger, fear, self-blame, sleep pattern disturbances, and phobias.
- • Monitor the client's verbal and nonverbal psychological state (e.g., crying, hand wringing, avoidance of interactions or eye contact with staff, silence and denial). **EB:** *The most depressed victims are those most concerned with being stigmatized and blamed for the crime (Frable, Blackstone, & Sherbaum, 1990).*
- ▲ Stay with (or have a trusted person stay with) the client initially. If a law enforcement interview is permitted, provide support by staying with the client, but only at the client's request. **EBN:** *Allow the client to make the decision about whom the client wishes to have present during any interviews or examinations to allow a return of control to the client (Ledray, 1998a).*
- • Explain the entire medical/legal examination to the client before beginning any procedures. **EBN:** *Explain to the client that the injuries or symptoms may require hospitalization and that the care provider in the hospital will be aware of their special needs. (Sommers, 2004). Obtain written permission to perform the examination but explain to the client that at any time during the examination the client may withdraw consent. Discuss with the client the importance of participating in the entire examination and the importance of the collection of evidence. The examination will include several procedures that might be uncomfortable or painful and the client should know this in advance. Before moving on to each procedure, repeat the explanation and offer the client the right to skip any part of the examination in which the client feels unable to fully participate. Discuss the importance of performing a speculum examination rather than a pelvic examination. If it is the client's first examination, explain the instruments and let the client know when and where you will touch. Encourage the presence of either an advocate or a person the client trusts during any physical examination. Do this with the client's permission. Most often the examiner is busy collecting evidence and photographs and cannot offer the emotional support the client may need during this portion of the examination.* **EBN:** *This returns control to the client. Explain that a speculum examination will be performed for the purpose of identifying any injury and collecting evidence (Hutson, 2002).*

- • Do not wait for the client to ask questions; explain everything you are doing, clarify why it must be done, and describe when and where you will touch. *Eye contact is very important because it helps the client feel worthy and alive (Ruckman, 1992).*
- ▲ Observe for signs of physical injury as you are asking the client to undress and collecting the client's clothing for evidence. Ask the client where it hurts without asking leading questions. Do not ask specific questions but allow the client to give you a history of the sexual assault in the client's own words. If the examiner needs further clarification, ask the client to point to areas that were injured or touched. Inform the client that photographs of any injuries are necessary for forensic evidence. Obtain specific written permission for photographs to be taken and released to law enforcement personnel. **EBN:** *The aforementioned nonleading questions are recommended. Do not ask questions that could indicate to the defense attorney and the jury that the examiner was leading the client and may have influenced the client's report of the assault (Ledray, 1998b).*
- ▲ Instruct the client to return for additional photographs either to the medical facility or to law enforcement personnel if bruises become more pronounced in a few days. It is recommended that all medical treatment be completed at the initial encounter due to the difficulty in getting clients to return for follow-up medical care. **EBN:** *Clients are reluctant to return for any medical evaluation and have a poor history of doing so (Dandino-Abbott, 1999). Sore areas can be visible using the new technology employed in these examinations (Sommers et al, 2001).*
- • Documentation of a sexual assault examination is critical to evidentiary reports. It is important to document the client's exact description of the assault and then to collect evidence and photographs that validate the history the client reports. **EBN:** *It is very important that the examiner not offer any subjective information on the documentation (Ledray, 1998a).*
- • It is also very important for the examiner not to offer any opinions in the documentation about whether or not the assault occurred according to the physical findings. **EBN:** *These opinions should be offered to the legal system only when they are requested for prosecution (Ledray, 1998b).*
- ▲ Document a one- or two-sentence summary of what happened. The chief complaint of the client reporting sexual assault should always be listed as "reported sexual assault"; obtaining the details of the sequence of events is the police officer's job. **EBN:** *The chief complaint of the client reporting sexual assault should always be listed as* reported sexual assault. *Other terms, such as* alleged sexual assault, rape, *or* sexual assault, *imply an opinion by the person taking the history (Hutson, 2002). It is important to remember that sexual assault clients are often very traumatized in the acute phase of the assault and may give several different histories of the event. They may remember certain aspects of the assault at different times. If the details given during the medical/legal examination differ from the details given to law enforcement personnel, the law enforcement agency will obtain the information needed to support or contradict the client's history of events (Ledray, 1998a). If some details that are not in the nurse's notes were told to the police, the defense attorney may attempt to make this look like a discrepancy in facts, which can cause reasonable doubt and result in an acquittal (Ledray, 1992).*
- • Encourage the client to verbalize feelings. *Listening to clients helps them gain self-control by feeling acceptance from others (Ruckman, 1992).*

R

- Escort the client to the treatment room immediately to remove the client from the general population; do not question the client in the triage area, close curtains and door, and avoid other interruptions during contact with the client (e.g., telephone calls, absence from the room, outside stimuli such as radios). **EB and EBN:** *It is preferable that the client have a dedicated caregiver such as a sexual assault nurse examiner (SANE) specially trained in sexual assault medical/forensic examinations so that interruptions can be avoided. This not only serves the client but allows for the accurate collection and preservation of evidence (Ledray, 1999; McGregor, DuMont, & Myhr, 2002).*
- ▲ Provide a sexual assault response team that includes a SANE, rape counseling advocate, and representative of law enforcement. **EBN:** *This team maximizes care to the client. In many cases, the advocate will be the person to assist the client through the legal system up to and including accompaniment to the courtroom. The quality of care the client receives from "first responders" may determine the client's willingness to continue with long-term treatment (Ledray, 1998a). Evidence-based practice indicates that this model brings quality care to women (Selig, 2000). Comparing a baseline group of 130 sexual assault victims with 39 clients who were evaluated after the SANE approach was implemented indicated that the SANE approach increased clinical interaction and completeness of evaluation and information gathered (Derhammer et al, 2000).* **EB:** *A multidisciplinary approach addresses both the needs of the survivor and the availability of resources to meet those needs.(Ratner, 2003).*
- ▲ The rape crisis center advocate should be part of the sexual assault response team (SART) and respond when the SANE responds. *This person can encourage follow-up at the rape crisis center. The advocate can talk with the client during the acute phase; the client does not need to make an immediate decision about whether the client would like the advocate called for follow-up. Because advocates are better trained and prepared to talk to clients of acute sexual assault, they are usually more successful in encouraging further follow-up than the medical/nursing staff.* **EB:** *Clients want control but may have difficulty making decisions during the initial visit to the emergency department. Involvement of social service agencies will help to guarantee a timely follow-up home visit (Jones, 1994).*
- Provide items for self-care after examination (e.g., for cleansing the vaginal and rectal area). **EBN:** *Many facilities that provide care for sexual assault clients have "survivor packs" available for post-treatment care. These include items for personal hygiene (i.e., shampoo, soap, toothbrush, toothpaste, new underwear and outer clothing to replace those secured for evidential purposes, and so on) (Hutson, 2002).*
- ▲ Most states provide sexual assault evidence collection kits that have been reviewed by the SART members to provide adequate evidence for analysis by the forensic laboratory. Explain to the client that all or some of the client's clothing may be kept for evidential purposes. Also explain that the client will receive replacement clothing or that the client can request that a friend or family member bring clothing from home to replace the clothing kept for evidence. Explain to the client that, if the clothing worn during the assault is still at the scene, the client should disclose this information to law enforcement officials so that law enforcement personnel can go to the scene and collect the evidence appropriately. **EBN:** *If the client arrives at the medical facility with the evidentiary clothing already in a bag, explain to the client that you will notify law enforcement personnel to pick it up directly from the client (Hutson, 2002). No clothing or evi-*

R

*dence should be placed in a plastic bag because of the potential for deterioration or destruction. SANEs are specifically trained in the appropriate procedure.*

- • An alternative light source will be used for direct inspection of the body for the presence of body fluids. *This is part of the examination and should be explained by the SANE (Ledray, 1999; O'Brien, 1998).*
- ▲ Discuss the possibility of pregnancy and sexually transmitted diseases (STDs) and the treatments available. *Administering a urine pregnancy test is routine before giving medications to prevent pregnancy or treat STDs. Most clients prefer to prevent pregnancy rather than face the possibility of terminating it in the future. The risk of human immunodeficiency virus (HIV) exposure is a special concern to rape victims; the nurse should bring up this issue and inform the client of locations and schedules for HIV testing.*
- ▲ Encourage the client to report the rape to a law enforcement agency. **EBN:** *It is important for rape victims to recognize that they are victims of a crime that is not their fault (Ledray, 1992). Reporting is an issue separate from prosecution; if victims report, they will not be forced to appear as a witness.*
- • Discuss the client's support system. Involve the support system if appropriate and if the client grants permission. *Unsupportive and victim-blaming attitudes by significant others are common responses.* **EB:** *Research indicates that significant others are coping with their own responses to the trauma and may be incapable of supporting the victim (Mackey et al, 1992).*
- ▲ Obtaining blood alcohol levels or levels of any drug should be discussed thoroughly with the medical director of your facility and the SART members. *Often alcohol or drug levels are used to prove that the client was unable to give consent for sexual contact. However, often levels are used by defense attorneys to destroy the client's credibility (Hutson, 2002).*

## Geriatric

- • Build a trusting relationship with the client. **EBN:** *Recognize the attitudes and values of an older generation; stigmatization may cause victims to view themselves with disgust and shame (Delorey & Wolf, 1993).*
- ▲ Explain reporting and encourage the client to report. **EB and EBN:** *Embarrassment may prevent reporting; respect the client's choice. Older rape victims have reported having a greater fear that people will find out about their rape than do younger women (Tyra, 1993). Timely reporting within 72 hours is necessary to document injuries and collect evidence that would be valuable in prosecution (Crowley, 1999; Adams, Girardin, & Faugno, 2000).* **EB:** *Timely reporting, although important, should not determine whether a client receives appropriate medical care. Clients requesting medical treatment, prophylactic antibiotics, and contraception are similar whether they report the incident to the police or not (Schei, et al, 2003).*
- • Observe for psychosocial distress (e.g., memory impairment, sleep disturbances, regression, changes in bodily functions). *Exacerbation of a chronic illness may be a major consequence of sexual assault.*
- ▲ All examinations should be done on the elderly as they would be done on any adult client after sexual assault. Evidence should be collected and consent for collection, photography, and law enforcement contact should be obtained as in all cases. Special

R

attention should be given to the explanation of the genital examination, especially as it relates to the use of a speculum. **EBN:** *Many elderly clients will not allow the use of a speculum. If this is the case the SANE should collect specimens by using only the collection swabs. The external genitalia should be thoroughly examined and photographs should be taken with the client's understanding and permission. Because of the altered levels of awareness in the elderly, it is important for members of the SART to evaluate the client's ability to give informed consent. Obtain information about whether the client is competent to make these decisions or whether the client has legal representation that signs and takes responsibility for consent (Hutson, 2002).*

- • Modify the rape protocol to promote comfort for the geriatric client. Consider positioning female clients with pillows rather than stirrups and consider using a smaller speculum. *Aging results in decreased muscle tone and thinning of the vaginal wall.*
- • Assess for mobility limitations and cognitive impairment. *Elicit information from family or caregivers to verify the level of functioning before sexual assault.*
- • Respect the client's need for privacy. *Older clients may be reluctant to have their children or younger family members present during the examination and treatment; give clients a choice.*
- ▲ Consider arrangements for temporary housing. *Most sexual assaults of older clients occur in the home (or nursing home).* **EBN:** *Older age increases the powerlessness of a person, especially if the individual is isolated as a result of living alone. Physical injury can have a much greater effect on older victims, and they may experience a compound reaction because they are older. Sexual violence against an older woman is a reflection of antiage and antiwoman attitudes. Of older sexually assaulted females, 43% are beaten, 7% are stabbed, 60% are severely injured, and 10% are murdered (Delorey & Wolf, 1993).*

### Male Rape

- • Reactions to male rape are often either disbelief or an assumption that the man who was raped is gay. **EBN:** *Most women are aware of the possibility that they may be raped, but many men are not. The care required is very similar to the care of women who have been raped (Laurent, 1993). Approximately 10% of rape victims who go to rape crisis centers are men (Dunn & Gilchrist, 1993).*

R

### Multicultural

- • Assess for the influence of cultural beliefs, norms, and values on the client's ability to cope with the trauma of the rape experience. **EBN:** *What the client views as healthy coping may be based on cultural perceptions (Cochran, 1998; Doswell & Erlen, 1998; Leininger & McFarland, 2002).*
- • Assess to determine if physically abused women are also victims of sexual assault. **EB:** *Sexual assault is experienced by most physically abused women and associated with significantly higher levels of post-traumatic stress disorder (PTSD) compared with women physically abused only. The risk of reassault is decreased if contact is made with health or justice agencies (McFarlane et al, 2005).*
- • Provide opportunities by which the family and individual can save face when working with Asian-American clients. **EBN:** *Asian-American families may avoid situations and*

*discussion of issues that they perceive will bring shame on the family unit (D'Avanzo et al, 2001).*

- Assure the client of confidentiality. **EBN:** *Many Indo-Chinese women will not discuss rape if they think that other staff members, their families, their husbands, or their community may find out (Mollica & Lavelle, 1988).*
- Validate the client's feelings regarding the rape and allow the client to tell his or her rape story. **EBN:** *Validation lets the client know that the nurse has heard and understood what was said, and it promotes the nurse-client relationship (Heineken, 1998). Through the trauma story, the clinician can bridge the disrupted social connection that exists between the client, family, and community (Mollica & Lavelle, 1988). Interventions should reaffirm therapeutic strategies that emphasize effective listening, based on speech styles appropriate to the cultural experiences of the women in question (Bletzer & Koss, 2004).*
- A culturally sensitive approach should be part of the training of all sexual assault response team teams and members of the teams. *Compassion and familiarity in a care plan will allow all care providers to provide a comfortable environment for the client (McCleary, 1994).*

### Home Care

- Some of the interventions described previously may be adapted for home care use.
- Interact with the client supportively and nonjudgmentally; this supports the client's self-worth. *Rape victims usually experience a loss of self-worth.*
- Assist the client with realistically assessing the home setting for safety and/or selecting a safe environment in which to live. *Rape clients may be unable to make a realistic assessment of home safety both immediately after the rape and during long-term recovery.*

▲ Ensure that the client has a support system in place for long-term support. Instruct the family that recovery may take a long time. Refer for medical social work services to assist in setting up a support system if necessary. Refer for counseling if necessary. *The long-term response to rape (up to 4 years) requires ongoing support for the client to reorganize and reintegrate.*

▲ Make sure that physical symptoms from the rape or other physical conditions are followed up. Follow-up should include a visit to the primary care physician or the local health department in 3 to 4 weeks for repeat pregnancy testing and STD testing. Explain to the client that additional medication may be necessary for the treatment of STDs or pregnancy (Ohio Chapter of the International Association of Forensic Nurses [IAFN], 2002*). Stress response to rape can precipitate reemergence of other physical conditions that may be ignored because of the rape.*

▲ If the client is homebound, refer for psychiatric home health care services for client reassurance and implementation of a therapeutic regimen. *Psychiatric home care nurses can address issues relating to the client's rape-trauma syndrome. Behavioral interventions in the home can help the client to participate more effectively in the treatment plan (Patusky, Rodning, & Martinez-Kratz, 1996).*

## Client/Family Teaching

▲ Provide information on prophylactic antibiotic therapy, hepatitis B vaccination, and

R

tetanus prophylaxis for nonimmunized clients with trauma. *Prophylactic treatment for STDs should be provided as part of the initial examination (Ohio Chapter of the IAFN, 2002).*

- • Discharge instructions should be written out for the client. *Anxiety can hamper comprehension and retention of information; repeat instructions and provide them in a written form.*
- • Give instructions to significant others. *Significant others need many of the same supportive and caring interventions as the client; suggest that they too might benefit from counseling.*
- • Explain the purpose of the "morning-after pill." *The morning-after pill (norgestrel [Ovral]) often prevents pregnancy and is used only in emergencies. It must be taken within 72 hours (3 days) of sexual contact to be effective. It will not cause a miscarriage if the client is already pregnant, but it could harm the fetus.*
- ▲ Explain the potential for common side effects related to treatment with norgestrel, such as breast swelling or nausea and vomiting. (Call the emergency department if the client vomits within 1 hour of taking the pill because the pill may need to be taken again.) (Discuss any issues about prophylactic medications at the follow-up visit in 3 to 4 weeks.) It may take 3 to 30 days for the menstrual period to start; if menstruation has not begun in 30 days, contact a physician.
- ▲ Explain the potential for severe side effects related to treatment with norgestrel, such as severe leg or chest pain, trouble breathing, coughing up of blood, severe headache or dizziness, and trouble seeing or talking.
- • Advise the client to call or return if new problems develop. *Physical injuries may not be recognized because of the client's emotional numbness during the initial examination or because the client may have forgotten or not understood some of the instructions.*
- • Teach relaxation techniques.
- • Discuss practical lifestyle changes within the client's control to reduce the risk of future attacks. *A client's financial situation may limit some options, such as moving to another home. Provide other alternatives such as keeping doors locked, checking the car before getting in, not walking alone at night, keeping someone informed of whereabouts, asking someone to check if the client has not arrived at a destination within a reasonable amount of time, keeping lights on in an entryway, having keys in hand when approaching the car or house, and having a remote key entry car or garage.*
- ▲ Teach the client to use self-defense techniques to surprise an attacker and create an opportunity to run for help. Refer the client to a self-defense school.
- • Teach the client appropriate outlets for anger. *Encourage the significant other to direct anger at the event and the attacker, not at the client.*
- • Emphasize the vulnerability of the client and ensure that reactions are appropriate for the victim of sexual assault. *Females are at higher risk for depression than males, and the risk is significantly higher between the ages of 18 and 44 (Mackey et al, 1992).*

NOTE: Post-traumatic stress disorder (PTSD) has a high probability of being a psychological sequela to rape. Research demonstrated two effective treatments for improvement of PTSD in rape victims—prolonged exposure and stress inoculation training (Foa et al, 1991). Prolonged exposure involves reliving the rape experience by imagining it as vividly as possible, describing it aloud in the present tense, taping this description, and listening to the tape at least once daily. Stress inoculation training uses breathing exercises to diminish anxiety and instruction in coping skills, thought stopping, cognitive restructuring, self-dialogue, and role playing. Research suggests that a combination of both treatments may provide the optimal effect.

## evolve WEBSITES FOR EDUCATION

See the EVOLVE website for World Wide Web resources for client education.

## REFERENCES

Adams JA, Girardin B, Faugno D: Signs of genital trauma in adolescent rape victims examined acutely, *J Pediatr Adolesc Gynecol* 13(2):88, 2000.

Bletzer KV, Koss MP: Narrative constructions of sexual violence as told by female rape survivors in three populations of the southwestern United States: scripts of coercion, scripts of consent, *Med Anthropol* 23(2):113-156, 2004.

Cochran M: Tears have no color, *Am J Nurs* 98(6):53, 1998.

Crowley SA: *Sexual assault: the medical-legal examination,* ed 1, Stamford, Conn, 1999, Appleton and Lange.

Dandino-Abbott D: Sexual assault: clinical issues: birth of a sexual assault response team: the first year of the Lucas County/Toledo, Ohio SART program, *J Emerg Nurs* 25(4):333, 1999.

D'Avanzo CE et al: Developing culturally informed strategies for substance-related interventions. In Naegle MA, D'Avanzo CE, editors: *Addictions and substance abuse: strategies for advanced practice nursing,* St Louis, 2001, Mosby.

Delorey C, Wolf KA: Sexual violence and older women, *AWHONNS Clin Issues Perinat Womens Health Nurs* 4:173, 1993.

Derhammer F, Lucente V, Reed JF III et al: Using a SANE interdisciplinary approach to care of sexual assault victims, *Joint Comm J Qual Improv* 26(8):488, 2000.

Doswell W, Erlen J: Multicultural issues and ethical concerns in the delivery of nursing care interventions, *Nurs Clin North Am* 33(2):353, 1998.

Dunn SF, Gilchrist VJ: Sexual assault, *Prim Care* 20(2):359, 1993.

Foa EB, Rothbaum BO, Riggs DS et al: Treatment of posttraumatic stress disorder in rape victims: a comparison between cognitive-behavioral procedures and counseling, *J Consult Clin Psychol* 59(5):715, 1991.

Frable D, Blackstone T, Sherbaum C: Marginal and mindful: deviants in social interaction, *J Pers Soc Psychol* 59:140, 1990.

Heineken J: Patient silence is not necessarily client satisfaction: communication in home care nursing, *Home Healthcare Nurse* 16(2):115, 1998.

Hutson L: Development of sexual assault nurse examiner programs, *Nurs Clin North Am* 35:79, 2002.

Jones J: Elder abuse and neglect: responding to a national problem, *Ann Emerg Med* 23:845, 1994.

Laurent C: Male rape, *Nurs Times* 89(6):18, 1993.

Ledray L: The sexual assault nurse clinician: a 15-year experience in Minneapolis, *J Emerg Nurs* 18(3):217, 1992.

Ledray L: Sexual assault: clinical issues. SANE development and operation guide, *J Emerg Nurs* 24(2):197, 1998a.

Ledray L: Sexual assault: clinical issues. SANE expert and factual testimony, *J Emerg Nurs* 24(3):284, 1998b.

Ledray LE: Sexual assault: clinical issues. IAFN Sixth Annual Scientific Assembly highlights, *J Emerg Nurs* 25(1):63, 1999.

Leininger MM, McFarland MR: *Transcultural nursing: concepts, theories, research and practices,* ed 3, New York, 2002, McGraw-Hill.

Ludwick R, Silva M: Nursing around the world: cultural values and ethical conflicts, *Online J Issues Nurs,* August 14, 2000. Available at www.nursingworld.org/ojin/ethcol/ethics_4.htm, accessed on June 19, 2003.

Mackey T, Sereika SM, Weissfeld LA et al: Factors associated with long-term depressive symptoms of sexual assault victims, *Arch Psychiatr Nurs* 6:10, 1992.

McCleary PH: Female genitalia mutilation and childbirth: a case report, *Birth* 21(4):221, 1994.

McFarlane J, Malecha A, Watson K et al: Intimate partner sexual assault against women: frequency, health consequences, and treatment outcomes, *Obstet Gynecol* 105(1):99-108, 2005.

McGregor MJ, DuMont J, Myhr TL: Sexual assault forensic medical examination: is evidence related to successful prosecution? *Ann Emerg Med* 39:6, 2002.



R

Mollica RF, Lavelle J: Southeast Asian refugees. In Comas-Diaz L, Griffith EEH, editors: *Clinical guidelines in cross-cultural mental health,* New York, 1988, John Wiley and Sons.
O'Brien C: Light staining microscope: clinical experience in a Sexual Assault Nurse Examiner (SANE) program, *Emerg Nurs* 24(1):95, 1998.
Ohio Chapter of the International Association of Forensic Nurses, *The Ohio adolescent and adult sexual assault nurse examiner training manual,* Cleveland, Ohio, 2002, Ohio Office of the Attorney General.
Patusky KL, Rodning C, Martinez-Kratz M: Clinical lessons in psychiatric home care: a case study approach, *J Home Health Case Manag* 9:18, 1996.
Ratner E, Botello, S: Forward for sexual assault, *Top Emerg Med* 25(3):197-198, 2003.
Ruckman LM: Rape: how to begin the healing, *Am J Nurs* 92:48, 1992.
Schei B, Sidenius K, Lundvall L et al: Adult victims of sexual assault: acute medical response and police reporting among women consulting a center for victims of sexual assault, *Acta Obstet Gynecol Scand* 82(8):750, 2003.
Selig C: Sexual assault nurse examiner and sexual assault response team (SANE/SART) program, *Nurs Clin North Am* 35(2):311, 2000.
Sommers M, Buschur C: Injury in women who are raped: what every critical care nurse needs to know, *Dimens Crit Care Nurs* 23(2):62-68, 2004.
Sommers M, Schafer J, Zink T et al: Injury patterns in women resulting from sexual assault, *Trauma Viol Abuse* 2(3):240-258, 2001.
Tyra PA: Older women: victims of rape, *J Gerontol Nurs* 19(5):7, 1993.
Vontress CE, Epp LR: Historical hostility in the African American client: implications for counseling, *J Multicult Counseling Dev* 25:170, 1997.

# Rape-trauma syndrome: compound reaction

*Linda Hutson*

**NANDA**

## Definition

Forced violent sexual act (penetration may not actually occur) (Ohio Revised Code) against victim's will and consent resulting in a trauma syndrome that includes an acute phase of disorganization of victim's lifestyle and a long-term process or reorganization of lifestyle

R

## Defining Characteristics

Change in lifestyle (e.g., changing residence, dealing with repetitive nightmares and phobias, seeking family support, seeking social network support in long-term phase); emotional reaction (e.g., anger, embarrassment, fear of physical violence and death, humiliation, desire for revenge, self-blame in acute phase); multiple physical symptoms (e.g., gastrointestinal irritability, genitourinary discomfort, muscle tension, sleep pattern disturbance in acute phase); reactivated symptoms of previous conditions (i.e., physical illness, psychiatric illness in acute phase); reliance on alcohol and/or drugs (acute phase)

## Related Factors (r/t)

Rape, sexual assault, abuse

**NOC**

## Outcomes (Nursing Outcomes Classification)

### Suggested NOC Outcomes

Abuse Cessation; Abuse Protection; Abuse Recovery: Emotional, Sexual; Coping; Impulse Self-Control; Self-Mutilation Restraint

**Example NOC Outcome with Indicators**

**Abuse Recovery: Sexual** as evidenced by the following indicators: Acknowledgment of right to disclose abusive situation/Expression of right to have been protected from abuse (Rate each indicator of **Abuse Recovery: Sexual:** 1 = none, 2 = limited, 3 = moderate, 4 = substantial, 5 = extensive [see Section I].)

## Client Outcomes

### Client Will (Specify Time Frame):

- Share feelings, concerns, and fears
- Recognize that the rape or attempt was not client's own fault
- State that, no matter what the situation, no one has the right to assault another
- Describe medical/legal treatment procedures and reasons for treatment
- Report absence of physical complications or pain
- Identify support people and be able to ask them for help in dealing with this trauma
- Function at same level as before crisis, including sexual functioning
- Recognize that it is normal for full recovery to take a minimum of 1 year

**NIC**

## Interventions (Nursing Interventions Classification)

### Suggested NIC Interventions

Counseling, Rape-Trauma Treatment

**Example NIC Activities—Counseling**

Encourage expression of feelings; help client to identify strengths and reinforce these

## Nursing Interventions and Rationales

- Refer to the care plans for **Rape-trauma syndrome, Powerlessness, Ineffective Coping, Dysfunctional Grieving, Anxiety, Fear, Risk for self-directed Violence,** and **Sexual dysfunction.**

### Geriatric

▲ A new subgroup of rape victims resides in nursing homes. *Treatment is necessary. Nursing home victims can suffer both compound and silent rape trauma (Burgess, Dowdell, & Prentky, 2000).*

R

## Risk for Compound Reaction

See the care plan for **Rape-trauma syndrome**.

### Multicultural

- Assess for the influence of cultural beliefs, norms, and values on the client's ability to cope with the trauma of the rape experience. **EBN:** *What the client views as healthy coping may be based on cultural perceptions (Cochran, 1998; Doswell & Erlen, 1998; Leininger & McFarland, 2002).*
- Assess to determine if physically abused women are also victims of sexual assault. **EB:** *Sexual assault is experienced by most physically abused women and associated with significantly higher levels of PTSD compared with women physically abused only. The risk of reassault is decreased if contact is made with health or justice agencies (McFarlane et al, 2005).*
- Provide opportunities by which the family and individual can save face when working with Asian-American clients. **EBN:** *Asian-American families may avoid situations and discussion of issues that they perceive will bring shame on the family unit (D'Avanzo et al, 2001).*
- Assure the client of confidentiality. **EBN:** *Many Indo-Chinese women will not discuss rape if they think that other staff members, their families, their husbands, or their community may find out (Mollica & Lavelle, 1988).*
- Validate the client's feelings regarding the rape and allow the client to tell his or her rape story. **EBN:** *Validation lets the client know that the nurse has heard and understood what was said, and it promotes the nurse-client relationship (Heineken, 1998). Through the trauma story, the clinician can bridge the disrupted social connection that exists between the client, family, and community (Mollica & Lavelle, 1988). Interventions should reaffirm therapeutic strategies that emphasize effective listening, based on speech styles appropriate to the cultural experiences of the women in question (Bletzer & Koss, 2004).*
- A culturally sensitive approach should be part of the training of all sexual assault response team teams and members of the teams. *Compassion and familiarity in a care plan will allow all care providers to provide a comfortable environment for the client (McCleary, 1994).*

R

### Home Care

▲ If the client has pursued psychiatric counseling, monitor and encourage attendance. *Reliving the rape experience and the accompanying feelings is painful. The client may need additional support to continue.*

▲ If the client is receiving medication, assess the client's knowledge of its purpose, side effects, and interactions with medications for other diagnoses. Monitor for effectiveness, side effects, and interactions. *Ongoing stress may leave the client overwhelmed and less able to cope with the impact of changing medical status.*

▲ Establish an emergency plan including use of hotlines. Contract with the client to use the emergency plan. Role play using the hotlines. *Having an emergency plan reassures the client and decreases the risk of suicide.*

- For other home care and hospice considerations, refer to the care plan for **Rape-trauma syndrome.**

## Client/Family Teaching

- Teach the client what reactions to expect during the acute and long-term phases: acute phase—anger, fear, self-blame, embarrassment, vengeful feelings, physical symptoms, muscle tension, sleeplessness, stomach upset, genitourinary discomfort; long-term phase—changes in lifestyle or residence, nightmares, phobias, seeking of family and social network support. *Of assessed rape victims, 16.5% were diagnosed with PTSD an average of 17 years after the assault (Mackey et al, 1992).* **EB:** *Past experiences of sexual assault/abuse and current age have an effect on whether or not the client identifies the current incident to be a rape or sexual assault (Kahn, et al, 2003).*
- ▲ Encourage psychiatric consultation if the client is suicidal, violent, or unable to continue activities of daily living (ADLs). *Rape victims are four times more likely than the general population to attempt suicide, which is an 8.7% higher rate than that of nonrape victims (Mackey et al, 1992).*
- ▲ Discuss any of the client's current stress-relieving medications that may result in substance abuse. *The initial response to trauma is for the noradrenergic system to maintain the arousal state, increase vigilance, and be protective to prevent subsequent trauma. Following massive trauma, neurotransmitters are depleted at the synapse level, which is associated with long-term depression and numbing. This depletion also leaves clients with a different threshold of sensitivity to their medications, which increases vulnerability to subsequent stress (Mackey et al, 1992).*

## evolve WEBSITES FOR EDUCATION

See the EVOLVE website for World Wide Web resources for client education.

## REFERENCES


Bletzer KV, Koss MP: Narrative constructions of sexual violence as told by female rape survivors in three populations of the southwestern United States: scripts of coercion, scripts of consent, *Med Anthropol* 23(2):113-156, 2004.

Burgess AW, Dowdell EB, Prentky RA: Sexual abuse of nursing home residents, *J Psychosoc Nurs Ment Health Serv* 38(6):10, 2000.

Cochran M: Tears have no color, *Am J Nurs* 98(6):53, 1998.

D'Avanzo CE et al: Developing culturally informed strategies for substance-related interventions. In Naegle MA, D'Avanzo CE, editors: *Addictions and substance abuse: strategies for advanced practice nursing,* St Louis, 2001, Mosby.

Doswell W, Erlen J: Multicultural issues and ethical concerns in the delivery of nursing care interventions, *Nurs Clin North Am* 33(2):353, 1998.

Heineken J: Patient silence is not necessarily client satisfaction: communication in home care nursing, *Home Healthc Nurs* 16(2): 115, 1998.

Kahn AS, Jackson J, Kully C et al: Calling it rape: differences in experiences of women who do or do not label their sexual assault as rape, *Psychol Women Q* 27(3):233, 2003.

Leininger MM, McFarland MR: *Transcultural nursing: concepts, theories, research and practices,* ed 3, New York, 2002, McGraw-Hill.

Mackey T, Sereika SM, Weissfeld LA et al: Factors associated with long-term depressive symptoms of sexual assault victims, *Arch Psychiatr Nurs* 6(1):10, 1992.

McCleary PH: Female genitalia mutilation and childbirth: a case report, *Birth* 21(4):221, 1994.

McFarlane J, Malecha A, Watson K et al: Intimate partner sexual assault against women: frequency, health consequences, and treatment outcomes, *Obstet Gynecol* 105(1):99-108, 2005.

Mollica RF, Lavelle J: Southeast Asian refugees. In Comas-Diaz L, Griffith EEH, editors: *Clinical guidelines in cross-cultural mental health,* New York, 1988, John Wiley and Sons.


R

# Rape-trauma syndrome: silent reaction

*Linda Hutson*

## NANDA

### Definition

Forced violent sexual act (penetration may not actually occur) (Ohio Revised Code) against victim's will and consent resulting in a trauma syndrome that includes an acute phase of disorganization of victim's lifestyle and a long-term process of reorganization of lifestyle

### Defining Characteristics

Increased anxiety during interview (e.g., blocking of associations, long periods of silence, minor stuttering, physical distress); sudden onset of phobic reactions; lack of verbalization about the rape; abrupt changes in relationships with males; increased nightmares; pronounced changes in sexual behavior

### Related Factors (r/t)

Rape; sexual assault; abuse

## NOC

### Outcomes (Nursing Outcomes Classification)

#### Suggested NOC Outcomes

Abuse Cessation; Abuse Protection; Abuse Recovery: Emotional, Sexual; Coping; Impulse Self-Control; Self-Mutilation Restraint

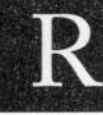

**Example NOC Outcome with Indicators**

**Abuse Recovery: Emotional** as evidenced by the following indicators: Demonstration of confidence/ Demonstration of self-esteem (Rate each indicator of **Abuse Recovery: Emotional:** 1 = none, 2 = limited, 3 = moderate, 4 = substantial, 5 = extensive [see Section I].)

### Client Outcomes

**Client Will (Specify Time Frame):**

- Resume previous level of relationships with significant others
- State improvement in sleep and fewer nightmares
- Express feelings about and discusses the rape (Nondisclosure about a sexual assault may arise out of self-protection, but this defensive coping style acts as a pressure cooker and is associated with more intense depressive symptoms. Clients should be as-

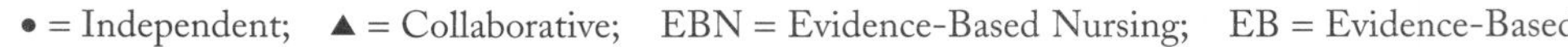

sured that disclosure of an incident of sexual assault to a care provider or advocate has guaranteed confidentiality and does necessitate notification of law enforcement [Mackey et al, 1992].)
- Return to usual pattern of sexual behavior (Women who are sexually active after the assault report lower levels of depression [Mackey et al, 1992]. However, being sexually active cannot be construed to mean that the client has adjusted to or resolved the sexual trauma.)
- Remain free of phobic reactions
- Refer to the care plan for **Rape-trauma syndrome.**

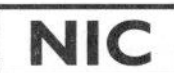

## Interventions (Nursing Interventions Classification)

### Suggested NIC Interventions

Counseling, Support System Enhancement

**Example NIC Activities—Counseling**

Encourage expression of feelings; help client to identify strengths and reinforce these

## Nursing Interventions and Rationales

- Refer to the care plans for **Rape-trauma syndrome, Powerlessness, Ineffective Coping, Dysfunctional Grieving, Anxiety, Fear, Risk for self-directed Violence, Sexual dysfunction,** and **Impaired verbal Communication.**
- Observe for disruptions in relationships with significant others. *Poorly adjusted clients may elicit nonsupportive behavior from others or perceive the actions of others in a negative way.*
- Monitor for signs of increased anxiety (e.g., silence, stuttering, physical distress, irritability, unexplained crying spells).
- Focus on the client's coping strengths.
- Observe for changes in sexual behavior. *More than 80% of sexually active victims reported some sexual dysfunction as a result of the assault (Mackey et al, 1992). Some victims engage in sexual intimacy to prove to themselves and their partners that they are normal or unaffected by the assault.*
- Identify phobic reactions to persons or objects in the environment (e.g., strangers, doorbells, groups of people, knives).
- Provide support by listening when the client is ready to talk. **EB:** *In one study, delayed disclosure of childhood rape was very common and long delays were typical. Close friends are the most common confidants (Smith et al, 2000).*
- Be nonjudgmental when feelings are expressed. Explain that anger is normal and needs to be verbalized. Reassure the client with phrases such as, "I'm sorry this happened to you."
- Remain with an anxious client even if the client is silent. Use gentle speech and actions; move slowly.

- Evaluate somatic complaints. *Women are at higher risk for depression than men (Mackey et al, 1992).*

### Geriatric

- A new subgroup of rape victims resides in nursing homes. Treatment is necessary. **EBN:** *Nursing home victims can suffer both compound and silent rape trauma (Burgess, Dowdell, & Prentky, 2000).*
- Refer to the care plan for **Rape-trauma syndrome.**

### Multicultural

- Assess for the influence of cultural beliefs, norms, and values on the client's ability to cope with the trauma of the rape experience. **EBN:** *What the client views as healthy coping may be based on cultural perceptions (Cochran, 1998; Doswell & Erlen, 1998; Leininger & McFarland, 2002).*
- Assess to determine if physically abused women are also victims of sexual assault. **EB:** *Sexual assault is experienced by most physically abused women and associated with significantly higher levels of PTSD compared with women physically abused only. The risk of reassault is decreased if contact is made with health or justice agencies (McFarlane et al, 2005).*
- Provide opportunities by which the family and individual can save face when working with Asian-American clients. **EBN:** *Asian-American families and individuals may avoid situations and discussion of issues that they perceive will bring shame on the family unit (D'Avanzo et al, 2001).*
- Assure the client of confidentiality. **EBN:** *Many Indo-Chinese women will not discuss rape if they think that other staff members, their families, their husbands, or their community may find out (Mollica & Lavelle, 1988).*
- Allow the client to tell his or her rape story without probing. **EBN:** *Through the rape story, the clinician can bridge the disrupted social connection that exists between the client, family, and community (Mollica & Lavelle, 1988). Interventions should reaffirm therapeutic strategies that emphasize effective listening, based on speech styles appropriate to the cultural experiences of the women in question (Bletzer & Koss, 2004).*

### Home Care

Refer to the care plan for **Rape-trauma syndrome.**

## Client/Family Teaching

- Reassure the client that he or she is not bad and is not at fault. Avoid questions beginning with "why." *"Why" questions may sound judgmental and feed into self-blame.*
- ▲ Refer the client to a sexual assault counselor. Long-term counseling may be necessary.
- Offer information about testing, treatment, and procedures related to pregnancy, hepatitis B, and sexually transmitted infection. Do not wait for the client to request information.
- Refer to the care plan for **Rape-trauma syndrome.**

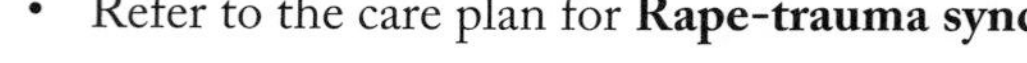

## evolve WEBSITES FOR EDUCATION

See the EVOLVE website for World Wide Web resources for client education.

## REFERENCES


Bletzer KV, Koss MP: Narrative constructions of sexual violence as told by female rape survivors in three populations of the southwestern United States: scripts of coercion, scripts of consent, *Med Anthropol* 23(2):113-156, 2004.

Burgess AW, Dowdell EB, Prentky RA: Sexual abuse of nursing home residents, *J Psychosoc Nurs Ment Health Serv* 38(6):10, 2000.

Cochran M: Tears have no color, *Am J Nurs* 98(6):53, 1998.

D'Avanzo CE et al: Developing culturally informed strategies for substance-related interventions. In Naegle MA, D'Avanzo CE, editors: *Addictions and substance abuse: strategies for advanced practice nursing,* St Louis, 2001, Mosby.

Doswell W, Erlen J: Multicultural issues and ethical concerns in the delivery of nursing care interventions, *Nurs Clin North Am* 33(2):353, 1998.

Leininger MM, McFarland MR: *Transcultural nursing: concepts, theories, research and practices,* ed 3, New York, 2002, McGraw-Hill.

Mackey T, Sereika SM, Weissfeld LA et al: Factors associated with long-term depressive symptoms of sexual assault victims, *Arch Psychiatr Nurs* 6(1):10, 1992

McFarlane J, Malecha A, Watson K et al: Intimate partner sexual assault against women: frequency, health consequences, and treatment outcomes, *Obstet Gynecol* 105(1):99-108, 2005.

Mollica RF, Lavelle J: Southeast Asian refugees. In Comas-Diaz L, Griffith EEH, editors: *Clinical guidelines in cross-cultural mental health,* New York, 1988, John Wiley and Sons.

Smith DW, Letourneau EJ, Saunders BEet al: Delay in disclosure of childhood rape: results from a national survey, *Child Abuse Negl* 24(2):273, 2000.


# Impaired Religiosity evolve

*Lisa Burkhart*

**NANDA**

### Definition

Impaired ability to exercise reliance on beliefs and/or participate in rituals of a particular faith tradition

### Defining Characteristics

Demonstrates or explains difficulty adhering to prescribed religious beliefs and rituals: religious ceremonies, dietary regulations, clothing, prayer, worship/religious services, private religious behaviors/reading religious materials/media, holiday observances, meetings with religious leaders; expresses emotional distress because of separation from faith community; expresses emotional distress regarding religious beliefs and/or religious social network; expresses a need to reconnect with previous belief patterns and customs; questions religious belief patterns and customs

## Related Factors (r/t)

*Physical*: sickness/illness; *psychological*: ineffective support/coping, personal disaster/crisis, lack of security, anxiety, fear of death, ineffective coping with disease, use of religion to manipulate; *sociocultural*: barriers to practicing religion, lack of social integration, lack of social/cultural interaction; *spiritual*: spiritual crises, suffering; *environmental:* barriers to practicing religion; *developmental and situational:* end-stage life crises, life transitions, aging

NOC

## Outcomes (Nursing Outcomes Classification)

### Suggested NOC Outcome

Client Satisfaction: Cultural Needs Fulfillment

**Example NOC Outcome with Indicators**

**Client Satisfaction: Cultural Needs Fulfillment** as evidenced by the following indicators: Respect for religious beliefs/Respect for cultural health behaviors/Incorporation of cultural beliefs in health teaching/Respect for personal values (Rate each indicator of **Client Satisfaction: Cultural Needs Fulfillment:** 1 = not at all satisfied, 2 = somewhat satisfied, 3 = moderately satisfied, 4 = very satisfied, 5 = completely satisfied [see Section I].)

## Client Outcomes

**Client Will (Specify Time Frame):**

- Express satisfaction with the ability to express of religious practices
- Express satisfaction with access to religious materials and rituals
- Demonstrate balance between religious practices and healthy lifestyles
- Avoid high risk controlling religious relationships that inflict physical, sexual, or emotional harm and/or exploitation

NIC

## Interventions (Nursing Interventions Classification)

### Suggested NIC Interventions

Religious Ritual Enhancement, Cultural Brokerage, Religious Addiction Prevention, Abuse Protection: Religious

**Example NIC Activities—Impaired Religiosity**

Encourage and assist use of religious resources if desired; avoid harmful religious practices

## Nursing Interventions and Rationales

- Identify patient's concerns regarding religious expression. **EBN:** *In a survey of primary care clinics in six academic centers, one third of patients wanted to be asked about their re-*

*ligious beliefs during an office visit, and two thirds felt their physician should be aware of their religious beliefs (MacLean et al, 2003). Most nurse practitioners do not believe religious practices hinder health (Stranahan, 2001). Respecting the client's beliefs promotes trust and connectedness (Engebretson, 1996). Individuals who have a religious faith tend to use that tradition in times of stress, but individuals without a religious faith do not turn to religion during times of stress (McGrath, 2003).*

- • Encourage and/or coordinate the use of and participation in usual religious rituals or practices that are not detrimental to health. **EBN:** *Religiosity is associated with more social support, fewer depressive symptoms, higher cognitive status, more cooperativeness, and better physical health (Koenig, George, & Titus, 2004). In a survey of battered women, church attendance and reading the Bible were rated highly in promoting spiritual well-being (Humphreys, 2000). In a survey of parish nurses, religious rites and rituals (e.g., ministering, offering communion, laying on of hands, and anointing) supported clients spiritually (Tuck, Wallace, & Pullen, 2001). Helping a client incorporate religious rites and rituals can enhance meaning in life and promote a sense of connectedness with a faith community and/or a higher power (Conrad, 1985; Lauver, 2000). Oncology nurses frequently pray with patients, refer patients to chaplains or clergy, and provide religious materials (Taylor, Amenta, & Highfield, 1995). Religious coping is associated with better mental health status and spiritual growth (Pargament, 1990; Pargament, 1997).*
- • Coordinate or provide transportation to worship site, particularly for the elderly and in meeting the needs of the disabled or ill. **EBN:** *Religious well-being is significantly correlated to greater social support and hope for institutionalized elderly women (Zorn & Johnson, 1997). Widows and widowers who participate in organized religion demonstrate higher levels of psychological well-being (Fry, 2001). Religion is a protective factor in depression for African-American women who live in poor urban areas (van Olpjen et al, 2003). Religiousness was associated with perceived well-being and fewer psychiatric symptoms in a sample of mentally ill individuals (Corrigan et al, 2003).*
- • Identify individuals at risk for an excessive dependence upon religion, religious leaders, or religious practices. **EBN:** *Challenges to traditional beliefs are anxiety provoking and can produce distress (Charron, 1998).*
- ▲ Refer to religious leader, professional counseling, or support group as needed. **EBN:** *The number one need expressed by clients who had been hospitalized, which was declared by persons of all denominations and faiths, was for their pastor/rabbi/spiritual advisor to not abandon them. For those who did not belong to a religious/spiritual group, the number one need was at least to be asked about some type of religious/spiritual preference (Moller, 1999).*

R

## Geriatric

- • Promote established religious practices in the elderly. **EBN:** *Older adults often identify religiosity as a source of hope (Gaskins & Forte, 1995). Religious belief has been associated with higher levels of well-being and lower levels of depression and suicide (Van Ness & Larson, 2002). Religious well-being is significantly correlated to greater social support and hope for institutionalized elderly women (Zorn & Johnson, 1997). Widows and widowers who participate in organized religion demonstrate higher levels of psychological well-being (Fry, 2001).*

### Multicultural

- Promote religious practices that are culturally appropriate. **EBN:** *How the client copes with spiritual distress may be based on cultural perceptions (Cesario, 2001; Cochran, 1998; Doswell & Erlen, 1998; Leininger & McFarland, 2002; Zapata & Shippee-Rice, 1999).* **EBN:** *African-Americans and Latinos may identify spirituality, religiousness, prayer, and church-based approaches as coping resources (Bourjolly, 1998; Mapp & Hudson, 1997; Samuel-Hodge et al, 2000). Religion is a protective factor in depression for African-American women who live in poor urban areas (van Olpjen et al, 2003).*

## evolve WEBSITES FOR EDUCATION

See the EVOLVE website for World Wide Web resources for client education.

## REFERENCES


Bourjolly JN: Differences in religiousness among black and white women with breast cancer, *Soc Work Health Care* 28(1):21, 1998.

Burkhart L, Solari-Twadell PA: Spirituality and religiousness: differentiating the diagnoses through a review of the nursing literature, *Nurs Diagn* 12:45, 2001.

Cesario S: Care of the Native American woman: strategies for practice, education, and research, *J Obstet Gynecol Neonatal Nurs* 30(1):13, 2001.

Charron HS: Anxiety disorders. In Varcarolis EM, editor: *Foundations of psychiatric mental health nursing,* ed 3, Philadelphia, 1998, WB Saunders.

Cochran M: Tears have no color, *Am J Nurs* 98(6):53, 1998.

Conrad NJ: Spiritual support for the dying, *Nurs Clin North Am* 20:415, 1985.

Corrigan P, McCorkle B, Schell B et al: Religion and spirituality in the lives of people with serious mental illness, *Community Ment Health J* 39(6):487:2003.

Doswell W, Erlen J: Multicultural issues and ethical concerns in the delivery of nursing care interventions, *Nurs Clin North Am* 33(2):353, 1998.

Engebretson J: Considerations in diagnosing in the spiritual domain, *Nurs Diagn* 7:100, 1996.

Fry PS: The unique contribution of key existential factors to the prediction of psychological well-being of older adults following spousal loss, *Gerontologist* 41(1):69, 2001.

Gaskins S, Forte L: The meaning of hope: implications for nursing practice and research, *J Gerontol Nurs* 21:17, 1995.

Humphreys J: Spirituality and distress in sheltered battered women, *J Nurs Scholarsh* 32:273, 2000.

Koenig HG, George LK, Titus P: Religion, spirituality, and health in medically ill hospitalized older patients, *J Am Geriatr Soc* 52: 554, 2004.

Lauver D: Commonalities in women's spirituality and women's health, *Adv Nurs Sci* 22:76, 2000.

Leininger MM, McFarland MR: *Transcultural nursing: concepts, theories, research and practices,* ed 3, New York, 2002, McGraw-Hill.

Mapp I, Hudson R: Stress and coping among African American and Hispanic parents of deaf children, *Am Ann Deaf* 142(1):48, 1997.

MacLean CD, Susi B, Phifer N et al: Patient preference for physician discussion and practice of spirituality: results from a multicenter patient survey, *J Gen Intern Med* 18:38, 2003.

McGrath P: Religiosity and the challenge of terminal illness, *Death Stud*, 27:881, 2003.

Moller MD: Meeting spiritual needs on an inpatient unit, *J Psychosoc Nurs Ment Health Serv* 37(11):5, 1999.

Pargament KL, Ensing DS, Falgout K et al: God help me (I): Religious coping efforts as predictors of the outcomes to significant negative life events. *Am J Community Psychol* 18:793, 1990.

Pargament KL: *The psychology of religion and coping: theory, research, practice,* New York, 1997, Guilford Press.

Samuel-Hodge CD, Headen SW, Skelly AH et al: Influences on day-to-day self-management of type 2 diabetes among African-American women: spirituality, the multi-caregiver role, and other social context factors, *Diabetes Care* 23(7):928, 2000.


R

Stranahan S: Spiritual perception, attitudes about spiritual care, and spiritual care practices among nurse practitioners, *West J Nurs Res* 23(1):90, 2001.
Taylor EJ, Amenta M, Highfield M: Spiritual care practices of oncology nurses, *Oncol Nurs Forum* 22(1):31, 1995.
Tuck I, Wallace D, Pullen L: Spirituality and spiritual care provided by parish nurses, *West J Nurs Res* 23:144, 2001.
Van Ness PH, Larson DB: Religion, senescence, and mental health: the end of life is not the end of hope, *Am J Geriatr Psychiatry* 10:386, 2002.
Van Olphen J, Schulz A, Isreal B et al: Religious involvement, social support, and health among African-American women on the east side of Detroit, *J Gen Intern Med* 18:549, 2003.
Zapata J, Shippee-Rice R: The use of folk healing and healers by six Latinos living in New England, *J Transcult Nurs* 10(2):136, 1999.
Zorn CR, Johnson MT: Religious well-being in noninstitutionalized elderly women, *Health Care Women Int* 18(3):209, 1997.

# Readiness for enhanced Religiosity

*Lisa Burkhart*

**NANDA**

## Definition

Ability to increase reliance on religious beliefs and/or participate in rituals of a particular faith tradition

## Defining Characteristics

Expresses desire to strengthen religious belief patterns and customs that had provided comfort/religion in the past; request for assistance to increase participate in prescribed religious beliefs through religious ceremonies, dietary regulations/rituals, clothing, prayer, worship/religious services, private religious behaviors, reading religious materials/ media, holiday observances; requests assistance expanding religious options; expresses meeting with religious leaders/facilitators; requests forgiveness, reconciliation; questions or rejects belief patterns and customs that are harmful

R

## Related Factors (r/t)

Health-seeking behaviors to express one's chosen faith tradition or to reject harmful belief patterns and customs

**NOC**

## Outcomes (Nursing Outcomes Classification)

### Suggested NOC Outcomes

Client Satisfaction: Cultural Needs Fulfillment, Spiritual Health

**Example NOC Outcome with Indicators**

**Client Satisfaction: Cultural Needs Fulfillment** as evidenced by the following indicators: Respect for religious beliefs/Respect for cultural health behaviors/Incorporation of cultural beliefs in health teaching/Respect for personal values (Rate each indicator of **Client Satisfaction: Cultural Needs Fulfillment:** 1 = not at all satisfied, 2 = somewhat satisfied, 3 = moderately satisfied, 4 = very satisfied, 5 = completely satisfied [see Section I].)

## Client Outcomes

**Client Will (Specify Time Frame):**

- Express satisfaction with an enhanced ability to express of religious practices
- Express satisfaction with access to religious materials and rituals
- Demonstrate balance between religious practices and healthy lifestyles
- Avoid high risk controlling religious relationships that inflict physical, sexual, or emotional harm and/or exploitation

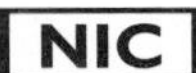

## Interventions (Nursing Interventions Classification)

### Suggested NIC Interventions

Religious Ritual Enhancement, Cultural Brokerage, Spiritual Growth Facilitation

**Example NIC Activities—Religious Ritual Enhancement**

Encourage and assist use of religious resources; avoid harmful religious practices

## Nursing Interventions and Rationales

- Identify patient's desire regarding religious expression. **EBN:** *In a survey of primary care clinics in six academic centers, one third of patients wanted to be asked about their religious beliefs during an office visit, and two thirds felt their physician should be aware of their religious beliefs (MacLean et al, 2003). Most nurse practitioners do not believe religious practices hinder health (Stranahan, 2001). Respecting the client's beliefs promotes trust and connectedness (Engebretson, 1996). Individuals who have a religious faith tend to use that tradition in times of stress, but individuals without a religious faith do not turn to religion during times of stress (McGrath, 2003).*
- Encourage and/or coordinate the use of and participation in usual religious rituals or practices that are not detrimental to health. **EBN:** *Religiosity is associated with more social support, fewer depressive symptoms, higher cognitive status, more cooperativeness, and better physical health (Koenig, George, & Titus, 2004). In a survey of battered women, church attendance and reading the Bible were rated highly in promoting spiritual well-being (Humphreys, 2000). In a survey of parish nurses, religious rites and rituals (e.g., ministering, offering communion, laying on of hands, and anointing) supported clients spiritually (Tuck, Wallace, & Pullen, 2001). Helping a client incorporate religious rites and rituals can enhance meaning in life and promote a sense of connectedness with a faith community and/or*

*a higher power (Conrad, 1985; Lauver, 2000). Oncology nurses frequently pray with patients, refer patients to chaplains or clergy, and provide religious materials (Taylor, Amenta, & Highfield, 1995). Religious coping is associated with better mental health status and spiritual growth (Pargament, 1990, 1997).*

- • Coordinate or provide transportation to worship site, particularly for the elderly and in meeting the needs of the disabled or ill. **EBN:** *Religious well-being is significantly correlated to greater social support and hope for institutionalized elderly women (Zorn & Johnson, 1997). Widows and widowers who participate in organized religion demonstrate higher levels of psychological well-being (Fry, 2001). Religion is a protective factor in depression for African-American women who live in poor urban areas (van Olpjen et al, 2003). Religiousness was associated with perceived well-being and fewer psychiatric symptoms in a sample of mentally ill individuals (Corrigan et al, 2003).*
- ▲ Refer to religious leader, as appropriate. **EBN:** *The number one need expressed by clients who had been hospitalized, which was declared by persons of all denominations and faiths, was for their pastor/rabbi/spiritual advisor to not abandon them. For those who did not belong to a religious/spiritual group, the number one need was at least to be asked about some type of religious/spiritual preference (Moller, 1999).*

## Pediatric

- • Provide spiritual care for children based on developmental level. *When nurses are comfortable providing spiritual care, they can implement numerous spiritual care activities and interventions to meet the spiritual needs of the child and family. After determining the child's spiritual beliefs and spiritual needs, a plan of care is developed based on the child's developmental age (Elkins & Cavendish, 2004).*
  - ■ **Infants:** Have the same nurse care for the child on a daily basis, hold, cuddle, rock play with and sing to the infant. *The primary needs of the infant are love and trust. Minimizing the separation of the child from family and having the same nurse care for the child on a daily basis can initiate spiritual care. Continuity of care will promote the establishment of trust because nurses provide much of the needed ongoing support. The infant who is ill or dying still needs to be sung and talked to played with, held, cuddled, and rocked (Elkins & Cavendish, 2004).*
  - ■ **Toddlers:** Provide consistency in care and familiar toys, music, stories, clothing blankets, pillows, and any other individual object of contentment. Schedule home religious routines into the plan of care and support home routines regarding good and bad behavior. *Toddlers and preschoolers need to feel safe and secure, and develop a trusting relationship with caretakers. The importance of consistency in care and routine with this age group cannot be overemphasized. The nurse should support parent's home routines during hospitalization as much as possible and encourage them to continue to have the same expectations regarding good and bad behavior. If particular religious routines are carried out at certain times of the day, the nurse should schedule them in the plan of care (Elkins & Cavendish, 2004).*
  - ■ **School-age children and adolescents**: Encourage both groups to express their feelings regarding spirituality. Ask them, "Do you wish to pray and what do want to pray about?" Children of all ages can express feelings in story telling. Offer age-appropriate complimentary therapies such as music, art, videos, connectedness with

R

peers through cards, letters, and visits. *School-age children and adolescents should be encouraged to express their feelings, concerns, and needs regarding spirituality. For the adolescent, nurses need to accept their beliefs and wishes even if they are different from their caregiver's. The nurse needs to facilitate the child's participation in religious rituals and spiritual practices. Referrals to clergy and other spiritual support may be necessary (Elkins & Cavendish, 2004).*

## Geriatric

- Promote established religious practices in the elderly. **EBN:** *Older adults often identify religiosity as a source of hope (Gaskins & Forte, 1995). Religious belief has been associated with higher levels of well-being and lower levels of depression and suicide (Van Ness & Larson, 2002). Religious well-being is significantly correlated to greater social support and hope for institutionalized elderly women (Zorn & Johnson, 1997). Widows and widowers who participate in organized religion demonstrate higher levels of psychological well-being (Fry, 2001).*

## Multicultural

- Promote religious practices that are culturally appropriate. **EBN:** *How the client copes with spiritual distress may be based on cultural perceptions (Cesario, 2001; Cochran, 1998; Doswell & Erlen, 1998; Leininger & McFarland, 2002; Zapata & Shippee-Rice, 1999).* **EBN:** *African-Americans and Latinos may identify spirituality, religiousness, prayer, and church-based approaches as coping resources (Bourjolly, 1998; Mapp & Hudson, 1997; Samuel-Hodge et al, 2000). Religion is a protective factor in depression for African-American women who live in poor urban areas (van Olpjen et al, 2003).*

## evolve WEBSITES FOR EDUCATION

See the EVOLVE website for World Wide Web resources for client education.

## REFERENCES

R

Bourjolly JN: Differences in religiousness among black and white women with breast cancer, *Soc Work Health Care* 28(1):21, 1998.

Burkhart L, Solari-Twadell PA: Spirituality and religiousness: differentiating the diagnoses through a review of the nursing literature, *Nurs Diagn* 12:45, 2001.

Cesario S: Care of the Native American woman: strategies for practice, education, and research, *J Obstet Gynecol Neonatal Nurs* 30(1):13, 2001.

Charron HS: Anxiety disorders. In Varcarolis EM, editor: *Foundations of psychiatric mental health nursing,* ed 3, Philadelphia, 1998, WB Saunders.

Cochran M: Tears have no color, *Am J Nurs* 98(6):53, 1998.

Conrad NJ: Spiritual support for the dying, *Nurs Clin North Am* 20:415, 1985.

Corrigan P, McCorkle B, Schell B et al: Religion and spirituality in the lives of people with serious mental illness, *Community Ment Health J* 39(6):487:2003.

Doswell W, Erlen J: Multicultural issues and ethical concerns in the delivery of nursing care interventions, *Nurs Clin North Am* 33(2):353, 1998.

Elkins M, Cavendish R: Developing a plan for pediatric spiritual care, *Holist Nurs Pract* 18(4):179. 2004.

Engebretson J: Considerations in diagnosing in the spiritual domain, *Nurs Diagn* 7:100, 1996.

Fry PS: The unique contribution of key existential factors to the prediction of psychological well-being of older adults following spousal loss, *Gerontologist* 41(1):69, 2001.

Gaskins S, Forte L: The meaning of hope: implications for nursing practice and research, *J Gerontol Nurs* 21:17, 1995.
Humphreys J: Spirituality and distress in sheltered battered women, *J Nurs Scholarsh* 32:273, 2000.
Koenig HG, George LK, Titus P: Religion, spirituality, and health in medically ill hospitalized older patients, *J Am Geriatr Soc* 52: 554, 2004.
Lauver D: Commonalities in women's spirituality and women's health, *Adv Nurs Sci* 22:76, 2000.
Leininger MM, McFarland MR: *Transcultural nursing: concepts, theories, research and practices,* ed 3, New York, 2002, McGraw-Hill.
Mapp I, Hudson R: Stress and coping among African American and Hispanic parents of deaf children, *Am Ann Deaf* 142(1):48, 1997.
MacLean, CD, Susi B, Phifer N et al: Patient preference for physician discussion and practice of spirituality: results from a multicenter patient survey, *J Gen Intern Med* 18:38, 2003.
McGrath P: Religiosity and the challenge of terminal illness, *Death Stud* 27:881, 2003.
Moller MD: Meeting spiritual needs on an inpatient unit, *J Psychosoc Nurs Ment Health Serv* 37(11):5, 1999.
Pargament KL: *The psychology of religion and coping: theory, research, practice.* New York: Guilford Press, 1997.
Pargament KL, Ensing DS, Falgout K et al: God help me (I): religious coping efforts as predictors of the outcomes to significant negative life events, *Am J Community Psychol* 18:793, 1990.
Samuel-Hodge CD, Headen SW, Skelly AH et al: Influences on day-to-day self-management of type 2 diabetes among African American women: spirituality, the multi-caregiver role, and other social context factors, *Diabetes Care* 23(7):928, 2000.
Stranahan S: Spiritual perception, attitudes about spiritual care, and spiritual care practices among nurse practitioners, *West J Nurs Res* 23(1):90, 2001.
Taylor EJ, Amenta M, Highfield M: Spiritual care practices of oncology nurses, *Oncol Nurs Forum* 22(1):31, 1995.
Tuck I, Wallace D, Pullen L: Spirituality and spiritual care provided by parish nurses, *West J Nurs Res* 23:144, 2001.
Van Ness PH, Larson DB: Religion, senescence, and mental health: the end of life is not the end of hope, *Am J Geriatr Psychiatry* 10:386, 2002.
Van Olphen J, Schulz A, Isreal B et al: Religious involvement, social support, and health among African-American women on the east side of Detroit, *J Gen Intern Med* 18:549, 2003.
Zapata J, Shippee-Rice R: The use of folk healing and healers by six Latinos living in New England, *J Transcult Nurs* 10(2):136, 1999.
Zorn CR, Johnson MT: Religious well-being in noninstitutionalized elderly women, *Health Care Women Int* 18(3):209, 1997.

# Risk for impaired Religiosity

*Lisa Burkhart*

R

**NANDA**

## Definition

At risk for impaired ability to exercise reliance on religious beliefs and/or participate in rituals of a particular faith tradition

## Risk Factors (r/t)

*Physical*: illness/hospitalization, pain; *psychological*: ineffective support/coping/caregiving, depression, lack of security; *sociocultural*: lack of social integration, cultural barriers to practicing religion, social isolation; *spiritual*: suffering; *environmental*: lack of transportation, barriers to practicing religion; *developmental*: life transitions

**NOC**

## Outcomes (Nursing Outcomes Classification)

### Suggested NOC Outcomes

Client Satisfaction: Cultural Needs Fulfillment, Spiritual Health

**Example NOC Outcome with Indicators**

**Client Satisfaction: Cultural Needs Fulfillment** as evidenced by the following indicators: Respect for religious beliefs/Respect for cultural health behaviors/Incorporation of cultural beliefs in health teaching/Respect for personal values (Rate each indicator of **Client Satisfaction: Cultural Needs Fulfillment:** 1 = not at all satisfied, 2 = somewhat satisfied, 3 = moderately satisfied, 4 = very satisfied, 5 = completely satisfied [see Section I].)

## Client Outcomes

### Client Will (Specify Time Frame):

- Express satisfaction with the ability to express of religious practices
- Express satisfaction with access to religious materials and rituals
- Demonstrate balance between religious practices and healthy lifestyles
- Avoid high risk controlling religious relationships that inflict physical, sexual, or emotional harm and/or exploitation

**NIC**

## Interventions (Nursing Interventions Classification)

### Suggested NIC Interventions

Religious Ritual Enhancement, Cultural Brokerage, Religious Addiction Prevention, Abuse Protection: Religious

**Example NIC Activities—Religious Ritual Enhancement**

Encourage and assist use of religious resources if desired; avoid harmful religious practices

## Nursing Interventions and Rationales

- Identify patient's concerns regarding religious expression. **EBN:** *In a survey of primary care clinics in six academic centers, one third of patients wanted to be asked about their religious beliefs during an office visit, and two thirds felt their physician should be aware of their religious beliefs (MacLean et alt, 2003). Most nurse practitioners do not believe religious practices hinder health (Stranahan, 2001). Respecting the client's beliefs promotes trust and connectedness (Engebretson, 1996). Individuals who have a religious faith tend to use that tradition in times of stress, but individuals without a religious faith do not turn to religion during times of stress (McGrath, 2003).*
- Encourage and/or coordinate the use of and participation in usual religious rituals or

practices that are not detrimental to health. **EBN:** *Religiosity is associated with more social support, fewer depressive symptoms, higher cognitive status, more cooperativeness, and better physical health (Koenig, George, & Titus, 2004). In a survey of battered women, church attendance and reading the Bible were rated highly in promoting spiritual well-being (Humphreys, 2000). In a survey of parish nurses, religious rites and rituals (e.g., ministering, offering communion, laying on of hands, and anointing) supported clients spiritually (Tuck, Wallace, & Pullen, 2001). Helping a client incorporate religious rites and rituals can enhance meaning in life and promote a sense of connectedness with a faith community and/or a higher power (Conrad, 1985; Lauver, 2000). Oncology nurses frequently pray with patients, refer patients to chaplains or clergy, and provide religious materials (Taylor, Amenta, & Highfield, 1995). Religious coping is associated with better mental health status and spiritual growth (Pargament, 1990, 1997).*

- • Coordinate or provide transportation to worship site, particularly for the elderly and in meeting the needs of the disabled or ill. **EBN:** *Religious well-being is significantly correlated to greater social support and hope for institutionalized elderly women (Zorn & Johnson, 1997). Widows and widowers who participate in organized religion demonstrate higher levels of psychological well-being (Fry, 2001). Religion is a protective factor in depression for African-American women who live in poor urban areas (van Olpjen et al, 2003). Religiousness was associated with perceived well-being and fewer psychiatric symptoms in a sample of mentally ill individuals (Corrigan et al, 2003).*
- • Identify individuals at risk for an excessive dependence upon religion, religious leaders, or religious practices. **EBN:** *Challenges to traditional beliefs are anxiety provoking and can produce distress (Charron, 1998).*
- ▲ Refer to religious leader, professional counseling, or support group as needed. **EBN:** *The number one need expressed by clients who had been hospitalized, which was declared by persons of all denominations and faiths, was for their pastor/rabbi/spiritual advisor to not abandon them. For those who did not belong to a religious/spiritual group, the number one need was at least to be asked about some type of religious/spiritual preference (Moller, 1999).*

## Geriatric

- • Promote established religious practices in the elderly. **EBN:** *Older adults often identify religiosity as a source of hope (Gaskins & Forte, 1995). Religious belief has been associated with higher levels of well-being and lower levels of depression and suicide (Van Ness & Larson, 2002). Religious well-being is significantly correlated to greater social support and hope for institutionalized elderly women (Zorn & Johnson, 1997). Widows and widowers who participate in organized religion demonstrate higher levels of psychological well-being (Fry, 2001).*

## Multicultural

- • Promote religious practices that are culturally appropriate. **EBN:** *How the client copes with spiritual distress may be based on cultural perceptions (Cesario, 2001; Cochran, 1998; Doswell & Erlen, 1998; Leininger & McFarland, 2002; Zapata & Shippee-Rice, 1999).* **EBN:** *African-Americans and Latinos may identify spirituality, religiousness, prayer, and church-based approaches as coping resources (Bourjolly, 1998; Mapp & Hudson,*

*1997; Samuel-Hodge et al, 2000). Religion is a protective factor in depression for African-American women who live in poor urban areas (van Olpjen et al, 2003).*

## evolve WEBSITES FOR EDUCATION

See the EVOLVE website for World Wide Web resources for client education.

## REFERENCES


Bourjolly JN: Differences in religiousness among black and white women with breast cancer, *Soc Work Health Care* 28(1):21, 1998.

Burkhart L, Solari-Twadell PA: Spirituality and religiousness: differentiating the diagnoses through a review of the nursing literature, *Nurs Diagn* 12:45, 2001.

Cesario S: Care of the Native American woman: strategies for practice, education, and research, *J Gynecol Neonat Nurs* 30(1):13, 2001.

Charron HS: Anxiety disorders. In Varcarolis EM, editor: *Foundations of psychiatric mental health nursing,* ed 3, Philadelphia, 1998, WB Saunders.

Cochran M: Tears have no color, *Am J Nurs* 98(6):53, 1998.

Conrad NJ: Spiritual support for the dying, *Nurs Clin North Am* 20:415, 1985.

Corrigan P, McCorkle B, Schell B et al: Religion and spirituality in the lives of people with serious mental illness, *Community Ment Health J* 39(6):487:2003.

Doswell W, Erlen J: Multicultural issues and ethical concerns in the delivery of nursing care interventions, *Nurs Clin North Am* 33(2):353, 1998.

Engebretson J: Considerations in diagnosing in the spiritual domain, *Nurs Diagn* 7:100, 1996.

Fry PS: The unique contribution of key existential factors to the prediction of psychological well-being of older adults following spousal loss, *Gerontologist* 41(1):69, 2001.

Gaskins S, Forte L: The meaning of hope: implications for nursing practice and research, *J Gerontol Nurs* 21:17, 1995.

Humphreys J: Spirituality and distress in sheltered battered women, *J Nurs Scholarsh* 32:273, 2000.

Koenig HG, George LK, Titus P: Religion, spirituality, and health in medically ill hospitalized older patients, *J Am Geriatr Soc* 52:554, 2004.

Lauver D: Commonalities in women's spirituality and women's health, *Adv Nurs Sci* 22:76, 2000.

Leininger MM, McFarland MR: *Transcultural nursing: concepts, theories, research and practices,* ed 3, New York, 2002, McGraw-Hill.

Mapp I, Hudson R: Stress and coping among African American and Hispanic parents of deaf children, *Am Ann Deaf* 142(1):48, 1997.

MacLean, CD, Susi B, Phifer N et al: Patient preference for physician discussion and practice of spirituality: results from a multicenter patient survey, *J Gen Intern Med* 18:38, 2003.

McGrath P: Religiosity and the challenge of terminal illness, *Death Stud*, 27:881, 2003.

Moller MD: Meeting spiritual needs on an inpatient unit, *J Psychosoc Nurs Ment Health Serv* 37(11):5, 1999.

Pargament KL: *The psychology of religion and coping: theory, research, practice.* New York: Guilford Press, 1997.

Pargament KL, Ensing DS, Falgout K et al: God help me (I): religious coping efforts as predictors of the outcomes to significant negative life events. *Am J Community Psychol* 18:793, 1990.

Pullen L, Modrcin-Talbott MA, West WR et al: Spiritual high vs high on spirits: is religiosity related to adolescent alcohol and drug abuse? *J Psychiatr Ment Health Nurs* 6(1):3, 1999.

Samuel-Hodge CD, Headen SW, Skelly AH et al: Influences on day-to-day self-management of type 2 diabetes among African American women: spirituality, the multi-caregiver role, and other social context factors, *Diabetes Care* 23(7):928, 2000.

Stranahan S: Spiritual perception, attitudes about spiritual care, and spiritual care practices among nurse practitioners, *West J Nurs Res* 23(1):90, 2001.

Taylor EJ, Amenta M, Highfield M: Spiritual care practices of oncology nurses, *Oncol Nurs Forum* 22(1):31, 1995.

Tuck I, Wallace D, Pullen L: Spirituality and spiritual care provided by parish nurses, *West J Nurs Res* 23:144, 2001.

Van Ness PH, Larson DB: Religion, senescence, and mental health: the end of life is not the end of hope, *Am J Geriatr Psychiatry* 10:386, 2002.

Van Olphen J, Schulz A, Isreal B et al: Religious involvement, social support, and health among African-American women on the east side of Detroit, J *Gen Intern Med* 18:549, 2003.

Zapata J, Shippee-Rice R: The use of folk healing and healers by six Latinos living in New England, *J Transcult Nurs* 10(2):136, 1999.
Zorn CR, Johnson MT: Religious well-being in noninstitutionalized elderly women, *Health Care Women Int* 18(3):209,1997.

# Relocation stress syndrome

*Betty J. Ackley and Gail B. Ladwig*

**NANDA**

## Definition

Physiological and/or psychosocial disturbances that result from transfer from one environment to another

## Defining Characteristics

Temporary and/or permanent move; voluntary and/or involuntary move; aloneness, alienation, or loneliness; depression; anxiety (e.g., separation); sleep disturbance; withdrawal; anger; loss of identity, self-worth, or self-esteem; increased verbalization of needs, unwillingness to move or concern over relocation; increased physical symptoms/illness (e.g., gastrointestinal disturbance, weight change); dependency; insecurity; pessimism; frustration; worry; fear

## Related Factors (r/t)

Unpredictability of experience/isolation from family/friends; passive coping; language barrier; decreased health status; impaired psychosocial health; past, concurrent, and recent losses; feeling of powerlessness; lack of adequate support system/group; lack of predeparture counseling

**NOC**

## Outcomes (Nursing Outcomes Classification)

### Suggested NOC Outcomes

Anxiety Self-Control; Child Adaptation to Hospitalization; Coping; Depression Level; Depression Self-Control; Loneliness Severity; Psychosocial Adjustment: Life Change; Quality of Life

**Example NOC Outcome with Indicators**

**Anxiety Self-Control** as evidenced by the following indicators: Seeks information to reduce anxiety/Plans coping strategies for stressful situations/Uses effective coping strategies/Uses relaxation techniques to reduce anxiety/Maintains social relationships/Maintains adequate sleep/Controls anxiety response (Rate each indicator of **Anxiety Self-Control:** 1 = never demonstrated, 2 = rarely demonstrated, 3 = sometimes demonstrated, 4 = often demonstrated, 5 = consistently demonstrated [see Section I].)

## Client Outcomes

**Client Will (Specify Time Frame):**

- Recognize and know the name of at least one staff member
- Express concern about move when encouraged to do so during individual contacts
- Carry out activities of daily living (ADLs) in usual manner
- Maintain previous mental and physical health status (e.g., nutrition, elimination, sleep, social interaction)

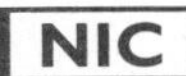

## Interventions (Nursing Interventions Classification)

### Suggested NIC Interventions

Anxiety Reduction, Coping Enhancement, Discharge Planning, Hope Instillation, Self-Responsibility Facilitation

**Example NIC Activities—Anxiety Reduction**

Stay with client to promote safety and reduce fear; provide objects that symbolize safeness

## Nursing Interventions and Rationales

- Obtain a history, including the reason for the move, the client's usual coping mechanisms, history of losses, and family support for the client. *A history helps the nurse determine the amount of support needed and appropriate interventions to decrease relocation stress.*
- Consider the clients' and families cultural and ethnic values as much as possible when choosing roommates, foods, and other aspects of care. *Nurses need to be aware of the differences in values and practices of different cultures and ensure they give culturally appropriate care (Spector, 2000).*
- Observe the following procedures if the client is being transferred to an extended care facility or assisted living facility:
  - Allow the client to have a choice of placement and arrange a preadmission visit if possible. *Having some control over the event strengthens problem-solving and coping strategies (Nypaver, Titus, & Brugler, 1996) and may help reduce mortality (Thorson & Davis, 2000).* **EB:** *Research has shown a link between the loss of indepence with transfer to a nursing home and depression (Loeher et al, 2004).*
  - If the client cannot choose placement, arrange for a visit or telephone call by a member of the staff to welcome the client and show a videotape or at least provide pictures of the new care facility.
  - Have a familiar person accompany the client to the new facility. *This lessens client and family anxiety, confusion, and dissatisfaction.*
  - Validate the caregiver's feelings of difficulty with putting a loved one in a different environment. *This is a distressing experience, and caregivers feel responsible. Validating the caregivers feelings will help establish a trusting relationship (Dellasega & Mastrian, 1995).*

- Identify previous routines for ADLs. Try to maintain as much continuity with the previous schedule as possible. *Continuity of routines has been shown to be a crucial factor in positively influencing adjustment to a new environment (Manion & Rantz, 1995; Kao, Travis, & Acton, 2004).*
- Bring in familiar items from home (e.g., pictures, clocks, afghans).
- Establish the way the client would like to be addressed (Mr., Mrs., Miss, first name, nickname). *Calling clients by the desired name shows respect.*
- Thoroughly orient the client and the family to the new environment and routines; repeat directions as needed. *The stress of the move may interfere with the client's ability to remember directions. A progressive introduction and orientation for both the client and the family should be done (Kao, Travis, & Acton, 2004).*
- Spend one-on-one time with the client. Allow the client to express feelings and convey acceptance of them; emphasize that the client's feelings are real and individual and that it is acceptable to be sad or angry about moving. *Expressing feelings can help the client deal with the change and facilitate grief work that accompanies loss of independence (Tracy & DeYoung, 2004).*
- Assign the same staff members to the client if compatible with client; maintain consistency in the personnel the client interacts with. *Consistency hastens adjustment and increases quality of care (Iwasiw et al, 2003).*
- Ask the client to state one positive aspect of the new living situation each day. *Helping the client focus on the positive aspects of the move can help change attitude and reframe the situation in a positive fashion.*
- Monitor the client's health status and provide appropriate interventions for problems with social interaction, nutrition, sleep, new onset of infection, or elimination problems. *Stress from the transfer can cause physiological and psychological disturbances (Lander, Brazill, & Ladrigan, 1997).* **EB and EBN:** *Clients who moved showed lower natural killer cell immunity 1 month after moving than was shown by a control group of elderly who did not move (Lutgendorf et al, 1999). Another study demonstrated that older adults who were relocated had lower natural killer cell cytotoxicity than control subjects who did not move, but the clients generally recovered normal immune function by 3 months (Lutgendorf et al, 2001).*
- If the client is being transferred within a facility, have staff members from the new unit visit the client before transfer.
- Work with the caregivers family members helping them deal with stages of "making the best of it," "making the move," and "making it better." **EBN:** *A study demonstrated that relatives of clients entering a nursing home can work in partnership with health care staff to ease the transition for their loved one more effectively (Davies & Nolan, 2004).*
- If a client is being transferred from the intensive care unit (ICU), have previous staff make occasional visits until the client is comfortable in the new surroundings. Ensure that the family is told relevant information. **EBN:** *Participants in one study discussed a desire for normality and indicated that leaving the ICU staff was the most negative component of transfer (McKinney & Deeny, 2002). A review of the literature in this area demonstrated that information needs were most important to families of clients transferred out of ICU (Mitchell, Courtney, & Coyer, 2003).*

R

- Watch for coping problems (e.g., withdrawal, regression, angry behavior, impaired sleeping, refusal to eat, flat affect) and intervene immediately. **EB:** *Research has shown a link between the loss of independence with transfer to a nursing home and depression (Loeher et al, 2004).*
- Allow the client to grieve for the loss of the old situation; explain that it is normal to feel sadness over change and loss.
- Encourage the client to participate in care as much as possible and make own decisions when possible (e.g., placement of the bed, choice of roommate, bathing routines).
- Make an effort to accommodate the client. *Having choices helps prevent feelings of powerlessness that may lead to depression.*

### Pediatric

- Provide support for a child and family who must relocate to be near a transplant center. **EBN:** *Recognizing the unique needs of parents who must relocate for a child's transplantation procedure supports the delivery of individualized nursing care and the effective allocation of program resources (Stubblefield & Murray, 2002).*
- If the client is an adolescent, try to avoid a move in the middle of the school year, find a newcomers' club for the adolescent to join, and refer for counseling if needed. *An adolescent who is relocating can experience emotional, social, and cognitive dysfunctions. The interventions listed can be helpful (Puskar & Dvorsak, 1991).*

### Geriatric

- Monitor the need for transfer and transfer only when necessary. *Elderly clients often adapt poorly to transfer; they can lose normal functioning in areas such as self-care (Lander, Brazill, & Ladrigan, 1997), and relocation may even cause death (Rantz & Egan, 1987; Thorson & Davis, 2000).*
- Protect the client from injuries such as falls. *An increase in the number of accidents in frail elderly can occur with relocation (Lander, Brazill, & Ladrigan, 1997).*
- After the transfer, determine the client's mental status. Document and observe for any new onset of confusion. *Confusion can follow relocation because of the overwhelming stress and sensory overload.*
- ▲ Refer for music therapy. **EBN:** *One case study indicated that music therapy may facilitate a resident's adjustment to life in a long-term-care facility (Kydd, 2001).*
- Use reality orientation if needed (e.g., "Today is . . . ," "The date is . . . ," "You are at . . . facility"). Repeat the information as needed and provide a clock or calendar. *Reality orientation can be helpful to prevent new onset of confusion (Manion & Rantz, 1995).*

R

## Client/Family Teaching

- Teach family members about relocation stress syndrome. Encourage them to monitor for signs of the syndrome. *Acceptance of the new living situation begins within 6 to 8 weeks after institutionalization, and adjustment is usually complete within 3 to 6 months (Manion & Rantz, 1995).*
- Help significant others learn how to support the client in the move by setting up a schedule of visits, arranging for holidays, bringing familiar items from home, and establishing a system for contact when the client needs support.

## evolve WEBSITES FOR EDUCATION

See the EVOLVE website for World Wide Web resources for client education.

## REFERENCES


Davies S, Nolan M: Making the move: relatives' experiences of the transition to a care home, *Health Soc Care Community*, 12(6): 517, 2004.

Dellasega C, Mastrian K: The process and consequences of institutionalizing an elder, *West J Nurs Res* 17(2):123, 1995.

Iwasiw C, Goldenberg D, Bol N et al: Resident and family perspectives: the first year in a long-term care facility, *J Gerontol Nurs* 29(1):45, 2003.

Kao HF, Travis SS, Action GH: Relocation to a long-term facility: working with patients and families before, during, and after, *J Psychos Nurs Ment Health Serv* 42(3):10, 2004.

Kydd P: Using music therapy to help a client with Alzheimer's disease adapt to long-term care, *Am J Alzheimers Dis Other Demen* 16(2):103, 2001.

Lander SM, Brazill AL, Ladrigan PM: Intrainstitutional relocation: effects on residents' behavior and psychosocial functioning, *J Gerontol Nurs* 23(4):35, 1997.

Loeher KE, Bank AL, MacNeill SE et al: Nursing home transition and depressive symptoms in older medical rehabilitation patients, *Clin Gerontol* 27(1/2):59-70, 2004.

Lutgendorf SK, Reimer TT, Harvey JH et al: Effects of housing relocation on immunocompetence and psychosocial functioning in older adults, *J Gerontol A Biol Sci Med Sci* 56(2):M97, 2001.

Lutgendorf SK, Vitaliano PP, Tripp-Reimer T et al: Sense of coherence moderates the relationship between life stress and natural killer cell activity in healthy older adults, *Psychol Aging* 14(4):552, 1999.

Mallick MJ, Whipple TW: Validity of the nursing diagnosis of relocation stress syndrome, *Nurs Res* 49(2):97, 2000.

Manion PD, Rantz MJ: Relocation stress syndrome: a comprehensive plan for long-term care admissions, *Geriatr Nurs* 16(3):108, 1995.

McKinney AA, Deeny P: Leaving the intensive care unit: a phenomenological study of the patients' experience, *Intensive Crit Care Nurs* 18(6):320, 2002.

Mitchell ML, Courtney M, Coyer F: Understanding uncertainty and minimizing families' anxiety at the time of transfer from intensive care, *Nurs Health Sci* 5(3):207, 2003.

Nypaver JM, Titus M, Brugler CJ: Patient transfer to rehabilitation: just another move? Relocation stress syndrome, *Rehabil Nurs* 21(2):94, 1996.

Puskar KR, Dvorsak KG: Relocation stress in adolescents: helping teenagers cope with a moving dilemma, *Pediatr Nurs* 17(3):295, 1991.

Rantz M, Egan K: Reducing death from translocation syndrome, *Am J Nurs* 87(9):1351, 1987.

Spector RE: The transcultural nursing society, *Nurs Spectr* 10(14), 2000.

Stubblefield C, Murray RL: Waiting for lung transplantation: family experiences of relocation, *Pediatr Nurs* 28(5):501, 2002.

Thorson JA, Davis RE: Relocation of the institutionalized aged, *J Clin Psychol* 56(1):131, 2000.

Tracy JP, DeYoung S: Moving to an assisted living facility: exploring the transitional experience of elderly individuals, *J Gerontol Nurs* 30(10):26, 2004.


R

# Risk for Relocation stress syndrome

*Betty J. Ackley*

**NANDA**

### Definition

At risk for physiological and/or psychosocial disturbances that result from transfer from one environment to another

• = Independent; ▲ = Collaborative; EBN = Evidence-Based Nursing; EB = Evidence-Based

## Risk Factors

Moderate to high degree of environmental change (e.g., physical, ethnic, cultural); temporary and/or permanent move; voluntary and/or involuntary move; lack of adequate support system/group; feelings of powerlessness; moderate mental competence (e.g., alert enough to experience changes); unpredictability of experiences; decreased psychosocial or physical health status; lack of predeparture counseling; passive coping; past, current, or recent losses

**NOC**

## Outcomes (Nursing Outcomes Classification)

### Suggested NOC Outcomes

Anxiety Self-Control; Child Adaptation to Hospitalization; Coping; Loneliness Severity; Psychosocial Adjustment: Life Change; Quality of Life

**Example NOC Outcome with Indicators**

**Anxiety Self-Control** as evidenced by the following indicators: Seeks information to reduce anxiety/Plans coping strategies for stressful situations/Uses effective coping strategies/Uses relaxation techniques to reduce anxiety/Maintains social relationships/Maintains adequate sleep/Controls anxiety response (Rate each indicator of **Anxiety Self-Control:** 1 = never demonstrated, 2 = rarely demonstrated, 3 = sometimes demonstrated, 4 = often demonstrated, 5 = consistently demonstrated [see Section I].)

## Client Outcomes, Nursing Interventions and Rationales, Client/Family Teaching

Refer to the care plan for **Relocation stress syndrome.**

# Ineffective Role performance

R

*Gail B. Ladwig*

**NANDA**

## Definition

Patterns of behavior and self-expression that do not match the environmental context, norms, and expectations

## Defining Characteristics

Change in self-perception of role, role denial, inadequate external support for role enactment, inadequate adaptation to change or transition, system conflict, change in usual patterns of responsibility, discrimination, domestic violence, harassment uncertainty, altered role perceptions, role strain, inadequate self-management, role ambivalence, pessimistic attitude, inadequate motivation, inadequate confidence, inadequate role competency and skills, inadequate knowledge, inappropriate developmental expectations, role conflict, role confusion, powerlessness, inadequate coping, anxiety or depression, role overload, change in other's perception or role, role dissatisfaction, inadequate opportunities for role enactment

## Related Factors (r/t)

### Social

Inadequate or inappropriate linkage with the health care system; job schedule demands; young age; developmental level; lack of rewards; poverty; family conflict; inadequate support system; inadequate role socialization (e.g., role model, expectations responsibilities); low socioeconomic status; stress and conflict; domestic violence; lack of resources

### Knowledge

Inadequate role preparation (e.g., role transition, skill, rehearsal, validation); lack of knowledge about role, role skills; role transition; lack of opportunity for role rehearsal; developmental transitions; unrealistic role expectations; education attainment level; lack of or inadequate role model

### Physiological

Inadequate/inappropriate linkage with health care system; substance abuse; mental illness; body image alteration; physical illness; cognitive deficits; health alterations (e.g., physical health, body image, self-esteem, mental health, psychosocial health, cognitive, learning style, neurological health); depression; low self-esteem; pain; fatigue

NOTE: The typology of roles includes sociopersonal (friendship, family, marital, parenting, community), home management intimacy (sexuality, relationship building), leisure/exercise/recreation, self-management, socialization (developmental transitions), community contributor, and religious.

**NOC**

## Outcomes (Nursing Outcomes Classification)

### Suggested NOC Outcomes

Coping; Psychosocial Adjustment: Life Change; Role Performance

**Example NOC Outcome with Indicators**

**Role Performance** as evidenced by the following indicators: Ability to meet role expectations/Knowledge of role transition periods/Reported strategies for role change(s) (Rate each indicator of **Role Performance:** 1 = Not adequate, 2 = Slightly adequate, 3 = Moderately adequate, 4 = Substantially adequate, 5 = Totally adequate [see Section I].)

## Client Outcomes

**Client Will (Specify Time Frame):**

- Identify realistic perception of role



R

- State personal strengths
- Acknowledge problems contributing to inability to carry out usual role
- Accept physical limitations regarding role responsibility and consider ways to change lifestyle to accomplish goals associated with role performance
- Demonstrate knowledge of appropriate behaviors associated with new or changed role
- State knowledge of change in responsibility and new behaviors associated with new responsibility
- Verbalize acceptance of new responsibility

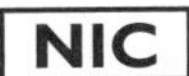

## Interventions (Nursing Interventions Classification)

### Suggested NIC Intervention

Role Enhancement

**Example NIC Activities—Role Enhancement**

Assist the client to identify behaviors needed for new or changed roles; assist the client to identify positive strategies for managing role changes

## Nursing Interventions and Rationales

### Social

- Observe the client's knowledge of behaviors associated with role. *Ability to perform perceived roles is easily hampered by illness. It is important to note whether or not the client feels capable of functioning in the usual role.*
- Ask the client direct questions regarding new roles and how the health care system can help him or her continue in roles. **EBN:** *This article suggests that best practice with regard to communication in palliative care could be achieved by using a sensitive assessment of how each client chooses to cope with his or her situation rather than a uniform approach to care (Dean, 2002).*
- Allow the client to express feelings regarding the role change. **EBN:** *In a study to determine how cancer affects men's role as a father, this central theme—change in self-image as a man and as a parent—was generated. This theme consists of the subthemes gaining control, balancing emotions, subjective well-being, being open or not toward the family, and challenges in family life and to family well-being (Elmberger & Bolund, 2002).*
- Reinforce the client's strengths, have the client identify past coping skills, and support the continued use of these skills. **EB:** *Behavioral change is facilitated by a personal sense of control. If people believe that they can take action to solve a problem instrumentally, they become more inclined to do so and feel more committed to this decision (Schwarzer & Fuchs, 1995).*
- Have the client make a list of strengths that are needed for the new role. Acknowledge which strengths the client has and which strengths need to be developed. Work with the client to set goals for desired role. *In setting valued goals, people adapt their world*

R

*to self-generated needs and projects rather than adapting themselves to a given world (Nuttin, 1992).*

- Have the client list problems associated with the new role and identify ways of overcoming them (e.g., if pain is worse late in day, have the client complete necessary role tasks early in day). *There are many ways to accomplish tasks; help the client recognize this and make the appropriate accommodations.*
- Support the client's religious practices. **EB:** *Religion plays a role in helping clients cope with illness and the outcomes of illness (Koenig, Larson, & Larson, 2001).*

## Physiological

▲ Identify ways to compensate for physical disabilities (e.g., have a ramp built to provide access to house, put household objects within the client's reach from wheelchair) and provide technological assistance when available. **EB:** *Among people with disability, use of assistive technology was associated with use of fewer hours of personal assistance. (Hoenig, Taylor, & Sloan, 2003)*

- Refer to the care plans for **Readiness for enhanced family Coping, Impaired Home maintenance, Impaired Parenting, Risk for Loneliness, Readiness for enhanced community Coping,** and **Ineffective Sexuality patterns.**

## Pediatric

- Assist new parents to adjust to changes in workload associated with childbirth. **EB:** *Expectant parents in this study anticipated increase in workload after childbirth. Work increases were greater for women than men (Gjerdingen, 2000).*
- Assist parents in coping with infants with colic, a condition common in infants. **EBN:** *Even though nursing interventions do not cure infant colic, the amount of crying may be reduced and life made easier for the families if the parents are offered help in coping with the situation (Helseth et al, 2002).*

▲ Refer to home health agency for home visits when there is an infant who has excessive crying. **EBN:** *Almost every aspect of family life was disrupted when there was an infant who cried excessively, resulting in strained relationships, feelings of guilt, and concerns about losing control. This study showed the benefit of a health visitor to support parents. This visitor needed to visit frequently, stay for a prolonged period, demonstrate engagement with the family and its difficulties, and impart specific messages with conviction and sincerity (Long & Johnson, 2001).*

- Provide parents with coping skills when the role change is associated with a critically ill child. **EBN:** *Results from mothers who received the Creating Opportunities for Parent Empowerment (COPE) program indicate the need to educate parents regarding their children's responses as they recover from critical illness and how they can assist their children in coping with the stressful experience (Melnyk et al, 1997).*
- Assist families with life beyond the hospital when living with the illness of a child. Teach family members to value the small things children do, connect with other families, locate community resources, and understand the short- and long-term needs of the child. *Family-focused activities can help families cope better with the hospital experience. To promote optimal healing, health care providers must recognize that a family's life goes on*

R

*after the hospital stay. Many stresses make life difficult for families. Most families are resilient, but many can benefit from help with managing the transition from hospital to home (Worthington, 1995).*

- ▲ Consider the use of media-based behavioral treatments for children with behavioral disorders. **EBN:** *Prevalence studies show that behaviors problems in children are quite common (10% to 15% in preschoolers). For straightforward cases media-based interventions may be enough to make clinically significant changes in a child's behavior. Media-based therapies appear to have both clinical and economic implications as regards the treatment of children with behavioral problems (Montgomery, 2005).*

## Geriatric

- ▲ Provide support for grandparents raising grandchildren. **EBN:** *Most grandparents raising grandchildren reported that their health was compromised (Gibbons & Jones, 2003).*
- ▲ Support the client's religious beliefs and activities and provide appropriate spiritual support persons. **EB:** *The findings from this study suggest that religious coping is a common behavior that is inversely related to depression in hospitalized elderly men (Koenig et al, 1992).*
- • Encourage the use of humor by family caregivers to describe their role reversal. **EB:** *This study suggested that humor is a useful communication tool for family caregivers that release nervous energy (Bethea et al, 2000).*
- • Explore community needs after assessing the client's strengths. Suggest functional activities (e.g., being a foster grandparent or a mentor for small businesses). *If physical strength is declining, activities that require less physical prowess and more mental expertise are sometimes appropriate (Ringsven & Bond, 1991).*
- ▲ Refer to appropriate support groups for adjustment to role changes. **EBN:** *Health care professionals should provide information on PD symptom management, identify appropriate resources to reduce caregiver burden, and use of support groups (Edwards et al, 2002).* **EBN:** *Significant differences were found for distress levels and quality of life, with the mutual support group having greater improvements than the control group for dementia family caregivers (Fung & Chien, 2002).*
- ▲ Refer to therapy to improve memory for patients with Alzheimer's disease. **EB:** *The available evidence shows that alternative and innovative ways of memory rehabilitation for Alzheimer's patients can indeed be clinically effective or pragmatically useful with a great potential for use within the new culture of a more graded and proactive type of Alzheimer's disease care (De Vreese et al, 2001).* **EB:** *Facing an inevitable decline, persons with early-stage dementia and their care partners found it helpful to talk with one another and with peers in the same circumstances about the disease and its effects in this memory club (Zarit et al, 2004).*

R

## Multicultural

- • Assess for the influence of cultural beliefs, norms, values, and expectations on the individual's role. **EBN:** *The individual's role may be based on cultural perceptions (Cochran, 1998; Doswell & Erlen, 1998; Leininger & McFarland, 2002).*
- • Assess for conflicts between the caregiver's cultural role obligations and competing factors like employment or school. **EBN:** *Conflicts between cultural expectations and*

*competing factors can increase role stress (Jones, 1996). Mexican immigrant children provide essential help to their families, including translating, interpreting, and caring for siblings (Orellana, 2003). A recent study found that African-American caregivers experienced a wide range of caregiver role strain (Wallace Williams, Dilworth-Anderson, & Goodwin, 2003).*

- Negotiate with the client regarding the aspects of their role that can be modified and still honor cultural beliefs. **EBN:** *Give and take with the client will lead to culturally congruent care (Leininger & McFarland, 2002).*
- Encourage family to use support groups or other service programs to assist with role changes. **EBN:** *Studies indicate that minority families of clients with dementia use few support programs even though these programs could have a positive impact on caregiver well-being (Cox, 1999).*
- Validate the individual's feelings regarding the impact of role changes on family and personal lifestyle. **EBN:** *Validation lets the client know that the nurse has heard and understands what was said (Heineken, 1998).*

### Home Care

- Above interventions may be adapted for home care use.
- Determine the anticipated duration of role change. *Knowing the anticipated duration of role change helps the client and significant others determine the acceptability of role change, role conflict, and changes in communication patterns.*
- Assess family's ability to physically or psychologically assume responsibilities of decrease or change in the client's role function. *The health, abilities, or other role expectations of caregivers or significant others may prohibit the assumption of responsibilities once held by the client.*
- ▲ Offer a referral to medical social services to assist with assessing the short- and long-term impacts of role change. *Social workers may assist clients with life care planning (Rice et al, 2000). Collaboration with specialists provides the client with greater resources for adaptation. Terminally ill clients may see the transition of role responsibilities as a task that must be completed before dying. Resolution of role transition will reassure the client, allow remaining energy to be focused elsewhere, and may give the client permission to die.*

## Client/Family Teaching

- Provide educational materials to family members on patient behavior management plus caregiver stress-coping management. **EB:** *Data in this study suggest that brief primary care interventions as described above may be effective in reducing caregiver distress and burden in the long-term management of the dementia patient (Burns et al, 2003).*
- Help the client identify resources for assistance in caring for a disabled or aging parent (e.g., adult day care). **EBN:** *The wives of men with chronic obstructive pulmonary disease (COPD) in this phenomenological study were dissatisfied with their lack of recreation, as well as support from friends, families, and health care providers (Bergs, 2002).*
- ▲ Refer to appropriate community agencies to learn skills for functioning in the new or changed role (e.g., vocational rehabilitation, parenting classes, hospice, respite care). *As one person changes, other family members need to alter their patterns of communication and behavior to maintain balance. Family members also need assistance with developing these new skills (Barry, 1994).*

## evolve WEBSITES FOR EDUCATION

See the EVOLVE website for World Wide Web resources for client education.

## REFERENCES


Barry P: *Mental health and mental illness,* ed 5, Philadelphia, 1994, JB Lippincott.

Bergs D: "The Hidden Client"—women caring for husbands with COPD: their experience of quality of life, *J Clin Nurs* 11(5): 613, 2002.

Bethea LS, Travis SS, Pecchioni L: Family caregivers' use of humor in conveying information about caring for dependent older adults, *Health Commun* 12(4):361, 2000.

Burns R, Nichols LO, Martindale-Adams J et al: Primary care interventions for dementia caregivers: 2-year outcomes from the REACH study, *Gerontologist* 43(4):547-555, 2003.

Cochran M: Tears have no color, *Am J Nurs* 98(6):53, 1998.

Cox C: Race and caregiving: patterns of service use by African American and white caregivers of persons with Alzheimer's, *J Gerontol Soc Work* 32(2):5, 1999.

De Vreese LP, Neri M, Fioravanti M et al: Memory rehabilitation in Alzheimer's disease: a review of progress, *Int J Geriatr Psychiatry* 16(8):794, 2001.

Dean A: Talking to dying clients of their hopes and needs, *Nurs Times* 98(43):34, 2002.

Doswell W, Erlen J: Multicultural issues and ethical concerns in the delivery of revising care interventions, *Nurs Clin North Am* 33(2):353, 1998.

Edwards NE, Scheetz PS: Predictors of burden for caregivers of patients with Parkinson's disease, *J Neurosci Nurs* 34(4):184, 2002.

Elmberger E, Bolund C: Men with cancer. Changes in attempts to master the self-image as a man and as a parent, *Cancer Nurs* 25(6):477, 2002.

Fleury J: The application of motivational theory to cardiovascular risk reduction, *Image J Nurs Sch* 24:229, 1992.

Fung WY, Chien WT: The effectiveness of a mutual support group for family caregivers of a relative with dementia, *Arch Psychiatr Nurs* 16(3):134, 2002.

Gibbons C, Jones TC: Kinship care: health profiles of grandparents raising their grandchildren, *J Fam Soc Work* 7(1):1-14, 2003.

Gjerdingen D: Expectant parents' anticipated changes in workload after the birth of their first child, *J Fam Pract* 49(11):993, 2000.

Heineken J: Patient silence is not necessarily client satisfaction: communication in home care nursing, *Home Healthc Nurs* 16(2): 115, 1998.

Helseth S: Help in times of crying: nurses' approach to parents with colicky infants, *J Adv Nurs* 40(3):267, 2002.

Hoenig H, Taylor DH Jr, Sloan FA: Does assistive technology substitute for personal assistance among the disabled elderly? *Am J Public Health* 93(2):330-337, 2003.

Jones PS: Asian American women caring for elderly parents, *J Fam Nurs* 2(1):56, 1996.

Koenig HG, Larson DB, Larson SS: Religion and coping with serious medical illness, *Ann Pharmacotherapy* 35(3): 352, 2001.

Koenig HG, Cohen HJ, Blazer DG et al: Religious coping and depression among elderly, hospitalized medically ill men, *Am J Psychiatry* 149(12):1693, 1992.

Leininger MM, McFarland MR: *Transcultural nursing: concepts, theories, research and practices,* ed 3, New York, 2002, McGraw-Hill.

Long T, Johnson M: Living and coping with excessive infantile crying, *J Adv Nurs* 34(2):155, 2001.

Mann WC, Llanes C, Justiss MD et al: Frail older adults' self-report of their most important assistive device, *Occup Ther J Res* 24(1):4-12, 2004.

Melnyk BM, Alpert-Gillis LJ, Hensel PB et al: Helping mothers cope with a critically ill child: a pilot test of the COPE intervention, *Res Nurs Health* 20(1):3, 1997.

Montgomery M: Media-based behavioural treatments for behavioural disorders in children, *Cochrane Database Syst Rev* (1): CD002206, 2005

Orellana MF: Responsibilities of children in Latino immigrant homes, *New Dir Youth Dev* (100):25-39, 2003.

Rice J, Hicks PB, Wiehe V: Life care planning: a role for social workers, *Soc Work Health Care* 31(1):85, 2000.

Ringsven M, Bond D: *Gerontology and leadership skills for nurses,* Albany, NY, 1991, Delmar.

Schwarzer R, Fuchs R: Self-efficacy and health behaviors. In Conner M, Norman P, editors: *Predicting health behaviour: research and practice with social cognition models,* Buckingham, UK, 1995, Open University Press.

Wallace Williams S, Dilworth-Anderson P, Goodwin PY: Caregiver role strain: the contribution of multiple roles and available resources in African-American women, *Aging Ment Health* 7(2):103-12, 2003.


R

Worthington R: Effective transitions for families: life beyond the hospital, *Pediatr Nurs* 21(1):86, 1995.
Zarit SH, Femia EE, Watson J et al: Memory Club: a group intervention for people with early-stage dementia and their care partners, *Gerontologist* 44(2):262-9, 2004.

# Bathing/hygiene Self-care deficit

evolve

*Linda S. Williams*

NANDA

## Definition

Impaired ability to perform or complete bathing/hygiene activities for oneself

## Defining Characteristics

Inability to wash body or body parts, obtain or get to water source, regulate temperature or flow of bath water, get bath supplies, dry body, get in and out of bathroom

Impaired physical mobility-functional level classification:
0—Completely independent
1—Requires use of equipment or device
2—Requires help from another person for assistance, supervision, or teaching
3—Requires help from another person and equipment or device
4—Dependent (does not participate in activity)

## Related Factors (r/t)

Decreased or lack of motivation, weakness and tiredness, severe anxiety, inability to perceive body part or spatial relationship, perceptual or cognitive impairment, pain, neuromuscular impairment, musculoskeletal impairment, environmental barriers

NOC

## Outcomes (Nursing Outcomes Classification)

### Suggested NOC Outcomes

Self-Care: Activities of Daily Living (ADLs), Bathing, Hygiene

**Example NOC Outcome with Indicators**

**Self-Care: Activities of Daily Living (ADLs)** as evidenced by the following indicators: Bathing/Hygiene (Rate each indicator of **Self-Care: Activities of Daily Living (ADLs):** 1 = severely compromised, 2 = substantially compromised, 3 = moderately compromised, 4 = mildly compromised, 5 = not compromised [see Section I].)

## Client Outcomes

**Client Will (Specify Time Frame):**

- Remain free of body odor and maintain intact skin



S

- Bathe with assistance of caregiver as needed and report sense of dignity is maintained
- Bathe with assistance of caregiver as needed without exhibiting aggressive behaviors
- State satisfaction with ability to use adaptive devices to bathe
- Use methods to bathe safely with minimal difficulty

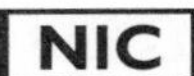

## Interventions (Nursing Interventions Classification)

### Suggested NIC Interventions

Bathing; Self-Care Assistance: Bathing/Hygiene

**Example NIC Activities—Self-Care Assistance: Bathing/Hygiene**

Monitor the client's ability for independent self-care; provide assistance until the client is fully able to assume self-care

## Nursing Interventions and Rationales

- If in a typical bathing setting for the client, assess the client's ability to bathe self via direct observation using physical performance tests for ADLs. *Observation of bathing performed in an atypical bathing setting may result in false data for which use of a physical performance test compensates to provide more accurate ability data.*
- Ask the client for input on bathing habits and cultural bathing preferences. **EB:** *Creating opportunities for guiding personal care honors long-standing routines, increases control, and makes bath time more pleasant for caregiver (Perimutter & Camberg, 2004).*
- Develop a bathing care plan based on the client's own history of bathing practices that addresses skin needs, self-care needs, client response to bathing, and equipment needs. *Bathing is a healing rite and should be a comforting experience that concentrates on the client's needs, rather than being a routinely scheduled task (Rasin & Barrick, 2004).*
- Individualize bathing by identifying function of bath (e.g., odor, urine removal), frequency required to achieve function, and best bathing form (e.g., towel bathing, tub, shower) to meet client preferences, preserve client dignity, make bathing a soothing experience, and reduce client aggression. **EB:** *Individualized bathing produces a more positive bathing experience and preserves client dignity. Client aggression is increased with shower (especially) and tub bathing. Towel bathing increases privacy and eliminates need to move the client to central bathing area; therefore it is a more soothing experience than either showering or tub bathing (Perimutter & Camberg, 2004).*
- ▲ Request referrals for occupational and physical therapy. *Collaboration and correlation of activities with interdisciplinary team members increases the client's mastery of self-care tasks.*
- Plan activities to prevent fatigue during bathing; seat the client with feet supported. *Energy conservation increases activity tolerance and promotes self-care.*
- Provide pain relief measures: ice packs, heat, and analgesics 45 minutes before bathing if needed. *Pain relief promotes participation in self-care, and preserves dignity.*
- Consider environmental and human factors that may limit bathing ability, such as

S

bending to get into tub, reaching required for bathing items, grasping force needed for faucets, and lifting of self. Adapt environment by placing items within easy reach, lowering faucets, and using a hand held shower. *Environmental factors affect task performance. Function can be improved based on engineering principles that adapt environmental factors to the meet the client's capabilities.*

- Teach use of adaptive bathing equipment (e.g., long-handled brushes, soap-on-a-rope, washcloth mitt, wall bars, tub bench, shower chair, commode chair without pan in shower) and follow up in the home. **EB:** *Adaptive devices extend the client's reach, increase speed and safety, and decrease exertion and reduce caregiver burden (Chen et al, 2000). Follow-up teaching in the home increases device use and safety of bathing (Chiu & Man, 2004). Identification of the client's likelihood of using devices such as the long-handled brush allows for alternate device planning (Rogers et al, 2002).*
- Ensure bathing assistance preserves client dignity through conveyance of honor and recognition of the deservedness of respect and esteem of all persons regardless of their dependency and infirmity. **EB:** *Needing assistance with bathing, being hospitalized, and having pain, were among the most significant issues fracturing a sense of the terminally ill client's dignity (defined as being worthy of honor, respect, or esteem), which resulted in a higher desire for death and loss of will to live; thus dignity-conserving care should be part of palliative care for all clients near death (Chochinov et al, 2002).*
- Provide privacy: have only one caregiver providing bathing assistance, encourage a traffic-free bathing area, and postprivacy signs. *The client perceives less privacy if more than one caregiver participates or if bathing takes place in a central bathing area in a high-traffic location that allows staff to enter freely during care (Calkins, 2005).*
- Keep the client warmly covered. *Clients, especially elderly clients who are prone to hypothermia, may experience evaporative cooling during and after bathing, which produces an unpleasant cold sensation.*
- Enhance communication during bathing. Allow the client to participate as able in bathing. Smile and provide praise for accomplishments in a relaxed manner. **EB:** *Improved communication decreases aggression during bathing and individualizes care (Perimutter & Camberg, 2004).*
- Inspect skin condition during bathing. *Observation of skin allows detection of skin problems. Towel bathing facilitates inspection of skin.*
- Use or encourage caregiver to use an unhurried, caring touch. *The basic human need of touch offers reassurance and comfort.*
- If the client is bathing alone, place assistance call light within reach. *A readily available signaling device promotes safety and provides reassurance for the client.*
- Bathe cognitively impaired clients before bedtime. *Bathing a cognitively impaired client in the evening helps improve symptoms of dementia (Deguchi et al, 1999).*
- Nurture personal attributes such as humor, positive attitude, faith, and hope. Control stress for clients with multiple sclerosis. **EBN:** *For those with multiple sclerosis, personal attributes intervene between emotional distress and ADL functioning by decreasing a stress appraisal response (Gulick, 2001).* **EBN:** *Continue rehabilitation efforts with post-stroke client's long-term to achieve optimal functioning. Client improvement may continue 6 months or longer poststroke (Cavanagh et al, 2002).*

S

## Geriatric

- Assess client's ability to perform ADLs independently with the Katz Index of Independence in Activities of Daily Living. *The Katz Index is the most appropriate instrument for assessing client's ADL abilities (Shelkey & Wallace, 1998).*
- Assess self-efficacy (The Self-Efficacy for Functional Activities scale); assess outcome expectations (Outcome Expectations for Functional Activities scale). Based on assessment, promote motivation and self-efficacy for ADL functioning by role modeling via videotape or partnering; verbal encouragement; individualize care using humor, kindness, joy, and excitement with achievements; social supports; and decrease unpleasant sensations with the ADL function. **EBN:** *Assessment and interventions for self-efficacy strengthen client efficacy expectations and improve functional performance (Resnick, 2002).*
- Assess for grieving resulting from loss of function. *Grief resulting from loss of function can inhibit relearning of self-care.*
- Develop client muscle strength building plan through exercise to build the client's physiological capacity and prevent decline in ADLs. **EB:** *Older adults who live in assisted living may have declines in their ADLs that access to a physical activity program can reverse. Maintaining independence in ADLs is vital to a sense of dignity and autonomy (Taylor et al, 2003).*
- Include exercise and walking program in plan of care. **EB:** *Exercise for flexibility, strengthening, and a walking program in the hospital promotes ADLs, prevents injury, increases quality of life, and may delay admission to a long-term care facility (Hart et al, 2002; Penninx, 2001).*
- Provide same type of bathrobe and bathing articles, such as scented dusting powder and bath oil, that the client used previously. *Use of sensory channels to stimulate memory may help foster understanding of bathing and self-care.*
- Emphasize how client experiences the bathing setting with secondary focus on ways environment can support caregiver. *Recognizing and supporting cognitive, emotional, psychological, spiritual, and physical needs of individuals should be reflected in spaces where the most personal care—such as bathing—is provided, which demonstrates the quality of a care setting (Calkins, 2005).*
- ▲ Design bathing environment for comfort: *Visual.* Reduce clutter and use partitions to hide equipment storage. Consider what bather looks at as he/she enters room and bathes. Reduce institutional signs and blend into background. Laminate and put artwork or decorative objects in bather's view, or cue cards to bathing process (wall, ceiling, shower). Stand or sit in bather's position to experience what he/she see. Decrease glare from tiles, white walls, and artificial lights. Use contrasting colors and soft but adequate lighting on a dimming switch for adjustment. *Bathing rooms are sterile, institutional, and frightening spaces filled with unfamiliar equipment—tubs with sides that open up and look like they might swallow you or gurneys with arms that look like construction cranes. Overhead lights can be bright and shine into the bather's eyes. Glare can cause visual discomfort, especially in clients with visual changes or cataracts (Calkins, 2005).*
- Arrange bathing environment to promote sensory comfort: *Auditory.* Reduce noise of voices and water. Do not allow traffic into bathing room. Add fabric to absorb sound

S

(three to four times the width of the opening for sound absorbing folds). Play soft music. *Noise discomfort can result from high-echo tiled walls, loud voices, and running water. Traffic can compromise privacy. Absorb negative sounds, and add positive sounds through music. (Calkins, 2005).*

- Design bathing environment for comfort: *Tactile.* Use heat lamps or radiant heat panels to keep room warm. Use warmed towels. Use powder-coated grab bars in decorative colors with non-slip grip. Provide soft rug to stand on. Ensure flooring is not slippery (a high coefficient of friction, ideally above 80, is desired and obtained through flooring coatings). *If caregiver is warm, to point of sweating, room temperature is about right for older person being bathed. Warm towels and soft rugs make bathing a much more luxuriant experience. Appealing stable grab bars are needed for balance. Preventing slippery floor from water is essential (Calkins, 2005).*
- Teach caregivers to use behaviors that validate client's feelings, reassure, segment tasks, and explain the care process while bathing Alzheimer's clients. **EBN:** *Caregivers should work to make bathing more therapeutic for individuals with Alzheimer's disease (Somboontanont et al, 2004).*
- Advise caregivers to initiate shower spray or touch during bathing carefully with verbal prompts beforehand. **EBN:** *Assaults are particularly likely to occur when caregivers spray water on a resident without letting the individual know in advance or when they touch resident's feet, axilla, or perineum possibly due to the startle reflex (Somboontanont et al, 2004).*
- Train caregivers bathing those with Alzheimer's disease to avoid behaviors that can trigger assault: confrontational communication, invalidation of resident's feelings, failure to prepare a resident for a task, speaking disrespectfully to the client, and a hurried pace of the bath. **EBN:** *Assaults by nursing home residents with Alzheimer's disease during bathing arc frequently triggered by caregiver actions that frighten, hurt, or upset the resident (Somboontanont et al, 2004).*
- When bathing a cognitively impaired client, have all bathing items ready for the client's needs before bathing begins. *Injury often occurs when cognitively impaired client is left alone while forgotten items are obtained.*
- Teach caregiver to use massage for frail elderly clients during bathing. *Massage is desired by clients to reduce pain or agitation (Perimutter & Camberg, 2004).*
- Bathe elderly clients before bedtime to improve sleep. *An evening bath helps elderly clients sleep better (Kanda et al, 1999).*
- Limit bathing to once or twice a week; provide a partial bath at other times. Frequent bathing promotes skin dryness. *Reducing frequency of bathing decreases aggressive behavior in cognitively impaired clients.*
- Allow the client or caregiver adequate time to complete the bathing activity. *Significant aging increases the time required to complete a task; therefore elderly individuals with a self-care deficit require more time to complete a task.*
- Use a nondetergent, no-rinse cleanser for bed bathing rather than soap and water. **EBN:** *Nondetergent, no-rinse cleanser bathing reduces skin tears and saves money for skin tear treatment costs, reduces bathing time, and eliminates soap residue on the skin (Burch & Coggins, 2003).*
- Avoid soap or use only mild soap on genital and axillary areas; rinse well. *Soap can alter*

*skin pH and thus skin defenses, and it may increase skin dryness that results from decreased oil and perspiration production in the elderly.*

- Use tepid water. *Hot water promotes skin dryness.*
- Test water temperature before use with thermometer. *With assistive bathing, temperature changes are not felt by the person controlling them (Fathers, 2004).*
- Recommend use of water temperature–sensing shower valve to prevent scalding. *Older or disabled people have slower reflexes to respond to hot water, yet may be left unattended although they are unable to regulate water temperature; water at 130° F takes 20 seconds to produce a first-degree burn; at 135–140° F, 5–6 seconds causes third-degree burns (Fathers, 2004).*
- Use a gentle touch when bathing; avoid vigorous scrubbing motions. *Aging skin is thinner, more fragile, and less able to withstand mechanical friction than younger skin.*
- Add hydrating bath oils to tub bath water 15 minutes after the client immerses in water. *Client's skin is coated with oil rather than being hydrated if bath oil is placed in water before the client's skin is moistened with water.*

### Home Care

- ▲ Based on functional assessment and rehabilitation capacity, refer for home health aide services to assist with bathing and hygiene. *Support by home health aides preserves the energy of the client and provides respite for caregivers.*
- Turn down temperature of hot water heater. **EBN:** *Prevent accidental scalding by reducing thermostat on water heater (Gerdner, 2002).*
- Show caregiver videotape of caregiver self-care activities (organizing day, talking when frustrated, self-time, and nonjudgmental person with whom to talk) followed by a discussion. **EBN:** *Videotape intervention and discussion can model self-care activities and buffer caregiver stress (Clark & Lester, 2000).*
- Cue cognitively impaired clients in steps of hygiene. *Cognitively impaired clients can successfully participate in many activities with cueing, and participation in self-care can enhance their self-esteem.*
- Respect the preference of terminally ill clients to refuse or limit hygiene care. *Maintaining hygiene, even with assistance, may require excessive energy demands from terminally ill clients. Pain on touch or movement may be intractable and not resolved by medication.*
- If a terminally ill client requests hygiene care, make an extra effort to meet request and provide care when client and family will most benefit (e.g., before visitors, at bedtime, in the early morning). *When desired, improved hygiene greatly boosts the morale of terminally ill clients.*
- Maintain temperature of home at a comfortable level when providing hygiene care to terminally ill clients. *Terminally ill clients may have difficulty with thermoregulation, which will add to the energy demand or decrease comfort during hygiene care.*

S

### Client/Family Teaching

- Teach the client and family how to use adaptive devices for bathing, and teach bathing techniques that promote safety and prevent burns (e.g., getting into tub before filling it with water if temperature sensor valve used, testing water with thermometer, emptying water before getting out, using an antislip mat, wall-grab bars, tub bench). *Adaptive devices can provide independence, safety, and speed. Burns can be prevented with the use of water temperature sensor valve (Fathers, 2004).*

- Teach the client and family an individualized bathing routine that includes a schedule, privacy, skin inspection, soap or lubricant, and chill prevention. *Teaching methods to meet the client's needs increases client's satisfaction with the bathing experience.*

## evolve WEBSITES FOR EDUCATION

See the EVOLVE website for World Wide Web resources for client education.

## REFERENCES


Burch S, Coggins T: No rinse, one step bed bath: the effects on the occurrence of skin tears in a long-term care setting, *Ostomy Wound Manag* 49(1):64, 2003.

Calkins M: Designing bathing rooms that comfort, *Nurs Homes* 54(1):54-55, 2005.

Cavanagh S Hogan K, Fairfax J et al: Assessing cognitive function after stroke using the FIM instrument, *J Neurosci Nurs* 34(2):99, 2002.

Chen T-Y A., Mann W, Tomita M et al: Caregiver involvement in the use of assistive devices by frail older persons, *OTJR* 20: 179-199, 2000.

Chochinov H, Hack T, Hassard T et al: Dignity in the terminally ill: a cross-sectional, cohort study, *Lancet* 360(9350):2026-2030, 2002.

Chiu C, Man D: The effect of training older adults with stroke to use home-based assistive devices, *OTJR* 24(3):113-120, 2004.

Clark M, Lester J: The effect of video-based interventions on self-care, *West J Nurs Res* 22(8):895, 2000.

Deguchi A, Nakamura S, Yoneyama S et al: Improving symptoms of senile dementia by a night time spa bathing, *Arch Gerontol Geriatr* 29(3):267, 1999.

Fathers B: Bathing safety for the elderly and disabled, *Nurs Homes* 53(9):50-52, 2004.

Gerdner LA, Buckwalter KC, Reed D: Impact of a psychoeducational intervention on caregiver response to behavioral problems, *Nurs Res* 51(6):363, 2002.

Gulick E: Emotional distress and activities of daily living functioning in persons with multiple sclerosis, *Nurs Res* 50(3):147, 2001.

Hart BD, Birkas J, Lachmann M et al: Promoting positive outcomes for elderly persons in the hospital: prevention and risk factor modification, *AACN Clin Issues* 13(1):22, 2002.

Kanda K, Tochihara Y, Ohnaka T: Bathing before sleep in the young and in the elderly, *Eur J Appl Physiol* 80:71, 1999.

Penninx BW, Messier SP, Rejeski WJ et al: Physical exercise and the prevention of disability in activities of daily living in older persons with osteoarthritis, *Arch Intern Med* 161(19):2309, 2001.

Perimutter J, Camberg L: Better bathing for residents with Alzheimer's, *Nurs Homes* 53(4):40-42, 2004.

Rasin J, Barrick AL: Bathing patients with dementia, *Am J Nurs* 104(3):30-34, 2004.

Resnick B: The impact of self-efficacy and outcome expectations on functional status in older adults, *Top Geriatr Rehabil* 17(4):1, 2002.

Rogers J, Holm M, Perkins L: Trajectory of assistive device usage and user and non-user characteristics: long-handled bath sponge, *Arthritis Rheum* 47(6):645, 2002.

Shelkey M, Wallace M: Katz Index of Independence in Activities of Daily Living. In *Try this: best practices in nursing care to older adults*, Issue 2, October 1998, The Hartford Institute for Geriatric Nursing.

Somboontanont W, Sloane P, Floyd F et al: Assaultive behavior in Alzheimer's disease: identifying immediate antecedents during bathing, *J Gerontol Nurs* 30(9):22-29, 2004.

Taylor L, Whittington F, Hollingsworth C et al: A comparison of functional outcomes following a physical activity intervention for frail older adults in personal care homes, *J Geriatr Phys Ther* 26(1):7-11, 2003.


S

# Dressing/grooming Self-care deficit

*Linda S. Williams*

**NANDA**

## Definition

Impaired ability to perform or complete dressing and grooming activities for self

## Defining Characteristics

Impaired ability to put on or take off necessary items of clothing, impaired ability to fasten clothing, impaired ability to obtain or replace articles of clothing, inability to clothe upper body, inability to clothe lower body, inability to choose clothing, inability to use assistive devices, inability to use zippers, inability to remove clothes, inability to put on socks, inability to maintain appearance at a satisfactory level, inability to pick up clothing, inability to put on shoes

## Related Factors (r/t)

Decreased or lack of motivation, pain, severe anxiety, perceptual or cognitive impairment, weakness or tiredness, neuromuscular impairment, musculoskeletal impairment, discomfort, environmental barriers

NOTE: See suggested Functional Level Classification in care plan for **Impaired physical Mobility.**

**NOC**

## Outcomes (Nursing Outcomes Classification)

### Suggested NOC Outcomes

Self-Care: Activities of Daily Living (ADLs), Dressing, Hygiene, Grooming

S

**Example NOC Outcome with Indicators**

**Self-Care: Dressing** as evidenced by the following indicators: Gets clothes from closet and puts on upper body, lower body (Rate each indicator of **Self-Care: Dressing:** 1 = severely compromised, 2 = substantially compromised, 3 = moderately compromised, 4 = mildly compromised, 5 = not compromised [see Section I].)

## Client Outcomes

### Client Will (Specify Time Frame):

- Dress and groom self to optimal potential
- Use adaptive devices to dress and groom

- Explain and use methods to enhance strengths during dressing and grooming
- Dress and groom with assistance of caregiver as needed

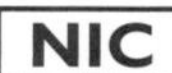

## Interventions (Nursing Interventions Classification)

### Suggested NIC Interventions

Dressing; Hair Care; Self-Care Assistance: Dressing/Grooming

**Example NIC Activities—Self-Care Assistance: Dressing/Grooming**

Be available for assistance in dressing as necessary; reinforce efforts to dress, groom self

## Nursing Interventions and Rationales

- • Observe the client's ability to dress and groom self through direct observation and from the client/caregiver report, noting specific deficits and their causes. **EB:** *Presence of a chronic disease alters dressing routines, and understanding these routines can allow development of energy conservation methods for dressing (Poole & Cordova, 2004).* **EB:** *Older adults with cerebral palsy often lost the ability to dress themselves, whereas other skill performance remained (Strauss et al, 2004).*
- • Consider and remove environmental barriers and human factors that may limit dressing/grooming ability, such as reaching for clothes or grooming aids in closets or drawers. Help the client arrange clothing and grooming devices within easy reach. Installing turntables and closet rods or drawers between eye and hip level is helpful. **EB:** *Reducing barriers to improve client's capabilities can improve function (Stark, 2004).*
- • Ask the client for input on clothing choices and how to increase the ease of dressing. **EBN:** *Client's task performance may be affected by a loss of individual control due to frustration from not being able to anticipate timing of care events, an inability to predict if nurse or client would perform tasks, and perception that nurse permission is necessary before performing a task (Brubaker, 1996).*
- ▲ Request referrals for occupational and physical therapy. *Collaboration with interdisciplinary team members increases the client's mastery of self-care tasks.* **EBN:** *Approaches to morning care for clients after a stroke differed between occupational therapists who used prompting/instructing commands and facilitation techniques and nurses who used supervision interactions during this care (Booth et al, 2001).*
- ▲ Provide medication for pain 45 minutes before dressing and grooming if needed. *Pain relief promotes participation in self-care.*
- • Plan activities to prevent fatigue while dressing and grooming. *Energy conservation increases activity tolerance and promotes self-care.*
- • Provide privacy and limit people/caregivers in room. **EBN:** *Privacy conveys respect and increases dressing ability (Beck et al, 1997).*
- • Select larger-sized clothing, clothing with elastic waistbands, wide sleeves and pant legs, dresses that open down the back for wheelchair-bound women, and Velcro fas-

S

teners or larger buttons. *Simplifying clothing facilitates dressing for those with impaired mobility.*

- Use adaptive dressing and grooming equipment as needed (e.g., long-handled brushes, grasping devices, Velcro closures, zipper pulls, button hooks, elastic shoelaces, large buttons, soap-on-a-rope, suction holders). *Adaptive devices increase speed and safety and decrease exertion.*
- Lay clothing out in the order that it will be put on by the client. Dress bottom half, then top half of body. **EBN:** *Simplifying dressing tasks increases self-care ability (Beck et al, 1997).*
- Encourage the client to dress appropriately for time of day. Perform dressing and grooming activities in a consistent sequence each day. *An established routine of waking and dressing provides a sense of normalcy and increases motivation to perform self-care.*
- Teach CNAs to use graduated verbal prompting for clients with dementia to complete dressing task and provide positive reinforcement immediately for accomplished steps of task. **EB:** *Client independence in dressing increased and range of motion improved when CNAs were taught to use graduated verbal prompting to allow client to participate in the dressing task (Engleman et al, 2002).*
- Encourage participation; guide the client's hand through task if necessary. **EBN:** *Experiencing the normal process of a task through guided practice facilitates optimal relearning (Beck et al, 1997).*
- If the client does not groom self, sit side-by-side with the client, put your hand over the client's hand, support the client's elbow with your other hand, and help the client comb hair. *This technique increases client mobility, range of motion, and independence (Pedretti, 1996).*
- Nurture personal attributes such as humor, positive attitude, faith, and hope and control of stress for clients with multiple sclerosis. **EBN:** *For those with multiple sclerosis, personal attributes intervene between emotional distress and ADL functioning by decreasing a stress appraisal response (Gulick, 2001).*
- Allow clients with a spinal cord injury to maximize control over activities and teach them how to direct their caregivers. **EB:** *Those with a spinal cord injury who were responsible for directing their caregivers felt more self-control, reported greater satisfaction with care, life, and better physical health and had fewer social handicaps.*
- Encourage family caregivers for clients with spinal cord injury. **EB:** *Satisfaction was higher with family member caregivers than home health agencies.*
- If client has had a cerebrovascular accident (CVA) with hemiparesis, consider use of constraint-induced movement therapy (CIMT), where the functional extremity is purposely constrained and the client is forced to use the involved extremity. *Constraint therapy is estimated to benefit about half of the total CVA population (Barker, 2005).* **EB:** *The plasticity of the brain allows the brain to rewire and reroute neural connections to take up the work of the injured area of the brain (National Institute of Neurological Disorders and Stroke, 2004; Liepert et al, 2000).*

S

## Geriatric

- Assess for grieving resulting from loss of function. *Grief resulting from loss of function can inhibit relearning of self-care tasks.*

- ▲ Provide medication for pain if needed and plan activities to prevent fatigue before dressing/grooming. **EBN:** *Level of functioning is increased for older adults with chronic medical conditions if pain and fatigue are controlled (Bennett et al, 2002).*
- • Assess self-efficacy (The Self-Efficacy for Functional Activities scale); assess outcome expectations (Outcome Expectations for Functional Activities scale). Based on assessment, promote motivation and self-efficacy for ADL functioning by role modeling via videotape or partnering; verbal encouragement; individualize care using humor, kindness, joy, and excitement with achievements; social supports; and decrease unpleasant sensations with the ADL function. *Assessment and interventions for self-efficacy strengthen client efficacy expectations and improve functional performance (Resnick, 2002).*
- • Assess tasks the client can complete, noting areas of independence and difficulty to make adaptations. **EBN:** *Some areas of a task can be performed independently but certain dressing tasks are reported as most difficult: tying shoelaces, fastening pants, and buttoning shirts; difficult grooming tasks are applying toothpaste and hair combing at the top and back of the head (Johnson et al, 1992).*
- • Allow the client or caregiver adequate time to complete dressing (e.g., do not insist that the client is dressed at an early hour). *Significant aging increases the time required to complete a task; elderly clients with a self-care deficit require more time than others to complete a task.*
- • For clients with dementia, maintain a specific routine for dressing to prevent increase in dressing time required. **EBN:** *Stage of dementia does not affect time required for dressing or undressing unless caregivers failed to keep to a specific routine (Kobayashi & Yamamoto, 2004).*
- ▲ Request referral for older women with cardiac disease to rehabilitation programs for strength training. *Older women with CHD demonstrated that an intense resistance-training program improved their performance with dressing and other daily activities (Ades et al, 2003).*
- • Telehomecare can be an effective way to assess and monitor ADL performance for older adults. **EBN:** *Telehomecare improves patient education and self-management outcomes (Bowles & Dansky, 2002). Telehealth is a cost-effective opportunity for gerontological home nursing practice for frequent monitoring and reassurance (Wakefield et al, 2001).*

## Home Care

- • Involve the client in planning of informal care and provide access to health professionals and financial support for the care. **EBN:** *Clients receiving informal care including dressing assistance reported concerns showing a need to increase their involvement in planning services related to informal care (McCann & Evans, 2002).*
- ▲ Based on functional assessment and rehabilitation capacity, refer for home health aide services to assist with dressing and grooming. *Support by home health aides preserve the energy of the client and provides respite for caregivers.*
- • Have caregiver view videotape showing caregiver self-care activities (organizing day, talking when frustrated, self-time, and nonjudgmental person with whom to talk) followed by a discussion. **EBN:** *Videotape intervention and discussion can model self-care activities and buffer caregiver stress (Clark & Lester, 2000).*
- • Cue cognitively impaired clients in steps of dressing and grooming. *Cognitively im-*

*paired clients can participate successfully in many activities with cueing, and participation in self-care can enhance their self-esteem.*

- Respect the preference of the terminally ill client to refuse dressing and limit grooming. *Dressing and grooming, even with assistance, may require excessive energy demands from the terminally ill. Pain on touch or movement may be intractable and not resolved by medication.*
- If terminally ill clients request dressing and grooming, make an extra effort to meet the request and provide care when the client and family will most benefit (e.g., before visitors, in early morning). *When desired, dressing and grooming are a great boost to the morale of terminally ill clients and their families.*
- Maintain the temperature of the home at a comfortable level when dressing terminally ill client. *Terminally ill clients may have difficulty with thermoregulation, which will add to the energy demand or decrease comfort during hygiene activities.*

## Client/Family Teaching

- Teach the client to dress the affected side first, then the unaffected side. *Dressing the affected side first allows for easier manipulation of clothing.*
- Teach the simplest step in a task until mastered, and then proceed to more complicated steps. Give praise. **EBN:** *Simplifying dressing and grooming tasks that consist of many small steps promotes mastery (Beck et al, 1997).*
- Teach the client how to use adaptive devices for dressing and grooming. *Adaptive devices can provide independence and safety and promote speed (Ryan & Cole, 2003).*
- Teach the client and family to select clothes appropriate for the season, temperature, and weather. *Clients with altered sensation need to understand the factors that influence body temperature and the environment.*

## evolve WEBSITES FOR EDUCATION

See the EVOLVE website for World Wide Web resources for client education.

## REFERENCES


Ades P, Savage P, Cress M et al: Resistance training on physical performance in disabled older female cardiac patients, *Med Sci Sports Exerc* 35(8):1265-1270, 2003.

Barker E: New hope for stroke patients, *RN* 68(2):38, 2005.

Beck C, Heacock P, Mercer SO et al: Improving dressing behavior in cognitively impaired nursing home residents, *Nurs Res* 46(3):126, 1997.

Bennett JA, Stewart AL, Kayser-Jones J et al: The mediating effect of pain and fatigue on level of functioning in older adults, *Nurs Res* 51(4):254, 2002.

Booth J, Davidson I, Winstanley J: Observing washing and dressing of stroke patients: nursing intervention compared with occupational therapists. What is the difference? *J Adv Nurs* 33(1):98-105, 2001.

Bowles K, Dansky K: Teaching self-management of diabetes via telehomecare, *Home Healthc Nurse* 20(1):36, 2002.

Brubaker B: Self care in nursing home residents, *J Gerontol Nurs* 22(7):22, 1996.

Chase B, Cornille T, English R: Life satisfaction among persons with spinal cord injuries, *J Rehabil* 66(3):14-20, 2000.

Clark M, Lester J: The effect of video-based interventions on self-care, *West J Nurs Res* 22(8):895, 2000.

Engleman K, Mathews R, Altus D: Restoring dressing independence in persons with Alzheimer's disease: a pilot study, *Am J Alzheimers Dis Other Demen* 17(1):37-43, 2002.

Gulick E: Emotional distress and activities of daily living functioning in persons with multiple sclerosis, *Nurs Res* 50(3):147, 2001.

Johnson PA, Stone MA, Larson AM et al: Applying nursing diagnosis and nursing process to activities of daily living and mobility, *Geriatric Nurs* 13:25, 1992.

Kobayashi N, Yamamoto M: Impact of the stage of dementia on the time required for bathing-related care: a pilot study in a Japanese nursing home, *Int J Nurs Stud* 41(7):767-774, 2004.

Liepert J, Bauder H, Wolfgang HR et al: Treatment-induced cortical reorganization after stroke in humans, *Stroke* 31(6):1210-1216, 2000.

McCann S, Evans D: Informal care: the views of people receiving care, *Health Soc Care Community* 10(4):221, 2002.

National Institute of Neurological Disorders and Stroke: *Stroke: hope through research*. Available at www.ninds.nih.gov/disorders/stgroke/detail_stroke.htm, accessed March 5, 2005.

Pedretti LW: *Occupational therapy: practice skills for physical dysfunction*, ed 4, St Louis, 1996, Mosby.

Poole J, Cordova J: Dressing routines in women with chronic disease: a pilot study, *N Z J Occup Ther* 51(1):30-35, 2004.

Resnick B: The impact of self-efficacy and outcome expectations on functional status in older adults, *Top Geriatr Rehabil* 17(4):1, 2002.

Ryan L, Cole M: Reaching your goals: low-tech patient aids can make all the difference in performing daily activities, *Rehab Manage* 16(7):42, 44-46, 2003.

Stark S: Removing environmental barriers in the homes of older adults with disabilities improves occupational performance, *OTJR* 24(1):32, 2004.

Strauss D, Ojdana K, Shavelle R et al: Decline in function and life expectancy of older persons with cerebral palsy, *Neuro Rehabil* 19(1):69-78, 2004.

Wakefield B, Flanagan J, Specht JK: Telehealth: an opportunity for gerontological nursing practice, *J Gerontol Nurs* 27(1):10-14, 2001.


# Feeding Self-care deficit

*Linda S. Williams*

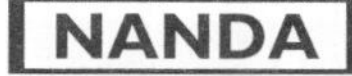

## Definition

Impaired ability to perform or complete feeding activities

## Defining Characteristics

Inability to swallow food, inability to prepare food for ingestion, inability to handle utensils, inability to chew food, inability to use assistive device, inability to get food onto utensils, inability to open containers, inability to ingest food safely, inability to manipulate food in mouth, inability to bring food from a receptacle to the mouth, inability to complete a meal, inability to ingest food in a socially acceptable manner, inability to pick up cup or glass, inability to ingest sufficient food

## Related Factors (r/t)

Weakness or tiredness, severe anxiety, neuromuscular impairment, pain, perceptual or cognitive impairment, discomfort, environmental barriers, decreased or lack of motivation, musculoskeletal impairment

NOTE: See suggested Functional Level Classification in the care plan **Impaired physical Mobility.**

NOC

## Outcomes (Nursing Outcomes Classification)

### Suggested NOC Outcomes

Self-Care: Activities of Daily Living (ADLs), Eating

**Example NOC Outcome with Indicators**

**Self-Care: Eating** as evidenced by the following indicators: Opens containers/Uses utensils/Completes a meal (Rate each indicator of **Self-Care: Eating:** 1 = severely compromised, 2 = substantially compromised, 3 = moderately compromised, 4 = mildly compromised, 5 = not compromised [see Section I].)

## Client Outcomes

**Client Will (Specify Time Frame):**

- Feed self safely
- State satisfaction with ability to use adaptive devices for feeding
- Use assistance with feeding when necessary (caregiver)

NIC

## Interventions (Nursing Interventions Classification)

### Suggested NIC Interventions

Feeding; Self-Care Assistance: Feeding

**Example NIC Activities—Self-Care Assistance: Feeding**

Provide adaptive devices to facilitate the client's feeding self (e.g., long handles, handle with large circumference, small strap on utensils) as needed; provide frequent cueing and close supervision as appropriate.

## Nursing Interventions and Rationales

S

- Assess the client's ability to feed self and note specific deficits. *Functional assessment provides ADL task analysis data for matching the client's ability to feed self with caregiver's level of assistance (Van Ort & Phillips, 1995).*
- Observe for cause of inability to feed self independently (see Related Factors). *Self-care requires multisystem competence. Restorative program planning is specific to problems that interfere with self-care (Phaneuf, 1996).*
- Ask the client for input on methods to facilitate eating and feeding (e.g., cultural foods, other food, and fluid preferences), and provide four entrée choices, including ethnic choice. *When clients are given a choice, food intake and quality of life increase (American Dietetic Association, 2002).*

▲ Consult speech-language pathologist for individualized feeding care plans. **EB:** *Those who are dependent for feeding develop aspiration pneumonia about 20 times more than those who are independent (Langmore et al, 1998). Speech-language pathologists design* *feeding plans to feed clients adequate nutrition in a safe, dignified manner (Pelletier, 2004).*

▲ Request referral for occupational and physical therapy; request a dietician. *Collaboration and correlation of activities with interdisciplinary team members increases the client's mastery of self-care tasks.*

• Ensure that the client has dentures, hearing aids, and glasses in place. *Adaptive devices increase opportunity for self-care.*

• Use any necessary adaptive feeding equipment (e.g., rocker knives, plate guards, suction mats, built-up handles on utensils, scoop dishes, large-handled cups). *Adaptive devices increase independence.*

• Seat the client at table using name card and place mat with meal in visual range next to role model who can eat, if applicable. *Familiar feeding patterns and cues increase self-feeding (Van Ort & Phillips, 1995).*

• Before feeding the client with brain trauma or dementia: provide oral hygiene; for dry mouth give tart or sour foods/fluids before meals; give proteolytic enzymes before meals if thick oral secretions are a problem. **EB:** *Oral hygiene stimulates saliva flow and taste, and tart/sour foods stimulate saliva production (The Joanna Briggs Institute for Evidence Based Nursing and Midwifery, 2000).*

• Positioning the client with brain trauma or dementia for feeding: help client sit upright with hips and knees flexed, feet supported, trunk and head in midline position, and head slightly flexed with chin down; for immobilized client in bed, use high Fowler's position and support the head and neck with neck slightly flexed; with unilateral paralysis, tilt head slightly to unaffected side and rotate the head toward the affected side. **EBN:** *Gravity assists with swallowing, and aspiration is decreased when sitting upright. (The Joanna Briggs Institute for Evidence Based Nursing and Midwifery, 2000).*

• Prepare meal items before the client begins eating. *Preparing items for the client conserves energy for hand-to-mouth activities.*

• Provide small portions of favorite foods, one entrée at a time, at proper serving temperature with unnecessary items, utensils removed. **EB:** *Food intake is increased when meal appeals to the client (Kayser-Jones & Schell, 1997);* **EBN:** *and is simplified to avoid distraction for those with brain trauma or dementia (The Joanna Briggs Institute for Evidence Based Nursing and Midwifery, 2000).*

• Provide consistency in caregiver and meal activities. *Assigning caregivers to clients rather than dining areas allows caregiver to learn the client's needs and promotes a positive attitude between caregiver and the client (Kennedy-Holzapfel et al, 1996).*

• To increase oral intake use feeding assistance intervention protocol: individual assistance, proper positioning, dining location preferences, and meal tray substitutions; use graduated prompting to enhance self-feeding ability as needed: (1) social stimulation and encouragement; (2) nonverbal cueing; (3) verbal cueing; (4) physical guidance; and (5) full physical assistance. **EB:** *Individualized nutritional care increased client daily oral intake for 90% of participants with one or both of the feeding assistance intervention protocol or the between meal snack (Simmons & Schnelle, 2004).*

• To increase oral intake use a three times a day between-meal snack, alone or if intake is not increased 15% with the feeding assistance intervention protocol (discussed previ-

S

ously), delivered to the client on a movable cart with a variety of food/fluid choices. **EB:** *Individualized nutritional care increased client daily oral intake for 90% of participants with one or both of the feeding assistance intervention protocol or the between meal snack (Simmons & Schnelle, 2004).*

- Caregiver should sit beside the client (on the client's unaffected side) at eye level. *Sitting at eye level with the client increases eye contact and promotes a relaxed atmosphere that increases consumed food (Kennedy-Holzapfel et al, 1996).*
- Caregiver can sit at a half circle table if interacting with a group of clients and should remain with clients until meal is completed. *Environmental strategies that reduce interruptions and distractions increase food intake (Van Ort & Phillips, 1995).*
- Allow the client to participate in feeding as able; provide verbal/visual cues with paced prompting; provide praise for all feeding attempts; increase tasks as able. *The client should be an active participant in feeding instead of a passive recipient of food (Osburn & Marshall, 1993); verbal and visual cues and/or paced prompting increase feeding.*
- Presentation of feeding: Provide 1/2–1 teaspoon of solid food or 10–15 mL of liquid at a time; wait until client has swallowed prior food/liquid. **EBN:** *Small feeding volume is best practice for brain trauma or dementia feeding (The Joanna Briggs Institute for Evidence Based Nursing and Midwifery, 2000).* **EB:** *Large volumes and fast rate of presentation occurred commonly likely due to lack of knowledge this could exacerbate dysphagia and increase the risk of health problems (Pelletier, 2004).*
- Provide the client with a pleasant, quiet meal environment with no distractions. **EBN:** *Food intake is increased when concentration on eating occurs (The Joanna Briggs Institute for Evidence Based Nursing and Midwifery, 2000).*
- Keep the environment free of toileting devices and odors, avoid painful procedures before meals, remove lids from tray, and provide clean utensils for separate courses. *Attention to the aesthetics of feeding increases food intake (Kayser-Jones & Schell, 1997).*
- Do not mix different foods together when assisting the client with eating. *Mixing foods together decreases client dignity and reduces appeal of food, decreasing food intake (Kayser-Jones & Schell, 1997).*
- Play slow-tempo, quiet music during meals. *Agitated behaviors may communicate anxiety from a noisy, overwhelming environment; quiet music can mask this, resulting in relaxed and smiling clients (Denney, 1997).*
- If client will not eat, provide 30 mL of nutritional supplement such as Ensure in a medication cup every hour while awake. *Clients who will not eat will often take medications so by placing supplement in a medication cup clients will often drink it. In 8 hours, the client will have ingested a can of supplement.*
- Encourage the client to keep food on the unaffected side of mouth with a rocking motion to deposit the food, if applicable. *Keeping food away from the affected side of the mouth prevents pocketing of food (The Joanna Briggs Institute for Evidence Based Nursing and Midwifery, 2000).*
- Be prepared to intervene if choking occurs; have suction equipment readily available and know the Heimlich maneuver. **EBN:** *Dysphagia increases the risk of choking (The Joanna Briggs Institute for Evidence Based Nursing and Midwifery, 2000).*
- For clients with conditions such as Parkinson's or myasthenia gravis, ensure that their medications are given so that peak drug action occurs during meal times. **EBN:** *Peak*

S

*action of medications promotes safety in eating and self-care ability (The Joanna Briggs Institute for Evidence Based Nursing and Midwifery, 2000).*

- ▲ Continue rehabilitation efforts with poststroke clients long-term to achieve optimal functioning. **EBN:** *Client improvement may continue 6 months or longer poststroke (Cavanagh et al, 2002).*
- • If client has had a cerebrovascular accident (CVA) with hemiparesis, consider use of constraint-induced movement therapy (CIMT) where the functional extremity is purposely constrained and the client is forced to use the involved extremity. *Constraint therapy is estimated to benefit about half of the total CVA population (Barker, 2005).* **EB:** *The plasticity of the brain allows the brain to rewire and reroute neural connections to take up the work of the injured area of the brain (National Institute of Neurological Disorders and Stroke, 2004; Liepert et al, 2000).*
- • If the client does not feed self, sit side-by-side with the client, put your hand over the client's hand, support the client's elbow with your other hand, and help the client feed self. *This feeding technique increases client mobility, range of motion, and independence, and clients often eat more food (Pedretti, 1996).*
- • Provide oral hygiene after every meal eating and check for pocketing of food. **EB:** *The incidence of pneumonia is reduced when clients receive oral care after every meal (Yoneyama et al, 2002).*

## Geriatric

- • Provide nutrition care that honors the individual client and enhances, rather than detracts from, each client's quality of life. *Principles to guide quality assurance for nutrition in nursing homes include meeting quality-of-life and nutrient needs of clients and implementing processes to provide high-quality nutrition care (Castellanos, 2004).*
- • Develop client muscle strength building plan to build the client's physiological capacity. **EBN:** *Elders may have little reserve capacity but building physiological capacity may allow continued functioning during periods of illness or stress (Leidy & Haase, 1999).*
- ▲ Implement Hospital Elder Life Program, a model of care to prevent functional and cognitive decline of older persons during hospitalization. *The Hospital Elder Life Program successfully prevents cognitive and functional decline in at-risk older patients (Inouye et al, 2000).*
- ▲ Implement the Wellspring model, which advocates education and empowerment of CNAs to solve problems without direct administrative oversight. **EB:** *Feeding techniques of nursing assistants can be improved with use of the Wellspring model (Stone et al, 2002).*
- ▲ Ensure CNAs know the signs/symptoms of dysphagia such as choking, coughing, oral/chewing problems, throat clearing, wet voice, gurgly voice, or pneumonia; if exhibited during feeding, report them promptly during feeding. **EB:** *CNAs knowledgeable of symptoms and who indicated they would report them did not acknowledge or report symptoms during feeding other than to generally feed clients slower or with smaller volumes (Pelletier, 2004).*
- ▲ Seek CNA input on feeding concerns to discussion possible actions and share techniques beneficial to specific clients. **EB:** *Collaborative communication may result in better feeding practices because CNAs will feel that their concerns are heard (Pelletier, 2004).*

- ▲ Ensure CNA feeding training includes the need to decrease command statements to clients being fed and instead offer encouraging statements. **EB:** *Improved intake and enjoyment during meals may occur with this type of communication (Pelletier, 2004).*
- ▲ Suggest CNAs learn 3–5 personal details about client being fed during the feeding. **EB:** *CNA communication skills while feeding and clients' psychosocial needs may increase by requiring the learning of personal data (Pelletier, 2004).*
- ▲ Provide medication for pain before meals if needed and plan activities to prevent fatigue before meals. **EBN:** *Level of functioning is increased for older adults with chronic medical conditions if pain and fatigue are controlled (Bennett et al, 2002).*
- • Assess and maintain documentation about poststroke client's eating and nutrition (include weight) upon admission to long-term care. **EBN:** *Poststroke clients may have multiple nutritional deficits that require early and ongoing assessment to enable appropriate care and promotion of health (Kumlien & Axelsson, 2002).*
- • Serve meals "family style" with food in serving bowls and an empty plate to be filled by patient. **EBN:** *Institutional practices foster "excess disability," with eating often the first skill to go, family-style meal serving rather than prepared meal plates allows opportunity for food and portion size selection, self-serving, passing serving bowls, selecting seconds, and social engagement. An added benefit is that less staff time is needed to prepare plates (Altus et al, 2002).*
- • Obtain and value patient's view of agency's food selection and presentation. Present views to administration. **EBN:** *Patient barriers to eating are the dislike of presented foods, feeling that the food is not appetizing and nonvaluing of patient's food reports from nursing assistants and the need for administration to value these reports (Crogan et al, 2001).*
- ▲ Ensure adequate staffing at meal times. **EBN:** *Short staffing results in decreased time for feeding (Crogan et al, 2001).*
- • Choose soft foods rather than liquids, or use dietary thickeners. *Choking occurs more easily with clear liquids than with solid or soft foods.*
- • Assess for intolerance to food texture and, if found, reverse food texture pattern as tolerated, progressing finally to texture stage of thick liquids. *Dementia clients lose ability to tolerate texture-pattern reverses from regular to soft to mechanical soft to mechanical soft with chopped meat to puree to thick liquids, and pocketing of food is seen, along with statements of choking and spitting of food (Boylston et al, 1995).*
- • Provide finger foods for clients with Alzheimer's disease and place in hands as needed to cue. *Finger foods attract patient attention and increase involvement in meal. They are easier to handle than utensils, and as a result, weight is maintained (Slotesz & Dayton, 1995). Finger foods can be nutritious and can allow independence and the choice of what and when to eat (Kennedy-Holzapfel et al, 1996).*
- • Allow the client with dentures adequate time to chew. *Chewing with dentures takes four times longer to reach a certain level of mastication than chewing with natural teeth.*
- • Provide emotionally neutral nonverbal cues to improve table-sitting behavior if patient rises from table early, such as a firm hand on dominant shoulder indicating to resit. **EBN:** *Wanderers often receive positive social engagement from staff when leaving the table early, so emotionally neutral behavior-extinguishing cues are useful to increase table sitting and food intake (Beattie & Algase, 2002).*

S

### Home Care

- ▲ Based on functional assessment and rehabilitation capacity, refer for home health aide services to assist with feeding. *Support by home health aides preserves the energy of the client and provides respite for caregivers.*
- • Telehomecare can be an effective way to assess and monitor ADL performance for older adults. **EBN:** *Telehomecare improves patient education and self-management outcomes (Bowles & Dansky, 2002). Telehealth is a cost-effective opportunity for gerontological home nursing practice for frequent monitoring and reassurance (Wakefield et al, 2001).*
- • Cue cognitively impaired client when feeding. *Cognitively impaired clients can participate successfully in many activities with cueing. Participation in self-care can enhance the self-esteem of cognitively impaired clients.*
- • Respect the preference of terminally ill clients to refuse nutrition or assistance with eating. Refer to care plans for **Imbalanced Nutrition: less than body requirements** and **Impaired Swallowing.**
- • If terminally ill client requests nutrition, take special care to provide foods and assistive devices that protect the client from aspiration, minimize energy requirements, and meet the client's taste preferences. *Terminally ill clients have altered taste and other sensations, which affects their willingness to eat or to invest time or energy in eating.*

### Client/Family Teaching

- • Teach the client how to use adaptive devices. *Adaptive devices increase independence.*
- • Teach the client with hemianopsia to turn head so that the plate is in the line of vision. *Compensation for hemianopsia is done by turning head to place items in line of vision (Needham, 1993).*
- • Teach visually impaired client to locate foods according to numbers on a clock. *Teach caregiver feeding techniques that prevent choking (e.g., sitting beside the client on the unaffected side, feeding the client slowly, checking food temperature, providing fluid between bites, establishing a method to communicate readiness for next bite, limiting conversation while chewing).*

## evolve WEBSITES FOR EDUCATION

See the EVOLVE website for World Wide Web resources for client education.

S

## REFERENCES


Altus DE, Engelman KK, Mathews RM: Using family-style meals to increase participation and communication in persons with dementia, *J Gerontol Nurs* 28(9):47, 2002.

American Dietetic Association: Liberalized diets for older adults in long-term care, *J Am Diet Assoc* 102:1316-1323, 2002.

Barker E: New hope for stroke patients, *RN* 68(2):38, 2005.

Beattie E, Algase D: Improving table-sitting behavior of wanderers, *J Gerontol Nurs* 28(10):6, 2002.

Bennett JA, Stewart AL, Kayser-Jones J et al: The mediating effect of pain and fatigue on level of functioning in older adults, *Nurs Res* 51(4): 254, 2002.

Bowles K, Dansky K: Teaching self-management of diabetes via telehomecare, *Home Healthc Nurse* 20(1):36, 2002.

Boylston E Ryan C, Brown C et al: Increase oral intake in dementia patients by altering food texture, *Am J Alzheimers Dis Other Dimen* 10(6):37, 1995.

Castellanos V: Food and nutrition in nursing homes, *Generations* 28(3):65-71, 2004.
Cavanagh S, Hogan K, Fairfax J et al: Assessing cognitive function after stroke using the FIM instrument, *J Neurosci Nurs* 34(2): 99, 2002.
Crogan NL, Shultz JA, Adams CE et al: Barriers to nutrition care for nursing home residents, *J Gerontol Nurs* 27(12):25, 2001.
Denney A: Quiet music: an intervention for mealtime agitation, *J Gerontol Nurs* 23(7):16, 1997.
Inouye SK, Bogardus ST Jr, Baker DI et al: The Hospital Elder Life Program: a model of care to prevent cognitive and functional decline in older hospitalized patients, *J Am Geriatr Soc* 48(12):1697, 2000.
Kayser-Jones J: Inadequate staffing at mealtime: implications for nursing and health policy, *J Gerontol Nurs* 23(8):4, 1997.
Kayser-Jones J, Schell E: The mealtime experience of a cognitively impaired elder: ineffective and effective strategies, *J Gerontol Nurs* 23(7):33, 1997.
Holzapfel SK, Ramirez RF, Layton MS et al: Feeder position and food and fluid consumed by nursing home residents, *J Gerontol Nurs* 22(4):6, 1996.
Kumlien S, Axelsson K: Stroke patients in nursing homes: eating, feeding, nutrition and related care, *J Clin Nurs* 11(4):498, 2002.
Langmore S, Terpenning M, Schork A et al: Predictors of aspiration pneumonia: how important is dysphagia? *Dysphagia* 73(2): 69-81, 1998.
Leidy N, Haase J: Functional status from the patient's perspective: the challenge of preserving personal integrity, *Res Nurs Health* 22:67, 1999.
Liepert J, Bauder H, Wolfgang HR et al: Treatment-induced cortical reorganization after stroke in humans, *Stroke* 31(6):1210, 2000.
National Institute of Neurological Disorders and Stroke: Stroke: hope through research. Available at www.ninds.nih.Gov/disorders/stgroke/detail_stroke.htm, accessed March 5, 2005.
Needham J: *Gerontological nursing: a restorative approach*, Albany, NY, 1993, Delmar.
Osburn C, Marshall M: Self-feeding performance in nursing home residents, *J Gerontol Nurs* 19:7, 1993.
Pedretti LW: *Occupational therapy: practice skills for physical dysfunction*, ed 4, St Louis, 1996, Mosby.
Pelletier C: What do certified nurse assistants actually know about dysphagia and feeding nursing home residents? *Am J Speech Lang Pathol* 13(2):99-113, 2004.
Phaneuf C: Screening elders for nutritional deficits, *Am J Nurs* 96:58, 1996.
Sharkey J: The influence of nutritional health on physical function: a critical relationship for homebound older adults, *Generations* 28(3):34-38, 2004.
Simmons S, Schnelle J: Individualized feeding assistance care for nursing home residents: staffing requirements to implement two interventions, *J Gerontol A Biol Sci Med Sci* 59(9):M966-973, 2004.
Slotesz KS, Dayton JH: The effects of menu modification to increase dietary intake and maintain the weight of Alzheimer's residents, *Am J Alzheimers Dis Other Dimen* 10(6):20, 1995.
Stone R, Reinhard S, Bowers B et al: *Evaluation of the Wellspring model for improving nursing home quality*, Washington, DC, 2002, The Commonwealth Fund.
The Joanna Briggs Institute for Evidence Based Nursing and Midwifery: Identification and nursing management of dysphagia in individuals with neurological impairment. *Best Practice*, 4(2):1-6, 2000. Available at http://www.joannabriggs.edu.au, accessed March 15, 2005.
Van Ort S, Phillips L: Nursing interventions to promote functional feeding, *J Gerontol Nurs* 21:6, 1995.
Wakefield B et al: Telehealth: an opportunity for gerontological nursing practice, *J Gerontol Nurs* 27(1):10, 2001.
Yoneyama T, Yoshida M, Ohrui T et al: Oral care reduces pneumonia in older patients in nursing homes, *J Am Geriatr Soc* 50: 430-433, 2002.



# Toileting Self-care deficit

*Linda S. Williams*

**NANDA**

## Definition

Impaired ability to perform or complete own toileting activities

## Defining Characteristics

Inability to get to toilet or commode, inability to sit on or rise from toilet or commode, inability to manipulate clothing for toileting, inability to carry out proper toilet hygiene, inability to flush toilet or commode

## Related Factors (r/t)

Environmental barriers, weakness or tiredness, decreased or lack of motivation, severe anxiety, impaired mobility status, impaired transfer ability, musculoskeletal impairment, neuromuscular impairment, pain, perceptual or cognitive impairment

NOTE: See suggested Functional Level Classification in care plan for **Impaired physical Mobility.**

**NOC**

## Outcomes (Nursing Outcomes Classification)

### Suggested NOC Outcomes

Self-Care: Activities of Daily Living (ADLs), Toileting

**Example NOC Outcome with Indicators**

**Self-Care: Toileting** as evidenced by the following indicators: Recognizes and responds to a full bladder and urge to have a bowel movement in a timely manner/Gets to and from toilet (Rate each indicator of **Self-Care: Toileting:** 1 = severely compromised, 2 =substantially compromised, 3 = moderately compromised, 4 = mildly compromised, 5 = not compromised [see Section I].)

## Client Outcomes

**Client Will (Specify Time Frame):**

- Remain free of incontinence and impaction with no urine or stool on skin
- State satisfaction with ability to use adaptive devices for toileting
- Explain and use methods to be safe and independent in toileting

S

**NIC**

## Interventions (Nursing Interventions Classification)

### Suggested NIC Interventions

Environmental Management; Self-Care Assistance: Toileting

**Example NIC Activities—Self-Care Assistance: Toileting**

Assist the client to toilet/commode/bedpan/fracture pan/urinal at specified intervals; institute a toileting schedule as appropriate

## Nursing Interventions and Rationales

- Observe cause of inability to toilet independently (see Related Factors). *Self-care requires multisystem competence. Restorative program planning is specific to problems that interfere with self-care.*
- Assess ability to toilet; note specific deficits. *Functional assessment provides analysis data for ADL tasks for use in goal and intervention planning.*
- Ask the client for input on toileting methods and timing and how to better provide toileting activity assistance. **EBN:** *Client's task performance may be affected by a loss of individual control due to frustration from not being able to anticipate timing of care events, an inability to predict if nurse or client would perform tasks, and perception that nurse permission is necessary before performing a task (Brubaker, 1996).*
- Assess the client's usual bowel and bladder toileting patterns and the terminology used for toileting. *Individuals develop a unique pattern of toileting over time for faster, normal elimination.*
- ▲ Request referral for occupational and physical therapy for help in working with the client to transfer from bed to commode. *Collaboration and correlation of activities with interdisciplinary team members increase the client's mastery of self-care tasks.*
- Use any necessary assistive toileting equipment (e.g., raised toilet seat, suction mats, spill-proof urinals, support rails next to toilet, toilet safety frames, Sanifems [allows a woman to void standing], fracture bedpans, long-handled toilet paper holders). *Adaptive devices promote independence and safety.*
- Provide privacy. *Privacy can prevent suppression of elimination resulting from embarrassment about noise and odor.*
- Assess barriers to implementation of a toileting program. **EBN:** *Barriers to successful implementation of toileting programs can include extra physical/cognitive demands on staff, perceived workload increase, lack of value to staff, and lack of incentives (Mueller & Bakas, 2002). Additionally, inadequate communication, lack of ownership, belief incontinence is part of aging, and unwillingness to alter routine affect implementation (Mather & Cain, 2002).*
- Assess client's voiding patterns and if consistent place on an individualized toileting schedule that is documented and allows the client to use the toilet/commode. **EBN:** *Improved bowel and bladder hygiene, skin care, and client dignity along with reduced frustration, agitation, and violence toward staff occurs with scheduled toileting (Frantz et al, 2003).*
- Develop toileting schedule using clocks, written schedules, or verbal prompting as cues for the client and provide assistance at scheduled times. *Toileting schedules convey continence is valued and maintain continence (Hart et al, 2002).*
- Schedule toileting to occur when defecation urge is strongest or voiding is likely (e.g., in the morning, every 2 hours, after meals, at bedtime). Assist the client until self-care ability increases. *The defecation urge is strongest in the morning or within 1 hour after meals or warm beverages. Approximately 50–75 mL of urine is produced hourly, and the urge to void occurs when 200 mL has accumulated.* **EBN:** *Medications (e.g., laxatives), briefs, linens, and enema use can be reduced with a scheduled toileting program (Engst et al, 2004).*
- Allow the client to participate as able in toileting, and provide praise for accomplish-

S

ments. Increase tasks as the client is able, and work with the client to aim toward independence in toileting. *Client's expenditure of energy provides caregiver the opportunity to convey respect for a well-done task, which increases self-esteem.*

- Obtain a bedside commode if necessary and adapt it for the client's needs; avoid bedpans if possible. If the client is acutely ill, provide bedpan at appropriate intervals. *A sitting position uses gravity and is more conducive to normal elimination than a lying position.*
- Make assistance call button readily available to the client and answer call light promptly. *To decrease incontinence, the client needs rapid access to toileting facilities.*
- Assess and remove physical barriers to toilet, such as cluttered walkways. *Environmental assessment identifies barriers that can increase incontinence episodes (Penn et al, 1996).*
- For clients with spinal cord injury select self-propelled commode-shower chair designed to enhance safety, ease of use, and caregiver access, marketed by Everest & Jennings. **EB:** *Research shows self-propelled commode-shower chair eliminates problems in previous chairs, allows safe transfers, has a foot-lift for foot washing, and has weight distributive seat padding and rounded heel cups to prevent pressure ulcers; tubular frame and smaller wheels allow positioning over toilet and caregiver access (Malassign et al, 2000).*
- Keep toilet paper and hand-washing items within easy reach of the client. Provide prompt skin care and linen changes after incontinence episodes. *The presence of urine or stool on the skin leads to skin breakdown.*

## Geriatric

▲ Remove barriers to toileting, support client's cultural beliefs, and preserve dignity. **EB:** *Physical/sociocultural environment in long-term care required older clients to overcome greater physical and cognitive challenges to maintain their participation, autonomy, and dignity in toileting than if residing at home (Sacco-Peterson & Borell, 2004).*

▲ Develop client muscle strength building plan to build the client's physiological capacity. **EBN:** *Elderly clients may have little reserve capacity but building physiological capacity may allow continued functioning during periods of illness or stress (Leidy & Haase, 1999).* **EBN:** *Trunk function training (strength, range of motion, balance) can be useful to increase bed/chair rising abilities (Alexander et al, 2000).*

▲ Include regular exercise and walking program in plan of care. **EB:** *Regular exercise improves functional abilities in clients in long-term care (de Carvalho & Filho, 2004). Exercise for flexibility, strengthening, and a walking program in the hospital promotes ADLs, prevents injury, increases quality of life, and may delay admission to a long-term care facility (Hart et al, 2002).*

▲ Assist client (especially frail older clients) to exercise (walk 2 minutes, push wheelchair, sit-stand repetitions) for several minutes every time up to toilet. **EBN:** *After 8 weeks of incidental exercise with toileting, ADL function increased (Schnelle et al, 1995).*

▲ Provide equipment routinely that allows elevation of seat/head of bed to enhance bed/chair rising ability. **EBN:** *Chair/bed designs allowing elevation of seat/head of bed enhance rising ability and could be more universally adopted in older adult care settings (Alexander et al, 2000).*

▲ Upper extremity use for disabled clients is an important consideration in equipment choice to facilitate use of hands in chair/bed rising abilities. **EBN:** *Equipment de-*

S

*signs (arm rest style and placement) can aid in the client in using upper extremities to facilitate rising, which is demonstrated to be essential in successful rising in disabled clients (Alexander et al, 2000).*

- ▲ Implement Hospital Elder Life Program, a model of care to prevent functional and cognitive decline of older persons during hospitalization. **EB:** *The Hospital Elder Life Program successfully prevents cognitive and functional decline in at-risk older patients (Inouye et al, 2000).*
- • Assess self-efficacy (The Self-Efficacy for Functional Activities scale); assess outcome expectations (Outcome Expectations for Functional Activities scale). Based on assessment, promote motivation and self-efficacy for ADL functioning by role modeling via videotape or partnering; providing verbal encouragement; individualizing care using humor, kindness, joy, and excitement with achievements; providing social supports; and decreasing unpleasant sensations with the ADL function. *Assessment and interventions for self-efficacy strengthen client efficacy expectations and improve functional performance (Resnick, 2002).*
- • Assess self-efficacy of nursing assistants who provide restorative care activities (Self-Efficacy for Restorative Care Nursing Activities), and assess their outcome expectations (Outcome Expectancy for Restorative Care Activities). **EBN:** *Establishes weaknesses in nursing assistants' expectations for implementation of interventions to increase self-efficacy and outcome expectations leading to improved adherence in nursing assistants. (Resnick & Simpson, 2002).*
- • After hip fracture, focusing on hospital-based multidisciplinary interventions and discharge planning. **EBN:** *The inability to recover ADL function, including toileting, 1 year postfracture in the elderly can be predicted by inability to independently walk outdoors before fracture, so discharge planning should focus on methods to promote functional recovery (Lin & Chang, 2004).*
- • Monitor clients with dementia for behavioral toileting cues (e.g., pacing, restlessness, fidgeting) and assist with prompt toileting, or use an individualized scheduled toileting for memory impaired elderly. **EBN:** *An individual toileting schedule helps prevent incontinence in moderately cognitively impaired elders (Jirovec & Templin, 2001).*
- • Assess the client's mobility status and speed of movement. **EBN:** *Elderly women with slower mobility have more incontinent episodes than others (Wyman & Eiswick, 1993).*
- • Reassure the client that call light will be answered promptly. *The elderly cannot respond quickly to the urge to void because of limited functional ability and environmental barriers; they are also unable to delay voiding because of decreased muscle tone and neurological changes (Palmer, 1994).*
- • Provide a small footstool in front of toilet or commode. *Elevating knees above the hips increases intraabdominal pressure, which facilitates elimination in elderly persons with weak abdominal muscles.*
- • Assess the client's functional ability to manipulate clothing for toileting. If necessary, modify clothing with Velcro fasteners and elastic waists. *Delays caused by having to manipulate zippers and buttons may cause functional incontinence (Penn et al, 1996).*
- • Avoid use of indwelling or condom catheters if possible. *An indwelling urinary catheter is a source of infection and keeps the bladder empty, which reduces bladder capacity and decreases the opportunity for independent toileting.*



• = Independent; ▲ = Collaborative; EBN = Evidence-Based Nursing; EB = Evidence-Based

### Home Care

- • Have caregiver view videotape showing caregiver self-care activities (organizing day, talking when frustrated, self-time, and nonjudgmental person with whom to talk) followed by a discussion. **EBN:** *Videotape intervention and discussion can model self-care activities and buffer caregiver stress (Clark & Lester, 2000).*
- ▲ Based on functional assessment and rehabilitation capacity, refer for home health aide services to assist with toileting. *Support by home health aides preserves the energy of the client and provides respite for caregivers.*
- • Cue cognitively impaired clients in steps of toileting. *Cognitively impaired persons can participate successfully in many activities with cueing, and participation in self-care can enhance their self-esteem.*
- ▲ Avoid the use of medications that place undue toileting stress on the client who is terminally ill.
- ▲ Provide pain medication for terminally ill clients 20–45 minutes before toileting in anticipation of possible pain (e.g., in coordination with a bowel stimulation program). See care plan for **Constipation.** *Pain from touch or movement may be intractable and not resolved by medication, but medication may decrease the pain enough to allow limited movement and passing of stool.*
- ▲ Consider use of an indwelling catheter for terminally ill clients in too much pain to move when hygiene and skin integrity are difficult to maintain. *The goal of hospice care is to promote comfort and dignity in the dying process.*

### Client/Family Teaching

- • Teach the client and family how to toilet the client with adaptive and safety devices. *Adaptive devices can provide independence and safety and promote speed.*
- • Have family install toilet seat of a contrasting color. **EBN:** *Visualization of toilet is aided by installing toilet seat of a contrasting color (Gerdner, 2002).*
- • Prepare the client for toileting needs by teaching the action of medications such as diuretics. *Medications that promote elimination require prompt responses to toileting needs.*
- • Help the visually impaired client to develop a plan for locating bathrooms in new environments. *Clients with visual impairments may find locating bathrooms in unfamiliar settings difficult.*

S

## evolve WEBSITES FOR EDUCATION

See the EVOLVE website for World Wide Web resources for client education.

## REFERENCES

Alexander N, Galecki L, Nyquist M et al: Chair and bed rise performance in ADL-impaired congregate housing residents, *J Am Geriatr Soc* 48(5):526-533, 2000.

Brubaker B: Self care in nursing home residents, *J Gerontol Nurs* 22(7):22, 1996.

Clark M, Lester J: The effect of video-based interventions on self-care, *West J Nurs Res* 22(8):895, 2000.

de Carvalho B, Filho W: Effect of an exercise program on functional performance of institutionalized elderly, *J Rehabil Res Dev* 41(5):659-668, 2004.

Engst C, Chhokar R, Robinson D et al: Implementation of a scheduled toileting program in a long term care facility, *AAOHN J* 52(10):427-435, 2004.
Frantz R., Xakellis G Jr, Harvey P et al: Implementing an incontinence management protocol in long-term care: clinical outcomes and costs, *J Gerontol Nurs* 29(8):46-53, 2003.
Gerdner LA, Buckwalter KC, Reed D: Impact of a psychoeducational intervention on caregiver response to behavioral problems, *Nurs Res* 51(6):363, 2002.
Hart BD, Birkas J, Lachmann M et al: Promoting positive outcomes for elderly persons in the hospital: prevention and risk factor modification, *AACN Clin Issues* 13(1):22, 2002.
Inouye SK, Bogardus ST Jr, Baker DI et al: The Hospital Elder Life Program: a model of care to prevent cognitive and functional decline in older hospitalized patients, *J Am Geriatr Soc* 48(12):1697, 2000.
Jirovec MM, Templin T: Predicting success using individualized scheduled toileting for memory-impaired elders at home, *Res Nurs Health* 24:1, 2001.
Leidy N, Haase J: Functional status from the patient's perspective: the challenge of preserving personal integrity, *Res Nurs Health* 22:67, 1999.
Lin P, Chang S: Functional recovery among elderly people one year after hip fracture surgery, *J Nurs Res* 12(1):72-82, 2004.
Malassign P, Nelson A, Cors M et al: Design of the advanced commode-shower chair for spinal cord-injured individuals, *J Rehabil Res Dev* 37(3):373-382, 2000.
Mather K, Bakas T: Nursing assistants' perceptions of their ability to provide continence care, *Geriatr Nurs* 23(2):76-81, 2002.
Mueller C, Cain H: Comprehensive management of urinary incontinence through quality improvement efforts, *Geriatr Nurs* 23(2):82-87, 2002.
Palmer M: Level 1: basic assessment and management of urinary incontinence in nursing homes, *Nurs Pract Forum* 5:152, 1994.
Penn C, Lekan-Rutledge D, Joers AM et al: Assessment of urinary incontinence, *J Gerontol Nurs* 22:8, 1996.
Resnick B: The impact of self-efficacy and outcome expectations on functional status in older adults, *Top Geriatr Rehabil* 17(4):1, 2002.
Sacco-Peterson M, Borell L: Struggles for autonomy in self-care: the impact of the physical and socio-cultural environment in a long-term care setting, *Scand J Caring Sci* 18(4):376-86, 2004.
Schnelle J, MacRae P, Ouslander J et al: Functional incidental training, mobility performance and incontinence with nursing home residents, *J Am Geriatr Soc* 43(12):1356-1362, 1995.
Wyman J, Eiswick R: Influence of functional, urological, and environmental characteristics on urinary incontinence in community-dwelling older women, *Nurs Res* 42:270, 1993.

# Readiness for enhanced Self-concept

*Gail B. Ladwig*

S

**NANDA**

## Definition

A pattern of perceptions or ideas about the self that is sufficient for well-being and can be strengthened

## Defining Characteristics

Expresses willingness to enhance self-concept; expresses satisfaction with thoughts about self, sense of worthiness, role performance, body image, and personal identity; actions are congruent with expressed feelings and thoughts; expresses confidence in abilities; accepts strengths and limitations

## Related Factors (r/t)

To be developed

**NOC**

## Outcomes (Nursing Outcomes Classification)

### Suggested NOC Outcome

Self-Esteem

**Example NOC Outcome with Indicators**

**Self-Esteem** as evidenced by the following indicators: Verbalizations of self-acceptance/Open communication/Confidence level/Description of pride in self (Rate each indicator of **Self-Esteem:** 1 = never positive, 2 = rarely positive, 3 = sometimes positive, 4 = often positive, 5 = consistently positive [see Section I].)

## Client Outcomes

**Client Will (Specify Time Frame):**

- State willingness to enhance self-concept
- State satisfaction with thoughts about self, sense of worthiness, role performance, body image, and personal identity
- Demonstrate actions that are congruent with expressed feelings and thoughts
- State confidence in abilities
- Accept strengths and limitations

**NIC**

## Interventions (Nursing Interventions Classification)

### Suggested NIC Intervention

Self-Esteem Enhancement

**Example NIC Activities—Self-Esteem Enhancement**

Encourage the client to identify strengths; assist the client in setting realistic goals to achieve higher self-esteem

S

## Nursing Interventions and Rationales

- Assess and support activities that promote self-concept developmentally. **EB:** *High self-esteem is associated with high academic achievement, involvement in sport and physical activity, and development of effective coping and peer pressure resistance skills (Gurney et al, 1987, in King, 2002).* **EBN:** *Social support, self-esteem, and optimism were all positively related to positive health practices (McNicholas, 2002).*

▲ Support the client's choice of alternative therapies and provide information on appropriate therapies (e.g., using a certified massage therapist when massage is the treatment of choice). *Nurses need to instruct the client to report special considerations, such as the presence of neutropenia or thrombocytopenia.*

- ▲ Clients with cancer often use massage therapy as an adjunct treatment. *Safe and effective massage therapy to clients with cancer only is achieved when the client, health care providers, and licensed massage therapist (LMT) collaborate effectively (Gecsedi, 2002).*
- ▲ Support establishing a church-based community health promotion programs (CBHPPs) with the following key elements: partnerships, positive health values, availability of services, access to church facilities, community-focused interventions, health behavior change, and supportive social relationships. *CBHPPs have effectively promoted health behaviors within certain communities. To promote health and wellness in light of our diverse society and health needs, health promotion professionals and churches can be dynamic partners (Peterson, Atwood, & Yates, 2002).*
- ▲ For clients who have had breast surgery and need prosthesis, provide the appropriate prosthesis before the client leaves the health care facility. *A diagnosis of breast cancer carries enormous implications for the client in terms of physical and psychological health. For this reason, it is vital that nurses respond sensitively to these needs and assist women to cope with the changes in body image and have the appropriate knowledge to fit the soft breast prosthesis (Keeton & McAloon, 2002).*

## Pediatric

- ▲ Consider the development of a Healthy Kids mentoring program that has four components: (1) relationship building, (2) self-esteem enhancement, (3) goal setting, and (4) academic assistance (tutoring). Mentors met with students twice each week for 1½ hours each session on school grounds. During each meeting, mentors devoted time to each program component. **EB:** *Paired sample* t *tests were conducted to assess The Healthy Kids Mentoring Program effect on mentored students' self-esteem and connectedness scores from pretest to posttest. Results indicated students' overall self-esteem, school connectedness, peer connectedness, and family connectedness were significantly higher at posttest than at pretest (King et al, 2002).*
- ▲ Assess and provide referrals to mental health professionals for clients with unresolved worries associated with terrorism. **EBN:** *National Association of Pediatric Nurse Practitioners (NAPNAP) initiated a new national campaign entitled Keep Your Children/Yourself Safe and Secure (KySS). The first phase of this campaign was to conduct a national survey. Results of this survey indicated that interventions are urgently needed to assist children and teens in coping with the multitude of stressors related to growing up in today's society (Melnyk et al, 2002).*
- ▲ Provide an alternative school-based program for pregnant and parenting teenagers. **EBN:** *Analysis of the data revealed four major themes: (1) nurture and positive regard, (2) sisterhood and belonging, (3) mentoring and sense of family, and (4) proactive learning environment and academic pride. The girls who attended the program developed close relationships with their peers and teachers. Many of them experienced academic success for the first time and reported that pregnancy and impending motherhood motivated them to do better in school (Spear, 2002).*

S

### Geriatric

▲ Encourage clients to consider a Web-based support program when they are in a caregiving situation. **EBN:** *In this study of caregivers of clients' with stroke, the caregivers came together and provided support for each other via a Web-based support program (Pierce et al, 2004).*

### Multicultural

- Carefully assess each client and allow families to participate in providing care that is acceptable based on the client's cultural beliefs; silent presence, quiet prayers (Hasidic Jewish families), telling stories, and singing songs in their native language. *Health services in a pluralistic society require interventional approaches that recognize the significance of culture in shaping a person's conception of self, as well as mental health and illness (Carnevale, 1999).*
- Provide support for health promoting behaviors and self-concept for clients from diverse cultures. **EBN:** *In this convenience sample, regression analyses demonstrated that the internalization racial identity stage (beta = 0.12; $p < 0.001$) and self-esteem (beta = 0.50; $p < 0.001$) contributed to the variance in health-promoting lifestyles (Johnson, 2002).*
- Refer to care plans **Disturbed Body image**; **Chronic low Self-esteem**; and **Readiness for enhanced Spiritual well-being.**

### Home Care

- Previously discussed interventions may be used in the home care setting.

## evolve WEBSITES FOR EDUCATION

See the EVOLVE website for World Wide Web resources for client education.

## REFERENCES


Carnevale FA: Toward a cultural conception of the self, *J Psychosoc Nurs Ment Health Serv* 37(8):26, 1999.

Cole DA, Maxwell SE, Martin JM et al: The development of multiple domains of child and adolescent self-concept: a cohort sequential longitudinal design, *Child Dev* 72(6):1723, 2001.

Gecsedi RA: Massage therapy for patients with cancer, *Clin J Oncol Nurs* 6(1):52, 2002.

Keeton S, McAloon L: The supply and fitting of a temporary breast prosthesis, *Nurs Stand* 16(41):43, 2002.

King K, Vidourek R, Davis B: Increasing self-esteem and school connectedness through a multidimensional mentoring program, *J School Health* 72(7):294, 2002.

McNicholas SL: Social support and positive health practices, *West J Nurs Res* 24(7):772, 2002.

Melnyk BM, Feinstein NF, Tuttle J et al: Mental health worries, communication, and needs in the year of the U.S. terrorist attack: national KySS survey findings, *J Pediatr Health Care* 16(5):222, 2002.

Peterson J, Atwood JR, Yates B: Key elements for church-based health promotion programs: outcome-based literature review, *Public Health Nurs* 19(6):401, 2002.

Pierce LL, Steiner V, Govoni AL: Caregivers dealing with stroke pull together and feel connected, *J Neurosci Nurs* 36(1):32-9, 2004.

Spear HJ: Reading, writing, and having babies: a nurturing alternative school program, *J School Nurs* 18(5):293, 2002.

Walter R, Davis K, Glass N: Discovery of self: exploring, interconnecting and integrating self (concept) and nursing, *Collegian* 6(2):12, 1999.


S

# Chronic low Self-esteem

Judith R. Gentz

## NANDA

### Definition

Long-standing negative self-evaluation/feelings about self or self-capabilities

### Defining Characteristics

Rationalizes away/rejects positive feedback and exaggerates negative feedback about self (long-standing or chronic), self-negating verbalization (long-standing or chronic), hesitant to try new things/situations (long-standing or chronic), expressions of shame/guilt (long-standing or chronic), evaluates self as unable to deal with events (long-standing or chronic), lack of eye contact, nonassertive/passive, frequent lack of success in work or other life events, excessively seeks reassurance, overly conforming, dependent on others' opinions, indecisive

### Related Factors (r/t)

Chronic illness (specify), persistent mental illness (specify), ongoing relationship problems (specify), ongoing social problems (specify)

## NOC

### Outcomes (Nursing Outcomes Classification)

#### Suggested NOC Outcomes

Self-Esteem

**Example NOC Outcome with Indicators**

Demonstrates improved **Self-Esteem** as evidenced by the following indicators: Verbalizations of acceptance of self and limitations/Open communication (Rate each indicator of **Self-Esteem:** 1 = never positive, 2 = rarely positive, 3 = sometimes positive, 4 = often positive, 5 = consistently positive [see Section I].)

S

### Client Outcomes

**Client Will (Specify Time Frame):**

- Demonstrate improved ability to interact with others (e.g., maintains eye contact, engages in conversation, expresses thoughts/feelings)
- Verbalize increased self-acceptance through positive self-statements about self
- Identify personal strengths, accomplishments, and values
- Identify and works on small, achievable goals
- Improve independent decision-making and problem-solving skills

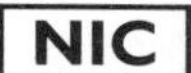

## Interventions (Nursing Interventions Classification)

### Suggested NIC Intervention

Self-Esteem Enhancement

| Example NIC Activities—Self-Esteem Enhancement |
| --- |
| Encourage client to identify strengths; assist client in setting realistic goals to achieve higher self-esteem |

## Nursing Interventions and Rationales

- Actively listen to and respect the client. *Listening and respect increase the development of a therapeutic relationship with the client.* **EBN:** *Listening and nurturing were identified as important aspects of care by clients (George, 2002).*
- Assess the client's environmental and everyday stressors, including physical health concerns and the potential of abusive relationships. *What clients face in their day-to-day lives is crucial to understanding their problems and goals.* **EBN:** *High everyday stress and a history of abuse in relationships are associated with low self-esteem and depressive symptoms (Lutenbacher, 2002).*
- Assess existing strengths and coping abilities, and provide opportunities for their expression and recognition. Self-esteem is enhanced by the ability to perform competently. **EBN:** *Nursing home residents supported in completing ADLs by nursing staff had significantly higher self-esteem than residents who were overly assisted (Blair, 1999).*
- Reinforce the personal strengths and positive self-perceptions that client identifies. Maintaining optimism may decrease anger and negative life events. **EBN:** *Lower levels of depressive symptoms were associated with higher optimism scores in rural adolescents (Puskar et al, 1999).*
- Identify and limit client's negative self-assessments. *Negative thinking increases depressive symptoms. Negative thinking had a greater effect on depressive symptoms than self-esteem (Peden, et al, 2000).*
- Encourage realistic and achievable goal setting, resources, and impediments to achievement. **EBN:** *Persons with higher self-esteem focus on resources and perceive fewer threats (Anderson, 2000).*
- Demonstrate and promote effective communication techniques; spend time with the client. **EBN:** *This study demonstrated the importance of presence and caring during communication (Sundin et al, 2002).*
- Encourage independent decision making by reviewing options and their possible consequences with client. **EBN:** *Perceived autonomy and control in nursing home residents increased motivation and self-esteem (Blair, 1999). Decision-making capacity is vital to a sense of autonomy (Hickman, 2004).*
- Assist client to challenge negative perceptions of self and performance. *Reduction in negative thinking is correlated with increase in self-esteem (Peden et al, 2000).*
- Use failure as an opportunity to provide valuable feedback. *This allows clients to change*

S

*expectations of what would happen given the reality of what did happen (Pierce & Hicks, 2001).*

- Promote a positive environment and activities that enhance self-esteem. *Self-esteem is positively correlated with the ability to meet self-care requirements (Blair, 1999).*
- Assist client with evaluating the effect of family and peer group on feelings of self-worth. *Strong negative societal messages may decrease self-esteem and increase depression (Peden, et al, 2000).*
- Support socialization and communication skills. **EBN:** *Social support increases the client's ability to cope with problems (Beebe, 2002).*
- Encourage journal/diary writing as a safe way of expressing emotions. **EBN:** *Journal writing prompts mood elevating activities and reduce reactive depression (Smith et al, 2003).*
- Help client to increase sense of belonging. *A sense of belonging reduces vulnerability to depression, effecting self-esteem (Haggerty & Williams, 1999).*

## Geriatric

- Support client in identifying and adapting to functional changes. *Accurate evaluation allows client to establish realistic expectations of self.*
- Use reminiscence therapy to identify patterns of strength and accomplishment. *Identifying strengths and accomplishments counteracts pervasive negativity.*
- Encourage participation in peer group activities. **EBN:** *Withdrawal and social isolation are detrimental to feelings of self-worth (Stuart-Shor, Buselli, & Carrol, 2003).*
- Encourage activities in which client can support/help others. **EBN:** *Helping others increases self-esteem in older adults. (Krause & Shaw, 2000).*

## Multicultural

- Assess for the influence of cultural beliefs, norms, and values on the client's sense of self-esteem. **EBN:** *How the client values self may be based on cultural perceptions (Cochran, 1998; Doswell & Erlen, 1998; Leininger & McFarland, 2002). Asian-American youths demonstrate lower levels of self-esteem than their non-Asian peers (Rhee, Chang, & Rhee, 2003).*
- Assess for evidence of patient financial strain. **EB:** *A recent study of Mexican origin individuals showed that financial strain was associated with cognitive self-esteem (Angel et al, 2003).*
- Assess for drug and alcohol use in individuals with low self-esteem. **EB:** *Among Mexican-American female adolescents, poor self-confidence predicts higher levels of alcohol use (Swaim & Wayman, 2004).*
- Validate the client's feelings regarding ethnic or racial identity. **EBN:** *Validation lets the client know that the nurse has heard and understands what was said, and it promotes the nurse-client relationship (Heineken, 1998). Individuals with strong ethnic affiliation have higher levels of self-esteem than others (Phinney, 1995; Greig, 2003).*

## Home Care

- Assess client's immediate support system/family for relationship patterns and content of communication. *Knowledge of client relationships helps the nurse to individualize care.*

- • Encourage family to provide support and feedback regarding client value or worth. *The family is a socially significant cultural group that generates behavior, defines roles, and promotes values.*
- ▲ Refer to medical social services to assist the family in pattern changes that could benefit the client. *The best nursing plan may be to access specialty services for the client and family.*
- ▲ If client is involved in counseling or self-help groups, monitor and encourage attendance. Help client identify value of group participation after each group encounter. *Discussion about group participation clarifies and reinforces group feedback and support.*
- ▲ If client is taking prescribed psychotropic medications, assess for knowledge of medication side effects and reasons for taking medication. Teach as necessary. *Understanding the medical regimen supports compliance.*
- ▲ Assess medications for effectiveness and side effects and monitor client for compliance. *Clients with poor ego strength may have difficulty adhering to a medication regimen. Clients who experience negative side effects are less likely than others to adhere to medication regimen.*

## Client/Family Teaching

- ▲ Refer to community agencies for psychotherapeutic counseling.
- ▲ Refer to psychoeducational groups on stress reduction and coping skills.
- ▲ Refer to self-help support groups specific to needs.

## evolve WEBSITES FOR EDUCATION

See the EVOLVE website for World Wide Web resources for client education.

## REFERENCES


Anderson E: Self-esteem and optimism in men and women infected with HIV: *Nurs Res* 49(5):262, 2000.

Angel RJ, Frisco M, Angel JL et al: Financial strain and health among elderly Mexican-origin individuals, *J Health Soc Beh* 44(4): 536-551, 2003.

Beebe LH: Problems in community living identified by people with schizophrenia, *J Psychosoc Nurs Ment Health Serv* 40(2):38, 2002.

Blair C: Effects of self-care ADL's on self-esteem of intact nursing home residents, *Issues Ment Health Nurs* 20:559-570, 1999.

Cochran M: Tears have no color, *Am J Nurs* 98(6):53, 1998.

Doswell W, Erlen J: Multicultural issues and ethical concerns in the delivery of revising care interventions, *Nurs Clin North Am* 33(2):353, 1998.

Giger JN, Davidhizar RE: *Transcultural nursing,* ed 2, St Louis, 1995, Mosby.

Greig R: Ethnic identity development: implications for mental health in African-American and Hispanic adolescents, *Issues Ment Health Nurs* 24(3):317-331, 2003.

Hagerty BM, Williams RA: The effects of sense of belonging, social support, conflict and loneliness on depression, *Nurs Res* 48(4):215, 1999.

Heineken J: Patient silence is not necessarily client satisfaction: communication in home care nursing, *Home Healthc Nurse* 16(2): 115, 1998.

Krause N, Shaw BA: Giving social support to others: socioeconomic status and self-esteem in late life, *J Gerontol B Psychol Sci Soc Sci* 55(6):S323, 2000.

Leininger MM: *Transcultural nursing: theories, research and practices,* ed 2, Hilliard, Ohio, 1996, McGraw-Hill.

Lutenbacher M: Relationships between psychosocial factors and abusive parenting attitudes in low-income single mothers, *Nurs Res* 51(3):158, 2002.

Maynard C: Psychoeducational approach to depression in women, *J Psychosoc Nurs Ment Health Serv* 31(12):9, 1993.
Peden AR, Hall LA, Rayens MK et al: Negative thinking mediates the effects of self-esteem on depressive symptoms in college women, *Nurs Res* 49(4):201, 2000.
Phinney JS: Ethnic identity and self-esteem. In Padilla A, editor: *Hispanic psychology: critical issues in theory and research,* Thousand Oaks, Calif, 1995, Sage.
Pierce P, Hicks F: Patient decision-making behavior: an emerging paradigm for nursing science, *Nurs Res* 50(5):267, 2001.
Puskar KR, Sereika SM, Lamb J et al: Optimism and its relationship to depression, coping, anger and life events in rural adolescents, *Issues Ment Health Nurs* 20(2):115, 1999.
Rhee S, Chang J, Rhee J: Acculturation, communication patterns, and self-esteem among Asian and Caucasian American adolescents, *Adolescence* 38(152):749-768, 2003.
Smith CE, Leenerts MH, Gajewski BJ: A systematically tested intervention for managing reactive depression, *Nurs Res* 52(6):401, 2003.
Stuart-Shor EM, Buselli EF, Carroll DL et al: Are psychosocial factors associated with the pathogenesis and consequences of cardiovascular disease in the elderly? *J Cardiovasc Nurs* 18(3):169, 2003.
Stuart GW, Laraia MT: Therapeutic nurse-patient relationship. In Stuart GW, Laraia MT, editors: *Principles and practice of psychiatric nursing,* St Louis, 2001, Mosby.
Swaim RC, Wayman JC: Multidimensional self-esteem and alcohol use among Mexican American and White non-Latino adolescents: concurrent and prospective effects, *Am J Orthopsychiatry* 74(4):559-570, 2004.

# Situational low Self-esteem

*Judith R. Gentz*

## NANDA

### Definition

Development of a negative perception of self-worth in response to a current situation (specify)

### Defining Characteristics

Verbally reports current situational challenge to self-worth; self-negating verbalizations; indecisive, nonassertive behavior; evaluation of self as unable to deal with situations or events; expressions of helplessness and uselessness

S

### Related Factors (r/t)

Developmental changes (specify); disturbed body image; functional impairment (specify); loss (specify); social role changes (specify); history of learned helplessness; history of abuse, neglect, or abandonment; unrealistic self-expectations; lack of recognition/rewards; behavior inconsistent with values; failures/rejections; decreased power/control; change in health status

## NOC

### Outcomes (Nursing Outcomes Classification)

#### Suggested NOC Outcomes

Decision Making, Self-Esteem

**Example NOC Outcome with Indicators**

Demonstrates **Self-Esteem** as evidenced by the following indicators: Verbalizations of acceptance of self and limitations/Open communication (Rate each indicator of **Self-Esteem:** 1 = never positive, 2 = rarely positive, 3 = sometimes positive, 4 = often positive, 5 = consistently positive [see Section I].)

## Client Outcomes

### Client Will (Specify Time Frame):

- State effect of life events on feelings about self
- State personal strengths
- Acknowledge presence of guilt and not blame self if an action was related to another person's appraisal
- Seek help when necessary
- Demonstrate self-perceptions are accurate given physical capabilities
- Demonstrate separation of self-perceptions from societal stigmas

**NIC**

## Interventions (Nursing Interventions Classification)

### Suggested NIC Interventions

Self-Esteem Enhancement

**Example NIC Activities—Self-Esteem Enhancement**

Encourage client to identify strengths; assist client in setting realistic goals to achieve higher self-esteem.

## Nursing Interventions and Rationales

- ▲ Assess the client for signs and symptoms of depression and potential for suicide and/or violence. If present, immediately notify the appropriate personnel of symptoms. See care plans for **Risk for other-directed Violence** and **Risk for Suicide.** *Nursing plays a vital role in assessing safety issues, managing the clients, and supervising other staff (Barloon, 2003).*
- Actively listen to, demonstrate respect for, and accept client. *Clarification of thoughts and feelings promotes self-acceptance (LeMone, 1991).*
- Assist in the identification of problems and situational factors that contribute to problems, offering options for resolution. **EBN:** *Clients often expect professionals to recommend remedies to problems and need encouragement to participate in selecting treatment options (Pierce & Hicks, 2001).*
- Mutually identify strengths, resources, and previously effective coping strategies. **EBN:** *Acknowledgment of competence reinforces previously intact self-esteem (Anderson, 1995). Knowledgeable clients make better decisions regarding their health care (Pierce & Hicks, 2001).*
- Have client list strengths. **EBN:** *Patients were found to use a variety of self-care strategies, medication management techniques, and emotional supports to alleviate symptoms of chronic heart failure (CHF) (Bennett et al, 2000).*

S

- Accept client's own pace in working through grief or crisis situations. *Maladjustment to loss or change can have detrimental effects on the entire concept of self (Drench, 1994).*
- Accept the client's own defenses in dealing with the crisis. *Denial protects the self-concept by distorting reality in a self-enhancing way (Russell, 1993). Decision-making behaviors adapt and change with time and experience (Pierce & Hicks, 2001).*
- Assess for unhealthy coping mechanisms such as substance abuse. *More than 50% of patients with mental illness also have substance abuse, and low self-esteem increases the risk further (NAMI online fact sheet, 2004).*
- Provide information about support groups of people who have common experiences or interests. **EBN:** *Social support was a strong predictor of resourcefulness, self-esteem, and well-being of postmastectomy patients (Dirsken, 2000).*
- Teach the client mindfulness techniques to cope more effectively with strong emotional responses. **EBN:** *Development of mindfulness strategies increased resolution of internal conflicts (Horton-Deutsch & Horton, 2003).*
- Support problem-solving strategies but discourage decision making when in crisis. *Crisis is a time of increased tension and disorganization.* **EBN:** *Uncertainty is a significant negative predictor of resourcefulness (Dirsken, 2000).*
- Assess client's environmental and everyday stressors, including evidence of abusive relationships. **EBN:** *High everyday stressors and a history of abuse in relationships are associated with low self-esteem and depression (Lutenbacher, 2002).*
- Encourage objective appraisal of self and life events and challenge negative or perfectionist expectations of self. *A positive adjustment to illness may be the result of the ability to lower ideal self-expectations (Heidrich & Ward, 1992).*
- Provide psychoeducation to client and family. **EB:** *Psychoeducation decreases symptomatology of client and increases support by care providers (Bigel, et al, 2000). Knowledge provides empowerment, which will increase self-esteem (Merrell, 2001).*
- Validate confusion when feeling ill but looking well. *Validation will decrease shame and guilt and invites further verbalization (Gordon et al, 1998).*
- Acknowledge the presence of societal stigma. Teach management tools. **EBN:** *Stigma was reported as a major influence on whether depressed and/or suicidal clients sought treatment (Raingruber, 2002).*
- Validate the effect of past experiences on self-esteem and work on corrective measures. *Family dysfunction, child abuse, and other childhood stressors may lead to low self-esteem (Harter, 2000).*
- See care plan for **Chronic low Self-esteem**.

S

### Geriatric

- Support the client in identifying and adapting to functional changes associated with aging. **EBN:** *Changes in physical well-being decrease emotional resources to cope with stress/grief (Talerico, 2003).*
- Use reminiscence therapy to identify patterns of strength and accomplishment. *Identifying strengths and accomplishments counteracts pervasive negativity.*
- Encourage participation in peer group activities. **EBN:** *Peer support provides an opportunity for sharing social modeling and reduces physiological arousal (Stuart-Shor, Buselli, & Carroll, 2003).*

- Encourage activities in which the client can support/help others. **EBN:** *Helping others increases self-esteem in older adults (Krause & Shaw, 2000).*

### Multicultural

- Assess for the influence of cultural beliefs, norms, and values on the client's sense of self-esteem. **EBN:** *How the client values self may be based on cultural perceptions (Cochran, 1998; Doswell & Erlen, 1998; Leininger & McFarland, 2002).*
- Validate the client's feelings regarding ethnic or racial identity. **EBN:** *Validation lets the client know that the nurse has heard and understands what was said, and it promotes the nurse-client relationship (Heineken, 1998). Individuals with strong ethnic affiliation have higher levels of self-esteem than others (Phinney, 1995).*

### Home Care

- Establish an emergency plan and contract with the client for its use. *Having an emergency plan is reassuring to the client. Establishing a contract validates the worth of the client and provides a caring link between the client and society.*
- Access supplies that support client's success at independent living.
- See care plan for **Chronic low Self-esteem**.

## Client/Family Teaching

- Assess person's support system (family, friends, community) and involve if desired.
- Educate client and family regarding the grief process. *Understanding this process normalizes responses of sadness, anger, guilt, and helplessness.*
- Teach client and family that the crisis is temporary. *Knowing that the crisis is temporary provides a sense of hope for the future.*

▲ Refer to appropriate community resources or crisis intervention centers.
▲ Refer to resources for handicap and/or disability services.
▲ Refer to illness-specific consumer support groups.
▲ Refer to self-help support groups specific to needs.

## evolve WEBSITES FOR EDUCATION

See the EVOLVE website for World Wide Web resources for client education.

S

## REFERENCES

Anderson K: The effect of chronic obstructive pulmonary disease on quality of life, *Res Nurs Health* 18:547, 1995.

Barloon, LF: Legal aspects of psychiatric nursing, *Nurs Clin North Am* 38(1):9, 2003.

Biegel DE, Robinson EM, Kennedy M: A review of empirical studies of interventions of families of persons with mental illness. In Morrisey J, editor: *Research in community mental health: social facets in mental health and illness,* vol 2, Greenwich, Conn, 2000, JAI Press.

Cochran M: Tears have no color, *Am J Nurs* 98(6):53, 1998.

Dirsken SR: Predicting well being among breast cancer survivors, *J Adv Nurs* 32(4):937, 2000.

Doswell W, Erlen J: Multicultural issues and ethical concerns in the delivery of revising care interventions, *Nurs Clin North Am* 33(2):353, 1998.

Drench ME: Changes in body image secondary to disease and injury, *Rehabil Nurs* 19:31, 1994.

Giger JN, Davidhizar RE: *Transcultural nursing,* ed 2, St Louis, 1995, Mosby.

Gordon PA, Feldman D, Crose R: The meaning of disability: how women with chronic illness view their experiences, *J Rehabil* 64:3, 1998.
Harter SL: Psychosocial adjustment of adult children of alcoholics, *Clin Psychol Rev* 20(3):311, 2000.
Heidrich SM, Ward SE: The role of the self in adjustment to cancer in elderly women, *Oncol Nurs Forum* 19:1491, 1992.
Heineken J: Patient silence is not necessarily client satisfaction: communication in home care nursing, *Home Healthc Nurse* 16(2): 115, 1998.
Horton-Deutsch S, Horton S: Mindfulness: overcoming intractable conflict, Arch *Psychiatr Nurs* 17(4):186, 2003.
Leininger MM: *Transcultural nursing: theories, research and practices,* ed 2, Hilliard, Ohio, 1996, McGraw-Hill.
LeMone P: Analysis of a human phenomenon: self-concept, *Nurs Diag* 2:126, 1991.
Merrell J: Social support for victims of domestic violence, *J Psychosoc Nurs* 39(11):30, 2001.
Miller JF: *Coping with chronic illness: overcoming powerlessness,* Philadelphia, 1983, FA Davis.
NAMI online fact sheet: *Dual disorders and integrated treatment.* Available at www.nami.org/content/contentgroups/helpline1/dual_diagnosis_and_integrated_treatment_of, accessed October 3, 2004.
Phinney JS: Ethnic identity and self-esteem. In Padilla A, editor: *Hispanic psychology: critical issues in theory and research,* Thousand Oaks, Calif, 1995, Sage.
Pierce P, Hicks F: Patient decision-making behavior: an emerging paradigm for nursing science, *Nurs Res* 50(5):267, 2001.
Puskar KR, Sereika SM, Lamb J et al: Optimism and its relationship to depression, coping, anger and life events in rural adolescents, *Issues in Ment Health Nurs* 20(2):115-130, 1999.
Raingruber B: Client and provider perspectives regarding the stigma of and non-stigmatizing interventions for depression. *Arch Psychiatr Nurs* 16(5):201, 2002.
Russell GC: The role of denial in clinical practice, *J Adv Nurs* 18:938, 1993.
Stuart GW, Laraia MT: Therapeutic nurse-patient relationship. In Stuart GW, Laraia MT, editors: *Principles and practice of psychiatric nursing,* St Louis, 2001, Mosby, p 30.
Stuart-Shor EM, Buselli EF, Carroll DL et al: Are psychosocial factors associated with the pathogenesis and consequences of cardiovascular disease in the elderly? *J Cardiovasc Nurs* 18(3):169, 2003.
Talerico K: Grief and older adults: differences, issues, and clinical approaches, *J Psychosoc Nurs* 41(7):12, 2003.

# Risk for situational low Self-esteem

evolve

*Judith R. Gentz*

## NANDA Definition

At risk for developing negative perception of self-worth in response to a current situation (specify)

S

## Risk Factors

Developmental changes (specify); disturbed body image; functional impairment (specify); loss (specify); social role changes (specify); history of learned helplessness; history of abuse, neglect, or abandonment; unrealistic self-expectations; behavior inconsistent with values; lack of recognition/rewards; failures/rejections; decreased power/control over environment; physical illness (specify)

## NOC Outcomes (Nursing Outcomes Classification)

### Suggested NOC Outcomes

Decision Making, Self-Esteem

**Example NOC Outcome with Indicators**

Demonstrates **Self-Esteem** as evidenced by the following indicators: Verbalizations of self-acceptance/ Acceptance of self-limitations/Open communication (Rate each indicator of **Self-Esteem:** 1 = never positive, 2 = rarely positive, 3 = sometimes positive, 4 = often positive, 5 = consistently positive [see Section I].)

## Client Outcomes

**Client Will (Specify Time Frame):**

- State accurate self-appraisal
- Demonstrate the ability to self-validate
- Demonstrate the ability to make decisions independent of primary peer group
- Express effects of media on self-appraisal
- Express influence of substances on self-esteem
- Identify strengths and healthy coping skills
- State life events and change as influencing self-esteem

## NIC Interventions (Nursing Interventions Classification)

### Suggested NIC Intervention

Self-Esteem Enhancement

**Example NIC Activities—Self-Esteem Enhancement**

Encourage client to identify strengths; help client to set realistic goals to achieve higher self-esteem

## Nursing Interventions and Rationales

- Help client to identify environmental and/or developmental factors that increase risk for low self-esteem. *Identification is an early stage of problem-solving process.* **EB:** *Preadolescence is a high-risk time for low self-esteem (McGee & Williams, 2000). Primary prevention includes community education in the schools (Merrell, 2001).*
- Assess the client's previous experiences with health care and coping with illness to determine the level of education and support needed. **EBN:** *Experienced patients report needing a different level of support than nonexperienced patients (Edwards et al 2001).*
- Help client to identify current behaviors resulting from low self-esteem. *Low self-esteem increases risk for unhealthy behaviors (Mcgee & Williams, 2000).*
- Encourage creative problem solving through writing exercises. **EBN:** *Creative writing increased self-efficacy and self-esteem among adolescents studied. Giving positive feedback can increase self-esteem (Chandler, 1999).*
- Encourage client to maintain highest level of functioning, including work schedule. **EBN:** *Social involvement and work were predictors of higher self-esteem among persons with mental illness (VanDongen, 1998). Encourage client to verbalize thoughts and feelings about the current situation, individually or in groups.* **EBN:** *Allowing the client to clarify*

S

*thoughts and feelings promotes self-acceptance (LeMone, 1991). Validation by others promotes acceptance of self (Linehan, 1993).*

- Help the client to identify what has helped maintain positive self-esteem thus far. *Identifying what works empowers the client and encourages positive outcomes.*
- Help the client to identify the resources and social support network available at this time. **EBN:** *Greater resourcefulness positively affected feelings of self-worth in breast cancer patients (Dirksen, 2000).*
- Assess for unhealthy coping mechanism such as substance abuse. *More than 50% of people with mental illness also have substance abuse, and low self-esteem increases the risk further (NAMI online fact sheet, 2004).*
- Encourage the client to find a self-help or therapy group that focuses on self-esteem enhancement. **EBN:** *Group therapy provides a safe place for feeling exploration, validation, positive role models, and gaining knowledge (Merrell, 2001).*
- Teach the client mindfulness techniques to cope with strong emotional responses and to prevent decreases in self-esteem. **EBN:** *Mindfulness strategies increase resolution of internal conflict and promote relaxation (Horton-Deutsch & Horton, 2003).* **EBN:** *Social support was a strong predictor of resourcefulness, self-esteem, and well-being in postmastectomy patients (Dirsken, 2000).*
- Encourage the client to create a sense of competence through short-term goal setting and goal achievement. **EB:** *Sense of competence is related to global self-esteem (Willoughby et al, 2000).*
- Educate female clients about self-esteem differences between genders, and encourage exploration. **EB:** *Females tend to have lower self-esteem than males no matter what domain is measured (Bolognini et al, 1996).*
- ▲ Assess the client for symptoms of depression and anxiety. Refer to specialist as needed. *Prompt and effective treatment can prevent exacerbation of symptoms or safety risks.*
- Teach client a systematic problem-solving process. *Crisis provides an opportunity for effective change in coping skills.*
- See care plans for **Disturbed personal Identity** and **Situational low Self-esteem**.

## Geriatric

- Help the client to identify age-related and/or developmental factors that may be affecting self-esteem. *Self-esteem levels vary with the normal aging process and tend to decrease with older age (Dietz, 1996).*
- Assist the client in life review and identifying positive accomplishments. *Life review is a developmental task that increases a person's sense of peace and serenity.*
- Help client to establish a peer group and structured daily activities. *Social isolation and lack of structure increase a client's sense of feeling lost and worthless.*

## Home Care

- Assess current environmental stresses and identify community resources. *Accessing resources to help decrease environmental stress will increase the client's ability to cope.*
- Encourage family members to acknowledge and validate the client's strengths. *Validation allows the client to increase self-reliance and to trust personal decisions.*

- Assess the need for establishing an emergency plan. *Openly assessing safety risks increases the client's sense of limits, boundaries, and safety.*
- See care plans for **Situational low Self-esteem** and **Chronic low Self-esteem**.

## Client/Family Teaching

▲ Refer the client/family to community-based self-help and support groups.
▲ Refer to educational classes on stress management, relaxation training, etc.
▲ Refer to community agencies that offer support and environmental resources.

## evolve WEBSITES FOR EDUCATION

See the EVOLVE website for World Wide Web resources for client education.

## REFERENCES


Bolognini M, Plancherel B, Bettschart W et al: Self-esteem and mental health in early adolescence: developmental and gender differences, *J Adolesc* 19(3):233, 1996.

Chandler GE: A creative writing program to enhance self-esteem and self-efficacy in adolescence, *J Child Adolesc Psychiatr Nurs* 12(2):70, 1999.

Dietz BE: The relationship of aging to self-esteem: the relative effects of maturation and role accumulation, *Int J Aging Hum Dev* 3:43, 1996.

Dirksen SR: Predicting well being among breast cancer survivors, *J Adv Nurs* 4:32, 2000.

Edwards J, Mulherin D, Ryan S et al: The experience of patients with rheumatoid arthritis admitted to the hospital, *Arthritis Care Res* 45:1-7, 2001.

Horton-Deutsch S, Horton S: Mindfulness: overcoming intractable conflict, *Arch Psych Nurs* 17(4):186, 2003.

LeMone P: Analysis of a human phenomenon: self-concept, *Nurs Diagn* 2:126, 1991.

McGee R, Williams S: Does low self-esteem predict health compromising behaviours among adolescents? *J Adolesc* 5:23, 2000.

Merrell J: Social support for victims of domestic violence, *J Psychos Nurs* 39(11):30, 2001.

NAMI online fact sheet: *Dual disorders and integrated treatment*. Available at www.nami.org/content/contentgroups/helpline1/dual_diagnosis_and_integrated_treatment_of, accessed October 3, 2004.

Van Dongen CJ: Self-esteem among persons with severe mental illness, *Issues Ment Health Nurs* 19(1):29, 1998.

Willoughby C, Polatajko H, Currado C et al: Measuring the self-esteem of adolescents with mental health problems: theory meets practice, *Can J Occup Ther* 67(4):230, 2000.


# Self-mutilation

*Kathleen L. Patusky*

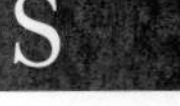

**NANDA**

## Definition

Deliberate self-injurious behavior causing tissue damage with the intent of causing nonfatal injury to attain relief of tension

## Defining Characteristics

Cuts/scratches on body; picking at wounds; self-inflicted burns (e.g., eraser, cigarette); ingestion/inhalation of harmful substances/objects; biting; abrading; severing; insertion of object(s) into body orifice(s); hitting; constricting a body part

## Related Factors (r/t)

Psychotic state (command hallucinations); inability to express tension verbally; childhood sexual abuse; violence between parental figures; family divorce; family alcoholism; family history of self-destructive behaviors; adolescence; peers who self-mutilate; isolation from peers; perfectionism; substance abuse; eating disorders; sexual identity crisis; low or unstable self-esteem; low or unstable body image; labile behavior (mood swings); history of inability to plan solutions or see long-term consequences; use of manipulation to obtain nurturing relationship with others; chaotic/disturbed interpersonal relationships; emotionally disturbed, battered child; feels threatened with actual or potential loss of significant relationship (e.g., loss of parent/parental relationship); experiences dissociation or depersonalization; mounting tension that is intolerable; impulsivity; inadequate coping; irresistible urge to cut/damage self; needs quick reduction of stress; childhood illness or surgery; foster, group, or institutional care; incarceration; character disorder; borderline personality disorder; developmentally delayed or autistic individual; history of self-injurious behavior; feelings of depression, rejection, self-hatred, separation anxiety, guilt, depersonalization; poor parent-adolescent communication; lack of family confidant

**NOC**

## Outcomes (Nursing Outcomes Classification)

### Suggested NOC Outcomes

Aggression Self-Control, Distorted Thought Self-Control, Impulse Self-Control, Mood Equilibrium, Risk Detection, Self-Mutilation Restraint

**Example NOC Outcome with Indicators**

**Self-Mutilation Restraint** as evidenced by the following indicators: Refrains from gathering means for self-injury/Seeks help when feeling urge to injure self/Upholds contract not to harm self/Maintains self-control without supervision/Refrains from injuring self (Rate each indicator of **Self-Mutilation Restraint:** 1 = never demonstrated, 2 = rarely demonstrated, 3 = sometimes demonstrated, 4 = often demonstrated, 5 = consistently demonstrated [see Section I].)

S

## Client Outcomes

### Client Will (Specify Time Frame):

- Have injuries treated
- Refrain from further self-injury
- State appropriate ways to cope with increased psychological or physiological tension
- Express feelings
- Seek help when having urges to self-mutilate
- Maintain self-control without supervision
- Use appropriate community agencies when caregivers are unable to attend to emotional needs

NIC

## Interventions (Nursing Interventions Classification)

### Suggested NIC Interventions

Active Listening; Anger Control Assistance; Behavior Management: Self-Harm; Calming Technique; Environmental Management: Safety; Limit Setting; Mood Management; Mutual Goal Setting; Risk Identification; Self-Responsibility Facilitation

**Example NIC Activities—Behavior Management: Self-Harm**

Anticipate trigger situations that may prompt self-harm and intervene to prevent; teach and reinforce effective coping behaviors and appropriate expression of feelings

## Nursing Interventions and Rationales

NOTE: Before implementation of interventions in the face of self-mutilation, nurses should examine their own emotional responses to incidents of self-harm to ensure that interventions will not be based on countertransference reactions. **EBN:** *A study of emergency department nurses encountering individuals who self-mutilate showed that nurses may experience negative feelings toward such clients. More positive feelings were associated with perceived confidence in assessment and referral, belief in the ability to deal effectively with clients, empathy toward self-mutilating clients, and confidence in the ability to cope with legal and hospital regulations guiding care of the clients (McAllister et al, 2002).*

- ▲ Provide medical treatment for injuries. Use careful aseptic technique when caring for wounds. Care for the wounds in a matter-of-fact manner. *A significant impediment to wound healing is infection. A matter-of-fact approach avoids promoting inappropriate attention-getting behavior and may decrease repetition of behavior.*
- • Assess for risk of suicide. **EB:** *Although self-mutilation should not be viewed simply as failed suicide, it is a significant indicator of suicide risk (Guertin et al, 2001; Milnes, Owens, & Blenkiron, 2002). A study of suicide attempters showed that individuals who mutilate themselves are at greater risk for suicide than those who do not (Stanley et al, 2001). Refer to the care plan for* **Risk for Suicide.**
- • Assess for signs of depression, anxiety, and impulsivity. *These behaviors are identified in clients with a history of self-mutilation (Stanley et al, 2001).*
- • Assess for presence of hallucinations. Ask specific questions such as, "Do you hear voices that other people do not hear? Are they telling you to hurt yourself?" *Command hallucinations occurring with schizophrenia or brief psychotic episodes may direct the client to hurt himself or herself, or others (Kress, 2003). An accurate assessment of the client's contact with reality is important in planning care. Acknowledging that the client may hear something that others do not may open up communication and help establish trust. The presence of hallucinations may also indicate use of specific medications (i.e., antipsychotics) that can reduce the hallucinations more effectively than antianxiety medications.*
- ▲ Assure the client that he or she will not be alone and will be safe during hallucinations. Provide referrals for medication. *Hallucinations can be very frightening; therefore clients need reassurance that they will not be left alone.*

S

▲ Assess for the presence of medical disorders, mental retardation, medication effects, or psychiatric disorders that may include self-mutilation. Initiate referral for evaluation and treatment as appropriate. **EB:** *Self-mutilation has been reported as a presenting symptom with medical disorders, such as the genetic Lesch-Nyhan disease (multiple types of behaviors; Robey et al, 2003); as a behavior initiated or aggravated by medications, such as certain serotonin reuptake inhibitors (skin picking; Denys, van Megan, & Westenberg, 2003) or amphetamines (genital mutilation; Israel & Lee, 2002); and as a sign of overt or incipient schizophrenia (autocastration; Myers & Nguyen, 2001). Children have demonstrated self-mutilative behavior in the presence of mental retardation (Zafeiriou et al, 2004) and spinal cord injury (biting and skin picking; Vogel & Anderson, 2002).*

- Differentiate between self-mutilation due to other causes and Munchausen syndrome. *Munchausen syndrome is a psychiatric factitious disorder in which individuals may create self-inflicted injuries as a means of assuming the sick role (de Fontaine et al, 2001).*
- Monitor the client's behavior using 15-minute checks at irregular times so that the client does not notice a pattern. *When lack of control exists, client safety is an important issue and close observation is essential. Avoiding a pattern prevents clients from being self-abusive when they know a caregiver will not be present.*
- Establish trust. *Establishing trust appears to be the most critical component of assessing and treating the client who self-mutilates (Derouin & Bravender, 2004; Machoian, 2001). Discussing feelings of self-harm with a trusted person provides relief for the client.*
- Be extremely cautious about touching the client when he or she is experiencing an abreaction (reenactment of precipitating trauma). Sometimes physically holding a client is necessary to prevent self-injury. *Reexperiencing of a traumatic event may initiate self-mutilation behavior in individuals with this behavior pattern. Touch may be interpreted as coming from an abuser and could result in aggressive acting out. Even well-intentioned or consoling touching may further upset the client. A therapist who is attempting to be consoling should always ask abreacting clients whether they may be touched. Clients may initially refuse, but they generally appreciate the offer. An offer may be repeated several times and clients may eventually agree to be touched or held. If clients must be held to prevent self-injury, explain why it is necessary before touching them (Weber, 2002).*
- Assess the client's ability to enter into a no-suicide contract. Secure a written or verbal contract from the client to notify staff when experiencing the desire to self-mutilate. *Discussing feelings of self-harm with a trusted person provides relief for the client. A contract gets the subject out in the open and places some of the responsibility for safety with the client. Some clients are not appropriate for a contract: those under the influence of drugs or alcohol or unwilling to abstain from substance use; those who are isolated or alone without assistance to keep the environment safe (Hauenstein, 2002). If the client will not contract, the risk of suicide should be considered higher. The lack of willingness for self-disclosure has been shown to discriminate the serious suicide attempter from clients with suicidal ideation or mild attempts (Apter et al, 2001).* **EBN:** *Contracting is a common practice in the psychiatric care setting. However, research has suggested that self-harm is not prevented by contracts (Drew, 2001). The researcher concluded that thorough, ongoing assessment of suicide risk is necessary, whether or not the client has a no self-harm contract.*

S

- ▲ Use a collaborative approach for care. *A collaborative approach to care is more helpful to the client (Clarke & Whittaker, 1998).*
- ▲ Refer for medication such as clozapine. **EB:** *In a study of seven subjects known to have a personality disorder and severe self-mutilation, there was a statistically significant reduction in incidents of self-mutilation with the use of medication (Chengappa et al, 1999).*
- ▲ Consider partial hospitalization with individual and group therapy. **EB:** *Psychoanalytically oriented partial hospitalization is superior to standard psychiatric care for clients with borderline personality disorder. These clients had a decrease in self-mutilation (Bateman & Fonagy, 1999).*
- • Refer to care plan for **Risk for Self-mutilation** for additional information.

### Home Care

See care plan for **Risk for Self-mutilation**.

## Client/Family Teaching

See care plan for **Risk for Self-mutilation**.

## evolve WEBSITES FOR EDUCATION

See the EVOLVE website for World Wide Web resources for client education.

## REFERENCES

Apter A, Horesh N, Gothelf D et al: Relationship between self-disclosure and serious suicidal behavior, *Comp Psychiatry* 42(1):70, 2001.

Bateman A, Fonagy P: Effectiveness of partial hospitalization in the treatment of borderline personality disorder: a randomized controlled trial, *Am J Psychiatry* 156(10):1563, 1999.

Chengappa KN, Ebeling T, Kang JS et al: Clozapine reduces severe self-mutilation and aggression in psychotic patients with borderline personality disorder, *J Clin Psychiatry* 60(7):477, 1999.

Clarke L, Whittaker M: Self-mutilation: culture, contexts and nursing responses, *J Clin Nurs* 7(2):129, 1998.

De Fontaine S, Van Geertruyden J, Preud'homme X, et al: Munchausen syndrome, *Ann Plast Surg* 46(2):153, 2001.

Denys D, van Megen HG, Westenberg HG: Emerging skin-picking behaviour after serotonin reuptake inhibitor treatment in patients with obsessive-compulsive disorder: possible mechanisms and implications for clinical care, *J Psychopharm* 17(1):127, 2003.

Derouin A, Bravender T: Living on the edge: the current phenomenon of self-mutilation in adolescents, *MCN Am J Matern Child Nurs* 29(1):12, 2004.

Drew BL: Self-harm behavior and no-suicide contracting in psychiatric inpatient settings, *Arch Psychiatr Nurs* 15:99, 2001.

Guertin T, Lloyd-Richardson E, Spirito A et al: Self-mutilative behavior in adolescents who attempt suicide by overdose, *J Am Acad Child Adolesc Psychiatry* 40(9):1062, 2001.

Hauenstein EJ: Case finding and care in suicide: children, adolescents, and adults. In Boyd MA, editor: *Psychiatric nursing: contemporary practice,* ed 2, Philadelphia, 2002, Lippincott.

Israel JA, Lee K: Amphetamine usage and genital self-mutilation, *Addiction* 97:1213, 2002.

Kress, VEW: Self-injurious behaviors: assessment and diagnosis, *J Counsel Develop* 81(4):490, 2003.

Machoian L: Cutting voices: self-injury in three adolescent girls, *J Psychosoc Nurs Ment Health Serv* 39(11):22, 2001.

McAllister M, Creedy D, Moyle W et al: Nurses' attitudes towards clients who self-harm, *J Adv Nurs* 40(5):578, 2002.

Milnes D, Owens D, Blenkiron P: Problems reported by self-harm patients. Perception, hopelessness, and suicidal intent, *J Psychosom Res* 53:819, 2002.

Myers WC, Nguyen M: Autocastration as a presenting sign of incipient schizophrenia, *Psychiatric Serv* 52(5):685, 2001.

S

Robey KL, Reck JF, Giacomini KD et al: Modes and patterns of self-mutilation in persons with Lesch-Nyhan disease, *Dev Med Child Neurol* 45:167, 2003.
Stanley B, Gameroff MJ, Michalsen V et al: Are suicide attempters who self-mutilate a unique population? *Am J Psychiatry* 158(3): 427, 2001.
Vogel LC, Anderson CJ: Self-injurious behavior in children and adolescents with spinal cord injuries, *Spinal Cord* 40:666, 2002.
Weber MT: Triggers for self-abuse: a qualitative study, *Arch Psychiatr Nurs* 16:118, 2002.
Zafeiriou DI, Vargiami E, Economou M et al: Self-mutilation and mental retardation: clues to congenital insensitivity to pain with anhidrosis, *J Pediatr* 144:284, 2004.

# Risk for Self-mutilation

*Kathleen L. Patusky*

**NANDA**

## Definition

At risk for deliberate self-injurious behavior causing tissue damage with the intent of causing nonfatal injury to attain relief of tension

## Risk Factors

Psychotic state (command hallucinations); inability to express tension verbally; childhood sexual abuse; violence between parental figures; family divorce; family alcoholism; family history of self-destructive behaviors; adolescence; peers who self-mutilate; isolation from peers; perfectionism; substance abuse; eating disorders; sexual identity crisis; low or unstable self-esteem; low or unstable body image; history of inability to plan solutions or see long-term consequences; use of manipulation to obtain nurturing relationship with others; chaotic/disturbed interpersonal relationships; emotionally disturbed and/or battered child; feels threatened with actual or potential loss of significant relationship; loss of parent/parental relationships; experiences dissociation or depersonalization; experiences mounting tension that is intolerable; impulsivity; inadequate coping; experiences irresistible urge to cut/damage self; needs quick reduction of stress; childhood illness or surgery; foster, group, or institutional care; incarceration; character disorders; borderline personality disorders; loss of control of problem-solving situations; developmentally delayed or autistic individual; history of self-injurious behavior; feelings of depression, rejection, self-hatred, separation anxiety, guilt, and depersonalization

**NOC**

## Outcomes (Nursing Outcomes Classification)

### Suggested NOC Outcomes

Abuse Recovery: Emotional; Aggression Self-Control; Distorted Thought Self-Control; Impulse Self-Control; Mood Equilibrium; Risk Detection; Self-Mutilation Restraint



S

**Example NOC Outcome with Indicators**

**Self-Mutilation Restraint** as evidenced by the following indicators: Refrains from gathering means for self-mutilation/Seeks help when feeling urge to injure self (Rate each indicator of **Self-Mutilation Restraint:** 1 = never demonstrated, 2 = rarely demonstrated, 3 = sometimes demonstrated, 4 = often demonstrated, 5 = consistently demonstrated [see Section I].)

## Client Outcomes

### Client Will (Specify Time Frame):

- Refrain from self-injury
- Identify triggers to self-mutilation
- State appropriate ways to cope with increased psychological or physiological tension
- Express feelings
- Seek help when having urges to self-mutilate
- Maintain self-control without supervision
- Use appropriate community agencies when caregivers are unable to attend to emotional needs

**NIC**

## Interventions (Nursing Interventions Classification)

### Suggested NIC Interventions

Active Listening; Anger Control Assistance; Behavior Management: Self-Harm; Calming Technique; Counseling; Environmental Management: Safety; Limit Setting; Mood Management; Mutual Goal Setting; Risk Identification; Self-Awareness Enhancement; Self-Esteem Enhancement; Self-Modification Assistance; Self-Responsibility Facilitation

**Example NIC Activities—Behavior Management: Self-Harm**

Anticipate trigger situations that may prompt self-harm and intervene to prevent; teach and reinforce effective coping behaviors and appropriate expression of feelings

S

## Nursing Interventions and Rationales

NOTE: Before implementation of interventions in the face of self-mutilation, nurses should examine their own emotional responses to incidents of self-harm to ensure that interventions will not be based on countertransference reactions. **EBN:** *A study of emergency department nurses encountering individuals who self-mutilate showed that nurses may experience negative feelings toward such clients. More positive feelings were associated with perceived confidence in assessment and referral, belief in the ability to deal effectively with clients, empathy toward self-mutilating clients, and confidence in the ability to cope with legal and hospital regulations guiding care of the clients (McAllister et al, 2002).*

- Assessment data from the client and family members may have to be gathered at different times; allowing a family member or trusted friend with whom the client is comfortable to be present during the assessment may be helpful. *Self-mutilation sometimes occurs if clients have been victims of abuse. Clients or family members may be more willing to disclose the presence of abuse if greater privacy is afforded them. Presence of a trusted family member or friend may help clients to respond more comfortably to the interview situation.*

- • Assess for risk factors of self-mutilation, including the categories of psychiatric disorders (particularly borderline personality disorder, psychosis, eating disorders, autism); psychological precursors (e.g., low tolerance for stress, impulsivity, perfectionism); psychosocial dysfunction (e.g., presence of sexual abuse, divorce or alcoholism in the family, manipulative behavior to gain nurturing, chaotic interpersonal relationships); coping difficulties (e.g., inability to plan solutions or see long-term consequences of behavior); personal history (e.g., childhood illness or surgery, past self-injurious behavior); and peer influences (e.g., friends who mutilate, isolation from peers). *All of the risk factors listed previously have been found to be associated with self-mutilation. A study of self-injurious behavior in women with eating disorders concluded that the occurrence of an eating disorder was sufficient to indicate the need for routine screening for self-injury (Paul et al, 2002).*
- ▲ Assess for the presence of medical disorders, mental retardation, medication effects, or psychiatric disorders that may include self-mutilation. Initiate referral for evaluation and treatment as appropriate. **EB:** *Self-mutilation has been reported as a presenting symptom with medical disorders, such as the genetic Lesch-Nyhan disease (multiple types of behaviors; Robey et al, 2003), Tourette's syndrome, autism, and temporal lobe epilepsy (Kress, 2003); as a behavior initiated or aggravated by medications, such as certain serotonin reuptake inhibitors (skin picking; Denys, van Megan, & Westenberg, 2003) or amphetamines (genital mutilation; Israel & Lee, 2002); and as a sign of overt or incipient schizophrenia (autocastration; Myers & Nguyen, 2001). Children have demonstrated self-mutilative behavior in the presence of mental retardation (Zafeiriou et al, 2004) and spinal cord injury (biting and skin picking; Vogel & Anderson, 2002).*
- • Differentiate between self-mutilation due to other causes, such as Munchausen syndrome. *Munchausen syndrome is a psychiatric factitious disorder in which individuals may create self-inflicted injuries as a means of assuming the sick role (de Fontaine et al, 2001).*
- • Assess family dynamics and need for family therapy, community supports. *Treatment generally focuses on increasing support for the client, improving family communication, and enhancing the client's sense of control over the environment (Derouin & Bravender, 2004).*
- • Assess for presence of hallucinations. Ask specific questions such as, "Do you hear voices that other people do not hear? Are they telling you to hurt yourself?" *Command auditory hallucinations occurring with schizophrenia or with brief psychotic episodes may direct the client to hurt himself, herself, or others (Kress, 2003). An accurate assessment of the client's contact with reality is important in planning care. Acknowledging that the client may hear something that others do not may open up communication and help establish trust. The presence of hallucinations may also indicate use of specific medications (i.e., antipsychotics) that can reduce the hallucinations more effectively than antianxiety medications.*
- ▲ Assure the client that he or she will not be alone and will be safe during hallucinations. Provide referrals for medication. *Hallucinations can be very frightening; therefore clients*

S

*need reassurance that they will not be left alone. Significantly reduced rates of further self-harm were observed for depot flupentixol versus placebo in multiple repeaters (Hawton et al, 1998).*

- Be alert to other risk factors of self-mutilation in clients with psychosis, including acute intoxication, dramatic changes in body appearance, preoccupation with religion and sexuality, and anticipated or perceived object loss. **EB:** *A case study of a client with bipolar disorder who self-mutilated revealed the previous list of risk factors, along with more usual risk factors of self-mutilation history and command auditory hallucinations. The client shaved his head, voiced literal interpretations of the Bible and profound feeling of guilt about his sexuality, and experienced rejection by his mother (Green et al, 2000).*
- Monitor clients with obsessive-compulsive disorder for possible self-mutilation. *Clients with high levels of obsessive-compulsive symptoms may self-mutilate (McKay et al, 2000).*
- Assess clients who have issues with gender identity or men who were molested as children for possible self-mutilation. *A study suggested that clients attending gender dysphoria clinics were at risk for self-mutilation (Wylie, 2000).* **EB:** *Another study of men who experienced child sexual abuse found that all forms of sexual molestation were predictive of self-harming behavior (King, Coxell, & Mezey, 2002).*
- Maintain ongoing surveillance of the client and environment. Monitor the client's behavior using 15-minute checks at irregular times so that the client does not notice a pattern. *When lack of control exists, client safety is an important issue and close observation is essential. Not following a pattern prevents clients from being self-abusive when they know a caregiver will not be present.*
- ▲ When the client is experiencing extreme anxiety, use one-to-one staffing. Offer activities that will serve as a distraction. **EBN:** *The presence of a trusted individual may calm fears about personal safety. Distraction was reported by self-abusing women as one way of preventing a self-injury episode (Weber, 2002).*
- Implement active listening and early intervention. **EBN:** *In one study, adolescent girls with a history of trauma found that cutting themselves communicated psychological distress when others would not listen to their verbal grievances but lead to a pattern of self-harm when intervention was not forthcoming (Machoian, 2001).*
- ▲ Refer to mental health counseling. Multiple therapeutic modalities are available for treatment. **EBN:** *Solution-focused brief therapy has been shown to be an effective treatment option for reducing repetitive self-harm (Wiseman, 2003).*
- When working with self-mutilative clients with borderline personality disorder, develop an effective therapeutic relationship by avoiding labeling, seeking to understand the meaning of the self-mutilation, and advocating for adequate opportunities for care. **EBN:** *The lived experience of clients with borderline personality disorder identified despair, estrangement, and inadequacy as elements of that experience. Living with the diagnosis resulted in the following experiences: being labeled rather than diagnosed, leading to preconceived and unfavorable opinions by all health care providers and a sense of being marginalized and potentially mistreated; having self-mutilation viewed as deliberate attempts to manipulate others rather than a means of controlling emotional pain; and limited access to care when health care providers conclude nothing will help and clients should "help themselves" (Moffat, 1999; Nehls, 1999).*



S

- When working with self-mutilative clients with a diagnosis of a Cluster B Personality Disorder (borderline, antisocial, narcissistic, or histrionic), carefully assess suicidal ideation. **EB:** *A study showed that Cluster B suicide attempters who also had a history of self-mutilation tended to be more depressed, anxious, and impulsive than those who did not self-mutilate. The Cluster B participants also tended to underestimate the lethality of their suicide attempt; as a result, clinicians could unintentionally underestimate the suicide risk (Stanley et al, 2001).*
- Maintain a consistent relational distance from the client with borderline personality disorder who self-mutilates: neither too close nor too distant, neither rewarding unacceptable behavior nor trying to control or avoid the client. *Clients with borderline personality disorder recreate the chaos of their previous relationships in dealing with health care providers. Clients fear that they will be overwhelmed by or abandoned in relationships, and their reactions can change rapidly. The most effective posture is one that is consistent, allowing clients to react as they need to, while assuring clients that they will not be abandoned (Horsfall, 1999).*
- Inform the client of unit expectations for appropriate behavior and consequences. Emphasize that the client must comply with the rules of the unit. Contract with the client for no self-harm. Give positive reinforcement for compliance and minimize attention paid to disruptive behavior while setting limits. *Clients benefit from clear guidance regarding behavioral expectations and consequences, providing much-needed structure. The process emphasizes client responsibility for his or her own behavior. It is important to reinforce appropriate behavior to encourage repetition. The unit serves as a microcosm of client's outside world, so adherence to social norms while on the unit models adherence upon discharge, while providing the client with staff support to learn appropriate coping skills and alternate behaviors.*
- Assess the client's ability to enter into a no-suicide contract. Secure a written or verbal contract from the client to notify staff when experiencing the desire to self-mutilate. *Discussing feelings of self-harm with a trusted person provides relief for the client. A contract gets the subject out in the open and places some of the responsibility for safety with the client. Some clients are not appropriate for a contract: those under the influence of drugs or alcohol or unwilling to abstain from substance use; those who are isolated or alone without assistance to keep the environment safe (Hauenstein, 2002). If the client will not contract, the risk of suicide should be considered higher. The lack of willingness for self-disclosure has been shown to discriminate the serious suicide attempter from clients with suicidal ideation or mild attempts (Apter et al, 2001).* **EBN:** *Contracting is a common practice in psychiatric care setting. However, research has suggested that self-harm is not prevented by contracts (Drew, 2001). The researcher concluded that thorough, ongoing assessment of suicide risk is necessary, whether or not the client has a no self-harm contract. Assist the client to identify and express the feelings that are being acted out in self-mutilation.*
- Clients need to learn to recognize distress as it occurs and express it verbally rather than as a physical action against the self. *Self-mutilation serves to act out feeling states that the client cannot express or process. Such acts may attempt to relieve pain or punish the self. Therapy helps the client to articulate emotions and needs (Derouin et al, 2004).*
- Assist the client to identify the motives/reasons for self-mutilation that have been perceived as positive. *Favazza (1989) identified the following gains of self-mutilation: ten-*

S

*sion release, returning to reality, regaining control of some aspect of self, expressing forbidden anger, escaping self-hatred associated with incest, aiming to decrease alienation from or influence others, relieve pressure from multiple personalities, sexual gratification, the sight of blood provides emotional release, the pain and the blood stop feelings of emptiness. The client must learn alternative ways of securing these gains if they are to give up self-mutilation as a means of obtaining the gains. The nurse should ask the client directly what is gained from continued self-mutilation, rather than assuming the motivation is already known (McAllister, 2001).*

- Help the client identify cues that precede impulsive behavior. *Early recognition of triggers permits the client to initiate self-calming procedures, such as relaxation techniques.* **EB:** *Dialectical behavior therapy (DBT) was found to be superior to non-DBT treatment in reducing self-mutilation among individuals with borderline personality disorder (Verheul et al, 2003).* **EBN:** *The DBT technique of behavioral chain analysis was found to reduce self-harm behaviors by 50% over a 4-week period, by processing events that precipitate self-mutilation (Alper & Peterson, 2001).*
- Give praise when the client identifies urges and delays self-destructive behavior. *Delaying destructive behavior and increasing awareness of urges to be self-destructive should both be acknowledged as progress.*
- Assist clients to identify ways to sooth themselves and generate hopefulness when faced with painful emotions. **EBN:** *Women with a history of childhood abuse may not have developed the internal ability to comfort themselves, or self-soothe, resulting in neurobiological disruptions that lead to self-harm as a means of relieving pain (Gallop, 2002). Generating hopefulness is an important self-comforting intervention (Weber, 2002).*
- Be extremely cautious about touching the client when he or she is experiencing an abreaction (reenactment of precipitating trauma). Sometimes physically holding a client is necessary to prevent self-injury. *Reexperiencing of a traumatic event, such as physical or sexual abuse, may initiate self-mutilative behavior in individuals with this behavior pattern. Touch may be interpreted as coming from an abuser and could result in aggressive acting out. Even well-intentioned or consoling touching may further upset the client. A therapist who is attempting to be consoling should always ask the reacting clients whether they might be touched. Clients may initially refuse, but they generally appreciate the offer. An offer may be repeated several times, and clients may eventually agree to be touched or held. If clients must be held to prevent self-injury, explain why it is necessary before touching them (Weber, 2002).*
- Reinforce alternative ways of dealing with depression and anxiety such as exercise, engaging in unit activities, or talking about feelings. *A study testing response to exercise, sertraline, or exercise plus sertraline found that the exercise-only group experienced the lowest depression levels, with the benefit of exercise continuing after the intervention period (Babyak et al, 2000).*
- Keep environment safe; remove all harmful objects from the area. Use of unbreakable glass is recommended for the client at risk for self-injury. *Client safety is a nursing priority. Unbreakable glass would eliminate this type of injury.*
- Encourage the client to seek out care providers to talk as urge to harm self occurs. Develop positive therapeutic relationship. *When the client seeks out staff, he or she is exercising self-responsibility and self-care management.* **EBN:** *Even with a contract in*

S

*place, clients are reassured that staff really do want to help. Self-abusing women have reported that caring relationships have kept them from hurting themselves, and that feeling comforted, supported, and believed would be helpful (Weber, 2002).*

- • Anticipate trigger situations and intervene to assist the client in applying alternatives to self-mutilation. *When triggers occur, client stress level may obstruct ability to apply new learning. Assistance facilitates the ability to practice new skills in real situations.*
- • Reduce or eliminate use of caffeine, alcohol, or street drugs. *Caffeine can increase anxiety, leading to a triggering of self-mutilation. Alcohol and street drugs alter mood and increase impulsivity while decreasing inhibitions (Derouin et al, 2004).*
- • If self-mutilation does occur, use a calm, nonpunitive approach. Whenever possible, assist the client to assume responsibility for consequences (e.g., dress self-inflicted wound). Refer to care plan for **Self-mutilation.** *This approach does not promote inappropriate attention-getting behavior, may decrease repetition of behavior, and reinforces self-responsibility and self-care management.*
- • If the client is unable to control behavior, provide interactive supervision, not isolation. *Isolation and deprivation take away individuals' coping abilities and place them at risk for self-harm. Implementing seclusion for clients who have injured themselves in the past may actually facilitate self-injury. Clients are extraordinarily resourceful at identifying environmental objects with which to self-mutilate.*
- ▲ Refer for medication such as clozapine. **EB:** *In a study of seven subjects known to have a personality disorder and severe self-mutilation, there was a statistically significant reduction in incidents of self-mutilation with use of medication (Chengappa et al, 1999).*
- • Involve the client in planning of care and problem solving, and emphasize that the client makes choices. *Individuals who self-mutilate can become caught up in power struggles with staff. A self-care management approach can circumvent such problems while emphasizing client responsibility and promoting active participation in therapeutic regimen. Individuals who self-mutilate also tend toward emotional impulsivity.* **EB:** *Problem solving is a way to gain better emotional control by assisting clients with seeing the connection between problems and emotions. A study of problem-solving therapy with self-mutilators indicated that the therapy significantly decreased depression, hopelessness, and perceived problems (Townsend et al, 2001). Individuals who self-mutilate were found to use more problem avoidance behaviors and to perceive that they had less control over problem-solving options (Haines & Williams, 2003).*
- ▲ Involve the client in group therapy. *Through interaction with others, group members learn to identify patterns of behavior that were acquired as a result of painful past events. The past is not trivialized but acknowledged as leading to patterns that now influence all interactions.*
- ▲ Use group therapy to exchange information about methods of coping with loneliness, self-destructive impulses, and interpersonal relationships, as well as housing, employment, and health care system issues directly and noninterpretively. *The group's focus should be here and now, supportive and psychoeducative, while providing a comforting level of structure.*
- ▲ Refer to protective services if evidence of abuse exists. *It is the nurse's legal responsibility to report abuse.*
- ▲ Discharge planning: Provide follow-up to ensure clients attend mental health appoint-

S

ments. *Only a small fraction of people who present in general health care settings with self-mutilation actually follow through with mental health specialist appointments (Tobin et al, 2001).*

- Monitor the client for self-harm impulses that may progress to suicidal ideation. *Self-mutilation is a significant indicator of suicide risk (Guertin et al, 2001; Milnes, Owens, & Blenkiron, 2002).*

## Pediatric

- Be aware of increasing incidence of self-mutilation, especially among teens and young adults. *The developmental stressors of adolescence, along with depression, play a role in the increased incidence of self-mutilation, especially among teens who do not have the usual risk factors of schizophrenia, severe depression, history of abuse, chemical dependency, or incarceration (Derouin et al, 2004).* **EBN:** *Teens who self-mutilate may be academically and socially successful, high-achieving, and outgoing, managing to hide evidence of problems or ineffective coping skills (Machoian, 2001).*
- Conduct a thorough physical examination, being alert for superficial scars that may be patterned, although in most cases scabbing or infection is not evident. *Apart from obvious sites, evidence of cutting or burning may be hidden in areas such as the axilla, abdomen, inner thighs, feet, and under breasts (Derouin et al, 2004).*
- Maintaining a therapeutic relationship with teens requires explicit assurances of confidentiality, consistency of clinical routines, and a nonjudgmental communication style. *Even adolescents younger than age 18 need assurances that confidentiality will be maintained unless there is a serious risk of harm to themselves or others (Bravender, 2002). However, teens of all ages should be advised that parental notification will be made to ensure the teen's safety and to implement a treatment plan (Derouian et al, 2004).*
- Attend to behavioral clues of self-mutilation; a brief self-report assessment can be useful. *Self-mutilators can exhibit mood swings, low self-esteem, poor impulse control, anxiety, self-disappointment, or an inability to identify positive elements in their lives (Machoian, 2001). The American Medical Association's Guidelines for Adolescent Preventive Services (GAPS) can be helpful, and is available at www.ama-assn.org/ama/pub/category/2280.html (Derouin et al, 2004).*
- Assess for the presence of an eating disorder or substance abuse. Attend to the themes that preoccupy teens with eating disorders who self-mutilate. **EB:** *Self-mutilation was shown to be more common among adolescents with dependence issues (drug abuse and eating disorders) (Bolognini et al, 2003). The thought processes of adolescents with eating disorders were found to center on themes of feeling undeserving of receiving help, feeling helpless and hopeless in dealing with the eating disorder itself, difficulty with recognizing and expressing feelings, and ambivalence regarding treatment along with mistrust of health care providers (Manley & Leichner, 2003).*
- Evaluate for suicidal ideation/suicide risk. Refer to care plan for **Risk for Suicide** for additional information. **EB:** *A study of adolescents who attempted suicide by overdose revealed that over one third of participants admitted to some method of self-mutilation. The self-mutilators were significantly more likely than non-self-mutilators to be diagnosed with oppositional defiant disorder, major depression, and dysthymia, and had higher scores on measures of hopelessness, loneliness, anger, risk taking, and alcohol use (Guertin et al, 2001).*

S

- Be aware that complete overlap does not exist between self-mutilation and suicidal behavior. The motivation may be different (coping with difficult feelings rather than ending life), and the method is usually different. **EB:** *In one study, about half of the participants reported both attempted suicide and self-mutilation; the other half there was no overlap in types of acts (Bolognini et al, 2003).*
- Use treatment approaches detailed previously, with modifications as appropriate for this age group.

## Geriatric

- Provide hand or back rubs and calming music when elderly client experiences symptoms of anxiety. **EBN:** *In a study of older adults in nursing homes, calming music and hand massage were found to soothe agitation for up to 1 hour. No additional benefit was found from combining the two interventions (Remington, 2002).*
- Provide soft objects for elderly clients to hold and manipulate when self-mutilation occurs as a function of delirium or dementia. Apply mitts, splints, helmets, or restraints as appropriate. *Delirious or demented clients may unconsciously scratch or pick at themselves. Soft objects may provide a substitute object to pick at; mitts or restraints ay be necessary if the client is unable to exercise self-restraint.*
- Older adults who show self-destructive behaviors should be evaluated for dementia. **EB:** *In a study of nursing home residents, self-destructive behaviors were common and more likely related to dementia than to depression (Draper et al, 2002).*

## Home Care

- Communicate degree of risk to family/caregivers; assess the family and care-giving situation for ability to protect the client and to understand the client's self-mutilative behavior. Provide family and caregivers with guidelines on how to manage self-harm behaviors in the home environment. *Client safety between home visits is a nursing priority. Family/caregivers may become frightened by the client's self-mutilation or may be angry with the client's perceived lack of self-control. Appropriate family/caregiver support is important to the client. Appropriate support will only be forthcoming if all parties understand the basis of the behavior and how to respond to it.*
- Establish an emergency plan, including when to use hotlines and 911. Develop a contract with the client and family for use of the emergency plan. Role play access to the emergency resources with the client and caregivers. *Having an emergency plan reassures the client and caregivers and promotes client safety. Contracting gives guided control to the client and enhances self-esteem.*
- Assess the home environment for harmful objects. Have family remove or lock objects as able. *Client safety is a nursing priority.*

▲ If client behaviors intensify, institute emergency plan for mental health intervention. *The degree of disturbance and the ability to manage care safely at home determines the level of services needed to protect the client.*

▲ Refer for homemaker or psychiatric home health care services for respite, client reassurance, and implementation of therapeutic regimen. *Responsibility for a person at high risk for self-mutilation provides high caregiver stress. Respite decreases caregiver stress. The presence of caring individuals is reassuring to both the client and caregivers, especially*

S

*during periods of client anxiety. Self-mutilative behavior, especially if accompanied by depression, can make use of the interventions described previously, modified for the home setting.*

- ▲ If the client is on psychotropic medications, assess client and family knowledge of medication administration and side effects. Teach as necessary. *Knowledge of the medical regimen promotes compliance and promotes safe use of medications.*
- ▲ Evaluate the effectiveness and side effects of medications. *Accurate clinical feedback improves physician ability to prescribe an effective medical regimen specific to client needs.*

## Client/Family Teaching

- Explain all relevant symptoms, procedures, treatments, and expected outcomes for self-mutilation that is illness based (e.g., borderline personality disorder, autism). *By increasing knowledge and adapting new behaviors, clients learn that they have some control over their health (Hennessy-Harstad, 1999). Clients are more amenable to therapy and better able to initiate appropriate self-care if they know what to expect.*
- Assist family members to understand the complex issues of self-mutilation. Provide instruction on relevant developmental issues, and on actions parents can take to avoid media that glorify self-harm behaviors. *Family members need to understand the behaviors with which they are dealing, need to receive positive reinforcement that will promote their patience and perseverance, and need to know that they can take positive action to remove media triggers for self-mutilation (Derouin et al, 2004).*
- Provide written instructions for treatments and procedures for which the client will be responsible. *A written record provides a concrete reference so that the client and family can clarify any verbal information that was given.*
- Instruct the client in coping strategies (assertiveness training, impulse control training, deep breathing, progressive muscle relaxation). *Clients who self-mutilate have difficulty dealing with stress and painful emotions, which serve as triggers to self-harm. Once clients are able to identify these triggers, they need to learn how to respond to them more effectively through assertiveness, impulse control, or relaxation, as appropriate.*
- Role play (e.g., say, "Tell me how you will respond if someone ignores you"). *Role playing is the most commonly used technique in assertiveness training. It deconditions the anxiety that arises from interpersonal encounters by allowing the client to practice how they might respond in a given situation. Anxiety levels tend to be higher in situations that are unfamiliar.*
- Teach cognitive-behavioral activities, such as active problem solving, reframing (reappraising the situation from a different perspective), or thought-stopping (in response to a negative thought, picture a large stop sign and replace the image with a prearranged positive alternative). Teach the client to confront his or her own negative thought patterns (or cognitive distortions), such as catastophizing (expecting the very worst), dichotomous thinking (perceiving events in only one of two opposite categories), or magnification (placing distorted emphasis on a single event). *Clients who self-mutilate have a low tolerance for stress. Individuals with borderline personality disorder commonly engage in self-talk that is invalid and self-deprecating. Cognitive-behavioral activities address clients' assumptions, beliefs, and attitudes about their situations, fostering modification of these elements to be as realistic and optimistic as possible. Persons with*

S

*negative cognitive styles tend to perceive situations as overwhelming, resistant to improvement, and all-encompassing. Through cognitive-behavioral interventions, clients become more aware of their cognitive choices in adopting and maintaining their belief systems, thereby exercising greater control over their own reactions (Hagerty & Patusky, 2003; Sinclair et al, 1998).*

▲ Provide the client and family with phone numbers of appropriate community agencies for therapy and counseling. *Continuous follow-up care should be implemented; therefore the method to access this care must be given to the client.*

▲ Give the client positive things on which to focus by referring to appropriate agencies for job-training skills or education. *Alternative coping skills and the means to access them are essential for continued good mental health.*

## evolve WEBSITES FOR EDUCATION

See the EVOLVE website for World Wide Web resources for client education.

## REFERENCES


Alper G, Peterson SJ: Dialectical behavior therapy for patients with borderline personality disorder, *J Psychosoc Nurs Ment Health Serv* 39(10):38, 52, 2001.

Apter A, Horesh N, Gothelf D et al: Relationship between self-disclosure and serious suicidal behavior, *Comp Psychiatry* 42(1):70, 2001.

Babyak M, Blumenthal JA, Herman S et al: Exercise treatment for major depression: maintenance of therapeutic benefit at 10 months, *Psychosom Med* 62:633, 2000.

Bolognini M, Plancherel B, Laget J et al: Adolescents' self-mutilation: relationship with dependent behaviour, *Swiss J Psychol* 62(4):241, 2003.

Bravender T: *Adolescent medicine,* Monograph ed. No. 279, Laewood, Kan, 2002, American Academy of Family Physicians.

Chengappa KN, Ebeling T, Kang JS et al: Clozapine reduces severe self-mutilation and aggression in psychotic patients with borderline personality disorder, *J Clin Psychiatry* 60(7):477, 1999.

De Fontaine S, Van Geertruyden J, Preud'homme X et al: Munchausen syndrome, *Ann Plast Surg* 46(2):153, 2001.

Denys D, van Megen HG, Westenberg HG: Emerging skin-picking behaviour after serotonin reuptake inhibitor treatment in patients with obsessive-compulsive disorder: possible mechanisms and implications for clinical care, *J Psychopharm* 17(1):127, 2003.

Derouin A, Bravender T: Living on the edge: the current phenomenon of self-mutilation in adolescents, *MCN Am J Matern Child Nurs* 29(1):12, 2004.

Draper B, Brodaty H, Lee-Fay L et al: Self-destructive behaviors in nursing home residents, *J Am Geriatr Soc* 50(2):354, 2002.

Drew BL: Self-harm behavior and no-suicide contracting in psychiatric inpatient settings, *Arch Psychiatr Nurs* 15:99, 2001.

Favazza A: Why patients mutilate themselves, *Hosp Commun Psychiatry* 40:137, 1989.

Gallop R: Failure of the capacity for self-soothing in women who have a history of abuse and self-harm, *J Am Psychiatr Nurses Assoc* 8:20, 2002.

Green CS, Knysz W, Tsuang MT: A homeless person with bipolar disorder and a history of serious self-mutilation, *Am J Psychiatry* 157:1392, 2000.

Guertin T, Lloyd-Richardson E, Spirito A et al: Self-mutilative behavior in adolescents who attempt suicide by overdose, *J Am Acad Child Adolesc Psychiatry* 40(9):1062, 2001.

Hagerty B, Patusky K: Mood disorders: depression and mania. In Fortinash KM, Holoday-Worret PA, editors: *Psychiatric mental health nursing,* ed 3, St Louis, 2003, Mosby.

Haines J, Williams CL: Coping and problem solving of self-mutilators, *J Clin Psychol* 59(10):1097, 2003.

Hauenstein EJ: Case finding and care in suicide: children, adolescents, and adults. In Boyd MA, editor: *Psychiatric nursing. Contemporary practice,* ed 2, Philadelphia, 2002, Lippincott.

Hawton K, Arensman E, Townsend E et al: Deliberate self-harm: systematic review of efficacy of psychosocial and pharmacological treatments in preventing repetition, *BMJ* 317(7156):441, 1998.


S

Hennessy-Harstad EB: Empowering adolescents with asthma to take control through adaptation, *J Pediatr Health Care* 13:273, 1999.
Horsfall J: Towards understanding some complex borderline behaviors, *J Psychiatr Ment Health Nurs* 6:425, 1999.
Israel JA, Lee K: Amphetamine usage and genital self-mutilation, *Addiction* 97:1213, 2002.
King M, Coxell A, Mezey G: Sexual molestation of males: associations with psychological disturbance, *Br J Psychiatry* 181:153, 2002.
Kress, VEW: Self-injurious behaviors: assessment and diagnosis, *J Counsel Develop* 81(4):490, 2003.
Machoian L: Cutting voices: self-injury in three adolescent girls, *J Psychosoc Nurs Ment Health Serv* 39(11):22, 2001.
Manley RS, Leichner P: Anguish and despair in adolescents with eating disorders: helping to manage suicidal ideation and impulses, *Crisis* 24(1):32, 2003.
McAllister MM: In harm's way: a postmodern narrative inquiry, *J Psychiatr Ment Health Nurs* 8:391, 2001.
McAllister M, Creedy D, Moyle W et al: Nurses' attitudes towards clients who self-harm, *J Adv Nurs* 40(5):578, 2002.
McKay D, Kulchycky S, Danyko S: Borderline personality and obsessive-compulsive symptoms, *J Personal Disord* 14(1):57, 2000.
Milnes D, Owens D, Blenkiron P: Problems reported by self-harm patients. Perception, hopelessness, and suicidal intent, *J Psychosom Res* 53:819, 2002.
Moffat C: Wound care. Self-inflicted wounding. I. Psychosomatic concepts and physical conditions, *Br J Community Nurs* 4:502, 1999.
Myers WC, Nguyen M: Autocastration as a presenting sign of incipient schizophrenia, *Psychiatric Serv* 52(5):685, 2001.
Nehls N: Borderline personality disorder: the voice of patients, *Res Nurs Health* 22:285, 1999.
Paul T, Schroeter K, Dahme B et al: Self-injurious behavior in women with eating disorders, *Am J Psychiatry* 159:408, 2002.
Remington R: Calming music and hand massage with agitated elderly, *Nurs Res* 51:317, 2002.
Robey KL, Reck JF, Giacomini KD et al: Modes and patterns of self-mutilation in persons with Lesch-Nyhan disease, *Dev Med Child Neurol* 45:167, 2003.
Sinclair VG, Wallston KA, Dwyer KA et al: Effects of a cognitive-behavioral intervention for women with rheumatoid arthritis, *Res Nurs Health* 21:315, 1998.
Stanley B, Gameroff MJ, Michalsen V et al: Are suicide attempters who self-mutilate a unique population? *Am J Psychiatry* 158(3): 427, 2001.
Tobin MJ, Clarke AR, Buss R et al: From efficacy to effectiveness: managing organizational change to improve health services for young people with deliberate self harm behaviour, *Aust Health Rev* 24:143, 2001.
Townsend E, Hawton K, Altman DG et al: The efficacy of problem-solving treatments after deliberate self-harm: meta-analysis of randomized controlled trials with respect to depression, hopelessness and improvement in problems, *Psychol Med* 31:979, 2001.
Verheul R, Van den Bosch LMC, Koeter MWJ et al: Dialectical behaviour therapy for women with borderline personality disorder, *Br J Psychiatry* 182:135, 2003.
Vogel LC, Anderson CJ: Self-injurious behavior in children and adolescents with spinal cord injuries, *Spinal Cord* 40:666, 2002.
Weber MT: Triggers for self-abuse: a qualitative study, *Arch Psychiatr Nurs* 16:118, 2002.
Wiseman S: Brief intervention: reducing the repetition of deliberate self-harm, *Nurs Times* 99:35, 2003.
Wylie KR: Suction to the breasts of a transsexual male, *J Sex Marital Ther* 26(4):353, 2000.
Zafeiriou DI, Vargiami E, Economou M et al: Self-mutilation and mental retardation: clues to congenital insensitivity to pain with anhidrosis, *J Pediatr* 44:284, 2004.



# Disturbed Sensory perception (specify: visual, auditory, kinesthetic, gustatory, tactile, olfactory) evolve

*Betty J. Ackley*

**NANDA**

## Definition

Change in the amount or patterning of incoming stimuli accompanied by a diminished, exaggerated, distorted, or impaired response to such stimuli

## Defining Characteristics

Poor concentration; auditory distortions; change in usual response to stimuli; restlessness; reported or measured change in sensory acuity; irritability; disoriented in time, in place, or with people; change in problem-solving abilities; change in behavior pattern; altered communication patterns; hallucinations; visual distortions

## Related Factors (r/t)

Altered sensory perception; excessive environmental stimuli; psychological stress; altered sensory reception, transmission, and/or integration/insufficient environmental stimuli; biochemical imbalances for sensory distortion (e.g., illusions, hallucinations); electrolyte imbalance; biochemical imbalance

**NOC**

## Outcomes (Nursing Outcomes Classification) for Disturbed Sensory Perception: Visual

### Suggested NOC Outcomes

Body Image; Cognitive Orientation; Sensory Function: Vision; Vision Compensation Behavior

**Example NOC Outcome with Indicators**

**Vision Compensation Behavior** as evidenced by the following indicators: Uses adequate light for activity being performed/Wears eyeglasses correctly/Uses vision assistive devices/Uses computer assistive devices/Uses support services for low vision (Rate each indicator of **Vision Compensation Behavior:** 1 = never demonstrated, 2 = rarely demonstrated, 3 = sometimes demonstrated, 4 = often demonstrated, 5 = consistently demonstrated [see Section I].)

**NOC**

## Outcomes (Nursing Outcomes Classification) for Disturbed Sensory Perception: Auditory

### Suggested NOC Outcomes

Cognitive Orientation; Communication: Receptive; Distorted Thought Self-Control; Hearing Compensation Behavior

**Example NOC Outcome with Indicators**

**Hearing Compensation Behavior** as evidenced by the following indicators: Reminds others to use techniques that advantage hearing/Eliminates background noise/Uses sign language/Uses lip reading/Uses hearing assistive devices/Uses hearing aid(s) correctly/Uses support services for hearing impaired (Rate each indicator of **Hearing Compensation Behavior:** 1 = never demonstrated, 2 = rarely demonstrated, 3 = sometimes demonstrated, 4 = often demonstrated, 5 = consistently demonstrated [see Section I].)

## Client Outcomes

**Client Will (Specify Time Frame):**

- Demonstrate understanding by a verbal, written, or signed response
- Demonstrate relaxed body movements and facial expressions
- Explain plan to modify lifestyle to accommodate visual or hearing impairment
- Remain free of physical harm resulting from decreased balance or a loss of vision, hearing, or tactile sensation
- Maintain contact with appropriate community resources

**NIC**

## Interventions (Nursing Interventions Classification)

### Suggested NIC Interventions

Cognitive Stimulation; Communication Enhancement: Hearing Deficit, Visual Deficit; Environmental Management

**Example NIC Activities—Communication Enhancement: Visual Deficit**

Identify yourself when you enter the patient's space; build on patient's remaining vision, as appropriate

## Nursing Interventions and Rationales

### Visual—Loss of Vision

- Identify name and purpose when entering the client's room. *Identification when entering the room helps the client feel secure and decreases social isolation.*
- Orient to time, place, person, and surroundings. Provide a radio or talking books. *These actions help the client remain oriented and provide sensory stimulation.*
- Keep doors completely open or closed. Keep furniture out of path to bathroom and do not rearrange furniture. *Consistency in placement of furniture and doors aids in location and decreases chances of injury (Houde & Huff, 2003).*
- Feed the client at mealtimes if blindness is temporary.
- Keep side rails up using half rails, maintain bed in a low position, keep call light readily available, and designate client a Fall Risk. **EB:** *Clients with visual impairment have increased risk for sustaining a fractured hip from a fall (Ivers, 2000).*
- Converse with and touch the client frequently during care if frequent touch is within the client's cultural norm. *Appropriate touch can decrease social isolation.*
- Walk the client by having the client grasp nurse's elbow and walk partly behind nurse.
- Walk a frightened or confused client by having the client put both hands on nurse's shoulders; nurse backs up in desired direction while holding the client around the waist. *These methods help the client feel secure and ensure safety.*
- Keep call light button within client's reach, and check location of call light button before leaving the room.

▲ For blind client, consider referring to a clinic for use of a blind mobility aid device that

S

uses ultrasound. *These devices can be helpful to the blind client to increase acuity to the environment and movement of objects in the environment (Bitjoka & Pourcelot, 1999).*

- Ensure access to eyeglasses or magnifying devices as needed.
- Pay attention to the client's emotional needs. Encourage expression of feelings and expect grieving behavior. *Blind people grieve the loss of vision and experience a loss of identity and control over their lives.* **EB:** *A study of 114 elderly age-related macular degeneration (AMD) clients indicated that 49 patients met Diagnostic and Statistical Manual of Mental Disorders (DSM-IV) criteria for syndromal depression and that visual acuity was the only variable significantly associated with vision-specific function. Although no effective treatments exist for restoring vision in AMD, depression is treatable. Both psychotherapy and antidepressants are efficacious and may indirectly improve function among older people with vision loss (Casten et al, 2002).*

▲ Refer to optometrist, ophthalmologist, or specialist in vision loss for vision care if needed. **EB:** *Photodynamic therapy for neovascular age-related changes is effective in preventing vision loss (Wormald et al, 2003).*

## Auditory—Hearing Loss

- Keep background noise to a minimum. Turn off television and radio when communicating with the client. If noisy environment, take the client to a private room and shut the door. *Background noise significantly interferes with hearing in the hearing-impaired client (Sommer & Sommer, 2002). Communication failure between health professionals and hearing-impaired clients is common (King, 2004).*
- Stand or sit directly in front of the client when communicating. Make sure adequate light is on nurse's face, avoid chewing gum or covering mouth or face with hands while speaking, establish eye contact, and use nonverbal gestures. *These measures make it easier to read lips and see nonverbal communication, which is a large component of all communication (Sommer & Sommer, 2002).*
- Speak distinctly in lower voice tones if possible. Do not overenunciate or shout at the client. *In many kinds of hearing loss, clients lose the ability to hear higher-pitched tones but can still hear lower-pitched tones. Overenunciating makes it difficult to read lips. Shouting makes the words less clear and may be painful (Jupiter & Spiver, 1997). Communication failure between health professionals and clients is common (King, 2004).*
- State the topic of conversation before begin the conversation; make it clear when you change conversation topics. *This helps give the client a clear context for interpreting what you are speaking about (Sommer & Sommer, 2002).*
- Verify the client understands critical information by asking the client to repeat the information back. *Hearing-impaired clients will often smile or nod when asked if they understand to avoid embarrassment; asking them to repeat the information back is the only way to verify they understand what is being said (Sommer & Sommer, 2002).*
- If necessary, provide a communication board or personnel who know sign language. *Health care institutions are required to provide and pay for qualified interpreters under the Americans with Disabilities Act; an interpreter can be found through the Registry of Interpreters for the Deaf (Sommer & Sommer, 2002).*

▲ Refer to appropriate resources such as a speech and hearing clinic; audiologist; or ear, nose, and throat physician. Refer children early for help. *Hearing loss can be treated with medical or surgical interventions or use of a hearing aid. Research demonstrates the positive effects of early diagnosis and intervention on the social and cognitive development of hearing-impaired children (Meadow-Orland et al, 1997).*

- • Encourage the client to wear hearing aid if available. **EB:** *A large study demonstrated that hearing-impaired persons who wore hearing instruments, compared with those who did not, were more socially active; experienced more interpersonal warmth and less interpersonal negativity; communicated more effectively; had less self-criticism, frustration, anger, and depression; and better health (Kochkin & Rogin, 2000).*
- ▲ Refer to hearing clinics.
- • Observe emotional needs and encourage expression of feelings. *Hearing impairments may cause frustration, anger, fear, and self-imposed isolation.*
- • For **Disturbed Sensory perception: kinesthetic, tactile,** see care plan for **Risk for Injury** or **Risk for Falls**. For **Disturbed Sensory perception: olfactory, gustatory,** see care plan for **Imbalanced Nutrition: less than body requirements.**

## Pediatric

- ▲ Test hearing of infants and begin treatment/therapy early as needed. *Early treatment of a hearing loss can decrease the effects of a hearing loss on social, emotional, and academic development of a child (Smith, Bale, & White, 2005).*
- • For classroom learning, ensure that ambient noise is minimized and devices are used to decrease reverberation in the environment. *For the hearing-impaired child, it is important that background noise is minimized and reverberation is controlled to increase the child's ability to hear and learn (Boothroyd, 2004; Crandell et al, 2004).*
- • Recommend the child use a frequency-modulated system along with a hearing aid in school. **EB:** *For classroom learning, use of a frequency-modulated system in combination with a personal hearing aid substantially improved speech recognition (Anderson & Goldstein, 2004).*
- ▲ Refer the child to the use of a language wizard player with Baldi, a computer-animated tutor for teaching vocabulary. **EB:** *A study demonstrated that use of the computer system resulted in excellent retention of learned words 4 weeks after the end of the experiment (Massaro & Light, 2004).*

## Geriatric

- • Keep environment quiet, soothing, and familiar. Use consistent caregivers. *These measures are comforting to the elderly and help decrease confusion.*
- • Avoid providing extremely hot or cold foods or using hot bath water if the client has decreased sensation in mouth, hands, or feet.
- • If the client has a sensory deprivation, encourage family to provide sensory stimulation with music, voices, photographs, touch, and familiar smells.
- • Increase the amount of light in the environment for elderly eyes; ensure it is nonglare lighting. *Increased lighting can help compensate for some of the visual changes of aging including reduced visual acuity, reduced contrast sensitivity, and reduced color discrimination (Boyce, 2003).*
- ▲ Refer to low-vision clinics, or the Independent Living Program, which is designed for older individuals who are blind to help maintain independence (Moore et al, 2001;

S

Houde & Huff, 2003). *Clients with vision loss should be referred to clinics early, preferably before vision is gone, for help dealing with the loss (Brown, 1998).* **EB:** *A research demonstrated that mobility function improved after blind rehabilitation training for a group of older veterans (Kuyk et al, 2004).*

- For a hearing impairment in the elderly, use the Hearing Handicap Inventory for the Elderly (HHIE-S) to determine how individuals perceive the emotional and social problems associated with a hearing loss. **EB:** *The HHIE-S is a valid and reliable questionnaire to predict social and emotional effects of hearing loss (Demers, 2001).*
- If the client has a hearing or vision loss, work with the client to ensure contact with others and to strengthen the social network. **EBN and EB:** *Severe loneliness can accompany vision loss in the elderly as a result of self-imposed isolation (Foxall et al, 1992). Loss of hearing has a negative effect on psychosocial function with loneliness and increased rate of depression (Wallhagen, 2001; Wallhagen 2002; Mullins 2004).*

### Home Care

- The listed interventions are applicable in the home care setting.

## Client/Family Teaching

### Low Vision

- Teach the client how to use a lighted magnification device to increase the ability to read text or see details.
- Teach the client to put a sheet of yellow acetate over text to make the text more visible. An alternative method is to highlight the text with a green or yellow highlighter (Beaver & Mann, 1995).
- Put red or yellow identifiers on important items that need to be seen, such as a red strip at the edge of steps, red behind a light switch, or a red dot on a stove or washing machine to indicate how far to turn knob. **EB:** *Color cues can improve the legibility of the environment and increase the ability to target objects quickly (Cooper, 1999).*
- Use a watch or clock that verbally tells time and a phone with large numbers and emergency numbers programmed into it.
- Teach blind client how to feed self; associate food on plate with hours on a clock so that the client can identify location of food.
- Use low-vision aids including magnifying devices for near vision and telescopes for seeing objects at a distance, a closed-circuit television that magnifies print, guides for writing checks and envelopes. *Low vision aids can improve vision in clients with limited sight (Derrington, 2002).*
- Teach the client with vision loss to do the following:
  - Use a magnifying mirror to shave, apply makeup. Use electric razor only.
  - Put personal care products in brightly colored pump containers (red, yellow, or orange) for identification.
  - Use tactile clues such as safety pins or buttons placed in hems to help client match clothing.
  - Use prefilled medication organizer with large lettering or three-dimensional (3D) markers.

*These methods can help maintain the independence of the client (McGrory, Remington, & Secrest, 2004).*

- Increase lighting in the home to help vision in the following ways:
  - Ensure adequate illumination of entire home, adding light fixtures and increasing wattage of existing bulbs as needed.
  - Decrease glare where light reflects on shiny surfaces, move or cover object.
  - Use nonglare wax on the floor.
  - Use motion lights that come on automatically when a person enters the room for nighttime use.
  - Add indoor strip or "runway" type of lighting to baseboards.

  *Visual acuity can be improved by taking steps to overcome age-related changes to vision (Slay, 2002; Smith, 1998).* **EB:** *Illumination can increase mobility in clients with age-related macular degeneration (Kuyk & Elliott, 1999).*

## Hearing Loss

- Suggest installation of devices such as ring signalers for the telephone and doorbell, sensors that detect an infant's cry, alarm clocks that vibrate the bed, and closed caption decoders for television sets. Other helpful devices include telephone amplifiers, speakerphones, pocket talker personal listening system, and FM and infrared amplification systems that connect directly to a TV or audio output jack. Also available is a telecommunication device—a typewriter keyboard with an alphanumeric display that allows the hearing-impaired person to send typed messages over the telephone line; software and modems are available that allow a home computer to be used in this fashion. Use of a hearing ear dogs—dogs specially trained to alert their owners to specific sound—may also be helpful. *These devices and the dogs can be helpful to increase communication and safety for the hearing-impaired client (Jupiter & Spiver, 1997; Zazove et al, 2004).*
- Teach client to avoid excessive noise at work or at home, wearing hearing protection when necessary. Any noise that hurts the ears or is above 90 decibels is excessive. *Hearing loss from excessive noise is common and preventable (Lusk, 2002; Smith, Bale, & White, 2005). The goal is to protect existing level of hearing.*
- Teach family how to provide appropriate stimuli in the home environment to prevent disturbed sensory perception.



## evolve WEBSITES FOR EDUCATION

See the EVOLVE website for World Wide Web resources for client education.

## REFERENCES

Anderson KL, Goldstein H: Speech perception benefits of FM and infrared devices to children with hearing aids in a typical classroom, *Lang Speech Hear Serv Sch* 35(2):169, 2004.

Beaver KA, Mann WC: Overview of technology for low vision, *Am J Occup Ther* 49:913, 1995.

Bitjoka L, Pourcelot L: New blind mobility aid devices based on the ultrasonic Doppler effect, *Int J Rehabil Res* 22(3):227, 1999.

Boothroyd A: Room acoustics and speech perception, *Seminars in Hearing* 25(2):155, 2004.

Boyce PR: Lighting for the elderly, *Technol Disabil* 15(3):165, 2003.

Casten RJ, Rovner BW, Edmonds SE: The impact of depression in older adults with age-related macular degeneration, *J Vis Impair Blindness* 96(6):399, 2002.
Cooper BA: The utility of functional colour cues: seniors' views, *Scand J Caring Sci* 13(3):186, 1999.
Crandell CC et al: Room acoustics intervention efficacy measures, *Seminars in Hearing* 25(2):201, 2004.
Demers K: Best practices in nursing care to older adults: hearing screening, *J Gerontol Nurs* 27(11):8, 2001.
Derrington D: Aids to low vision, *Nurs Res Care* 4:5, 2002.
Foxall MJ et al: Predictors of loneliness in low vision adults, *West J Nurs Res* 14:86, 1992.
Houde SC, Huff MA: Age-related vision loss in older adults: a challenge for gerontological nurses, *J Gerontol Nurs* 29(4):25, 2003.
Ivers RQ et al: Visual impairment and hip fracture, *Am J Epidemiol* 152(7): 633, 2000.
Jupiter T, Spiver V: Perception of hearing loss and hearing handicap on hearing aid use by nursing home residents: geriatric nursing, *Am J Care Aging* 18(5):201, 1997.
King A: Hearing and the elderly: a simple cure, *Geriatr Med* 34(6):9, 2004.
Kochkin W, Rogin CM: Quantifying the obvious: the impact of hearing instruments on quality of life, *Hearing Rev* 7:1, 2000.
Kuyk T, Elliott JL: Visual factors and mobility in persons with age-related macular degeneration, *J Rehabil Res Dev* 36(4):303, 1999.
Kuyk T et al: Mobility function in older veterans improves after blind rehabilitation, *J Rehabil Res Dev* 41(3):337, 2004.
Lusk SL: Preventing noise-induced hearing loss, *Nurs Clin North Am* 37(2):257, 2002.
Massaro DW, Light, J: Improving the vocabulary of children with hearing loss, *Volta Rev* 104(3):141, 2004.
McGrory A, Remington R, Secrest JA: Optimizing the functionality of clients with age-related macular degeneration, *Rehabil Nurs* 29(3):90, 2004.
Meadow-Orland KP et al: Support services for parents and their children who are deaf or hard of hearing, *Am Ann Deaf* 142(4): 278, 1997.
Moore JE, Giesen JM, Weber JM: Functional outcomes reported by consumers of the Independent Living Program for Older Individuals who are blind, *J Visual Impairment Blindness* 95:7, 2001.
Mullins T: Depression in older adults with hearing loss, *ASHA Leader* 9(1):12, 2004.
Slay DH: Home-based environmental lighting assessments for people who are visually impaired: developing techniques and tools, *J Visual Impairment Blindness* 96:2, 2002.
Smith SD: Aging, physiology, and vision, *Nurse Pract Forum* 9(1):19, 1998.
Smith RJ, Bale JF, White KR: Sensorineural hearing loss in children, *Lancet* 365(9462):879, 2005.
Sommer SK, Sommer NW: When your patient is hearing impaired, *RN* 65(12):28, 2002.
Wallhagen MI: Hearing impairment, *Annu Rev Nurs Res* 20:341, 2002.
Wallhagen MI, Strawbridge WJ, Kaplan GA: Five-year impact of hearing impairment on physical functioning, mental health and social relationships, *Br Soc Audiol News* 32:9, 2001.
Wormald R et al: Photo dynamic therapy for neovascular age-related macular degeneration, *Cochrane Database Syst Rev* (2): CD002030, 2003.
Zazove P et al: Deaf persons and computer use, *Am Ann Deaf* 148(5):376, 2004.

S

# Sexual dysfunction

*Gail B. Ladwig*

**NANDA**

## Definition

Change in sexual function that is viewed as unsatisfying, unrewarding, inadequate

## Defining Characteristics

Change of interest in self and others, conflicts involving values, inability to achieve desired satisfaction, verbalization of problem, alteration in relationship with significant other, alteration in achieving sexual satisfaction, actual or perceived limitation imposed by disease and/or therapy, seeking confirmation of desirability, alteration in achieving perceived sex role

## Related Factors (r/t)

Misinformation or lack of knowledge; vulnerability; values conflict; psychosocial abuse (e.g., harmful relationships); physical abuse; lack of privacy; ineffectual or absent role models; altered body structure of function (e.g., pregnancy, recent childbirth, drugs, surgery, anomalies, disease process, trauma, radiation); lack of significant other; biopsychosocial alteration of sexuality

**NOC**

## Outcomes (Nursing Outcomes Classification)

### Suggested NOC Outcomes

Abuse Recovery: Sexual; Physical Aging; Risk Control: Sexually Transmitted Diseases (STDs); Sexual Functioning, Sexual Identity

**Example NOC Outcome with Indicators**

**Sexual Functioning** as evidenced by the following indicators: Expresses comfort with sexual expression/ Expresses comfort with body/Expresses sexual interest (Rate each indicator of **Sexual Functioning:** 1= never demonstrated, 2 = rarely demonstrated, 3 = sometimes demonstrated, 4 = often demonstrated, 5 = consistently demonstrated [see Section I].)

## Client Outcomes

**Client Will (Specify Time Frame):**

- Identify individual cause of sexual dysfunction
- Identify stressors that contribute to dysfunction
- Discuss alternative, satisfying, and acceptable sexual practices for self and partner
- Discuss with partner concerns about body image and sex role

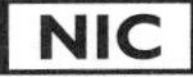

## Interventions (Nursing Interventions Classification)

### Suggested NIC Intervention

Sexual Counseling

**Example NIC Activities—Sexual Counseling**

Provide privacy and ensure confidentiality; discuss necessary modifications in sexual activity, as appropriate; provide referral/consultation with other members of the health care team, as appropriate

## Nursing Interventions and Rationales

- Gather the client's sexual history, noting normal patterns of functioning and the client's vocabulary. **EB:** *Health care professionals in urologic, gynecologic, and family practice* *offices and clinics are in key roles to identify females experiencing sexual dysfunction. Sexual identity is shaped throughout our life. It depends on religious and cultural beliefs and is strongly related to early sexual experiences (Brassil & Keller, 2002). Documentation of sexual function after all local treatments, including prostate brachytherapy, may help to clarify the cause of treatment-induced erectile dysfunction (ED) (Stipetich et al, 2002).*

- Determine the client's and partner's current knowledge and understanding. **EB:** *This survey indicated that in clinical practice and for those who have a partner, sexual disabilities and distress caused by them should be regarded from the partner relationship perspective (Fugl-Meyer & Fugl-Meyer, 2002).*
- ▲ Assess and provide treatment for ED. Involve the person's partner in the process. Consider pharmacologic and nonpharmacological interventions. **EB:** *Of equal value—and necessity—is the involvement of the man's partner in both the assessment and treatment processes of ED. Nonpharmacologic interventions should be considered as means to support and augment the effects of phosphodiesterase type 5 (PDE5) inhibitors (Dunn, 2004). ED affects the lives of up to 30 million American men and their partners (Mayo Foundation for Medical Education and Research, 2003).*
- Observe for stress, anxiety, and depression as possible causes of dysfunction. **EB:** *Sexual dysfunction can be attributed to many psychological factors. Sexual problems are common in chronic-pain patients. Patients who reported symptoms of depression and distress had more sexual problems than others (Monga et al, 1998). Recognition of sexual dysfunction associated with depression and its treatment is critical for client satisfaction and medication compliance (Clayton, 2001).*
- Observe for grief related to loss (e.g., amputation, mastectomy, ostomy). *A change in body image often precedes sexual dysfunction (see care plan for* **Disturbed Body image***). The trauma of being diagnosed and treated for breast cancer can greatly affect women's psychosexual functioning and intimate relationships. Survivors of breast cancer report that issues of body image, sexuality, and partner communication are rarely addressed by traditional health care providers (Anllo, 2000). Sexuality concerns should be addressed with all clients undergoing ostomy placement (Sprunk & Alteneder, 2000).*
- Explore physical causes such as diabetes, arteriosclerotic heart disease, arthritis, drug or medication side effects, or smoking (males). **EBN:** *Sexual difficulties often occur as a result of cardiovascular disease (Papadopoulos, 1995). In this research study, women with arthritis and a high degree of morning stiffness worried more about their bodies and reported significantly more problems with sexuality than others (Gutweniger et al, 1999). EBN: The literature review of 18 studies revealed the detrimental effect of smoking on erectile function. Smokers were 1.5 times more likely to suffer ED than were nonsmokers (Dorey, 2001a).*
- Provide privacy and be verbally and nonverbally nonjudgmental. *Privacy is important to ensure confidentiality. To facilitate communication, it is also vital that the nurse clarify personal values and remain nonjudgmental.*
- Provide privacy to allow sexual expression between the client and partner (e.g., private room, "Do Not Disturb" sign for a specified length of time). *The hospital setting has little opportunity for privacy, so the nurse must ensure that it is available.*
- Explain the need for the client to share concerns with partner. **EBN:** *This literature re-*



S

*view demonstrated increasing recognition that the partner should be involved in the assessment, diagnosis, patient education, counseling, and choice of treatment for long-term treatment to be successful, unless the informed patient is unwilling (Dorey, 2001b).*

- • Validate the client's feelings, let the client know that he or she is normal, and correct misinformation. **EB:** *Because men see the primary care physician's office as a natural and expected place in which to address issues of sexual health, those health care professionals who are prepared to initiate discussion of ED can offer patients and their partners the possibility of effective and enduring treatment success and the restoration of a satisfying relationship (Dunn, 2004).*
- ▲ Refer to appropriate medical providers for consideration of medication with premature ejaculation. **EB:** *This study examined the efficacy of citalopram, an SSRI, to 26 married patients diagnosed with premature ejaculation according to Diagnostic and Statistical Manual of Mental Disorders Third Revised Version (DSM-III-R). The patients were randomly assigned to two groups. The patients treated with citalopram showed significantly greater improvement compared with the patients receiving placebo (Atmaca et al, 2002).*
- ▲ Refer women for possible pharmacological intervention when sexual dysfunction is present. **EB:** *For women with sexual dysfunction pharmacotherapy may augment desire, arousability, and genital congestion, and lessen the pain of chronic dyspareunia (Basson, 2004).*

## Geriatric

- ▲ Carefully assess the sexuality needs of the elderly client and refer for counseling if needed. **EB:** *Older adults face several barriers to sexual expression, ranging from societal beliefs, to problems arising from aging, disease, and medications, to changes in social circumstances, particularly in nursing home placement. Because sexual issues are seldom volunteered, questions regarding sexuality and intimacy may have to be raised by the clinician, who can help his or her patients with sexual expression by providing appropriate assessment and counseling (Messinger-Rapport, Sandhu, & Hujer, 2003).*
- ▲ Carefully assess sexual functioning needs of clients with dementia and provide privacy for them and their spouse. **EBN:** *The author argues, from a relationship-centered perspective, that although women with dementia are particularly vulnerable to abuse, certainly some, if not most, sexual activity between loving spouses may be morally permissible even when one partner has dementia and cannot consent (Lingler, 2003).*
- • Teach about normal changes that occur with aging: Female—reduction in vaginal lubrication, decrease in the degree and speed of vaginal expansion, reduction in duration and resolution of orgasm. Male—increase in time required for erection, increase in erection time without ejaculation, less firm erection, decrease in volume of seminal fluid, increase in time before another erection can occur (12–24 hours). **EBN:** *The older adult experiences a number of physiological changes; however, these changes are gradual and vary from person to person (Shell & Smith, 1994). Erectile dysfunction may affect 1 in 10 men as they age (Sounes, 2001).*
- ▲ Suggest the following to enhance sexual functioning: Female—use water-based vaginal lubricant, increase foreplay time, avoid direct stimulation of the clitoris if painful (clitoris may be exposed because of atrophy of the labia), practice Kegel exercises (alternately contracting and relaxing the muscles in the pelvic area), urinate immedi-

S

ately after coitus to prevent irritation of the urethra and bladder, and consult with a physician about use of systemic estrogen therapy or topical estrogen cream. Male—have female partner try a new coital position by bending her knees and placing a pillow under her hips to elevate pelvis (will more easily accommodate a partially erect penis); massage penis down using pressure at base, which puts pressure on major blood vessel and keeps blood in the penis; ask the female partner to push the penis into the vagina herself and flex her vaginal muscles that have been strengthened by Kegel exercises. If one of the partners has a protruding abdomen, experiment to find a position that allows the penis to reach the vagina (e.g., have woman lie on her back with legs apart and knees sharply bent while the man places himself over her with his hips under the angle formed by the raised knees). **EBN:** *These gender-specific sexual interventions for the elderly may help maintain sexual functioning (Shell & Smith, 1994).*

- • Explore various sexual gratification alternatives (e.g., caressing, sharing feelings) with the client and partner. *Many satisfying alternatives are available for expressing sexual feelings. The many losses associated with aging leave the elderly with special needs for love and affection.*
- • Discuss the difference between sexual function and sexuality. *All individuals possess sexuality from birth to death, regardless of the changes that occur over the life span.*
- ▲ If prescribed, teach how to use nitroglycerin before sexual activity. *Pain inhibits satisfying sexual activity.*
- • See care plan for **Ineffective Sexuality pattern**.

## Multicultural

- • Assess for the influence of cultural beliefs, norms, and values on the client's perceptions of normal sexual functioning. **EBN:** *What the client considers normal sexual functioning may be based on cultural perceptions (Cochran, 1998; Doswell & Erlen, 1998; Leininger & McFarland, 2002). Hasidic (ultraorthodox) Jews believe that male ejaculation must be vaginally contained. This belief will influence choice of interventions for certain sexual dysfunctions (Ribner, 2004). Most research on the sexual health of ethnic minority populations is typically focused on preventive sexual health without examination of the racial or ethnic aspects of sexual health (Lewis, 2004).*
- • Discuss with the client those aspects of sexual health/lifestyle that remain unchanged by his or her health status. **EBN:** *Aspects of the client's life that are valuable to him or her should be understood and preserved without change (Leininger & McFarland, 2002).*
- • Validate the client's feelings and emotions regarding the changes in sexual behavior. **EBN:** *Validation lets the client know the nurse has heard and understands what was said, and it promotes the nurse-client relationship (Heineken, 1998). A recent study found that African-American men also had more positive attitudes than did Caucasian men toward seeking help for sexual problems and were more likely to report seeking past help and intending to seek future help. African-American men reported more problems with sexual desire ($p = .0003$), although their sexual function scores did not differ significantly from those of Caucasians (Jenkins et al, 2004).*

## Home Care

- • Previously discussed interventions may be adapted for home care use.

- Identify specific sources of concern over sexual activity. Provide reassurance and instruction on appropriate expectations as indicated. **EBN:** *In a study of heart transplantation clients' spouses (Bohachick et al, 2001), both clients and spouses reported large improvements in sexual function after transplant. A psychological influence before transplant was identified as concern over finding a donor.*
- Help the client and significant other to identify a place and time in the home and daily living for privacy to share sexual or relationship activity. If necessary, help the client to communicate the need for privacy to other family members. Consider periodic escapes to desirable surroundings. *The home setting can be one that affords little, if any, privacy without conscious effort on the part of members of the home.*
- ▲ Confirm that physical reasons for dysfunction have been addressed. Encourage participation in support groups or therapy if appropriate. **EBN:** *Alterations in physical appearance can significantly influence people's perceptions of their sexual identities, attractiveness, and worthiness. Patients with lung cancer receiving chemotherapy may need sexual counseling. Therefore patients and health care providers should create an environment that allows adequate time to discreetly discuss the effect that chemotherapy treatment may have on appearance, self-esteem, and sexuality (Schwartz & Plawecki, 2002).*
- Reinforce or teach the client about sexual functioning, alternative sexual practices, and necessary sexual precautions. Update teaching as the client status changes. **EBN:** *In this descriptive, qualitative study of the experiences of couples living with prostate cancer, participants demonstrated a need for information and support. Both men and spouse-caregivers felt unprepared to manage treatment effects (Harden et al, 2002).*

## Client/Family Teaching

- Provide accurate information for clients concerning sexual activity after a myocardial infarction (MI); consider use of a videotape. **EBN:** *This study of 110 patients found all 110 had insufficient information about their future sexual functioning after an MI. Unnecessary limitations in sexual activities and mistakes in the reorganization of activities, such as resumption of sexual activity and frequency and positions of sexual intercourse, were identified (Akdolun & Terakye, 2001).* **EBN:** *Significant improvements in knowledge were found in clients who had a videotape to view at home on return to sexual activity. This intervention provides an alternative method for education to facilitate recovery post-MI (Steinke & Swan, 2004).*
- Teach the client to resume intimate physical contact by using mutual touching 3–6 weeks after a MI. **EBN:** *Sexual activity after a MI should not be demanding; therefore mutual touching is recommended (Papadopoulos, 1995).*
- Teach the client to begin vigorous sexual activity after a MI when the client can walk rapidly for 10 minutes and then climb two flights of stairs in 10 seconds. **EBN:** *If this can be done without shortness of breath or other symptoms, then the client is ready to begin preestablished levels of sexual activity (Papadopoulos, 1995). The causes of erection problems after an MI can be physical, psychological, a result of medication, or a combination of these factors (Jones & Nugent, 2001).*
- Provide written educational materials that address sexual issues for clients and families of clients with implantable cardiac defibrillators (ICDs). **EBN:** *Addressing the fears and concerns related to sexual function of ICD patients and partners is an essential aspect of*

*rehabilitation and recovery. Study results suggest a need for written patient education tools specific to sexual issues for patients and partners, as well as educational resources for health professionals (Steinke, 2003).*

- ▲ Refer to appropriate community resources, such as a clinical specialist, family counselor, or sexual counselor. If appropriate, include both partners in the discussion. *A high percentage of women report a need for more information after a cancer surgery that affected their sexual response. They also express a need for partners to be included in the discussions (Corney et al, 1992). Changes in the sexual relationship were described in the context of the effects of having interstitial cystitis and the centrality of maintaining relationships. Participation in support groups has a healing potential related to the woman's desire to maintain independence and to help others with the disease (Webster, 1997).*
- • Teach vaginal dilation to prevent stenosis. Inform the client to expect a bit of spotting after first session of intercourse. *In this Cochrane review of women who had pelvic radio therapy, the use of vaginal dilators to prevent the development of vaginal stenosis is supported by grade IIC evidence (Denton & Maher, 2004).*
- • Teach how drug therapy affects sexual response (e.g., the possible side effects and the need to report them). **EBN:** *SSRI-induced sexual dysfunction affects 30%–50% or more of individuals who take these drugs for depression (Keltner et al, 2002).*
- • Teach the importance of diabetic control and its effect on sexuality to clients with insulin-dependent diabetes. *Sexual functioning may be changed by alterations in glucose levels, infections that affect comfort during sexual intercourse, changes in vaginal lubrication and penile erection, and changes in sexual desire and arousal (Lemone, 1993).*
- ▲ Refer for medical advice for ED that lasts longer than 2 months or is recurring. *ED can be treated, and underlying causes need to be investigated (Mayo Foundation for Medical Education and Research, 2003).*
- • Teach the following interventions to decrease the likelihood of ED: limit or avoid the use of alcohol, stop smoking, exercise regularly, reduce stress, get enough sleep, deal with anxiety or depression, and see doctor for regular checkups and medical screening tests. *These interventions may prevent ED (Mayo Foundation for Medical Education and Research, 2003).*
- ▲ Refer for medication to treat ED if necessary. **EB:** *The oral agent sildenafil is now widely used, but not without concern about specific health risks (Mulhall, 2000). This study of 10 patients suggests that sildenafil use is effective and well-tolerated in patients with olanzapine-induced ED (Atmaca et al, 2002). In this prospective, parallel-group, randomized, double-blind, placebo-controlled trial, sildenafil effectively improved erectile function and other aspects of sexual function in men with sexual dysfunction associated with the use of SRI antidepressants (Nurnberg et al, 2003).*
- • Teach specifics if the client has a stoma: do not substitute the stoma for an anus. *If a stoma is abused in this way, it can become traumatized and need further surgery (Taylor, 1994).*
- • See Geriatric Interventions if a problem with erection is associated with stoma surgery.

S

## evolve WEBSITES FOR EDUCATION

See the EVOLVE website for World Wide Web resources for client education.

## REFERENCES


Akdolun N, Terakye G: Sexual problems before and after myocardial infarction: patients' needs for information, *Rehabil Nurs* 26(4):152, 2001.

Anllo LM: Sexual life after breast cancer, *J Sex Marital Ther* 26(3):241, 2000.

Atmaca M, Kuloglu M, Tezcan E: Sildenafil use in patients with olanzapine-induced erectile dysfunction, *Int J Impot Res* 14(6): 547, 2002.

Atmaca M, Kuloglu M, Tezcan E et al: The efficacy of citalopram in the treatment of premature ejaculation: a placebo-controlled study, *Int J Impot Res* 14(6):502, 2002.

Basson R: Pharmacotherapy for sexual dysfunction in women, *Expert Opin Pharmacother* 5(5):1045-59, 2004.

Bohachick P, Reeder S, Taylor MV et al: Psychosocial impact of heart transplantation on spouses, *Clin Nurs Res* 10(1):6, 2001.

Brassil DF, Keller M: Female sexual dysfunction: definitions, causes, and treatment, *Urol Nurs* 22(4):237, 284; quiz 245, 248, 2002.

Clayton AH: Recognition and assessment of sexual dysfunction associated with depression, *J Clin Psychiatry* 62(suppl 3):5, 2001.

Cochran M: Tears have no color, *Am J Nurs* 98(6):53, 1998.

Corney R, Everett H, Howells A et al: The care of patients undergoing surgery for gynecological cancer: the need for information, emotional support and counseling, *J Adv Nurs* 17:667, 1992.

Denton AS, Maher EJ: Interventions for the physical aspects of sexual dysfunction in women following pelvic radiotherapy, Cochrane Database Sys Rev, 2004.

Dorey G: Is smoking a cause of erectile dysfunction? A literature review, *Br J Nurs* 10(7):455, 2001a.

Dorey G: Partners' perspective of erectile dysfunction: literature review, *Br J Nurs* 10(3):187, 2001b.

Doswell W, Erlen J: Multicultural issues and ethical concerns in the delivery of revising care interventions, *Nurs Clin North Am* 33(2):353, 1998.

Dunn ME: Restoration of couple's intimacy and relationship vital to reestablishing erectile function, *J Am Osteopath Assoc* 104(3): S6-10, S16, 2004.

Dupont S: Multiple sclerosis and sexual functioning: a review, *Clin Rehabil* 9:135, 1995.

Fugl-Meyer K, Fugl-Meyer AR: Sexual disabilities are not singularities, *Int J Impot Res* 14(6):487, 2002.

Gutweniger S, Kopp M, Mur E et al: Body image of women with rheumatoid arthritis, *Clin Exp Rheumatol* 17(4):413, 1999.

Harden J, Schafenacker A, Northouse L et al: Couples' experiences with prostate cancer: focus group research, *Oncol Nurs Forum* 29(4):701, 2002.

Heineken J: Patient silence is not necessarily client satisfaction: communication in home care nursing, *Home Healthc Nurse* 16(2): 115, 1998.

Jones C, Nugent P: The problem of erectile dysfunction following myocardial infarction, *Prof Nurse* 17(3):161, 2001.

Keltner NL, McAfee KM, Taylor CL: Mechanisms and treatments of SSRI-induced sexual dysfunction, *Perspect Psychiatr Care* 38(3):111, 2002.

Leininger MM, McFarland MR: *Transcultural nursing: concepts, theories, research and practices,* ed 3, New York, 2002, McGraw-Hill.

Lemone P: Human sexuality in adults with insulin-dependent diabetes mellitus, *Image* 25:101, 1993.

Lingler JH: Ethical issues in distinguishing sexual activity from sexual maltreatment among women with dementia, *J Elder Abuse Neglect* 15(2):85-102, 2003.

Mayo Foundation for Medical Education and Research: *Erectile dysfunction.* Available at www.mayohealth.org/home?id=DS00162, accessed February 27, 2003.

Messinger-Rapport BJ, Sandhu SK, Hujer ME: Sex and sexuality: is it over after 60? *Clin Geriatr* 11(10): 45-55, 2003.

Monga TN, Tan G, Ostermann HJ et al: Sexuality and sexual adjustment of patients with chronic pain, *Disabil Rehabil* 20(9):317, 1998.

Mulhall JP: Current concepts in erectile dysfunction, *Am J Manag Care* 6(suppl 12):S641-S643, 2000.

Nurnberg HG, Hensley PL, Gelenberg AJ et al: Treatment of antidepressant-associated sexual dysfunction with sildenafil: a randomized controlled trial, *JAMA* 289(1):56, 2003.

Papadopoulos C: Sex and the cardiac patient, 1991, *Med Aspects Hum Sexuality* 24:55, 1991.

Quadagno D, Nation AJ, Johnson D et al: Cardiovascular disease and sexual functioning, Appl *Nurs Res* 8:143, 1995.

Schwartz S, Plawecki HM: Consequences of chemotherapy on the sexuality of patients with lung cancer, *Clin J Oncol Nurs* 6(4): 212, 2002.

Shell J, Smith C: Sexuality and the older person with cancer, *Oncol Nurs Forum* 21:553, 1994.

Steinke EE: Sexual concerns of patients and partners after an implantable cardioverter defibrillator, *Dimen Crit Care Nurs* 22(2): 89-96, 2003.




S

Steinke EE, Swan JH: Effectiveness of a videotape for sexual counseling after myocardial infarction, *Res Nurs Health* 27(4):269-280, 2004.
Stipetich RL, Abel LJ, Blatt HJ et al: Nursing assessment of sexual function following permanent prostate brachytherapy for patients with early-stage prostate cancer, *Clin J Oncol Nurs* 6(5):271, 2002.
Sounes P: Providing nursing care for erectile dysfunction, *Prof Nurse* 16(9):1374, 2001.
Sprunk E, Alteneder RR: The impact of an ostomy on sexuality, *Clin J Oncol Nurs* 4(2):85, 2000.
Taylor P: Beating the taboo, stoma and sexual difficulty, *Nurs Times* 90:51, 1994.
Webster DC: Recontextualizing sexuality in chronic illness: women and interstitial cystitis, *Health Care Women Int* 18(6):575, 1997.

# Ineffective Sexuality pattern

*Gail B. Ladwig*

**NANDA**

## Definition

Expressions of concern regarding own sexuality

## Defining Characteristics

Reported difficulties, limitations, or changes in sexual behaviors or activities

## Related Factors (r/t)

Lack of significant other; conflicts with sexual orientation or variant preferences; fear of pregnancy or of acquiring a sexually transmitted disease; impaired relationship with significant other; ineffective or absent role models; knowledge/skill deficit about alternative responses to health-related transitions; altered body function or structure; illness or medical treatment; lack of privacy

**NOC**

## Outcomes (Nursing Outcomes Classification)

### Suggested NOC Outcomes

Abuse Recovery: Sexual; Child Development: Middle Childhood/Adolescence; Risk Control: Sexually Transmitted Diseases (STDs); Role Performance; Self-Esteem; Risk Control: Unintended Pregnancy

**Example NOC Outcome with Indicators**

**Risk Control: Sexually Transmitted Diseases (STDs)** as evidenced by the following indicators: Acknowledges individual risk for STD; Uses methods to control STD transmission (Rate each indicator of **Risk Control: Sexually Transmitted Diseases (STDs):** 1= never demonstrated, 2 = rarely demonstrated, 3 = sometimes demonstrated, 4 = often demonstrated, 5 = consistently demonstrated [see Section I].)



S

## Client Outcomes

**Client Will (Specify Time Frame):**

- State knowledge of difficulties, limitations, or changes in sexual behaviors or activities
- State knowledge of sexual anatomy and functioning
- State acceptance of altered body structure or functioning
- Describe acceptable alternative sexual practices
- Identify importance of discussing sexual issues with significant other
- Describe practice of safe sex with regard to pregnancy and avoidance of STDs

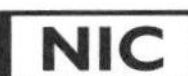

## Interventions (Nursing Interventions Classification)

### Suggested NIC Intervention

Sexual Counseling

**Example NIC Activities—Sexual Counseling**

Provide privacy and ensure confidentiality; provide information about sexual functioning, as appropriate

## Nursing Interventions and Rationales

- After establishing rapport or therapeutic relationship, give the client permission to discuss issues dealing with sexuality. Ask the client specifically, "Have you been or are you concerned about functioning sexually because of your health status?" **EBN:** *When taking a sexual history, the health care professional aims to achieve a clear understanding of both the nature of the problem and the effect that this is having on the patient and the patient's partner if he or she has one. The history may also give a strong indication of the cause of the problem and will help ascertain what the person and his or her partner are expecting from treatment. Men may find it difficult or embarrassing to discuss such an intimate subject, so the health professional must be open and nonjudgmental with excellent communication skills (Ashford, 2003).*
- Determine the client's and partner's current knowledge and understanding. **EB:** *This survey indicated that in clinical practice and for those who have a partner, sexual disabilities and distress caused by them should be regarded from the partner relationship perspective (Fugl-Meyer & Fugl-Meyer, 2002).*
- Encourage the client to discuss concerns with his or her partner. *Carefully assess a client's sexuality. A sexual relationship may be heterosexual or homosexual, and nurses must not lose sight of this (Silenzio, 2003).*
- Discuss alternative sexual expressions for altered body functioning or structure. Closeness and touching are other forms of expression. *Extensive touching, hugging, holding, huddling, and cuddling (3HC) in intimate (committed, close, and prolonged) relationships is important couple and family therapy (L'Abate, 2001).*
- Some clients choose masturbation for sexual release. **EB:** *Nearly 50% of staff who worked with clients with intellectual disability identified more training and clear policy guidelines as the two means of increasing their confidence in dealing with issues of client sexuality such as masturbation (McConkey & Ryan, 2001).*

S

- If mutual masturbation is a choice of expression, provide latex gloves. *Latex gloves prevent possible exposure to infection through cuts on hands (Tucker et al, 1996).*
- The following are guidelines for sexual activity for clients who have had hip replacement surgery:
  - Do not bend the affected leg more than 90 degrees at the hip.
  - When lying on your back, do not turn or roll your affected leg toward the other leg.
  - Do not turn the toes of the affected leg inward.
  - When lying on your side, keep both legs separated with pillows between them. Do not let your knees touch and do not let the toes of your affected leg turn downward.
- The following are recommended sexual positions for clients who have had hip replacement surgery:
  - Bottom position for the male or female patient
    - Place one or two pillows under your affected thigh for support and comfort and to reduce friction on your skin, which may still be healing. Keep the toes of your affected leg pointed upward and slightly outward—but never inward.
  - Top position for male patients only
    - Do not bend your affected hip more than 90 degrees while getting into position. Keep your affected leg out to the side with your toes pointed slightly outward. (Female patients: Do not assume this position because it will require that you bend more than 90 degrees at the hip).
  - Side-lying position for the male patient
    - Lie on your unaffected side. Both you and your partner should face the same direction. You should be behind your partner in a "spooning" position. Your partner should place at least two pillows between her legs and your affected leg should rest on top of hers during intercourse. Do not bend your affected leg more than 90 degrees, and do not let the toes of your affected leg dangle or turn downward.
  - Side-lying position for the female patient
    - Lie on your unaffected side and place enough pillows between your legs to support the affected leg. Make sure the affected leg does not drop off the pillows during intercourse. Your partner should assume the spooning position behind you. Do not bend your affected hip more than 90 degrees, and do not let the toes of your affected leg turn downward.

  Caution: If you dislocate your hip during sexual intercourse, you will experience pain, your affected leg will appear shorter, and your foot will turn inward. Lie down, do not move, and tell your partner to call an ambulance. *Clients who have had total hip replacement surgery need to follow some basic advice about how to protect the hip joint. The goal of rehabilitation after THR is to sustain and, if possible, increase patients' ability to function, and that includes sexual function (FN5). Addressing issues about sexual activity should therefore be made a part of the standard instructions given to THR patients on how to protect the new hip (Rogers, 2003).*
- Provide client privacy for sexual expression (e.g., closed door when significant other visits, "Do Not Disturb" sign on door). *The hospital environment needs to allow for sexual expression between partners.*

S

## Pediatric

- Provide age-appropriate information for adolescents regarding human immunodeficiency virus (HIV) or the acquired immunodeficiency syndrome (AIDS) and sexual behavior. **EB:** *Although teens acquire HIV/AIDS knowledge in school and are aware of positive and negative outcomes of engaging in sexual behavior, many times the information does not seem salient or personally relevant and thus is not used in making decisions related to having sex. Attempts should be made to make HIV education more relevant for teens so that they use the information they have when making decisions about safer sexual behavior (Hoppe et al, 2004).* **EBN:** *Pregnant adolescents and young mothers living in Los Angeles County are vulnerable to acquiring HIV/AIDS through sexual transmission because they lack the resources, social status, and power to protect themselves (Lesser et al, 2003).*
- Provide support for the client's chosen ways to cope with HIV or AIDS. **EBN:** *This descriptive study was designed to assess coping strategies of female adolescents infected with HIV/AIDS (N = 30). Results from the Adolescent Coping Orientation for Problem Experiences Questionnaire (ACOPES) revealed that the most often used coping strategies identified by the adolescents were listening to music, thinking about good things, making your own decisions, being close to someone you care about, sleeping, trying on your own to deal with problems, eating, watching television, daydreaming, and praying (Lewis & Brown, 2002).*

## Geriatric

▲ Carefully assess the sexuality needs of the elderly client and refer for counseling if needed. *Being a sexual being and having sexual feelings is a part of what it is to be a human being—no age limits exist to enjoying a healthy sex life and having the ability to love and be loved. Nurses need to demonstrate empathy and understanding if the patient is to disclose intimate feelings concerning his or her sexual health (Peate, 2004).* **EB:** *Older adults face several barriers to sexual expression, ranging from societal beliefs, to problems arising from aging, disease, and medications, to changes in social circumstances, particularly in nursing home placement. Because sexual issues are seldom volunteered, questions regarding sexuality and intimacy may have to be raised by the clinician, who can help his or her patients with sexual expression by providing appropriate assessment and counseling (Messinger-Rapport, Sandhu, & Hujer, 2003).*

- Explore possible changes in sexuality related to menopause. **EB:** *Evidence from existing research suggests a decline in sexual interest, frequency of sexual intercourse, and vaginal lubrication in association with menopause. Findings for variables such as capacity for orgasm, satisfaction with sex partner, and vaginal pain or discomfort are few and mixed (McCoy, 1998).*
- Allow the client to verbalize feelings regarding loss of sexual partner or significant other. Acknowledge problems such as disapproval of children, lack of available partner for women, and environmental variables that make forming new relationships difficult. **EBN:** *Many individuals face loneliness when they lose a partner, and the loss of interpersonal intimacy is a sensitive problem. After a loss of this magnitude, elderly persons often*

S

*find that forming new relationships is difficult. Privacy is also a problem (Shell & Smith, 1994).*

- Provide a milieu that allows for discussion of sexual issues and a higher level of sexual satisfaction. Allow couples to room together and bring in double beds from home. Place signs on the door to ensure privacy. *Sexuality among adults in long-term care facilities is a difficult issue for staff to address. A need exists for education programs for staff on promoting privacy, independence, and confidentiality for nursing home residents (Lantz, 2004).*
- Provide clients with the following information:
  - Exercise, such as walking, swimming, cycling, and riding a stationary bike, will help control flabby thighs and weak musculature and make people feel more sexually attractive.
  - Overindulgence in food or alcohol can affect sexual activity (see care plan for **Imbalanced Nutrition: more than body requirements**).
  - Resting and sleeping on a firm mattress may augment sexual desire.
  - Femininity and masculinity are still important.
  - Pay attention to cleanliness, skin care, and clothing.
  - Change environment.
  - Experiment with position changes.

  *Because the majority of the elderly population maintains sexual interest, desire, and functioning, these interventions may be helpful during the rehabilitation process. Older adults may exercise aerobically 3–5 times a week for 15–30 minutes depending on physical status and treatment regimen (Steinke et al, 1986).*
- See care plan for **Sexual dysfunction**.

## Multicultural

- Assess for the influence of cultural beliefs, norms, and values on client's perceptions of normal sexual behavior. **EBN:** *What the client considers normal sexual behavior may be based on cultural perceptions (Leininger & McFarland, 2002; Cochran, 1998; Doswell & Erlen, 1998). Religion may also influence one's perception of sexual behavior (Lazoritz & McDermott, 2002). Common cultural beliefs and behaviors of South Asian Indian patients around sexuality include the role of the individual patient's duty to society, the patient's sense of place in society, lack of formal sexual education, prearranged marriages, little premarital contraceptive education, and the dominance of the husband in contraceptive decisions (Fisher, Bowman, & Thomas, 2003).*
- Discuss with the client those aspects of his or her sexual health/lifestyle that remain unchanged by health status. **EBN:** *Aspects of the client's life that are valuable to him or her should be understood and preserved without change (Leininger & McFarland, 2002).*
- Validate the client's feelings and emotions regarding the changes in sexuality patterns. **EBN:** *Validation lets the client know the nurse has heard and understands what was said and promotes the nurse-client relationship (Heineken, 1998).*

## Home Care

- Previously discussed interventions may be adapted for home care use.
- Help the client and significant other to identify a place and time in the home and daily

living for privacy in sharing sexual or relationship activity. If necessary, help the client to communicate the need for privacy to other family members. Consider periodic escapes to desirable surroundings. *The home setting can be one that affords little, if any, privacy without a conscious effort made by members of the home.*

- ▲ Confirm that physical reasons for dysfunction have been addressed. Encourage participation in support groups or therapy if appropriate. **EB:** *Clients express embarrassment at continuing medical intervention or participation in groups once they are back in the community and know that peers may judge their activities. However, 22 female psychiatric outpatients with experience of childhood sexual abuse took part in a 2-year group therapy, and at the end of the 2 years, group members evaluated their relationships as having improved (Lundquist & Ojehagen, 2001).*
- • Reinforce or teach about sexual functioning, alternative sexual practices, and necessary sexual precautions. Update teaching as client status changes. *If the client or significant other has received information during an institutional stay, other stressors may have made the information a temporarily low priority or may have impaired learning. Depending on the cause for dysfunction, the client may experience changing status or feelings about the problem.*

## Client/Family Teaching

- ▲ Refer to appropriate community agencies (e.g., certified sex counselor, Reach to Recovery, Ostomy Association). **EBN:** *Sexuality concerns should be addressed with all clients undergoing ostomy placement (Sprunk & Alteneder, 2000).*
- • Provide information regarding self-care and sexuality for the woman who has cancer and her partner. **EBN:** *Couples may hesitate to change their routines. Providing this kind of information in a sensitive way often gives permission to change (Shell & Smith, 1994).*
- ▲ Sexuality education is important to all populations, whether hearing or deaf, sighted or blind, disabled, or not disabled. Discuss contraceptive choices. Refer to appropriate health professional (e.g., gynecologist, nurse practitioner [NP]). *The need for accurate, comprehensive, current sexuality education is present in all cultures and at all socioeconomic levels. The spread of myths, opinions, and stereotypes can be reduced by correctly educating children. Sexuality education enables an individual to make the most appropriate decisions to advance his or her sexual and interpersonal health (Getch et al, 2001).*
- • Teach safe sex to all clients including the elderly, which includes using latex condoms, washing with soap immediately after sexual contact, not ingesting semen, avoiding oral-genital contact, not exchanging saliva, avoiding multiple partners, abstaining from sexual activity when ill, and avoiding recreational drugs and alcohol when engaging in sexual activity. Contrary to previously published information, the use of a spermicide containing nonoxynol-9 (N-9) should not be recommended as a preventative strategy for HIV infection. **EB:** *In a study of 1000 women it was determined that N-9 has now been proven ineffective against HIV transmission. The possibility of risk, with no benefit, indicates that N-9, a product widely used in spermicides, should not be recommended as an effective means of HIV prevention (US Department of Health and Human Services, 2003).* **EBN:** *Interventions that focus on self-efficacy are most likely to reduce anxiety related to condom use, increase positive perceptions about condoms, and increase the*

S

*likelihood of adopting condom use behaviors (Dilorio et al, 2000).* **EB:** *Older adults can and will acquire new information regarding AIDS-related information when it is presented to them (Falvo & Norman, 2004).*

## evolve WEBSITES FOR EDUCATION

See the EVOLVE website for World Wide Web resources for client education.

## REFERENCES


Ashford L: Erectile dysfunction, *J Pract Nurs* 25(1):18-19, 23-24, 26-27, 2003.

Cochran M: Tears have no color, *Am J Nurs* 98(6):53, 1998.

Dilorio C, Dudley WN, Soet J et al: A social cognitive-based model for condom use among college students, *Nurs Res* 49(4):208, 2000.

Doswell W, Erlen J: Multicultural issues and ethical concerns in the delivery of revising care interventions, *Nurs Clin North Am* 33(2):353, 1998.

Falvo N, Norman S: Never too old to learn: the impact of an HIV/AIDS education program on older adults' knowledge, *Clin Gerontol* 27(1/2):103-117, 2004.

Fisher JA, Bowman M, Thomas T: Issues for South Asian Indian patients surrounding sexuality, fertility, and childbirth in the US health care system, *J Am Board Fam Pract* 16(2):151-155, 2003.

Fugl-Meyer K, Fugl-Meyer AR: Sexual disabilities are not singularities, *Int J Impot Res* 14(6):487, 2002.

Getch YQ, Branca DL, Fitz-Gerald D: A rationale and recommendations for sexuality education in schools for students who are deaf, *Am Ann Deaf* 146(5):401, 2001.

Heineken J: Patient silence is not necessarily client satisfaction: communication in home care nursing, *Home Healthc Nurs* 16(2): 115, 1998.

Hoppe MJ, Graham L, Wilsdon A: Teens speak out about HIV/AIDS: focus group discussions about risk and decision-making, *J Adolesc Health* 35(4):345-346, 2004.

L'Abate L: Hugging, holding, huddling and cuddling (3HC): a task prescription in couple and family therapy, *J Clin Activities Assignments Handouts Psychother Pract* 1(1):5, 2001.

Lantz MS: Consenting adults: sexuality in the nursing home, *Clin Geriatr* 12(6):33-36, 2004.

Lazoritz S, McDermott RT: Adolescent sexuality, cultural sensitivity and the teachings of the Catholic Church, *J Reprod Med* 47(8):603, 2002.

Leininger MM, McFarland MR: *Transcultural nursing: concepts, theories, research and practices,* ed 3, New York, 2002, McGraw-Hill.

Lesser J, Oakes R, Koniak-Griffin D: Vulnerable adolescent mothers' perceptions of maternal role and HIV risk, *Health Care Women Int* 24(6):513-528, 2003.

Lewis CL, Brown SC: Coping strategies of female adolescents with HIV/AIDS, *ABNF J* 13(4):72, 2002.

Lewis JH: Treatment options for men with sexual dysfunction, *J ET Nurs* 19:131, 1992.

Lundquist G, Ojehagen A: Childhood sexual abuse: an evaluation of a two-year group therapy in adult women, *Eur Psychiatry* 16(1):64, 2001.

McConkey R, Ryan D: Experiences of staff in dealing with client sexuality in services for teenagers and adults with intellectual disability, *J Intellectual Disabil Res* 45(1):83 2001.

McCoy N: Methodological problems in the study of sexuality and menopause, *Maturitas* 29(1):51, 1998.

Messinger-Rapport BJ, Sandhu SK, Hujer ME: Sex and sexuality: is it over after 60? *Clin Geriatr* 11(10):45-55, 2003.

Peate I: Sexuality and sexual health promotion for the older person, *Br J Nurs* 13(4):188-193, 2004.

Rogers D: New meaning for safe sex, *RN* 66(1):38-42, 2003.

Shell J, Smith C: Sexuality and the older person with cancer, *Oncology* 21:553, 1994.

Silenzio VMB: Anthropological assessment for culturally appropriate interventions targeting men who have sex with men, *Am J Pub Health* 93(6):867-871, 2003.

Sprunk E, Alteneder RR: The impact of an ostomy on sexuality, *Clin J Oncol Nurs* 4(2):85, 2000.

Steinke EE et al: Sexuality and aging, *J Gerontol Nurs* 12(6):6, 1986.

Tucker M et al: *Patient care standards: collaborative practice planning,* ed 6, St Louis, 1996, Mosby.


S

US Department of Health and Human Services: *AIDS info.* Available at http://aidsinfo.nih.gov/rwscripts/rwisapi.dll/@aidsinfo.env, accessed Feb 27, 2003.

# Impaired Skin integrity

evolve

*Sharon Baranoski*

**NANDA**

## Definition

Altered epidermis and/or dermis

## Defining Characteristics

Invasion of body structures, destruction of skin layers (dermis), disruption of skin surface (epidermis)

## Related Factors (r/t)

### External

Hyperthermia; hypothermia; chemical substance (e.g., incontinence); mechanical factors (e.g., friction, shearing forces, pressure, restraint); physical immobilization; humidity; extremes in age; moisture; radiation; medications

### Internal

Altered metabolic state; altered nutritional state (e.g., obesity, emaciation); altered circulation; altered sensation; altered pigmentation; skeletal prominence; developmental factors; immunological deficit; alterations in skin turgor (change in elasticity); altered fluid status

**NOC**

## Outcomes (Nursing Outcomes Classification)

### Suggested NOC Outcomes

Tissue Integrity: Skin and Mucous Membranes; Wound Healing: Primary Intention, Secondary Intention

**Example NOC Outcome with Indicators**

**Tissue Integrity: Skin and Mucous Membranes** will be intact as evidenced by the following indicators: Skin intactness/Skin lesions/Tissue perfusion/Skin temperature (Rate each indicator of **Tissue Integrity: Skin and Mucous Membranes:** 1 = severely compromised, 2 = substantially compromised, 3 = moderately compromised, 4 = mildly compromised, 5 = not compromised [see Section I].)



S

## Client Outcomes

**Client Will (Specify Time Frame):**

- Regain integrity of skin surface
- Report any altered sensation or pain at site of skin impairment
- Demonstrate understanding of plan to heal skin and prevent reinjury
- Describe measures to protect and heal the skin and to care for any skin lesion

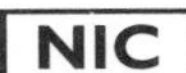

## Interventions (Nursing Interventions Classification)

### Suggested NIC Interventions

Incision Site Care; Pressure Ulcer Care; Skin Care: Topical Treatments; Skin Surveillance; Wound Care

| Example NIC Activities—Pressure Ulcer Care |
| --- |
| Monitor color, temperature, edema, moisture, and appearance of surrounding skin; note characteristics of any drainage |

## Nursing Interventions and Rationales

- Assess site of skin impairment and determine cause (e.g., acute or chronic wound, burn, dermatological lesion, pressure ulcer, skin tear). **EB:** *The cause of the wound must be determined before appropriate interventions can be implemented. This will provide the basis for additional testing and evaluation to start the assessment process (Baranoski & Ayello, 2003).*
- Determine that skin impairment involves skin damage only (e.g., partial-thickness wound, stage I or stage II pressure ulcer). The following classification system is for pressure ulcers:
  - Stage I: Observable pressure-related alteration of intact skin with indicators as compared with the adjacent or opposite area on the body that may include changes in one or more of the following: skin temperature (warmth or coolness), tissue consistency (firm or boggy feel), and/or sensation (pain, itching). The ulcer appears as a defined area of persistent redness in lightly pigmented skin, whereas in darker skin tones, the ulcer may appear with persistent red, blue, or purple hues (National Pressure Ulcer Advisory Panel, 1998).
  - Stage II: Partial-thickness skin loss involving epidermis or dermis superficial ulcer that appears as an abrasion, blister, or shallow crater (National Pressure Ulcer Advisory Panel, 1998).

S

NOTE: For wounds deeper into subcutaneous tissue, muscle, or bone (stage III or stage IV pressure ulcers), see the care plan for **Impaired Tissue integrity.**

- Monitor site of skin impairment at least once a day for color changes, redness, swelling, warmth, pain, or other signs of infection. Determine whether the client is experiencing changes in sensation or pain. Pay special attention to high-risk areas such as bony prominences, skinfolds, the sacrum, and heels. *Systematic inspection can identify impending problems early (Ayello & Braden 2002).*

- • Monitor the client's skin care practices, noting type of soap or other cleansing agents used, temperature of water, and frequency of skin cleansing.
- • Individualize plan according to the client's skin condition, needs, and preferences. **EBN:** *Avoid harsh cleansing agents, hot water, extreme friction or force, or cleansing too frequently (Panel for the Prediction and Prevention of Pressure Ulcers in Adults, 1992; WOCN Clinical Practice Guideline series 2, 2003).*
- • Monitor the client's continence status, and minimize exposure of skin impairment and other areas to moisture from incontinence, perspiration, or wound drainage. **EBN:** *Moisture from incontinence contributes to pressure ulcer development by macerating the skin (WOCN Clinical Practice Guideline series 2, 2003).*
- ▲ If the client is incontinent, implement an incontinence management plan to prevent exposure to chemicals in urine and stool that can strip or erode the skin. Refer to a continence care specialist, urologist, or gastroenterologist for incontinence assessment (WOCN Clinical Practice Guideline series 2, 2003). **EB:** *Implementing an incontinence prevention plan with the use of a skin protectant or a cleanser protectant can significantly decrease skin breakdown and pressure ulcer formation (Clever et al, 2003; Fantl et al, 1996; Warshaw et al, 2002).*
- • For clients with limited mobility, use a risk assessment tool to systematically assess immobility-related risk factors (Ayello & Braden, 2002). *A validated risk assessment tool such as the Norton or Braden scale should be used to identify clients at risk for immobility-related skin breakdown (Ayello & Braden, 2002).* **EB:** *Targeting variables (such as age and Braden Scale Risk Category) can focus assessment on particular risk factors (e.g. pressure) and help guide the plan of prevention and care (Panel for the Prediction and Prevention of Pressure Ulcers in Adults, 1992; WOCN Clinical Practice Guideline series 2, 2003; Young et al, 2002).*
- • Do not position the client on site of skin impairment. If consistent with overall client management goals, turn and position the client at least every 2 hours. Transfer the client with care to protect against the adverse effects of external mechanical forces such as pressure, friction, and shear.
- • Evaluate for use of specialty mattresses, beds, or devices as appropriate. Maintain the head of the bed at the lowest possible degree of elevation to reduce shear and friction, and use lift devices, pillows, foam wedges, and pressure-reducing devices in the bed (WOCN Clinical Practice Guideline series 2, 2003; Panel for the Prediction and Prevention of Pressure Ulcers in Adults, 1992).
- ▲ Implement a written treatment plan for topical treatment of the site of skin impairment. *A written plan ensures consistency in care and documentation (Baranoski & Ayello, 2003; Maklebust & Sieggreen, 2001).*
- ▲ Select a topical treatment that will maintain a moist wound-healing environment and that is balanced with the need to absorb exudate. **EBN:** *Choose dressings that provide a moist environment, keep periwound skin dry and control exudate and eliminate dead space (WOCN Clinical Practice Guideline series 2, 2003).*

S

- Avoid massaging around the site of skin impairment and over bony prominences. *Research suggests that massage may lead to deep-tissue trauma (Panel for the Prediction and Prevention of Pressure Ulcers in Adults, 1992).*
- ▲ Assess the client's nutritional status. Refer for a nutritional consult and/or institute dietary supplements as necessary. *Optimizing nutritional intake, including calories, fatty acids, protein, and vitamins, is needed to promote wound healing (Russell, 2001).* **EB:** *The benefit of nutritional evaluation and intensive nutritional support in patients at risk for and with pressure ulcers is not supported by rigorous clinical trials. Despite this "lack of evidence," NPUAP endorses the application of reasonable nutritional assessment and treatment for patients at risk for and with pressure ulcers (www.npuap.org, accessed January 2005).*
- Identify the patient/client's phase of wound healing (inflammation, proliferation, maturation) and stage of injury. *Accurate understanding of tissue status combined with knowledge of underlying diagnoses and product validity provide a basis for determining appropriate treatment objectives). No single wound dressing is appropriate for all phases of wound healing (Ovington, 1999).*

### Home Care

- Some of the interventions described previously may be adapted for home care use.
- Instruct and assist the client and caregivers in understanding how to change dressings and the importance of maintaining a clean environment. Provide written instructions and observe them completing the dressing change.
- Educate client and caregivers on proper nutrition, signs and symptoms of infection, and when to call the agency and or physician with concerns.
- ▲ It may be beneficial to initiate a consultation in a case assignment with a wound, ostomy, continence (WOC) nurse (or wounds specialist) to establish a comprehensive plan for complex wounds.

## Client/Family Teaching

- Teach skin and wound assessment and ways to monitor for signs and symptoms of infection, complications, and healing. *Early assessment and intervention help prevent serious problems from developing.*
- ▲ Teach the client why a topical treatment has been selected. **EBN:** *The type of dressing needed may change over time as the wound heals and/or deteriorates (WOCN Clinical Practice Guideline series 2, 2003).*
- ▲ If consistent with overall client management goals, teach how to turn and reposition at least every 2 hours. **EB:** *If the goal of care is to keep a client (e.g., terminally ill client) comfortable, turning and repositioning may not be appropriate (Krasner et al, 2001; Panel for the Prediction and Prevention of Pressure Ulcers in Adults, 1992).*
- Teach the client to use pillows, foam wedges, and pressure-reducing devices to prevent pressure injury. **EB:** *The use of effective pressure-reducing seat cushions for elderly wheelchair users significantly prevented sitting-acquired pressure ulcers (Geyer et al, 2001).*

## evolve WEBSITES FOR EDUCATION

See the EVOLVE website for World Wide Web resources for client education.

## REFERENCES


Ayello EA, Braden B: How and why to do pressure ulcer risk assessment, *Adv Skin Wound Care* 15(3):125, 2002.

Baranoski S, Ayello EA, editors: *Wound care essentials: practice principles,* Springhouse, Penn, 2003, Lippincott, Williams, & Wilkins.

Bergstrom N et al: *Treatment of pressure ulcers,* Clinical Practice Guideline No. 15, Agency for Health Care Policy and Research, Pub No 95, Rockville, Md, 1994, Public Health Service, US Department of Health and Human Services.

Clever K, Smith G, Bowser C et al: Evaluating the efficacy of a uniquely delivered skin protectant and its effect on the formation of sacral/buttock pressure ulcers, *Ostomy Wound Manag* 48(12):60, 2002.

Fantl JA et al: *Urinary incontinence in adults: acute and chronic management,* Clinical Practice Guideline No 2, 1996 Update, Agency for Health Care Policy and Research, Pub No 96, Rockville, Md, 1996, Public Health Service, US Department of Health and Human Services.

Geyer MJ, Brienza DM, Karg P et al: A randomized control trial to evaluate pressure-reducing seating cushions for elderly wheelchair users, *Adv Skin Wound Care* 14(3):120, 2001.

Krasner D, Rodeheaver G, Sibbald RG: *Chronic wound care: a clinical source book for healthcare professionals,* ed 3, Wayne, Penn, 2001, HMP Communications.

Maklebust J, Sieggreen M: *Pressure ulcers: guidelines for prevention and nursing management,* ed 3, Springhouse, Penn, 2001, Springhouse.

National Pressure Ulcer Advisory Panel, 1998. Available at www.npuap.org, accessed January 2005.

Ovington L: Dressings and adjunctive therapies: AHCPR guidelines revisited, *Ostomy Wound Manag* 45(suppl 1A):94-106S, 1999.

van Rijswijk L: Wound assessment and documentation. In Krasner D, Rodeheaver G, Sibbald RG, editors: *Chronic wound care: a clinical source book for healthcare professionals,* ed 3, Wayne, Penn, 2001, HMP Communications.

Warshaw E, Nix D, Kula J et al: Clinical and cost effectiveness of a cleanser protectant lotion for treatment of perineal skin breakdown in low-risk patients with incontinence, *Ostomy Wound Manag* 48(6):44, 2002.

Wound, Ostomy, and Continence Nurses Society: *Guideline for prevention and management of pressure ulcers. WOCN clinical practice guideline series No 2,* Glenview, Ill, 2003, The Society.

Young J, Nikoletti S, McCaul K et al: Risk factors associated with pressure ulcer development at a major Western Australia teaching hospital from 1998 to 2000, *J Wound Ostomy Continence Nurs* 29(5):234, 2002.


# Risk for impaired Skin integrity

*Sharon Baranoski*

**NANDA**

### Definition

At risk for skin being adversely altered

### Risk Factors

#### External

Hypothermia; hyperthermia; chemical substance; excretions and/or secretions; mechanical factors (e.g., shearing forces, pressure, restraint); radiation; physical immobilization; humidity; moisture; extremes of age

### Internal

Medication; altered nutritional state (e.g., obesity, emaciation); altered metabolic state; altered circulation; altered sensation; altered pigmentation; skeletal prominence; developmental factors; immunological deficit; alterations in skin turgor (change in elasticity); psychogenetic, immunological factors

NOTE: Risk should be determined by the use of a risk assessment tool (e.g., Norton scale, Braden scale).

## Related Factors (r/t)

See Risk Factors

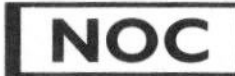

## Outcomes (Nursing Outcomes Classification)

### Suggested NOC Outcomes

Immobility Consequences: Physiological; Tissue Integrity: Skin and Mucous Membranes

**Example NOC Outcome with Indicators**

**Tissue Integrity: Skin and Mucous Membranes** will be intact as evidenced by the following indicators: Skin intactness/Skin lesions/Tissue perfusion/Skin temperature (Rate each indicator of **Tissue Integrity: Skin and Mucous Membranes:** 1 = severely compromised, 2 = substantially compromised, 3 = moderately compromised, 4 = mildly compromised, 5 = not compromised [see Section I].)

## Client Outcomes

### Client Will (Specify Time Frame):

- Report altered sensation or pain at risk areas
- Demonstrate understanding of personal risk factors for impaired skin integrity
- Verbalize a personal plan for preventing impaired skin integrity



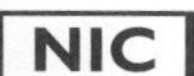

## Interventions (Nursing Interventions Classification)

### Suggested NIC Interventions

Positioning, Pressure Management, Pressure Ulcer Care, Pressure Ulcer Prevention, Skin Surveillance

**Example NIC Activities—Pressure Ulcer Care**

Monitor color, temperature, edema, moisture, and appearance of surrounding skin; note characteristics of any drainage

## Nursing Interventions and Rationales

- • Monitor skin condition at least once a day for color or texture changes, dermatological conditions, or lesions. Determine whether the client is experiencing loss of sensation or pain. *Systematic inspection can identify impending problems early (Ayello & Braden 2002; Krasner, Rodeheaver, & Sibbald, 2001).*
- • Identify clients at risk for impaired skin integrity as a result of immobility, chronological age, malnutrition, incontinence, compromised perfusion, immunocompromised status, or chronic medical condition such as diabetes mellitus, spinal cord injury, or renal failure. **EB:** *These patient populations are known to be at high risk for impaired skin integrity (Maklebust & Sieggreen, 2001; Stotts & Wipke-Tevis, 2001). Targeting variables (such as age and Braden Scale Risk Category) can focus assessment on particular risk factors (e.g., pressure) and help guide the plan of prevention and care (Young et al, 2002).*
- • Monitor the client's skin care practices, noting type of soap or other cleansing agents used, temperature of water, and frequency of skin cleansing. *Individualize plan according to the client's skin condition, needs, and preferences (Baranoski, 2001).*
- • Avoid harsh cleansing agents, hot water, extreme friction or force, or too-frequent cleansing (Panel for the Prediction and Prevention of Pressure Ulcers in Adults, 1992).
- ▲ Monitor the client's continence status and minimize exposure of the site of skin impairment and other areas to moisture from incontinence, perspiration, or wound drainage. If the client is incontinent, implement an incontinence management plan to prevent exposure to chemicals in urine and stool that can strip or erode the skin; refer to a physician (e.g., continence care specialist, urologist, gastroenterologist) for an incontinence assessment (WOCN Clinical Practice Guideline series 2, 2003; Fantl et al, 1996). **EB:** *Implementing an incontinence prevention plan with the use of a skin protectant or a cleanser protectant can significantly decrease skin breakdown and pressure ulcer formation (Clever et al, 2003; Warshaw et al, 2002).*
- • For clients with limited mobility, monitor condition of skin covering bony prominences. *Pressure ulcers usually occur over bony prominences, such as the sacrum, coccyx, trochanter, and heels, as a result of unrelieved pressure between the prominence and support surface (WOCN Clinical Practice Guideline series 2, 2003; Maklebust & Sieggreen, 2001).*
- • Use a risk assessment tool to systematically assess immobility-related risk factors. *A validated risk assessment tool such as the Norton or Braden scale should be used to identify clients at risk for immobility-related skin breakdown (Ayello & Braden, 2002; Panel for the Prediction and Prevention of Pressure Ulcers in Adults, 1992; Sussman & Bates-Jensen, 1998).*
- • Implement a written prevention plan. **EB:** *A written plan ensures consistency in care and documentation (Baranoski & Ayello, 2003; Maklebust & Sieggreen, 2001).* **EBN:** *Implementing a prevention protocol can significantly reduce costs and incidence of skin breakdown and pressure ulcers in the long-term care setting (Lyder et al, 2002).*
- • If consistent with overall client management goals, turn and position the client at least every 2 hours. Transfer the client with care to protect against the adverse effects of external mechanical forces (e.g., pressure, friction, shear) (WOCN Clinical Practice Guideline series 2, 2003).

S

- ▲ Evaluate for use of specialty mattresses, beds, or devices as appropriate (Geyer, 2001; Fleck, 2001). *If the goal of care is to keep the client (e.g., a terminally ill client) comfortable, turning and repositioning may not be appropriate. Maintain the head of the bed at the lowest possible degree of elevation to reduce shear and friction and use lift devices, pillows, foam wedges, and pressure-reducing devices in the bed (WOCN Clinical Practice Guideline series 2, 2003; Krasner et al, 2001; Panel for the Prediction and Prevention of Pressure Ulcers in Adults, 1992).*
- • Avoid massaging over bony prominences. *Research suggests that massage may lead to deep-tissue trauma (WOCN Clinical Practice Guidelines Series 2, 2003; Panel for the Prediction and Prevention of Pressure Ulcers in Adults, 1992).*
- ▲ Assess the client's nutritional status; refer for a nutritional consult, and/or institute dietary supplements. **EB:** *The benefit of nutritional evaluation and intensive nutritional support in patients at risk for and with pressure ulcers is not supported by rigorous clinical trials. Despite this "lack of evidence" NPUAP endorses the application of reasonable nutritional assessment and treatment for patients at risk for and with pressure ulcers (www.npuap.org, accessed January 2005).*

## Geriatric

- • Limit number of complete baths to two or three per week, and alternate them with partial baths. Use a tepid water temperature (between 90° and 105° F) for bathing. **EB:** *Excessive bathing, especially in hot water, depletes aging skin of moisture and increases dryness. The ability to retain moisture is decreased in aging skin due to diminished amounts of dermal proteins. One of the most common age-related changes to the skin is damage to the stratum corneum (Baranoski & Ayello, 2003; Baranoski, 2001).*
- • Use lotions and moisturizers to prevent skin from drying out, especially in the winter (Sibbald & Cameron, 2001). *Avoid skin care products that contain allergens such as lanolin, latex, and dyes (Sibbald & Cameron, 2001).*
- • Increase fluid intake within cardiac and renal limits to a minimum of 1500 mL per day. *Dry skin is caused by loss of fluid; increasing fluid intake hydrates the skin.*
- • Increase humidity in the environment, especially during the winter, by using a humidifier or placing a container of water on a warm object. *Increasing the moisture in the air helps keep moisture in the skin (Sibbald & Cameron, 2001).*

S

## Home Care

- • Assess caregiver vigilance and ability. *In a limited study of the Braden Scale, caregiver vigilance and ability were recognized as potentially significant variables for determining the risk of developing pressure sores (Ramundo, 1995).*
- • Initiate a consultation in a case assignment with a wound care specialist or wound, ostomy, and continence (WOC) nurse to establish a comprehensive plan as soon as possible.
- • See the care plan for **Impaired Skin integrity**.

## Client/Family Teaching

- • Teach the client skin assessment and ways to monitor for impending skin breakdown. *Early assessment and intervention help prevent the development of serious problems.* **EB:**

*Basic elements of a skin assessment are assessment of temperature, color, moisture, turgor, and intact skin (Baranoski & Ayello, 2003).*

- If consistent with overall client management goals, teach how to turn and reposition the client at least every 2 hours. **EB:** *If the goal of care is to keep the client (e.g., a terminally ill client) comfortable, turning and repositioning may not be appropriate (Panel for the Prediction and Prevention of Pressure Ulcers in Adults, 1992).*
- Teach the client to use pillows, foam wedges, and pressure-reducing devices to prevent pressure injury (WOCN Clinical Practice Guidelines series 2, 2003; Krasner & Sibbald, 1999). **EB:** *The use of effective pressure-reducing seat cushions for elderly wheelchair users significantly prevented sitting-acquired pressure ulcers (Geyer et al, 2001).*

## evolve WEBSITES FOR EDUCATION

See the EVOLVE website for World Wide Web resources for client education.

## REFERENCES


Ayello EA, Braden B: How and why to do pressure ulcer risk assessment, *Adv Skin Wound Care* 15(3):125, 2002.

Baranoski S: Skin tears: the enemy of frail skin, *Adv Skin Wound Care* 13(3 Pt 1):123-126, 2000.

Baranoski S, Ayello EA: Skin an essential organ. In Baranoski S, Ayello EA, editors: *Wound care essentials: practice principles,* Springhouse, Penn, 2003, Lippincott, Williams, & Wilkins.

Clever K, Smith G, Bowser C et al: Evaluating the efficacy of a uniquely delivered skin protectant and its effect on the formation of sacral/buttock pressure ulcers, *Ostomy Wound Manag* 48(12):60, 2002.

Colburn L: Prevention for chronic wounds. In Krasner D, Rodeheaver G, Sibbald RG, editors: *Chronic wound care: a clinical source book for healthcare professionals,* ed 3, Wayne, Penn, 2001, HMP Communications.

Fantl JA et al: *Urinary incontinence in adults: acute and chronic management,* Clinical Practice Guideline No 2, 1996 Update, Agency for Health Care Policy and Research, Pub No 96, Rockville, Md, 1996, Public Health Service, US Department of Health and Human Services.

Fleck C: Support surfaces: criteria and selection. In Krasner D, Rodeheaver G, Sibbald RG, editors: *Chronic wound care: a clinical source book for healthcare professionals,* ed 3, Wayne, Penn, 2001, HMP Communications.

Geyer MJ, Brienza DM, Karg P et al: A randomized control trial to evaluate pressure-reducing seating cushions for elderly wheelchair users, *Adv Skin Wound Care* 14(3):120, 2001.

Krasner D, Rodeheaver G, Sibbald RG: Advanced wound caring for a new millennium. In Krasner D, Rodeheaver G, Sibbald RG, editors: *Chronic wound care: a clinical source book for healthcare professionals,* ed 3, Wayne, Penn, 2001, HMP Communications.

Krasner D, Sibbald RG: Moving beyond the AHCPR guidelines: wound care evolution over the last five years, *Ostomy Wound Manag Spec Suppl* 45(1A):1SS, 1999.

Lyder CH, Shannon R, Empleo-Frazier O et al: A comprehensive program to prevent pressure ulcers in long-term care: exploring costs and outcomes, *Ostomy Wound Manage* 48(4):52, 2002.

Maklebust J, Sieggreen M: *Pressure ulcers: guidelines for prevention and nursing management,* ed 3, Springhouse, Penn, 2001, Springhouse.

National Pressure Ulcer Advisory Panel, 1998. Available at www.npuap.org, accessed January 2005.

Panel for the Prediction and Prevention of Pressure Ulcers in Adults: *Pressure ulcers in adults: prediction and prevention,* Clinical Practice Guideline No 3, Agency for Health Care Policy and Research, Pub No 92, Rockville, Md, 1992, Public Health Service, US Department of Health and Human Services.

Ramundo J: Reliability and validity of the Braden Scale in the home care setting, *J Wound Ostomy Cont Nurs* 22:3, 1995.

Sibbald RG, Cameron J: Dermatological aspects of wound care. In Krasner D, Rodeheaver G, Sibbald RG, editors: *Chronic wound care: a clinical source book for healthcare professionals,* ed 3, Wayne, Penn, 2001, HMP Communications.

Stotts NA, Wipke-Tevis: Co-factors in impaired wound healing. In Krasner D, Rodeheaver G, Sibbald RG, editors: *Chronic wound care: a clinical source book for healthcare professionals,* ed 3, Wayne, Penn, 2001, HMP Communications.


S

Sussman C, Bates-Jensen BM: *Wound care: a collaborative practice manual for physical therapists and nurses,* Gaithersburg, Md, 1998, Aspen.

Warshaw E, Nix D, Kula J et al: Clinical and cost effectiveness of a cleanser protectant lotion for treatment of perineal skin breakdown in low-risk patients with incontinence, *Ostomy Wound Manag* 48(6):44, 2002.

Wound, Ostomy, and Continence Nurses Society: *Guideline for prevention and management of pressure ulcers. II. WOCN clinical practice guideline series*, Glenview, Ill, 2003.

Young J, Nikoletti S, McCaul K et al: Risk factors associated with pressure ulcer development at a major Western Australia teaching hospital from 1998 to 2000, *J WOCN* 29(5):234, 2002.

# Sleep deprivation

*Judith A. Floyd*

## NANDA

### Definition

Prolonged periods without sleep (sustained natural, periodic suspension of relative consciousness)

### Defining Characteristics

Daytime drowsiness; decreased ability to function; malaise; tiredness; lethargy; restlessness; irritability; heightened sensitivity to pain; listlessness; apathy; slowed reaction; inability to concentrate; perceptual disorders (e.g., disturbed body sensation, delusions, feeling afloat); hallucinations; acute confusion; transient paranoia; agitated or combative; anxious; mild, fleeting nystagmus; hand tremors

### Related Factors (r/t)

Prolonged physical discomfort; prolonged psychological discomfort; sustained inadequate sleep hygiene; prolonged use of pharmacological or dietary antisoporifics; aging-related sleep stage shifts; sustained circadian asynchrony; inadequate daytime activity; sustained environmental stimulation; sustained unfamiliar or uncomfortable sleep environment; non–sleep-inducing parenting practices; sleep apnea; periodic limb movement (e.g., restless leg syndrome, nocturnal myoclonus); sundowner's syndrome; narcolepsy; idiopathic central nervous system hypersomnolence; sleep walking; sleep terror; sleep-related enuresis; nightmares; familial sleep paralysis; sleep-related painful erections; dementia



## NOC

### Outcomes (Nursing Outcomes Classification)

#### Suggested NOC Outcomes

Rest, Sleep, Symptom Severity

**Example NOC Outcome with Indicators**

**Sleep** as evidenced by the following indicators: Hours of sleep/Sleep pattern/Sleep quality/Sleep efficiency/ Feels rejuvenated after sleep/Napping appropriate for age (Rate each indicator of **Sleep:** 1 = severely compromised, 2 = substantially compromised, 3 = moderately compromised, 4 = mildly compromised, 5 = not compromised [see Section I].)

## Client Outcomes

### Client Will (Specify Time Frame):

- Wake up less frequently during night
- Awaken refreshed and be less fatigued during day
- Fall asleep without difficulty
- Verbalize plan that provides adequate time for sleep
- Identify actions that can be taken to improve quality of sleep

**NIC**

## Interventions (Nursing Interventions Classification)

### Suggested NIC Intervention

Sleep Enhancement

**Example NIC Activities—Sleep Enhancement**

Monitor/record patient's sleep pattern and number of sleep hours; encourage patient to establish a schedule that allows for adequate amounts of sleep

## Nursing Interventions and Rationales

- Obtain a sleep-wake history including work and other scheduled activities, history of sleep problems, changes in sleep with present illness, and use of medications and stimulants. *Assessment of sleep behavior and patterns are an important part of any health status examination (Landis, 2002).*
- Ask the client to keep a sleep-wake diary for several weeks, which includes bedtime, rise time, number of awakenings, naps, and scheduled daytime events that may be depriving the client of adequate sleep time. *Often the client can find the cause of the sleep deprivation when the pattern of sleeping is examined (Pagel et al, 1997). A sleep diary is a necessary component of a behavioral assessment of sleep problems (Landis, 2002).* **EBN:** *A study demonstrated that a daily sleep diary provided reliable and valid measurement of insomnia (Coates et al, 1982).*

▲ Observe for underlying physiological illnesses causing sleep loss (e.g., cardiovascular, pulmonary, gastrointestinal, hyperthyroidism, nocturia occurring with benign hypertrophic prostatitis or pain). *Symptomatology of disease states can cause insomnia (Sateia et al, 2000).*

▲ Determine level of anxiety. If the client is anxious, use relaxation techniques. See further Nursing Interventions and Rationales for **Anxiety. EBN and EB:** *The use of relax-*

S

*ation techniques to promote sleep in people with chronic insomnia has been shown to be effective (Floyd et al, 2000; Johnson, 1991a; Morin et al, 1994).*

- ▲ Assess for signs of depression: depressed mood state, flat affect, statements of hopelessness, poor appetite. Refer for counseling/treatment as appropriate. *Many symptoms associated with sleep deprivation probably arise from central nervous system hyperarousal in the depressed client (Sateia et al, 2000).*
- ▲ Assess the client for other symptoms of bipolar disorder (mania, hypomania). Refer for mental health services as indicated. *Sleep loss is part of the syndrome of bipolar disorder. Resumption of a normal sleep pattern is unlikely unless the underlying bipolar disorder is treated (Morris, 2003).*
- ▲ Monitor for presence of nocturnal symptoms of restless leg syndrome with uncomfortable restless sensations in legs that occur before sleep onset or during the night. In addition, monitor for nocturnal panic attacks, presence of headaches, or gastroesophageal reflux disease. Refer for treatment as appropriate. *Numerous nocturnal events and symptoms can contribute to sleep loss (Sateia et al, 2000).*
- • Observe the client's medication, diet, and caffeine intake. Look for hidden sources of caffeine, such as over-the-counter medications. *Difficulty sleeping can be a side effect of medications such as bronchodilators; caffeine can also interfere with sleep (Benca, 2005).* **EB:** *Caffeine use after 2 PM is associated within poor sleep (Ellis et al, 2002).*
- ▲ Provide pain relief shortly before bedtime, and position the client comfortably for sleep. *Clients have reported that uncomfortable positions and pain are common factors in sleep loss (Sateia et al, 2000).*
- ▲ Monitor for presence of sleep disordered breathing as evidenced by loud snoring with periods of apnea, or other sleep disorders such as restless leg syndrome or periodic limb movement disorder. Refer to an accredited sleep disorder center. *Up to 15% of all chronic poor sleep is associated with breathing disturbances (Sateia et al, 2000). Polysomnography evaluation is recommended if a sleep disorder exists (Epstein & Bootzin, 2002).*
- • Keep environment quiet for sleeping (e.g., avoid use of intercoms, lower the volume on radio and television, keep beepers on nonaudio mode, anticipate alarms on intravenous (IV) pumps, talk quietly on unit) (Barr, 1993). **EBN:** *Healthy volunteers exposed to recorded critical care noise levels experienced poor quality sleep (Topf et al, 1996). Excessive noise disrupts sleep (Floyd, 1999).*
- • Use soothing sound generators with sounds of the ocean, rainfall, or waterfall to induce sleep, or use "white noise" such as a fan to block out other sounds. Also consider the use of earplugs. **EBN:** *Ocean sounds promoted sleep for a group of postoperative open-heart surgery clients (Williamson, 1992). Earplugs have been found to decrease the effects of simulated intensive care unit noise on sleep (Wallace et al, 1999).*
- • Encourage the client to use soothing music to facilitate sleep. **EBN:** *Music results in better sleep quality, longer sleep duration, greater sleep efficiency, shorter sleep latency, less sleep disturbance, and less daytime dysfunction (Lai & Good, 2005).*

S

## Geriatric

- ▲ Determine if the client has a physiological problem that could result in sleep loss such as pain, cardiovascular disease, pulmonary disease, neurological problems such as dementia, or urinary problems. *Sleep disturbances in the elderly may represent a complex interaction of age-related changes and pathological causes (Sateia et al, 2000).*

- Observe elimination patterns. Have the client decrease fluid intake in the evening, and ensure that diuretics are taken early in the morning. *Many elderly people void during the night. Increasing water intake at night or taking diuretics late in the day increases nocturia, which results in sleep loss (Avidan, 2005).*
- ▲ If the client is waking frequently during the night with periods of apnea or increased leg movement, consider the presence of sleep apnea problems or periodic leg movements disorder and refer to a sleep clinic for evaluation. *Sleep apnea and periodic limb movement disorders interfere more with sleep as clients age (Floyd, 2002).*
- Suggest light reading or TV viewing that does not excite as an evening activity. *Soothing activities decrease stimulation of the reticular activating system and help sleep come naturally.*
- Help the client take a warm bath in the evening. **EBN:** *Passive heating by using a warm bath has been shown to increase deep sleep in the elderly (Dorsey et al, 1996).*
- ▲ If the client continues to have sleep loss despite developing good sleep hygiene habits, refer to a sleep clinic for further evaluation (Pagel et al, 1997).

## Home Care

- Previously discussed interventions may be adapted for home care use.
- Obtain a full current assessment and history of sleep activity, sleep disturbance, and sleep disturbance–related behaviors. *A complete assessment promotes accurate determination of the client's needs.*
- Instruct the client/family in expectations for normal sleep. Elicit expectations for sleep, previous sleep patterns; correct misconceptions that influence emotional responses to deviation from expectations. *Client/family may be unduly disturbed by normal changes in sleep patterns. Disturbances in sleep or frequent awakening may be misconstrued as lack of sleep.* **EBN:** *As persons age, increased time is needed to fall asleep; frequency of waking after sleep onset increases; length of waking after sleep onset increases (which may be related to unrecognized sleep apnea); and nighttime sleep amount tends to decrease (Floyd et al, 2000).* **EB:** *A study found that older adults often have insomnia, with frequent nocturnal awakenings, snoring, restlessness, and periodic limb movements during sleep; daytime sleepiness often is a symptom (Piani et al, 2004).*
- Have the client maintain a sleep diary, describing daily activity levels, use of stimulants, activities or physical sensations around bedtime. Assess diary for potential areas of intervention. *Details about daily activities may yield clues to change sleep pattern (e.g., exercise timing or excessive coffee use, meals before bedtime, acid indigestion while lying flat).*
- Assess environment for possible hazards to the client during period of deprivation (e.g., appliances, stairs). Ensure that, if client awakens during the night, there will be sufficient light (consider a night light), with passageways clear of obstruction between bed and bathroom. *Client safety is a primary goal of care in the home setting.* **EB:** *Older adults frequently wake during the night with an urge to void (Piani et al, 2004).*

S

- • Obtain a listing of expected daily behaviors, before and since the onset of deprivation (e.g., mowing lawn, shaving, cooking). Identify tasks that may be delegated. Establish level of client participation in tasks. Use short task periods for the client. *Role changes may be necessary to protect client and family safety. Continued participation in family activities promotes sense of belonging.*
- • Assess client support system for availability of psychological and task-related support.
- ▲ Refer to chore, homemaker, or home health aide services as necessary. *Home health aides can assist with ADLs; homemakers can do household tasks and shopping to support the family. Chore services can do major household cleaning and yard work.*
- ▲ Assess family/caregiver response to client status. Provide nursing support; refer to medical social services or mental health services/support groups as necessary. *Support of the family/caregiver structure can decrease caregiver burden.*
- ▲ If the client is taking medication, assess for effectiveness and safety in administration.
- ▲ Identify person administering medication if not the client. *Sleep-deprived persons may not be consistent in self-administration of medications.*
- • Assist the family to arrange for supervision if the client presents confusion or perceptual dysfunction. *Client supervision provides for client safety and may provide additional caregiver respite if obtained from outside the usual support system.*
- ▲ Refer the client to medical social services or mental health/group support services such as I Can Cope. *Venting validates feelings of the client. Groups allow the client to recognize the love and caring of others and provide alternative ways of problem solving.*
- ▲ In the presence of a psychiatric disorder, refer for psychiatric home health care services for client reassurance and implementation of therapeutic regimen. **EBN:** *Psychiatric home care nurses can address issues relating to the client's sleep deprivation and bipolar disorder. Behavioral interventions in the home can assist the client to participate more effectively in treatment plan (Patusky et al, 1996).*

## Client/Family Teaching

- • Encourage the client to avoid coffee and other caffeinated foods and liquids and to avoid eating large high-protein or high-fat meals close to bedtime. *Caffeine intake increases the time it takes to fall asleep and increases awake time during the night (Evans & Rogers, 1994).*
- • Advise the client to avoid use of alcohol or hypnotics to induce sleep. Avoid alcohol ingestion 4–6 hours before bedtime. *Sleep induced by alcohol is often disrupted later in the night (Epstein & Bootzin, 2002).*
- • Encourage the client to develop a bedtime ritual that includes quiet activities such as reading, television, or crafts. **EBN:** *The use of a bedtime routine has been shown to be effective in inducing and maintaining sleep in a population of older women (Johnson, 1991).*
- • Teach the following sleep hygiene guidelines for improving sleep habits:
  - ■ Go to bed only when sleepy.
  - ■ When awake in the middle of the night, go to another room, do quiet activities, and go back to bed only when sleepy.
  - ■ Use the bed only for sleeping—not for reading or snoozing in front of the television.

S

- Avoid afternoon and evening naps.
- Get up at the same time every morning.
- Recognize that not everyone needs 8 hours of sleep.
- Do not associate lulls in performance with sleeplessness; sleeplessness should not be blamed for everything that goes wrong during the day.

**EB:** *These guidelines on sleep hygiene have been shown to effectively improve quality of sleep (Morin et al, 1994).*

## evolve WEBSITES FOR EDUCATION

See the EVOLVE website for World Wide Web resources for client education.

## REFERENCES


Avidan AY: Sleep in the geriatric patient population, *Semin Neurol* 25(1):52, 2005.

Barr WJ: Noise notes: working smart, *Am J Nurs* 93:16, 1993.

Benca RM: Diagnosis and treatment of chronic insomnia: review, *Psychiatr Serv* 56(3):334, 2005.

Coates TJ, Killen JD, George J et al: Discriminating good sleepers from insomniacs using all-night polysomnograms conducted at home, *J Nerv Ment Dis* 170(4):224, 1982.

Dorsey CM, Lukas SE, Teicher MH et al: Effects of passive body heating on the sleep of older female insomniacs, *J Geriatr Psychiatry Neurol* 9(2):83, 1996.

Ellis J, Hampson SE, Cropley M: Sleep hygiene or compensatory sleep practices: an examination of behaviours affecting sleep in older adults, *Psychol Health Med* 7(2):156-161, 2002.

Epstein DR, Bootzin RR: Insomnia, *Nurs Clin North Am* 37(4):611, 2002.

Evans BD, Rogers AE: 24-hour sleep/wake patterns in healthy elderly persons, *Appl Nurs Res* 7:75, 1994.

Floyd JA: Sleep promotion in adults, *Annu Rev Nurs Res* 17:27, 1999.

Floyd JA: Sleep and aging, *Nurs Clin North Am* 37:719, 2002.

Floyd JA, Falahee ML, Fhobir RH: Creation and analysis of a computerized database of interventions to facilitate adult sleep, *Nurs Res* 49(4):236, 2000.

Johnson JE: Progressive relaxation and the sleep of older noninstitutionalized women, *Appl Nurs Res* 4(4):165, 1991a.

Johnson JE: A comparative study of the bedtime routines and sleep of older adults, *J Community Health Nurs* 8(3):129, 1991b.

Lai HL, Good M: Music improves sleep quality in older adults, *J Adv Nurs* 49(3):234, 2005.

Landis CA: Sleep and methods of assessment, *Nurs Clin North Am* 37:583, 2002.

Morin CM, Culbert JP, Schwartz SM: Nonpharmacological interventions for insomnia: a meta-analysis of treatment efficacy, *Am J Psychiatry* 151(8):1172, 1994.

Morris CM: Managing depression in primary care, *Physician Assist* 27(1):20, 2003.

Pagel JF et al: How to prescribe a good night's sleep, *Patient Care* 31(4):87, 1997.

Patusky KL et al: Clinical lessons in psychiatric home health care: a case study approach, *Home Healthc Manag Pract* 9(1):8, 1996

Piani A, Brotini S, Dolso P et al: Sleep disturbances in elderly: a subjective evaluation over 65, *Arch Gerontol Geriatr* 9(Suppl):325, 2004.

Sateia MJ, Doghramji K, Hauri PJ et al: Evaluation of chronic insomnia. An American Academy of Sleep Medicine review, *Sleep* 23(2):243, 2000.

Topf M, Bookman M, Arand D: Effects of critical care unit noise on the subjective quality of sleep, *J Adv Nurs* 24(3):545, 1996.

Wallace CJ, Robins J, Alvord LS et al: The effect of earplugs on sleep measures during exposure to simulated intensive care unit noise, *Am J Crit Care* 8(4):210, 1999.

Williamson J: The effect of ocean sounds on sleep after coronary artery bypass graft surgery, *Am J Crit Care* 1(1):91, 1992.


S

# Disturbed Sleep pattern

evolve

*Judith A. Floyd*

NANDA

## Definition

Time-limited disruption of sleep (natural, periodic suspension of consciousness) amount and quality

## Defining Characteristics

Prolonged awakenings; sleep maintenance insomnia; self-induced impairment of normal pattern; sleep onset greater than 30 minutes; early morning insomnia; awakening earlier or later than desired; verbal complaints of difficulty falling asleep; verbal complaints of not feeling well-rested; increased proportion of stage 1 sleep; dissatisfaction with sleep; less than age-normed total sleep time; three or more nighttime awakenings; decreased proportion of stages 3 and 4 sleep (e.g., hyporesponsiveness, excess sleepiness, decreased motivation); decreased proportion of REM sleep (e.g., REM rebound, hyperactivity, emotional lability, agitation and impulsivity, atypical polysomnographic features); decreased ability to function

## Related Factors (r/t)

Ruminative presleep thoughts; daytime activity pattern; thinking about home; body temperature; temperament; dietary; childhood onset; inadequate sleep hygiene; sustained use of antisleep agents; circadian asynchrony; frequently changing sleep-wake schedule; depression; loneliness; frequent travel across time zones; daylight/darkness exposure; grief; anticipation; shift work; delayed or advanced sleep phase syndrome; loss of sleep partner, life change; preoccupation with trying to sleep; periodic gender-related hormonal shifts; biochemical agents; fear; separation from significant others; social schedule inconsistent with chronotype; aging-related sleep shifts; anxiety; medications; fear of insomnia; maladaptive conditioned wakefulness; fatigue; boredom



### Environmental

Noise; unfamiliar sleep furnishings; ambient temperature, humidity; lighting; other-generated awakening; excessive stimulation; physical restraint; lack of sleep privacy/control; interruptions for therapeutics, monitoring, lab tests; sleep partner; noxious odors

### Parental

Mother's sleep-wake pattern, parent-infant interaction, mother's emotional support

### Physiological

Urinary urgency, incontinence; fever; nausea; stasis of secretions; shortness of breath; position; gastroesophageal reflux

NOC

## Outcomes (Nursing Outcomes Classification)

### Suggested NOC Outcomes

Comfort Level; Pain Level; Personal Well-Being; Psychosocial Adjustment: Life Change; Quality of Life; Rest; Sleep

**Example NOC Outcome with Indicators**

**Sleep** as evidenced by the following indicators: Hours of sleep/Sleep pattern/Sleep quality/Sleep efficiency/Feels rejuvenated after sleep/Napping appropriate for age (Rate each indicator of **Sleep:** 1 = severely compromised, 2 = substantially compromised, 3 = moderately compromised, 4 = mildly compromised, 5 = not compromised [see Section I].)

## Client Outcomes

### Client Will (Specify Time Frame):

- Wake up less frequently during night
- Awaken refreshed and not be fatigued during day
- Fall asleep without difficulty
- Verbalize plan to implement sleep promoting routines

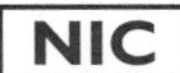

## Interventions (Nursing Interventions Classification)

### Suggested NIC Intervention

Sleep Enhancement

**Example NIC Activities—Sleep Enhancement**

Monitor/record patient's sleep pattern and number of sleep hours; encourage patient to establish a bedtime routine to facilitate transition from wakefulness to sleep

## Nursing Interventions and Rationales

S

- Obtain a sleep history including bedtime routines, history of sleep problems, changes in sleep with present illness, and use of medications and stimulants. *Assessment of sleep behavior and patterns are an important part of any health status examination (Landis, 2002).*
- Ask the client to keep a sleep diary for several weeks, which includes bedtime, rise time, number of awakenings and naps. *A sleep diary is a necessary component of a behavioral assessment of sleep problems (Landis, 2002).* **EB:** *A study demonstrated that a daily sleep diary provided reliable and valid measurement of insomnia (Coates et al, 1982).*

▲ Assess level of pain and use available pharmacological and nonpharmacological approaches to pain management. *Pain leads to sleep disruption and sleep disruption increases the perception of pain (Stiefel & Stagno, 2004; Roehrs & Roth, 2005).*

- • Determine level of anxiety. If the client is anxious, use relaxation techniques. See further Nursing Interventions and Rationales for **Anxiety. EBN and EB:** *The use of relaxation techniques to promote sleep in people with chronic insomnia has been shown to be effective (Johnson, 1991a; Morin et al, 1994; Floyd et al, 2000).*
- ▲ Assess for signs of new onset of depression: depressed mood state, statements of hopelessness, poor appetite. Refer for counseling as appropriate. *Many symptoms associated with sleep disruption probably arise from central nervous system hyperarousal in the depressed client (Sateia et al, 2000).*
- • Observe the client's medication, diet, and caffeine intake. Look for hidden sources of caffeine, such as over-the-counter medications. *Difficulty sleeping can be a side effect of medications such as bronchodilators; caffeine can also interfere with sleep (Benca, 2005).* **EB:** *Caffeine use after 2 PM is associated with poor sleep (Ellis et al, 2002).*
- • Provide measures to take before bedtime to assist with sleep (e.g., quiet time to allow the mind to slow down, carbohydrates such as crackers). *Simple measures can increase quality of sleep. Carbohydrates cause release of the neurotransmitter serotonin, which helps induce and maintain sleep (Somer, 1999).*
- • Provide a back massage before bedtime. *Use of a back massage has been shown effective for promoting relaxation, which likely leads to improved sleep (Richards et al, 2003).*
- • Provide pain relief shortly before bedtime and position the client comfortably for sleep. *Clients have reported that uncomfortable positions and pain are common factors of sleep disturbance (Sateia et al, 2000).*
- • Keep environment quiet for sleeping (e.g., avoid use of intercoms, lower the volume on radio and television, keep beepers on nonaudio mode, anticipate alarms on IV pumps, talk quietly on unit) (Barr, 1993). **EBN:** *Healthy volunteers exposed to recorded critical care noise levels experienced poor quality sleep (Topf et al, 1992). Excessive noise disrupts sleep (Floyd, 1999).*
- • Use soothing sound generators with sounds of the ocean, rainfall, or waterfall to induce sleep, or use "white noise" such as a fan to block out other sounds. Also consider the use of earplugs. **EBN:** *Ocean sounds promoted sleep for a group of postoperative open-heart surgery clients (Williamson, 1992). Earplugs have been found to decrease the effects of simulated intensive care unit noise on sleep (Wallace et al, 1999).*
- • Encourage the client to use soothing music to facilitate sleep. **EBN:** *Music results in better sleep quality, longer sleep duration, greater sleep efficiency, shorter sleep latency, less sleep disturbance, and less daytime dysfunction (Lai & Good, 2005).*
- • For hospitalized stable clients, consider instituting the following sleep protocol to foster sleep:
  - ■ Night shift: Give the client the opportunity for uninterrupted sleep from 1 AM–5 AM. Keep environmental noise to a minimum.
  - ▲ Evening shift: Limit napping between 4 PM and 9 PM. At 10 PM turn lights off, provide sleep medication according to individual assessment, and keep noise and conversation on the unit to a minimum.

S

- ▲ Day shift: Encourage short naps before 11 AM. Enforce a physical activity regimen as appropriate. Schedule newly ordered medications to avoid waking the client between 1 AM and 5 AM.

**EBN:** *The high frequency of nocturnal care interaction have been found to leave patients with few uninterrupted periods for sleep (Edwards & Schuring, 1993a; Tamburri et al, 2004). Critical care nurses can take effective actions to promote sleep (Edwards & Schuring, 1993b).*

## Geriatric

- ▲ Determine if the client has new onset of a physiological problem that could result in insomnia, such as pain, cardiovascular disease, pulmonary disease, neurological problems such as dementia, or urinary problems. *Sleep disturbances in the elderly may represent a complex interaction of age-related changes and pathological causes (Sateia et al, 2000).*
- • Observe elimination patterns. Have the client decrease fluid intake in the evening and ensure that diuretics are taken early in the morning unless contraindicated. *Many elderly people awaken to void during the night. Increasing water intake at night or taking diuretics late in the day increases nocturia, which results in disrupted sleep (Avidan, 2005).*
- • Do a careful history of all medications including over-the-counter medications and alcohol intake. *Alcohol intake and medication effects are common causes of insomnia in the elderly. Rebound insomnia associated with the use of shorter-acting hypnotics may perpetuate a cycle of sleep disturbance and chronic hypnotic use (Sateia et al, 2000).*
- ▲ If the client is waking frequently during the night, consider the presence of sleep apnea problems and refer to a sleep clinic for evaluation. *Sleep apnea in the elderly may be caused by changes in the respiratory drive of the central nervous system or may be obstructive and associated with obesity (Foyt, 1992).*
- ▲ Evaluate the client for presence of depression or anxiety, which can result in insomnia. Refer for treatment as appropriate. *Anxiety and depression are common in the elderly and can result in insomnia (Sateia et al, 2000).*
- • Encourage social activities. Help elderly get outside for increased light exposure and to enjoy nature. *Exposure to natural light and social interactions influence the circadian rhythms that control sleep (Labyak, 2002).*
- • Suggest light reading or TV viewing that does not excite as an evening activity. *Soothing activities decrease stimulation of the reticular activating system and help sleep come naturally (Labyak, 2002).*
- • Increase daytime physical activity and social activities. Encourage walking as the client is able. **EBN:** *Increasing activity during the day is effective in promoting sleep in residential care (Richards et al, 2001).*
- ▲ Recommend avoidance of hypnotics and alcohol to induce sleep. Avoid alcohol ingestion 4–6 hours before bedtime. *Long-term use of hypnotics can induce a drug-related insomnia. Alcohol also disrupts sleep and can exacerbate sleep apnea (Evans & Rogers, 1994). Sleep induced by alcohol is often disrupted later in the night (Epstein & Bootzin, 2002).* **EB:** *In nonalcoholic sleepers, bedtime alcohol use decreased sleep latency but increased wakefulness during the latter part of the sleep period (Roehrs & Roth, 1997).*

S

- Reduce daytime napping in the late afternoon; limit naps to short intervals as early in the day as possible. *The majority of elderly nap during the day (Evans & Rogers, 1994). Avoiding naps in the late afternoon makes it easier to fall asleep at night.* **EBN:** *Naps longer than 50 minutes were associated with increased nighttime awakening (Floyd, 1995).* **EB:** *Napping short intervals early in the day enhanced cognitive and psychomotor performance (Campbell et al, 2005).*
- Help the client take a warm bath in the evening. **EBN and EB:** *Passive heating by using a warm bath has been shown to increase deep sleep in the elderly (Dorsey et al, 1996; Liao, 2002).*
- Help the client recognize that changes in length of sleep occur with aging. *Client may not be able to sleep for 8 hours as when younger, and more frequent awakening is part of the aging process (Floyd, 2002).*

▲ If the client continues to have disturbed sleep despite developing good sleep hygiene habits, refer to a sleep clinic for further evaluation (Pagel et al, 1997).

## Home Care

- Previously discussed interventions may be adapted for home care use.
- Provide support to the family of the client with chronic sleep pattern disturbance. *Ongoing sleep pattern disturbances can disrupt family patterns and cause sleep deprivation in client or family members, which creates increased stress on the family.*
- Instruct the client/family in expectations for normal sleep. Elicit expectations for sleep, previous sleep patterns; correct misconceptions that influence emotional responses to deviation from expectations. **EBN:** *Client/family may be unduly disturbed by normal changes in sleep patterns. As persons age, increased time is needed to fall asleep; frequency of waking after sleep onset increases; length of waking after sleep onset increases (which may be related to unrecognized sleep apnea); and nighttime sleep amount tends to decrease (Floyd et al, 2000).* **EBN:** *A study found that older adults often have insomnia, frequent nocturnal awakenings, snoring, restlessness, and periodic limb movements during sleep; daytime sleepiness often is a symptom (Piani et al, 2004).*

▲ Assess the client for sleep apnea, particularly poststroke (e.g., interview partner regarding the client's sleep pattern and behaviors, have the client maintain sleep log). *Perceived sleep disturbance may be an indication of sleep apnea, which tends to increase with age. In one study poststroke, 59% of participants met criteria for sleep apnea. More clients with sleep apnea than without were delirious, depressed, or ADL dependent; and had a higher frequency of ischemic heart disease and latency in reaction and in response to verbal stimuli. Clients may benefit from continuous positive airway pressure (CPAP) treatment (Sandberg et al, 2001).*

▲ Assess the client for depression or other psychiatric disorder. Refer for mental health services as indicated. *Sleep disturbance is part of the syndrome of depression and other psychiatric disorders. Improvement in sleep pattern is unlikely unless the underlying disorder is treated.*

- Have the client maintain a sleep diary, describing daily activity levels, use of stimulants, activities, or physical sensations around bedtime. Assess diary for potential areas of intervention. *Details about daily activities may yield clues to change sleep pattern (e.g., exercise timing or excessive coffee use, meals before bedtime, acid indigestion while lying flat).*

S

- Assess environment for possible hazards to the client during periods of disturbance (e.g., appliances, stairs). Ensure that, if client awakens during the night, there will be sufficient light (consider a night light), with passageways clear of obstruction between bed and bathroom. *Client safety is a primary goal of care in the home setting.* **EB:** *Older adults frequently wake during the night with an urge to void (Piani et al, 2004).*
- Initiate nonpharmacological interventions for insomnia: stimulus control, sleep restriction, relaxation techniques, increasing sunlight exposure, acupuncture, cognitive and educational interventions to address dysfunctional attitudes about sleep. **EBN and EB:** *Nonpharmacological interventions can improve sleep efficiency and continuity and increase satisfaction with sleep pattern while reducing hypnotic use (Morin et al, 1999; Woodward, 1999). Nursing interventions are directed at making environments conducive to sleep, relaxing the client, or entraining the circadian sleep-wake cycle (Floyd, 1999).*
- In the presence of a cognitive disorder, reassure family regarding sleep expectations for the client and address potential problems (e.g., enuresis will require frequent cleansing of client and changes of bed linens); procurement of a hospital bed with side rails may be necessary to prevent falling out of bed. **EB:** *A study showed that older adults with cognitive disorders had fewer nighttime awakenings than those without a cognitive disorder but were the only participants to be enuretic or to fall out of bed. Individuals with cognitive dysfunctions had more daytime sleepiness and more difficulty maintaining attention and concentration; sleep attacks were much more common in participants with cognitive disorders (Piani et al, 2004).*

▲ In the presence of a psychiatric disorder, refer for psychiatric home health care services for client reassurance and implementation of therapeutic regimen. *Psychiatric home care nurses can address issues relating to client's sleep disturbance. Behavioral interventions in the home can assist client to participate more effectively in treatment plan (Patusky et al, 1996).*

- Provide support to the family of the client with chronic sleep pattern disturbance. *Ongoing sleep pattern disturbances can disrupt family patterns and cause sleep deprivation in the client or family members, which creates increased stress on the family.*

## Client/Family Teaching

- Encourage the client to avoid coffee and other caffeinated foods and liquids and also to avoid eating large high-protein or high-fat meals close to bedtime. *Caffeine intake increases the time it takes to fall asleep and increases awake time during the night (Evans & Rogers, 1994).*
- Advise the client to avoid use of alcohol or hypnotics to induce sleep. Avoid alcohol ingestion 4–6 hours before bedtime. *Sleep induced by alcohol is often disrupted later in the night (Epstein & Bootzin, 2002). Clients can easily become dependent on hypnotics for sleep and develop rebound insomnia if they are discontinued. Nonpharmacological interventions to maintain sleep are more effective than pharmacological treatments in the long-term (Epstein & Bootzin, 2002).*
- Ask the client to keep a sleep diary for several weeks. *Often the client can find the cause of the sleep deprivation when the pattern of sleeping is examined (Pagel et al, 1997).*
- Teach somatic and cognitive relaxation techniques to induce the relaxation response and facilitate sleep. **EBN and EB:** *The use of relaxation techniques to promote sleep in peo-*

S

*ple with chronic insomnia has been shown to be effective (Floyd et al, 2000; Johnson, 1991; Morin et al, 1994).*

- Teach the client need for increased exercise. Encourage to take a daily walk 5–6 hours before retiring. *Moderate activity such as walking can increase the quality of sleep (King et al, 1997).*
- Encourage the client to develop a bedtime ritual that includes quiet activities such as reading, television, or crafts. **EBN:** *The use of a bedtime routine has been shown to be effective in inducing and maintaining sleep in a population of older women (Johnson, 1991).*
- Teach the following guidelines for good sleep hygiene to improve sleep habits:
  - Go to bed only when sleepy.
  - When awake in the middle of the night, go to another room, do quiet activities, and go back to bed only when sleepy.
  - Use the bed only for sleeping—not for reading or snoozing in front of the television.
  - Avoid afternoon and evening naps.
  - Get up at the same time every morning.
  - Recognize that not everyone needs 8 hours of sleep.
  - Move the alarm clock away from the bed so that it cannot be seen.
  - Do not associate lulls in performance with sleeplessness; sleeplessness should not be blamed for everything that goes wrong during the day.

  **EB:** *These guidelines on sleep hygiene have been shown to effectively improve quality of sleep (Morin et al, 1994).*

## evolve WEBSITES FOR EDUCATION

See the EVOLVE website for World Wide Web resources for client education.

## REFERENCES

Avidan AY: Sleep in the geriatric patient population, *Semin Neurol* 25(1):52, 2005.
Barr WJ: Noise notes: working smart, *Am J Nurs* 93:16, 1993.
Benca RM: Diagnosis and treatment of chronic insomnia: review, *Psychiatr Serv* 56(3):334, 2005.
Campbell SS, Murphy PJ, Stauble TN: Effects of a nap on nighttime sleep and waking function in older subjects, *J Am Geriatr Soc* 53(1):48, 2005.
Coates TJ, Killen JD, George J et al: Discriminating good sleepers from insomniacs using all-night polysomnograms conducted at home, *J Nerv Ment Dis* 170(4):224, 1982.
Dorsey CM, Lukas SE, Teicher MH et al: Effects of passive body heating on the sleep of older female insomniacs, *J Geriatr Psychiatry Neurol* 9(2):83, 1996.
Edwards GB, Schuring LM: Pilot study: validating staff nurses' observations of sleep and wake states among critically ill patients using polysomnography, *Am J Crit Care* 2(2):125, 1993a.
Edwards GB, Schuring LM: Sleep protocol: a research-based practice change, *Crit Care Nurse* 13:84, 1993b.
Ellis J, Hampson SE, Cropley M et al: Sleep hygiene or compensatory sleep practices: an examination of behaviours affecting sleep in older adults, *Psychol Health Med* 7(2):157, 2002.
Epstein DR, Bootzin RR: Insomnia, *Nurs Clin North Am* 37(4):611, 2002.
Evans BD, Rogers AE: 24-hour sleep/wake patterns in healthy elderly persons, *Appl Nurs Res* 7:75, 1994.
Floyd JA: Another look at napping in the older adult, *Geriatr Nurs* 16(3):136, 1995.
Floyd JA: Sleep promotion in adults, *Annu Rev Nurs Res* 17:27, 1999.
Floyd JA: Sleep and aging, *Nurs Clin North Am* 37(4):719, 2002.

Floyd JA, Falahee ML, Fhobir RH: Creation and analysis of a computerized database of interventions to facilitate adult sleep, *Nurs Res* 49(4):236, 2000.
Floyd JA, Medler SM, Ager JW et al: Age-related changes in initiation and maintenance of sleep: a meta-analysis, *Res Nurs Health* 23(2):106, 2000.
Foyt MM: Impaired gas exchange in the elderly, *Geriatr Nurs* 13:262, 1992.
Johnson JE: Progressive relaxation and the sleep of older noninstitutionalized women, *Appl Nurs Res* 4(4):165, 1991a.
Johnson JE: A comparative study of the bedtime routines and sleep of older adults, *J Commun Nurs* 8(3):129, 1991b.
King AC, Oman RF, Brassington GS et al: Moderate-intensity exercise and self-rated quality of sleep in older adults, *JAMA* 277(1):32, 1997.
Labyak S: Sleep and circadian schedule disorders, *Nurs Clin North Am* 37:599, 2002.
Lai HL, Good M: Music improves sleep quality in older adults, *J Adv Nurs* 49(3):234, 2005.
Landis CA: Sleep and methods of assessment, *Nurs Clin North Am* 37:583, 2002.
Liao WC: Effects of passive body heating on body temperature and sleep regulation in the elderly: a systematic review, *Int J Nurs Stud* 39(8):803, 2002.
Morin C: Cognitive behavior therapy for late-life insomnia, *J Consult Clin Psychol* 61(1):137, 1993.
Morin CM, Culbert JP, Schwartz SM: Nonpharmacological interventions for insomnia, *Am J Psychiatry* 151(8):1172, 1994.
Morin CM, Mimeault V, Gagne A: Nonpharmacologic treatment of chronic insomnia, *J Psychosom Res* 46(2):103, 1999.
Pagel JF et al: How to prescribe a good night's sleep, *Patient Care* 31(4):87, 1997.
Patusky KL et al: Clinical lessons in psychiatric home health care: a case study approach, *Home Healthc Manag Pract* 9(1):18, 1996.
Piani A, Brotini S, Dolso P et al: Sleep disturbances in elderly: a subjective evaluation over 65, *Arch Gerontol Geriatr* 9(Suppl): 325, 2004.
Richards K et al: Use of complementary and alternative therapies to promote sleep in critical ill patients, *Crit Care Nurs Clin North Am* 15(3):329, 2003.
Richards KC et al: The effect of individualized activities on the sleep of nursing home residents who are cognitively impaired: a pilot study, *J Gerontol Nurs* 27(9):30, 2001.
Roehrs T, Roth T: Hypnotics, alcohol, and caffeine: relation to insomnia. In Pressman MR, Orr WC, editors: *Understanding sleep: the evaluation and treatment of sleep disorders,* Washington, DC, 1997, American Psychological Association.
Roehrs T, Roth T: Sleep and pain: interaction of two vital functions, *Semin Neurol* 25(1):106, 2005.
Sandberg O et al: Sleep apnea, delirium, depressed mood, cognition, and ADL ability after stroke, *J Am Geriatr Soc* 49:391, 2001.
Sateia MJ et al: Evaluation of chronic insomnia, *Sleep* 23(2):243, 2000.
Somer E: *Food and mood: the complete guide to eating well and feeling your best,* ed 2, New York, 1999, Henry Holt.
Stiefel F, Stagno D: Management of insomnia in patients with chronic pain conditions, *CNS Drugs* 18(5):285, 2004.
Tamburri et al: Nocturnal care interactions with patients in critical care units, *Am J Crit Care* 13(2):102, 2004.
Topf M: Effects of personal control over hospital noise on sleep, *Res Nurs Health* 15:19, 1992.
Wallace CJ et al: The effect of earplugs on sleep measures during exposure to simulated intensive care unit noise, *Am J Crit Care* 8:210, 1999.
Williamson J: The effect of ocean sounds on sleep after coronary artery bypass graft surgery, *Am J Crit Care* 1(1):91, 1992.
Woodward M: Insomnia in the elderly, *Aust Fam Phys* 28:653, 1999.



# Readiness for enhanced Sleep

*Judith A. Floyd*

**NANDA**

## Definition

A pattern of natural, periodic suspension of consciousness that provides adequate rest, sustains a desired lifestyle, and can be strengthened

• = Independent; ▲ = Collaborative; EBN = Evidence-Based Nursing; EB = Evidence-Based

## Defining Characteristics

Expresses willingness to enhance sleep, amount of sleep and REM sleep is congruent with developmental needs, expresses a feeling of being rested after sleep, follows sleep routines that promote sleep habits, occasional or infrequent use of medications to induce sleep

## Related Factors (r/t)

Desire to improve sleep

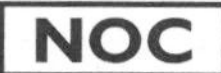

## Outcomes (Nursing Outcomes Classification)

### Suggested NOC Outcomes

Personal Well-Being, Rest, Sleep

**Example NOC Outcome with Indicators**

**Sleep** as evidenced by the following indicators: Hours of sleep/Sleep pattern/Sleep quality/Sleep efficiency/Feels rejuvenated after sleep/Napping appropriate for age (Rate each indicator of **Sleep:** 1 = severely compromised, 2 = substantially compromised, 3 = moderately compromised, 4 = mildly compromised, 5 = not compromised [see Section I].)

## Client Outcomes

**Client Will (Specify Time Frame):**

- Awaken refreshed and is not fatigued during day
- Fall asleep without difficulty
- Verbalize plan to implement sleep promotion routines

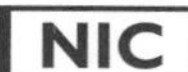

## Interventions (Nursing Interventions Classification)

S

### Suggested NIC Intervention

Sleep Enhancement

**Example NIC Activities—Sleep Enhancement**

Determine patient's sleep/activity pattern; encourage patient to establish a bedtime routine to facilitate transition from wakefulness to sleep

## Nursing Interventions and Rationales

- Obtain a sleep history including bedtime routines, sleep patterns, and use of medications and stimulants. *Assessment of sleep behavior and patterns is an important part of any health status examination (Landis, 2002).*
- Ask the client to keep a sleep diary for several weeks, which includes bedtime, rise

time, number of awakenings, naps, and energy-using activities. *A sleep-wake diary is a necessary component of a behavioral assessment of sleep problems (Landis, 2002).* **EB:** *A study demonstrated that a daily sleep diary provided reliable and valid measurement of insomnia (Coates et al, 1982).*

- Determine level of anxiety. If the client is anxious, use relaxation techniques. See further Nursing Interventions and Rationales for **Anxiety. EBN and EB:** *The use of relaxation techniques to promote sleep in people with chronic insomnia has been shown to be effective (Johnson, 1991a; Morin et al, 1994; Floyd et al, 2000a).*
- Observe the client's medication, diet, and caffeine intake. Look for hidden sources of caffeine, such as over-the-counter medications. *Difficulty sleeping can be a side effect of medications such as bronchodilators; caffeine can also interfere with sleep (Benca, 2005).* **EB:** *Caffeine use after 2 PM is associated within poor sleep (Ellis et al, 2002).*
- Provide measures to take before bedtime to assist with sleep (e.g., quiet time to allow the mind to slow down, carbohydrates such as crackers). *Simple measures can increase quality of sleep. Carbohydrates cause release of the neurotransmitter serotonin, which helps induce and maintain sleep (Somer, 1999).*
- Provide a back massage before bedtime. *Use of a back massage has been shown effective for promoting relaxation, which likely leads to improved sleep (Richards et al, 2003).*
- Initiate nonpharmacological interventions for improved sleep: stimulus control, sleep restriction, increasing sunlight exposure, acupuncture, and cognitive and educational interventions to address dysfunctional attitudes about sleep. **EBN and EB:** *Nonpharmacological interventions have been shown to improve sleep efficiency and continuity, increase satisfaction with sleep pattern, while reducing hypnotic usage (Morin et al, 1999; Woodward, 1999). Nursing interventions have been directed at making environments conducive to sleep, relaxing the client, or entraining the circadian sleep-wake cycle (Floyd, 1999).*

## Geriatric

- Encourage the client to develop a bedtime ritual that includes quiet activities such as reading, television, or crafts. **EBN:** *The use of a bedtime routine has been shown to be effective in inducing and maintaining sleep in a population of older women (Johnson, 1991b).*
- Encourage the client take a warm bath in the evening. **EBN:** *Passive heating by using a warm bath has been shown to increase deep sleep in the elderly (Dorsey et al, 1996; Liao, 2002).*
- Observe elimination patterns. Have the client decrease fluid intake in the evening and ensure that diuretics are taken early in the morning unless contraindicated. *Many elderly people awaken to void during the night. Increasing water intake at night or taking diuretics late in the day increases nocturia, which results in disrupted sleep (Avidan, 2005).*
- Encourage social activities. Help elderly get outside for increased light exposure and to enjoy nature. *Exposure to natural light and social interactions influence the circadian rhythms that control sleep (Labyak, 2002).*
- Increase daytime physical activity. Encourage walking as the client is able. **EB:** *Research focusing on older adults suggested significant sleep benefits resulting from exercise (Lichstein & Morin, 2000).*

- Recommend avoidance of hypnotics and alcohol to induce sleep. Avoid alcohol ingestion 4–6 hours before bedtime. *Long-term use of hypnotics can induce a drug-related insomnia. Alcohol also disrupts sleep and can exacerbate sleep apnea (Evans & Rogers, 1994). Sleep induced by alcohol is often disrupted later in the night (Epstein & Bootzin, 2002).* **EB:** *In nonalcoholic sleepers, bedtime alcohol use decreased sleep latency but increased wakefulness during the latter part of the sleep period (Roehrs & Roth, 1997).*
- Reduce daytime napping in the late afternoon; limit naps to short intervals as early in the day as possible. *The majority of elderly nap during the day (Evans & Rogers, 1994). Avoiding naps in the late afternoon makes it easier to fall asleep at night.* **EBN:** *Naps longer than 50 minutes were associated with increased nighttime awakening (Floyd, 1995).* **EB:** *Napping short intervals early in the day enhanced cognitive and psychomotor performance (Campbell et al, 2005).*
- Help the client recognize that changes in length of sleep occur with aging. *Client may not be able to sleep for 8 hours as when younger, and more frequent awakening is part of the aging process (Floyd et al, 2000b).*
- Teach somatic and cognitive relaxation techniques to induce the relaxation response and facilitate sleep. **EBN and EB:** *The use of relaxation techniques to promote sleep in people with chronic insomnia has been shown to be effective (Johnson, 1991a; Morin et al, 1994; Floyd et al, 2000).*
- Teach the following guidelines for good sleep hygiene to improve sleep habits:
  - Go to bed only when sleepy.
  - When awake in the middle of the night, go to another room, do quiet activities, and go back to bed only when sleepy.
  - Use the bed only for sleeping—not for reading or snoozing in front of the television.
  - Avoid afternoon and evening naps.
  - Get up at the same time every morning.
  - Recognize that not everyone needs 8 hours of sleep.
  - Move the alarm clock away from the bed so that it cannot be seen.
  - Do not associate lulls in performance with sleeplessness; sleeplessness should not be blamed for everything that goes wrong during the day.

  **EB:** *These guidelines on sleep hygiene have been shown to effectively improve quality of sleep (Morin et al, 1994; Benca, 2005).*
- Encourage the client to develop a bedtime ritual that includes quiet activities such as reading, television, or crafts. **EBN:** *The use of a bedtime routine has been shown to be effective in inducing and maintaining sleep in a population of older women (Johnson, 1991b).*
- Encourage the client to use soothing music to facilitate sleep. **EBN:** *Music results in better sleep quality, longer sleep duration, greater sleep efficiency, shorter sleep latency, less sleep disturbance, and less daytime dysfunction (Lai & Good, 2005).*

S

## Home Care

- Previously discussed interventions may be adapted for home care use.
- Obtain a full current assessment and history of sleep activity, sleep disturbance, and sleep disturbance–related behaviors. *A complete assessment promotes accurate determination of the client's needs.*

- Instruct the client/family in expectations for normal sleep. Elicit expectations for sleep, previous sleep patterns; correct misconceptions that influence emotional responses to deviation from expectations. *Client/family may be unduly disturbed by normal changes in sleep patterns. Disturbances in sleep or frequent awakening may be misconstrued as lack of sleep. Reassurance may calm concerns.* **EBN:** *As people age, increased time is needed to fall asleep; frequency of waking after sleep onset increases; length of waking after sleep onset increases (which may be related to unrecognized sleep apnea); and nighttime sleep amount tends to decrease (Floyd et al, 2000).*
- Have the client maintain a sleep diary, describing daily activity levels, use of stimulants, activities, or physical sensations around bedtime. Assess diary for potential areas of intervention. *Details about daily activities may yield clues to change sleep pattern (e.g., exercise timing or excessive coffee use, meals before bedtime, acid indigestion while lying flat).*
- Assess environment for possible hazards to the client during period of deprivation (e.g., appliances, stairs). Ensure that, if client awakens during the night, there will be sufficient light (consider a night light), with passageways clear of obstruction between bed and bathroom. *Client safety is a primary goal of care in the home setting.* **EB:** *Older adults frequently wake during the night with an urge to void (Piani et al, 2004).*

▲ Assess client support system for availability of psychological and task-related support. Refer to chore, homemaker, or home health aide services as necessary to relieve client of overexertion. *Home health aides can assist with ADLs; homemakers can do household tasks and shopping to support the family. Chore services can do major household cleaning and yard work.*

▲ Assess family/caregiver response to client status. Provide nursing support; refer to medical social services or mental health services/support groups as necessary. *Support of the family/caregiver structure can decrease caregiver burden.*

- If the client is taking medication, assess for effectiveness and safety in administration. Identify person administering medication if not the client. *If sleep difficulties exist, persons may not be consistent in self-administration of medications or may take them beyond need, leading to dependence.*
- Assist the family to arrange for supervision if the client presents confusion or perceptual dysfunction. *Client supervision provides for client safety and may provide additional caregiver respite if obtained from outside the usual support system.*

▲ Refer the client to medical social services or mental health/group support services such as I Can Cope. *Venting validates feelings of the client. Groups allow the client to recognize the love and caring of others and provide alternative ways of problem solving.*

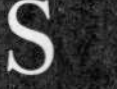

## evolve WEBSITES FOR EDUCATION

See the EVOLVE website for World Wide Web resources for client education.

## REFERENCES


Avidan AY: Sleep in the geriatric patient population, *Semin Neurol* 25(1):52, 2005.

Benca RM: Diagnosis and treatment of chronic insomnia: review, *Psychiatr Serv* 56(3):334, 2005.

Campbell et al: Effects of a nap on nighttime sleep and waking function in older subjects, *J Am Geriatr Soc* 53(1):48, 2005

Coates TJ et al: Discriminating good sleepers from insomniacs using all-night polysomnograms conducted at home, *J Nerv Ment Dis* 170, 1982.
Dorsey CM et al: Effects of passive body heating on the sleep of older female insomniacs, *J Geriatr Psychiatry Neurol* 9:83, 1996.
Ellis J et al: Sleep hygiene or compensatory sleep practices: an examination of behaviours affecting sleep in older adults, *Psychol Health Med* 7(2):157, 2002.
Epstein DR, Bootzin RR: Insomnia, *Nurs Clin North Am* 37:4, 2002.
Evans BD, Rogers AE: 24-hour sleep/wake patterns in healthy elderly persons, *Appl Nurs Res* 7:75, 1994.
Floyd JA: Another look at napping in the older adult, *Geriatr Nurs* 16:136, 1995.
Floyd JA: Sleep promotion in adults, *Annu Rev Nurs Res* 17:27, 1999.
Floyd JA et al: Creation and analysis of a computerized database of interventions to facilitate adult sleep, *Nurs Res* 49:4, 2000a
Floyd JA et al: Age-related changes in initiation and maintenance of sleep: a meta-analysis, *Res Nurs Health* 23:106, 2000b.
Johnson JE: Progressive relaxation and the sleep of older noninstitutionalized women, *Appl Nurs Res* 4, 1991a.
Johnson JE: A comparative study of the bedtime routines and sleep of older adults, *J Commun Nurs,* 1991b.
Labyak S: Sleep and circadian schedule disorders, *Nurs Clin North Am* 37:599, 2002.
Lai HL, Good M: Music improves sleep quality in older adults, *J Adv Nurs* 49(3):234, 2005.
Landis CA: Sleep and methods of assessment, *Nurs Clin North Am* 37:583, 2002.
Liao WC: Effects of passive body heating on body temperature and sleep regulation in the elderly: a systematic review, *Int J Nurs Stud* 39(8): 803, 2002.
Lichstein KL, Morin, CM: *Treatment of late-life insomnia,* Thousand Oaks, Calif, 2000, Sage Publications.
Morin C et al: Nonpharmacological interventions for insomnia, *Am J Psychiatry* 151:1172, 1994.
Morin CM et al: Nonpharmacological treatment of late-life insomnia, *J Psychosom Res* 46:103, 1999.
Piani A, Brotini S, Dolso P et al: Sleep disturbances in elderly: a subjective evaluation over 65, *Arch Gerontol Geriatr* 9(Suppl):325, 2004.
Richards K et al: Use of complementary and alternative therapies to promote sleep in critical ill patients, *Crit Care Nurs Clin North Am* 15(3):329, 2003.
Roehrs T, Roth T: Hypnotics, alcohol, and caffeine: relation to insomnia. In Pressman MR, Orr WC, editors: *Understanding sleep: the evaluation and treatment of sleep disorders,* Washington, DC, 1997, American Psychological Association.
Somer E: *Food and mood: the complete guide to eating well and feeling your best,* ed 2, New York, 1999, Henry Holt.
Woodward M: Insomnia in the elderly, *Aust Fam Physician* 28:653, 1999.

# Impaired Social interaction

*Gail B. Ladwig*

**NANDA**

## Definition

S

Insufficient or excessive quantity or ineffective quality of social exchange

## Defining Characteristics

Verbalized or observed inability to receive or communicate a satisfying sense of belonging, caring, interest, or shared history; verbalized or observed discomfort in social situations; observed use of unsuccessful social interaction behaviors; dysfunctional interaction with peers, family and/or others; family report of change of style or pattern of interaction

## Related Factors (r/t)

Knowledge/skill deficit regarding ways to enhance mutuality, therapeutic isolation, sociocultural dissonance, limited physical mobility, environmental barriers, communication barriers, altered thought processes, absence of available significant others or peers, self-concept disturbance

**NOC**

## Outcomes (Nursing Outcomes Classification)

### Suggested NOC Outcomes

Child Development: Middle Childhood, Adolescence; Play Participation; Role Performance; Social Interaction Skills; Social Involvement

**Example NOC Outcome with Indicators**

**Social Involvement** as evidenced by the following indicator: Interacts with close friends, neighbors, family members, and members of work groups (Rate each indicator of **Social Involvement:** 1 = never demonstrated, 2 = rarely demonstrated, 3 = sometimes demonstrated 4 = often demonstrated, 5 = consistently demonstrated [see Section I].)

## Client Outcomes

### Client Will (Specify Time Frame):

- Identify barriers that cause impaired social interactions
- Discuss feelings that accompany impaired and successful social interactions
- Use available opportunities to practice interactions
- Use successful social interaction behaviors
- Report increased comfort in social situations
- Communicate, state feelings of belonging, demonstrate caring and interest in others
- Report effective interactions with others

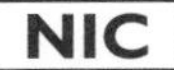

## Interventions (Nursing Interventions Classification)

### Suggested NIC Intervention

Socialization Enhancement



**Example NIC Activities—Socialization Enhancement**

Encourage patience in developing relationships; help the client increase awareness of strengths and limitations in communicating with others

## Nursing Interventions and Rationales

- Observe for cause of discomfort in social situations; ask the client to explain when discomfort began and identify any losses (e.g., loss of health, job, or significant other; aging) and changes (e.g., marriage, birth or adoption of a child, change in body appearance). *Individualized assessment indicates specific interventions (Warren, 1993).*

- Assess the client's social support system. **EBN:** *Use a social support tool or validated assessment tool if possible (e.g., UCLA Loneliness Scale for Adolescents [Mahon et al, 1995]).*
- Spend time with the client. **EBN:** *In this study being truly present was listed as one behavior that demonstrated caring (Yonge & Molzahn, 2002).*
- Use active listening skills including assessment and clarification of the client's verbal and nonverbal responses and interactions. **EBN:** *This article suggests that best practice with regard to communication in palliative care could be achieved by using a sensitive assessment of how each client chooses to cope with his or her situation rather than a uniform approach to care (Dean, 2002).*
- Encourage social support for patients with visual impairments. **EB:** *A large, nationwide study, conducted 1994 at the University of Amsterdam, on the meaning of personal networks and social support for Dutch adolescents with visual impairments indicate that social support, especially the support of peers, is important to adolescents with visual impairments (Kef, 2002).*
- Have the client list behaviors that are associated with being disconnected, and discuss alternative responses that may increase comfort. *Connections occur when a person is actively involved with another person, object, group, or environment; such involvement promotes a sense of comfort, well-being, and anxiety reduction (Hagerty et al, 1993).*
- Monitor the client's use of defense mechanisms, and support healthy defenses (e.g., the client focuses on present and avoids placing blame on others for personal behavior). *Solution-focused techniques have been demonstrated to be beneficial. Therapy focuses on client's present and future, capitalizing on the strengths and resources of the client and significant others around them (Bowles, 2002; University of Central Lancashire Department of Nursing, 2003).*
- Have the client list behaviors that cause discomfort. Discuss alternative ways to alleviate discomfort (e.g., focusing on others and their interests, practicing making caring statements such as, "I understand you are feeling sad"). Encourage the client to express feelings to others (e.g., "I feel sad also"). *Self-expression invites involvement and increases connectedness (Hagerty et al, 1993).*
- Identify client strengths. Have the client make a list of strengths and refer to it when experiencing negative feelings. He or she may find it helpful to put the list on a note card to carry at all times. **EBN:** *Extra stress in this study was reduced by positive thinking (Mkinen et al, 2000).*
- Have group members identify each other's strengths in a group setting. *This exercise encourages individuals to practice relating to each other on a more intimate level (Drew, 1991).*
- Role play comfortable and uncomfortable social interactions with the client and appropriate responses (e.g., acknowledging a friendly greeting, responding to rude remarks with an "I" statement, such as, "I understand you may feel that way, but this is how I feel"). *Role plays may help the client develop social interaction skills and identify feelings associated with isolation (Warren, 1993).*
- Model appropriate social interactions. Give positive verbal and nonverbal feedback for appropriate behavior (e.g., make statements such as, "I'm proud that you made it to work on time and did all the tasks assigned to you without saying that your supervisor was picking on you"; make eye contact). If not contraindicated, touch the client's arm

S

or hand when speaking. *One way to learn social skills is to observe the productive interactions of others (Drew, 1991).* **EBN:** *Shared feelings increased communication with stroke and aphasia clients without words (Sundin et al, 2000).*

- Use humor as appropriate. **EBN:** *Humor is important for helping clients cope mentally (Makinen et al, 2000).*
- Consider use of "animal" therapy; arrange for visitation. **EBN:** *Equine-facilitated psychotherapy, although not a new idea, is a little-known experiential intervention that offers the opportunity to achieve healing (Vidrine et al, 2002).*
- Consider the use of the Internet to promote socialization. **EBN:** *Use of the Internet was effective in providing social support and education for isolated rural women with chronic illness (Hill & Weinert, 2004).*

## Pediatric

- Provide computers and the Internet access to children with chronic disabilities that limit socialization. **EB:** *Established information technology was used in an attempt to reduce social isolation by providing each family who had a child with Duchenne's muscular dystrophy with a personal computer and e-mail and Internet connectivity. Results from quantitative and qualitative interviews with parents indicated that benefits accrued to the families and to the boys themselves: social isolation was felt to have been reduced, and an occupation, interest, and enjoyment provided (Soutter et al, 2004).*

▲ Consider use of RAP Therapy in groups to advance social skills of urban adolescents. **EB:** *Findings were unequivocally in favor of the RAP therapy as a tool for advancing prosocial behavior in three adolescent groups: violent offenders, status offenders, and a control condition of high school students with no criminal history (DeCarlo & Hoffman, 2003).*

## Geriatric

- Avoid assuming that social isolation is normal for elderly client. **EBN:** *Socialization is important throughout the life span. It provides a mode for enhancing a person's quality of life (Gosline, 2003).*

▲ Assess the client's potential or actual sensory problems with hearing and vision and make appropriate referrals if a problem is identified. **EB:** *Sensory problems are common experiences within the older US population. Of people age 70 years, 18% reported blindness in one or both eyes or some other trouble seeing, 33.2% reported problems with hearing, and 8.6% reported problems with both hearing and seeing (FN1). Precisely because these experiences are so common, they are often overlooked or dismissed. Older people with both hearing loss and vision impairment reported substantial difficulty sustaining social participation activities (Crews & Campbell, 2004).*

- Monitor for depression, a particular risk in the elderly. *Age and its associated losses may cause formerly socially active people to be alone. Loneliness contributes to depression and social withdrawal (Warren, 1993).*
- Provide group situations for the client. *Group settings are necessary for the client to practice new skills.*
- Encourage physical activity such as aerobics or stretching and toning in a group. *These activities decreased loneliness in former sedentary adults (N = 174, median age = 65.5 years) (McAuley et al, 2000).* **EBN:** *Extra stress was reduced for clients in this study (Makinen*

*et al, 2000).* **EB:** *This article reports an evaluation of a football project that was established to promote the social well-being of service users with enduring mental health problems. Participation was perceived as very beneficial by all interviewed. Specifically, the project offered the opportunity for social interaction within the context of a normalizing activity and was used as a process for challenging auditory hallucinations and delusional beliefs. The authors conclude that where appropriate, the development of sport and physical activity opportunities for service users should be considered by mental health professionals (Carter-Morris & Faulkner, 2003).*

- Have clients reminisce. **EBN:** *Through the process of reminiscence, older adults can actively evaluate life experiences and explore the meaning of memorable events (Harrand & Bollstetter, 2000).*

## Multicultural

- Acknowledge racial/ethnic differences at the onset of care. **EBN:** *Acknowledgement of race/ethnicity issues will enhance communication, establish rapport, and promote positive treatment outcomes (D'Avanzo et al, 2001; Ludwick & Silva, 2000; Vontress & Epp, 1997).*
- Assess for the influence of cultural beliefs, norms, and values on the client's perception of social activity and relationships. **EBN:** *What the client considers normal social interaction may be based on cultural perceptions (Cochran, 1998; Doswell & Erlen, 1998; Leininger & McFarland, 2002).*
- Assess for the effect of racism on the client's perceptions of social interactions. **EB:** *Accumulated experiences of racial discrimination by African-American women constitute an independent risk factor for preterm delivery (Collins et al, 2004).*
- Approach individuals of color with respect, warmth, and professional courtesy. **EBN:** *Instances of disrespect and lack of caring have special significance for individuals of color and may impede efforts to increase social outlets (D'Avanzo et al, 2001; Vontress & Epp, 1997). Physicians were 23% more verbally dominant and engaged in 33% less patient-centered communication with African-American patients than with Caucasian patients (Johnson et al, 2004). Minorities were significantly more likely to report being treated with disrespect or being looked down upon in the patient-provider relationship (Blanchard & Lurie, 2004).*
- Assess the use of personal space needs, communication styles, acceptable body language, eye contact, perception of touch, and paraverbals when communicating with the client. **EBN:** *Nurses need to consider these when interpreting verbal and nonverbal messages (Purnell, 2000). Native Americans may consider avoidance of direct eye contact as a sign of respect and asking questions to be rude and intrusive (Seiderman et al, 1996).*
- Validate the client's feelings regarding social interaction. **EBN:** *Validation lets the client know that the nurse has heard and understands what was said, and it promotes the nurse-client relationship (Heineken, 1998). Research suggests that an increased risk of health pessimism among African-American adults is due in part to race differences in the perception of interpersonal maltreatment (Boardman, 2004).*
- Use interpreters as needed. **EB:** *Primary care nurses act as gatekeepers to interpreting services (Gerrish et al, 2004).*

S

## Home Care

- • Previously discussed interventions may be adapted for home care use.
- ▲ Assess family and living environment for social dynamics. Refer for medical social services to assist with family dynamics if appropriate. *The family is a socially significant cultural group that generates behavior, defines roles, and promotes values.*
- ▲ Assess the client for a psychiatric disorder. Refer for mental health services as indicated. *Impaired social interaction can occur with a number of psychiatric disorders (depression, bipolar disorder, schizophrenia). Improved social interaction is unlikely unless the underlying disorder is treated.*
- • Assess the client's social skills; provide feedback regarding maladaptive skills, and opportunities to role play alternative communication styles. *Social interaction is likely to be impaired if the client uses ineffective social skills. Experiencing how to interact with others differently is influential in creating new behaviors.*
- • Suggest that the client avoid contact with negative persons. *Negative interactions reinforce undesired patterns.*
- • Identify activities that the client does alone and assist the client with balancing solitary and social activities. *A healthy balance of social and private time supports positive coping.*
- • Establish pattern of care and daily activities that involve the client socially (e.g., Meals on Wheels, home health aide visits). Give supportive feedback for positive and appropriate interactions. *The assumption of new patterns of interaction requires practice in safe situations. Feedback reinforces desired behaviors.*
- ▲ Refer to or support involvement with supportive groups and counseling. **EB:** *Cognitive behavioral group therapy was effective for social phobia in this group of 11 adolescent girls (Hayward et al, 2000). Group settings provide the opportunity to practice new skills. Counseling helps the client to define appropriate actions, and it is a source of support.*
- ▲ In the presence of a psychiatric disorder, refer for psychiatric home health care services for the client reassurance and implementation of therapeutic regimen. *Psychiatric home care nurses can address issues relating to the client's impaired social interaction. Behavioral interventions in the home can assist the client to participate more effectively in the treatment plan (Patusky et al, 1996).*

## Client/Family Teaching

- • Help the client accept responsibility for own behavior. Have the client keep a journal, and review it together at prescheduled intervals. Give the client positive feedback for appropriate behaviors, and suggest alternative approaches for behaviors that do not enhance social interaction. Positive reinforcement perpetuates appropriate behaviors. Teach social interaction skills for use in actual situations the client is faced with daily. *Through productive connections with others, social skills are learned and a repertoire of roles for many social situations is developed, which leads to an increase in self-esteem and the capacity to interact with others (Drew, 1991).*
- • Practice social skills one to one and, when the client is ready, practice in group sessions. *Practice improves performance and comfort level.*
- ▲ Refer to appropriate social agencies for assistance (e.g., family therapy, self-help groups, crisis intervention).



S

## evolve WEBSITES FOR EDUCATION

See the EVOLVE website for World Wide Web resources for client education.

## REFERENCES


Blanchard J, Lurie N: R-E-S-P-E-C-T: patient reports of disrespect in the health care setting and its impact on care, *J Fam Pract* 53(9):721-730, 2004.

Boardman JD: Health pessimism among black and white adults: the role of interpersonal and institutional maltreatment, *Soc Sci Med* 59(12):2523-2533, 2004.

Bowles N: A solution-focused approach to engagement in acute psychiatry, *Nurs Times* 98(48):26, 2002.

Carter-Morris P, Faulkner G: A football project for service users: the role of football in reducing social exclusion, *J Ment Health Promot* 2(1):7, 2003.

Cochran M: Tears have no color, *Am J Nurs* 98(6):53, 1998.

Collins JW Jr, David RJ, Handler A et al: Very low birthweight in African American infants: the role of maternal exposure to interpersonal racial discrimination, *Am J Public Health* 94(12):2132-2138, 2004.

Crews JE, Campbell VA: Vision impairment and hearing loss among community-dwelling older Americans: implications for health functioning, *Am J Pub Health* 94(5):823-829, 2004.

D'Avanzo CE et al: Developing culturally informed strategies for substance-related interventions. In Naegle MA, D'Avanzo CE, editors: *Addictions and substance abuse: strategies for advanced practice nursing,* St Louis, 2001, Mosby.

Dean A: Talking to dying clients of their hopes and needs, *Nurs Times* 98(43):34, 2002.

DeCarlo A, Hockman E: RAP therapy: a group work intervention method for urban adolescents, *Soc Work Groups* 26(3):45-59, 2003.

Doswell W, Erlen J: Multicultural issues and ethical concerns in the delivery of revising care interventions, *Nurs Clin North Am* 33(2):353, 1998.

Drew N: Combating the social isolation of chronic mental illness, *J Psychosoc Nurs Ment Health Serv* 29:14, 1991.

Gerrish K, Chau R, Sobowale A et al: Bridging the language barrier: the use of interpreters in primary care nursing, *Health Soc Care Community* 12(5):407-413, 2004.

Gosline MB: Client participation to enhance socialization for frail elders, *Geriatr Nurs* 24(5):286-289, 2003.

Hagerty BM, Lynch-Sauer J, Patusky KL et al: An emerging theory of human relatedness, *Image* 25:291, 1993.

Harrand AG, Bollstetter JJ: Developing a community-based reminiscence group for the elderly, *Clin Nurse Spec* 14(1):17, 2000.

Hayward C, Varady S, Albano AM et al: Cognitive-behavioral group therapy for social phobia in female adolescents: results of a pilot study, *J Am Acad Child Adolesc Psychiatry* 39(6):721, 2000.

Heineken J: Patient silence is not necessarily client satisfaction: communication in home care nursing, *Home Healthc Nurse* 16(2): 115, 1998.

Hill WG, Weinert C: An evaluation of an online intervention to provide social support and health education, *Comput Inform Nurs* 22(5):282-288, 2004.

Johnson RL, Roter D, Powe NR et al: Patient race/ethnicity and quality of patient-physician communication during medical visits, *Am J Public Health* 94(12):2084-2090, 2004.

Kef S: Psychosocial adjustment and the meaning of social support for visually impaired adolescents, *J Visual Impairment Blindness* 96(1):22, 2002.

Leininger MM, McFarland MR: *Transcultural nursing: concepts, theories, research and practices,* ed 3, New York, 2002, McGraw-Hill.

Ludwick R, Silva M: Nursing around the world: cultural values and ethical conflicts, *Online J Issues Nursing,* August 14, 2000. Available at www.nursingworld.org/ojin/ethcol/ethics_4.htm, accessed June 19, 2003.

Mahon NE, Yarcheski T, Yarcheski A: Validation of the revised UCLA loneliness scale for adolescents, *Res Nurs Health* 18:263, 1995.

McAuley E, Blissmer B, Marquez DX et al: Social relations, physical activity, and well-being in older adults, *Prev Med* 31(5):608, 2000.

Makinen S, Suominen T, Lauri S: Self-care in adults with asthma: how they cope, *J Clin Nurs* 9(4):557, 2000.

Patusky KL, Rodning C, Martinez-Kratz M: Clinical lessons in psychiatric home care: a case study approach, *J Home Healthc Manag* 9:18, 1996.

Purnell L: A description of the Purnell model for cultural competence, *J Transcult Nurs* 11(1):40, 2000.


S

Seideman RY, Jacobson S, Primeaux M et al: Assessing American Indian families, *MCN Am J Matern Child Nurs* 21(6):274, 1996.

Soutter J, Hamilton N, Russell P: The golden freeway: a preliminary evaluation of a pilot study advancing information technology as a social intervention for boys with Duchenne muscular dystrophy and their families, *Health Soc Care Community* 12(1): 25-33, 2004.

Sundin K, Jansson L, Norberg A: Communicating with people with stroke and aphasia: understanding through sensation without words, *J Clin Nurs* 9(4):481, 2000.

University of Central Lancashire: Department of Nursing: Available at www.uclan.ac.uk/courses/factsheets/health/nursing/3284.pdf, accessed January 18, 2003.

Vidrine M, Owen-Smith P, Faulkner P et al: Equine-facilitated group psychotherapy: applications for therapeutic vaulting, *Ment Health Nurs* 23(6):587, 2002.

Vontress CE, Epp LR: Historical hostility in the African American client: implications for counseling, *J Multicult Counseling Dev* 25:170, 1997.

Warren BJ: Explaining social isolation through concept analysis, *Arch Psychiatr Nurs* 7:270, 1993.

Yonge O, Molzahn A: Exceptional nontraditional caring practices of nurses, *Scand J Caring Sci* 16(4):399, 2002.

# Social isolation

*Gail B. Ladwig*

**NANDA**

## Definition

Aloneness experienced by the individual and perceived as imposed by others and as a negative or threatening state

## Defining Characteristics

### Objective

Absence of supportive significant others (e.g., family, friends, group); projection of hostility in voice and behavior; withdrawal; uncommunicativeness; demonstration of behavior unaccepted by dominant cultural group; desire to be alone or exist in a subculture; repetitive and meaningless actions; preoccupation with own thoughts; lack of eye contact; inappropriate or immature activities for developmental age/stage; evidence of physical/mental handicap or altered state of wellness; sad, dull affect

### Subjective

Expression of feelings of aloneness imposed by others, expression of feelings of rejection, inappropriate or immature interests for developmental age/stage, inadequate or absent significant purpose in life, inability to meet expectations of others, expression of values acceptable to subculture but unacceptable to dominant cultural group, expression of interest inappropriate to developmental age/stage, feelings of differences from others, insecurity in public

## Related Factors (r/t)

Alterations in mental status, inability to engage in satisfying personal relationships, unacceptable social values, unacceptable social behavior, inadequate personal resources, immature interests, factors contributing to absence of satisfying personal relationships (e.g., delay in accomplishing developmental tasks), alterations in physical appearance, altered state of wellness

**NOC**

## Outcomes (Nursing Outcomes Classification)

### Suggested NOC Outcomes

Loneliness Severity, Mood Equilibrium, Personal Well-Being, Play Participation, Social Interaction Skills, Social Involvement, Social Support

**Example NOC Outcome with Indicators**

**Social Involvement** as evidenced by the following indicator: Interacts with close friends, neighbors, family members, and members of work groups (Rate the indicator of **Social Involvement:** 1 = never demonstrated, 2 = rarely demonstrated, 3 = sometimes demonstrated, 4 = often demonstrated, 5 = consistently demonstrated [see Section I].)

## Client Outcomes

### Client Will (Specify Time Frame):

- Identify feelings of isolation
- Practice social and communication skills needed to interact with others
- Initiate interactions with others; set and meet goals
- Participate in activities and programs at level of ability and desire
- Describe feelings of self-worth

**NIC**

## Interventions (Nursing Interventions Classification)

S

### Suggested NIC Intervention

Socialization Enhancement

**Example NIC Activities—Socialization Enhancement**

Encourage patience in developing relationships; help client increase awareness of strengths and limitations in communicating with others

## Nursing Interventions and Rationales

- Establish a therapeutic relationship by being emotionally present and authentic. *Being emotionally present and authentic fosters growth in relationships and decreases isolation*

*(Jordan, 2000).* **EBN:** *In one study, being truly present was listed as one behavior that demonstrated caring (Yonge & Molzahn, 2002).*

- • Observe for barriers to social interaction (e.g., illness; incontinence; decreasing ability to form relationships; lack of transportation, money, support system, or knowledge). **EBN:** *Causes of social isolation may be different for each individual; therefore adequate information must be gathered so that appropriate interventions can be planned (Badger, 1990).*
- • Note risk factors (e.g., membership in ethnic/cultural minority, chronic physiological or psychological illness or deformities, advanced age). **EBN:** *Clients with these risk factors may be at risk for social isolation (Warren, 1993).*
- • Discuss causes of perceived or actual isolation. **EBN:** *The individual's experience of illness; the circumstances of everyday living that influence quality of life; and emotions, fears, and concerns all have a bearing on the way illness is managed (Anderson, 1991).*
- ▲ Promote social interactions. Support the expression of feelings. Consider the use of music therapy. **EB:** *This study of terminally ill clients discusses the role music plays in accessing emotion. The goals set for these patients were to decrease depressive symptoms and social isolation, increase communication and self-expression, stimulate reminiscence and life review, and enhance relaxation. The clients were all successful in reaching their individual goals (Clement, 2004).*
- • Establish trust one on one and then gradually introduce the client to others. Allow the client opportunities to introduce issues and to describe his or her daily life. **EBN:** *Individualization of care, or tailoring of care, involves taking into account the client's individuality and allowing that individuality to determine interpersonal approaches and health-illness management actions (Brown, 1994).*
- • Involve clients in writing specific outcomes such as identifying what is most important from their viewpoint and lifestyle. **EBN:** *In this study of women diagnosed with early breast cancer the understanding of factors that are important to women when they are making decisions for medical treatment is a mandatory step in designing customized evidence-based decision support (Budden et al, 2003).*
- • Provide positive reinforcement when the client seeks out others. **EBN:** *Receiving instrumental social support such as practical help, advice, and feedback significantly contributes to positive well-being (White, 1992).*
- • Help the client identify appropriate diversional activities to encourage socialization. *Active participation by the client is essential for behavioral changes.*
- • Encourage physical closeness (e.g., use touch) if appropriate. **EBN:** *Touch helps with integration and fosters social relatedness. Tactile stimulation benefits the older adult's psychological well-being (Jamison, 1997).*
- • Identify available support systems and involve these individuals in the client's care. **EBN:** *Clients cope more successfully with stressful life events if they have support (White, 1992).*
- ▲ Refer clients to support groups. **EB:** *Clients who are victims of domestic violence often endure social isolation imposed by significant others and benefit from support groups (Larance & Porter, 2004).*
- • Encourage liberal visitation for a client who is hospitalized or in an extended care

S

facility. **EB:** *Visits from those in an emotionally close network were associated with perceived support, and this was associated with a decrease in depression (Oxman & Hull, 2001).*

- Help the client identify role models and others with similar interests. *Sometimes the client needs someone to model the appropriate behavior.*
- See the care plan for **Risk for Loneliness.**

## Geriatric

- Assess physical and mental status to establish a firm basis for planning social activities. **EBN:** *Socialization is important throughout the life span. It provides a mode for enhancing a person's quality of life. Older adults living alone and with spouses continue to desire social interaction at levels similar to their participation in earlier life stages (Gosoline, 2003).*
- Assess for hearing deficit. Provide aids and use adaptive techniques such as facing the individual when speaking, speaking slowly, lowering the pitch of the voice, and enunciating clearly. **EB:** *A relationship exists between hearing acuity and loneliness. Hearing loss is one of the most prevalent chronic health problems of older adults, especially the very old. Adaptive techniques that facilitate communication must be used (Dugan & Kivett, 1994).*
- Involve client in goal setting and planning activities. Have them write down five activities in which they would like to participate. **EBN:** *In this study of frail older adults, involving participation of clients in goal setting and planning of social activities enhanced both their anticipation and their participation in the activities (Gosoline, 2003).*
- If the client is in a health care facility, visit him or her for at least 10 minutes every 2–3 hours. *The presence of a trusted individual provides emotional security for the client.*
- ▲ Involve nonprofessionals in activities, projects, and goal setting with the client. Practice interdisciplinary management for unit-based activities: engaging in arts and crafts projects, sewing, watching videos, reading large-print books, reading magazines, playing games, playing musical instruments, and using assistive listening devices. **EBN:** *Nursing assistants are commonly concerned about the social support of residents; therefore they can be a valuable resource for generating intervention ideas. (Alterations in job descriptions would be required.) Residents with visual, hearing, cognitive, and mobility impairments will participate more readily in events that involve a smaller number of people and in which the staff takes initiative and establishes rapport with each resident (Windriver, 1993).* **EBN:** *In a study of the use of calming music and hand massage, physically nonaggressive behaviors decreased during each of the interventions. At 1 hour after either intervention, agitated verbal behavior decreased (Remington, 2002).*
- Offer the client a choice of activities and persons with whom to sit and socialize. Introductions to strangers may need to be repeated several times. **EBN:** *A recognized intervention for loneliness is to provide opportunities and assistance for making choices, setting goals, and making decisions. Cognitively impaired clients may require several repetitions (Windriver, 1993).*
- Put clients in groups according to activity preferences, abilities, age, life situations, personal and cultural characteristics, and social networks. **EBN:** *Positive social interactions are enhanced by the aforementioned interventions (Windriver, 1993).*
- Develop and display a seating chart for the common areas of each personal care unit and develop a process for both identifying needed changes and executing them

promptly. **EBN:** *Personality factors that are difficult to predict affect the success of social groupings (Windriver, 1993).*

- Provide physical activity, either aerobic or stretching and toning. **EB:** *Physical activity increased social support in a group of older, formerly sedentary adults (McAuley et al, 2000).*
- Provide music with active participation; drumming, rhythm circle. **EBN:** *There is no active participation for many residents when the music programs they experience are limited to attendance at concerts and sing-alongs. Drum circles and rhythm circles actively involve residents, even those who are cognitively impaired (Rozon, Hagens, & Martin, 2004).*
- Consider the use of simulated presence therapy (see the care plan for **Hopelessness**). **EBN:** *Simulated presence therapy appears to be the most effective therapy for treating social isolation (Woods & Ashley, 1995).*

▲ Refer to programs such as Foster Grandparents and Senior Companions. **EB:** *Emotional isolation leads to social isolation. Social programs help increase contact with peers and decrease isolation. Programs to alleviate emotional isolation should focus on attachment loss (Dugan & Kivett, 1994).*

- Consider using computers and the Internet to alleviate or reduce loneliness and social isolation. **EBN:** *A descriptive qualitative study used a Web page questionnaire and chat room interviews with online participants age 65 years and older living alone. Seven of the 10 participants used the computer to combat loneliness (Clark, 2002). In another study, Internet use was found to decrease loneliness and depression significantly, while perceived social support and self-esteem increased significantly (Shaw & Gant, 2002).*

## Multicultural

- Acknowledge racial/ethnic differences at the onset of care. **EBN:** *Acknowledgment of race/ethnicity issues will enhance communication, establish rapport, and promote positive treatment outcomes (D'Avanzo et al, 2001; Ludwick & Silva, 2000; Vontress & Epp, 1997).*
- Assess for the influence of cultural beliefs, norms, and values on the client's perception of social activity and relationships. **EBN:** *What the client considers normal social interaction may be based on cultural perceptions (Cochran, 1998; Doswell & Erlen, 1998; Leininger & McFarland, 2002).*
- Approach individuals of color with respect, warmth, and professional courtesy. **EBN:** *Instances of disrespect and lack of caring have special significance for individuals of color and may impede efforts to increase social outlets (D'Avanzo et al, 2001; Vontress & Epp, 1997).*
- Assess personal space needs, communication styles, acceptable body language, attitude toward eye contact, perception of touch, and paraverbal messages when communicating with the client. **EBN:** *Nurses need to consider these aspects when interpreting verbal and nonverbal messages (Purnell, 2000). Native-American clients may consider avoiding direct eye contact to be a sign of respect and asking questions to be rude and intrusive (Seideman et al, 1996).*
- Use a family-centered approach when working with Latino, Asian, African-American, and Native-American clients. **EBN:** *Latinos may perceive the family as source of support, solver of problems, and source of pride. Asian Americans may regard the family as the primary decision maker and influence on individual family members (D'Avanzo et al, 2001).*

- Promote a sense of ethnic attachment. **EBN:** *Older Korean clients with strong ethnic attachments had higher levels of social involvement than others (Kim, 1999).*
- Validate the client's feelings regarding social isolation. **EBN:** *Validation lets the client know that the nurse has heard and understood what was said, and it promotes the nurse-client relationship (Heineken, 1998). A study of African-American men found a sense of family in the AIDS dedicated nursing home, making it potentially a valuable source of needed social support, which decreased social isolation (Fields & Jemmot, 2003).*

## Home Care

- The interventions described previously may be adapted for home care use.
- ▲ Assess the client for depression or other psychiatric disorder. Refer for mental health services as indicated. *Social isolation is part of the syndrome of depression or other psychiatric disorders. Increase in social activities is unlikely unless the underlying disorder is treated.*
- Confirm that the home setting has a telephone. Obtain one if necessary for medical safety. If the client lives alone, set up a Lifeline safety system that requires the client to answer the telephone. *The telephone can be used to achieve continuity of care and successful client/family interaction (Skinner, 2001). A Lifeline system can be a safety net for physical and psychological safety.*
- Consider the use of the computer and Internet to decrease isolation. **EBN:** *In a qualitative exploratory, descriptive investigation of pregnant women on home bed rest for preterm labor, the women stated that their participation in a virtual online peer support group was valuable and beneficial in helping them to cope with the hardships of bed rest (Adler & Zarchin, 2002). A study of homebound older adults found that the Internet and e-mail were excellent sources of support and enjoyment, and their use resulted in an improved quality of life (Nahm & Resnick, 2001).*
- Encourage family involvement in daily life in small, nonthreatening activities such as short outings, assistance with shopping, and solicitation of input from the isolated person in decision making. *Reversing social isolation is a gradual process.*
- Establish a pattern of care and daily activities that involves the client socially (e.g., Meals-on-Wheels, home health aide visits). *Pattern changes encourage new behaviors.*
- Have the client keep a diary of social experiences. Discuss the diary during visits. *A review of social experiences helps the client identify those that are most comfortable.*
- Identify activities that the client does alone. Assist the client with balancing solitary and social activities, keeping alone time to a minimum. *A healthy balance of social and private time supports positive coping.*
- ▲ Refer for visiting volunteer services. *Spending time with the client enhances client self-esteem.*
- When the client is ready, encourage him or her to volunteer for short periods at community agencies in which contact is positive and nonthreatening (e.g., with hospitalized older adults for 1 hr/wk). *Contributing to the welfare of others enhances self-esteem.*
- ▲ Assess options for living that allow the client privacy but not isolation (e.g., boarding home, congregate living, assertive community treatment programs). **EB:** *An exploratory qualitative study examined contexts and processes of social relationship development as experienced by adults with schizophrenia participating in assertive community treatment pro-*

S

*grams. Participants described their relationships with other mental health clients in primarily positive terms, yet several participants expressed dissatisfaction and desired greater integration into mainstream social networks (Angell, 2003).*

▲ In the presence of a psychiatric disorder, refer for psychiatric home health care services for client reassurance and implementation of a therapeutic regimen. **EBN:** *Psychiatric home care nurses can address issues relating to the client's social isolation. Behavioral interventions in the home can help the client to participate more effectively in the treatment plan (Patusky, Rodning, & Martinez-Kratz, 1996).*

## Client/Family Teaching

- Teach skills related to problem solving, communication, social interaction, ADL, and positive self-esteem. *All of these skills are necessary to change isolating behavior.*
- Consider the use of telecommunication and group support via the Internet. **EB:** *One study delivered diabetes education and social support to rural women with diabetes. The women declared the computer-based social support to have positive effects (Smith & Weinert, 2000).*
- Teach role playing (practicing communication skills in specific situations). **EB:** *Role playing may help clients develop social interaction skills and identify feelings associated with their isolation (Warren, 1993).*

▲ Encourage the client to initiate contacts with self-help groups, counselors, and therapists. **EBN:** *If adjustment is to be successful and maintained, management of a chronic illness cannot occur in isolation; it requires a complex interaction of resources (White, 1992).*

- Provide information to the client about senior citizen services, house sharing, pets, day care centers, churches, and community resources. **EBN:** *The well-documented negative effect of social isolation suggests that clients without confidants and supportive others must be referred to alternative sources, such as cardiac rehabilitation programs, support groups, and community agencies (McCauley, 1995).*

▲ Refer socially isolated caregivers to appropriate support groups as well. *Identification and recognition of the overwhelming task of caregiving are needed so that caregivers do not suffer in silence. Alzheimer's disease support groups offer participants an opportunity to share troubles and triumphs with others who truly understand the turmoil of caregiving (Bergman-Evans, 1994). (See the care plan for* **Caregiver role strain.**)

- Teach caregivers methods to deal with troublesome behaviors related to memory disturbances, restlessness and agitation, catastrophic reactions, day/night disturbances, delusions, wandering, and physical violence. A general method for clinicians to manage these problems involves the identification of the behavior and its antecedent and consequent events. Stressors that may cause behavioral problems include fatigue, a change of routine, excessive demands, overwhelming stimuli, and acute illness or pain. **EB:** *Caregivers can be taught to identify these stressors to prevent or alleviate troublesome behaviors (Alessi, 1991).*

S

## evolve WEBSITES FOR EDUCATION

See the EVOLVE website for World Wide Web resources for client education.

## REFERENCES


Adler CL, Zarchin YR: The "virtual focus group": using the Internet to reach pregnant women on home bed rest, *J Obstet Gynecol Neonatal Nurs* 31(4):418, 2002.

Alessi C: Managing the behavioral problems of dementia in the home, *Clin Geriatr Med* 7(4):787, 1991.

Anderson JM: Immigrant women speak of chronic illness: the social construction of the devalued self, *J Adv Nurs* 16:710, 1991.

Angell B: Contexts of social relationship development among assertive community treatment clients, *Ment Health Serv Res* 5(1): 13, 2003.

Badger VT: Men with cardiovascular diseases and their spouses, coping health and marital adjustment, *Arch Psychiatr Nurs* 4:319, 1990.

Bergman-Evans BF: Alzheimer's and related disorders: loneliness, depression, and social support of spousal caregivers, *J Gerontol Nurs* 20:6, 1994.

Brown S: Communication strategies used by an expert nurse, *Clin Nurs Res* 3(1):43, 1994.

Budden LM, Pierce PF, Hayes BA et al: Australian women's prediagnostic decision-making styles, relating to treatment choices for early breast cancer treatment, *Res Theory Nurs Pract* 17(2):117-136, 2003.

Clark DJ: Older adults living through and with their computers, *Comput Inform Nurs* 20(3):117, 2002.

Clements-Cortes A: The use of music in facilitating emotional expression in the terminally ill, *Am J Hosp Palliat Care* 21(4):255-260, 2004.

Cochran M: Tears have no color, *Am J Nurs* 98(6):53, 1998.

D'Avanzo CE et al: Developing culturally informed strategies for substance-related interventions. In Naegle MA, D'Avanzo CE, editors: *Addictions and substance abuse: strategies for advanced practice nursing,* St Louis, 2001, Mosby.

Doswell W, Erlen J: Multicultural issues and ethical concerns in the delivery of nursing care interventions, *Nurs Clin North Am* 33(2):353, 1998.

Dugan E, Kivett V: The importance of emotional and social isolation to loneliness among very old rural adults, *Gerontologist* 34: 340, 1994.

Fields SD, Jemmott LS: The love and belonging healthcare needs of HIV infected African-American men upon admission to an AIDS dedicated nursing home, *J Natl Black Nurses Assoc* 14(1):38-44, 2003.

Gosline MB: Client participation to enhance socialization for frail elders, *Geriatr Nurs* 24(5):286-289, 2003.

Heineken J: Patient silence is not necessarily client satisfaction: communication in home care nursing, *Home Healthc Nurse* 16(2): 115, 1998.

Jamison M: Failure to thrive in older adults, *J Gerontol Nurs* 23(2):13, 1997.

Jordan JV: The role of mutual empathy in relational/cultural therapy, *J Clin Psychol* 56(8):1005, 2000.

Kim O: Mediation effect of social support between ethnic attachment and loneliness in older Korean immigrants, *Res Nurs Health* 22(2):169, 1999.

Larance LY, Porter ML: Observations from practice: support group membership as a process of social capital formation among female survivors of domestic violence, *J Interpers Violence* 19(6):676-690, 2004.

Leininger MM, McFarland MR: *Transcultural nursing: concepts, theories, research and practices,* ed 3, New York, 2002, McGraw-Hill.

Ludwick R, Silva M: Nursing around the world: cultural values and ethical conflicts, *Online J Issues Nurs,* August 14, 2000. Available online at www.nursingworld.org/ojin/ethcol/ethics_4.htm, accessed June 19, 2003.

McAuley E, Blissmer B, Marquez DX et al: Social relations, physical activity, and well-being in older adults, *Prev Med* 31(5):608, 2000.

McCauley K: Assessing social support in patients with cardiac disease, *J Cardiovasc Nurs* 10:73, 1995.

Nahm ES, Resnick B: Homebound older adults' experiences with the Internet and e-mail, *Comput Nurs* 19(6): 257, 2001.

Oxman TE, Hull JG: Social support and treatment response in older depressed primary care patients, *J Gerontol B Psychol Sci Soc Sci* 56(1):P35, 2001.

Patusky KL, Rodning C, Martinez-Kratz M: Clinical lessons in psychiatric home care: a case study approach, *J Home Health Case Manag* 9:18, 1996.

Purnell L: A description of the Purnell model for cultural competence, *J Transcult Nurs* 11(1):40, 2000.

Remington R: Calming music and hand massage with agitated elderly, *Nurs Res* 51(5):317, 2002.

Rozon L, Hagens C, Martin LS: Music programs that create a sense of community: music therapy for even the most severe cognitively impaired resident, *Can Nurs Home* 15(1):57-59, 2004.

Seideman RY, Jacobson S, Primeaux M et al: Assessing American Indian families, *MCN Am J Matern Child Nurs* 21(6):274, 1996.


S

Shaw LH, Gant LM: In defense of the Internet: the relationship between Internet communication and depression, loneliness, self-esteem, and perceived social support, *Cyberpsychol Behav* 5(2):157, 2002.
Skinner D: Intimacy and the telephone, *Caring* 20(2):28, 2001.
Smith L, Weinert C: Telecommunication support for rural women with diabetes, *Diabetes Educ* 26:645, 2000.
Vontress CE, Epp LR: Historical hostility in the African American client: implications for counseling, *J Multicult Counseling Dev* 25:170, 1997.
Warren B: Explaining social isolation through concept analysis, *Arch Psychiatr Nurs* 7:270, 1993; 14(2):211-212, 1992.
Windriver W: Social isolation: unit-based activities for impaired elders, *J Gerontol Nurs* 19:15, 1993.
Woods P, Ashley J: Simulated presence therapy: using selected memories to manage problem behaviors in Alzheimer's disease patients, *Geriatr Nurs* 16:9, 1995.
Yonge O, Molzahn A: Exceptional nontraditional caring practices of nurses, *Scand J Caring Sci* 16(4):399, 2002.

# Chronic Sorrow

*Betty J. Ackley and Gail B. Ladwig*

**NANDA**

## Definition

Cyclical, recurring, and potentially progressive pattern of pervasive sadness that is experienced (by client, parent or caregiver, or individual with chronic illness or disability) in response to continual loss throughout the trajectory of an illness or disability

## Defining Characteristics

Feelings that vary in intensity, are periodic, may progress and intensify over time, and may interfere with client's ability to reach his or her highest level of personal and social well-being; expression of periodic, recurrent feelings of sadness; expression of one or more of the following feelings: anger, being misunderstood, confusion, depression, disappointment, emptiness, fear, frustration, guilt/self-blame, helplessness, hopelessness, loneliness, low self-esteem, recurring loss, being overwhelmed

## Related Factors (r/t)

Death of a loved one; experience of chronic physical or mental illness or disability such as mental retardation, multiple sclerosis, prematurity, spina bifida or other birth defects, chronic mental illness, infertility, cancer, Parkinson's disease; experience of one or more trigger events (e.g., crises in management of illness, crises related to developmental stages and missed opportunities or milestones that bring comparisons with developmental, social, or personal norms); unending caregiving as constant reminder of loss

S

**NOC**

## Outcomes (Nursing Outcomes Classification)

### Suggested NOC Outcomes

Acceptance: Health Status; Depression Level; Depression Self-Control; Grief Resolution; Hope; Mood Equilibrium

**Example NOC Outcome with Indicators**

**Grief Resolution** with plans for a positive future as evidenced by the following indicators: Resolves feelings about loss/Verbalizes acceptance of loss/Describes meaning of loss or death/Reports decreased preoccupation with loss/Expresses positive expectations about the future (Rate each indicator of **Grief Resolution:** 1 = never demonstrated, 2 = rarely demonstrated, 3 = sometimes demonstrated, 4 = often demonstrated, 5 = consistently demonstrated [see Section I].)

## Client Outcomes

### Client Will (Specify Time Frame):

- Express appropriate feelings of guilt, fear, anger, or sadness
- Identify problems associated with sorrow (e.g., changes in appetite, insomnia, nightmares, loss of libido, decreased energy, alteration in activity levels)
- Seek help in dealing with grief-associated problems
- Plan for future one day at a time
- Function at normal developmental level

NIC

## Interventions (Nursing Interventions Classification)

### Suggested NIC Interventions

Grief Work Facilitation; Grief Work Facilitation: Perinatal Death

**Example NIC Activities—Grief Work Facilitation**

Encourage client to verbalize memories of loss, both past and current; assist client in identifying personal coping strategies

## Nursing Interventions and Rationales

S

- Assess the client's degree of sorrow. Use the Burke/NCRS Chronic Sorrow Questionnaire for the individual or caregiver as appropriate. *This questionnaire is designed to determine the occurrence of chronic sorrow, cues that trigger sorrow, coping strategies, and factors that direct health care personnel to deal with the sorrowful client or caregiver (Hainsworth, Eakes, & Burke, 1994; Hobdell, 2004).*
- Identify problems of eating and sleeping; ensure that basic human needs are being met. **EBN:** *One study indicated that bereaved individuals, irrespective of whether they had counseling for grief resolution or not, had a moderate risk for poor nutrition. The implication is that food issues need to be included in grief resolution interventions (Johnson, 2002).*
- Spend time with the client and family. **EB:** *The main suggestion in a study of families who have a child with a chronic illness and are facing loss in their lives was the provision of an empathetic presence (Langridge, 2002).*
- Develop a trusting relationship with the client by using empathetic therapeutic communication techniques. **EB:** *An empathetic person who takes the time to listen, offers support and reassurance, recognizes and focuses on feelings, and appreciates the uniqueness of*

*each individual and family is helpful to clients experiencing chronic sorrow (Eakes, Burke, & Hainsworth, 1998).*

- Help the client to understand that sorrow may be ongoing. No timetable exists for grieving, despite popular thought. After loss, life is characterized by good times and bad times when sorrow is triggered by events. **EBN:** *Studies have demonstrated that feelings of sadness, guilt, anger, frustration, and fear occur periodically throughout the lives of people experiencing chronic loss resulting in chronic sorrow (Eakes, Burke, & Hainsworth, 1998). In an analysis of 85 mourners' narratives, the most prominent theme was feeling the absence of the decedent (Gamino, Hogan, & Sewell, 2002).*
- Help the client recognize that, although sadness will occur at intervals for the rest of his or her life, it will become bearable. *In time the client may develop a relationship with grief that is lifelong but livable, and as much filled with comfort as it is with sorrow (Moules, 1998). The sadness associated with chronic sorrow is permanent, but as the grief resolves there can be times of satisfaction and even happiness (Clements, 2004).*
- Encourage the use of positive coping techniques:
  - Taking action: Suggested strategies include keeping busy, keeping personal interests, going away, getting out of the house, doing something to gain a feeling of control over life.
  - Cognitive coping: Techniques include concentrating on the positive aspects of life, having a "can do" attitude, taking 1 day at a time, and taking responsibility for the quality of one's own life. Encourage the client to write about the experience.
  - Interpersonal coping: Techniques include talking to a close friend, a health care professional, or someone with the same condition or circumstance. Joining a support group can also help the sorrowful person to cope.
  - Emotional coping: Encourage the client to express feelings, cry as desired, give thanks, and pray if desired.

  *Clients with chronic sorrow have found these coping techniques helpful. The techniques are arranged in order of effectiveness (Hainsworth, Eakes, & Burke, 1994).* **EB:** *A group of 26 individuals with traumatic memories were instructed to write about the negative events they had experienced during five 45-minute sessions over a period of 2 weeks. The trauma-writing participants experienced fewer intrusions and showed less avoidance behavior from pretreatment to follow-up, whereas a waiting list control group did not change significantly (Schoutrop et al, 2002).*
- Review past experiences, role changes, and coping skills. Use music if appropriate. *One study revealed the theme of a need to remember and to hold onto the memory. Participants in this study found comfort in knowing that they were not alone (Hentz, 2002). One article presented four case studies that demonstrate the use of music therapy in assisting palliative care clients and families to cope with grief and loss (Hilliard, 2001b).* **EB:** *One investigator concluded that participation of grieving children in music therapy–based bereavement groups served to reduce grief symptoms among the participants as evaluated in the home (Hilliard, 2001a).*
- Expect the client to meet responsibilities; give positive reinforcement.

▲ Refer the client to spiritual counseling if desired. **EB:** *A prospective cohort study included people about to be bereaved, with follow-up continuing for 14 months after the death. Those who professed stronger spiritual beliefs seemed to resolve their grief more rapidly and com-*

S

*pletely after the death of a close person than people with no spiritual beliefs (Walsh et al, 2002).*

- ▲ Encourage the client to make time to talk to family members about the loss with the help of professional support as needed and without criticizing or belittling each other's feelings about the loss. *Once these feelings are shared, family members can better begin to accept the chronic loss and develop coping strategies.* **EBN:** *In a study of adolescents dealing with the death of a loved one, the most important factors that helped adolescents cope with the grief were self-help and support from parents, relatives, and friends (Rask, Kaunonen, & Paunonen-Ilmonen, 2002). A study analyzing the grief and coping of mothers who had lost children under the age of 7 years found that the spouse, children, grandparents, next of kin, friends, and colleagues were the main sources of support (Laakso & Paunonen-Ilmonen, 2002).*
- • Recognize that a stimulus for reactivation of sorrow in women is when a developmentally disabled child develops a health care crisis. *In men, reactivation of sorrow is more associated with comparison with social norms (Mallow & Bechtel, 1999).*
- • Help the client determine the best way and place to find social support. *Social support is shown to help bereaved individuals as they reconstruct their lives and find new meaning in life (Hogan & Schmidt, 2002).*
- ▲ Identify available community resources, including grief counselors or support groups available for specific losses (e.g., Multiple Sclerosis Society). *Support groups can serve as a helpful means to improve interpersonal coping strategies to deal with the loss (Hainsworth, Eakes, & Burke, 1994).*
- ▲ Encourage the client to become active in interests such as volunteer work, service projects, or church activities. *When a grieving person can express caring for another, he or she gains a sense of being needed and an increased sense of purpose, which results in increased engagement in the world (Fischer & Hegge, 2000).*
- ▲ Identify whether the client is experiencing depression, suicidal tendencies, or other emotional disorders. Refer for counseling as appropriate. *Counseling with therapeutic goal setting has been shown to be helpful (Clements et al, 2004).*

## Pediatric/Parent

- • Treat the child with respect, give him or her the opportunity to talk about their concerns, and answer questions honestly. *Children know much more than adults realize. They are very observant and generally know if a parent or loved one is dying, or cause of death, even if they have not been told (Schuurman, 2005).*
- • Listen to the child's expression of grief. *The best thing to be done to help a child is to listen with our ears, eyes, hearts, and souls, and recognize that we do not have to have answers (Schuurman, 2005).*
- • Help parents recognize that the child does not have to be "fixed," instead they need support going through an experience of grieving just as adults. *The role of the nurse, parent, and friends is to support and assist, not to help them "get over it" (Schuurman, 2005).*
- • Encourage children to listen to music that they enjoy. **EB:** *The investigator concluded that participation of grieving children in music therapy–based bereavement groups served to reduce grief symptoms among the subjects as evaluated in the home (Hilliard, 2001a).*

- ▲ Consider the use of art for children in hospice care who are dying or dealing with the death of a parent, sibling, or other family member. **EBN:** *The arts are being recognized as a powerful tool for psychological, emotional, and spiritual support. Through an "ART is the heART" approach, children learn to use the arts as a healthy and effective coping strategy (Rollins & Riccio, 2002).*
- ▲ Refer grieving children and parents to a program to help facilitate grieving if desired, especially if the death was traumatic. **EB:** *A study demonstrated treatment for children and parents with grief associated with trauma helped decrease symptoms of post-traumatic stress disorder (PTSD) (Cohen, 2004).* **EBN:** *A program designed for grieving children involving riding horses was shown to increase self-confidence and self-esteem (Glazer, Clark, & Stein, 2004).*
- • Help the adolescent determine sources of support and how to use them effectively. **EBN:** *In a study of adolescents dealing with the death of a loved one, the most important factors that helped adolescents cope with the grief were self-help and support from parents, relatives, and friends (Rask, Kaunonen, & Paunonen-Ilmonen, 2002).*
- ▲ Encourage parents to seek mental health services as needed, learn stress reduction, and take good care of their health. **EB:** *A study demonstrated that there was a modest association between chronic sorrow and situational depression (Hobdell, 2004). Research has demonstrated that the loss of a child for a mother results in an increased loss of life within 18 years, either due to disease or suicide (Lawson, 2003).* **EBN:** *A study analyzing the grief and coping of mothers who had lost children under the age of 7 years found that the spouse, remaining children, grandparents, next of kin, friends, and colleagues were the main sources of support (Laakso & Paunonen-Ilmonen, 2002).*

## Geriatric

- ▲ Use reminiscence therapy in conjunction with the expression of emotions. Refer to a reminiscence group if available. **EBN and EB:** *Two studies demonstrated that participation in a reminiscence group reduced symptoms of depression (Jones, 2003; Zauszniewski et al, 2004).*
- • Identify previous losses and assess the client for depression. *In older age, losses and changes often occur in rapid succession without adequate recovery time.*
- • Evaluate the social support system of the elderly client. If the support system is minimal, help the client determine how to increase available support. *The elderly who have poor grieving outcomes often do not live with family members and have a minimal support system. The support of family (especially children) and friends is a common way for elderly widows to cope with a loss (Hegge & Fischer, 2000).*

S

## Multicultural

- • Assess for the influence of cultural beliefs, norms, and values on the client's expressions of sorrow. **EBN:** *Expressions of sorrow may be based on cultural perceptions (Cochran, 1998; Doswell & Erlen, 1998; Leininger & McFarland, 2002). African Americans may be expected to act "strong" and go on with the business of life after a death; Native Americans may not talk about the death because of beliefs that such talk will detract from spirituality and bring bad luck; Latinos may wear black and act subdued during their* luto *(mourning) period; Southeast Asian families may wear white when mourning*

*(McQuay, 1995). Korean family caregivers' experiences in making the decision to place a family member with dementia in a long-term care facility showed a pattern of deep sorrow (Park, Butcher, & Moss, 2004). Sorrow is one of the seven emotions identified by Eastern philosophies of Buddhism, Taoism, and traditional Chinese medicine (Chan, Ho, & Chow, 2001).*

- • Identify whether the client had been notified of the health status of the deceased and was able to be present during death and illness. **EBN:** *Not being present during terminal illness and death can disrupt the grieving process and contribute to chronic sorrow (McQuay, 1995).*
- • Validate the client's feelings regarding the loss. **EBN:** *Validation is a therapeutic communication technique that lets the client know that the nurse has heard and understood what was said, and it promotes the nurse-client relationship (Heineken, 1998).*

## Home Care

- • The interventions described previously may be adapted for home care use. Identify causes for chronic sorrow and observe the client's expression of this sorrow. *A clinician's ability to understand a client's perception of the affect of the illness is crucial to the clinician's ability to be therapeutic. Knowledge of a client's perceptions of chronic illness will help nurses intervene sensitively and effectively (Yuen-Juen, 1995).*
- ▲ Assess the client for depression. Refer for mental health services as indicated. *Sadness is part of the syndrome of depression. Increase in mood is unlikely unless the underlying depression is treated. Counseling services provide an opportunity for expression of feelings, increase coping skills, and provide respite for caregivers.*
- ▲ When sorrow is focused around loss of a pregnancy, encourage the client to follow through on a counseling referral. **EBN and EB:** *Parents with a history of perinatal loss are at higher risk for depressive symptoms and pregnancy-specific anxiety during subsequent pregnancies, particularly before the third trimester. Mothers had a higher level of symptoms than fathers (Armstrong, 2002; Franche & Mikail, 1999).*
- • Encourage the client to participate in activities that are diversionary and uplifting as tolerated (e.g., outdoor activities, hobby groups, church-related activities, pet care). *Diversionary activities decrease the time spent in sorrow, can give meaning to life, and provide a sense of well-being.*
- • Encourage the client to participate in support groups appropriate to the area of loss or illness (e.g., Crohn's disease support group or Widow to Widow). *Support groups can increase an individual's sense of belonging. Group activity helps the client to identify alternative ways to problem solve and experience feelings.*
- • Provide psychological support for family/caregivers. *Family/caregivers who feel supported are often able to provide greater and more consistent support to the affected person.*
- ▲ In the presence of a psychiatric disorder, refer for psychiatric home health care services for client reassurance and implementation of a therapeutic regimen. *Psychiatric home care nurses can address issues relating to the client's depression. Behavioral interventions in the home can help the client to participate more effectively in the treatment plan (Patusky, Rodning, & Martinez-Kratz, 1996).*
- • See the care plans for **Impaired Adjustment**, **Chronic low Self-esteem**, **Risk for Loneliness**, and **Hopelessness.**

S

• = Independent; ▲ = Collaborative; EBN = Evidence-Based Nursing; EB = Evidence-Based

## evolve WEBSITES FOR EDUCATION

See the EVOLVE website for World Wide Web resources for client education.

## REFERENCES


Armstrong DS: Emotional distress and prenatal attachment in pregnancy after perinatal loss, *J Nurs Scholarsh* 34:339, 2002.

Chan C, Ho PS, Chow E: A body-mind-spirit model in health: an Eastern approach, *Soc Work Health Care* 34(3-4):261-282, 2001.

Clements PT, DeRanieri JT, Vigil GJ et al: Life after death: grief therapy after the sudden traumatic death of a family member, *Perspect Psychiatr Care* 40(4):149, 2004.

Cochran M: Tears have no color, *Am J Nurs* 98(6):53, 1998.

Cohen JA, Mannarino AP, Knudsen K: Treating childhood traumatic grief: a pilot study, *J Am Acad Child Adolesc Psychiatry* 43(10):171, 2004.

Doswell W, Erlen J: Multicultural issues and ethical concerns in the delivery of nursing care interventions, *Nurs Clin North Am* 33(2):353, 1998.

Eakes GG, Burke ML, Hainsworth MA: Middle-range theory of chronic sorrow, *Image J Nurs Sch* 30:179, 1998.

Fischer C, Hegge M: The elderly woman at risk, *Am J Nurs* 100(6):54, 2000.

Franche R, Mikail S: The impact of perinatal loss on adjustment to subsequent pregnancy, *Soc Sci Med* 48:1613, 1999.

Gamino LA, Hogan NS, Sewell KW: Feeling the absence: a content analysis from the Scott and White grief study, *Death Stud* 26(10):793, 2002.

Glazer HR, Clark MD, Stein DS: The impact of hypnotherapy on grieving children, *J Hosp Palliat Nurs* 6(3):171, 2004.

Hainsworth MA, Eakes GG, Burke ML: Coping with chronic sorrow, *Issues Ment Health Nurs* 15:59, 1994.

Hegge M, Fischer C: Grief responses of senior and elderly widows: practice implications, *J Gerontol Nurs* 26(2):35, 2000.

Heineken J: Patient silence is not necessarily client satisfaction: communication in home care nursing, *Home Healthc Nurse* 16(2): 115, 1998.

Hentz P: The body remembers: grieving and a circle of time, *Qual Health Res* 12(2):161, 2002.

Hilliard RE: The effects of music therapy-based bereavement groups on mood and behavior of grieving children: a pilot study, *J Music Ther* 38(4):291, 2001a.

Hilliard RE: The use of music therapy in meeting the multidimensional needs of hospice patients and families, *J Palliat Care* 17(3):161, 2001b.

Hobdell E: Chronic sorrow and depression in parents of children with neural tube defects, *J Neurosci Nurs* 36(2):82, 2004.

Hogan NS, Schmidt LA: Testing the grief to personal growth model using structural equation modeling, *Death Stud* 26(8):615, 2002.

Johnson CS: Nutritional considerations for bereavement and coping with grief, *J Nutr Health Aging* 6(3):171, 2002.

Jones ED: Reminiscence therapy for older women with depression: effects of nursing intervention classification in assisted-living long-term care, *J Gerontol Nurs* 29(7), 2003.

Laakso H, Paunonen-Ilmonen M: Mothers' experience of social support following the death of a child, *J Clin Nurs* 11(2):176, 2002.

Langridge P: Reduction of chronic sorrow: a health promotion role for children's community nurses? *J Child Health Care* 6(3):157, 2002.

Lawson W: Grieving mothers suffer early deaths, *Psychology Today*, 36(3):18, 2003.

Leininger MM, McFarland MR: *Transcultural nursing: concepts, theories, research and practices*, ed 3, New York, 2002, McGraw-Hill.

Mallow GE, Bechtel GA: Chronic sorrow: the experience of parents with children who are developmentally disabled, *J Psychosoc Nurs* 37(7):31, 1999.

McQuay JE: Cross-cultural customs and beliefs related to health crises, death, and organ donation/transplantation: a guide to assist health care professionals understand different responses and provide cross-cultural assistance, *Crit Care Nurs Clin North Am* 7(3):581, 1995.

Park M, Butcher HK, Maas ML: A thematic analysis of Korean family caregivers' experiences in making the decision to place a family member with dementia in a long-term care facility, *Res Nurs Health* 27(5):345-356, 2004.

Patusky KL, Rodning C, Martinez-Kratz M: Clinical lessons in psychiatric home care: a case study approach, *J Home Health Case Manag* 9:18, 1996.


S

Rask K, Kaunonen M, Paunonen-Ilmonen M: Adolescent coping with grief after the death of a loved one, *Int J Nurs Pract* 8(3): 137, 2002.
Rollins JA, Riccio LL: ART is the heART: a palette of possibilities for hospice care, *Pediatr Nurs* 28(4):355, 2002.
Schoutrop MJ, Lange A, Hanewald G et al: Structured writing and processing major stressful events: a controlled trial, *Psychother Psychosom* 71(3):151, 2002.
Schuurman DL: The club no one wants to join: a dozen lessons I've learned from grieving children and adolescents. Available at www.grief.org.au/child_support.html, accessed March 7, 2005.
Steen KF: A comprehensive approach to bereavement, *Nurse Pract* 23(3):54, 1998.
Walsh K, King M, Jones L et al: Spiritual beliefs may affect outcome of bereavement: prospective study, *BMJ* 324(7353):1551, 2002.
Yuen-Juen H: The impact of chronic illness on patients, *Rehabil Nurs* 20:221, 1995.
Zauszniewski JA, Eggenschwiler K, Preechawong S et al: Focused reflection reminiscence group for elders: implementation and evaluation, *Appl Gerontol* 23(4):429, 2004.

# Spiritual distress

evolve

*Lisa Burkhart and Ann Solari-Twadell*

**NANDA**

## Definition

Impaired ability to experience and integrate meaning and purpose in life through the individual's connectedness with self, others, art, music, literature, nature, or a power greater than oneself

## Defining Characteristics

*Connections to self:* Expresses lack of hope, meaning, and purpose in life, peace/serenity, acceptance, love, forgiveness of self, courage; expresses anger, guilt, poor coping
*Connections with others:* Refuses interactions with spiritual leaders; refuses interactions with friends and family; verbalizes being separated from their support system, expresses alienation
*Connections with art, music, literature, nature:* Demonstrates inability to express previous state of creativity (singing, listening to music, writing), disinterest in nature, and disinterest in reading spiritual literature
*Connections with power greater than self:* Demonstrates inability to pray, inability to participate in religious activities, expressions of being abandoned by or having anger toward God; requests to see a religious leader; demonstrates sudden changes in spiritual practices, inability to be introspective/inward turning; expresses being hopeless and suffering, inability to experience the transcendent

## Related Factors (r/t)

Self-alienation, loneliness/social isolation, anxiety, sociocultural deprivation, death and dying of self or others, pain, life change, chronic illness of self or others

S

NOC

## Outcomes (Nursing Outcomes Classification)

### Suggested NOC Outcomes

Acceptance: Health Status; Dignified Life Closure; Grief Resolution; Hope; Spiritual Health; Suffering Severity

**Example NOC Outcome with Indicators**

**Spiritual Health** as evidenced by the following indicators: Quality of faith and hope/Meaning and purpose in life/Connectedness with inner-self and with others/Interaction with others to share thoughts, feelings, and beliefs (Rate each indicator of **Spiritual Health:** 1 = severely compromised, 2 = substantially compromised, 3 = moderately compromised, 4 = mildly compromised, 5 = not compromised [see Section I].)

## Client Outcomes

### Client Will (Specify Time Frame):

- Express sense of connectedness with self, others, arts, music, literature, or power greater than oneself
- Express meaning and purpose in life
- Express sense of hope in the future
- Express ability to forgive
- Express acceptance of health status
- Discuss personal response to dying
- Discuss personal response to grieving

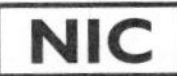

## Interventions (Nursing Interventions Classification)

### Suggested NIC Interventions

Active Listening; Forgiveness Facilitation; Grief Work Facilitation; Hope Instillation; Humor; Music Therapy; Presence; Referral; Reminiscence Therapy; Self-Awareness Enhancement; Simple Guided Imagery; Simple Massage; Simple Relaxation Therapy; Spiritual Support; Therapeutic Touch; Touch



**Example NIC Activities—Spiritual Support**

Encourage use of spiritual resources if desired; Be available to listen to client's expression of feelings

## Nursing Interventions and Rationales

- Observe the client for loss of meaning, purpose, and hope in life. **EBN:** *A qualitative study of mental health nursing professionals found that it is important for health care providers to identify and assess for spiritual needs (Greasley, Chiu, & Gartland, 2001). Spirituality is associated with meaning and purpose in life and hope (Burkhart & Solari-Twadell,*

*2001). Nelson and colleagues (2002) found that spirituality had a significant negative correlation with depression and meaning and peace. McGrath (2003) found that individuals in crisis express strong spiritual beliefs. Ferrell and colleagues (2003) found in an ethnographic study of 21,805 ovarian cancer survivors that spirituality was used to derive meaning in the life experience. McClain, Rosenfeld, and Breitart (2003) found that spiritual well-being was a better predictor that depression for end-of-life patients in terms of hopelessness and suicidal ideation.*

- Respect the client's beliefs; avoid imposing your own spiritual beliefs on the client. Be aware of your own belief systems and accept the client's spirituality. Allow for self-disclosure. Promote a sense of love, caring, and compassion. **EBN:** *Respecting the client's beliefs promotes trust and connectedness (Engebretson, 1996). In a literature study of AIDS clients in pain, Newshan (1998) found that disclosure of the self could be comforting and healing. In a study of mental health nursing professionals, Greasley, Chiu, and Gartland (2001) found that love, caring, and compassion are interpersonal values that promote spiritual care.*
- Monitor and promote supportive social contacts. **EBN:** *Coward (1995) found in a study of self-transcendence in women with AIDS that successful nursing interventions include preventing emotional and environmental isolation. In a phenomenological study, clients found spiritual support from family and friends (Smucker, 1996). Also, by definition, spirituality, or the expression of the spirit, is enhanced through a sense of connectedness with other people (Burkhart & Solari-Twadell, 2001). Social supports are positively correlated with spiritual well-being (Coyle, 2002). Corrigan and colleagues (2003) found that spirituality was associated with social inclusion in individuals with mental illness. Coleman (2003) found that in a sample of African-American men and women living with HIV/AIDS, spirituality significantly correlated with social functioning. Keeley (2004) found that spirituality was an important theme in final conversations with loved ones.*

▲ Refer the client to a support group. **EBN:** *In a study of battered women, the women participated in spiritual discussion and other practices once a week (Humphreys, 2000). The findings indicated that, among these sheltered battered women, spirituality may be associated with greater internal resources that buffer distressing feelings and calm the mind. Cultivating relationships that promote transformation, empowerment, and healing promotes spiritual well-being (Lauver, 2000).*

S

- Be physically present and actively listen to the client. **EBN:** *In a phenomenological study, Smucker (1996) found that listening is an important nursing intervention. Another study demonstrated that the client's faith and trust in nurses produces a positive effect on the client and family. Listening attentively and being physically present can be spiritually nourishing (Berggren-Thomas & Griggs, 1995). Physical presence can decrease separation and aloneness, which clients often fear (Dossey et al, 1995). Being present and actively listening to the client promotes nurse-client connectedness and helps the client feel valued (Lauver, 2000). A survey of parish nurses demonstrated that listening and presence support clients spiritually (Tuck, Wallace, & Pullen, 2001).*
- Support meditation, guided imagery, therapeutic touch, journaling, relaxation, and involvement in art, music, or poetry. Support outdoor activities. **EBN:** *All these techniques have been used to promote spiritual well-being (Newshan, 1998). Sowell and colleagues (2000) found a significant correlation between spiritual activities and emotional*

*distress and quality of life for HIV-positive African-American women. In a survey of parish nurses, the nurses were found to use guided imagery to support clients spiritually (Tuck, Wallace, & Pullen, 2001). By definition, spirituality includes connectedness with art, music, literature, and nature (Burkhart & Solari-Twadell, 2001).*

- Offer or suggest visits with spiritual and/or religious advisors. **EBN:** *The number one need expressed by clients who had been hospitalized, which was declared by persons of all denominations and faiths, was for their pastor/rabbi/spiritual advisor to not abandon them. For those who did not belong to a religious/spiritual group, the number one need was at least to be asked about some type of religious/spiritual preference (Moller, 1999). Clients are experts on their own paths, and knowing their values helps in exploring their uniqueness (Dossey et al, 1995).*
- Help the client make a list of important and unimportant values. **EBN:** *In a survey of parish nurses, the nurses were found to implement values clarification to support clients spiritually (Tuck, Wallace, & Pullen, 2001). Corrigan and colleagues (2003) found that spirituality was associated with empowerment in individuals with mental illness.*
- Assist the client in identifying and creating his or her own meaningful experiences. Help the client develop skills to deal with illness or lifestyle changes. Include the client in care planning. **EBN:** *Clients perceived the experience of healing as an active process and expressed a desire to take conscious control (Criddle, 1993). In a phenomenological study, Smucker (1996) found that nurses assist clients in finding clients' own strategies to meet their spiritual needs. Meaningful experiences promote spiritual well-being (Lauver, 2000). Fry (2003) found that spirituality accounted for 28% of the variance of psychological well-being.*
- Ask how to be most helpful; encourage the client to look inward, look outward, reflect, and seek clarification. **EBN:** *Tuck, Pullen, and Lynn (1997) suggested that spiritual interventions include doing things for clients and encouraging inward and outward reflection.*
- If the client is comfortable with touch, hold the client's hand or place a hand gently on the client's arm. **EBN:** *A survey of parish nurses found that touch supports clients spiritually (Tuck, Wallace, & Pullen, 2001).*
- Help the client find a reason for living and be available for support. Promote hope. **EBN:** *In one study, "the need for a positive attitude for optimum healing was by far the most commonly mentioned subtheme by these participants and the strongest area of literature" (Criddle, 1993). Instilling hope is a common strategy to promote spiritual well-being (Baldacchino & Draper, 2001). Corrigan and colleagues (2003) found that spirituality was associated in hope with individuals with mental illness. Gibson and Parker (2003) found that in a study of 116 African-American breast cancer survivors, spirituality had a significant correlation with hope.*
- Listen to the client's feelings about suffering and/or death. Be nonjudgmental and allow time for grieving. *Being with the person who is suffering gives meaning to his or her experience (O'Brien, 1999).*
- Provide appropriate religious materials, artifacts, or music as requested. **EBN:** *In a survey of battered women, church attendance and reading the Bible were rated highly in promoting spiritual well-being (Humphreys, 2000). Helping a client incorporate religious rites and rituals can enhance meaning in life and promote a sense of connectedness with a faith community and/or a higher power (Conrad, 1985; Lauver, 2000). In a survey of parish*

*nurses, religious rites and rituals (e.g., ministering, offering communion, laying on of hands, anointing) supported clients spiritually (Tuck, Wallace, & Pullen, 2001). McGrath (2003) found that individuals who have a history of religious beliefs turn to those beliefs in crisis.*

- Promote forgiveness. **EBN:** *In a survey of battered women, forgiveness was rated as an important part of spirituality (Humphreys, 2000). In a survey of parish nurses, the nurses promoted forgiveness (Tuck, Wallace, & Pullen, 2001).*
- Provide privacy or a "sacred space." *Sacred spaces promote spiritual well-being by enhancing a sense of connectedness with self and/or others (Lauver, 2000).*
- Allow time and a place for prayer. **EBN:** *In a double-blind experiment, Byrd (1988) found that intercessory prayer improved clinical outcomes in coronary bypass clients. Engebretson (1996) also supported prayer, or looking upward, to promote spiritual well-being. In a survey of battered women, prayer was highly rated in promoting spiritual well-being (Humphreys, 2000). A survey of parish nurses found that prayer supports clients spiritually (Tuck, Wallace, & Pullen, 2001). Meraviglia (2004) found that in a sample of 60 adults with non–small cell lung cancer, meaning in life and prayer significantly predicted the variance of symptom distress.*
- Encourage the use of humor, as appropriate, to promote spiritual well-being. **EBN:** *Johnson (2002) found that in breast cancer survivors, humor promoted spirituality and helped them find meaning and purpose in life.*

## Geriatric

- Discuss personal definitions of spiritual wellness with the client. *Listening attentively and helping elderly clients identify past coping strategies is part of helping with life review and finding meaning in life (Berggren-Thomas & Griggs, 1995). Daaleman, Perera, and Studenski (2004) found in a sample of 277 geriatric outpatients, those who rated themselves in good health reported significantly higher levels of spirituality, controlling for functional health, race, and ethnicity.*
- Identify the client's past sources of spirituality. Help the client explore his or her life and identify those experiences that are noteworthy. Clients may want to read the Bible or other religious text or have it read to them. *Older adults often identify spirituality as a source of hope (Gaskins & Forte, 1995). Religious belief has been associated with higher levels of well-being and lower levels of depression and suicide (Van Ness & Larson, 2002). Kirby, Coleman, and Daley (2004) studied the well-being of adults living in retirement housing estates in Britain and found that spirituality had a small significant correlation with psychological well-being, personal growth, and positive relations with others, and spirituality reduced the negative effects of frailty.*

S

## Multicultural

- Assess for the influence of cultural beliefs, norms, and values on the client's ability to cope with spiritual distress. **EBN:** *How the client copes with spiritual distress may be based on cultural perceptions (Cesario, 2001; Cochran, 1998; Doswell & Erlen, 1998; Leininger & McFarland, 2002; Zapata & Shippee-Rice, 1999).*
- Acknowledge the value conflicts from acculturation stresses that may contribute to spiritual distress. **EBN:** *Challenges to traditional beliefs are anxiety provoking and can produce distress (Charron, 1998; Mazanec & Tyler, 2003).*

- Encourage spirituality as a source of support. **EBN:** *African Americans and Latinos may identify spirituality, religiousness, prayer, and church-based approaches as coping resources (Bourjolly, 1998; Mapp & Hudson, 1997; Samuel-Hodge et al, 2000). A study of battered women showed that African-American women were significantly more likely to report using prayer as a coping strategy and significantly less likely to seek help from mental health counselors (El-Khoury et al, 2004). A recent study showed religion and spirituality are associated with health-seeking behaviors of African-American women (Dessio et al, 2004).*
- Identify, develop and implement culturally appropriate spiritual nursing interventions. **EBN:** *A study of Christian African Americans examining spiritual perspectives, spiritual needs, and desired nursing interventions during hospitalization identified participating in spiritual activities and recognizing the spiritual caregiver role as desired nursing interventions (Connor & Eller, 2004). Spiritual coping may serve as a moderator of health among Native-American women (Walters & Simoni, 2002).*
- Validate the client's spiritual concerns and convey respect for his or her beliefs. **EBN:** *Validation is a therapeutic communications technique that lets the client know the nurse has heard and understood what was said (Heineken, 1998).*

### Home Care

- All of the nursing interventions described previously apply in the home setting.
- Assist client to examine past and present risk factors, concentrating on the identification of capabilities, assets, and positive attributes, and how they relate to perceptions of the home setting. *Perspective counseling has been suggested as a means of enhancing resiliency and spirituality. Dialogue can address the following:*
  - Identification of spiritual resources that have offered strength and energy to overcome stresses, losses.
  - How these resources have changed across the life span.
  - How these resources have given life meaning or purpose.
  - Identification of activities that still give meaning or purpose to life.

  *Identification of family or friends contributes to strength for living and energy to overcome obstacles (Langer, 2004).*

## evolve WEBSITES FOR EDUCATION

See the EVOLVE website for World Wide Web resources for client education.

S

## REFERENCES

Baldacchino D, Draper P: Spiritual coping strategies: a review, *J Adv Nurs* 34:83, 2001.

Berggren-Thomas P, Griggs M: Spirituality in aging: spiritual need or spiritual journey? *J Gerontol Nurs* 21:5, 1995.

Bourjolly JN: Differences in religiousness among black and white women with breast cancer, *Soc Work Health Care 28(1):21, 1998.*

Burkhart L, Solari-Twadell PA: Spirituality and religiousness: differentiating the diagnoses through a review of the nursing literature, *Nurs Diagn* 12:45, 2001.

Byrd RC: Positive therapeutic effects of intercessory prayer in a coronary care unit population, *South Med J* 81: 826, 1988.

Cavendish R, Konecny L, Mitzeliotis CR et al: Spiritual care activities of nurses using nursing interventions classification (NIC) labels, *Nurs Diag* 14(4):113-124, 2003.

Cesario S: Care of the Native American woman: strategies for practice, education, and research, *J Gynecol Neonat Nurs* 30(1):13, 2001.

Charron HS: Anxiety disorders. In Varcarolis EM, editor: *Foundations of psychiatric mental health nursing,* ed 3, Philadelphia, 1998, WB Saunders.
Cochran M: Tears have no color, *Am J Nurs* 98(6):53, 1998.
Coleman CL: Spirituality and sexual orientation: relationship to mental well-being and functional health status, *J Adv Nurs* 43(5): 457-464, 2003.
Conner NE, Eller LS: Spiritual perspectives, needs and nursing interventions of Christian African-Americans, *J Adv Nurs* 46(6): 624-632, 2004.
Conrad NJ: Spiritual support for the dying, *Nurs Clin North Am* 20:415, 1985.
Corrigan P, McCorkle B, Schell B et al: Religion and spirituality in the lives of people with serious mental illness, *Community Ment Health J* 39(6):487-499, 2003.
Coward DD: The lived experience of self-transcendence in women with AIDS, *J Obstet Gynecol Neonat Nurs* 24:314, 1995.
Coyle J: Spirituality and health: towards a framework for exploring the relationship between spirituality and health, *J Adv Nurs* 37: 589, 2002.
Criddle L: Healing from surgery: a phenomenological study, *Image* 25:208, 1993.
Daaleman TP, Perera S, Studenski SA: Religion, spirituality, and health status in geriatric outpatients, *Ann Fam Med* 2(1):49-53, 2004.
Dessio W, Wade C, Chao M et al: Religion, spirituality, and healthcare choices of African-American women: results of a national survey, *Ethn Dis* 14(2):189-197, 2004.
Dossey BM et al: *Holistic nursing: a handbook for practice,* ed 1, Rockville, Md, 1988, Aspen.
Dossey BM et al: *Holistic nursing: a handbook for practice,* ed 2, Gaithersburg, Md, 1995, Aspen.
Doswell W, Erlen J: Multicultural issues and ethical concerns in the delivery of nursing care interventions, *Nurs Clin North Am* 33(2):353, 1998.
El-Khoury MY, Dutton MA, Goodman LA et al: Ethnic differences in battered women's formal help-seeking strategies: a focus on health, mental health, and spirituality, *Cultur Divers Ethnic Minor Psychol* 10(4):383-393, 2004.
Engebretson J: Considerations in diagnosing in the spiritual domain, *Nurs Diagn* 7:100, 1996.
Ferrell BR, Smith SL, Juarez G et al: Meaning of illness and spirituality in ovarian cancer survivors, *Oncol Nurs Forum* 30(2):249-257, 2003.
Fry PS: The unique contribution of key existential factors to the prediction of psychological well-being of older adults following spousal loss, *Gerontologist* 41(1):69-81, 2001.
Gaskins S, Forte L: The meaning of hope: implications for nursing practice and research, *J Gerontol Nurs* 21:17, 1995.
Gibson LMR, Parker V: Inner resources as predictors of psychological well-being in middle-income African American breast cancer survivors, *Cancer Control* 10(5):52-58, 2003.
Greasley P, Chiu LF, Gartland RM: The concept of spiritual care in mental health nursing, *J Adv Nurs* 33:629, 2001.
Heineken J: Patient silence is not necessarily client satisfaction: communication in home care nursing, *Home Healthc Nurse* 16(2): 115, 1998.
Humphreys J: Spirituality and distress in sheltered battered women, *J Nurs Scholarsh* 32:273, 2000.
Johnson P: The use of humor and its influences on spirituality and coping in breast cancer survivors, *Oncol Nurs Forum* 29(4):691-695, 2002.
Keeley MP: Final conversations: survivors' memorable messages concerning religious faith and spirituality, *Health Commun* 16(1): 87-104, 2004.
Kirby SE, Coleman PG, Daley D: Spirituality and well-being in frail and nonfrail older adults, *J Gerontol* 59B(3):P123-P129, 2004.
Langer N: Resiliency and spirituality: foundations of strengths perspective counseling with the elderly, *Educat Gerontol* 30:611, 2004.
Lauver D: Commonalities in women's spirituality and women's health, *Adv Nurs Sci* 22:76, 2000.
Leininger MM, McFarland MR: *Transcultural nursing: concepts, theories, research and practices,* ed 3, New York, 2002, McGraw-Hill.
Mapp I, Hudson R: Stress and coping among African American and Hispanic parents of deaf children, *Am Ann Deaf* 142(1):48, 1997.
Mazanec P, Tyler MK: Cultural considerations in end-of-life care: how ethnicity, age, and spirituality affect decisions when death is imminent, *Am J Nurs* 103(3):50-58, 2003.
McClain CS, Rosenfeld B, Breitbart W: Effect of spiritual well-being on end-of-life despair in terminally-ill cancer patients, *Lancet* 361:1603-1607, 2003.

McGrath P: Religiosity and the challenge of terminal illness, *Death Stud* 27:881-899, 2003.
Meraviglia MG: The effects of spirituality on well-being of people with lung cancer, *Oncol Nurs Forum* 31(1):89-94, 2004.
Moller MD: Meeting spiritual needs on an inpatient unit, *J Psychosoc Nurs Ment Health Serv* 37(11):5, 1999.
Nelson CJ, Rosenfeld B, Breitbart W et al: Spirituality, religion, and depression in the terminally ill, *Psychosomatics* 43(3):213-220, 2002.
Newshan G: Transcending the physical: spiritual aspects of pain in patients with HIV and/or cancer, *J Adv Nurs* 28:1236, 1998.
O'Brien ME: *Spirituality in nursing: standing on holy ground,* Boston, 1999, Jones and Bartlett.
Samuel-Hodge CD, Headen SW, Skelly AH et al: Influences on day-to-day self-management of type 2 diabetes among African American women: spirituality, the multi-caregiver role, and other social context factors, *Diabetes Care* 23(7):928, 2000.
Sowell R, Moneyham L, Hennessy M et al: Spiritual activities as a resistance resource for women with human immunodeficieny virus, *J Nurs Res* 49(2):73-82, 2000.
Smucker C: A phenomenological description of the experience of spiritual distress, *Nurs Diagn* 7:81, 1996.
Tuck I, Pullen L, Lynn C: Spiritual interventions provided by mental health nurses, *West J Nurs Res* 19:351, 1997.
Tuck I, Wallace D, Pullen L: Spirituality and spiritual care provided by parish nurses, *West J Nurs Res* 23:144, 2001.
Van Ness PH, Larson DB: Religion, senescence, and mental health: the end of life is not the end of hope, *Am J Geriatr Psychiatry* 10:386, 2002.
Walters KL, Simoni JM: Reconceptualizing native women's health: an "indigenist" stress-coping model, *Am J Public Health* 92(4): 520-524, 2002.
Zapata J, Shippee-Rice R: The use of folk healing and healers by six Latinos living in New England, *J Transcult Nurs* 10(2):136, 1999.

# Risk for Spiritual distress

*Lisa Burkhart and Ann Solari-Twadell*

**NANDA**

## Definition

At risk for impaired ability to experience and integrate meaning and purpose in life through the individual's connectedness with self, others, art, music, literature, nature, and/or a power greater than oneself

S

## Risk Factors

*Physical:* Physical illness, substance abuse/excessive drinking, chronic illness
*Psychosocial:* Low self-esteem, depression, anxiety, stress, poor relationships, separate from support systems, blocks to experiencing love, inability to forgive, loss
*Sociocultural:* Racial/cultural conflict, change in religious rituals
*Spiritual:* Change in spiritual practices
*Developmental:* Life transitions
*Environmental:* Environmental changes, natural disasters

# NOC

## Outcomes (Nursing Outcomes Classification)

### Suggested NOC Outcomes

Acceptance: Health Status; Dignified Life Closure; Health Beliefs; Hope; Grief Resolution; Quality of Life; Spiritual Health; Suffering Severity

#### Example NOC Outcome with Indicators

**Spiritual Health** as evidenced by the following indicators: Quality of faith and hope/Meaning and purpose in life/Connectedness with inner self and with others/Interaction with others to share thoughts, feelings, and beliefs (Rate each indicator of **Spiritual Health:** 1 = severely compromised, 2 = substantially compromised, 3 = moderately compromised, 4 = mildly compromised, 5 = not compromised [see Section I].)

## Client Outcomes

### Client Will (Specify Time Frame):

- Express sense of connectedness with self, others, arts, music, literature, or power greater than oneself
- Express meaning and purpose in life
- Express sense of optimism and hope in the future
- Express ability to forgive
- Express desire to discuss health state and integrate care in lifestyle
- Discuss personal response to dying
- Discuss personal response to grieving
- Express satisfaction with life circumstances

# NIC

## Interventions (Nursing Interventions Classification)

### Suggested NIC Interventions

Active Listening; Forgiveness Facilitation; Grief Work Facilitation; Hope Instillation; Humor; Music Therapy; Presence; Referral; Reminiscence Therapy; Self Awareness Enhancement; Simple Guided Imagery; Simple Massage; Simple Relaxation Therapy; Spiritual Support; Touch; Therapeutic Touch

S

#### Example NIC Activities—Spiritual Support

Encourage use of spiritual resources if desired; be available to listen to client's feelings

## Nursing Interventions and Rationales

- Observe the client for loss of meaning, purpose, and hope in life. **EBN:** *Spirituality is associated with meaning and purpose in life and with hope (Burkhart & Solari-Twadell, 2001). A qualitative study of mental health nursing professionals found that it is important for health care providers to identify and assess for spiritual needs (Greasley, Chiu, &*

*Gartland, 2001). McGrath (2003) found that individuals in crisis express strong spiritual beliefs. Nelson and colleagues (2002) found that spirituality had a significant negative correlation with depression and meaning and peace. Ferrell and colleagues (2003) found in an ethnographic study of 21,805 ovarian cancer survivors that spirituality was used to derive meaning in the life experience. McClain, Rosenfeld, and Breitart (2003) found that spiritual well-being was a better predictor that depression for end-of-life patients in terms of hopelessness and suicidal ideation.*

- Respect the client's beliefs; avoid imposing your own spiritual beliefs on the client. Be aware of your own belief systems and accept the client's spirituality. Allow for self-disclosure. Promote a sense of love, caring, and compassion. **EBN:** *Respecting the client's beliefs promotes trust and connectedness (Engebretson, 1996). In a literature study of AIDS clients in pain, Newshan (1998) found that disclosure of self could be comforting and healing. In a study of mental health nursing professionals, Greasley, Chiu, and Gartland (2001) found that love, caring, and compassion are interpersonal values that promote spiritual care.*
- Monitor and promote supportive social contacts. **EBN:** *Coward (1995) found in a study of self-transcendence in women with AIDS that successful nursing interventions include preventing emotional and environmental isolation. In a phenomenological study, clients found spiritual support from family and friends (Smucker, 1996). In addition, by definition, spirituality, or the expression of the spirit, is enhanced through a sense of connectedness with other people (Burkhart & Solari-Twadell, 2001). Social supports are positively correlated with spiritual well-being (Coyle, 2002). Corrigan and colleagues (2003) found that spirituality was associated with social inclusion in individuals with mental illness. Coleman (2003) found that in a sample of African-American men and women living with HIV/AIDS, spirituality significantly correlated with social functioning. Keeley (2004) found that spirituality was an important theme in final conversations with loved ones.*
- Inform the client about available support groups. **EBN:** *In a study of battered women, the women participated in spiritual discussion and other practices once a week (Humphreys, 2000). Cultivating relationships that promote transformation, empowerment, and healing promotes spiritual well-being (Lauver, 2000).*
- Be physically present and actively listen to the client. **EBN:** *Listening attentively and being physically present can be spiritually nourishing (Berggren-Thomas & Griggs, 1995). Physical presence can decrease separation and aloneness, which clients often fear (Dossey et al, 1995). In a phenomenological study, Smucker (1996) found that listening is an important nursing intervention. Being present and actively listening to the client promotes nurse-client connectedness and helps the client feel valued (Lauver, 2000). A survey of parish nurses found that listening and presence support clients spiritually (Tuck, Wallace, & Pullen, 2001).*
- Support meditation, guided imagery, therapeutic touch, journaling, relaxation, and involvement in art, music, or poetry. Support outdoor activities. **EBN:** *All these techniques have been used to promote spiritual well-being (Newshan, 1998). Sowell and colleagues (2000) found a significant correlation between spiritual activities and emotional distress and quality of life for HIV-positive African-American women. By definition, spirituality includes connectedness with art, music, literature, and nature (Burkhart &*

S

*Solari-Twadell, 2001). In a survey of parish nurses, the nurses were found to use guided imagery to support clients spiritually (Tuck, Wallace, & Pullen, 2001).*

- Offer or suggest visits with spiritual and/or religious advisors. **EBN:** *Clients are experts on their own paths and knowing their values helps in exploring their uniqueness (Dossey et al, 1995). The number one need expressed by clients who had been hospitalized, which was declared by persons of all denominations and faiths, was for their pastor/rabbi/spiritual advisor to not abandon them. For those who did not belong to a religious/spiritual group, their number one need was at least to be asked for some type of religious/spiritual preference (Moller, 1999).*
- Help the client make a list of important and unimportant values. **EBN:** *In a survey of parish nurses, the nurses implemented values clarification to support clients spiritually (Tuck, Wallace, & Pullen, 2001).*
- Assist the client in identifying and creating his or her own meaningful experiences. Help the client develop skills to deal with illness or lifestyle changes. Include the client in care planning. **EBN:** *In a phenomenological study, Smucker (1996) found that nurses help clients to find their own strategies to meet their spiritual needs. Clients perceived the experience of healing as an active process and expressed a desire to take conscious control (Criddle, 1993). Meaningful experiences promote spiritual well-being (Lauver, 2000). Corrigan and colleagues (2003) found that spirituality was associated with empowerment in individuals with mental illness. Fry (2003) found that spirituality accounted for 28% of the variance of psychological well-being.*
- Ask how to be most helpful; encourage the client to look inward, look outward, reflect, and seek clarification. **EBN:** *Tuck, Pullen, and Lynn (1997) suggested that spiritual interventions include doing things for clients and encouraging inward and outward reflection.*
- If the client is comfortable with touch, hold the client's hand or place a hand gently on the client's arm. **EBN:** *A survey of parish nurses found that touch supports clients spiritually (Tuck, Wallace, & Pullen, 2001).*
- Help the client find a reason for living and be available for support. Promote hope. **EBN:** *In one study, "the need for a positive attitude for optimum healing was by far the most commonly mentioned subtheme by these participants and the strongest area of literature" (Criddle, 1993). Instilling hope is a common strategy to promote spiritual well-being (Baldacchino & Draper, 2001). Corrigan and colleagues (2003) found that spirituality was associated in hope with individuals with mental illness. Gibson and Parker (2003) found that in a study of 116 African-American breast cancer survivors, spirituality had a significant correlation with hope.*
- Listen to the client's feelings about suffering and/or death. Be nonjudgmental and allow time for grieving. *Being with the person who is suffering gives meaning to his or her experience (O'Brien, 1999).*
- Provide appropriate religious materials, artifacts, or music as requested. **EBN:** *In a survey of battered women, church attendance and reading the Bible were rated highly in promoting spiritual well-being (Humphreys, 2000). In a survey of parish nurses, religious rites and rituals (e.g., ministering, offering communion, laying on of hands, anointing) supported clients spiritually (Tuck, Wallace, & Pullen, 2001). Helping a client incorporate reli-*

S

*gious rites and rituals can enhance meaning in life and promote a sense of connectedness with a faith community and/or a higher power (Conrad, 1985; Lauver, 2000). Corrigan and colleagues (2003) found that spirituality was associated in hope with individuals with mental illness. Gibson and Parker (2003) found that in a study of 116 African-American breast cancer survivors, spirituality had a significant correlation with hope.*

- Promote forgiveness. **EBN:** *In a survey of battered women, forgiveness was rated as an important part of spirituality (Humphreys, 2000). In a survey of parish nurses, the nurses promoted forgiveness (Tuck, Wallace, & Pullen, 2001).*
- Provide privacy or a "sacred space." *Sacred spaces promote spiritual well-being by enhancing a sense of connectedness with self and/or others (Lauver, 2000).*
- Allow time and a place for prayer. **EBN:** *Byrd (1988) found that intercessory prayer significantly improved clinical outcomes of coronary bypass clients. Engebretson (1996) also supported prayer, or looking upward, to promote spiritual well-being. In a survey of battered women, prayer was highly rated in promoting spiritual well-being (Humphreys, 2000). A survey of parish nurses found that prayer supports clients spiritually (Tuck, Wallace, & Pullen, 2001).*
- Use humor, as appropriate, to promote spiritual well-being. **EBN:** *Johnson (2002) found that in breast cancer survivors, humor promoted spirituality and helped them find meaning and purpose in life.*

## Multicultural

- Assess for the influence of cultural beliefs, norms, and values on the client's ability to cope with spiritual distress. **EBN:** *How the client copes with spiritual distress may be based on cultural perceptions (Cesario, 2001; Cochran, 1998; Doswell & Erlen, 1998; Leininger & McFarland, 2002; Zapata & Shippee-Rice, 1999).*
- Acknowledge the value conflicts from acculturation stresses that may contribute to spiritual distress. **EBN:** *Challenges to traditional beliefs are anxiety provoking and can produce distress (Charron, 1998; Mazanec & Tyler, 2003).*
- Encourage spirituality as a source of support. **EBN:** *African Americans and Latinos may identify spirituality, religiousness, prayer, and church-based approaches as coping resources (Bourjolly, 1998; Mapp & Hudson, 1997; Samuel-Hodge et al, 2000). A study of battered women showed that African-American women were significantly more likely to report using prayer as a coping strategy and significantly less likely to seek help from mental health counselors (El-Khoury et al, 2004). A recent study showed religion and spirituality are associated with health-seeking behaviors of African-American women (Dessio et al, 2004).*
- Identify, develop, and implement culturally appropriate spiritual nursing interventions. **EBN:** *A study of Christian African-Americans examining spiritual perspectives, spiritual needs, and desired nursing interventions during hospitalization identified participating in spiritual activities and recognizing the spiritual caregiver role as desired nursing interventions (Connor & Eller, 2004). Spiritual coping may serve as a moderator of health among Native-American women (Walters & Simoni, 2002).*
- Validate the client's spiritual concerns and convey respect for his or her beliefs. **EBN:** *Validation is a therapeutic communication technique that lets the client know the nurse has heard and understood what was said (Heineken, 1998).*

S

### Home Care

- Interventions mentioned under other subheadings in this nursing diagnosis also apply to home care.

## evolve WEBSITES FOR EDUCATION

See the EVOLVE website for World Wide Web resources for client education.

## REFERENCES


Baldacchino D, Draper P: Spiritual coping strategies: a review, *J Adv Nurs* 34:83, 2001.

Berggren-Thomas P, Griggs M: Spirituality in aging: spiritual need or spiritual journey? *J Gerontol Nurs* 21:5, 1995.

Bourjolly JN: Differences in religiousness among black and white women with breast cancer, *Soc Work Health Care* 28(1):21, 1998.

Burkhart L, Solari-Twadell PA: Spirituality and religiousness: differentiating the diagnoses through a review of the nursing literature, *Nurs Diagn* 12:45, 2001.

Byrd RC: Positive therapeutic effects of intercessory prayer in a coronary care unit population, *South Med J* 81: 826, 1988.

Cavendish R, Konecny L, Mitzeliotis CR et al: Spiritual care activities of nurses using nursing interventions classfication (NIC) labels, *Nurs Diag* 14(4):113-124, 2003.

Cesario S: Care of the Native American woman: strategies for practice, education, and research, *J Gynecol Neonat Nurs* 30(1):13, 2001.

Charron HS: Anxiety disorders. In Varcarolis EM, editor: *Foundations of psychiatric mental health nursing,* ed 3, Philadelphia, 1998, WB Saunders.

Cochran M: Tears have no color, *Am J Nurs* 98(6):53, 1998.

Coleman CL: Spirituality and sexual orientation: relationship to mental well-being and functional health status, *J Adv Nurs* 43(5): 457-464, 2003.

Conner NE, Eller LS: Spiritual perspectives, needs and nursing interventions of Christian African-Americans, *J Adv Nurs* 46(6): 624-632, 2004.

Conrad NJ: Spiritual support for the dying, *Nurs Clin North Am* 20:415, 1985.

Corrigan P, McCorkle B, Schell B et al: Religion and spirituality in the lives of people with serious mental illness, *Community Ment Health J* 39(6):487-499, 2003.

Coward DD: The lived experience of self-transcendence in women with AIDS, *J Obstet Gynecol Neonat Nurs* 24:314, 1995.

Coyle J: Spirituality and health: towards a framework for exploring the relationship between spirituality and health, *J Adv Nurs* 37: 589, 2002.

Criddle L: Healing from surgery: a phenomenological study, *Image* 25:208, 1993.

Daaleman TP, Perera S, Studenski SA: Religion, spirituality, and health status in geriatric outpatients, *Ann Fam Med* 2(1):49-53, 2004.

Dessio W, Wade C, Chao M et al: Religion, spirituality, and healthcare choices of African-American women: results of a national survey, *Ethn Dis* 14(2):189-197, 2004.

Dossey BM et al: *Holistic nursing: a handbook for practice,* ed 1, Rockville, Md, 1988, Aspen.

Dossey BM et al: *Holistic nursing: a handbook for practice,* ed 2, Gaithersburg, Md, 1995, Aspen.

Doswell W, Erlen J: Multicultural issues and ethical concerns in the delivery of nursing care interventions, *Nurs Clin North Am* 33(2):353, 1998.

El-Khoury MY, Dutton MA, Goodman LA et al: Ethnic differences in battered women's formal help-seeking strategies: a focus on health, mental health, and spirituality, *Cultur Divers Ethnic Minor Psychol* 10(4):383-393, 2004.

Engebretson J: Considerations in diagnosing in the spiritual domain, *Nurs Diagn* 7:100, 1996.

Ferrell BR, Smith SL, Juarez G et al: Meaning of illness and spirituality in ovarian cancer survivors, *Oncol Nurs Forum* 30(2):249-257, 2003.

Fry PS: The unique contribution of key existential factors to the prediction of psychological well-being of older adults following spousal loss, *Gerontologist* 41(1):69-81, 2001.

Gaskins S, Forte L: The meaning of hope: implications for nursing practice and research, *J Gerontol Nurs* 21:17, 1995.

Gibson LMR, Parker V: Inner resources as predictors of psychological well-being in middle-income African American breast cancer survivors, *Cancer Control* 10(5):52-58, 2003.

Greasley P, Chiu LF, Gartland RM: The concept of spiritual care in mental health nursing, *J Adv Nurs* 33:629, 2001.
Heineken J: Patient silence is not necessarily client satisfaction: communication in home care nursing, *Home Healthc Nurse* 16(2): 115, 1998.
Humphreys J: Spirituality and distress in sheltered battered women, *J Nurs Scholarsh* 32:273, 2000.
Johnson P: The use of humor and its influences on spirituality and coping in breast cancer survivors, *Oncology Nursing Forum* *29*(4):691-695, 2002.
Keeley MP: Final conversations: survivors' memorable messages concerning religious faith and spirituality, *Health Commun* 16(1): 87-104, 2004.
Kirby SE, Coleman PG, Daley D: Spirituality and well-being in frail and nonfrail older adults, *J Gerontol* 59B(3):P123-P129, 2004.
Lauver D: Commonalities in women's spirituality and women's health, *Adv Nurs Sci* 22:76, 2000.
Leininger MM, McFarland MR: *Transcultural nursing: concepts, theories, research and practices,* ed 3, New York, 2002, McGraw-Hill.
Mapp I, Hudson R: Stress and coping among African American and Hispanic parents of deaf children, *Am Ann Deaf* 142(1):48, 1997.
Mazanec P, Tyler MK: Cultural considerations in end-of-life care: how ethnicity, age, and spirituality affect decisions when death is imminent, *Am J Nurs* 103(3):50-58, 2003.
McClain CS, Rosenfeld B, Breitbart W: Effect of spiritual well-being on end-of-life despair in terminally-ill cancer patients, *Lancet* 361:1603-1607, 2003.
McGrath P: Religiosity and the challenge of terminal illness, *Death Stud* 27:881-899, 2003.
Meraviglia MG: The effects of spirituality on well-being of people with lung cancer, *Oncol Nurs Forum* 31(1):89-94, 2004.
Moller MD: Meeting spiritual needs on an inpatient unit, *J Psychosoc Nurs Ment Health Serv* 37(11):5, 1999.
Nelson CJ, Rosenfeld B, Breitbart W et al: Spirituality, religion, and depression in the terminally ill, *Psychosomatics* 43(3):213-220, 2002.
Newshan G: Transcending the physical: spiritual aspects of pain in patients with HIV and/or cancer, *J Adv Nurs* 28:1236, 1998.
O'Brien ME: *Spirituality in nursing: standing on holy ground,* Boston, 1999, Jones and Bartlett.
Samuel-Hodge CD, Headen SW, Skelly AH et al: Influences on day-to-day self-management of type 2 diabetes among African American women: spirituality, the multi-caregiver role, and other social context factors, *Diabetes Care* 23(7):928, 2000.
Sowell R, Moneyham L, Hennessy M et al: Spiritual activities as a resistance resource for women with human immunodeficieny virus, *J Nurs Res* 49(2):73-82, 2000.
Smucker C: A phenomenological description of the experience of spiritual distress, *Nurs Diagn* 7:81, 1996.
Tuck I, Pullen L, Lynn C: Spiritual interventions provided by mental health nurses, *West J Nurs Res* 19:351, 1997.
Tuck I, Wallace D, Pullen L: Spirituality and spiritual care provided by parish nurses, *West J Nurs Res* 23:144, 2001.
Van Ness PH, Larson DB: Religion, senescence, and mental health: the end of life is not the end of hope, *Am J Geriatr Psychiatry* 10:386, 2002.
Walters KL, Simoni JM: Reconceptualizing native women's health: an "indigenist" stress-coping model, *Am J Public Health* 92(4): 520-524, 2002.
Zapata J, Shippee-Rice R: The use of folk healing and healers by six Latinos living in New England, *J Transcult Nurs* 10(2):136, 1999.



# Readiness for enhanced Spiritual well-being

*Ann Solari-Twadell and Lisa Burkhart*

**NANDA**

## Definition

Ability to experience and integrate meaning and purpose in life through connectedness with self, others, art, music, literature, nature, or a power greater than oneself

## Defining Characteristics

*Connections to self:* Desires enhanced connections; expresses hope, meaning and purpose in life, peace and serenity, acceptance, surrender, love, forgiveness of self, satisfying philosophy of life, joy, courage, heightened coping, and meditation

*Connections with others:* Provides service to others, requests interaction with spiritual leaders, requests forgiveness of others, requests interaction with friends and family

*Connections with art, music, literature, nature:* Displays creative energy (e.g., writing poetry), sings, listens to music, reads spiritual literature, spends time outdoors

*Connection with a power greater than self:* Prays, reports mystical experiences, participates in religious activities, expresses reverence and awe

## Related Factors (r/t)

Health-seeking behaviors, empathy, self-care, self-awareness, desire for harmonious interconnectedness, desire to find meaning and purpose in life

**NOC**

## Outcomes (Nursing Outcomes Classification)

### Suggested NOC Outcomes

Acceptance: Health Status; Adherence Behavior; Caregiver Emotional Health; Caregiver Well-Being; Caregiver-Patient Relationship; Comfort Level; Coping; Dignified Life Closure; Endurance; Family Integrity; Grief Resolution; Health Beliefs; Health-Promoting Behavior; Hope; Knowledge: Health Behavior; Leisure Participation; Personal Well-Being; Psychosocial Adjustment: Life Change; Quality of Life; Self-Esteem; Social Involvement; Spiritual Health

**Example NOC Outcome with Indicators**

**Hope** as evidenced by the following indicators: Expression of positive future orientation/Faith/Optimism/Belief in self/Sense of meaning in life/Belief in others/Inner peace (Rate each indicator of **Hope:** 1 = never demonstrated, 2 = rarely demonstrated, 3 = sometimes demonstrated, 4 = often demonstrated, 5 = constantly demonstrated [see Section I].)

S

## Client Outcomes

### Client Will (Specify Time Frame):

- Express hope
- Express sense of meaning and purpose in life
- Express peace and serenity
- Express acceptance
- Express surrender
- Express forgiveness of self and others
- Express satisfaction with philosophy of life
- Express joy
- Express courage

- Describe being able to cope
- Describe use of spiritual practices
- Describe providing service to others
- Describe interaction with spiritual leaders, friends, and family
- Describe appreciation for art, music, literature, and nature

**NIC**

## Interventions (Nursing Interventions Classification)

### Suggested NIC Interventions

Active Listening, Animal-Assisted Therapy, Anticipatory Guidance, Anxiety Reduction, Art Therapy, Coping Enhancement, Counseling, Crisis Intervention, Decision-Making Support, Dying Care, Emotional Support, Forgiveness Facilitation, Grief Work Facilitation, Guilt Work Facilitation, Hope Instillation, Humor, Meditation Facilitation, Music Therapy, Mutual Goal Setting, Presence, Religious Ritual Enhancement, Reminiscence Therapy, Security Enhancement, Self-Awareness Enhancement, Self-Esteem Enhancement, Simple Guided Imagery, Simple Relaxation Therapy, Socialization Enhancement, Spiritual Growth Facilitation, Spiritual Support, Support Group, Support System Enhancement, Touch, Truth Telling, Values Clarification

| Example NIC Activities—Spiritual Support |
| --- |
| Encourage use of spiritual resources if desired; be available to listen to client's feelings |

## Nursing Interventions and Rationales

- Perform a spiritual assessment that includes the client's relationship with God, meaning and purpose in life, religious affiliation, and any other significant beliefs. *Autonomy, the right of client self-determination, encompasses a client's needs whether physical, psychosocial, or spiritual. Autonomy requires nurses to assess what client's desire regarding spiritual care, setting aside personal beliefs and values to meet clients' needs from clients' own perspective of meaning (Wright, 1998).* **EBN:** *Meaning and purpose in life are associated with spirituality (Burkhart & Solari-Twadell, 2001). Many nurses feel they have assessed spiritual needs when in reality they have only determined religious affiliation. Spiritual assessment reveals clients' deeper feelings about the meaning of life, love, hope, and forgiveness (Newshan, 1998). McClain, Rosenfeld, and Breitbart (2003) found that spiritual well-being offered some protection against end-of-life despair.*
- Be present for the client. **EBN:** *Wisdom is required in practicing presence; the nurse strives to be a caregiver, not a caretaker (Montgomery, 1992). Eliminating expectations is essential to true presence (Bunkers, 1999). For staff to acknowledge spiritual issues, a more holistic approach to care is necessary that would entail multidisciplinary education and training in spiritual care (Greasely, Chiu, & Gartland, 2001). Presencing is effective not only for clients who are dying or in severe pain but also for those who are experiencing spiritual or emotional discomfort (Taylor, 2002). Walton (2002) found that presence of others was a theme in spirituality for individuals receiving hemodialysis.*
- Listen actively to the client. **EBN:** *In a phenomenological study, Smucker (1996) found*

S

*that listening is an important nursing intervention. A survey of parish nurses found that listening and presence were the most frequently used interventions (Tuck, Wallace, & Pullen, 2001). Listening attentively and being physically present can be spiritually nourishing (Berggren-Thomas & Griggs, 1995). Listening is an element of presencing (Taylor, 2002). Gibson & Parker (2003) found that engaging in discussions related to spirituality promote psychological well-being.*

- Encourage the client to pray, setting the example by praying with and for the client. **EBN:** *Frequent prayer is associated with high mental scores regardless of age and gender (Meisenhelder & Chandler, 2000). Prayer is considered an adjunct therapy in some critical care settings (Holt-Ashley, 2000). Shared prayer can be one of the deepest forms of communication (Shelly, 2000). Parish nurses reported prayer to be the intervention used most frequently with clients (Tuck, Wallace, & Pullen, 2001). Taylor and Outlaw (2002) found that prayer is associated with coping in persons with cancer. Gibson & Parker (2003) also found that prayer and spiritual study can promote psychological well-being. Meraviglia (2004) found that prayer was associated with higher psychological well-being.*
- Encourage involvement in group religious practices. **EBN:** *Socialization and support found through participation in personal and/or group religious practices may decrease feelings of withdrawal and isolation (Baldacchino & Draper, 2001). Gibson and Parker (2003) found that incorporating Bibles and other religious material can promote psychological well-being.*
- Encourage increased quality of life through social support. **EBN:** *Quality of life was potentially related to social support; physical, social, and functional well-being; and appraisal-focused coping in persons living with HIV (Tuck, McCain, & Elswick, 2001). Connectedness, beliefs, inner motivating factors, divine providence, and understanding the mystery are important elements that enhanced spirituality (Cavendish et al, 2000, 2001). Keeley (2004) found that spirituality was an important theme in final conversations with loved ones. Coleman (2003) found that in a sample of African-American men and women living with HIV/AIDS, spirituality significantly correlated with social functioning.*
- Assist the client in identifying religious or spiritual beliefs that encourage integration of meaning and purpose in the client's life. **EBN:** *Beliefs were identified as an important theme that enhanced spirituality (Cavendish et al, 2001). Religious and/or spiritual beliefs were presented as important in interviews conducted with focus groups of users, caregivers, and mental health nursing professionals (Greasely, Chiu, & Gartland, 2001).*
- Encourage the client to use music as a means of reducing stress. **EBN:** *Participants in one study used music listening as a means of stress reduction in the home. They were facilitated by a music therapist visit and a self-administered program using the same techniques with a phone call by the therapist. These subjects performed significantly better than controls on standardized tests of depression, distress, self-esteem, and mood (Hanser & Thompson, 1994). Music is known to relieve stress and promote an interest in the transcendent (O'Brien, 1999).*
- Encourage the client to engage regularly in bibliotherapy. *Reading spiritually uplifting materials, including sacred writings, enhances well-being (Taylor, 2002). Gibson and Parker (2003) found that incorporating the Bible and other religious reading material can promote psychological well-being.*

- Encourage storytelling. *This is an intervention nurses can use to promote spiritual health. Stories are a medium for assessment and intervention in areas that essentially reflect an individual's spirituality (Taylor, 1997).*
- Offer to read to the client. *Some clients cannot read because they are illiterate, have a pathological problem that prevents reading, or are taking medications that cause visual problems or drowsiness. Reading to clients, regardless of whether the material is religious or not, is an act of care because time is being spent with them (Bolander, 1994).*
- Support involvement in expressive art. *Sculpture, painting, knitting, and dance are all forms of expressive art that can boost the spirit (Taylor, 2002).*
- Support the use of humor by the client. *Laughter and humor increase physiological production of endorphins and shorten the distance between people (Dossey et al, 1995). Johnson (2002) found humor promoted coping in breast cancer survivors.*
- Encourage the client to use journal writing as a means of reflection on his or her life. *Journaling guides the client in tapping into inner realities through use of reflection and writing (Dossey et al, 1995).*
- Encourage the client to practice forgiveness. **EBN:** *Caregivers agreed that forgiveness is an important part of spirituality (Kaye & Robinson, 1994). In a survey of battered women, forgiveness was rated as an important part of spirituality (Humphreys, 2000). In a survey of parish nurses, the nurses promoted forgiveness (Tuck, Wallace, & Pullen, 2001).*
- Support the client in contemplating, viewing, and/or experiencing nature. **EBN:** *Postoperative hospital stay was shorter and use of analgesics was lower with natural surroundings than with an urban view (Travis & McCauley, 1998). Walton (2002) found that nature was a theme in spirituality for individuals receiving hemodialysis.*
- Encourage expressions of spirituality. **EBN:** *African Americans and Latinos may identify spirituality, religiousness, prayer, and church-based approaches as coping resources (Samuel-Hodge et al, 2000; Bourjolly, 1998; Mapp & Hudson, 1997).*
- Validate the client's spiritual concerns and convey respect for his or her beliefs. *Validation lets the client know that the nurse has heard and understood what was said (Giger & Davidhizar, 1995; Stuart & Laraia, 2001).* **EBN:** *Gibson and Parker (2003) found that presence and use of inner resources in creating a therapeutic environment can promote psychological well-being.*
- Help the client participate in religious rites or obtain spiritual guidance. *Support in spiritual beliefs (belief in a divine being or God) was identified as a factor that contributed to initiation and maintenance of behavior changes after an illness (McSweeney, 1993). The nurse is rarely the client's primary spiritual caregiver. No single approach to spiritual care is satisfactory for all clients; many kinds of resources are needed (Bolander, 1994).* **EBN:** *Kennedy, Abbott, and Rosenberg (2002) found that retreats increased spirituality, well-being, meaning in life, confidence in handling problems, and decreased tendency to become angry.*
- Assist the client in developing spirituality. List the most valuable qualities he or she can bring from within, the circumstances most helpful for unfolding these qualities, and the ways of incorporating these circumstances into the client's lifestyle. *Interventions assist clients in bringing forth courage, compassion, inner peace, and creative insight (spirituality) (Macrae, 1995).* **EBN:** *Walton (2002) found that receiving help and giving help was a theme in spirituality for individuals receiving hemodialysis.*

S

## Pediatric

- Provide spiritual care for children based on developmental level. *When nurses are comfortable providing spiritual care, they can implement numerous spiritual care activities and interventions to meet the spiritual needs of the child and family. After determining the child's spiritual beliefs and spiritual needs, a plan of care is developed based on the child's developmental age (Elkins & Cavendish, 2004).*
  - **Infants:** Have the same nurse care for the child on a daily basis, hold, cuddle, rock, play with and sing to the infant. *The primary needs of the infant are love and trust. Minimizing the separation of the child from family and having the same nurse care for the child on a daily basis can initiate spiritual care. Continuity of care will promote the establishment of trust because nurses provide much of the needed ongoing support. The infant who is ill or dying still needs to be sung and talked to played with, held, cuddled, and rocked (Elkins & Cavendish, 2004).*
  - **Toddlers:** Provide consistency in care and familiar toys, music, stories, clothing blankets, pillows, and any other individual object of contentment. Schedule home religious routines into the plan of care and support home routines regarding good and bad behavior. *Toddlers and preschoolers need to feel safe and secure and develop a trusting relationship with caretakers. The importance of consistency in care and routine with this age group cannot be overemphasized. The nurse should support parent's home routines during hospitalization as much as possible and encourage them to continue to have the same expectations regarding good and bad behavior. If particular religious routines are carried out at certain times of the day, the nurse should schedule them in the plan of care (Elkins & Cavendish, 2004).*
  - **School-age children and adolescents:** Encourage both groups to express their feelings regarding spirituality. Ask them, "Do you wish to pray and what do you want to pray about?" Children of all ages can express feelings in story telling. Offer age-appropriate complimentary therapies such as music, art, videos, connectedness with peers through cards, letters, and visits. *School-age children and adolescents should be encouraged to express their feelings, concerns, and needs regarding spirituality. For the adolescent, nurses need to accept their beliefs and wishes even if they are different from their caregiver's. The nurse needs to facilitate the child's participation in religious rituals and spiritual practices. Referrals to clergy and other spiritual support may be necessary (Elkins & Cavendish, 2004).*

S

## Geriatrics

- Discuss personal definitions of spiritual wellness with the client. *Listening attentively and helping elderly clients identify past coping strategies is part of helping with life review and finding meaning in life (Berggren-Thomas & Griggs, 1995).* **EBN:** *Daaleman, Perera, and Studenski (2004) found in a sample of 277 geriatric outpatients, those who rated themselves in good health reported significantly higher levels of spirituality, controlling for functional health, race, and ethnicity.*
- Identify the client's past sources of spirituality. Help the client explore his or her life and identify those experiences that are noteworthy. Clients may want to read the Bible or other religious text or have it read to them. *Older adults often identify spirituality as*

*a source of hope (Gaskins & Forte, 1995).* **EBN:** *Kirby, Coleman, and Daley (2004) studied the well-being of adults living in retirement housing estates in Britain and found that spirituality had a small significant correlation with psychological well-being, personal growth, and positive relations with others, and spirituality reduced the negative effects of frailty.*

## Multicultural

- Assess for the influence of cultural beliefs, norms, and values on the client's ability to cope with spiritual distress. **EBN:** *How the client copes with spiritual distress may be based on cultural perceptions (Cesario, 2001; Cochran, 1998; Doswell & Erlen, 1998; Leininger & McFarland, 2002; Zapata & Shippee-Rice, 1999).*
- Acknowledge the value conflicts from acculturation stresses that may contribute to spiritual distress. **EBN:** *Challenges to traditional beliefs are anxiety provoking and can produce distress (Charron, 1998; Mazanec & Tyler, 2003).*
- Encourage spirituality as a source of support. **EBN:** *African Americans and Latinos may identify spirituality, religiousness, prayer, and church-based approaches as coping resources (Bourjolly, 1998; Mapp & Hudson, 1997; Samuel-Hodge et al, 2000). A study of battered women showed that African-American women were significantly more likely to report using prayer as a coping strategy and significantly less likely to seek help from mental health counselors (El-Khoury et al, 2004). A recent study showed religion and spirituality are associated with health-seeking behaviors of African-American women (Dessio et al, 2004).*
- Identify, develop, and implement culturally appropriate spiritual nursing interventions. **EBN:** *A study of Christian African Americans examining spiritual perspectives, spiritual needs, and desired nursing interventions during hospitalization identified participating in spiritual activities and recognizing the spiritual caregiver role as desired nursing interventions (Connor & Eller, 2004). Spiritual coping may serve as a moderator of health among Native-American women (Walters & Simoni, 2002).*
- Validate the client's spiritual concerns and convey respect for his or her beliefs. **EBN:** *Validation is a therapeutic communications technique that lets the client know the nurse has heard and understood what was said (Heineken, 1998).*

## Home Care

▲ All of the nursing interventions mentioned previously apply in the home setting. Refer the client to parish nurses. **EBN:** *Parish nurses are experienced registered nurses committed to helping people meet the health needs of the mind, body, and spirit (Stewart, 2000).*

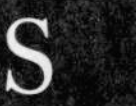


## evolve WEBSITES FOR EDUCATION

See the EVOLVE website for World Wide Web resources for client education.

## REFERENCES

Baldacchino D, Draper P: Spiritual coping strategies: a review, *J Adv Nurs* 34:83, 2001.
Berggren-Thomas P, Griggs M: Spirituality in aging: spiritual need or spiritual journey? *J Gerontol Nurs* 21:5, 1995.
Bolander V: *Sorensen and Luckmann's basic nursing: a psychophysiologic approach,* Philadelphia, 1994, WB Saunders.

Bourjolly JN: Differences in religiousness among black and white women with breast cancer, *Soc Work Health Care* 28(1):21, 1998.
Bunkers S: Learning to be still, *Nurs Sci Q* 12(2):172, 1999.
Burkhart L, Solari-Twadell A: Spirituality and religiousness: differentiating the diagnosis through a review of the literature, *Nurs Diagn* 12(2):45, 2001.
Cavendish R, Luise BK, Horne K et al: Opportunities for enhanced spirituality relevant to well adults, *Nurs Diagn*, 11(4):151-163, 2000.
Cavendish R et al: Recognizing opportunities for spiritual enhancement in young adults, *Nurs Diagn* 12(3):77, 2001.
Cesario S: Care of the Native American woman: strategies for practice, education, and research, *J Gynecol Neonat Nurs* 30(1):13, 2001.
Charron HS: Anxiety disorders. In Varcarolis EM, editor: *Foundations of psychiatric mental health nursing,* ed 3, Philadelphia, 1998, WB Saunders.
Cochran M: Tears have no color, *Am J Nurs* 98(6):53, 1998.
Coleman CL: Spirituality and sexual orientation: relationship to mental well-being and functional health status, *J Adv Nurs 43*(5): 457-464, 2003.
Conner NE, Eller LS: Spiritual perspectives, needs and nursing interventions of Christian African-Americans, *J Adv Nurs* 46(6): 624-632, 2004.
Daaleman TP, Perera S, Studenski SA: Religion, spirituality, and health status in geriatric outpatients, *Ann Fam Med* 2(1):49-53, 2004.
Dessio W, Wade C, Chao M et al: Religion, spirituality, and healthcare choices of African-American women: results of a national survey, *Ethn Dis* 14(2):189-197, 2004.
Dossey BM et al: *Holistic nursing: a handbook for practice,* ed 2, Gaithersburg, Md, 1995, Aspen.
Doswell W, Erlen J: Multicultural issues and ethical concerns in the delivery of nursing care interventions, *Nurs Clin North Am* 33(2):353, 1998.
El-Khoury MY, Dutton MA, Goodman LA et al: Ethnic differences in battered women's formal help-seeking strategies: a focus on health, mental health, and spirituality, *Cultur Divers Ethnic Minor Psychol* 10(4):383-393, 2004.
Elkins M, Cavendish R: Developing a plan for pediatric spiritual care, *Holistic Nurs Pract* 8(4):179, 2004
Gibson LMR, Parker V: Inner resources as predictors of psychological well-being in middle-income African American breast cancer survivors, *Cancer Control* 10(5):52-58, 2003.
Giger JN, Davidhizar RE: *Transcultural nursing,* ed 2, St Louis, 1995, Mosby.
Greasley P, Chiu LF, Gartland RM: The concept of spiritual care in mental health nursing, *J Adv Nurs* 33:629, 2001.
Hanser SB, Thompson L: Effects of a music therapy strategy on depressed older adults, *J Gerontol* 49(6):P265, 1994.
Heineken J: Patient silence is not necessarily client satisfaction: communication in home care nursing, *Home Healthc Nurse* 16(2): 115, 1998.
Holt-Ashley M: Nurses pray: use of prayer and spirituality as complementary therapy in the intensive care setting, *AACN Clin Issues* 11(1):60, 2000.
Humphreys J: Spirituality and distress in sheltered battered women, *Image J Nurs Sch* 32:273, 2000.
Johnson P: The use of humor and its influences on spirituality and coping in breast cancer survivors, *Oncol Nurs Forum* 29(4):691-695, 2002.
Kaye J, Robinson KM: Spirituality among caregivers, *Image J Nurs Sch* 26(3):218, 1994.
Keeley MP: Final conversations: survivors' memorable messages concerning religious faith and spirituality, *Health Commun* 16(1): 87-104, 2004.
Kirby SE, Coleman PG, Daley D: Spirituality and well-being in frail and nonfrail older adults, *J Gerontol* 59B(3):P123-P129, 2004.
Leininger MM, McFarland MR: *Transcultural nursing: concepts, theories, research and practices,* ed 3, New York, 2002, McGraw-Hill.
Macrae J: Nightingale's spiritual philosophy and its significance for modern nursing, *Image* 27:8, 1995.
Mapp I, Hudson R: Stress and coping among African American and Hispanic parents of deaf children, *Am Ann Deaf* 142(1):48, 1997.
Mazanec P, Tyler MK: Cultural considerations in end-of-life care: how ethnicity, age, and spirituality affect decisions when death is imminent, *Am J Nurs* 103(3):50-58, 2003.
McClain CS, Rosenfeld B, Breitbart W: Effect of spiritual well-being on end-of-life despair in terminally-ill cancer patients, *Lancet* 361:1603-1607, 2003.
McSweeney J: Making behavior changes after a myocardial infarction, *West J Nurs Res* 15:441, 1993.

Meisenhelder JB, Chandler EN: Prayer and health outcomes in church lay leaders, *West J Nurs Res* 22:706, 2000.
Meraviglia MG: The effects of spirituality on well-being of people with lung cancer, *Oncol Nurs Forum* 31(1):89-94, 2004.
Montgomery CL: The spiritual connection: nurses perceptions of the experience of caring. In Gaur DA, editor: *The presence of caring in nursing,* Pub No. 15-2465, New York, 1992, National League for Nursing.
Newshan G: Transcending the physical: spiritual aspects of pain in patients with HIV and/or cancer, *J Adv Nurs* 28(6):1236, 1998.
O'Brien ME: *Spirituality in nursing: standing on holy ground,* Boston, 1999, Jones and Bartlett.
Poindexter CC, Linsk NL: Sources of support in a sample of HIV-affected older minority caregivers, *Fam Soc J Contemp Hum Serv* Sep/Oct:491, 1998.
Samuel-Hodge CD, Headen SW, Skelly AH et al: Influences on day-to-day self-management of type 2 diabetes among African American women: spirituality, the multi-caregiver role, and other social context factors, *Diabetes Care* 23(7):928, 2000.
Shelly J: *Spiritual care: a guide for caregivers,* Downers Grove, Ill, 2000, InterVarsity Press.
Smucker C: A phenomenological description of the experience of spiritual distress, *Nurs Diagn* 7:81, 1996.
Stewart LE: Parish nursing: renewing a long tradition of caring, *Gastroenterol Nurs* 23(3):116, 2000.
Stuart GW, Laraia MT: Therapeutic nurse-patient relationship. In Stuart GW, Laraia MT, editors: *Principles and practice of psychiatric nursing,* St Louis, 2001, Mosby, p 30.
Taylor E: The story behind the story: the use of storytelling in spiritual caregiving, *Semin Oncol Nurs* 13(4):252, 1997.
Taylor E: *Spiritual care: nursing theory, research and practice,* Upper Saddle River, NJ, 2002, Prentice Hall.
Taylor EJ, Outlaw FH: Use of prayer among persons with cancer, *Holistic Nurs Pract* 16(3):46-60, 2002.
Travis S, McCauley W: Mentally restorative experience supporting rehabilitation of high functioning elders recovering from hip surgery, *J Adv Nurs,* 27:977, 1998.
Tuck I, McCain NL, Elswick RK: Spirituality and psychosocial factors in persons living with HIV, *J Adv Nurs* 33(6):776, 2001.
Tuck I, Wallace D, Pullen L: Spirituality and spiritual care provided by parish nurses, *West J Nurs Res* 23:144, 2001.
Walters KL, Simoni JM: Reconceptualizing native women's health: an "indigenist" stress-coping model, *Am J Public Health* 92(4): 520-524, 2002.
Walton: Finding a balance: a grounded theory study of spirituality in hemodialysis patients, *Nephrol Nurs J* 29(5), 447-457, 2002.
Wright KB: Professional, ethical and legal implications for spiritual care in nursing, *Image J Nurs Sch* 30(1):81, 1998.
Zapata J, Shippee-Rice R: The use of folk healing and healers by six Latinos living in New England, *J Transcult Nurs* 10(2):136, 1999.

# Risk for Suffocation

*Betty J. Ackley and T. Heather Herdman*

**NANDA**

## Definition

Accentuated risk of accidental suffocation (inadequate air available for inhalation)

## Risk Factors

### External

Vehicle warming in closed garage, use of fuel-burning heaters not vented to outside, smoking in bed, children's playing with plastic bags or inserting small objects into their mouths or noses, placement of propped bottle in infant's crib, placement of pillow in infant's crib, consumption of large mouthfuls of food, failure to remove doors on dis-

S

carded or unused refrigerators or freezers, leaving children unattended in bathtubs or pools, household gas leaks, low-strung clothesline, hanging of pacifier around infant's neck

### Internal

Reduced olfactory sensation, reduced motor abilities, cognitive or emotional difficulties, disease or injury process, lack of safety education, lack of safety precautions

## Related Factors (r/t)

See Risk Factors

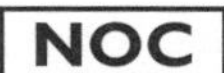

## Outcomes (Nursing Outcomes Classification)

### Suggested NOC Outcomes

Knowledge: Child Physical Safety, Personal Safety; Parenting: Adolescent Physical Safety, Early/Middle Childhood Physical Safety, Infant/Toddler Physical Safety; Risk Control; Risk Detection; Safe Home Environment; Substance Addiction Consequences

**Example NOC Outcome with Indicators**

**Knowledge: Child Physical Safety** as evidenced by the following indicators: Description of methods to prevent choking on objects/Description of appropriate activities for child's developmental level/Description of first aid techniques (Rate each indicator of **Knowledge: Child Physical Safety:** 1 = none, 2 = limited, 3 = moderate, 4 = substantial, 5=extensive [see Section I].)

## Client Outcomes

### Client Will (Specify Time Frame):

- Explain and undertake appropriate measures to prevent suffocation.
- Demonstrate correct techniques for emergency rescue maneuvers (e.g., Heimlich maneuver, rescue breathing, cardiopulmonary resuscitation [CPR]) and describe situations that require them.



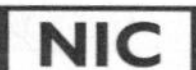

## Interventions (Nursing Interventions Classification)

### Suggested NIC Interventions

Aspiration Precautions; Environmental Management: Safety; Infant Care; Positioning; Security Enhancement; Surveillance; Surveillance: Safety; Teaching: Infant Safety

**Example NIC Activities—Environmental Management: Safety**

Identify safety hazards in environment (e.g., physical, biological, chemical); remove hazards from environment when possible

## Nursing Interventions and Rationales

- Identify hospitalized clients at particular risk for suffocation, including the following:
  - Clients with altered levels of consciousness
  - Infants or young children
  - Clients with developmental delays
  - Clients with mental illness, especially schizophrenia

  *Institute safety measures such as proper positioning and feeding precautions. See the care plans for* **Risk for Aspiration** *and* **Impaired Swallowing** *for additional interventions. Vigilance and special protective measures are necessary for clients at greater risk for suffocation.* **EB:** *Mental health clients have an increased incidence of choking and suffocation incidents (Corcoran & Walsh, 2003).*

### Pediatric

- Counsel families on the following:
  - Following general safety practices such as not smoking in bed, properly disposing of large appliances, using properly functioning heating systems and ventilation, having functional smoke detectors, and opening garage doors when warming up a car
  - Position infants on their back to sleep, do not position in the prone position. **EB:** *Research has demonstrated that the prone position for sleeping infants is a risk factor for SIDS (Li et al, 2003; Malloy and Freeman, 2004). Population studies have demonstrated a striking trend in decreased incidence of SIDS since parents have been taught to* ***not*** *place infants in the prone position (Ponsonby et al, 2002).*
  - Avoid use of loose bedding such as blankets and sheets for sleeping. If blankets are used, they should be tucked in around the crib mattress so the infant's face is less likely to become covered by bedding. "One strategy is to make up the bedding so that the infant's feet are able to reach the foot of the crib with the blankets tucked in around the crib mattress and reaching only the level of the infant's chest" (American Academy of Pediatrics, 2000, p. 650). **EB:** *Epidemiological studies have identified soft surfaces as a significant risk factor for SIDS, especially when these items are placed under the sleeping infant (Mitchell et al, 1998; Ponsonby et al, 1998).*
  - Teach parents not to sleep with an infant, especially if alcohol or medications/illicit drugs are used by the parents. **EB:** *A study demonstrated that parents who were under the influence of alcohol or illicit drugs or were smoking were more likely to have a SIDS result (James et al, 2003). Another study demonstrated that mothers who consumed three or more alcoholic drinks in the past 24 hours increased the risk of SIDS when bed sharing with an infant (Carpenter et al, 2004).*
- Conduct risk factor identification, noting special circumstances in which preventive or protective measures are indicated. Note the presence of environmental hazards, including the following:
  - Plastic bags (e.g., dry cleaner's bags, bags used for mattress protection)
  - Cribs with slats wider than 2³/₈ inches
  - Ill-fitting crib mattresses that can allow the infant to become wedged between the mattress and crib
  - Pillows in cribs
  - Abandoned large appliances such as refrigerators, dishwashers, or freezers



S

- Clothing with cords or hoods that can become entangled
- Bibs, pacifiers on a string, drapery cords, pull-toy strings

*Suffocation by airway obstruction is a leading cause of death in children younger than 6 years of age. Families need to be taught child protection.*

- Counsel families to not serve these foods to the child younger than 4 years of age: hot-dogs, popcorn, nuts, pretzels, chips, peanut butter, chunks of meat, hard pieces of fruit or vegetables, raisins, whole grapes, hard candies, marshmallows (Single Parent Central, 2005). *Hot dogs are the most common item associated with fatal choking incidences in children (Behrman, Kliegman, & Jenson, 2004).* **EB:** *Children between the ages of 4 and 36 months of age are at risk for suffocation by hollow, semirigid hemispherical/ellipsoidal objects through suction formation and complete airway obstruction (Nakamura, Pollack-Nelson, & Chidekel, 2003).*
- Provide information to parents about obtaining the "No-choke Test Tube" (No-choke tubes are sold at stores that sell baby items), or use of a toilet paper roll. If an object fits in the tube or the roll, it is too small to give to a child (Single Parent Central, 2005). **EB:** *Rigid items that are of a spherical or cylindrical shape can cause upper airway occlusion (Nakamura, Pollack-Nelson, & Chidekel, 2003).*
- Stress water and pool safety precautions, including vigilant, uninterrupted parental supervision. *An intense drive for exploration combined with a lack of awareness of danger makes drowning a threat to small children. A child's high center of gravity and poor coordination make buckets and toilets a threat because a child looking inside either can fall over and become lodged (Behrman, Kliegman, & Jenson, 2004).*
- Underscore the necessity of not allowing children to play with or near electric garage doors and of keeping garage door openers out of the reach of young children. *Children close to the ground may not be large enough to trigger reversal mechanisms on the door and may become trapped.*
- For adolescents, watch for signs of depression that could result in suicide by suffocation. **EB:** *For adolescents 10–19 years of age, suffocation by hanging is the second most common method of suicide (Centers for Disease Control and Prevention, 2004).*

## Geriatric

- Assess the status of the swallow reflex. Offer appropriate foods and beverages accordingly. *The elderly, especially those receiving antipsychotic medications, have an increased incidence of choking.*
- Observe the client for pocketing of food in the side of the mouth; remove food as needed.
- Position the client in high Fowler's position when eating and for 1 hour afterward. *Elderly clients may be at risk for suffocation that results from dysphagia.*
- Use care in pillow placement when positioning frail elderly clients who are on bed rest. *Frail elderly clients are at risk for suffocation if the head becomes lodged against pillows and the client cannot reposition them because of weakness.*

## Home Care

- Assess the home for potential safety hazards in systems that are not likely to be fixed (e.g., faulty pilot lights or gas leaks in gas stoves, carbon monoxide release from heat-

S

ing systems, kerosene fumes from portable heaters). Assist the family in having these areas assessed and making appropriate safety arrangements (e.g., installing detectors, making repairs). *Assessment and correction of system problems prevents accidental suffocation.*

## Client/Family Teaching

- ▲ Recommend that families who are seeking day care or in-home care for children, geriatric family members, or at-risk family members with developmental or functional disabilities inspect the environment for hazards and examine the first aid preparation and vigilance of providers. *Many working families must trust others to care for family members.*
- ▲ Involve family members in learning and practicing rescue techniques, including treatment of choking and lack of breathing, as well as CPR. Initiate referral to formal training classes. *Family members need adequate preparation to deal with emergency situations and should take part in the American Heart Association Basic Lifesaving Course or the American Red Cross Infant/Child CPR Course (MMWR Morb Mort Wkly Rep, 2002).*

## evolve WEBSITES FOR EDUCATION

See the EVOLVE website for World Wide Web resources for client education.

## REFERENCES


American Academy of Pediatrics, Task Force on Infant Sleep Position and Sudden Infant Death Syndrome: Changing concepts of sudden infant death syndrome: implications for infant sleeping environment and sleep position (RE9946), *Pediatrics* 105(3): 650, 2000.

Behrman RE, Kliegman RM, Jenson HB: *Nelson textbook of pediatrics*, ed 17, Philadelphia, 2004, Saunders.

Carpenter RG, Irgens LM, Blair PS et al: Sudden unexplained infant death in 20 regions in Europe: case control study, *Lancet* 363(9404):185, 2004.

Corcoran E, Walsh D: Obstructive asphyxia: a cause of excess mortality in psychiatric patients, *Ir J Psychol Med* 20(3):88-90, 2003.

Li DK, Petitti DB, Willinger M et al: Infant sleeping position and the risk of sudden infant death syndrome in California, 1997-2000, *Am J Epidemiol* 157(5):446, 2003.

James C, Klenka H, Manning D: Sudden infant death syndrome: bed sharing with mothers who smoke, *Arch Dis Child* 88(2):112, 2003.

Centers for Disease Control and Prevention (CDC): Methods of suicide among persons aged 10-19 years—United States, 1992-2001, *MMWR Morb Mort Wkly Rep* 53(22):471, 2004.

Malloy MS: Trends in postneonatal aspiration deaths and reclassification of sudden infant death syndrome: impact of the "Back to Sleep" program, *Pediatrics* 109(4):661, 2002.

Mitchell EA, Thompson JM, Ford RP et al: Sheepskin bedding and the sudden infant death syndrome, *J Pediatr* 133:701, 1998.

Nakamura S, Pollack-Nelson C, Chidekel A: Suction-type suffocation incidents in infants and toddlers, *Pediatrics* 111(1):12-16, 2003.

Nonfatal choking-related episodes among children—United States, 2001, *MMWR Morb Mort Wkly Rep* 51(42):945, 2002.

Person TL, Lavezzi WA, Wolf BC: Cosleeping and sudden unexpected death in infancy, *Arch Pathol Lab Med* 126(3):343, 2002.

Ponsonby A, Dwyer T, Cochrane JL: Population trends in sudden infant death syndrome, *Semin Perinatol* 26(4):296, 2002.

Ponsonby AL, Dwyer T, Couper D et al: Association between use of a quilt and sudden infant death syndrome: case-control study, *BMJ* 316(7126):195, 1998.

Single Parent Central: *Preventing choking in young children*. Available at http://library.adoption.com/Child-Safety/Preventing-Choking-in-Young-Children/article/2724/1.html, accessed March 29, 2005.


S

# Risk for Suicide

evolve

*Kathleen L. Patusky*

NANDA

## Definition

At risk for self-inflicted, life-threatening injury

## Related Factors (r/t)

### Behavioral

History of previous suicide attempt; impulsiveness; purchase of gun; stockpiling of medicines; making or changing of a will; giving away of possessions; sudden euphoric recovery from major depression; marked changes in behavior, attitude, or school performance

### Verbal

Threats of killing oneself, statement of desire to die/end it all

### Situational

Living alone; retirement; relocation, institutionalization; economic instability; loss of autonomy/independence; presence of gun in home; residence of adolescent in non-traditional setting (e.g., juvenile detention center, prison, half-way house, group home)

### Psychological

Family history of suicide; alcohol and substance use/abuse; psychiatric illness/disorder (e.g., depression, schizophrenia, bipolar disorder); abuse in childhood; guilt; gay or lesbian orientation in youth

### Demographic

Age: elderly, young adult male, adolescent; race: Caucasian, Native American; gender: male; marital status: divorced, widowed

### Physical

Physical illness, terminal illness, chronic pain

### Social

Loss of important relationship; disrupted family life; grief, bereavement; poor support systems; loneliness; hopelessness; helplessness; social isolation; legal or disciplinary problems; cluster suicides

**NOC**

## Outcomes (Nursing Outcomes Classification)

### Suggested NOC Outcomes

Depression Level, Distorted Thought Self-Control, Impulse Self-Control, Loneliness Severity, Mood Equilibrium, Risk Detection, Self-Mutilation Restraint, Suicide Self-Restraint

**Example NOC Outcome with Indicators**

**Suicide Self-Restraint** as evidenced by the following indicators: Expresses feelings/Seeks help when feeling self-destructive/Verbalizes suicidal ideas/Controls impulses (Rate each indicator of **Suicide Self-Restraint:** 1 = never demonstrated, 2 = rarely demonstrated, 3 = sometimes demonstrated, 4 = often demonstrated, 5 = consistently demonstrated [see Section I].)

## Client Outcomes

**Client Will (Specify Time Frame):**

- Not harm self
- Maintain connectedness in relationships
- Disclose and discuss suicidal ideas if present; seek help
- Express decreased anxiety and control of impulses
- Talk about feelings; express anger appropriately
- Refrain from using mood-altering substances
- Obtain no access to harmful objects
- Yield access to harmful objects
- Maintain self-control without supervision

**NIC**

## Interventions (Nursing Interventions Classification)

### Suggested NIC Interventions

Anger Control Assistance, Anxiety Reduction, Calming Technique, Coping Enhancement, Crisis Intervention, Delusion Management, Medication Administration, Mood Management, Substance Use Prevention, Suicide Prevention, Support System Enhancement, Surveillance

**Example NIC Activities—Suicide Prevention**

Determine presence and degree of suicide risk; encourage client to seek out care providers to talk when urge to harm self occurs

## Nursing Interventions and Rationales

NOTE: Before implementation of interventions in the face of suicidal behavior, nurses should examine their own emotional responses to incidents of suicide to ensure that interventions will not be based on countertransference reactions. **EBN:** *Suicidal behavior can lead to stigmatization and discrediting of the client, because it may tap into the nurse's fears about mental illness, concerns about being able to respond effectively, and expectations that persons with mental illness tend toward violence (Joachim & Acorn, 2000). In one study, medical nurses reported that they could not understand why people harm themselves, and they felt they did not have the skills to deal with suicidal clients (Hopkins, 2002).*

- Establish a therapeutic relationship with the client. Use a direct, nonjudgmental approach in discussing suicide. **EB:** *A study has demonstrated the importance of the therapeutic relationship in identifying risk for and preventing suicide (Rudd et al, 2000). Clients who perceive that nurses are responding negatively to suicidal behavior are less likely to self-disclose.*
- Monitor, document, and report the client's potential for suicide. *All members of the health care team need to be aware of a client's potential risk for suicide and to be prepared to respond in the event of suicidal behavior.*
- Be alert for warning signs of suicide:
  - Making statements such as, "I can't go on," "Nothing matters anymore," "I wish I were dead."
  - Becoming depressed or withdrawn
  - Behaving recklessly
  - Getting affairs in order and giving away valued possessions
  - Showing a marked change in behavior, attitudes, or appearance
  - Abusing drugs or alcohol
  - Suffering a major loss or life change

  *Suicide is rarely a spontaneous decision. In the days and hours before people kill themselves, clues and warning signs usually appear (Befrienders International, 2003).*
- Pay particular attention to clients manifesting a psychiatric disorder associated with suicidal behavior, including depression, substance abuse, bipolar disorder, schizophrenia, panic disorder, dissociative disorder, antisocial personality disorder, or borderline personality disorder. *All suicide threats should be recognized and taken seriously. The incidence of serious suicide attempts and completed suicide in clients with borderline or antisocial personality disorders is similar to that of clients with major depression without a personality disorder (Lambert, 2003; Kernberg, 2001). Suicidality in schizophrenic clients is highly prevalent, with the need for unique interventions including effective treatment of positive symptoms, reduction of substance abuse, avoidance of akathisia, reduction of demoralization, and instillation of hope (Tandon & Jibson, 2003). Clients with bipolar disorder are at high risk for suicide, especially early in the course of the illness, immediately posthospital discharge, when substance abuse is comorbid, and during periods of mood destabilization (Pies, 2004).* **EB:** *First episode psychosis is a particular risk factor for suicide; early intervention has been shown to be helpful (Power et al, 2003).*
- Take suicide notes seriously. Consider themes of notes in determining appropriate interventions. **EB:** *A study of suicide note themes found that a theme of "apology/shame" was present in 74% of notes, suggesting that alternative solutions to dilemmas may have been welcomed. The researcher concluded that cognitive therapy techniques, particularly problem*

*solving, would be useful. Individuals with major unipolar depression were more likely than individuals without (40% versus 11%, p = .049) to report "hopelessness, nothing to live for" (Foster, 2003).*

- Question family members regarding the preparatory actions mentioned. *Clinicians should be alert for suicide when these factors are present in asymptomatic persons (American Psychiatric Association, 2005). Family members may have noted preparatory actions.*
- Assess for suicidal ideation when the history reveals the following:
  - Depression, substance abuse, or other psychiatric disorders
  - Attempted suicide, current or past
  - Recent stressful life events (divorce and/or separation, relocation, problems with children)
  - Recent unemployment
  - Recent bereavement
  - Chronic pain or physical illness
  - Childhood physical or sexual abuse
  - Gay, lesbian, or bisexual gender orientation
  - Family history of suicide

  *Clinicians should be alert for suicide when the aforementioned factors are present in asymptomatic persons (American Psychiatric Association, 2005).* **EB:** *Studies have revealed that clients with chronic pain and depression expressed suicidal ideation (Fisher et al, 2001; Gilman et al, 2001). In one study, although only 32% of successful suicides had contact with mental health services in the preceding year, 75% had contact with primary care providers. The researchers concluded that primary care providers could be effective in preventing suicide, particularly among older adults and women (Luoma, Martin, & Pearson, 2002).*
- Use brief self-report measures to improve clinical management of at-risk cases. Suicide assessment may be aided by having the client complete screening instruments such as the Center for Epidemiological Studies Depression Scale (CES-D), which indicates degree of depressed mood, or the Beck Suicide Intent Scale, which identifies a strong intent to die. **EBN:** *The Nurses' Global Assessment of Suicide Risk (NGASR) has been developed and preliminary support for its use, especially by novice clinicians, has been reported (Cutcliffe & Barker, 2004).* **EB:** *The Suicide Assessment Checklist (SAC) has demonstrated strengths as part of a thorough protocol in evaluating suicidal risk (Rogers, Lewis, & Subich, 2002). One study identified a significant decrease in assessment errors of suicide risk when brief self-report measures were used (Brown et al, 2003).*
- Determine the presence and degree of suicidal risk. A number of questions will elicit the necessary information:
  - Have you been thinking about hurting or killing yourself?
  - How often do you have these thoughts and how long do they last?
  - Do you have a plan? What is it?
  - Do you have access to the means to carry out that plan?
  - How likely is it that you could carry out the plan?
  - Are there people or things that could prevent you from hurting yourself?
  - What do you see in your future a year from now? Five years from now?
  - What do you expect would happen if you died?
  - What has kept you alive up to now?

S

*Using the acronym SAL, the nurse can evaluate the client's suicide plan for its specificity (how detailed and clear is the plan?), availability (does the client have immediate access to the planned means?), and lethality (could the plan be fatal or does the client believe it would be fatal?). Assessment of reasons for living is another important part of evaluating suicidal clients (Malone et al, 2000).*

▲ Refer to mental health counseling and refer for possible hospitalization if evidence of suicidal intent exists, which may include evidence of preparatory actions (e.g., obtaining a weapon, making a plan, putting affairs in order, giving away prized possessions, preparing a suicide note).

- Assign a hospitalized client to a room located near the nursing station. *Close assignment increases ease of observation and availability for a rapid response in the event of a suicide attempt.*
- Search the newly hospitalized client and the client's personal belongings for weapons or potential weapons and hoarded medications during the in-patient admission procedure, as appropriate. *Clients intent on suicide may bring the means with them.*
- Initiate suicide precautions (e.g., ongoing observation and monitoring of the client, provision of a protective environment) for a client who is at serious risk of suicide.
- Place the client in the least restrictive environment that allows for the necessary level of observation. Assess suicidal risk at least daily. *Close observation of the client is necessary for safety as long as intent remains high. Suicide risk should be assessed at frequent intervals to adjust suicide precautions and limitations on the client's freedom of movement and to ensure that restrictions continue to be appropriate.*

▲ Assess the client's ability to enter into a no-suicide contract. Contract (verbally or in writing) with the client for no self-harm; recontract at appropriate intervals. *Discussing feelings of self-harm with a trusted person provides relief for the client. A contract gets the subject out in the open and places some of the responsibility for safety with the client. A contract is not appropriate for some clients: those who are under the influence of drugs or alcohol or are unwilling to abstain from substance use; those who are isolated or alone without assistance to keep the environment safe; those who are unwilling to dismantle a suicide plan or disclose alternative plans (Hauenstein, 2002). If the client will not contract, the risk of suicide should be considered higher.* **EB:** *The lack of willingness to self-disclose has been shown to discriminate the serious suicide attempter from the client with suicidal ideation or the mild attempter (Apter et al, 2001).* **EBN:** *Note: Contracting is a common practice in psychiatric care settings. However, research has suggested that self-harm is not prevented by contracts (Drew, 2001). The researcher concluded that thorough, ongoing assessment of suicide risk is necessary, whether or not the client has entered into a no-self-harm contract. Further discussion of contracts has advised that nurses should be clearer about the basis for their decision to contract (i.e., use of therapeutic rationale rather than staffing shortages), and that contracts may not be appropriate in community settings (Farrow, 2002, 2003).*

- Increase surveillance of a hospitalized client at times when staffing is predictably low (e.g., staff meetings, change of shift report, periods of unit disruption). *Clients who remain intent on suicide will be watchful of periods when staff surveillance lessens to permit completion of a suicide plan.*
- Consider strategies to decrease isolation and opportunity to act on harmful thoughts

S

(e.g., use of a sitter). **EBN:** *Clients have reported feeling safe and having their hope restored in response to close observation (Bowers & Park, 2001).*

- Observe, record, and report any changes in mood or behavior that may signify increasing suicide risk and document results of regular surveillance checks. *Suicidal ideation often is not continuous; it may decrease then increase in response to negative thinking or exposure to stressors (e.g., family visits). Documentation of surveillance will alert all members of the health care team to changes in the client's potential risk for suicide so they may be prepared to respond in the event of suicidal behavior.*
- Explain suicide precautions and relevant safety issues to the client and family (e.g., purpose, duration, behavioral expectations, and behavioral consequences). **EBN:** *Suicide precautions may be viewed as restrictive. Clients have reported the loss of privacy as distressing (Bowers & Park, 2001). Explanations will highlight the importance of taking suicidal behavior seriously, as well as emphasize that the client makes choices and is an integral part of his or her own care.*

▲ Refer for treatment and participate in the management of any psychiatric illness or symptoms that may be contributing to the client's suicidal ideation or behavior. *Psychiatric disorders have been associated with suicidal behavior. Symptoms of the disorder may require treatment with antidepressant, antipsychotic, or antianxiety medications.*

▲ Verify that the client has taken medications as ordered (e.g., conduct mouth checks after medication administration). *The client may attempt to hoard medications for a later suicide attempt.*

▲ Maintain increased surveillance of the client whenever use of an antidepressant has been initiated or the dose increased. Antidepressant medications take anywhere from 2 to 6 weeks to achieve full efficacy. *During that period the client's energy level may increase, although the depression has not yet lifted, which increases the potential for suicide.*

- Search the environment routinely and remove dangerous items. *Action is necessary to maintain a hazard-free environment and client safety. Controlling the environment may be a viable strategy for preventing suicide (Leenaars et al, 2000).*
- Limit access to windows and exits unless locked and shatterproof, as appropriate. *Suicidal behavior may include attempts to jump out of windows or to escape the unit to find other means of suicide (e.g., gaining roof access for a jump). Hospitals should ensure that exits are secure.*
- Monitor the client during the use of potential weapons (e.g., razor, scissors). *Clients with suicidal intent may take advantage of any opportunity to harm themselves.*
- Involve the client in treatment planning and self-care management of psychiatric disorders. *Self-care management promotes feelings of self-efficacy (Lorig et al, 2001), particularly for clients with depression (Allen & Hagerty, 2003; Ellis, 2004). Suicidal ideation may occur in response to a sense of hopelessness, a sense that the client has no control over life circumstances. The more clients participate in their own care, the less powerless and hopeless they feel. Refer to the care plan for* **Powerlessness.**
- Develop a positive therapeutic relationship with the client; do not make promises that may not be kept. *Clients will speak of their suicidal ideation more readily if they feel a connection with the nurse. Be aware that some clients may offer to self-disclose if the nurse will promise not to tell anyone what they have said. Clarify with the client that*

*anything they share will be communicated only to other staff, but that secrets cannot be kept.*

- Interact with the client at regular intervals to convey caring and openness and to provide opportunities for the client to talk about feelings. *Emotional safety is promoted when the nurse helps the client to become aware of feelings, name them, and develop strategies to express distress more constructively.*
- Explore with the client all circumstances and motivations related to the suicidality. *Interpersonal conflict is a frequent precipitating factor in suicidal ideation and should be addressed, even if the primary focus of treatment is to be an underlying psychiatric disorder (Isacsson & Rich, 2001).*
- Explore with the client all perceived consequences that could act as a barrier to suicide (e.g., affect on family, religious beliefs). Be aware that resources should not be assumed to be barriers to suicide without exploring the client's feelings toward them. **EBN:** *A study of older Caucasian men revealed that the most common barrier to suicide was consequences to family members (Bell, 2000). When familial relations are strained, however, consequences to family members may not be a barrier if the client perceives suicide as a way to punish others.*
- Encourage the client to seek out care providers to talk whenever the urge to harm himself or herself occurs. *Listening, being supportive, exploring antecedents to suicidal ideation, and helping the client verbalize pain and fear provide an alternative to suicide (Horsfall, 1999). Much of suicidality results from the client's frustrated efforts at affiliation (Schneidman, 2001); thus the nurse-client relationship provides needed empathetic contact.*
- Avoid repeated discussion of the client's suicide history by keeping discussion oriented to the present and future. *Clients under stress have difficulty focusing their thoughts, which leads to a sense of being overwhelmed by problems. Focusing on the present and future helps the client to address problem solving with regard to current stressors, while avoiding secondary gain from idealizing past behavior.*
- ▲ Discuss plans for dealing with suicidal ideation in the future (e.g., how to identify precipitating factors, whom to contact, where to go for help, how to respond to desire for self-harm) and for dealing with questions from friends and others about the client's hospitalization/suicide attempt. *Clients are supported in self-care management when they are helped to identify actions they can take if suicidal ideation recurs. However, the social stigma attached to the client's behavior can create stress and discomfort, potentially leading to additional feelings of alienation and suicidal ideation.*
- ▲ Assist the client in identifying a network of supportive persons and resources (e.g., clergy, family, care providers). *Clients who are suicidal often feel alienated from others and benefit from actions that facilitate support of the client by family and friends.*
- ▲ Refer family members and friends to local mental health agencies and crisis intervention centers if the client has suicidal ideation or a suspicion of suicidal thoughts exists. *Clients at risk should receive evaluation and help (American Psychiatric Association, 2005).*
- ▲ Consider outpatient commitment or an overnight psychiatric observation program for an actively suicidal client. *Involuntary outpatient commitment can improve treatment, reduce the likelihood of hospital readmission, and reduce episodes of violent behavior in persons with severe psychiatric illnesses (Torrey & Zdanowicz, 2001). Overnight psychiatric*

S

*observation followed by outpatient referral also can be an effective alternative to traditional hospitalization without leading to an increase in suicide gestures or attempts (Francis et al, 2000).*

- Cognitive behavioral techniques help the client to modify thinking styles that promote depression, hopelessness, and a belief that suicide is a valid means of escaping the current situation. *Suicide has been shown to be associated with constriction in cognitive style, leading to decreased problem solving and information processing (Sheehy & O'Connor, 2002).* **EBN:** *Cognitive behavioral techniques and the promotion of problem-solving skills, combined with the therapeutic relationship, have been posited as key interventions when dealing with the hopelessness inherent to suicidal ideation (Collins & Cutcliffe, 2003).*
- Group interventions can be useful to address recurrent suicide attempts. **EB:** *A study in progress incorporated the following principles: validation of the client's struggle, instillation of hope, framing the client as "expert" in his/her life experience, use of "solution talk," and identifying appropriate expectations about the group process. Thus far, findings support the willingness of participants to attend the group, and the clients' perceptions that their suicidal behaviors had decreased (Bergmans & Links, 2002).*

▲ If imminent suicide is suspected or an attempt has occurred, call for assistance and do not leave the client alone. *Client and staff safety will be served by assistance in the response. The client may attempt additional self-harm if left alone.*

▲ With the client's consent, facilitate family-oriented crisis intervention. *Family-oriented crisis intervention can clarify stresses and allow assessment of family dynamics.* **EB:** *A study of depressed adult inpatients revealed that the families of suicidal clients were considered more dysfunctional than the families of clients with no history of attempted suicide (McDermut et al, 2001).*

▲ Involve the family in discharge planning (e.g., illness/medication teaching, recognition of increasing suicidal risk, client's plan for dealing with recurring suicidal thoughts, community resources). *Suicidal clients often are ambivalent about hurting themselves; they may not want to die so much as to escape an intolerable situation. Consequently they often leave clues about their state of mind. Family members can learn to respond to clues early, support the treatment regimen, and encourage the client to initiate the emergency plan.*

▲ Before discharge from the hospital, ensure that the client has a supply of ordered medications, has a plan for outpatient follow-up, understands the plan or has a caregiver able and willing to follow the plan, and has the ability to access outpatient treatment. *With shortened hospital stays, clients may be discharged before they have recovered substantial functional ability and may have difficulty concentrating on the plan for follow-up. They may need the assistance of others to ensure that prescriptions are filled, that they attend appointments, or that they have transportation to the outpatient care setting.* **EB:** *Nonresponse to treatment of depression has been associated with the clinical factor of suicidal ideation, socioeconomic factors (unemployment) not usually addressed by medical intervention, and medication nonadherence (Sherbourne et al, 2004).*

▲ In the event of successful suicide, refer the family to a therapy group for survivors of suicide. Recommended clinical interventions include addressing psychological distress, normalizing denial as an effective coping strategy, working with concerns about family disintegration, and helping families deal with stigmatization (Kaslow & Aronson, 2004). **EBN:** *Survivors of suicide may be reluctant to contact health care professionals, out of*

S

*fear that they will be blamed or stigmatized. Group counseling addresses the blame, anger, guilt, shame, and search for a reason for the suicide that occurs in suicide survivors (Barlow & Morrison, 2002). Psychoeducational support group participants found relief in sharing a personal narrative of their suicide bereavement with others (Mitchell et al, 2003).*

- See the care plans for **Risk for self-directed Violence, Hopelessness,** and **Risk for Self-mutilation.** *Clients with suicidal ideation often are reacting to a feeling of hopelessness.*

## Pediatric

- Determine the presence and degree of suicidal risk. A number of questions will elicit the necessary information:
  - "Did you ever feel so upset that you wished you were not alive or wanted to die?"
  - "Did you ever do something that you knew was so dangerous that you could get hurt or killed by doing it?"
  - "Did you ever hurt yourself or try to hurt yourself?"
  - "Did you ever try to kill yourself?"
  - "Did you ever think about or try to commit suicide?"
- Use brief self-report measures to improve clinical management of at-risk cases. *The Risk of Suicide Questionnaire (RSQ) is available for children and adolescents (Horowitz et al, 2001).*
- Assess for both medical and psychiatric disturbances that may contribute to suicidality. *The process leading to suicide in young people often involves untreated depression (Houston, Hawton, & Shepperd, 2001). Epilepsy has a fourfold risk increase of suicide, particularly documented in children and adolescents (Muzina, 2004).*
- Recognize that the developmental issues of childhood and adolescence may heighten suicide risks and involve different issues from those with adults. *Assessment of suicidality in children is difficult because of cognitive and language immaturity. Until the concept of causality is mastered, young children have difficulty making connections between causal events or emotional states. Lethality of an action may be misperceived; motivation varies greatly between children. Reuniting with a lost loved one may be more dangerous than gaining attention or other motivations more common at an older age (Fritz, 2004). Physically aggressive behavior learned in early childhood may translate into suicide risk (Tremblay, 2004). The rates of attempted suicide are particularly higher during adolescence. Puberty, social, and cognitive changes can lead to greater unhappiness. Rage, hopelessness, despair, and guilt are common with suicide attempts, with greater variability of suicide timing, impulsivity, and mood (Spirito & Overholser, 2003).*
- Assess specific stressors for the adolescent client. *Adolescents tend to experience concerns about personal issues, school pressures, and relationships. Poor familial communications and lack of a parental confidant may be present. Key interventions include improving family communications, addressing psychosocial issues, teaching problem-solving skills, and fostering decreased impulsivity (Webb, 2002).*
- Evaluate for the presence of self-mutilation. Refer to care plan for **Risk for Self-mutilation** for additional information. **EB:** *A study of adolescents who attempted suicide by overdose revealed that over one third of participants admitted to some method of self-mutilation. The self-mutilators were significantly more likely than nonself-mutilators to be*

*diagnosed with oppositional defiant disorder, major depression, and dysthymia, and had higher scores on measures of hopelessness, loneliness, anger, risk taking, and alcohol use (Guertin et al, 2001).*

- Be aware that complete overlap does not exist between suicidal behavior and self-mutilation. The motivation may be different (ending life rather than coping with difficult feelings), and the method is usually different. **EB:** *In one study, about half of the participants reported both attempted suicide and self-mutilation; the other half there was no overlap in types of acts (Bolognini et al, 2003).*
- Assess for the presence of an eating disorder. Attend to the themes that preoccupy teens with eating disorders who have suicidal ideations. *Suicidal behavior was shown to be more common among adolescents with dependence issues (drug abuse and eating disorders) (Bolognini et al, 2003). The thought processes of adolescents with an eating disorder were found to center on themes of feeling undeserving of receiving help, feeling helpless and hopeless in dealing with the eating disorder itself, difficulty with recognizing and expressing feelings, and ambivalence regarding treatment along with mistrust of health care providers (Manley & Leichner, 2003).*
- Parental education groups can influence suicide risk factors. **EB:** *A program of parent education groups focused on improved communication skills and relationships with adolescents. Students in the intervention group reported increased maternal care, decreased conflict with parents, decreased substance abuse, and decreased delinquency (Toumbourou & Gregg, 2002).*
- Support the implementation of school-based suicide prevention programs. *School nurses can be key to early intervention.* **EBN:** *An intervention study by school nurses on providing coping skills training and emotional support yielded a 55% decrease in suicidal ideation, a 27% decrease in perceived stress, and a 26% decrease in family distress among participating students (Houck, Darnell, & Lussman, 2002).* **EB:** *A test of the effectiveness of the Signs of Suicide (SOS) prevention program found that suicide attempts decreased, knowledge-based awareness increased, and adaptive attitudes toward depression and suicide were observed (Aseltine & DeMartino, 2004).*
- Before discharge from the hospital, ensure that the client's parent has a supply of ordered medications, has a plan for outpatient follow-up, has a caregiver who understands the plan or is able and willing to follow the plan, and has the ability to access outpatient treatment. *Lack of adequate follow-up has been associated with repeated suicide attempts among adolescents (Hulten et al, 2001).* **EB:** *A compliance enhancement intervention (including contracting interview with parent and adolescent, and telephone contacts) improved attendance at follow-up appointments only when barriers to service were controlled (e.g., delays in getting appointments, placement on a waiting list, inability to switch therapists, problems with insurance coverage) (Spirito et al, 2002).*

S

## Geriatric

- Perform careful assessment and ongoing evaluation of the potential for suicidal ideation in the older adult, particularly the older Caucasian man. **EB:** *The highest incidence of completed suicide occurs in older Caucasian men (Erlangsen et al, 2004).*
- Evaluate the older client's mental and physical health status and financial stressors. The possibility of reversible/medical causes of depression, including medical or neuro-

logical disorders, as well as psychomimetic reactions to medications, should inform nursing observations (Hall, Hall, & Chapman, 2003). *Physical illness, particularly that accompanied by chronic or unremitting pain, as well as financial difficulties can precipitate suicide in older men (Uncapher et al, 1998).*

- Explore with client any concerns or pressures (physical and financial) regarding ability to secure support of medical care, especially perceived pressures about being a burden on family. **EB:** *The suicide notes of older adults were more likely than those of younger adults to contain the theme "burden to others" (40% versus 3%, p = .03) (Foster, 2003).*
- When assessing suicide risk factors, incorporate a higher degree of risk for older men and for some older adults who have lost a loved one in the previous year. **EB:** *Although mortality for oldest old adults (80+) has increased, the suicide mortality has not decreased. In one study, oldest old men had the highest increase in suicide risk after death of a partner (more so than oldest old women) and took a longer time to recover from the death of a spouse (Erlangsen et al, 2004).*
- Monitor the older adult for subtle signs of suicidal risk. *The elderly, who experience multiple losses and have fragile support systems, are at greatest risk for suicide. Assess death wishes and suicidal thoughts. Consider noncompliance with medical treatment to be a possible means of suicide.*
- Explore triggers of and barriers to suicidal behavior, with particular attention to real and perceived losses (e.g., professional role, health). **EB:** *For adults 75 years of age or older, predictors of suicide included family conflict, serious physical illness, and both major and minor depressions. For adults 65–74 years of age, but not for the older group, economic problems were predictive of suicide (Waern, Rubenowitz, & Wilhelmson, 2003).* **EBN:** *A study of older Caucasian men revealed that losing connections initiated a process of loss and depression and triggered a decision point that could include suicidal ideation. Triggers included death of a spouse, emotional pain, health problems, and feelings of uselessness or hopelessness. A strong barrier was consequences to family members. Religion and social isolation were not relevant (Bell, 2000).*
- An older adult who shows self-destructive behaviors should be evaluated for dementia. **EB:** *In a study of nursing home residents, self-destructive behaviors were common; these behaviors were more likely related to dementia than to depression and were only weakly associated with suicidal intent (Draper et al, 2002).*
- Anticipate overall responsiveness to treatment, but monitor for early relapse. **EB:** *Older adults had high remission rates after antidepressant treatment, whether they had suicidal ideation or not. However, older adults with suicidal ideation had a higher relapse rate and a greater need for adjunctive psychotropic medications (Szanto et al, 2001).*

▲ Advocate for the older client with other professionals in securing treatment for suicidal states. Primary care physicians have been noted to underrecognize and undertreat older adult clients with depression. **EB:** *A study of primary care providers reported that, although physicians recognized depression and suicidal risk in both adults and geriatric clients, they were less willing to treat or refer the older suicidal client, viewing the suicidal ideation as rational and normal (Uncapher & Arean, 2000). In another study, older adults above age 75 with major or minor depression were less likely than those age 65–74 to receive depression treatment (Waern et al, 2003).*

S

- Encourage physical activity in older adults. *Benefits to mood have been found with exercise. Activity therapy based on an ancient Chinese system of exercise (Qigong) has been proposed as a means of preventing disease, increasing strength, and resisting premature senility, as well as improving mood among depressed elders with chronic physical illnesses (Tsang, Cheung, & Lak, 2002).* **EB:** *A study testing response to exercise, sertraline, or exercise plus sertraline found that the exercise-only group experienced the lowest depression levels, with the benefit of exercise continuing after the intervention period (Babyak et al, 2000).*
- Assist the older adult to identify protective factors that serve as resources to mitigate against suicidal ideation. *Internal and external factors that can serve as resources for the older adult include the ability to learn from experience and accept help, a sense of humor and interest in social concerns, a sense of purpose or meaning in life, a history of successful coping, caring and available family and a supportive community network, and membership in a religious community (Holkup, Tang, & Titler, 2003).*
- Collaborative care management of older adults in primary care settings is a growing area for nursing intervention. **EB:** *In a study of older adults with late life depression, nurse collaboration in a primary care setting increased treatment response, remission of depressive symptoms, therapeutic adherence, and quality of life, while reducing functional impairment (Unutzer et al, 2002). A wide-scale study of individualized care provided by "depression care managers" (social workers, nurses, psychologists) in collaboration with physicians yielded faster decline of suicidal ideation in the intervention group, along with a greater degree and speed of depression symptom reduction (Bruce et al, 2004). A comparison of physician versus nurse practitioner (NP) patterns to the care of depressed and suicidal older clients found that NPs had a greater orientation toward psychosocial approaches than did physicians. The researchers concluded that the differing perspectives of NPs and physicians could enhance the mental health care of geriatric clients (Adamek & Kaplan, 2000).*

## Multicultural

- Assess for the influence of cultural beliefs, norms, and values on the individual's perceptions of suicide. **EBN:** *What the individual believes about suicide may be based on cultural perceptions (Cochran, 1998; Doswell & Erlen, 1998; Leininger & McFarland, 2002). Among Hispanics, the largest proportion of suicides occurred among young persons; suicide rates were higher among males; and the most common method of suicide was by firearms (Centers for Disease Control and Prevention, 2004).*
- Facilitate modeling and role playing for the client and family regarding healthy ways to start a discussion about the client's suicide attempt. *It is helpful for families and the client to practice communication skills in a safe environment before trying them in a real-life situation (Rivera-Andino & Lopez, 2000).*
- Identify and acknowledge the stresses unique to culturally diverse individuals. *Financial difficulties and maintaining cultural values are two of the most common family stressors cited by women of color (Majumdar & Ladak, 1998). Suicide rates among African-American male teenagers increased 105% from 1980 to 1986 (Surgeon General, 1999), with "suicide by cop" speculated to increase these rates (Daugherty, 1999). A high rate of suicidal ideation has been reported as a result of the social discrimination experienced by gay and bisexual Latino men in the United States (Diaz et al, 2001). There may be a relationship*

S

*between the possible relationship between rapid social change and the increasing rates of suicide among Alaska Natives (Richards, 2004).*

- Identify and acknowledge unique cultural responses to stressors in determining sensitive interventions to prevent suicide. **EBN:** *In a study of African-American, Hispanic/Latino, and Caucasian adolescent girls, the Hispanic/Latino girls had a significantly higher percentage of suicide attempts. Relationships were found between recent suicide attempts and family history of suicide attempts, friend's history of suicide attempt, history of physical or sexual abuse, and environmental stress. For all three groups, rate of recent suicide attempts was also associated with stress level, social connectedness, and religious influence (Rew et al, 2001). A recent study found African-American men committed suicide at rates much lower than those for Caucasians, but they do so at much younger ages (Garlow, Purselle, & Heninger, 2005).*
- Encourage physical activity as intervention to decrease suicidal behavior. **EB:** *Increased physical activity was associated with lower suicidal feelings and suicidal behaviors in Hispanic and non-Hispanic boys (Brosnahan et al, 2004).*
- Encourage family members to demonstrate and offer caring and support to each other. **EB:** *The familial characteristics of care and support may be associated with fostering resilience in African-American families. Resilience is the ability to experience adverse conditions and successfully overcome them (Calvert, 1997). Family closeness is strong resiliency factor of suicidal behavior in African-American and Hispanic youths (O'Donnell et al, 2004).*
- Encourage family meals. **EB:** *Frequency of family meals was inversely associated with tobacco, alcohol, and marijuana use; low grade point average; depressive symptoms; and suicide involvement (Eisenberg et al, 2004).*
- Foster the client's use of available family and religious supports. **EB:** *Christian religious roots and family closeness, although eroding among many young African Americans, traditionally have worked against suicidal behavior among African Americans (Neeleman, Wessely, & Lewis, 1998).*
- Validate the individual's feelings regarding concerns about the current crisis and family functioning. *Validation lets the client know that the nurse has heard and understood what was said, and it promotes the nurse-client relationship (Stuart & Laraia, 2001; Giger & Davidhizar, 1995).*

S

## Home Care

- Communicate the degree of risk to family/caregivers; assess the family and caregiving situation for ability to protect the client and to understand the client's suicidal behavior. Provide the family and caregivers with guidelines on how to manage self-harm behaviors in the home environment. *Client safety between home visits is a nursing priority. Family/caregivers may become frightened by the client's suicidal ideation, may be angry at the client's perceived lack of self-control, or may feel as if they are walking on eggshells awaiting another suicide attempt. Appropriate family/caregiver support is important to the client and will be forthcoming only if all parties understand the basis of the suicidal behavior and how to respond to it.*

▲ Establish an emergency plan, including when to use hotlines and 911. Develop a contract with the client and family for use of the emergency plan. Role play access to the emergency resources with the client and caregivers. *Having an emergency plan reassures the client and caregivers and promotes client safety. Contracting gives guided control to the client and enhances self-esteem.*

- Assess the home environment for harmful objects, especially guns. Have the family remove or lock up objects as possible. *Client safety is a nursing priority.*
- Counsel parents and homeowners to restrict unauthorized access to potentially lethal prescription drugs and firearms within the home. *Identifying teens at high risk of firearm suicide and limiting access to firearms is a type of public health intervention likely to be successful in preventing firearm suicides (Shah, 2000).*
- Identify the client's concerns and implement interventions to address the consequences of disability in a client with medical illness. **EB:** *In a study of cancer clients being cared for at home, primary factors influencing vulnerability to suicide were identified as real or feared loss of autonomy and independence, concerns about being a burden on others, hopelessness about the health condition, and fear of suffering (Filiberti et al, 2001). Hopelessness and demoralization in conjunction with dependence have been noted as precursors to suicidal ideation in palliative care clients (Kissane, Clarke, & Street, 2001). Refer to the care plans for* **Hopelessness** *and* **Powerlessness.**

▲ If the client's suicidal ideation intensifies, or if a suicide plan with access to means becomes evident, institute an emergency plan for mental health intervention. *The degree of disturbance and the ability to manage care safely at home determines the level of services needed to protect the client. Approximately 25% of clients who are hospitalized after a suicide attempt kill themselves within 3 months after hospitalization (Appleby et al, 1999).*

▲ Refer for homemaker or psychiatric home health care services for respite, client reassurance, and implementation of a therapeutic regimen. *Respite decreases the high degree of caregiver stress that goes with the responsibility of caring for a person at risk for suicide. The presence of caring individuals is reassuring to both the client and caregivers, especially during periods of client anxiety. A client with suicidal ideation, especially if the ideation is accompanied by depression or other psychiatric disorders, can benefit from use of the interventions described earlier, modified for the home setting.* **EB:** *In a study of community-integrated home-based treatment for depression, depressive symptoms were significantly reduced in elderly participants, and improved health status was noted in chronically medically ill older adults with minor depression and dysthymia (Ciechanowski et al, 2004).*

- Telephone contacts can serve as an effective intervention for suicidal older adults. **EBN:** *Nurse telehealth care, involving an average of 10 calls over 16 weeks to answer questions, offer support, and discuss overall health, reduced depressive symptoms better than usual physician care (Hunkeler et al, 2000).* **EB:** *A protocol of twice-weekly support calls resulted in significantly fewer suicide deaths among women, although not among men. The researchers concluded that outreach, continuity of care, and increased emotional support provided protection against suicide, at least for women (DeLeo, Dello Buono, & Dwyer, 2002).*

▲ If the client is on psychotropic medications, assess the client's and family's knowledge of medication administration and side effects. Teach as necessary. *Knowledge of the medical regimen promotes compliance and promotes safe use of medications.*

▲ Evaluate the effectiveness and side effects of medications, and adherence to the medi-

S

cation regimen. Review with the client and family all medications kept in the home; encourage discarding of old prescriptions. Monitor the amount of medications ordered/provided by the physician; limiting the amount of medications to which the client has access may be necessary. *Accurate clinical feedback improves the physician's ability to prescribe an effective medical regimen specific to the client's needs. At home, clients may have greater access to medications, including old prescriptions, that may be used to overdose.*

## Client/Family Teaching

- Establish a supportive relationship with family members. **EBN:** *When families with a suicidal member experienced mental health care personnel as reaching out to them, they reported an ability to trust the personnel, treatment, and care; a feeling of being trusted; and a sense of hope (Talseth, Gilje, & Norberg, 2001).*
- Explain all relevant symptoms, procedures, treatments, and expected outcomes for suicidal ideation that is illness based (e.g., depression, bipolar disorder). *Self-care management has been posited to empower clients with depression and suicidal ideation (Allen & Hagerty, 2003). By increasing knowledge and adapting new behaviors, clients learn that they have some control over their health (Hennessy-Harstad, 1999). Clients are more amenable to therapy and better able to initiate appropriate self-care if they know what to expect.*
- Teach the family how to recognize that the client is at increased risk for suicide (changes in behavior and verbal and nonverbal communication, withdrawal, depression, or sudden lifting of depression). *A client may be at peace because a suicide plan has been made and the client has the energy to carry it out. Therefore when depression lifts, increased vigilance is necessary.*
- Provide written instructions for treatments and procedures for which the client will be responsible. *A written record provides a concrete reference so that the client and family can clarify any verbal information that was given.*
- Instruct the client in coping strategies (assertiveness training, impulse control training, deep breathing, progressive muscle relaxation*). Suicidal ideation may be triggered by stress and painful emotions. Once clients are able to identify these triggers, they need to learn how to respond to them more effectively through assertiveness, impulse control, or relaxation techniques, as appropriate.*
- Role play (e.g., say, "Tell me how you will respond if a friend asks why you were in the hospital"). *Role playing is the most commonly used technique in assertiveness training. It deconditions the anxiety that arises from interpersonal encounters by allowing the client to practice how he or she might respond in a given situation. Anxiety levels tend to be higher in situations that are unfamiliar.*
- Teach cognitive behavioral activities, such as active problem solving, reframing (reappraising the situation from a different perspective), or thought stopping (in response to a negative thought, picturing a large stop sign and replacing the image with a prearranged positive alternative). Teach the client to confront his or her own negative thought patterns (or cognitive distortions), such as catastrophizing (expecting the very worst), dichotomous thinking (perceiving events in only one of two opposite categories), or magnification (placing distorted emphasis on a single event). *Depressed and suicidal clients often have negative perceptions of themselves, their circumstances, and their*

S

*future. Cognitive behavioral activities address clients' assumptions, beliefs, and attitudes about their situations, and foster modification of these elements to be as realistic and optimistic as possible. Persons with negative cognitive styles tend to perceive situations as overwhelming, resistant to improvement, and all encompassing. Through cognitive behavioral interventions, clients become more aware of their cognitive choices in adopting and maintaining their belief systems and thereby exercise greater control over their own reactions (Hagerty & Patusky, 2003).*

▲ Provide the client and family with phone numbers of appropriate community agencies for therapy and counseling. Continuous follow-up care should be implemented; therefore the method to access this care must be given to the client.

## evolve WEBSITES FOR EDUCATION

See the EVOLVE website for World Wide Web resources for client education.

## REFERENCES


Adamek ME, Kaplan MS: Caring for depressed and suicidal older patients: a survey of physicians and nurse practitioners, *Int J Psychiatry Med* 30(2):111, 2000.

Allen KS, Hagerty BM: Depression in primary care: empowering depressed patients to monitor their recurrent depression, article in preparation, 2003.

American Psychiatric Association—Medical Specialty Society: *Practice guideline for the assessment and treatment of patients with suicidal behaviors.* Available www.ngc.gov/summary/summary.aspx?doc_id=4529&nbr=3343&string=suicide, accessed January 10, 2005.

Appleby L, Shaw J, Amos T et al: Suicide within 12 months of contact with mental health services: national clinical survey, *BMJ* 318(7193):1235, 1999.

Apter A, Horesh N, Gothelf D et al: Relationship between self-disclosure and serious suicidal behavior, *Compr Psychiatry* 42(1):70, 2001.

Aseltine Jr RH, DeMartino R: An outcome evaluation of the SS suicide prevention program, *Am J Public Health* 94:446, 2004.

Babyak M, Blumenthal JA, Herman S et al: Exercise treatment for major depression: maintenance of therapeutic benefit at 10 months, *Psychosom Med* 62:633, 2000.

Barlow CA, Morrison H: Survivors of suicide. Emerging counseling strategies, *J Psychosoc Nurs Ment Health Serv* 40(1):28, 2002.

Befrienders International: *The warning signs of suicide.* Available at www.befrienders.org/suicide.htm, accessed June 22, 2003.

Bell MA: *Losing connections: a process of decision-making in late-life suicidality*, doctoral dissertation, Tucson, Ariz, 2000, University of Arizona.

Bergmans Y, Links PS: A description of a psychosocial/psychoeducational intervention for persons with recurrent suicide attempts, *Crisis* 23(4):156, 2002.

Bolognini M, Plancherel B, Laget J et al: Adolescents' self-mutilation: relationship with dependent behaviour, *Swiss J Psychol* 62(4):241, 2003.

Bowers L, Park A: Special observation in the care of psychiatric inpatients: a literature review, *Issues Ment Health Nurs* 22:769, 2001.

Brosnahan J, Steffen LM, Lytle L et al: The relation between physical activity and mental health among Hispanic and non-Hispanic white adolescents, *Arch Pediatr Adolesc Med* 158(8):818-823, 2004.

Brown GS, Jones ER, Betts E et al: Improving suicide risk assessment in a managed-care environment, *Crisis* 24(2):49, 2003.

Bruce ML, Ten Have TR, Reynolds CF III et al: Reducing suicidal ideation and depressive symptoms in depressed older primary care patients: a randomized controlled trial, *JAMA* 291:1081, 2004.

Calvert WJ: Protective factors within the family, and their role in fostering resiliency in African American adolescents, *J Cult Divers* 4(4):110, 1997.

Centers for Disease Control and Prevention (CDC): Suicide among Hispanics—United States, 1997-2001, *MMWR Morb Mort Wkly Rep* 53(22):478-81, 2004.

Ciechanowski P, Wagner E, Schmaling K et al: Community-integrated home-based depression treatment in older adults: a randomized controlled trial, *JAMA* 291(13):1569, 2004.


S

Cochran M: Tears have no color, *Am J Nurs* 98(6):53, 1998.
Collins S, Cutcliffe JR: Addressing hopelessness in people with suicidal ideation: building upon the therapeutic relationship utilizing a cognitive behavioural approach, *J Psychiatr Ment Health Nurs* 10:175, 2003.
Cutcliffe JR, Barker P: The Nurses' Global Assessment of Suicide Risk (NGASR): developing a tool for clinical practice, *J Psychiatr Ment Health Nurs* 11(4):393, 2004.
Daugherty M: Suicide by cop, *J Calif Alliance Ment Ill* 10(2):79, 1999.
De Leo D, Della Buono M, Dwyer J: Suicide among the elderly: the long-term impact of a telephone support and assessment intervention in northern Italy, *Br J Psychiatr* 181:226, 2002.
Diaz RM, Ayala G, Bein E et al: The impact of homophobia, poverty, and racism on the mental health of gay and bisexual Latino men: findings from 3 US cities, *Am J Public Health* 91:927, 2001.
Doswell W, Erlen J: Multicultural issues and ethical concerns in the delivery of nursing care interventions, *Nurs Clin North Am* 33(2):353, 1998.
Draper B, Brodaty H, Low LF et al: Self-destructive behaviors in nursing home residents, *J Am Geriatr Soc* 50:354, 2002.
Drew BL: Self-harm behavior and no-suicide contracting in psychiatric inpatient settings, *Arch Psychiatr Nurs* 15:99, 2001.
Eisenberg ME, Olson RE, Neumark-Sztainer D et al: Correlations between family meals and psychosocial well-being among adolescents, *Arch Pediatr Adolesc Med* 158(8):792-796, 2004.
Ellis TE: Collaboration and a self-help orientation in therapy with suicidal clients, *J Contemp Psychother* 34(1):41, 2004.
Erlangsen A, Jeune B, Bille-Brahe U et al: Loss of partner and suicide risks among oldest old: a population-based register study, *Age Ageing* 33:378, 2004.
Farrow TL: Owning their expertise: why nurses use "no suicide contracts" rather than their own assessments, *Int J Ment Health Nurs* 11:214, 2002.
Farrow TL: "No suicide contracts" in community crisis situations: a conceptual analysis, *J Psychiatr Ment Health Nurs* 10:199, 2003.
Filiberti A, Ripamonti C, Totis A et al: Characteristics of terminal cancer patients who committed suicide during a home palliative care program, *J Pain Symptom Manage* 22:544, 2001.
Fisher BJ, Haythornthwaite JA, Heinberg LJ et al: Suicidal intent in patients with chronic pain, *Pain* 89(2-3):199, 2001.
Foster T: Suicide note themes and suicide prevention, *Int J Psychiatry Med* 33(4):323, 2003.
Francis E, Marchand W, Hart M et al: Utilization and outcome in an overnight psychiatric observation program at a Veterans Affairs medical center, *Psychiatr Serv* 51:92, 2000.
Fritz GK: Suicide in young children (editorial), *Brown Univ Child Adolesc Behav Lett* 20(7):8, 2004.
Garlow SJ, Purselle D, Heninger M: Ethnic differences in patterns of suicide across the life cycle, *Am J Psychiatry* 162(2):319-323, 2005.
Gilman SE, Cochran SD, Mays VM et al: Risk of psychiatric disorders among individuals reporting same-sex sexual partners in the National Comorbidity Survey, *Am J Public Health* 91:933, 2001.
Graham TLC: Using reasons for living to connect to American Indian healing traditions, *J Sociol Soc Welfare* 29(1):55, 2002.
Guertin T, Lloyd-Richardson E, Spirito A et al: Self-mutilative behavior in adolescents who attempt suicide by overdose, *J Am Acad Child Adolesc Psychiatry* 40(9):1062, 2001.
Hagerty B, Patusky K: Mood disorders: depression and mania. In Fortinash KM, Holoday-Worret PA, editors: *Psychiatric mental health nursing,* ed 3, St Louis, 2003, Mosby.
Hall RCW, Hall RCW, Chapman MJ: Identifying geriatric patients at risk for suicide and depression, *Clin Geriatr* 11(10):36, 2003.
Hauenstein EJ: Case finding and care in suicide: children, adolescents, and adults. In Boyd MA, editor: *Psychiatric nursing: contemporary practice,* ed 2, Philadelphia, 2002, Lippincott.
Hennessy-Harstad EB: Empowering adolescents with asthma to take control through adaptation, *J Pediatr Health Care* 13:273, 1999.
Holkup PA, Tang JH, Titler MG: Evidence-based protocol elderly suicide—secondary prevention, *J Gerontol Nurs* 29(6):6, 2003.
Hopkins C: But what about the really ill, poor people? *J Psychiatr Ment Health Nurs* 9:147, 2002.
Horowitz LM, Wang PS, Koocher GP et al: Detecting suicide risk in a pediatric emergency department: development of a brief screening tool, *Pediatrics* 107:1133, 2001.
Horsfall J: Towards understanding some complex borderline behaviors, *J Psychiatr Ment Health Nurs* 6:425, 1999.
Houck GM, Darnell S, Lussman S: A support group intervention for at-risk female high school students, *J School Nurs* 18(4):212, 2002.
Houston K, Hawton K, Shepperd R: Suicide in young people aged 15-24: a psychological autopsy study, *J Affect Disord* 63(1-3):159, 2001.

Hulten A, Jiang GX, Wasserman D et al: Repetition of attempted suicide among teenagers in Europe: frequency, timing and risk factors, *Eur Child Adolesc Psychiatry* 10:161, 2001.
Hunkeler EM, Meresman JF, Hargreaves WA et al: Efficacy of nurse telehealth care and peer support in augmenting treatment of depression in primary care, *Arch Fam Med* 9:700, 2000.
Isacsson G, Rich CL: Management of patients who deliberately harm themselves, *BMJ* 322:213, 2001.
Joachim G, Acorn S: Stigma of visible and invisible chronic conditions, *J Adv Nurs* 32(1):243, 2000.
Kaslow NJ, Aronson SG: Recommendations for family interventions following a suicide, *Professional Psychol Res Pract* 35(3):240, 2004.
Kernberg OF: The suicidal risk in severe personality disorders: differential diagnosis and treatment, *J Pers Disord* 15(3), 2001.
Kissane DW, Clarke DM, Street AF: Demoralization syndrome—relevant psychiatric diagnosis for palliative care, *J Palliat Care* 17(1):12, 2001.
Lambert MT: Suicide risk assessment and management: focus on personality disorders, *Curr Opin Psychiatry* 16:71, 2003.
Leenaars A, Cantor C, Connolly J et al: Controlling the environment to prevent suicide: international perspectives, *Can J Psychiatry* 45(7):639, 2000.
Leininger MM, McFarland MR: *Transcultural nursing: concepts, theories, research and practices,* ed 3, New York, 2002, McGraw-Hill.
Lorig KR, Ritter P, Stewart AL et al: Chronic disease self-management program: 2-year health status and health care utilization outcomes, *Med Care* 39:1217, 2001.
Luoma JB, Martin CE, Pearson JL: Contact with mental health and primary care providers before suicide: a review of the evidence, *Am J Psychiatry* 159:909, 2002.
Majumdar B, Ladak S: Management of family and workplace stress experienced by women of color from various cultural backgrounds, *Can J Public Health* 89(1):48, 1998.
Malone KM, Oquendo MA, Haas GL et al: Protective factors against suicidal acts in major depression: reasons for living, *Am J Psychiatry* 157:1084, 2000.
Manley RS, Leichner P: Anguish and despair in adolescents with eating disorders: helping to manage suicidal ideation and impulses, *Crisis* 24(1):32, 2003.
McDermut W, Miller IW, Solomon D et al: Family functioning and suicidality in depressed adults, *Compr Psychiatry* 42:96, 2001.
Mitchell AM, Gale DD, Garand L et al: The use of narrative data to inform the psychotherapeutic group process with suicide survivors, *Issues Ment Health Nurs* 24:91, 2003.
Muzina DJ: What physicians can do to prevent suicide, *Cleveland Clinic J Med* 71(3):242, 2004.
Neeleman J, Wessely S, Lewis G: Suicide acceptability in African and white Americans: the role of religion, *J Nerv Ment Dis* 186: 12, 1998.
O'Donnell L, O'Donnell C, Wardlaw DM et al: Risk and resiliency factors influencing suicidality among urban African American and Latino youth, *Am J Community Psychol* 33(1-2):37-49, 2004.
Pies R: Bipolar disorder and suicide: an update, *Psychiatric Times Supplement, Bipolar Disorder and Impulsive Spectrum Letter*:1, February 2004.
Power PJR, Bell RJ, Mills R et al: Suicide prevention in first episode psychosis: the development of a randomized controlled trial of cognitive therapy for acutely suicidal patients with early psychosis, *Austr N Z J Psychiatry* 37:414, 2003.
Quan H, Arboleda-Florez J: Elderly suicide in Alberta: difference by gender, *Can J Psychiatry* 44:762, 1999.
Rew L, Thomas N, Horner SD et al: Correlates of recent suicide attempts in a triethnic group of adolescents, *J Nurs Scholarsh* 33: 361, 2001.
Richards B: From respect to rights to entitlement, blocked aspirations and suicidal behavior, *Int J Circumpolar Health* (Suppl 1):19-24, 2004.
Rivera-Andino J, Lopez L: When culture complicates care, *RN* 63(7):47, 2000.
Rogers JR, Lewis MM, Subich LM: Validity of the Suicide Assessment Checklist in an emergency crisis center, *J Counsel Develop* 80:493, 2002.
Rudd MD, Ellis TE, Rajab MH et al: Personality types and suicidal behavior: an exploratory study, *Suicide Life Threat Behav* 30(3):199, 2000.
Schneidman E: *Contemporary suicide,* Washington, DC, 2001, American Psychological Association.
Shah S, Hoffman RE, Wake L et al: Adolescent suicide and household access to firearms in Colorado: results of a case-control study, *J Adolesc Health* 26(3):157, 2000.
Sheehy N, O'Connor RC: Cognitive style and suicidal behaviour: implications for therapeutic intervention, research lacunae and priorities, *Br J Guidance Counsel* 30(4):353, 2002.

S

Sherbourne C, Schoenbaum M, Wells KB et al: Characteristics, treatment patterns, and outcomes of persistent depression despite treatment in primary care, *Genl Hosp Psychiatry* 26:106, 2004.

Spirito A, Boergers J, Donaldson D et al: An intervention trial to improve adherence to community treatment by adolescents after a suicide attempt, *J Am Acad Child Adolesc Psychiatry* 41(4):435, 2002.

Spirito A, Overholser J: The suicidal child: assessment and management of adolescents after a suicide attempt, *Child Adolesc Psychiatric Clin North Am* 12:649, 2003.

Stuart GW, Laraia MT: Therapeutic nurse-patient relationship. In Stuart GW, Laraia MT, editors: *Principles and practice of psychiatric nursing,* St Louis, 2001, Mosby.

Surgeon General: *The Surgeon General's call to action to prevent suicide, 1999.* Available at www.surgeongeneral.gov/library/calltoaction/fact3.htm, accessed Dec 1, 2002.

Szanto K, Mulsant BH, Houck PR et al: Treatment outcome in suicidal vs. non-suicidal elderly patients, *Am J Geriatr Psychiatry* 9(3):261, 2001.

Talseth A, Gilje F, Norberg A: Being met—a passageway to hope for relatives of patients at risk of committing suicide: a phenomenological hermeneutic study, *Arch Psychiatr Nurs* 15:249, 2001.

Tandon R, Jibson MD: Suicidal behavior in schizophrenia: diagnosis, neurobiology, and treatment implications, *Curr Opin Psychiatry* 16:193, 2003.

Torrey EF, Zdanowicz M: Outpatient commitment: what, why, and for whom, *Psychiatr Serv* 52(3):337, 2001.

Toumbourou JW, Gregg ME: Impact of an empowerment-based parent education program on the reduction of youth suicide risk factors, *J Adolesc Health* 31:277, 2002.

Tremblay RE: Physical aggression during early childhood: trajectories and predictors, *Pediatrics* 114(1):43, 2004.

Tsang HWH, Cheung L, Lak DCC: Qigong as a psychsocial intervention for depressed elderly with chronic physical illness, *Int J Geriatr Psychiatry* 17:1146, 2002.

Uncapher H, Arean PA: Physicians are less willing to treat suicidal ideation in older patients, *J Am Geriatr Soc* 48:188, 2000.

Uncapher H, Gallagher-Thompson D, Osgood NJ et al: Hopelessness and suicidal ideation in older adults, *Gerontologist* 38:62, 1998.

Unutzer J, Katon W, Callahan CM: Collaborative care management of late-life depression in the primary care setting: a randomized controlled trial, *JAMA* 288:2836, 2002.

Waern M, Rubenowitz E, Wilhelmson K: Predictors of suicide in the old elderly, *Gerontology* 49:328, 2003.

Webb L: Deliberate self-harm in adolescence: a systematic review of psychological and psychosocial factors, *J Adv Nurs* 38(3):235, 2002.

Zaloshnja E, Miller TR, Galbraith MS: Reducing injuries among Native Americans: five cost-outcome analyses, *Accident Anal Prevent* 35:631, 2003.

# Delayed Surgical recovery

evolve

*Gail B. Ladwig*

S

**NANDA**

## Definition

Extension in number of postoperative days required for individuals to initiate and perform on their own behalf activities that maintain life, health, and well-being

## Defining Characteristics

Evidence of interrupted healing of surgical area (e.g., redness, induration, draining, immobility); loss of appetite with or without nausea; difficulty in moving about; need for help to complete self-care; fatigue; report of pain or discomfort; postponement in resumption of employment activities; perception that more time is needed to recover

## Related Factors (r/t)

To be developed

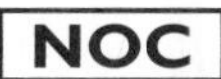

## Outcomes (Nursing Outcomes Classification)

### Suggested NOC Outcomes

Endurance; Infection Severity; Mobility; Pain Control; Self-Care: Activities of Daily Living (ADLs); Wound Healing: Primary Intention

#### Example NOC Outcome with Indicators

**Wound Healing: Primary Intention** as evidenced by the following indicators: Skin approximation/Scar formation (Rate each indicator of **Wound Healing: Primary Intention:** 1 = none, 2 = limited, 3 = moderate, 4 = substantial, 5 = extensive [see Section I].)

## Client Outcomes

**Client Will (Specify Time Frame):**

- Have surgical area that shows evidence of healing: no redness, induration, draining, or immobility
- State that appetite is regained
- State that no nausea is present
- Demonstrate ability to move about
- Demonstrate ability to complete self-care activities
- State that no fatigue is present
- State that pain is controlled or relieved after nursing interventions
- Resume employment activities/ADLs

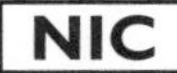

## Interventions (Nursing Interventions Classification)

### Suggested NIC Interventions

Incision Site Care, Nutrition Management, Pain Management, Self-Care Assistance

S

#### Example NIC Activities—Incision Site Care, Nutrition Management

Teach client and/or family how to care for the incision, including how to recognize signs and symptoms of infection; provide client with high-protein, high-calorie, nutritious finger foods and drinks that can be readily consumed, as appropriate

## Nursing Interventions and Rationales

- Perform a thorough assessment of the client, including risk factors. Allow time to be with the client. **EBN:** *Nursing interventions can either enhance or delay the healing process (King, 2001).* **EBN:** *In this study of clients in the perioperative period when the nurse made time to talk with them they felt eased, were made more confident, and gained faith in the* *success of their operation. The perioperative dialogue allowed the patients time with the nurse and was experienced by them as having a positive effect on the healing process and recovery (Rudolffson et al , 2004).*

- ▲ Assess for the presence of medical conditions and treat appropriately before surgery. If the client is diabetic, maintain normal blood glucose levels before surgery. **EB:** *Good blood glucose control promotes faster healing (Cavanaugh et al, 1999). Good diabetes control in the hospital is vital. High blood glucose levels slow healing and increase risk of infection. The American Diabetes Association recommends that blood glucose should be less than 180 mg/dL for people in the hospital or having surgery. For some, the goal is less than 110 mg/dL (Anonymous, 2005).*
- ▲ Carefully assess clients use of dietary supplements such as feverfew, ginkgo biloba, garlic, ginseng, ginger, valerian, kava, St. John's wort, ephedra (Ma huang or metabolite), and echinacea. It is recommended that all patients be advised to stop all dietary supplements at least 1 week before major surgical or diagnostic procedures. *Dietary supplements are commonly used by patients of all ages, yet few patients reveal use of these products to their medical providers. Certain dietary supplements can react or interact with frequently used surgical medications—including anesthesia—and may cause serious unforeseen consequences or complications. Arrhythmias, poor wound healing, bleeding, photosensitivity reaction, and prolonged sedation are among the serious reactions during and after surgical and diagnostic procedures that have been attributed to these products (Ciocon et al, 2004).*
- • Provide preoperative teaching by a nurse to decrease postoperative problems of anxiety, pain, nausea, and lack of independence. **EBN:** *One study showed a significant decrease in anxiety 24–72 hours postoperatively for the group who had preoperative teaching by a nurse. The author recommends that all surgical clients receive a visit from theater nurses before their operations (Martin, 1996).* **EBN:** *Those who displayed high fear wanted informational support from nurses more often than clients who showed lower fear. It was concluded that the fear and anxiety of clients awaiting coronary artery bypass grafting (CABG) are connected with their social support resources (Koivula et al, 2002).*
- • Provide preoperative information in verbal and written form. **EBN:** *Receipt of preparatory information of various types and in different forms appears to have positive effects on clients' ability to cope with and recover physically from a total hip replacement. Clients who received such information required significantly less postoperative intramuscular analgesia and were mobilized sooner with a Zimmer frame and walking sticks. In addition, their length of stay was, on average, 2 days shorter than that of the control group (Gammon & Mulholland, 1996).*
- • Play music of the client's choice preoperatively, intraoperatively, and postoperatively. **EBN:** *In this study in China it was demonstrated that the administration of self-selected music to day procedure patients in the preprocedure period can be effective in the reduction of physiological parameters and anxiety (Lee, Henderson, & Shum, 2004).* **EBN:** *Study results of these outpatient orthopedic clients indicate that participants overwhelmingly felt that music listening was a positive addition to traditional pain and anxiety management (Lukas, 2004).*
- ▲ Consider using healing touch in the perianesthesia setting and other mind body spirit interventions such as stress control and imagery. **EBN:** *Energy-medicine therapy such*

S

*as healing touch is a powerful way to promote relaxation and enhance the healing process in the perianesthesia setting (King, 2000).* **EBN:** *Many common medical, surgical, and diagnostic procedures performed for conscious patients can be accompanied by significant anxiety. Analysis of complete data from 108 patients showed that stress management, imagery, and touch therapy all produced reductions in reported worry, as compared with standard therapy (Seskevitch, 2004).*

- • For female premenopausal clients, assess the date when the menstrual cycle is most likely to occur and schedule surgery on alternate dates if possible. **EB:** *Menstruation at the time of surgery increases the likelihood of vomiting to four times higher than normal (Haynes & Bailey, 1996).*
- ▲ Consider the use of preoperative reflective hats and jackets to reduce heat loss during surgery. **EB:** *Mild perioperative hypothermia may delay awakening and increase recovery time. In this study the prevention of intraoperative heat loss was provided by preoperative reflective hats and jackets (Sheng et al, 2003).*
- • Consider the use of an adjustable recliner if not contraindicated for recovery. **EBN:** *Postsurgical laparoscopy clients who recovered in adjustable recliner-chairs reached home readiness sooner and experienced greater comfort levels than clients who recovered in traditional hospital beds. Furthermore, clients in the recliner-chair group had fewer adverse symptoms such as nausea, severe pain, and delayed voiding (Agodoa, Holder, & Fowler, 2002).*
- • Do not offer fluids in the immediate postoperative period. **EB:** *Early ingestion of fluids in the postoperative period contributes to emesis. Oral intake before discharge from an ambulatory surgery unit increased the incidence of vomiting to four times that of the control group and prolonged the hospital stay (Haynes & Bailey, 1996).*
- ▲ In a client with postoperative nausea and vomiting, consider the use of multiple antiemetic medications (double or triple combinations of antiemetic agents acting at different neuroreceptor sites), less emetogenic anesthesia techniques, and adequate intravenous hydration. **EB:** *The combination of antiemetic therapy and the other measures mentioned improved efficacy of prevention and treatment of postoperative nausea and vomiting (Kovac, 2000).*
- • The client should be provided with a complete, balanced therapeutic diet after the immediately postoperative period (24–48 hours). **EB:** *Evidence suggests that improvement in nutritional status can improve outcomes of wound healing (Thomas, 1996).* **EBN:** *Good nutrition is important for effective wound healing (Casey, 1998).*
- • The client should have a nutritious diet with adequate protein intake that restores normal weight for the client. **EB:** *In a study that examined restoration of weight loss and healing of a "nonhealing wound," the rate of wound healing was most prominent after 50% of the weight loss had been restored. This finding reflects the key relationship between restoration of body weight, body protein stores, and wound healing (Demling & De Santi, 1998).*
- • Use careful aseptic technique when caring for wounds. **EB:** *A significant impediment to wound healing is infection. Treatment of chronic wounds should be directed at the main causal factors responsible for the wound. Moreover, factors that may impede healing must be identified and corrected, if possible, for healing to occur (Stadelmann, Digenis, & Tobin, 1998).*
- ▲ Suggest the use of a semipermeable dressing and suction drainage for selected orthopedic clients. **EB:** *A combination of a semipermeable dressing and suction drainage was*

S

*used successfully in 20 orthopedic clients without any wound complication and with satisfactory comfort to the client. This form of postoperative wound management appears to retain the nursing and hygiene advantages of suction drainage while avoiding the client discomfort and possibilities of wound infection associated with deep internal drainage (Strover & Thorpe, 1997).*

- ▲ Promote mobility and deep breathing with the use of a transcutaneous electrical nerve stimulation (TENS) unit for pain relief. **EBN:** *The results of this study suggest TENS reduces pain intensity during walking and deep breathing and increases walking function postoperatively when used as a supplement to pharmacologic analgesia (Rakel & Franz, 2003).*
- ▲ Carefully consider the use of alternative therapy with a physician's order, such as application of aloe vera or aqueous cream to promote wound healing. **EBN:** *Aloe vera gel or aqueous cream was used in a randomized study involving 225 clients with breast cancer who required a course of radiation therapy after lumpectomy or partial mastectomy. Aloe vera gel did not significantly reduce radiation-induced skin side effects. Aqueous cream was useful in reducing dry desquamation and pain related to radiation therapy (Heggie et al, 2002).*
- • Clients should be allowed to shower after surgery to maintain cleanliness if not contraindicated because of the presence of pacemaker wires, etc. **EB:** *Clients undergoing open hernia repair who were allowed to shower showed no manifest infection and no difference in wound healing compared with those who were not allowed to shower (Riederer & Inderbitzi, 1997).*
- • Provide 20-minute foot and hand massage (5 minutes to each extremity), 1–4 hours after a dose of pain medication. **EBN:** *Physiological responses to pain create harmful effects that prolong the body's recovery after surgery. This study showed statistically significant decreases in sympathetic responses to pain (i.e., heart rate, respiratory rate). The patients experienced moderate pain after they received pain medications. This pain was reduced by the intervention, thus supporting the effectiveness of foot and hand massage in postoperative pain management (Wang & Keck, 2004).*
- • Provide supportive telephone calls from nurse to client as a means of decreasing anxiety and providing the psychosocial support necessary for recovery from surgery. **EB:** *Telephone calls are an effective method of providing supportive psychosocial care for individuals who may not be able to access this care because of geographic isolation, physical limitations, or discomfort with face-to-face interventions (Gotay & Bottomley, 1998).*
- ▲ Assess and treat for depression and anxiety in a client complaining of continuing fatigue after surgery. **EB:** *Level of fatigue at 30 days after coronary bypass surgery correlated with concurrent levels of depression and anxiety (Pick et al, 1994).*
- ▲ Consider the use of alternative therapies: hypnosis, aromatherapy, music, guided imagery, and massage. **EBN:** *Alternative therapies offer high-touch balance when integrated with high-tech surgical treatments and may decrease anxiety (Norred, 2000).*
- • Encourage the client to use prayer as a form of spiritual coping if this is comfortable for the client. **EB:** *Results of one study show that most clients pray about their postoperative problems and that private prayer appears to significantly decrease depression and general distress 1 year after CABG (Ai et al, 1998).*
- • See the care plans for **Anxiety, Acute Pain, Fatigue,** and **Impaired physical Mobility.**

S

### Pediatric

- Teach imagery and encourage distraction for children for postsurgical pain relief. **EBN:** *The results of this study of children aged 8–12 undergoing surgery indicated that all of the children used at least one self-initiated pain-relieving method (e.g., distraction, resting/sleeping), in addition to receiving assistance in pain relief from nurses (e.g., giving pain killers, helping with daily activities) and parents (e.g. distraction, presence) (Pikki et al, 2003).* **EBN:** *Imagery using distraction was helpful in decreasing the use of analgesics for pain in a group of 7 to 12-year-olds who had had tonsillectomy and/or adenoidectomy (Huth, 2002).*

### Geriatric

- Perform a thorough preoperative assessment including a cardiac assessment. **EB:** *Better preoperative risk assessment and preparation of the patient have helped to improve outcomes in geriatric patients (Dharmarajan et al, 2003).*

▲ Carefully assess the fluid and electrolyte status and glomerular filtration rate (GFR) of elderly clients before surgery. Provide fluid and electrolyte replacement per the physician's order. **EB:** *In many cases acute renal failure (ARF) can be prevented in older clients (e.g., by correcting any sodium deficit and hypovolemia before a surgical procedure and by considering the true GFR of a given client before prescribing a potentially nephrotoxic drug). Recovery is delayed in older clients and in those whose oliguric period is prolonged. The high cost of therapy for ARF justifies the use of all current preventive measures in clients at risk. The incidence of ARF is five times higher in elderly clients than in younger clients (Kleinknecht & Pallot, 1998).*

- Carefully evaluate the client's temperature. Know what is normal and abnormal for each client. Check baseline temperature and monitor trends. *Even a normal temperature (98.6° F [37° C]) can indicate an infection, because many older adults have subnormal body temperatures (averaging 96.8° F [36° C]) (Faherty, 1994).*
- To minimize risks of hypothermia, cover the patient with warmed forced-air blankets or blankets from a warmer, infuse only warm fluids and blood, and provide heated, humidified inspired gases. *Integumentary, cardiopulmonary, thermoregulatory, and metabolic changes in elderly patients make them more vulnerable to hypothermia than other adults. Hypothermia impairs renal concentrating ability, slows the drug clearance, causes lactic acidosis, produces arrhythmias, and precipitates acute delirium. It also prolongs prothrombin time and anesthetic agents' effects. Postoperatively hypothermia may delay healing and increase the risk of wound infections. In addition, if a hypothermic patient starts to shiver, his or her tissue oxygen requirements could increase 200%–500%, which increases his risk of myocardial infarction (Dunn, 2004).*
- Teach guided imagery for pain relief. **EBN:** *The management of postoperative pain in elderly orthopedic patients is critical for advancing patient outcomes Trends in this pilot study of elderly clients with hip replacements demonstrated positive outcomes for pain relief, decreased anxiety, and decreased length of stay (Antall & Kresevec, 2004).*
- Offer spiritual support. **EB:** *In a qualitative study, religion and spirituality were found to help older adults maintain and recover both physical and mental health (Mackenzie et al, 2000).*

S

## Client/Family Teaching

▲ To decrease postoperative nausea and vomiting, the client should be instructed to fast before surgery, with the period to be determined by the physician. **EBN:** *Fasting times for fluids should not normally be longer than 4 hours or less than 2 hours. Fasting times for solid food should not normally be longer than 6 hours or less than 4 hours. Inappropriately prolonged preoperative fasting might result in dehydration, electrolyte imbalance, hypoglycemia, discomfort, and confusion (Dean & Fawcett, 2002).* **EBN:** *Fasting overnight or up to 8 hours before surgery can cause dehydration, electrolyte imbalance, malnutrition, and general malaise. Evidence shows that clients can benefit from receiving clear liquids up to 3 hours before surgery (Watson & Rinombota, 2002).* **EB:** *Evidence is lacking that adults given fluids 1½–3 hours preoperatively have a greater risk of aspiration or regurgitation than those who have a standard fast (Power, 2003).*

• Teach systematic muscle relaxation for pain relief. **EBN:** *Unrelieved pain after surgery can lead to complications, prolonged hospital stay, and delayed recovery. Because of side effects from opioids and differences in response, it is important to use nonpharmacological methods in addition to analgesics to decrease patient discomfort and anxiety. Substantial reductions in the sensation and distress of pain were found when postoperative patients used systematic relaxation (Roykulcharoen & Good, 2004).*

▲ Provide individualized teaching plans for the client with an ostomy. Consider basic needs: (1) maintenance of a pouching seal for a consistent, predictable wear time; (2) maintenance of peristomal skin integrity; and (3) social and professional support of the patient. **EB:** *Ostomy surgery changes a person's life in observable, obvious, overt, physical ways. Before a patient can achieve a desired quality of life, however, basic needs must be met. Guiding the patient to the ostomy management system suited to his or her lifestyle can play a vital role toward achieving individual quality-of-life goals. Teaching plans should be individualized and customized to reflect and accommodate the phase of rehabilitation and patient-defined quality-of-life goals at the time the nurse interacts with the patient, whether during the preoperative or postoperative periods or years after (Turnbull, Colwell, & Erwin-Toth, 2004).*

## evolve WEBSITES FOR EDUCATION

S

See the EVOLVE website for World Wide Web resources for client education.

## REFERENCES


Agodoa SE, Holder MA, Fowler SM: Effects of recliner-chair versus traditional hospital bed on postsurgical diagnostic laparoscopic recovery time, *J Perianesth Nurs* 17(5):318, 2002.

Ai AL, Dunkle RE, Peterson C et al: The role of private prayer in psychological recovery among midlife and aged patients following cardiac surgery, *Gerontologist* 38(5):591, 1998.

Anonymous: Diabetes in the hospital: taking charge, *Diabetes Spectrum* 18(1):49, 2005.

Antall GF, Kresevic D: The use of guided imagery to manage pain in an elderly orthopaedic population, *Orthop Nurs* 23(5):335-340, 2004.

Casey G: The importance of nutrition in wound healing, *Nurs Stand* 13(3):51, 1998.

Cavanaugh P et al: Consensus development conference on diabetic wound foot care. Paper presented at the meeting of the American Diabetes Association, Boston, April 7-8, 1999. Available at http://care.diabetesjournals.org/cgi/reprint/22/8/1354.pdf?ijkey=ae4410ea6195e10bbe290d5ada6908966f5739d7, accessed June 22, 2003.
Ciocon JO, Ciocon DG, Galindo DJ: Dietary supplements in primary care. Botanicals can affect surgical outcomes and follow-up, *Geriatrics* 59(9):20-24, 2004.
Dharmarajan TS, Unnikrishnan D, Dharmarajan L: Preparing the older adult for surgery, *Hosp Physician* 39(11):45-54, 2003.
Dean A, Fawcett T: Nurses' use of evidence in pre-operative fasting, *Nurs Stand* 17(12):33, 2002.
Demling R, De Santi L: Closure of the "non-healing wound" corresponds with correction of weight loss using the anabolic agent oxandrolone, *Ostomy Wound Manage* 44(10):58, 1998.
Dunn D: Preventing perioperative complications in an older adult, *Nursing* 34(11):36, 2004.
Faherty B: Myths and facts about older adults, *Nursing* 24(4):75, 1994.
Gammon J, Mulholland CW: Effect of preparatory information prior to elective total hip replacement on postoperative physical coping outcomes, *Int J Nurs Stud* 33(6):589, 1996.
Gotay CC, Bottomley A: Providing psychosocial support by telephone: what is its potential in cancer patients? *Eur J Cancer Care* 7(4):225, 1998.
Haynes G, Bailey M: Postoperative nausea and vomiting: review and clinical approaches, *South Med J*, 89(10):940, 1996.
Heggie S, Bryant GP, Tripcony L et al: A phase III study on the efficacy of topical aloe vera gel on irradiated breast tissue, *Cancer Nurs* 25(6):442, 2002.
Huth MM: Imagery to reduce children's postoperative pain, doctoral dissertation, Cleveland, Ohio, 2002, Case Western Reserve University.
King CE: Healing pathways through energy work in the perianesthesia care setting, *CRNA* 11(4):180, 2000.
King L: Impaired wound healing in patients with diabetes, *Nurs Stand* 15(38):39, 2001.
Kleinknecht D, Pallot JL: Epidemiology and prognosis of acute renal insufficiency in 1997, *Nephrologie* 19(2):49, 1998.
Koivula M, Paunonen-Ilmonen M, Tarkka MT et al: Social support and its relation to fear and anxiety in patients awaiting coronary artery bypass grafting, *J Clin Nurs* 11(5):622, 2002.
Kovac AL: Prevention and treatment of postoperative nausea and vomiting, *Drugs* 59(2):213, 2000.
Lee D, Henderson A, Shum D: The effect of music on preprocedure anxiety in Hong Kong Chinese day patients, *J Clin Nurs* 13(3):297-303, 2004.
Lukas LK: Orthopedic outpatients' perception of perioperative music listening as therapy, *J Theory Construct Testing* 8(1):7-12, 2004
Mackenzie ER, Rajagopal DE, Meibohm M et al: Spiritual support and psychological well-being: older adults' perceptions of the religion and health connection, *Altern Ther Health Med* 6(6):37, 2000.
Martin D: Pre-operative visits to reduce patient anxiety: a study, *Nurs Stand* 10(23):33, 1996.
Norred CL: Minimizing preoperative anxiety with alternative caring-healing therapies, *AORN J* 72(5):838, 2000.
Pick B, Molloy A, Hinds C et al: Post-operative fatigue following coronary artery bypass surgery: relationship to emotional state and to the catecholamine response to surgery, *J Psychosom Res* 38(6):599, 1994.
Plkki T, Pietil A, Vehvilinen-Julkunen K: Hospitalized children's descriptions of their experiences with postsurgical pain relieving methods, *Int J Nurs Stud* 40(1):33-44, 2003.
Rakel B, Frantz R: Effectiveness of transcutaneous electrical nerve stimulation on postoperative pain with movement, *J Pain* 4(8):455-464, 2003.
Riederer SR, Inderbitzi R: Does a shower put postoperative wound healing at risk? *Chirurg* 68(7):715, 1997.
Roykulcharoen V, Good M: Systematic relaxation to relieve postoperative pain, *J Adv Nurs* 48(2):140-148, 2004.
Seskevich JE, Crater SW, Lane JD: Beneficial effects of noetic therapies on mood before percutaneous intervention for unstable coronary syndromes, *Nurs Res* 53(2):116-121, 2004.
Sheng Y, Zavisca F, Schonlau E: The effect of preoperative reflective hats and jackets, and intraoperative reflective blankets on perioperative temperature, *Internet J Anesthesiol* 6(2):8, 2003.
Stadelmann WK, Digenis AG, Tobin GR: Impediments to wound healing, *Am J Surg* 176(Suppl 2A):39S, 1998.
Strover AE, Thorpe R: Suction dressings: a new surgical dressing technique, *J R Coll Surg Edinb* 42(2):119, 1997.
Thomas DR: Nutritional factors affecting wound healing, *Ostomy Wound Manage* 42(5):40, 1996.
Turnbull GB, Colwell J, Erwin-Toth P: Quality of life: pre, post, and beyond ostomy surgery: clinician strategies for helping people with a stoma lead healthy, productive lives, *Ostomy Wound Manage* 50(7):S2, 2004.
Wang H, Keck JF: Foot and hand massage as an intervention for postoperative pain, *Pain Manage Nurs* 5(2):59-65, 2004.
Watson K, Rinomhota S: Preoperative fasting: we need a new consensus, *Nurs Times* 98(15):36, 2002.

S

# Impaired Swallowing

evolve

Betty J. Ackley and Roslyn Fine

NANDA

## Definition

Abnormal functioning of the swallowing mechanism associated with deficits in oral, pharyngeal, or esophageal structure or function

## Defining Characteristics

*Oral phase impairment:* Lack of tongue action to form bolus; weak suck resulting in inefficient nippling; incomplete lip closure; pushing of food out of mouth; slow bolus formation; falling of food from mouth; premature entry of bolus; nasal reflux; inability to clear oral cavity; long meals with little consumption; coughing, choking, or gagging before a swallow; abnormality in oral phase of swallow study; piecemeal deglutition; lack of chewing; pooling in lateral sulci; sialorrhea or drooling

*Pharyngeal phase impairment:* Altered head position; inadequate laryngeal elevation; food refusal; unexplained fever; delayed swallow; recurrent pulmonary infections; gurgly voice quality; nasal reflux; choking, coughing, or gagging; multiple swallows; abnormality in pharyngeal phase by swallowing study

*Esophageal phase impairment:* Heartburn or epigastric pain; acidic-smelling breath; unexplained irritability surrounding mealtime; vomitus on pillow; repetitive swallowing or ruminating; regurgitation of gastric contents or wet belches; bruxism; nighttime coughing or awakening; observed evidence of difficulty in swallowing (e.g., stasis of food in oral cavity, coughing, or choking); hyperextension of head, arching during or after meals; abnormality in esophageal phase by swallow study; odynophagia; food refusal or volume limiting; complaints of "something stuck"; hematemesis; vomiting

## Related Factors (r/t)

S

Congenital deficits; upper airway anomalies; failure to thrive; protein energy malnutrition; conditions with significant hypotonia; respiratory disorders; history of tube feeding; behavioral feeding problems; self-injurious behavior; neuromuscular impairment (e.g., decreased or absent gag reflex, decreased strength or excursion of muscles involved in mastication, perceptual impairment, or facial paralysis); mechanical obstruction (e.g., edema, tracheotomy tube, or tumor); congenital heart disease; cranial nerve involvement; neurological problems; upper airway anomalies; laryngeal abnormalities; achalasia; gastroesophageal reflux disease; acquired anatomic defects; cerebral palsy; internal or external traumas; tracheal, laryngeal, or esophageal defects; traumatic head injury; developmental delay; nasal or nasopharyngeal cavity defects; oral cavity or oropharynx abnormalities; prematurity

**NOC**

## Outcomes (Nursing Outcomes Classification)

### Suggested NOC Outcomes

Swallowing Status; Swallowing Status: Esophageal Phase, Oral Phase, Pharyngeal Phase

**Example NOC Outcome with Indicators**

**Swallowing Status** as evidenced by the following indicators: Delivery of bolus to hypopharynx is timed with swallow reflex/Ability to clear oral cavity/Number of swallows appropriate for bolus size and texture/Voice quality/Choking, coughing, gagging/Normal swallow effort (Rate each indicator of **Swallowing Status:** 1 = severely compromised, 2 = substantially compromised, 3 = moderately compromised, 4 = mildly compromised, 5 = not compromised [see Section I].)

## Client Outcomes

### Client Will (Specify Time Frame):

- Demonstrate effective swallowing without choking or coughing
- Remain free from aspiration (e.g., lungs clear, temperature within normal range)

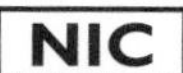

## Interventions (Nursing Interventions Classification)

### Suggested NIC Interventions

Aspiration Precautions; Swallowing Therapy

**Example NIC Activities—Swallowing Therapy**

Assist client to sit in erect position (as close to 90 degrees as possible) for feeding/exercise; instruct client not to talk during eating, if appropriate

## Nursing Interventions and Rationales

- • Determine the client's readiness to eat. The client needs to be alert, able to follow instructions, able to hold the head erect, and able to move the tongue in the mouth. *If one of these elements is missing, it may be advisable to withhold oral feeding and use enteral feeding for nourishment (Smith & Connolly, 2003).*
- ▲ If the swallowing impairment is of new onset, ensure that the client receives a diagnostic workup. *Swallowing impairment can have multiple causes, many of which are treatable (Smith & Connolly, 2003).*
- • Assess ability to swallow by positioning the thumb and index finger on the client's laryngeal protuberance. Ask the client to swallow; feel the larynx elevate. Ask the client to cough; test for a gag reflex on both sides of the posterior pharyngeal wall (lingual surface) with a tongue blade. Do not rely on the presence of a gag reflex to

determine when to feed. *Normally the time required for the bolus to move from the point at which the reflex is triggered to the esophageal entry (pharyngeal transit time) is less than 1 second (Logemann, 1983). Clients can aspirate even if they have an intact gag reflex (Smith & Connolly, 2003).* **EB:** *CVA clients with prolonged pharyngeal transit times (prolonged swallowing) have an increased chance of developing aspiration pneumonia (Marik & Kaplan, 2003).*

- • Consider the use of the Massey Bedside Swallowing Screen to screen for swallowing dysfunction. **EBN:** *The Massey Bedside Swallowing Screen demonstrated high sensitivity and specificity in predicting dysphagia, compared with assessment by experts in the field (Massey & Jedlicka, 2002).*
- • Observe for signs associated with swallowing problems (e.g., coughing, choking, spitting of food, drooling, difficulty handling oral secretions, double swallowing or major delay in swallowing, watering eyes, nasal discharge, wet or gurgly voice, decreased ability to move the tongue and lips, decreased mastication of food, decreased ability to move food to the back of the pharynx, slow or scanning speech). *These are all signs of swallowing impairment (Terrado, Russell, & Bowman, 2001).* **EB:** *A study demonstrated that voice analysis could accurately predict the clients with dysphagia by presence of perturbation, shimmer percentage, noise-to-harmonic ratio, and voice turbulence as tested by videofluoroscopic swallowing studies (Ryu, Park, & Choi, 2004).*
- ▲ If the client has impaired swallowing, refer to a speech pathologist for bedside evaluation as soon as possible. Ensure that the client is seen by a speech pathologist within 48 hours after admission if the client has had a CVA. *Speech pathologists specialize in impaired swallowing.* **EBN:** *Early referral of CVA clients to a speech pathologist, along with early initiation of nutritional support, can result in decreased length of hospital stay, shortened recovery time, and reduced overall health costs (Runions, Rodrigue, & White, 2004).*
- ▲ To manage impaired swallowing, use a dysphagia team composed of a rehabilitation nurse, speech pathologist, dietitian, physician, and radiologist who work together. *The dysphagia team can help the client learn to swallow safely and maintain a good nutritional status (Davies, 2002).*
- ▲ If the client has impaired swallowing, do not feed until an appropriate diagnostic workup is completed. Ensure proper nutrition by consulting with a physician regarding enteral feedings, preferably using a percutaneous endoscopic gastrostomy (PEG) tube in most cases. *Feeding a client who cannot adequately swallow results in aspiration and possibly death.* **EB:** *Enteral feedings via PEG tube are generally preferable to nasogastric tube feedings, but further studies are needed (Bath, Bath-Hextall, & Smithard, 2005).*
- • If client is not eating sufficient amount of food, recognize that the immune system may be impaired with resultant increased risk of infection. **EB:** *A study comparing elderly clients with dysphagia who were tube fed versus others who were orally fed, the orally fed clients had much lower CD4 cell counts, as well as a low CD4/CD8 ratio (Leibovitz et al, 2004).*
- • If the client has an intact swallowing reflex, attempt to feed. Observe the following feeding guidelines:
  - ■ Position the client upright at a 90-degree angle with the chin tucked forward at a 45-degree angle (Galvan, 2001). *The chin tuck is protective for most people with*

S

*dysphagia, because the epiglottis forms a protective shelf over the vocal folds as the client swallowed (West & Redstone, 2004).*

- ■ Ensure that the client is awake, alert, and able to follow sequenced directions before attempting to feed. *As the client becomes less alert, the swallowing response decreases, which increases the risk of aspiration.*
- ■ Begin by feeding the client one third of a teaspoon of applesauce. Provide sufficient time to masticate and swallow.
- ■ Place the food on the unaffected side of the tongue.
- ■ During feeding, give the client specific directions (e.g., "Open your mouth, chew the food completely, and when you are ready, tuck your chin to your chest and swallow").
- ■ Ensure client is kept in an upright posture for an hour after eating. *An upright posture after eating has been associated with a decreased incidence of pneumonia in the elderly (Coleman, 2004).*

▲ Watch for uncoordinated chewing or swallowing; coughing immediately after eating or delayed coughing, which may indicate silent aspiration; pocketing of food; wet-sounding voice; sneezing when eating; delay of more than 1 second in swallowing; or a change in respiratory patterns. If any of these signs is present, put on gloves, remove all food from the oral cavity, stop feedings, and consult with a speech and language pathologist and a dysphagia team. *These are signs of impaired swallowing and possible aspiration (Galvan, 2001).*

• If the client tolerates single-textured foods such as pudding, hot cereal, or strained baby food, advance to a soft diet with guidance from the dysphagia team. Avoid foods such as hamburgers, corn, and pastas that are difficult to chew. Also avoid sticky foods such as peanut butter and white bread. *The dysphagia team should determine the appropriate diet for the client based on progression in swallowing and need to ensure that the client is nourished and hydrated.*

• Avoid providing liquids until the client is able to swallow effectively. Add a thickening agent to liquids to obtain a soft consistency that is similar to nectar, honey, or pudding, depending on the degree of swallowing problems. *Liquids can be easily aspirated; thickened liquids form a cohesive bolus that the client can swallow with increased efficiency (Langmore & Miller, 1994; Poertner & Coleman, 1998).*

• Preferably use prepackaged thickened liquids, or use a viscosimeter to ensure appropriate thickness. *Often staff members overthicken liquids, which results in decreased palatability with decreased intake.* **EB:** *Using prepackaged thickened liquids or a viscosimeter to determine appropriate thickness can increase intake, which increases hydration and nutrition (Boczko, 2000; Goulding & Bakheit, 2000). A study of 252 skilled nursing facilities demonstrated that the majority of clients with swallowing difficulties received liquids thickened to nectar-syrup consistency (60%), 33% received honey consistency, and only 6% received pudding consistency thickened fluids (Castellanos et al, 2004).*

▲ Work with the client on swallowing exercises prescribed by the dysphagia team (e.g., touching the palate with the tongue, stimulating the tonsillar arch and soft palate with a cold metal examination mirror [thermal stimulation], labial/lingual range-of-motion exercises). *Swallowing exercises, including both motor and sensory stimulation, can improve the client's ability to swallow (Hagg & Larsson, 2004; Langmore & Miller, 1994).*

*Exercises need to be done at intervals, which necessitates nursing involvement (Poertner & Coleman, 1998).*

▲ For many adult clients, avoid the use of straws if recommended by the speech pathologist. *Use of straws can increase the risk of aspiration, because straws can result in spilling of a bolus of fluid in the oral cavity, as well as decrease control of the posterior transit of fluid to the pharynx (Travers, 1999).*

• Provide meals in a quiet environment away from excessive stimuli such as a community dining room. *A noisy environment can be an aversive stimulus and can decrease effective mastication and swallowing. Talking and laughing while eating increase the risk of aspiration (Galvan, 2001).*

• Ensure that there is adequate time for the client to eat. *Clients with swallowing impairments often take two to four times longer than others to eat, if they are being fed. Often, food is offered rapidly to speed up the task, and this can increase the chance of aspiration (Poertner & Coleman, 1998).*

▲ Have suction equipment available during feeding. If choking occurs and suctioning is necessary, discontinue oral feeding until the client is safely assessed with a videofluoroscopic swallow study. *Suctioning may be necessary if the client is choking on food and could aspirate.*

• Check the oral cavity for proper emptying after the client swallows and after the client finishes the meal. Provide oral care at the end of the meal. It may be necessary to manually remove food from the client's mouth. If this is the case, use gloves and keep the client's teeth apart with a padded tongue blade. *Food may become pocketed on the affected side and cause stomatitis, tooth decay, and possible later aspiration.*

• Praise the client for successfully following directions and swallowing appropriately. *Praise reinforces behavior and sets up a positive atmosphere in which learning takes place.*

• Keep the client in an upright position for 45 minutes to an hour after a meal. *Maintaining an upright position ensures that food stays in the stomach until it has emptied and decreases the chance of aspiration after meals (Galvan, 2001).* **EB:** *A study demonstrated that the number of elderly clients developing a fever was significantly reduced when clients were kept sitting upright after eating (Matsui et al, 2002).*

▲ Watch for signs of aspiration and pneumonia. Auscultate lung sounds after feeding. Note new crackles or wheezing, and note elevated temperature. Notify the physician as needed. *The presence of new crackles or wheezing, an elevated temperature or white blood cell count, and a change in sputum could indicate aspiration of food (Murray & Brzozowski, 1998). It could also indicate the presence of pneumonia (Galvan, 2001). Clients with dysphagia are at serious risk for aspiration pneumonia (Kedlaya & Brandstater, 2002; Langmore, 1999).* **EB:** *Bronchial auscultation of lung sounds was shown to be specific in identifying clients at risk for aspirating (Shaw et al, 2004).*

• Watch for signs of malnutrition and dehydration. Keep a record of food intake. *Malnutrition is common in dysphagic clients (Galvan, 2001). Clients with dysphagia are at serious risk for malnutrition and dehydration, which can lead to aspiration pneumonia resulting from depressed immune function and weakness, lethargy, and decreased cough (Langmore, 1999).*

• Weigh the client weekly to help evaluate nutritional status. Evaluate nutritional status daily. If the client is not adequately nourished, work with the dysphagia team to determine whether the client needs to avoid oral intake with therapeutic feeding only or needs enteral feedings until the client can swallow adequately. **EB:** *One study demonstrated that dysphagic stroke clients who received thickened fluid dysphagia diets failed to meet their needs for fluids, whereas a group receiving enteral feeding and IV fluid did meet fluid requirements (Finestone et al, 2001).* **EBN:** *Four independent risk factors for dysphagia—hypoglossal nerve dysfunction, National Institutes of Health Stroke Scale score, incomplete oral labial closure, and wet voice after swallowing water—predicted the need for tube feedings in stroke clients with dysphagia (Wojner & Alexandrov, 2000).*

▲ If client has a tracheostomy, ask for referral to speech pathologist for swallowing studies before attempting to feed. After evaluation, decision should be made to have cuff either inflated or deflated when client eats. **EBN and EB:** *The presence of a tracheostomy tube increases the incidence of aspiration (Elpern et al, 1993). One study demonstrated that clients who had aspiration after a tracheostomy had aspiration before the tracheostomy, and if the client did not aspirate before the tracheostomy, they also did not aspirate after the tracheostomy procedure was done (Leder & Ross, 2000). For some clients, inflating the cuff may help decrease aspiration; for others, the inflated cuff will interfere with swallowing. This decision should be made after swallowing studies for the safety of the client's airway (Murray & Brzozowski, 1998).*

## Pediatric

▲ Refer to a physician a child who has difficulty swallowing and symptoms such as difficulty manipulating food, delayed swallow response, and pocketing of a bolus of food. *Research has indicated that surgery should be used to correct structural deficits (e.g., those related to pyloric stenosis, neurological disorders that involve cranial nerve pathways, and disorders resulting in swallowing changes, such as brain injury and cerebral palsy) (Rosenthal, Sheppard, & Lotze, 1995). Respiratory and gastrointestinal system disorders (gastroesophageal reflux disease) and esophagitis can affect swallowing and nutrition. These systemic disorders are diagnosed by a physician and treated with medications.*

• When feeding an infant or child, place the infant/child in a 90-degree position with the head slightly flexed. Change the consistency of the diet as needed, and use a curly straw for young children to facilitate tucking the chin, which helps improve swallowing ability (Arvedson & Brodsky, 1993).

• Give oral motor stimulation that increases oral-sensory awareness by waking the mouth using exercises that focus on temperature, taste, and texture. *Many of these infants require supplemental tube feedings and special nipples or bottles to boost oral intake.*

• For infants with poor sucking and swallowing, do the following:
  ■ Support the cheeks and jaw to increase sucking skills.
  ■ Pace or rhythmically move the bottle, which encourages better suck-swallow-breath synchrony.

▲ Work with the dietitian. *Some infants may need a high-calorie formula so that food volume can be decreased (which requires the infant to expend less energy) while still meeting nutritional requirements (Klein & Tracey, 1994). Some infants may also need to have the tongue brushed, which provides tongue stimulation (tongue tip and tongue lateralization) and promotes lip seal and lip pursing.*

• Watch for indicators of aspiration: coughing, a change in web vocal quality while feed-



S

ing, perspiration and color changes during feeding, sneezing, and increased heart rate and breathing.

- Watch for warning signs of reflux: sour-smelling breath after eating, sneezing, lack of interest in feeding, crying and fussing extraordinarily when feeding, pained expressions when feeding, and excessive chewing and swallowing after eating. *Many premature and medically fragile children experience growth deficits and respiratory problems from an underlying dysphagia. Some infants may need to work harder to breathe than others and as a result develop a decreased tolerance for food intake. They also demonstrate inconsistent arousal and poor/uncoordinated suck-swallow-breath synchrony. Many of these infants require supplemental tube feedings and the use of special nipples or bottles to boost oral intake.*

### Geriatric

- Recognize that being elderly does not result in dysphagia, but having medical problems including such things as arthritis, hypertension, and other chronic medical problems can result in dysphagia. **EB:** *No delay in swallowing was found in elderly subjects, but clients with medical conditions did often have problems with dysphagia (Kendall, Leonard, & McKenzie, 2004).*
- ▲ Evaluate medications the client is presently taking, especially if elderly. Consult with the pharmacist for assistance in monitoring for incorrect doses and drug interactions that could result in dysphagia. *Most elderly clients take numerous medications, which when taken individually can slow motor function, cause anxiety and depression, and reduce salivary flow. When taken together, these medications can interact, resulting in impaired swallowing function. Drugs that reduce muscle tone for swallowing and can cause reflux include calcium channel blockers and nitrates. Drugs that can reduce salivary flow include antidepressants, antiparkinsonism drugs, antihistamines, antispasmodics, antipsychotic agents or major tranquilizers, antiemetics, antihypertensives, and drugs for treating diarrhea and anxiety (Schechter, 1998).*
- Recognize that the elderly client with dementia needs a longer time to eat. *The dementia client has decreased cognition, distractibility, and decreased efficiency in chewing and is likely to have problems with swallowing (Granville, 2002).*
- Recognize that the loss of teeth can cause problems with chewing and swallowing. *Without teeth, three to four times more effort may be required to chew food so that it is able to be swallowed (Granville, 2002).*



### Home Care

- ▲ Refer to speech therapy. Speech therapists can work with clients to enhance swallowing ability.

## Client/Family Teaching

- ▲ Teach the client and family exercises prescribed by the dysphagia team.
- Teach the client a systematic method of swallowing effectively as prescribed by the dysphagia team.
- Educate the client, family, and all caregivers about rationales for food consistency and choices. *It is common for family members to disregard necessary dietary restrictions and*

*give the client inappropriate foods that predispose to aspiration (Poertner & Coleman, 1998).*

- Teach the family how to monitor the client to prevent and detect aspiration during eating.

## evolve WEBSITES FOR EDUCATION

See the EVOLVE website for World Wide Web resources for client education.

## REFERENCES


Arvedson JC, Brodsky L: *Pediatric swallowing and feeding assessment and management,* San Diego, 1993, Singular.

Bath PM, Bath-Hextrall FJ, Smithard EG: Interventions for dysphagia in acute stroke, *Cochrane Database Syst Rev* (2): CD000323, DJ9, 2005.

Boczko T: Increasing liquid consumption in patients with dysphagia, *Adv Speech Language Pathol Audiol* 10(45), 2000.

Castellanos VH et al: Use of thickened liquids in skilled nursing facilities, *J ADA Assoc* 104(8):1222, 2004.

Coleman PR: Pneumonia in the long-term care setting: etiology, management, and prevention, *J Gerontol Nurs* 30(4):14, 2004.

Elpern EH, Jacobs ER, Bone RC: Incidence of aspiration in tracheally intubated adults, *Heart Lung* 16:527, 1993.

Davies S: An interdisciplinary approach to the management of dysphagia, *Prof Nurse* 18(1):22, 2002.

Finestone HM et al: Quantifying fluid intake in dysphagic stroke patients: a preliminary comparison of oral and nonoral strategies, *Arch Phys Med Rehabil* 82(12):1744, 2001.

Galvan TJ: Dysphagia: going down and staying down, *Am J Nurs* 101(1):37, 2001.

Goulding R, Bakheit A: Evaluation of the benefits of monitoring fluid thickness in the dietary management of dysphagic stroke patients, *Clin Rehabil* 14:119, 2000.

Granville L: Introduction to comprehensive geriatric assessment. Paper presented at the Florida Speech-Language Hearing Association Convention, Orlando, Fla, Sept 21-22, 2002.

Hagg, Larsson B: Effects of motor and sensory stimulation in stroke patients with long-lasting dysphagia, *Dysphagia* 19(4):219, 2004.

Kedlaya D, Brandstater ME: Swallowing, nutrition and hydration during acute stroke care, *Top Stroke Rehabil* 9(2):23, 2002.

Kendall KA, Leonard RJ, McKenzie S: Airway protection: evaluation with videofluoroscopy, *Dysphagia* 19(2):65, 2004a.

Kendall KA, Leonard RJ, McKenzie S: Common medical conditions in the elderly: impact on pharyngeal bolus transit, *Dysphagia* 19(2):71, 2004b.

Klein MD, Tracey A: *Feeding and nutrition for the child with special needs*, Tucson, Ariz, 1994, Therapy Skill Builders.

Langmore SE: Risk factors for aspiration pneumonia, *Nutr Clin Pract* 14(5):S41, 1999.

Langmore SE, Miller RM: Behavioral treatment for adults with oropharyngeal dysphagia, *Arch Phys Med Rehabil* 75:1154, 1994.

Leder SB, Ross DA: Investigation of the causal relationship between tracheostomy and aspiration in the acute care setting, *Laryngoscope* 100(4):641, 2000.

Leibovitz A et al: CD4 lymphocyte count and CD4/CD8 ratio in elderly long-term care patients with oropharyngeal dysphagia: comparison between oral and tube enteral feedings, *Dysphagia* 19(2):83, 2004.

Logemann JA: *Evaluation and treatment of swallowing disorders*, San Diego, 1983, College Hill.

Lugger KE: Dysphagia in the elderly stroke patient, *J Neurosci Nurs* 26:78, 1994.

Marik PE, Kaplan D: Aspiration pneumonia and dysphagia in the elderly, *Chest* 124(1):328, 2003.

Massey R, Jedlicka D: The Massey Bedside Swallowing Screen, *J Neurosci Nurs* 34(5):252, 2002.

Matsui T et al: Sitting position to prevent aspiration in bed-bound patients, *Gerontology* 48:194, 2002.

Murray KA, Brzozowski LA: Swallowing in patients with tracheotomies, *AACN Clin Issues* 9(3):416, 1998.

Poertner LC, Coleman RF: Swallowing therapy in adults, *Otolaryngol Clin North Am* 31(3):561, 1998.

Rosenthal WR, Sheppard JJ, Lotze M: *Dysphagia and the child with developmental disabilities*, San Diego, 1995, Singular.

Runions S, Rodrigue N, White C: Practice on an acute stroke until after implementation of a decision-making algorithm for dietary management of dysphagia, *J Neurosci Nurse* 36(4): 200, 2004.

Ryu JS, Park SR, Choi KH: Prediction of laryngeal aspiration using voice analysis, *Am J Phy Med Rehabil* 83(10):753, 2004.

Schechter GL: Systemic causes of dysphagia in adults, *Otolaryngol Clin North Am* 31(3):525, 1998.


S

Shaw JL et al: Bronchial auscultation: an effective adjunct to speech and language therapy bedside assessment when detecting dysphagia and aspiration? *Dysphagia* 19(4):211, 2004.
Smith HA, Connolly MJ: Evaluation and treatment of dysphagia following stroke, *Top Geriatr Rehabil* 19(1), 2003.
Terrado M, Russell C, Bowman JF: Dysphagia: an overview, *Medsurg Nurs* 10(5):233, 2001.
Travers P: Poststroke dysphagia: implications for nurses, *Rehabil Nurs* 24(2):69, 1999.
West JF, Redstone F: Feeding the adult with neurogenic disorders, *Top Geriatr Rehabil* 20(2):131-134, 2004.
Wojner AW, Alexandrov AV: Predictors of tube feeding in acute stroke patients with dysphagia, *AACN Clin Issues* 11(4):531, 2000.

# Effective Therapeutic regimen management

*Margaret Lunney*

## NANDA

### Definition

Pattern of regulating and integrating into daily living a program for treatment of illness and its sequelae that is satisfactory for meeting specific health goals

### Defining Characteristics

Appropriate choices of daily activities for meeting goals of a treatment or prevention program, illness symptoms within normal range of expectation, verbalization of desire to manage treatment of illness and prevention of sequelae, verbalization of intent to reduce risk factors for progression of illness and sequelae

### Related Factors (r/t)

None; related factors are not relevant with strength diagnoses.

## NOC

### Outcomes (Nursing Outcomes Classification)

#### Suggested NOC Outcomes

Knowledge: Treatment Regimen; Participation in Health Care Decisions; Risk Control; Symptom Control

T

**Example NOC Outcome with Indicators**

**Knowledge: Treatment Regimen** as evidenced by the following indicator: Description of prescribed medication, activity, exercise, and specific disease process (Rate each indicator of **Knowledge: Treatment Regimen**: 1 = none, 2 = limited, 3 = moderate, 4 = substantial, 5 = extensive [see Section I].)

### Client Outcomes

**Client Will (Specify Time Frame):**

- Acknowledge appropriateness of choices for meeting goals of treatment or prevention programs

- Agree to continue making appropriate choices
- Verbalize intent to contact health provider(s) for additional information, support, or resources as needed

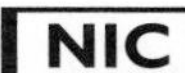

## Interventions (Nursing Interventions Classification)

### Suggested NIC Interventions

Anticipatory Guidance, Health Education, Health Screening, Health System Guidance, Learning Facilitation, Learning Readiness Enhancement, Risk Identification, Self-Modification Assistance

**Example NIC Activities—Learning Facilitation**

Relate information in a stimulating manner; encourage client's active participation

## Nursing Interventions and Rationales

NOTE: Little or no research is being done to investigate interventions to maintain strengths. For many interventions, theoretical rationales are provided as evidence rather than research findings.

- Review self-management strategies and related outcomes (e.g., changes in function and/or relief of symptoms such as pain). **EB:** *A review of 14 clinical trials to test self-management interventions for three chronic diseases showed that positive outcomes were generally associated with effective self-management strategies (Newman, Steed, & Mulligan, 2004).*
- Explore the meaning of the person's illness experience and identify uncertainties and needs through open-ended questions. **EB:** *This approach is necessary to know the person's perspective of self-management. Even though providers agree that self-management is the ideal approach to patient care, studies show that there are significant discrepancies between providers' and patients' views. Providers talk about self-management but may still expect compliance (Rogers et al, 2005).*
- Acknowledge the congruence of choices in activities of daily living (ADLs) with health-related goals. **EBN:** *Support from health provider(s) in efforts to self-manage therapeutic regimens motivates individuals to continue these efforts despite difficulties (Hibbard, 2004; Miller, 2000).*
- Support decisions regarding the person's methods of integrating therapeutic regimens into ADLs. **EBN:** *"A growing body of evidence shows that patients who are engaged, active participants in their own care have better health outcomes and measurable cost savings" (Hibbard, 2004, p. 134).*
- Provide information on possible illness trajectories to allow planning for future management. **EBN:** *Knowledge and awareness of illness trajectories enables the person to plan for future management of therapeutic regimens (Corbin, 1998; Lubkin & Larsen, 2002).*
- Assist the person to resolve ambivalent feelings about the illness and management of therapeutic regimens. **EBN:** *Wide variations may exist in attitudes and ambivalence*



T

*toward illness and management of illness regimens. Ambivalence interferes with effective decision making regarding illness care (Chinn et al, 2000).*

- Review methods of contacting health provider(s) for changes in therapeutic regimen and/or methods of incorporating therapeutic regimens into ADLs. **EBN:** *The partnership process includes continued contact as changes occur; people with chronic illnesses need to know how to obtain interventions that are needed in the future (Gallant, Beaulieu, & Carnevale, 2002; Lubkin and Larsen, 2002).*
- Record the effectiveness of managing the therapeutic regimens. **EBN:** *For clients who are at risk of ineffective management of therapeutic regimens, health providers may continue to assess and diagnose this phenomenon unnecessarily. It saves the health care system time, effort, and money if the assessment and diagnosis of effective management is communicated to other health providers.*

## Multicultural

- Assess for the influence of cultural beliefs, norms, and values on the individual's perceptions of the therapeutic regimen. **EBN:** *African Americans, Latinos born in the United States, and Latinos born in Mexico were less likely to adhere to all of the food group recommendations of the food pyramid (Sharma et al, 2004). A recent study showed that Hispanic outpatients experienced akathisia as an increase in* nerviosismo. *Addressing this issue, as well as using anxiolytics and low doses of antipsychotics when beginning treatment, led to an improvement in compliance (Opler et al, 2004).*
- Assess health literacy in patients of diverse backgrounds. **EB:** *Individuals with marginal or inadequate functional health literacy will have difficulty reading, understanding, and interpreting most written health texts and instructions. In addition, patients with marginal or inadequate health literacy scores are more likely to misunderstand directions for health care. Consequently, these patients are also more likely to take medications incorrectly and more likely to fail to follow a prescribed diet or treatment regimen (Georges, Bolton, & Bennett, 2004).*
- Assess cultural relevance of health information. **EB:** *A study of breast health information needs of women from minority ethnic groups found that health care professionals' lack of understanding about cultural beliefs, values and knowledge, together with racial stereotyping and misconceptions about cancer in minority ethnic groups, posed challenges to information dissemination (Watts, Merrell, Murphy, & Williams, 2004).*
- Assess for barriers that may interfere with compliance to follow-up treatment recommendations. **EB:** *Adherence and compliance to a treatment regimen is often compounded by variables like cost, availability of services, and convenience of accessing care. Knowledge of barriers to seeking health care is important when developing interventions to address adherence and compliance (Unzueta et al, 2004).*
- Discuss with the client their beliefs about medication and treatment in order to enhance medication and treatment adherence. **EB:** *A recent study of Hispanic and African-American women found that adherence was associated with recognition of the serious consequences of nonadherence, realization of the beneficial effects, and the belief that medicines are not harmful (Unson et al, 2003).*
- Use electronic monitoring to improve medication adherence. **EB:** *A recent study showed*

*that the use of electronic monitors had a positive effect on adherence for the minority women (Robbins, Rausch, Garcia, & Prestwood, 2004).*

- Validate the client's feelings regarding the ability to manage his or her own care and the impact on current lifestyle. **EB:** *A recent study that elicited the expectations of treatment in 93 hypertensive African-American patients. Patient expectations of treatment could serve as the basis for patient education and counseling about hypertension and its management in this patient population (Ogedegbe, Mancuso, & Allegrante, 2004).*

## Client/Family Teaching

- Teach about the disease trajectory and ways to manage disease symptoms as the trajectory changes.

## evolve WEBSITES FOR EDUCATION

See the EVOLVE website for World Wide Web resources for client education.

## REFERENCES


Becker G, Gates RJ, Newsom E: Self care among chronically ill African Americans: culture, health disparities, and health insurance status, *Am J Public Health* 94(12):2066-2073, 2004.

Chinn MH, Polonsky TS, Thomas VD et al: Developing a conceptual framework for understanding illness and attitudes in older, urban African Americans with diabetes, *Diabetes Educ* 26(3):439, 2000.

Corbin JM: The Corbin and Strauss chronic illness trajectory model: an update, *Sch Inq Nurs Pract* 12(1):33-41, 1998.

D'Avanzo CE et al: Developing culturally informed strategies for substance-related interventions. In Naegle MA, D'Avanzo CE, editors: *Addictions and substance abuse: strategies for advanced practice nursing,* St Louis, 2001, Mosby.

Gallant MH, Beaulieu MC, Carnevale FA: Partnership: an analysis of the concept within the nurse-client relationship, *J Adv Nurs* 40(2):149, 2002.

Georges CA, Bolton LB, Bennett C: Functional health literacy: an issue in African-American and other ethnic and racial communities, *J Natl Black Nurses Assoc* 15(1):1-4, 2004.

Leininger MM, McFarland MR: *Transcultural nursing: concepts, theories, research and practices,* ed 3, New York, 2002, McGraw-Hill.

Lubkin IM, Larsen PD: *Chronic illness: impact and interventions,* ed 5, Boston, 2002, Jones and Bartlett.

Miller JF: *Coping with chronic illness: overcoming powerlessness,* ed 3, Philadelphia, 2000, FA Davis.

Newman S, Steed L, Mulligan K: Self management interventions for chronic illness, *Lancet* 364(9444):1523-1537, 2004.

Opler LA, Ramirez PM, Dominguez LM et al: Rethinking medication prescribing practices in an inner-city Hispanic mental health clinic, *J Psychiatrc Pract* 10(2):134-140, 2004.

Ogedegbe G, Mancuso CA, Allegrante JP: Expectations of blood pressure management in hypertensive African-American patients: a qualitative study, *J Natl Med Assoc* 96(4):442-449, 2004.

Robbins B, Rausch KJ, Garcia RI et al: Multicultural medication adherence: a comparative study, *J Gerontol Nurs* 30(7):25-32, 2004.

Rogers A, Kennedy A, Nelson E et al: Uncovering the limits of patient centeredness. Implementing a self management trail for chronic illness, *Qual Health Res* 15(2):224-239, 2005.

Sharma S, Murphy SP, Wilkens LR et al: Adherence to the food guide pyramid recommendations among African Americans and Latinos: results from the Multiethnic Cohort, *J Am Diet Assoc* 104(12):1873-1877, 2004.

Stuart GW, Laraia MT: Therapeutic nurse-patient relationship. In Stuart GW, Laraia MT, editors: *Principles and practice of psychiatric nursing,* St Louis, 2001, Mosby.

Unson CG, Siccion E, Gaztambide J et al: Nonadherence and osteoporosis treatment preferences of older women: a qualitative study, *J Womens Health* 12(10):1037-1045, 2003.

Unzueta M, Globe D, Wu J et al: Los Angeles Latino Eye Study Group. Compliance with follow-up care in Latinos: the Los Angeles Latino Eye Study, *Ethn Dis* 14(2):285-291, 2004.

Watts T, Merrell J, Murphy F et al: Breast health information needs of women from minority ethnic groups, *J Adv Nurs* 47(5): 526-535, 2004.


T

# Ineffective Therapeutic regimen management

evolve

*Margaret Lunney*

NANDA

## Definition

Pattern of regulating and integrating into daily living a program for treatment of illness and its sequelae that is unsatisfactory for meeting specific health goals

## Defining Characteristics

Choices of daily living ineffective for meeting goals of a treatment or prevention program; verbalization that client did not take action to reduce risk factors for progression of illness and sequelae; verbalization of desire to manage treatment of illness and prevention of sequelae; verbalization of difficulty with regulation of one or more prescribed regimens for prevention of complications and treatment of illness or its effects; verbalization that client did not take action to include treatment regimens in daily routines

## Related Factors (r/t)

Perceived barriers, social support deficits, powerlessness, perceived susceptibility, perceived benefits, mistrust of regimen and/or health care personnel, knowledge deficit, family patterns of health care, family conflict, excessive demands made on individual or family, economic difficulties, decisional conflicts, complexity of therapeutic regimen, complexity of health care system, faulty perception of illness seriousness, inadequate number and types of cues to action

NOC

## Outcomes (Nursing Outcomes Classification)

### Suggested NOC Outcomes

Decision Making; Knowledge: Disease Process, Treatment Regimen; Participation in Health Care Decisions; Symptom Severity; Treatment Behavior: Illness or Injury

**Example NOC Outcome with Indicators**

**Knowledge: Treatment Regimen** as evidenced by the following indicator: Description of prescribed medication, activity, exercise, and specific disease process (Rate the indicator of **Knowledge: Treatment Regimen**: 1 = none, 2 = limited, 3 = moderate, 4 = substantial, 5 = extensive [see Section I].)

## Client Outcomes

### Client Will (Specify Time Frame):

- Describe daily food and fluid intake that meets therapeutic goals

- Describe activity/exercise patterns that meet therapeutic goals
- Describe scheduling of medications that meets therapeutic goals
- Verbalize ability to manage therapeutic regimens
- Collaborate with health providers to decide on therapeutic regimen that is congruent with health goals and lifestyle

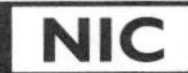

## Interventions (Nursing Interventions Classification)

### Suggested NIC Interventions

Anticipatory Guidance, Health Education, Health Screening, Health System Guidance, Learning Facilitation, Learning Readiness Enhancement, Risk Identification, Self-Modification Assistance

**Example NIC Activities—Learning Facilitation**

Relate information in a stimulating manner; encourage client's active participation

## Nursing Interventions and Rationales

NOTE: This diagnosis does not have the same meaning as the diagnosis **Noncompliance.** This diagnosis is made with the client, so if the client does not agree with the diagnosis, it should not be made. The emphasis is on helping the client to direct his or her own life and health, not on the client's compliance with the provider's instructions (Kastermans & Bakker, 1999).

- Refer to the care plans for **Effective Therapeutic regimen management** and **Ineffective family Therapeutic regimen management.**
- Establish a collaborative partnership with the client for purposes of meeting health-related goals. **EBN:** *Nurse-client partnerships reflect nursing models for practice (Gallant et al, 2002), and are consistent with national health care goals and objectives (www.healthypeople.gov). This approach differs from a traditional health care model in which the provider assumes authoritative and paternalistic roles. Nurse-consumer partnerships embody power sharing and negotiation (Gallant et al, 2002). In a grounded theory study, a caring partnership was used to control hypertension; the authors suggest that this model should also be used with other chronic illnesses (Mohammadi et al, 2002). In clinical trials, it was shown that self-efficacy was enhanced when people solved problems that they themselves identified (Bodenheimer et al, 2002).*
- Discuss all strategies with the client in the context of the client's culture. **EBN:** *Research studies involving culture, health behaviors and self-management show that culture significantly affects decision making for meeting therapeutic goals and is related to self-management strategies (Degazon, 2004; Thackerey et al, 2004).*
- Involve family members in knowledge development, planning for self-management and shared decision making. **EBN:** *In a study conducted in the United Kingdom of factors that influence adherence to a cardiac rehabilitation program for a convenience sample of 52 patients, family support and encouragement were found to be key predictors (Leong et al,*

T

*2004). Family support was shown to influence diet and exercise patterns of 138 older Mexican Americans with type 2 diabetes (Wen et al, 2004). Family support was one of two predictors of positive self-management strategies in a study of 53 women with type 2 diabetes (Whittemore et al, 2005).*

- Explore the meaning of the person's illness experience and identify uncertainties and needs through open-ended questions. **EB:** *This approach is necessary to know the person's perspective of self-management. Even though providers agree that self-management is the ideal approach to patient care, studies show that there are significant discrepancies between providers' and clients' views. Providers talk about self-management but may still expect compliance (Rogers et al, 2005).*
- Review factors of the Health Belief Model with the client (i.e., individual perceptions of seriousness and susceptibility, demographic and other modifying factors, and perceived benefits and barriers). **EBN:** *Studies using the Health Belief Model support the view that individual perceptions and a variety of modifying factors affect the likelihood of changing health behaviors (Pender, Murdaugh, & Parsons, 2002). In a study of 52 post–myocardial infraction patients, adherence to a physical activity regimen was associated with health motivation while adherance to smoking cessation was associated with self-efficacy (Leong et al, 2004).*
- Identify the reasons for actions that are not therapeutic and discuss alternatives. **EBN:** *Many possible reasons for actions do not meet therapeutic goals. Older women, for example, may not increase their activity levels because they have inaccurate perceptions of the related risks (Cousins, 2000). Fatigue and pain can have profound effects on the ability to perform therapeutic actions (Thorne & Paterson, 2000). Perceptions may differ according to diseases (e.g., people with pulmonary diseases are more likely than others to blame themselves for their condition) (Thorne & Paterson, 2000). In a longitudinal study of 7991 middle- and older-age adults, those who did not take medications as prescribed because the medications were too costly were 50% more likely to experience adverse events such as heart attacks (Heisler, 2004).*
- Provide in-depth explanations of the therapeutic regimen to meet health-related goals, including pathophysiology and scientific rationales. **EBN:** *In a prospective, randomized, controlled trial involving 77 clients with asthma, participants with moderate and severe asthma in the group that received additional client education experienced significant improvements in quality of life and symptoms (Marabini et al, 2002).*
- Use various formats to provide information about the therapeutic regimen (e.g., brochures, videotapes, written instructions, computer-based programs). **EBN:** *In a study with older adults using a three-group design, users of computer-based software for education about self-medication had significantly greater knowledge and self-efficacy scores, as well as fewer adverse self-medication behaviors over time than conventional education and control groups (Neafsey et al, 2002).*
- Help the client to develop a positive attitude toward the disease and therapeutic regimen management. **EBN:** *In a study of 29 adults with asthma, more positive attitudes were associated with higher knowledge and self-efficacy scores, and greater compliance with the use of peak flow meters (Scherer & Bruce, 2001). In a quasi-experimental study of the regi-*

T

*men adherence patterns of 249 people with osteoarthritis, self-efficacy and beliefs were contributing factors to adherence (Belza et al, 2002).*

- Deliberate with the client on changes that are possible to meet therapeutic goals. **EBN:** *Although decisions about actions to meet therapeutic goals are made by the client, the collaborative nature of the nurse-client interaction strengthens the relationship and contributes to the effectiveness of primary care (Wilkinson & Williams, 2002).*
- Help the client to self-manage his or her own health through teaching about strategies for changing habits such as overeating, sedentary lifestyle, and smoking. **EB:** *Evidence from controlled clinical trials indicates that teaching self-management skills is more effective for improving health outcomes than just providing information (Bodenheimer et al, 2002). In a review of 71 clinical trials of self-management education, it was shown that patients who participated in self-management achieved positive health outcomes such as reductions in glycosated hemoglobin levels and systolic blood pressure, as well as fewer asthmatic attacks (Warsi et al, 2004).* **EBN:** *In a quasi-experimental study involving 83 diabetic clients on a dialysis unit, the group that received self-management education showed a higher rate of significantly improved or maintained health outcomes than did those in the control group (McMurray et al, 2002).*
- Develop a contract with the client to maintain motivation for changes in behavior. **EBN:** *The nursing intervention of patient contracting provides a concrete means of keeping track of actions to meet health-related goals (Dochterman & Bulechek, 2004).*
- Help the client to maintain consistency in therapeutic regimen management for optimum results. **EBN:** *In a randomized quasi-experimental study of 249 adults with osteoarthritis, the group that consistently participated in the aquatic exercise program (attended 16 of 20 weeks) had improved quality of well-being, physical functioning, and changes in arthritis quality of life compared with those who were inconsistent in participation (Belza et al, 2002). In a study of 372 people on hemodialysis, self-management activities varied tremendously (Curtin et al, 2004).*
- Review how to contact health providers as needed to address issues and concerns regarding self-management. **EBN:** *The partnership process includes continued contact as changes occur; people with chronic illnesses need to know how to obtain interventions that are needed in the future (Gallant, Beaulieu, & Carnevale, 2002).*
- Implement organizational changes to facilitate shared decision making for self-management of chronic illnesses. **EB:** *Even with the goal of shared decision making and instructions on how to accomplish this goal, qualitative data from a quantitative clinical trail revealed that providers still approached patient care as if compliance was the goal. It was found that organizational structures and patterns contributed to the difficulty of adopting a patient-centered self-management approach (Rogers et al, 2005).*
- Use focus groups to evaluate the implementation of self-management programs. **EBN:** *In two studies using focus group methods, it was substantiated that the focus group format facilitated identification and understanding of themes that were important to self-management (Benavides-Vaello et al, 2004; Vijan et al, 2004). Themes identified were health maintenance, barriers to self-management, self-awareness, familial support, folk remedies, and confidence to mange diabetes (Benavides-Vaello et al, 2004). In a larger study*

T

*with quantitative and qualitative components, it was found that cost, portion size, and family support were majors issues of concern (Vijan et al, 2004).*

**Multicultural**

- Conduct a self-assessment of the relation of culture to ethically based care. **EBN:** *A tool was developed by the Midwest Bioethics Center Cultural Diversity Task Force (2001) to help providers conduct self-reflection and examination for ethically based care.*
- Assess for the influence of cultural beliefs, norms, and values on the individual's perceptions of the therapeutic regimen. **EBN:** *African Americans, Latinos born in the United States, and Latinos born in Mexico were less likely to adhere to all of the food group recommendations of the food pyramid (Sharma et al, 2004). A recent study showed that Hispanic psychiatric outpatients experienced akathisia as an increase in* nerviosismo. *Addressing this issue, as well as using anxiolytics and low doses of antipsychotics when beginning treatment, led to an improvement in compliance (Opler et al, 2004).*
- Assess health literacy in patients of diverse backgrounds. **EB:** *Individuals with marginal or inadequate functional health literacy will have difficulty reading, understanding, and interpreting most written health texts and instructions. In addition, patients with marginal or inadequate health literacy scores are more likely to misunderstand directions for health care. Consequently, these patients are also more likely to take medications incorrectly and more likely to fail to follow a prescribed diet or treatment regimen (Georges, Bolton, & Bennett, 2004).*
- Assess cultural relevance of health information. **EB:** *A study of breast health information needs of women from minority ethnic groups found that health care professionals lack of understanding about cultural beliefs, values, and knowledge, together with racial stereotyping and misconceptions about cancer in minority ethnic groups, posed challenges to information dissemination (Watts, Merrell, Murphy, & Williams, 2004).*
- Assess for barriers that may interfere with compliance to follow-up treatment recommendations. **EB:** *Adherence and compliance to a treatment regimen is often compounded by variables like cost, availability of services, and convenience of accessing care. Knowledge of barriers to seeking health care is important when developing interventions to address adherence and compliance (Unzueta et al, 2004).*
- Discuss with the client their beliefs about medication and treatment in order to enhance medication and treatment adherence. **EB:** *A recent study of Hispanic and African American women found that adherence was associated with recognition of the serious consequences of nonadherence, realization of the beneficial effects, and the belief that medicines are not harmful (Unson et al, 2003).*
- Utilize electronic monitoring to improve medication adherence. **EB:** *A recent study showed that the use of electronic monitors had a positive effect on adherence for the minority women (Robbins, Rausch, Garcia, & Prestwood, 2004).*
- Validate the client's feelings regarding the ability to manage his or her own care and the impact on current lifestyle. **EB:** *A recent study that elicited the expectations of treatment in 93 hypertensive African-American patients. Patient expectations of treatment could serve as the basis for patient education and counseling about hypertension and its management in this patient population (Ogedegbe, Mancuso, & Allegrante, 2004).*

T

- Assess temporal orientation and its relationship to the management of the therapeutic regimen. **EBN:** *Temporal orientation differs among cultures. The client's orientation to the present or the future was shown to affect management of hypertension and may also affect other therapeutic regimens (Brown & Segal, 1996).*
- Assess the effect of fatalism on the client's ability to adopt the therapeutic regimen. **EBN:** *Fatalistic perspectives, which involve the belief that one cannot control one's own fate, may influence health behaviors in some African American and Latino populations (Harmon, Castro, & Coe, 1996; Phillips, Cohen, & Moses, 1999).*

### Home Care

- Prepare and instruct clients/family members in the use of a medication box. Set up an appropriate schedule for filling of the medication box, and post medication times/doses in an accessible area (e.g., attached by magnet to a refrigerator). *Adherence to a medication regimen is increased through the use of cues and supports that assist clients to remember to take medications appropriately.*
- Monitor adherence to the medical regimen. **EBN:** *In elderly clients with diabetes mellitus living alone, home visits (both daily and weekly) were associated with reductions in fasting blood sugar, postmeal blood sugar, and hemoglobin A1c (Huang, Wu, Jeng, et al, 2004).*
- ▲ Consult with physician and/or pharmacist as questions arise. **EBN:** *A study demonstrated that nurses monitoring of medication regimen and appropriate referral for medication review helped to increase client's knowledge of medications and appropriate use of compliance aids (Griffiths, Johnson, Piper, et al, 2004).*

### Client/Family Teaching

- Identify what the client and/or family knows and adjust teaching accordingly. *Teach the client and family about all aspects of the therapeutic regimen, providing as much knowledge as the client and family will accept, in a culturally congruent manner.*
- Teach ways to adjust ADLs for inclusion of therapeutic regimens.
- Teach safety in taking medications.
- Teach the client to act as a self-advocate with health providers who prescribe therapeutic regimens.

## evolve WEBSITES FOR EDUCATION

See the EVOLVE website for World Wide Web resources for client education.

T

## REFERENCES


Belza B, Topolski T, Kinne S et al: Does adherence make a difference: results from a community-based aquatic exercise program, *Nurs Res* 51(5):285, 2002.

Benavides-Vaello S, Garcia AA, Brown SA et al: Using focus group to plan and evaluate diabetes self-management interventions for Mexican Americans, *Diabetes Educ* 30(2):238-256, 2004.

Bodenheimer T, Lorig K, Holman H et al: Patient self-management of chronic disease in primary care, *JAMA* 288(19):2469, 2002.

Brown CM, Segal R: Ethnic differences in temporal orientation and its implications for hypertension management, *J Health Soc Behav* 37:350, 1996.

Chinn MH et al: Developing a conceptual framework for understanding illness and attitudes in older, urban African Americans with diabetes, *Diabetes Educ* 26(3):439, 2000.

Cousins SO: "My heart can't take it": older women's beliefs about exercise benefits and risks, *J Gerontol B Psychol Sci Soc Sci* 55B(5): 283, 2000.

Curtin RB, Sitter DCB, Schatell D et al: Self-management, knowledge, and functioning and well being of patients on hemodialysis, *Neph Nurs J* 31(4):378-386, 2004.

Degazon C: Cultural diversity and community-oriented nursing practice. In Stanhope M, Lancaster J: *Community and public health nursing,* ed 6, St Louis, 2004, Mosby.

Dochterman JM, Bulechek GM: *Nursing interventions classification (NIC),* ed 6, St Louis, Mosby, 2004.

Gallant MH, Beaulieu MC, Carnevale FA: Partnership: an analysis of the concept within the nurse-client relationship, *J Adv Nurs* 40(2):149, 2002.

Georges CA, Bolton LB, Bennett C: Functional health literacy: an issue in African-American and other ethnic and racial communities, *J Natl Black Nurses Assoc* 15(1):1-4, 2004.

Goodwin JS, Black SA, Satish S: Aging versus disease: the opinions of older black, Hispanic, and non-Hispanic white Americans about the causes and treatment of common medical conditions, *J Am Geriatr Soc* 47(8):973, 1999.

Griffiths R, Johnson M, Piper M et al: A nursing intervention for the quality use of medicines by elderly community clients, *Intl J Nurs Pract* 10(4):166, 2004.

Harmon MP, Castro FG, Coe K: Acculturation and cervical cancer: knowledge, beliefs, and behaviors of Hispanic women, *Women Health* 24(3):37, 1996.

Heisler M: The health effects of restricting prescription medication use because of cost, *Med Care* 42(7):626-634, 2004.

Huang CL, Wu SC, Jeng CY et al: The efficacy of a home-based nursing program in diabetic control of elderly people with diabetes mellitus living alone, *Publ Health Nurse* 21(1):49, 2004.

Kastermans MC, Bakker RH: Managing the impact of health problems on daily living. In Ranz MJ, Lemone P, editors: *Classification of nursing diagnoses: proceedings of the thirteenth conference,* Glendale, Calif, 1999, CINAHL Information Systems.

Leininger MM: *Culture care diversity and universality: a theory of nursing,* Boston, 2001, Jones and Bartlett.

Leininger MM, McFarland MR: *Transcultural nursing: concepts, theories, research and practices,* ed 3, New York, 2002, McGraw-Hill.

Leong J, Molassiotis A, Marsh H: Adherence to health recommendations after a cardiac rehabilitation programme in post-myocardial infarction patients: the role of heath beliefs, locus of control and psychological status, *Clin Effectiveness in Nurs* 8(1):26-38, 2004.

Marabini A, Brugnami G, Curradi F et al: Short term effectiveness of an asthma educational program: results of a randomized controlled trial, *Respir Med* 96(12):933, 2002.

McMurray SD, Johnson G, Davis S et al: Diabetes education and care management significantly improve patient outcomes in a dialysis unit, *Am J Kidney Dis* 40(3):566, 2002.

Midwest Bioethics Center: Healthcare narratives from diverse communities—a self-assessment tool for health-care providers, *Bioethics Forum* 17(3-4):SS1, 2001.

Mohammadi E, Abedi HA, Gofranipour F et al: Partnership caring: a theory of high blood pressure control in Iranian hypertensives, *Int J Nurs Pract* 8(6):324, 2002.

Neafsey PJ, Strickler Z, Shellman J et al: An interactive technology approach to educate older adults about drug interactions arising from over-the-counter self medication practices, *Public Health Nurs* 19(4):255, 2002.

Opler LA, Ramirez PM, Dominguez LM et al: Rethinking medication prescribing practices in an inner-city Hispanic mental health clinic, *J Psychiatr Pract* 10(2):134-140, 2004.

Ogedegbe G, Mancuso CA, Allegrante JP: Expectations of blood pressure management in hypertensive African-American patients: a qualitative study, *J Natl Med Assoc* 96(4):442-449, 2004.

Pender NJ, Murdaugh CL, Parsons MA: *Health promotion in nursing practice,* ed 4, Upper Saddle River, NJ, 2002, Prentice Hall.

Phillips JM, Cohen MZ, Moses G: Breast cancer screening and African American women: fear, fatalism, and silence, *Oncol Nurs Forum* 26(3):561, 1999.

Robbins B, Rausch KJ, Garcia RI et al: Multicultural medication adherence: a comparative study, *J Gerontol Nurs* 30(7):25-32, 2004.

Rogers A, Kennedy A, Nelson E et al: Uncovering the limits of patient centeredness: implementing a self management trail for chronic illness, *Qual Health Res* 15(2):224-239, 2005.

Scherer YK, Bruce S: Knowledge, attitudes, and self-efficacy and compliance with medical regimen, number of emergency visits, and hospitalizations in adults with asthma, *Heart Lung* 30(4):250, 2001.
Sharma S, Murphy SP, Wilkens LR et al: Adherence to the food guide pyramid recommendations among African Americans and Latinos: results from the Multiethnic Cohort, *J Am Diet Assoc* 104(12):1873-1877, 2004.
Stuart GW, Laraia MT: Therapeutic nurse-patient relationship. In Stuart GW, Laraia MT, editors: *Principles and practice of psychiatric nursing,* St Louis, 2001, Mosby.
Thackeray R, Merrill RM, Neiger BL: Disparities in diabetes management practice between racial and ethnic groups in the United States, *Diabetes Educ* 30(4):665-675, 2004.
Thorne SE, Paterson BL: Two decades of insider research: what we know and don't know about chronic illness experience, *Annu Rev Nurs Res* 18:3, 2000.
Unson CG, Siccion E, Gaztambide J et al: Nonadherence and osteoporosis treatment preferences of older women: a qualitative study, *J Womens Health* 12(10):1037-1045, 2003.
Unzueta M, Globe D, Wu J et al: Los Angeles Latino Eye Study Group. Compliance with recommendations for follow-up care in Latinos: the Los Angeles Latino Eye Study, *Ethn Dis* 14(2):285-291, 2004.
Warsi A, Wang PS, LaValley MP et al: Self management education programs in chronic disease, *Arch Intern Med* 164:1641-1649, 2004.
Watts T, Merrell J, Murphy F et al: Breast health information needs of women from minority ethnic groups, *J Adv Nurs* 47(5): 526-535, 2004.
Wen LK, Shepard MD, Parchman ML: Family support, diet, and exercise among older Mexican Americans with type 2 diabetes, *Diabetes Educ* 30(6):980-993, 2004.
Whittemore R, Melkus GD, Grey M: Metabolic control, self management and psychosocial adjustment in women with type 2 diabetes, *J Clin Nurs* 14(2):195-204, 2005.
Wilkinson CR, Williams M: Strengthening patient-provider relationships, *Lippincott's Case Manag* 7(3):86, 2002.

# Readiness for enhanced Therapeutic regimen management

*Margaret Lunney*

**NANDA**

## Definition

Pattern of regulating and integrating into daily living a program(s) for treatment of illness and its sequelae that is sufficient for meeting health-related goals and can be strengthened

## Defining Characteristics

Expression of desire to manage treatment of illness and prevention of sequelae, choices of daily living that are appropriate for meeting goals of treatment or prevention, expression of little to no difficulty with regulation/integration of one or more prescribed regimens for treatment of illness or prevention of complications, reduction of risk factors for progression of illness and sequelae, lack of unexpected acceleration of illness symptoms



T

## NOC

## Outcomes (Nursing Outcomes Classification)

### Suggested NOC Outcomes

Health-Promoting Behavior; Health-Seeking Behavior; Knowledge: Health Behavior, Health Promotion, Health Resources, Illness Care, Medication, Prescribed Activity, Treatment Regimen

**Example NOC Outcome with Indicators**

**Health-Promoting Behavior** as evidenced by the following indicators: Monitors personal behavior for risks/Seeks balance among exercise, work, leisure, rest, and nutrition/Performs healthy behaviors routinely/Uses financial and physical resources to promote health (Rate each indicator of **Health-Promoting Behavior**: 1 = never demonstrated, 2 = rarely demonstrated, 3 = sometimes demonstrated, 4 = often demonstrated, 5 = consistently demonstrated [see Section I].)

## Client Outcomes

### Client Will (Specify Time Frame):

- Describe integration of therapeutic regimen into daily living
- Demonstrate continued commitment to integration of therapeutic regimen into daily living routines

## NIC

## Interventions (Nursing Interventions Classification)

### Suggested NIC Interventions

Anticipatory Guidance; Mutual Goal Setting; Patient Contracting; Self-Modification Assistance; Self-Responsibility Facilitation; Support System Enhancement; Teaching: Disease Process

**Example NIC Activities—Mutual Goal Setting**

Assist client in prioritizing identified goals; clarify roles of client and health care provider, respectively

T

## Nursing Interventions and Rationales

- Acknowledge the expertise that the patient and family bring to self-management. **EBN:** *In a study of older people diagnosed with asthma using three different methods—interviews, a questionnaire, and participatory action research—it was found that there are three different models of self-management: medical model, collaborative model, and self-agency model. To achieve optimum self-agency, it was recommended that health care professionals respect the expertise of patients (Koch, Jenkin, & Kralik, 2004).*
- Explore attitudes toward the illness/disease and the need for management of a therapeutic regimen. **EBN:** *In a qualitative study of 19 African-American clients 65 years of age and older, ambivalence toward illness care was an identified theme (Chinn et al, 2000).*

- Review factors that contribute to the likelihood of health promotion and health protection. Use Pender's Health Promotion Model and Becker's Health Belief Model to identify contributing factors (Pender, Murdaugh, & Parsons, 2002). **EBN:** *Many studies using both the Health Promotion Model and the Health Belief Model support the view that individual perceptions and a variety of modifying factors affect the likelihood of improving health behaviors (Pender, Murdaugh, & Parsons, 2002). For example, in a study of 52 post–myocardial patients in the United Kingdom, adhering to physical activity was associated with health motivation and adhering to smoking cessation was associated with self-efficacy (Leong, Molassiotis, & Marsh, 2004). Also, in the same study, 37.5% of the variance in adherence to healthy diet was accounted for by the extent that family members encouraged the patient to follow the therapeutic regimen.*
- Assess for depression. **EB:** *In a study of 168 diabetic patients in a Korean clinic, depression was an explanatory factor for those reporting low adherence with self-care (Park et al, 2004). In a study of 52 post–myocardial patients in the United Kingdom, more than 19% had symptoms of depression, which were thought to contribute to low adherence (Leong, Molassiotis, & Marsh, 2004)*
- Facilitate the patient and family to obtain health insurance and drug payment plans whenever needed and possible. **EB:** *In a qualitative study of 167 African Americans, those who had health insurance reported more frequently the influence of health providers on self-care (Becker, Gates, & Newsom, 2004). In a study of two prospective cohort studies with almost 8000 older Americans, it was found that underuse of prescription medications because of cost led to adverse health effects (Heisler, 2004).*
- Further develop and reinforce contributing factors that might change with ongoing management of the therapeutic regimen (e.g., knowledge, self-efficacy, self-esteem, and perceived benefits). **EBN:** *Illness care is associated with ongoing changes and, over time, management of therapeutic regimens can become increasingly tedious and difficult (Lubkin & Larsen, 2002). For example, in a study of the education of hypertensive clients and their compliance with the medication regimen (N = 40), a negative correlation was seen between duration of treatment and compliance.*
- Support all efforts to self-manage therapeutic regimens. **EBN:** *Ongoing support and assistance from health care providers is needed to identify and enhance factors that contribute to the likelihood of taking action for health promotion and health protection (Pender, Murdaugh, & Parsons, 2002). In a study examining whether adherence to regular aquatic exercise made a difference for 249 adults with osteoarthritis, it was found that exercise benefited the participants and that increased attention by health providers to improving clients' self-efficacy and belief systems would likely facilitate adherence (Belza et al, 2002).*
- Review the client's strengths in the management of the therapeutic regimen. **EBN:** *People who are doing the work of managing a therapeutic regimen may not even realize that they are doing it well (Lubkin & Larsen, 2002).*
- Collaborate with the client to identify strategies to maintain strengths and develop additional strengths as indicated. **EBN:** *The client and provider working in partnership can facilitate, support, and reinforce the client's strengths (Gallant, Beaulieu, & Carnevale, 2002).*
- Identify contributing factors that may need to be improved now or in the future. **EBN:** *Health promotion and protection are complex behaviors that are difficult to imple-*

T

*ment on a daily basis. Based on the complexity of achieving these behaviors and the perceived barriers to implementation (e.g., time, energy, money), usually one or more contributing factors would benefit from increased focus and attention (Pender, Murdaugh, & Parsons, 2002).*

- Provide knowledge as needed related to the pathophysiology of the disease/illness, prescribed activities, prescribed medications, and nutrition. **EBN:** *Knowledge is a factor that contributes significantly to the client's taking action for health promotion and protection (Pender, Murdaugh, & Parsons, 2002). It is important to remember, however, that knowledge is necessary but not sufficient to explain why people perform or do not perform actions for health promotion and protection (Pender, Murdaugh, & Parsons, 2002).*
- Use coaching strategies such as educational reinforcement, psychosocial support, and motivational guidance. **EBN:** *In a study involving individuals newly diagnosed with type 2 diabetes, nurse coaching yielded a modest increase in health-promoting behaviors and a decrease in fasting blood glucose level (Whittemore et al, 2001).*
- Support positive health-promotion and health-protection behaviors. **EBN:** *Ongoing support may be needed to maintain these behaviors (Pender, Murdaugh, & Parsons, 2002).*
- Help the client maintain existing support and seek additional supports as needed. **EBN:** *In numerous research studies, social support was shown to be a factor contributing to ongoing maintenance of positive health behaviors (Lubkin & Larsen, 2002; Pender, Murdaugh, & Parsons, 2002). For example, in a study of long-term survivors of cancer, social support and self-esteem were two of the three variables that explained 53% of the variance in health-related quality of life (Pedro, 2001).*

## Multicultural

- Manipulate community factors that may affect the management of the therapeutic regimen (e.g., barriers, supports, insurance, education about the illness, and provider-client relationships). **EBN:** *A study involving African-American clients with diabetes concluded that complex environmental factors can indirectly affect glycemic control and management of the therapeutic regimen (Brody et al, 2001).*
- Validate the client's feelings regarding the ability to manage his or her own care and the impact on current lifestyle. **EB:** *A recent study elicited the expectations of treatment in 93 hypertensive African-American patients. Patient expectations of treatment could serve as the basis for patient education and counseling about hypertension and its management in this patient population (Ogedegbe, Mancuso, & Allegrante, 2004).*
- Use electronic monitoring to improve medication adherence. **EB:** *A recent study showed that the use of electronic monitors had a positive effect on adherence for the minority women (Robbins, Rausch, Garcia, & Prestwood, 2004).*
- Discuss with the client their beliefs about medication and treatment in order to enhance medication and treatment adherence. **EB:** *A recent study of Hispanic and African-American women found that adherence was associated with recognition of the serious consequences of nonadherence, realization of the beneficial effects, and the belief that medicines are not harmful (Unson et al, 2003).*
- Use electronic monitoring to improve medication adherence. **EB:** *A recent study showed that the use of electronic monitors had a positive effect on adherence for the minority women (Robbins, Rausch, Garcia, & Prestwood, 2004).*

### Community Teaching

- Review therapeutic regimens and their optimum integration with daily living routines.
- Teach disease processes and therapeutic regimens for management of these disease processes.

## evolve WEBSITES FOR EDUCATION

See the EVOLVE website for World Wide Web resources for client education.

## REFERENCES

Becker G, Gates RJ, Newsom E: Self care among chronically ill African Americans: culture, health disparities, and health insurance status, *Am J Public Health* 94(12):2066-2073, 2004.
Belza B, Topolski T, Kinne S et al: Does adherence make a difference? Results from a community-based aquatic exercise program, *Nurs Res* 51(5):285, 2002.
Brody GH, Jack L Jr, Murry VM et al: Heuristic model linking contextual processes to self-management in African American adults with type 2 diabetes, *Diabetes Educ* 27(5):685, 2001.
Chinn MH et al: Developing a conceptual framework for understanding illness and attitudes in older, urban African Americans with diabetes, *Diabetes Educ* 26(3):439, 2000.
Gallant MH, Beaulieu MC, Carnevale FA: Partnership: an analysis of the concept within the nurse-client relationship, *J Adv Nurs* 40(2):149, 2002.
Heisler M: The health effects of restricting prescription medication use because of cost, *Med Care* 42(7):626-634, 2004.
Koch T, Jenkin P, Kralik D: Chronic illness self management: locating the self, *J Adv Nurs* 48(5):484-492, 2004.
Leininger MM: *Culture care diversity and universality: a theory of nursing,* Boston, 2001, Jones and Bartlett.
Leininger MM, McFarland MR: *Transcultural nursing: concepts, theories, research and practices,* ed 3, New York, 2002, McGraw-Hill.
Lubkin IM, Larsen PD: *Chronic illness: impact and interventions,* ed 5, Boston, 2002, Jones and Bartlett.
Ogedegbe G, Mancuso CA, Allegrante JP: Expectations of blood pressure management in hypertensive African-American patients: a qualitative study, *J Natl Med Assoc* 96(4):442-449, 2004.
Park H, Hong Y, Lee H et al: Individuals with type 2 diabetes and depressive symptoms exhibited low adherence with self care, *J Clin Epidemiol* 57:978-984, 2004.
Pedro LW: Quality of life for long-term survivors of cancer: influencing variables, *Cancer Nurs* 24(1):1, 2001.
Pender NJ, Murdaugh CL, Parsons MA: *Health promotion in nursing practice,* ed 4, Upper Saddle River, NJ, 2002, Prentice Hall.
Robbins B, Rausch KJ, Garcia RI et al: Multicultural medication adherence: a comparative study, *J Gerontol Nurs* 30(7):25-32, 2004.
Unson CG, Siccion E, Gaztambide J et al: Nonadherence and osteoporosis treatment preferences of older women: a qualitative study, *J Womens Health* 12(10):1037-1045, 2003.
Whittemore R, Chase S, Mandle CL et al: The content, integrity and efficacy of a nurse coaching intervention in type 2 diabetes, *Diabetes Educ* 27(6):887, 2001.

# Ineffective community Therapeutic regimen management

*Margaret Lunney*

T

**NANDA**

### Definition

Pattern of regulating and integrating into community processes programs for the treatment of illness and its sequelae that is unsatisfactory for meeting health-related goals

## Defining Characteristics

Illness symptoms above norm expected for number and type of population, unexpected acceleration of illness(es), number of health care resources insufficient for incidence or prevalence of illness(es), deficits in aggregates for specific groups, deficits in people and programs to be accountable for illness care of specific groups, deficits in community activities for secondary and tertiary prevention, unavailability of health care resources for illness care

## Related Factors (r/t)

To be developed.

**NOC**

## Outcomes (Nursing Outcomes Classification)

### Suggested NOC Outcomes

Community Competence; Community Health Status; Community Health Status: Immunity; Community Risk Control: Chronic Disease; Community Risk Control: Communicable Disease; Community Risk Control: Lead Exposure

**Example NOC Outcome with Indicators**

**Community Health Status** as evidenced by the following indicators: Participation rates in preventive health services and health promotion programs/Prevalence of health protection and health promotion programs/Mortality rates/Morbidity rates/Mental health illness rates/Chronic disease rates/Low birth weight rates/Injury rates (Rate each indicator of **Community Health**: 1 = poor, 2 = fair, 3 = good, 4 = very good, 5 = excellent [see Section I].)

## Community Outcomes

**Community members and leaders will (Specify Time Frame):**

- Secure community members and/or health providers who will be accountable for illness care of specific groups
- Remain involved in advocacy for illness care and prevention programs
- Develop health care plans for effective prevention and treatment of illnesses
- Make resources available for illness care and prevention
- Initiate or improve strategies for prevention of the sequelae of illness

T

**NIC**

## Interventions (Nursing Interventions Classification)

### Suggested NIC Interventions

Community Health Development; Case Management; Health Education; Environmental Management: Community; Health Policy Monitoring; Health Screening; Risk Identification

NOTE: NIC interventions that were developed for use with individuals can be adapted for use with communities.

**Example NIC Activities—Community Health Development**

Identify health concerns, strengths, and priorities with community partners; facilitate implementation and revision of community plans

## Nursing Interventions and Rationales

NOTE: Nursing interventions are conducted in collaboration with community leaders, community and public health nurses, and members of other disciplines (Anderson & McFarlane, 2003; Chinn, 2001).

- • Implement strategies to engage community members to be team members for health assessments and development of community programs. **EB:** *In a survey related to the conduct of community health assessments in 105 counties of Kansas, the researcher concluded that team building of health providers with community leaders was an important aspect of success (Curtis, 2002). The experiences of numerous other communities have shown that community participation is critical to the success of programs for illness prevention and control and reducing health disparities (e.g., Faust et al, 2005; Horowitz et al, 2004; Kieffer et al, 2004; Thacker, 2005).*
- • Request that a Clinical Nurse Specialist (CNS) in community health nursing work with coalitions of health providers and community leaders. **EBN:** *Community health nurses who are prepared as CNS have competencies in direct care of communities and community-based organizations and networks (Logan, 2005).*
- ▲ Recruit additional health providers as needed. **EB and EBN:** *Designing and implementing community-based programs requires the participation of providers from multiple disciplines working alongside community members (Anderson & McFarland, 2003). In applying the caring model to a community, Smith-Campbell (1999) was able to enlist additional health providers to participate in supplying community services.*
- • Examine the perceptions of community members regarding service needs. **EBN:** *In a study to determine the congruence of the perceptions of consumers (N =385) and case managers, the correlations were low between the perceptions of these two groups; consumers perceived that service needs were unmet, whereas case managers perceived that service needs were overly met (Crane-Ross, Roth, & Lauber, 2000).*
- • Establish Special Action Groups (SAGs) for specific problems and/or localities to address health policies and practices. **EB:** *After 3 years, two SAGs in Arizona with a focus on diabetes prevention and control successfully documented changes in local policies and practices (Meister et al, 2005).*
- • Evaluate community infrastructures for adequacy in serving community illness-related needs. **EB:** *Community infrastructures are important aspects of self-management, including health policies, illness-focused education, availability of services and resources, and so forth (Chaffee et al, 2002; Ingram et al, 2005).*
- • Apply the concept of caring to the community as client. **EBN:** *A systematic case study*

*approach illustrated a community model of caring and showed that the concept of caring applies to communities as well as individuals (Smith-Campbell, 1999).*

- Advocate for and with the community in multiple arenas (e.g., newspapers, television, legislative bodies, community boards). **EBN:** *Many communities have benefited from the advocacy of nurses and other health providers whose opinions are respected (Anderson & McFarlane, 2003).*
- Provide information to public and private sources about community assessment, diagnosis, and plans of care. **EBN:** *The commitment that is needed for improvements in health services can be obtained only when community members have adequate information (Anderson & McFarland, 2003).*
- Mobilize support for the community to obtain the resources necessary for illness care and prevention. **EB:** *In a study of the Cardiovascular Health Network Project using focus groups with women participants, lack of community resources and support were identified as barriers for women from some communities to practice health-promoting activities such as physical exercise (Eyler et al, 2002).*
- Establish culturally sensitive community health programs for self-management. **EB:** *In New York City, between 2001 and 2004, emergency room and unscheduled physician office visits for asthma-related problems were reduced from 35% to 8% after 18 months of a culturally sensitive community-based program (Centers for Disease Control and Prevention (CDC), 2005). Many other studies have shown that community-based programs for illness care and prevention have positive results (e.g., Garvin et al, 2004; Lee et al, 2004).*
- Provide coaching interventions in programs for chronic disease self-management. **EBN:** *The positive patient outcomes of a community-based nursing program with a focus on coaching showed that nursing programs such as this can successfully engage middle and older age adults in health promotion and protection activities (Tidwell, et al, 2004).*
- Integrate the Internet with community health programs. **EB:** *The internet is widely used by consumers of all ages and ethnicities (e.g., in a study of 208 church-based African-Americans, 47% used the Internet for health-related information (Laken et al, 2004).*
- Determine the cultural appropriateness of all programs. **EBN:** *The cultural appropriateness of a program is an indicator of the potential success of the program (Leininger & McFarland, 2002).*
- Support the population of family caregivers through implementation of the National Family Support Program. **EB:** *A study of community leaders in 10 states showed that programs to support family caregivers are under way and are sorely needed to relieve the burden of family caregiving (Feinberg & Newman, 2004).*
- Write grant proposals for the funding of new programs or the expansion of existing programs. (See Coley and Scheinberg [2000] for grant-writing methods.) **EB:** *Public and private sources of funds can often supply the financial bases of health care programs (Anderson & McFarlane, 2003).*
- Conduct research studies to convince others of the need to improve services or change policies. **EBN:** *Research findings may be needed to obtain broad support for needed changes (Anderson & McFarland, 2003). For example, in the last few decades, nurses have conducted research studies on the topic of battered women that were successful in influencing legislators to change laws and public policies in ways that positively affected the prevention*

T

*and treatment of violence against women. A recent example of this type of research showed that there is a definite link between abuse during pregnancy and attempted and completed femicide (homicide of females) (McFarlane et al, 2002).*

- Avoid victim-blaming stances in efforts to promote community responsibility for health. **EB:** *Based on 40 years of work with multiple agencies, Green & Kreuter (2005) identified multiple determinants of health besides local community participation. Some of these determinants include national health policy, media, resources, and organizations.*

## Multicultural

- Hire culturally diverse staff members for community agencies. **EB:** *In a study of 22 community agencies that provide end-of-life care in a southeastern state, the presence of more diverse staff members or volunteers was associated with more diverse clients. Culturally diverse services were more likely to be provided when directors provided leadership in welcoming diversity (Reese et al, 2004).*
- Identify the health services and information resources that are currently available in the community. **EBN:** *This will assist in focusing efforts and promote the wise use of valuable resources. Many communities of color lack access to culturally competent health care providers, pharmacies, and grocery stores (National Institutes of Health, 1998).*
- Identify cultural barriers such as acculturation issues, lack of community support, and lack of past experience with a health behavior. **EBN:** *Cultural barriers to exercise regimens were identified in a series of focus groups with women in the Cardiovascular Health Network Project (Eyler et al, 2002).*
- Work with members of the community to prioritize and target health goals specific to the community. **EBN:** *This will increase feelings of control and sense of ownership of programs and interventions (National Institutes of Health, 1998).*
- Approach community leaders and members of color with respect, warmth, and professional courtesy. **EBN:** *Instances of disrespect and lack of caring have special significance for individuals of color (D'Avanzo et al, 2001).*
- Establish and sustain partnerships with key individuals within the community in developing and implementing programs. **EBN:** *Local leaders are excellent sources of information, and their participation will enhance the credibility of the programs (National Institutes of Health, 1998).*
- Develop a health promotion directory that lists health resources for patients. **EB:** *A study that assessed utilization of a health promotion directory found that African-American group members were significantly more likely to contact one of the resources listed in the health directory (Haber & Looney, 2003).*
- Use community church settings as a forum for advocacy, teaching, and program implementation. **EBN:** *A review of church-based health promotion programs shows that they are successful in helping people to adopt health-promoting behaviors (Peterson, Atwood, & Yates, 2002). Church-based interventions have been very successful in communities of color (Kotecki, 2002).*

T

## evolve WEBSITES FOR EDUCATION

See the EVOLVE website for World Wide Web resources for client education.

## REFERENCES


Anderson ET, McFarlane J: *Community as partner: theory and practice in nursing,* ed 4, Philadelphia, 2003, JB Lippincott.

Centers for Disease Control and Prevention: Reducing childhood asthma through community-based service delivery, New York City, 2001-2004, *MMWR,* 54(1):11-14, 2005.

Chaffee MW, Mason DJ, Leavitt JK: *Policy and politics in nursing and health care,* ed 4, Philadelphia, 2002, WB Saunders.

Chinn PL: Making a difference in health care, *ANS Adv Nurs Sci* 24(1), 2001.

Coley SM, Scheinberg CA: *Proposal writing,* ed 2, Thousand Oaks, Calif, 2000, Sage.

Crane-Ross D, Roth D, Lauber BG: Consumers' and case managers' perceptions of mental health and community support service needs, *Community Ment Health J* 36(2):161, 2000.

Curtis DC: Evaluation of community health assessment in Kansas, *J Public Manage Pract* 8(4):20-25, 2002.

D'Avanzo CE et al: Developing culturally informed strategies for substance related interventions. In Naegle MA, D'Avanzo CE, editors: *Addictions and substance abuse: strategies for advanced practice nursing,* St Louis, 2001, Mosby, 59-104.

Eyler AA, Matson-Koffman D, Vest JR et al: Environmental, policy, and cultural factors related to physical activity in a diverse sample of women: the Women's Cardiovascular Health Network Project—summary and discussion, *Women Health* 36(2):123, 2002.

Faust LA, Blanchard LW, Breyfogle DA et al: Discussion suppers as a means for community engagement, *J Rural Health* 21(1): 92-95, 2005.

Feinberg LF, Newman SL: A study of 10 states since passage of the national family caregiver support program: policies, perceptions and program development, *Gerontologist* 44(6):760-769, 2004.

Garvin CC, Cheadle A, Chrisman N et al: A community-based approach to diabetes control in multiple cultural groups, *Ethn Dis* 14(3 Suppl 1): S83-92.

Green LW, Kreuter MW: *Health promotion planning: an education and ecological approach,* ed 4, New York, 2005, McGraw Hill.

Haber D, Looney C: Health promotion directory: development, distribution, and utilization, *Health Promotion Pract* 4(1):72-77, 2003.

Horowitz CR, Arniella A, James S et al: Using community-based participatory research to reduce health disparities in East and Central Harlem, *MT Sinai J Med* 71(6):368-374, 2004.

Ingram M, Gallegos G, Elenes J: Diabetes is a community issue: the critical elements of a successful outreach and education model on the U.S.-Mexico Border, *Prev Chronic Dis* 2(1):A15, 2005.

Jack L, Liburd L, Spencer T et al: Understanding the environmental issues in diabetes self management education research: a re-examination of 8 studies in community-based settings, *Ann Intern Med* 140(11):964-971, 2004.

Kieffer EC, Willis SK, Odoms-Young AM et al: Reducing disparities in diabetes among African American and Latino residents of Detroit: the essential role of community planning focus groups, E*thn Dis* 14(3 Suppl 1):S27-37, 2004.

Kotecki CN: Developing a health promotion program for faith-based communities, *Holist Nurs Pract* 16(3):61, 2002.

Laken MA, O'Rourke K, Duffy NG et al: Use of the Internet for health information by African Americans with modifiable risk factors for cardiovascular disease, *J E Health* 10(3):304-310, 2004.

Lee S, Naimark B, Porter MM et al: Effects of a long term, community-based cardiac rehabilitation program on middle aged and elderly cardiac patient, *Am J Geriatr Cardiol* 13(6):293-298, 2004.

Leininger MM, McFarland MR: *Transcultural nursing: concepts, theories, research and practices,* ed 3, New York, 2002, McGraw-Hill.

Logan L: The practice of certified community health CNSs, *Clin Nurse Spec* 19(1):43-48, 2005.

McFarlane J, Campbell JC, Sharps P et al: Abuse during pregnancy and femicide: urgent implications for women's health, *Obstet Gynecol* 100(1):27, 2002.

Meister JS, Guernsey de Zapien J: Bringing health policy issues front and center in the community: expanding the role of community health coalitions, *Prev Chronic Dis* 2(1):A16, 2005.

National Institutes of Health: *Salud para su corazo´n: bringing heart health to Latinos—a guide for building community programs,* DHHS Pub No. 98-3796, Washington, DC, 1998, U.S. Government Printing Office.

Peterson J, Atwood JR, Yates B: Key elements for church-based health promotion programs: outcome-based literature review, *Public Health Nurs* 19(6):401, 2002.

Reese DJ, Melton E, Ciaravino K: Programmatic barriers to providing culturally competent end-of-life care, *Am J Hosp Palliat Care* 21(5):357-364, 2004.

Smith-Campbell B: A case study on expanding the concept of caring from individuals to communities, *Public Health Nurs* 16(6): 405, 1999.

Thacker K: Academic-community partnerships: opening the doors to a nursing career, *J Transcult Nurs* 16(1):57-63, 2005.
Tidwell L, Holland SK, Greenberg J et al. Community-based nurse health coaching and its effect on fitness participation, *Lippincotts Case Manag* 9(6):267-279, 2004.

# Ineffective family Therapeutic regimen management

*Margaret Lunney*

## NANDA

### Definition

Pattern of regulating and integrating into family processes a program for treatment of illness and its sequelae that is unsatisfactory for meeting specific health goals

### Defining Characteristics

Inappropriate family activities for meeting goals of treatment or prevention program, acceleration of illness symptoms of family member, lack of attention to illness and its sequelae, verbalization of difficulty with regulation/integration of one or more activities or prevention of complications, verbalization of desire to manage treatment of illness and prevention of its sequelae, verbalization that family did not take action to reduce risk factors for progression of illness and sequelae

### Related Factors (r/t)

Complexity of health care system, complexity of therapeutic regimen, decisional conflicts, economic difficulties, excessive demands on individual or family, family conflict

## NOC

### Outcomes (Nursing Outcomes Classification)

#### Suggested NOC Outcomes

Health Orientation; Health-Promoting Behavior; Health-Seeking Behavior; Knowledge: Treatment Regimen; Participation in Health Care Decisions; Treatment Behavior: Illness or Injury

**Example NOC Outcome with Indicators**

**Knowledge: Treatment Regimen** as evidenced by the following indicator: Description of prescribed medication, activity, exercise, and specific disease process (Rate each indicator of **Knowledge: Treatment Regimen**: 1 = none, 2 = limited, 3 = moderate, 4 = substantial, 5 = extensive [see Section I].)

## Family Outcomes

**Family Will (Specify Time Frame):**

- Make adjustments in usual activities (e.g., diet, activity, stress management) to incorporate therapeutic regimens of its members
- Reduce illness symptoms of family members
- Desire to manage therapeutic regimens of its members
- Describe a decrease in the difficulties of managing therapeutic regimens
- Describe actions to reduce risk factors

**NIC**

## Interventions (Nursing Interventions Classification)

### Suggested NIC Interventions

Family Involvement Promotion; Family Mobilization; Family Process Maintenance; Teaching: Disease Process

**Example NIC Activities—Family Involvement Promotion**

Identify and respect family's coping mechanisms; provide information to family members about client in accordance with client's preference

## Nursing Interventions and Rationales

- Base family interventions on your knowledge of the family, family context, and family function. **EBN:** *Family research has established that families differ widely from one another, even within cultures (Denham, 2002; Friedman, Bowden, & Jones, 2002). Family context "includes all aspects of the larger societal systems. The context is the stage for interactive relationships and discourse, the place where functional relationships occur, and the settings for enacting family health routines" (Denham, 2002, p. 52).*
- Use a family approach when helping an individual with a health problem that requires therapeutic management. **EBN:** *In a family health model developed from three qualitative studies involving Appalachian families from Ohio, it was shown that health habits are largely taught and defined within the family, so therapeutic regimens need to be addressed with the family (Denham, 2002). In studies of self-management, it was found that family support is a predictor of positive self-management (Whittemore et al, 2005; Leong et al, 2004; Thackeray et al, 2004; Wen et al, 2004).*
- Ensure that all strategies for working with the family are congruent with the culture of the family. **EBN:** *Many nursing studies among people of a variety of cultures show that cultural variations exist in the management of therapeutic regimens, and these differences should be taken into account when working with families (Degazon, 2004; Leininger, 2001; Leininger & McFarland, 2002).*
- Support religious beliefs and the comfort role of religion. **EBN:** *Studies have shown that there is a strong relationship between religion and subjective health and that subjective health is predictive of health outcomes. There seems to be a stronger relationship between religion and subjective health for African Americans than for Caucasians (Kotecki, 2002; Musick, 1996).*

T

- Identify family interactions and their embedded contexts relative to specific health objectives. **EBN:** *Family-focused practice requires viewing each interaction to accomplish health objectives as an opportunity to address the household production of health or work toward health objectives (Denham, 2002).*
- Review with family members the congruence and incongruence of family behaviors and health-related goals. **EBN:** *To attain the motivation that is needed for changes in health habits, family members should understand the relationship of daily habits to health-related goals (Miller, 2000).*
- Help family members make decisions regarding ways to integrate therapeutic regimens into daily living. Provide advice or suggestions as solicited and accepted by the family. **EBN:** *Decisions made by the family rather than by health providers or others guide everyday actions (Denham, 2002; Friedman, Bowden, & Jones, 2002). The advice of others, including nurses, will not be followed unless it is valued and respected by the family.*
- Demonstrate respect for and trust in family decisions. **EBN:** *People make decisions that they believe are appropriate for them. Family members who are respected and trusted by health providers are more likely to collaborate effectively with them (Denham, 2002).*
- Acknowledge the challenge of integrating therapeutic regimens with family behaviors. **EBN:** *Therapeutic regimens require modifications of daily activities that have already been established based on family values and beliefs. Acknowledging the difficulty of changing family habits supports families through the process (Friedman, Bowden, & Jones, 2002).*
- Review the symptoms of specific illness(es) and work with the family toward development of greater self-efficacy in relation to these symptoms. **EBN:** *Knowledge of symptoms improves the ability of family members to adjust behaviors to prevent and manage symptoms (Lubkin & Larsen, 2002). In a study of 197 family caregivers of people with Alzheimer's disease, higher symptom management self-efficacy scores were associated with fewer depressive symptoms and fewer physical health symptoms (Fortinsky, Kercher, & Burant, 2002).*
- Selectively support family decisions to adjust therapeutic regimens as indicated. **EBN:** *Sometimes families do not have access to health providers and should make independent decisions because of side effects or adverse effects of therapeutic regimens. Family members need to make informed decisions that are in their best interests (Lubkin & Larsen, 2002). Providing support for appropriate decisions made by the family and caregivers improves the ability of the family to make such decisions.*
- Advocate for the family in negotiating therapeutic regimens with health providers. **EB:** *Illness regimens generally are neither arbitrary nor absolute; therefore modifications can be discussed as needed to fit with the family lifestyle (Lubkin & Larsen, 2002).*
- Help the family to mobilize social supports. **EBN:** *Increased social support helps families to meet health-related goals (Pender, Murdaugh, & Parsons, 2002).*
- Help family members to modify perceptions as indicated. **EBN:** *Individual perceptions of the seriousness of, susceptibility to, and threat of illness may be distorted or inaccurate and may be modified with new information (Pender, Murdaugh, & Parsons, 2002).*
- Use one or more theories of family dynamics to describe, explain, or predict family behaviors (e.g., theories of Bowen, Satir, & Minuchin). **EBN:** *Family systems may not be understood by the nurse without adequate knowledge of family theory (Denham, 2002; Friedman, Bowden, & Jones, 2002).*



T

▲ Collaborate with expert nurses or other consultants regarding strategies for working with families. **EBN:** *Family systems are complex and challenging (Freidman, Bowden & Jones, 2002).*

### Multicultural

- Acknowledge racial/ethnic differences at the onset of care. **EBN:** *Acknowledgment of race/ethnicity issues will enhance communication, establish rapport, and promote treatment outcomes (D'Avanzo et al, 2001).*
- Approach families of color with respect, warmth, and professional courtesy. **EBN:** *Instances of disrespect and lack of caring have special significance for families of color (D'Avanzo et al, 2001).*
- Give a rationale when assessing African-American families about sensitive issues. **EBN:** *Many African Americans expect white caregivers to hold negative and preconceived ideas about African Americans. Giving a rationale for questions asked will help reduce this perception (D'Avanzo et al, 2001).*
- Use a family-centered approach when working with Latino, Asian, African-American, and Native-American clients. **EBN:** *Latinos may perceive the family as a source of support, solver of problems and source of pride. Asian Americans may regard the family as the primary decision maker and influence on individual family members (D'Avanzo et al, 2001). Native-American families may have extended structures and exert powerful influences over functioning (Seideman et al, 1996).*
- Facilitate modeling and role-playing for the family regarding healthy ways to communicate and interact. **EBN:** *It is helpful for families and the client to practice communication skills in a safe environment before trying them in a real-life situation (Rivera-Andino & Lopez, 2000).*

## Client/Family Teaching

- Teach about all aspects of therapeutic regimens. Provide as much knowledge as family members will accept, adjust instruction to account for what the family already knows, and provide information in a culturally congruent manner.
- Teach ways to adjust family behaviors to include therapeutic regimens.

▲ Teach safety in taking medications.

▲ Teach family members to act as self-advocates with health providers who prescribe therapeutic regimens.



## evolve WEBSITES FOR EDUCATION

See the EVOLVE website for World Wide Web resources for client education.

## REFERENCES


D'Avanzo CE et al: Developing culturally informed strategies for substance related interventions. In Naegle MA, D'Avanzo CE, editors: *Addictions and substance abuse: strategies for advanced practice nursing,* St Louis, 2001, Mosby, 59-104.

Degazon C: Cultural diversity and community-oriented nursing practice. In Stanhope M, Lancaster J: *Community and public health nursing,* ed 6, St Louis, 2004, Mosby.

Denham SA: Family routines: a structural perspective for viewing family health, *ANS Adv Nurs Sci* 24(4):60, 2002.
Fortinsky RH, Kercher K, Burant CJ: Measurement and correlates of family caregiver self-efficacy for managing dementia, *Aging Ment Health* 6(2):153, 2002.
Friedman M, Bowden V, Jones E: *Family nursing: research, theory and practice,* ed 5, New York, 2002, Prentice Hall.
Kotecki CN: Developing a health promotion program for faith-based communities, *Holist Nurs Pract* 16(3):61, 2002.
Leininger MM: *Culture care diversity and universality: a theory of nursing,* Boston, 2001, Jones and Bartlett.
Leininger MM, McFarland MR: *Transcultural nursing: concepts, theories, research and practices,* ed 3, New York, 2002, McGraw-Hill.
Leong J, Molassiotis A, Marsh H: Adherence to health recommendations after a cardiac rehabilitation programme in post-myocardial infarction patients: the role of heath beliefs, locus of control and psychological status, *Clin Eff Nurs* 8(1):26-38, 2004.
Lubkin IM, Larsen PD: *Chronic illness: impact and interventions,* ed 5, Boston, 2002, Jones and Bartlett.
Miller JF: *Coping with chronic illness: overcoming powerlessness,* ed 3, Philadelphia, 2000, FA Davis.
Musick MA: Religion and subjective health among black and white elders, *J Health Soc Behav* 37:221, 1996.
Pender NJ, Murdaugh CL, Parsons MA: *Health promotion in nursing practice,* ed 4, Upper Saddle River, NJ, 2002, Prentice Hall.
Rivera-Andino J, Lopez L: When culture complicates care, *RN* 63(7):47, 2000.
Seideman RY et al: Assessing American Indian families, *MCN Am J Matern Child Nurs* 21(6):274, 1996.
Stetz KM, Lewis FM, Houck GM: Family goals as indicants of adaptation during chronic illness, *Public Health Nurs* 11:385, 1994.
Stuart GW, Laraia MT: Therapeutic nurse-patient relationship. In Stuart GW, Laraia MT, editors: *Principles and practice of psychiatric nursing,* St Louis, 2001, Mosby.
Thackeray R, Merrill RM, Neiger BL: Disparities in diabetes management practice between racial and ethnic groups in the United States, *Diabetes Educ* 30(4):665-675, 2004.
Wen LK, Shepard MD, Parchman ML: Family support, diet, and exercise among older Mexican Americans with type 2 diabetes, *Diabetes Educ* 30(6):980-993, 2004.
Whittemore R, Melkus GD, Grey M: Metabolic control, self management and psychosocial adjustment in women with type 2 diabetes, *J Clin Nurs* 14(2):195-204, 2005.

# Ineffective Thermoregulation

*Betty J. Ackley*

**NANDA**

## Definition

Temperature fluctuation between hypothermia and hyperthermia

T

## Defining Characteristics

Fluctuations in body temperature above or below normal range; cool skin; cyanotic nailbeds; flushed skin; hypertension; increased respiratory rate; pallor (moderate); piloerection; reduction in body temperature below normal range; seizures/convulsions; shivering (mild); slow capillary refill; tachycardia; warmth to touch

## Related Factors (r/t)

Trauma, illness, immaturity, aging, fluctuating environmental temperature

NOC

## Outcomes (Nursing Outcomes Classification)

### Suggested NOC Outcomes

Thermoregulation; Thermoregulation: Newborn

**Example NOC Outcome with Indicators**

**Thermoregulation** as evidenced by the following indicators: Body temperature/Skin temperature/Skin color changes/Hydration/Reported thermal comfort (Rate each indicator of **Thermoregulation:** 1 = severely compromised, 2 = substantially compromised, 3 = moderately compromised, 4 = mildly compromised, 5 = not compromised [see Section I].)

## Client Outcomes

**Client Will (Specify Time Frame):**

- Maintain temperature within normal range
- Explain measures needed to maintain normal temperature
- Explain symptoms of hypothermia or hyperthermia

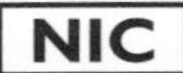

## Interventions (Nursing Interventions Classification)

### Suggested NIC Interventions

Temperature Regulation; Temperature Regulation: Inoperative

**Example NIC Activities—Temperature Regulation**

Institute use of a continuous core temperature–monitoring device, as appropriate; promote adequate fluid and nutritional intake

## Nursing Interventions and Rationales

- Monitor temperature every 1 to 4 hours or use continuous temperature monitoring as appropriate. *Normal adult temperature is usually identified as 98.6° F (37° C ), but in actuality the normal temperature fluctuates throughout the day. In the early morning it may be as low as 96.4° F (35.8° C ) and in the late afternoon or evening as high as 99.1° F (37.3° C ) (Bickley & Szilagyj, 2002). Disease, injury, or pharmacological agents may impair regulation of body temperature (Kasper et al, 2005).*
- If the client is awake, measure the oral temperature, instead of the tympanic or axillary temperature. **EBN:** *Oral temperature measurement provides a more accurate temperature reading than tympanic measurement (Fisk & Arcona, 2001; Giuliano et al, 2000; Lee, McKenzie, & Cathcart, 1999). Axillary temperatures are often inaccurate (Fulbrook, 1997). The oral temperature is usually accurate even in the intubated client (Fallis, 2000).*

*The SolarTherm and Data Therm devices correlated strongly with core body temperatures obtained from a pulmonary artery catheter (Smith, 2004).*

- Take vital signs every 1 to 4 hours, noting changes associated with hypothermia: first, increased blood pressure, pulse, and respirations; then, decreased values as hypothermia progresses (Kasper et al, 2005).
- Note changes in vital signs associated with hyperthermia: rapid, bounding pulse; increased respiratory rate; and decreased blood pressure, accompanied by orthostatic hypotension (Worfolk, 2000). *Consistent monitoring promotes prevention and early intervention in clients with altered cardiopulmonary status associated with hypothermia or hyperthermia.*
- Monitor the client for signs of hyperthermia (e.g., headache, nausea and vomiting, weakness, absence of sweating, delirium, and coma) (Worfolk, 2000). *Monitoring for the defining characteristics of hypothermia and hyperthermia allows for prevention and/or early intervention.*
- Note vital sign changes associated with hypothermia: first increased and then decreased blood pressure, pulse rate, and respiratory rate. *Mild hypothermia activates the sympathetic nervous system, which can increase the levels of vital signs; as hypothermia progresses, the heart becomes suppressed, with decreased cardiac output and lowering of vital sign readings (Ruffolo, 2002).*
- Monitor the client for signs of hypothermia (e.g., shivering, cool skin, piloerection, pallor, slow capillary refill, cyanotic nailbeds, decreased mentation, dysrhythmias) (Elliott, 2004).
- Maintain a consistent room temperature (72° F [22.2° C]). *A consistent temperature limits environmental effects on thermoregulation.*
- Promote adequate nutrition and hydration. *These measures help maintain a normal body temperature.*
- Adjust clothing to facilitate passive warming or cooling as appropriate. *This will help maintain a normal body temperature.*
- See the Nursing Interventions and Rationales for **Hypothermia** or **Hyperthermia** as appropriate.

## Pediatric

- Recognize that pediatric clients have a decreased ability to adapt to temperature extremes. Take the following actions to maintain body temperature in the infant/child:
  - Keep the head covered.
  - Use blankets to keep the client warm.
  - Keep the client covered during procedures, transport, and diagnostic testing.
  - Keep the room temperature at 72° F (22.2° C).

  *These measures can help prevent hypothermia in the child, which is a very possible occurrence, especially in the pediatric trauma client (Bernardo & Henker, 1999). The combination of a relatively larger body surface area, smaller body fluid volume, less well-developed temperature control mechanisms, and smaller amount of protective body fat limits the infant's and child's ability to maintain normal temperatures (Hockenberry, 2005).*
- Recognize that the infant and small child are vulnerable to develop heat stroke in hot weather and ensure they receive sufficient fluids and are protected from hot environ-

T

ments. *Infants and young children are at risk for heat stroke for many reasons including a decreased thermoregulatory ability in the young body and the inability to obtain their own fluids (Carroll, 2002).*

### Geriatric

- Do not allow an elderly client to become chilled or over heated. Keep the client covered when giving a bath and offer socks to wear in bed. Be aware of factors such as room temperature (heating/air conditioning), clothing (layered/loose), and fluid intake. *Older adults have a decreased ability to adapt to temperature extremes and need protection from extreme environmental temperatures. They also have a higher threshold of central temperature for sweating, diminished or absent sweating, impaired warmth or cold perception, an impaired shiver response, diminished thermogenesis, an abnormal peripheral blood flow response to warmth or cold, and a compromised cardiovascular reserve (Ballester & Harchelroad, 1999; Florez-Duquet & McDonald, 1998).*
- Ensure that elderly clients receive sufficient fluids during hot days and stay out of the sun. *The elderly may have trouble walking independently to obtain fluids, have decreased thirst sensation, and have chronic illnesses that predispose to heat stroke (Carroll, 2002).*
- ▲ Assess the medication profile for the potential risk of drug-related altered body temperature. *Anesthetics, barbiturates, salicylates, nonsteroidal anti-inflammatory drugs, diuretics, antihistamines, anticholinergics, beta-blockers, and thyroid hormones have been linked to altered body temperature (Elliott, 2004; Haskell et al, 1997).*

### Home Care

#### Prevention of Hypothermia in Cold Weather

- Instruct the client to avoid prolonged exposure outdoors. When outdoors, the client should wear gloves and a cap on the head. *Wool or fleece clothing can help to maintain body heat.*
- Keep the room temperature at 68° to 72° F (20° to 22.2° C).
- ▲ Ensure an adequate source of heat. Refer to social services if the client/family has a low income and the heat could be turned off.
- Help the elderly client locate a warm environment to which the client can go for safety in cold weather if the home environment is no longer warm.

#### Prevention of Hyperthermia in Hot Weather

T

- Encourage the client to wear lightweight cotton clothing. Help the elderly client remove the usual sweater.
- Ensure that the client drinks adequate amounts of fluids (2000 mL/day) and avoids caffeine and alcohol. *Adequate fluids are needed during hot weather to replace fluids lost from sweating. Fluids containing caffeine and alcohol can serve as a diuretic and decrease fluid volume in the body.*
- Help the client obtain a fan or an air conditioner to increase evaporation, as needed.
- Take the temperature of the elderly client in hot weather. *Elderly clients may not be able to tell that they are hot because of decreased sensation (Worfolk, 2000).*
- Help the elderly client locate a cool environment to which the client can go for safety in hot weather.

### Client/Family Teaching

- Teach the client and family the signs of hypothermia and hyperthermia and appropriate actions to take if either condition develops. *Adequate teaching improves compliance and reduces anxiety.*
- Teach the client and family an age-appropriate method for taking the temperature. *Optimal placement of the appropriate device is essential for accurate monitoring.*
- Teach the client to avoid alcohol and medications that depress cerebral function. *When the client is sedated or under the influence of alcohol, mentation is depressed, which results in decreased activities to maintain an adequate body temperature.*

## evolve WEBSITES FOR EDUCATION

See the EVOLVE website for World Wide Web resources for client education.

## REFERENCES

Ballester JM, Harchelroad FP: Hypothermia: an easy-to-miss, dangerous disorder in winter weather, *Geriatrics* 54(2):51, 1999.
Bernardo LM, Henker R: Thermoregulation in pediatric trauma: an overview, *Int J Trauma Nurs* 5(3):101, 1999.
Bickley LS, Szilagyj PJ: *Bate's guide to physical examination and history taking*, ed 8, Philadelphia, 2002, JB Lippincott.
Carroll P: The heat is on: protecting your patients from nature's silent killer, *Home Healthc Nurse* 20(6):376, 2002.
Elliott F: You'd better watch out, *Occup Health Saf* 73(11):76, 2004.
Fallis WM: Oral measurement of temperature in orally intubated critical care patients: state-of-the-science review, *Am J Crit Care* 9(5):334, 2000.
Fisk J, Arcona S: Comparing tympanic membrane and pulmonary artery catheter temperatures, *Dimens Crit Care Nurs* 20(2):44, 2001.
Florez-Duquet M, McDonald RB: Cold-induced thermoregulation and biological aging, *Physiol Rev* 78(2):339, 1998.
Fulbrook P: Core body temperature measurement: a comparison of axilla, tympanic membrane and pulmonary artery blood temperature, *Intens Crit Care Nurs* 13(5):1997.
Giuliano KK, Giuliano AJ, Scott SS et al: Temperature measurement in critically ill adults: a comparison of tympanic and oral methods, *Am J Crit Care* 9(4):254, 2000.
Haskell RM et al: Hypothermia, *AACN Clin Issues* 8(3):368, 1997.
Hockenberry MJ: *Wong's essentials of pediatric nursing*, ed 7, St. Louis, 2005, Mosby.
Kasper DL et al: *Harrison's principles of internal medicine*, ed 16, New York, 2005, McGraw Hill.
Lee VK, McKenzie NE, Cathcart M: Ear and oral temperatures under usual practice conditions, *Res Nurs Pract* 1(1):8, 1999.
Ruffolo D: Hypothermia in trauma: the cold hard facts, *RN* 65(2):2002.
Smith LS: Temperature measurement in critical care adults: a comparison of thermometry and measurement routes, *Biol Res Nurs* 6(2):117, 2004.
Worfolk JB: Heat waves: their impact on the health of elders, *Geriatr Nurs* 21(2):70, 2000.

T

# Disturbed Thought processes

evolve

*Judith R. Gentz*

**NANDA**

### Definition

Disruption in cognitive operations and activities

• = Independent; ▲ = Collaborative; EBN = Evidence-Based Nursing; EB = Evidence-Based

## Defining Characteristics

Cognitive dissonance, memory deficit/problems, inaccurate interpretation of environment, hypovigilance, hypervigilance, distractibility, egocentricity, inappropriate non–reality-based thinking

## Related Factors (r/t)

Organic brain changes (specify); changes in physical health (specify); mental illness (specify)

**NOC**

## Outcomes (Nursing Outcomes Classification)

### Suggested NOC Labels

Cognitive Ability; Cognitive Orientation; Concentration; Decision Making; Distorted Thought Self-Control; Identity; Information Processing; Memory; Neurological Status: Consciousness

**Example NOC Outcome**

Accomplishes **Distorted Thought Self-Control** as evidenced by the following indicators: Recognizes hallucinations or delusions are occurring/Refrains from attending to or responding to hallucinations or delusions/Exhibits reality-based thinking (Rate each indicator of **Distorted Thought Self-Control:** 1 = never demonstrated, 2 = rarely demonstrated, 3 = sometimes demonstrated, 4 = often demonstrated, 5 = consistently demonstrated [see Section I])

## Client Outcomes

- Remains oriented to time, place, person and circumstance; demonstrates improved cognitive function
- Remains free from actual and potential harm by self or others
- Performs activities of daily living (ADLs) adequately and independently
- Identifies community resources for help after discharge
- Understands the actions and side effects of medications

**NIC**

T

## Interventions (Nursing Interventions Classification)

### Suggested NIC Labels

Delusion Management, Dementia Management

**Example NIC Interventions—Delusion Management**

Provide an opportunity for client to discuss delusions with caregivers; focus discussion on the underlying feeling, rather than the content of the delusion ("It appears as if you may be feeling frightened.")

## Nursing Interventions and Rationales

- Observe for causes of altered thought processes (see Related Factors). *Differential diagnosis is important as physical and mental health problems, substance abuse, neoplasms and medication side effects may effect cognitive status (Ungvarski & Trzcianowska, 2000).*
- Monitor, record, and report changes in client's neurological status (level of consciousness, increased intracranial pressure), mental status (memory, cognition, judgment, concentration), vital signs, laboratory results, and ability to follow commands. *Assessing cognitive, physical and behavioral symptoms help to determine the relationship between brain anatomy, neurochemical systems, and symptoms (Garand, et al, 2000).*
- Obtain a medical history to rule out physical illness etiology for mental status changes. *Changes in behavior, cognitive functioning and functional level occur with organic brain disease and other physiological changes in the body (Garand, et al, 2000).* **EBN:** *Older adults are more likely to present with physical complaints than mental health complaints so both must be closely assessed (Antai-Otong, 2003).*
- Complete a mental status examination of client. **EB:** *A mental status examination is a recommended procedure in assessing any cognitive difficulties (Boise, et al, 1999).* **EBN:** *Determining the cause of psychosis will determine practical and effective treatment (Jensen, 2003).*
- Report any new onset or sudden increase in confusion. **EB:** *Postoperative acute confusional state is a significant problem among older surgical clients; its incidence is higher in orthopedic surgery than in general surgery (Wong, Wong, & Brooks, 2002).*
- Adjust communication style to client. Speak slowly and calmly; use short phrases and concrete, nontechnical words; use writing if appropriate; allow time for thinking; use face-to-face communication; listen carefully; and seek clarification. *Basic interactions provide the nurse with opportunity to assess patient agitation and response level (Kozub & Skidmore, 2001).*
- ▲ Assess pain and promptly provide comfort measures. **EBN:** *Confused clients cannot accurately report pain. Pain control reduces suffering and adverse health effects related to pain (Huffman & Kunik, 2000).*
- Identify and remove potentially dangerous items in the environment. **EBN:** *Interview clients in a private area while maintaining staff safety. Nursing staff should sit closest to the door (Jensen, 2003).*
- Limit use of sedatives and drugs affecting the nervous system. *Sedation, imbalance, slowed reaction time, hypotension, and Parkinsonian side effects all increase the risk of falls and confusion (Lieu et al, 1997).* **EB:** *Cognitive impairment can result in a number of problems, such as communication difficulties, compromised safety, self-care deficits, and behavioral problems (Day et al, 2000).*
- Use soft restraints with discretion and physician order. *Seclusion, restraint, and/or other behavioral management interventions must be used in accordance to the patient's plan of care and regulatory guidelines (Health Care Financing Administration [HCFA], 2000; Joint Commission on Accreditation of Healthcare Organizations [JCAHO], 2000).*
- Orient client and call client by name; introduce self on each contact; frequently mention time, date, and place; prominently display a clock and calendar that are easy to

T

read in room and refer to them; and request family to bring in familiar pictures and articles from home. **EB:** *These steps help reinforce reality and provide cues that maintain orientation. External, written reminders are more effective than verbal reinforcement for memory aids (Day, et al, 2000; Davis & Burgio, 1999).*

- Provide validation of thoughts and feelings of client. *Validation seeks to help the caregiver understand the care receiver, encouraging empathy (Linehan, 1993).*
- Stay with clients if they are agitated and likely to be injured. *A quiet environment with the presence of another person can calm an agitated client. One-on-one contact from staff to patient is the first step is successful de-escalation (Kozub & Skidmore, 2001).*
- Observe for therapeutic and side effects of psychotropic medications. *Side effects may mimic agitation, anxiety and other primary symptoms and are usually remedied by altering the dosage or otherwise changing the medication schedule in consultation with the prescriber.*
- Develop a therapeutic alliance to increase trust with the client. **EBN:** *Approaching the client in a nonjudgmental manner, acknowledging the client's experience, and not challenging the client's reality help develop a therapeutic alliance (Jensen, 2003).*
- Assess client's assault potential and maintain staff safety. *Patient resistance to staff direction requires immediate consideration of staff safety (Kozub & Skidmore, 2001).*
- Establish predictable care routines and maintain continuity of client's nursing staff. *Routines promote feelings of security.*
- Frequently check on client and have brief interactions to prevent sensory deprivation. Avoid an over-stimulated or a sensory-deprived environment. Provide adequate lighting that is not too bright. Alternate short, frequent visits with defined rest periods. Monitor noise levels. **EB:** *Excessive environmental stimuli can adversely affect client's level of orientation and increase disorganization (Day et al, 2000).*
- Assist client with daily hygiene as needed; encourage self-care. **EBN:** *Observe the client's ability to complete hygiene. Clients may minimize problems on self-reports and require staff observation for accurate assessment of self-care (Sousa & Frazier, 2004).*
- Observe for signs and symptoms of significant depression concomitant to altered thoughts. **EB:** *Severely depressed clients may also demonstrate declines in activities of daily living and cognitive functioning (McCall & Dunn, 2003).*
- Provide support and education to family during client's period of cognitive change. Involve family in current care and in planning of postdischarge care, recognizing the family members' strengths and needs. **EBN:** *Family members may also have cognitive symptoms related to age or mental illness (Wuerker, 2000). Family involvement promotes continuity of care.*



▲ Initiate a social service referral to find help for client following discharge. **EB:** *A client's level of supervision following discharge may reduce risk of readmission (Mercer et al, 1999).*

- Observe for evidence of auditory and/or visual hallucination experiences. Teach management techniques. **EBN:** *Behavioral techniques taught to clients with auditory hallucinations were found to reduce negative characteristics of hallucinations (Buccheri, Trygstad, & Dowling, 2004).*
- Ask empathic and direct questions such as, "What are you seeing (or hearing) now?" or "Do you sometimes hear or see things that other people don't hear or see?" **EBN:**

*Validation of symptoms increases empathy and client's perception of safety (Forchuk et al, 2000).*

- Do not attempt to argue or change the client's beliefs. Without implying agreement, focus on feelings that accompany hallucinations and delusions rather than content of delusions (e.g., "You look frightened."). **EBN:** *Acceptance promotes trust and understanding (Forchuk, et al, 2000).*
- Set limits on delusional conversations (e.g., "We discussed that; let's talk about what is happening on the unit."). **EBN:** *Balancing control versus caring behaviors fosters rapport between nurse and client (Forchuk et al, 2000).*
- Ask for clarification when necessary. **EB:** *There is a discrepancy between expression of emotion and experience of emotion in schizophrenia (Aghevli, Blanchard, & Horan, 2003).*
- Help client state needs and ask for assistance. *Establish that staff should not automatically know the client's needs and wants and that it is acceptable to ask.*
- Involve client in short activities. *Distraction is a positive coping skill (Linehan, 1993).*
- Refer to care plans for **Risk for self-and other-directed Violence** for further nursing interventions and rationales.

## Geriatric

- Monitor for dementia, as evidenced by its gradual onset and a progressive deterioration, or for delirium, as evidenced by its acute onset and generally reversible course. *States of confusion require careful assessment (Milisen et al, 1998; Vermeersch, 1990).*
- Focus on feelings associated with hallucinations and delusions rather than content. *Tuning into disoriented clients' feelings is more important than rigidly insisting that they share the nurse's reality. Be comforting and understanding when client has processing difficulties (Bleathman & Morton, 1992).*

## Multicultural

- Assess for the influence of cultural beliefs, norms, and values on the family's or caregiver's understanding of disturbed thought processes. **EBN:** *What the family considers normal and abnormal behavior may be based on cultural perceptions (Cochran, 1998; Doswell & Erlen, 1998; Guarnaccia, 1998). A recent study found that African-American families were unable to correctly identify early psychotic symptoms that led to delays for treatment (Compton, Kaslow, & Walker, 2004). A study in the United Kingdom found that perceived discrimination may induce delusional ideation (Janssen et al, 2003).*
- Inform the client's family or caregiver of the meaning of and reasons for common behaviors observed in client with disturbed thought processes. *An understanding of behavior will enable the client's family or caregiver to provide the client with a safe environment.*
- Validate the family members' feelings regarding the impact of the client's behavior on family lifestyle. **EBN:** *Validation is a therapeutic communication technique that lets the individual know that the nurse has heard and understood what was said, and it promotes the relationship between the nurse and the individual (Heineken, 1998).*

## Home Care

- The interventions described previously may be adapted for home care use.

- ▲ Assess the client for the presence of a psychiatric disorder. Refer for mental health services as indicated. *Disturbed thought processes are part of several psychiatric disorders. Improvement in thought processes is unlikely unless the underlying disorder is treated.*
- • Assess the family's knowledge of the disease process and plan of care; teach as necessary. Encourage participation. *Illnesses associated with thought process disorders generally affect the family and family life as much as they do the client. Misinterpretation of the client's behavior is common, and instruction regarding the disease process is necessary to secure understanding of and cooperation with the treatment plan.*
- • Identify the strengths of the caregiver and the caregiver's efforts to gain control of unpredictable situations. Help the caregiver to stay connected with a client who may be behaving differently than usual, to make life as routine as possible, to help the client set goals and sustain hope, and to allow the client space to experience progress. **EBN:** *Identifying and acknowledging positive caregiver responses to the client's illness will assist the caregiver in maintaining a positive relationship with the client. Family members of persons with severe mental illness have found it helpful to work at staying connected to the person with mental illness, finding a role that they can feel comfortable with, and helping the relative move forward (Rose, 1998).*
- ▲ Assess the client's functional status as it relates to the ability for self-care; refer to a physician for evaluation of medication levels as indicated. *Negative symptoms, abnormal movements, and use of antiparkinsonism agents may increase the likelihood of functional impairment in older adults with schizophrenia. These elements may be treatable with new antipsychotic medications and psychological approaches (e.g., social skills training) (Cohen & Talavera, 2000).*
- • Assess the home environment for the availability of distractions from hallucinations, such as playing music over headphones. **EB:** *One study showed that having schizophrenics listen to music produced beneficial effects (Glicksohn & Cohen, 2000).*
- ▲ If the client's condition deteriorates, seek acute medical or mental health intervention immediately, as appropriate. *Acute behavioral change could place the client or caregivers at risk; behavioral change often responds to sedation or increase in medications.*
- ▲ Identify an emergency plan and discuss criteria for its use with the family or caregivers. *An appropriate level of clinical intervention supports client and family well-being.*
- ▲ Assess the client's ability to manage his or her own medications. If the client is unable, identify a responsible caregiver for medication administration. Teach the purpose, administration, and side effects of medications based on level of knowledge. Identify a plan for response to side effects if they occur. **EBN:** *Assistance, such as the use of a medication box or reminder telephone calls, may be sufficient to allow the client to perform care activities independently (Beebe, 2001).*
- • Assess and modify environmental stimuli that could be misinterpreted (e.g., use a night light, evaluate placement of mirrors). *Clients may tend toward illusory experiences, misinterpreting actual stimuli. Nightlights help clients reorient themselves and decrease fear if clients awaken during the night.*
- • Allow the client control over aspects of his or her environment, as he or she is able. *Control enhances self-esteem, although sometimes only for a short time. Refer to the care plan for* **Powerlessness.**
- • Identify the client's interests and skills. Provide an opportunity for the client to pursue

T

interests and use skills without taxing the client's judgment and cognitive ability. *Diversionary activities decrease anxiety and give meaning to life.*

▲ Refer the client and family to community support groups (e.g., psychosocial rehabilitation programs for the client, National Alliance for the Mentally Ill for the client and family). Groups that include older adults with mental illness would be particularly useful. *Coping strategies described by older adults with mental illness were similar to those of younger clients but were used more effectively in conjunction with greater acceptance of the mental illness. Older adults may serve as a helpful resource to younger clients struggling with adjustment to their illness (Solano & Whitbourne, 2001).*

▲ In the presence of chronic thought process disorder, institute case management of frail elderly to support continued independent living. *Difficulties with thought disorder can lead to increasing needs for assistance in using the health care system effectively. Case management combines the nursing activities of client and family assessment, planning and coordination of care among all health care providers, delivery of direct nursing care, and monitoring of care and outcomes. These activities can address continuity of care, mutual goal setting, behavior management, and prevention of worsening health problems (Guttman, 1999).*

▲ When the client has a psychiatric disorder, pay special attention to the presence of comorbid medical conditions and the need for medical care. *Clients with schizophrenia have higher mortality rates and generally have received less than optimal health care. They are in particular need of assessment, health instruction, and involvement in their own care (Folsom & Jeste, 2001).*

▲ When the client has a psychiatric disorder, refer for psychiatric home health care services for client reassurance and implementation of a therapeutic regimen. **EBN:** *Psychiatric home care nurses can address issues relating to the client's thought process disorder. Behavioral interventions in the home can help the client to participate more effectively in the treatment plan (Patusky, Rodning, & Martinez-Kratz, 1996).*

## Client/Family Teaching

- Teach family members reorientation techniques and about the need to frequently repeat instructions.
- Teach client distraction techniques to manage hallucinations.
- Teach family members ways to support client without supporting delusional beliefs.
- Help family identify coping skills, environmental supports, and community services for dealing with chronically mentally ill clients.
- Discuss caregiver's need for respite. Offer support, encouragement, and information for meeting those needs.

T

## evolve WEBSITES FOR EDUCATION

See the EVOLVE web site for World Wide Web resources for client education.

## REFERENCES

Beebe LH: Community nursing support for clients with schizophrenia, *Arch Psychiatr Nurs* 15:214, 2001.

Bleathman C, Morton I: Validation therapy: extracts from 20 groups with dementia sufferers, *J Adv Nurs* 17:658, 1992.

Cochran M: Tears have no color, *Am J Nurs* 98(6):53, 1998.

Cohen CI, Talavera N: Functional impairment in older schizophrenic persons, *Am J Geriatr Psychiatry* 8:237, 2000.
Compton MT, Kaslow NJ, Walker EF: Observations on parent/family factors that may influence the duration of untreated psychosis among African American first-episode schizophrenia-spectrum patients, *Schizophr Res* 68(2-3):373-385, 2004.
Davis L, Burgio L: Planning cognitive behavioral management for long-term care, *Issues Ment Health Nurs* 20:587-601, 1999.
Day K, Carreon D, Stump C: The therapeutic design of environments for people with dementia: a review of the empirical research, *Gerontologist* 40:4, 2000.
Doswell W, Erlen J: Multicultural issues and ethical concerns in the delivery of nursing care interventions, *Nurs Clin North Am* 33(2):353, 1998.
Folsom DP, Jeste DV: Medical comorbidity in patients with schizophrenia, *Home Healthc Consult* 8(9):17, 2001.
Forchuk C, Westwell J, Martin ML et al: The developing nurse-client relationship: nurses' perspective, *J Am Psychiatr Nurses Assoc* 6(1):3, 2000.
Garand L, Buckwater K, Hall G: The biological basis of behavioral symptoms in dementia, *Iss Ment Health Nurs* 21:21-107, 2000.
Giger JN, Davidhizar RE: *Transcultural nursing,* ed 2, St Louis, 1995, Mosby.
Glicksohn J, Cohen Y: Can music alleviate cognitive dysfunction in schizophrenia? *Psychopathology* 33(1):43, 2000.
Guarnaccia P: Multicultural experiences of family caregiving: a study of African American, European American, and Hispanic American families, *New Dir Ment Health Serv* 77:45, 1998.
Guttman R: Case management of the frail elderly in the community, *Clin Nurs Spec* 13(4):174, 1999.
Heineken J: Patient silence is not necessarily client satisfaction: communication in home care nursing, *Home Healthc Nurse* 16(2):115, 1998.
Huffman J, Kunik M: Assessment and understanding of pain in patients with dementia, *Gerontologist* 40:5, 2000.
Janssen I, Hanssen M, Bak M et al: Discrimination and delusional ideation, *Br J Psychiatry* 182:71-76, 2003.
Kozub M, Skidmore R: Least to most restrictive interventions, *J Psychos Nurs* 39:3, 2001.
Leininger MM: *Transcultural nursing: theories, research and practices,* ed 2, Hilliard, Ohio, 1996, McGraw-Hill.
Lieu PK, Ismail N, Choo P et al: Prevention of fall in a geriatric ward, *Ann Acad Med* 29:872, 1997.
Linehan M: *Cognitive-behavioral treatment of borderline personality disorder,* New York, 1993, Guilford Press.
Mercer, G, Molinar V, Kunik M: Rehospitalization of older psychiatric inpatients: an investigation of predictors, *Gerontologist* 39:5, 1999.
Milisen K, Foreman MD, Godderis J et al: Delirium in the hospitalized elderly, *Nurs Clin North Am* 33:3, 1998.
Neelon VJ: Postoperative confusion, *Crit Care Nurs Clin North Am* 2:4, 1990.
Patusky KL, Rodning C, Martinez-Kratz M: Clinical lessons in psychiatric home care: a case study approach, *J Home Health Case Manag* 9:18, 1996.
Platzer H: Post-operative confusion in the elderly: a literature review, *Int J Nurs Stud* 26:367, 1989.
Rose LE: Gaining control: family members relate to persons with severe mental illness, *Res Nurs Health* 21:363, 1998.
Solano NH, Whitbourne SK: Coping with schizophrenia: patterns in later adulthood, *Int J Aging Hum Dev* 53:1, 2001.
Stuart GW, Laraia MT: Therapeutic nurse-patient relationship. In Stuart GW, Laraia MT, editors: *Principles and practice of psychiatric nursing,* St Louis, 2001, Mosby, p 30.
Stuart G, Sundeen S: *Pocket guide to psychiatric nursing,* ed 2, St Louis, 1991, Mosby.
Ungvarski P, Trzcianowski H: Neurocognitive disorders seen in HIV disease, *Issues Ment Health Nurs* 21:51-70, 2000.
Vermeersch PE: The clinical assessment of confusion, *Appl Nurs Res* 3(3):128-133, 1990.



# Impaired Tissue integrity

evolve

*Sharon Baranoski*

**NANDA**

### Definition

Damage to mucous membrane, corneal, integumentary, or subcutaneous tissues

## Defining Characteristics

Damaged or destroyed tissue (e.g., cornea, mucous membrane, integumentary or subcutaneous tissue)

## Related Factors (r/t)

Mechanical factors (e.g., pressure, shear, friction); radiation (including therapeutic radiation); nutritional deficit or excess; thermal factors (temperature extremes); knowledge deficit; chemical irritants (including body excretions, secretions, medications); impaired physical mobility; altered circulation; fluid deficit or excess

**NOC**

## Outcomes (Nursing Outcomes Classification)

### Suggested NOC Outcomes

Tissue Integrity: Skin and Mucous Membranes; Wound Healing: Primary Intention, Secondary Intention

**Example NOC Outcome with Indicators**

Intact **Tissue Integrity: Skin and Mucous Membranes** as evidenced by the following indicators: Skin intactness/Skin lesions absent/Tissue perfusion/Skin temperature (Rate each indicator of **Tissue Integrity: Skin and Mucous Membranes:** 1 = severely compromised, 2 = substantially compromised, 3 = moderately compromised, 4 = mildly compromised, 5 = not compromised [see Section I].)

## Client Outcomes

### Client Will (Specify Time Frame):

- Report any altered sensation or pain at site of tissue impairment
- Demonstrate understanding of plan to heal tissue and prevent injury
- Describe measures to protect and heal the tissue, including wound care
- Experience a wound that decreases in size and has increased granulation tissue

**NIC**

## Interventions (Nursing Interventions Classification)

### Suggested NIC Interventions

Incision Site Care; Pressure Ulcer Care; Skin Care: Topical Treatments; Skin Surveillance; Wound Care

**Example NIC Activities—Pressure Ulcer Care**

Monitor color, temperature, edema, moisture, and appearance of surrounding skin; note characteristics of any drainage

## Nursing Interventions and Rationales

- Assess the site of impaired tissue integrity and determine the cause (e.g., acute or chronic wound, burn, dermatological lesion, pressure ulcer, leg ulcer). **EB:** *The etiology or cause of the wound must be determined before appropriate interventions can be implemented. This will provide the basis for additional testing and evaluation to start the assessment process (Baranoski & Ayello, 2003).*
- Determine the size and depth of the wound (e.g., full-thickness wound, stage III or IV pressure ulcer). **EB:** *Serial wound assessments are more reliable when performed by the same caregiver, with the client in the same position, and using the same techniques (Sussman & Bates-Jensen, 1998).*
- Classify pressure ulcers in the following manner (National Pressure Ulcer Advisory Panel, available at www.npuap.org, accessed January 2005):
  - Stage III: Full-thickness skin loss involving damage to or necrosis of subcutaneous tissue that may extend down to but not through underlying fascia; ulcer appears as a deep crater with or without undermining of adjacent tissue
  - Stage IV: Full-thickness skin loss with extensive destruction; tissue necrosis; or damage to muscle, bone, or supporting structures (e.g., tendons, joint capsules)
- Monitor the site of impaired tissue integrity at least once daily for color changes, redness, swelling, warmth, pain, or other signs of infection. Determine whether the client is experiencing changes in sensation or pain. Pay special attention to all high-risk areas such as bony prominences, skin folds, sacrum, and heels. *Systematic inspection can identify impending problems early.* **EBN:** *Pain secondary to dressing changes can be managed by interventions aimed at reducing trauma and other sources of wound pain (Ayello & Braden 2002; Moffatt, 2002; European Wound Management Association, 2001; Krasner 2001).*
- Monitor the status of the skin around the wound. Monitor the client's skin care practices, noting type of soap or other cleansing agents used, temperature of water, and frequency of skin cleansing. *Individualize the plan according to the client's skin condition, needs, and preferences. Avoid harsh cleansing agents, hot water, extreme friction or force, or too frequent cleansing (Rodeheaver, 2001; Bergstrom et al, 1994; Panel for the Prediction and Prevention of Pressure Ulcers in Adults, 1992).*
- Monitor the client's continence status and minimize exposure of the skin impairment site and other areas to moisture from urine or stool, perspiration, or wound drainage. *If the client is incontinent, implement an incontinence management plan to prevent exposure to chemicals in urine and stool that can strip or erode the skin. Refer to a continence care specialist, urologist, or gastroenterologist for incontinence assessment (WOCN Clinical Practice Guideline Series 2, 2003).* **EB:** *Implementing an incontinence prevention plan with the use of a skin or cleanser protectant can significantly decrease skin breakdown and pressure ulcer formation (Clever et al, 2002; Warshaw et al, 2002; Fantl et al, 1996).*
- Monitor for correct placement of tubes, catheters, and other devices. Assess the skin and tissue affected by the tape that secures these devices. *Mechanical damage to skin and tissues as a result of pressure, friction, or shear is often associated with external devices (Faller & Beitz, 2001).*
- In an orthopedic client, check every 2 hours for correct placement of foot-boards, restraints, traction, casts, or other devices, and assess skin and tissue integrity. Be alert

T

for symptoms of compartment syndrome (refer to the care plan for **Risk for Peripheral neurovascular dysfunction**). *Mechanical damage to skin and tissues (pressure, friction, or shear) is often associated with external devices.*

- For a client with limited mobility, use a risk assessment tool to systematically assess immobility-related risk factors. **EBN and EB:** *A validated risk assessment tool such as the Norton or Braden scale should be used to identify clients at risk for immobility-related skin breakdown (Ayello & Braden, 2002; Panel for the Prediction and Prevention of Pressure Ulcers in Adults, 1992). Targeting variables (e.g., age and Braden Scale risk category) can focus assessment on particular risk factors (e.g., pressure) and help guide the plan of prevention and care (WOCN Clinical Pratice Guideline Series 2, 2003; Young et al, 2002).*
- Implement a written treatment plan for the topical treatment of the skin impairment site. *A written treatment plan ensures consistency in care and documentation (Baranoski & Ayello, 2003; Maklebust & Sieggreen, 2001).*
- ▲ Identify a plan for débridement if necrotic tissue (eschar or slough) is present and if consistent with overall client management goals. *Healing does not occur in the presence of necrotic tissue (Bergstrom et al, 1994; WOCN Clinical Practice Guideline Series 2, 2003; Panel for the Prediction and Prevention of Pressure Ulcers in Adults, 1992).*
- Select a topical treatment that maintains a moist wound-healing environment but that also allows absorption of exudate and filling of dead space. *No single wound care product provides the optimum environment for healing all wounds.* **EBN:** *Choose dressings that provide a moist environment, keep periwound skin dry, and control exudate and eliminate dead space. (WOCN Clinial Practice Guideline Series 2, 2003; Bergstrom et al, 1994; Panel for the Prediction and Prevention of Pressure Ulcers in Adults, 1992).*
- Do not position the client on the site of impaired tissue integrity. If it is consistent with overall client management goals, turn and position the client at least every 2 hours and transfer the client carefully to avoid adverse effects of external mechanical forces (i.e., pressure, friction, and shear) (WOCN Clinical Practice Guideline Series 2, 2003).
- Evaluate for the use of specialty mattresses, beds, or devices as appropriate (Fleck, 2001; Geyer, 2001).
- If the goal of care is to keep the client comfortable (e.g., for a terminally ill client), turning and repositioning may not be appropriate. Maintain the head of the bed at the lowest degree of elevation possible to reduce shear and friction, and use lift devices, pillows, foam wedges, and pressure-reducing devices in the bed (WOCN Clinical Practice Guideline Series 2, 2003; Krasner, Rodeheaver, & Sibbald, 2001; Panel for the Prediction and Prevention of Pressure Ulcers in Adults, 1992).
- Avoid massaging around the site of impaired tissue integrity and over bony prominences. *Research suggests that massage may lead to deep tissue trauma (Panel for the Prediction and Prevention of Pressure Ulcers in Adults, 1992).*
- Assess the client's nutritional status; refer for a nutritional consultation and/or institute use of dietary supplements. **EB:** *The benefit of nutritional evaluation and intensive nutritional support in patients at risk for and with pressure ulcers is not supported by rigorous clinical trials. Despite this "lack of evidence," NPUAP endorses the application of reasonable nutritional assessment and treatment for patients at risk for and with pressure ulcers. Available at www.npuap.org).*

▲ A comprehensive plan of care includes a through wound assessment, treatment interventions, support surfaces, nutritional products, adjunctive therapies and evaluation of the outcome of care. *Documentation of these essential elements is paramount to establishing a framework for quality care (Baranoski, 2003).*

## Home Care

- Some of the interventions described previously may be adapted for home care use.
- Assess the client's current phase of wound healing (i.e., inflammation, proliferation, maturation) and stage of injury; initiate appropriate wound management. **EB:** *Accurate understanding of tissue status combined with knowledge of underlying diagnoses and product validity provide a basis for determining appropriate treatment objectives (Ovington, 1999).*
- Instruct and assist the client and caregivers in understanding how to change dressings and the importance of maintaining a clean environment. Provide written instructions and observe them completing the dressing change (Ovington & Schaum, 2001).

▲ Initiate a consultation in a case assignment with a wound specialist or wound, ostomy, and continence nurse to establish a comprehensive plan as soon as possible. Plan case conferencing to promote optimal wound care. *Case conferencing ensures that cases are reviewed regularly to discuss and implement the most effective wound care management to meet client needs (Biala, 2002).*

▲ Consultation with other health care discipline will provide a through comprehensive assessment. *Consider referring to the dietitian, physical therapist, occupational therapist, and social worker as needed.*

## Client/Family Teaching

- Teach skin and wound assessment and ways to monitor for signs and symptoms of infection, complications, and healing. *Early assessment and intervention help prevent serious problems from developing.*
- Teach the client why a topical treatment has been selected. Explain wound bed changes that the caregiver can expect to see. Instruct on when the dressing needs to be changed. **EBN:** *The type of wound dressing needed may change over time as the wound heals and/or deteriorates. WOCN Clinical Practice Guideline Series 2, 2003).*
- If it is consistent with overall client management goals, teach how to turn and reposition the client at least every 2 hours. **EB:** *If the goal of care is to keep the client comfortable (e.g., for a terminally ill client), turning and repositioning may not be appropriate (Krasner, Rodeheaver, & Sibbald, 2001; Panel for the Prediction and Prevention of Pressure Ulcers in Adults, 1992).*
- Teach the use of pillows, foam wedges, and pressure-reducing devices to prevent pressure injury. *The use of effective pressure-reducing seat cushions for elderly wheelchair users significantly prevented sitting-acquired pressure ulcers (Geyer et al, 2001).*



## evolve WEBSITES FOR EDUCATION

See the EVOLVE website for World Wide Web resources for client education.

## REFERENCES


Ayello EA, Braden B: How and why to do pressure ulcer risk assessment, *Adv Skin Wound Care* 15(3):125, 2002.

Baranoski S, Ayello EA, editors: *Wound care essentials: practice principles,* Springhouse, Penn, 2003, Lippincott, Williams, & Wilkins.

Bergstrom N et al: *Treatment of pressure ulcers,* Clinical Practice Guideline No 15, Agency for Health Care Policy and Research Pub No 95-0652, Rockville, Md, 1994, Public Health Service, U.S. Department of Health and Human Services.

Biala KY: Case conferencing for wound care patients, *Home Healthcare Nurs* 20(2):120, 2002.

Clever K et al: Evaluating the efficacy of a uniquely delivered skin protectant and its effect on the formation of sacral/buttock pressure ulcers, *Ostomy Wound Manage* 48(12):60, 2002.

European Wound Management Association: *Pain at wound dressing changes,* position document, London, 2001, Medical Education Partnership. Available at www.tendra.com/index.htm, accessed on February 10, 2003.

Faller N, Beitz J: When a wound isn't a wound: tubes, drains, fistulas and draining wounds. In Krasner D, Rodeheaver G, Sibbald RG, editors: *Chronic wound care: a clinical source book for healthcare professionals,* ed 3, Wayne, Penn, 2001, HMP Communications.

Fleck D: Support surfaces: criteria and selection. In Krasner D, Rodeheaver G, Sibbald RG, editors: *Chronic wound care: a clinical source book for healthcare professionals,* ed 3, Wayne, Penn, 2001, HMP Communications.

Geyer MJ et al: A randomized control trial to evaluate pressure-reducing seating cushions for elderly wheelchair users, *Adv Skin Wound Care* 14(3):120, 2001.

Krasner D: Caring for the person experiencing chronic wound pain. In Krasner D, Rodeheaver G, Sibbald RG, editors: *Chronic wound care: a clinical source book for healthcare professionals,* ed 3, Wayne, Penn, 2001, HMP Communications.

Krasner D, Rodeheaver G, Sibbald RG, editors: *Chronic wound care: a clinical source book for healthcare professionals,* ed 3, Wayne, Penn, 2001, HMP Communications.

Maklebust J, Sieggreen M: *Pressure ulcers: guidelines for prevention and nursing management,* ed 3, Springhouse, Penn, 2001, Springhouse.

Moffatt CJ et al Understanding wound pain and trauma: An international perspective, *EWMA Position document: Pain at wound dressing changes 2-7,* 2002.

National Pressure Ulcer Advisory Panel. Available at www.npuap.org, accessed January 2005.

Ovington L: Dressings and adjunctive therapies: AHCPR guidelines revisited, *Ostomy Wound Manage* 45(Suppl 1A):94S-106S, 1999.

Ovington LG, Schaum KD: Wound care products: how to choose, *Home Healthcare Nurse* 19(4):224, 2001.

Panel for the Prediction and Prevention of Pressure Ulcers in Adults: *Pressure ulcers in adults: prediction and prevention,* Clinical Practice Guideline No 3, Agency for Health Care Policy and Research Pub No. 92-0047, Rockville, Md, 1992, US Department of Health and Human Services, Public Health Service.

Rodeheaver GT: Wound cleansing, wound irrigation wound disinfection. In Krasner D, Rodeheaver G, Sibbald RG, editors: *Chronic wound care: a clinical source book for healthcare professionals,* ed 3, Wayne, Penn, 2001, HMP Communications.

Sussman C, Bates-Jensen BM: *Wound care: a collaborative practice manual for physical therapists and nurses,* Gaithersburg, Md, 1998, Aspen.

van Rijswijk L: Wound assessment and documentation. In Krasner D, Rodeheaver G, Sibbald RG: *Chronic wound care: a clinical source book for healthcare professionals,* ed 3, Wayne, Penn, 2001, HMP Communications.

Warshaw E et al: Clinical and cost effectiveness of a cleanser protectant lotion for treatment of perineal skin breakdown in low-risk patients with incontinence, *Ostomy Wound Manage* 48(6):44, 2002.

Wound, Ostomy, and Continence Nurses Society: Guideline for prevention and management of pressure ulcers: WOCN Clinical Practice Guideline Series 2, Glenview, IL, 2003, The Society.

Young J et al: Risk factors associated with pressure ulcer development at a major Western Australia teaching hospital from 1998 to 2000, *J Wound Ostomy Continence Nurs* 29(5):234, 2002.


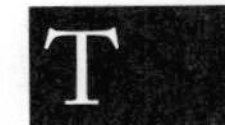

# Ineffective Tissue perfusion (specify type: renal, cerebral, cardiopulmonary, gastrointestinal, peripheral) evolve

*Betty J. Ackley*

**NANDA**

## Definition

Decrease in oxygen resulting in failure to nourish tissues at capillary level

## Defining Characteristics

### Renal

Altered blood pressure outside of acceptable parameters, hematuria, oliguria or anuria, elevation in blood urea nitrogen/creatinine ratio

### Cerebral

Speech abnormalities; changes in pupillary reactions, extremity weakness or paralysis, altered mental status, difficult in swallowing, changes in motor response, behavioral changes

### Cardiopulmonary

Altered respiratory rate outside of acceptable parameters, use of accessory muscles, capillary refill longer than 3 seconds, abnormal arterial blood gas levels, chest pain, sense of impending doom, bronchospasms, dyspnea, dysrhythmias, nasal flaring, chest retraction

### Gastrointestinal

Hypoactive or absent bowel sounds; nausea; abdominal distention; abdominal pain or tenderness

### Peripheral

Edema; positive Homans' sign; altered skin characteristics (hair, moisture) or nails; weak or absent pulses; skin discolorations; skin temperature changes; altered sensations; diminished arterial pulsations; pale skin color upon elevation of leg with color not returning upon lowering of leg; slow healing of lesions; cold extremities; dependent, blue, or purple skin color

## Related Factors (r/t)

Hypovolemia, interruption of arterial flow, hypervolemia, exchange problems, interruption of venous flow, mechanical reduction of venous and/or arterial blood flow, hypoventilation, impaired transport of oxygen across alveolar and/or capillary membrane, mismatch of ventilation with blood flow, decreased hemoglobin concentration in blood, enzyme poisoning, altered affinity of hemoglobin for oxygen

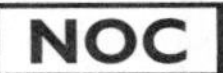

## Outcomes (Nursing Outcomes Classification)

### Suggested NOC Outcomes

Cardiac Pump Effectiveness; Circulation Status; Fluid Balance; Hydration; Tissue Perfusion: Cardiac, Cerebral, Peripheral; Urinary Elimination

**Example NOC Outcome with Indicators**

Demonstrates adequate **Circulation Status** as evidenced by the following indicators: Peripheral pulses strong/Peripheral pulses symmetrical/Peripheral edema not present (Rate each indicator of **Circulation Status:** 1 = severely compromised, 2 = substantially compromised, 3 = moderately compromised, 4 = mildly compromised, 5 = not compromised [see Section I].)

## Client Outcomes

### Client Will (Specify Time Frame):

- Demonstrate adequate tissue perfusion as evidenced by palpable peripheral pulses, warm and dry skin, adequate urinary output, and absence of respiratory distress
- Verbalize knowledge of treatment regimen, including appropriate exercise and medications and their actions and possible side effects
- Identify changes in lifestyle that are needed to increase tissue perfusion

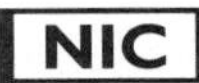

## Intervention (Nursing Interventions Classification)

### Suggested NIC Intervention

Circulatory Care: Arterial Insufficiency

**Example NIC Activities—Circulatory Care: Arterial Insufficiency**

Evaluate peripheral edema and pulses; inspect skin for arterial ulcers and tissue breakdown

## Nursing Interventions and Rationales

T

### Cerebral Perfusion

- • If the client experiences dizziness because of postural hypotension when getting up, teach methods to decrease dizziness, such as remaining seated for several minutes before standing, flexing feet upward several times while seated, rising slowly, sitting down immediately if feeling dizzy, and trying to have someone present when standing. *Postural hypotension can be detected in up to 30% of elderly clients. These methods can help prevent falls (Tinetti, 2003).*
- ▲ Monitor neurological status; perform a neurological examination; if symptoms of a cerebrovascular accident occur (e.g., hemiparesis, hemiplegia, or dysphasia), call 911

and send the client to the emergency department. **EB:** *New onset of these neurological symptoms can signify a stroke. If the stroke is caused by a thrombus and the client receives thrombolytic treatment within 3 hours, effects can often be reversed and function improved, although there is an increased risk of intracranial hemorrhage (Wardlaw et al, 2003).*

- ▲ If an ischemic stroke is present, consider keeping the head of the bed lower or flat as long as the airway is maintained, after consulting with the physician. **EBN:** *A pilot study examining the velocity of blood flow in the middle cerebral artery demonstrated increased flow when the head was lower than 30 degrees or flat (Wojner, El-Mitwalli, & Alexandrov, 2002). This study must be replicated before the change in position can be advocated for general practice.*
- • See the care plans for **Decreased Intracranial adaptive capacity, Risk for Injury**, and **Acute Confusion.**

## Peripheral Perfusion

- ▲ Check the dorsalis pedis, posterior tibial, and popliteal pulses bilaterally. If unable to find them, use a Doppler stethoscope and notify the physician immediately if new onset of pulses not present. *Diminished or absent peripheral pulses indicate arterial insufficiency with resultant ischemia (Kasirajan & Ouriel, 2002).*
- • Note skin color and feel the temperature of the skin. *Skin pallor or mottling, cool or cold skin temperature, or an absent pulse can signal arterial obstruction, which is an emergency that requires immediate intervention (Dillon, 2003). Rubor (reddish-blue color accompanied by dependency) indicates dilated or damaged vessels. Brownish discoloration of the skin indicates chronic venous insufficiency (Simon, Dix, & McCollum, 2004).*
- • Check capillary refill. *Nailbeds usually return to a pinkish color within 2 to 3 seconds after nailbed compression (Dillon, 2003).*
- • Note skin texture and the presence of hair, ulcers, or gangrenous areas on the legs or feet. *Thin, shiny, dry skin with hair loss; brittle nails; and gangrene or ulcerations on toes and anterior surfaces of the feet are seen in clients with arterial insufficiency. If ulcerations are on the side of the leg, they are usually associated with venous insufficiency (Bickley, Szilagyi, & Stackhouse, 2003).*
- • Note the presence of edema in the extremities and rate it on a four-point scale. Measure the circumference of the ankle and calf at the same time each day in the early morning.
- • Assess for pain in the extremities, noting severity, quality, timing, and exacerbating and alleviating factors. Differentiate venous from arterial disease. *In clients with venous insufficiency the pain lessens with elevation of the legs and exercise. In clients with arterial insufficiency the pain increases with elevation of the legs and exercise (Kasper et al, 2005). Some clients have both arterial and venous insufficiency. Arterial insufficiency is associated with pain when walking (claudication) that is relieved by rest. Clients with severe arterial disease have foot pain while at rest, which keeps them awake at night. Venous insufficiency is associated with aching, cramping, and discomfort (Kasper et al, 2005).*



## Arterial Insufficiency

- ▲ Monitor peripheral pulses. If there is new onset of loss of pulses with bluish, purple, or black areas and extreme pain, notify the physician immediately. *These are symptoms of arterial obstruction that can result in loss of a limb if not immediately reversed.*

- • Do not elevate the legs above the level of the heart. *With arterial insufficiency, leg elevation decreases arterial blood supply to the legs.*
- ▲ For early arterial insufficiency, encourage exercise such as walking or riding an exercise bicycle from 30 to 60 min/day as ordered by the physician. *Exercise therapy should be the initial intervention in nondisabling claudication (Zafar, Farkouh, & Chesebro, 2000; Treat-Jacobson & Walsh, 2003).* **EB:** *Participation in an exercise program was shown to increase walking times more effectively than angioplasty and antiplatelet therapy (Leng, Fowler, & Ernst, 2004).*
- • Keep the client warm and have the client wear socks and shoes or sheepskin-lined slippers when mobile. Do not apply heat. *Clients with arterial insufficiency complain of being constantly cold; therefore, keep extremities warm to maintain vasodilation and blood supply. Heat application can easily damage ischemic tissues.*
- ▲ Pay meticulous attention to foot care. Refer to a podiatrist if the client has a foot or nail abnormality. *Ischemic feet are very vulnerable to injury; meticulous foot care can prevent further injury.*
- • If the client has ischemic arterial ulcers, refer to the care plan for **Impaired Tissue integrity** but avoid use of occlusive dressings. *Occlusive dressings should be used with caution in clients with arterial ulceration because of the increased risk for cellulitis (Cahall & Spence, 1995).*
- ▲ If client smokes, aggressively counsel the client to stop smoking and refer to the physician for medications to support nicotine withdrawal and a smoking withdrawal program. **EB:** *A combination of psychosocial and pharmacological interventions was more effective than either intervention alone to stop smoking behavior (van der Meer et al, 2003).*

### Venous Insufficiency

- • Elevate edematous legs as ordered and ensure that there is no pressure under the knee. *Elevation increases venous return, helps decrease edema, and can help heal venous leg ulcers (Simon, Dix, & McCollum, 2004). Pressure under the knee decreases venous circulation.*
- • Apply graduated compression stockings as ordered. Ensure proper fit by measuring accurately. Remove the stocking at least twice a day, in the morning with the bath and in the evening, to assess the condition of the extremity, then reapply. **EBN and EB:** *A meta-analysis of 11 studies demonstrated that the use of graduated compression stockings reduced the incidence of deep vein thrombosis in a high-risk orthopedic surgical population and that implementation of additional antithrombotic measures along with stocking use decreased the incidence even further (Joanna Briggs Institute, 2001). Graduated compression stockings, alone or used in conjunction with other prevention modalities, help prevent deep vein thrombosis in hospitalized patients (Amarigiri & Lees, 2005).*
- • Encourage the client to walk with compression stockings on and perform toe-up and point-flex exercises. *Exercise helps increase venous return, build up collateral circulation, and strengthen the calf muscle pumps (Simon, Dix, & McCollum, 2004).*
- • If the client is overweight, encourage weight loss to decrease venous disease. *Obesity is a risk factor for development of chronic venous disease (Kunimoto et al, 2001).*

- If the client has venous leg ulcers, encourage the client to avoid prolonged sitting, standing, and elevation of the involved leg. **EBN:** *A study demonstrated that wound perfusion was lower when the client with venous leg ulcers was sitting, standing, or elevating the involved leg than when the client was lying supine (Wipke-Tevis et al, 2001).*
- Discuss lifestyle with the client to determine if the client's occupation requires prolonged standing or sitting, which can result in chronic venous disease (Kunimoto et al, 2001).
- If the client is mostly immobile, consult with the physician regarding use of a calf-high pneumatic compression device for prevention of deep vein thrombosis. *Pneumatic compression devices can be effective in preventing deep vein thrombosis in the immobile client (Roman, 2005; Van Gerpen & Mast, 2004).*
- Observe for signs of deep vein thrombosis, including pain, tenderness, swelling in the calf and thigh, and redness in the involved extremity. Take serial leg measurements of the thigh and calf circumferences. In some clients a tender venous cord can be felt in the popliteal fossa. Do not rely on Homans' sign. *Thrombosis with clot formation is usually first detected as swelling of the involved leg and then as pain. Homans' sign is not reliable (Kasper et al, 2005). Unfortunately, symptoms of existing deep vein thrombosis will not be found in 25% to 50% of client examinations even when a thrombus is present (Launius & Graham, 1998).*
- ▲ Note the results of a d-dimer test and ultrasounds. *High levels of d-dimer, a fibrin degradation fragment, are found in deep vein thrombosis and pulmonary embolism (Sadovsky, 2005) but results should be confirmed with a duplex venous ultrasonogram (Kasper et al, 2005).*
- ▲ If deep vein thrombosis is present, observe for symptoms of a pulmonary embolism including dyspnea, tachypnea, and tachycardia, especially if there is history of trauma. **EB:** *Based on data from 16 studies, fatal pulmonary embolisms are reported in one third of trauma clients (Agency for Healthcare Research and Quality, 2000).*
- If client is receiving heparin subcutaneously, do not change the needle after drawing up the dose. **EBN:** *A study concluded that changing the subcutaneous needle after withdrawing heparin from a vial did not reduce the size of ecchymoses at the injection site of study subjects (Klingman, 2000).*
- If client develops deep vein thrombosis, after treatment and hospital discharge, recommend client wear below the knee elastic compression stockings during the day in the involved extremity. **EB:** *A research study demonstrated that a group of clients who wore them had a 50% less likely incidence of developing post-thrombotic syndrome, than those clients who did not wear the stockings (Shaughnessy, 2005). A meta-analysis of research demonstrated that there is substantial evidence that compression stockings reduce the occurrance of postthrombotic syndrome after deep vein thrombosis (Kolbach et al, 2004).*

T

## Geriatric

- Change the client's position slowly when getting the client out of bed. *Postural hypotension can be detected in up to 30% of elderly clients (Tinetti, 2003).*
- Recognize that the elderly have an increased risk of developing pulmonary embolism and that, if it is present, the symptoms are nonspecific and often mimic those of heart failure or pneumonia (Berman, 2001).

### Home Care

- The interventions described previously may be adapted for home care use.
- Differentiate between arterial and venous insufficiency. *Accurate diagnostic information clarifies clinical assessment and allows for more effective care.*
- If arterial disease is present and the client smokes, aggressively encourage smoking cessation. See the care plan for **Health-seeking behaviors.**
- Examine the feet carefully at frequent intervals for changes and new ulcerations. *Lower Extremity Amputation Prevention Program (LEAP) documentation forms are available at www.bphc.hrsa.gov/leap/ (Feldman, 1998).*
- ▲ Assess the client's nutritional status, paying special attention to obesity, hyperlipidemia, and malnutrition. Refer to a dietitian if appropriate. *Malnutrition contributes to anemia, which further compounds the lack of oxygenation to tissues. Obese clients encounter poor circulation in adipose tissue, which can create increased hypoxia in tissue (Rolstad, 1990).*
- Monitor for development of gangrene, venous ulceration, and symptoms of cellulitis (redness, pain, and increased swelling in an extremity). *Cellulitis often accompanies peripheral vascular disease and is related to poor tissue perfusion (Marrelli, 1994).*

## Client/Family Teaching

- ▲ Explain the importance of good foot care. Teach the client and family to wash and inspect the feet daily. Recommend that the diabetic client wear padded socks, special insoles, and jogging shoes. *Use of cushioned footwear can decrease pressure on the feet, decrease callus formation, and help save the feet (Feldman, 1998; George, 1993).*
- ▲ Teach the diabetic client that he or she should have a comprehensive foot examination at least annually, including assessment of sensation using the Semmes-Weinstein monofilaments. If good sensation is not present, refer to a footwear professional for fitting of therapeutic shoes and inserts, the cost of which is covered by Medicare. **EB:** *Testing with Semmes-Weinstein monofilaments is effectively diagnostic of impaired sensation, especially when combined with clinical examination (Pham et al, 2000).*
- For arterial disease, stress the importance of not smoking, following a weight loss program (if the client is obese), carefully controlling a diabetic condition, controlling hyperlipidemia and hypertension, maintaining intake of anti-platelet therapy and reducing stress. *All of these risk factors for atherosclerosis can be modified (Treat-Jacobson, 2003).*
- Teach the client to avoid exposure to cold, to limit exposure to brief periods if going out in cold weather, and to wear warm clothing.
- For venous disease, teach the importance of wearing compression stockings as ordered, elevating the legs at intervals, and watching for skin breakdown on the legs (Shaughnessy, 2005).
- Teach the client to recognize the signs and symptoms that should be reported to a physician (e.g., change in skin temperature, color, or sensation, or the presence of a new lesion on the foot).

NOTE: If the client is receiving anticoagulant therapy, see the care plan for **Ineffective Protection.**



T

## evolve WEBSITES FOR EDUCATION

See the EVOLVE website for World Wide Web resources for client education.

## REFERENCES


Agency for Healthcare Research and Quality: *Prevention of venous thromboembolism after injury: summary,* Evidence Report/Technology Assessment Number 22, Rockville, Md, August 2000, The Agency. Available at www.ahrq.gov/clinic/epcsums/vtsumm.htm, accessed on March 11, 2005.

Amarigiri SV, Lees TA: Elastic compression stockings for prevention of deep vein thrombosis. *Cochrane Database Syst Rev* (3): CD001484, 2005.

Bickley LS, Szilagyi PG, Stackhouse JG: *Bates guide to physical examination and history taking,* ed 8, Philadelphia, 2003, Lippincott.

Beere PA, Russell SD, Morey MC et al: Aerobic exercise training can reverse age-related peripheral circulatory changes in healthy older men, *Circulation* 100(10):1085, 1999.

Berman AR: Pulmonary embolism in the elderly, *Clin Geriatr Med* 17(1):107, 2001.

Black SB: Venous stasis ulcers: a review, *Ostomy Wound Manage* 41:20, 1995.

Cahall E, Spence RK: Practical nursing measures for vascular compromise in the lower leg, *Ostomy Wound Manage* 41:16, 1995.

Dillon PM: *Nursing health assessment,* Philadelphia, 2003, FA Davis.

Feldman CB: Caring for feet: patients and nurse practitioners working together, *Nurse Pract Forum* 9(2):87, 1998.

Joanna Briggs Institute: Best practice: graduated compression stockings for the prevention of post-operative venous thromboembolism, *Evidence based practice information sheets for health professions* 5:2, 2001.

Kasirajan K, Ouriel K: Current options in the diagnosis and management of acute limb ischemia, *Prog Cardiovasc Nurs* 17(1):26, 2002.

Kasper DL et al: *Harrison's principles of internal medicine,* ed 16, New York, 2005, McGraw-Hill.

Klingman L: Effects of changing needles prior to administering heparin subcutaneously, *Heart Lung* 29(1):70, 2000.

Kolbach DN, Sandbrink MW, Hamulyak K et al: Non-pharmaceutical measures for prevention of post-thrombotic syndrome, *Cochrane Database Syst Rev* (1):CD004174, 2004.

Kunimoto B, Cooling M, Gulliver W et al: Best practices for the prevention and treatment of venous leg ulcers, *Ostomy Wound Manage* 47(2):34, 2001.

Leng GC, Fowler B, Ernst E: Exercise for intermittent claudication, *Cochrane Database Syst Rev* (2):CD000990, 2004.

Marrelli TM: *Handbook of home health standards and documentation guidelines for reimbursement,* ed 2, St Louis, 1994, Mosby.

Pham H, Armstrong DG, Harvey C et al: Screening techniques to identify people at high risk for diabetic foot ulceration: a prospective multicenter trial, *Diabetes Care* 23(5):606, 2000.

Rolstad BS: Treatment objectives in chronic wound care, *Home Healthc Nurse* 9:6, 1990.

Roman M: Deep vein thrombosis: an overview, *Med-Surg Matters* 14(1), 2005.

Sadovsky R: D-Dimer assays for prediction of venous thromboembolism, *Am Fam Physician* 71(4), 2005.

Shaughnessy AF: Compression stockings and post-thrombotic syndrome, *Am Family Physician* 71(1), 2005.

Simon DA, Dix FP, McCollum CN: Management of venous leg ulcers, *BMJ* 328(7452):1358, 2004.

Sullano ME, Ortiz EJ: Deep vein thrombosis and anticoagulant therapy, *Nurs Clin North Am* 36(4):645, 2001.

Tinetti ME: Preventing falls in elderly persons, *N Engl J Med* 348(1):421, 2003.

Treat-Jacobson D, Walsh ME: Treating patients with peripheral arterial disease and claudication, *J Vasc Nurs* 21(1):5, 2003.

van der Meer RM, Wagena EJ, Ostelo RWet al: Smoking cessation for chronic obstructive pulmonary disease, *Cochrane Database Syst Rev* (2):CD002999, 2003.

Van Gerpen RV, Mast ME: Thromboembolic disorders in cancer, *Clin J Oncol Nurs* 8(3):289, 2004.

Wardlaw JM, Zoppo G, Yamaguchi T et al: Thrombolysis for acute ischaemic stroke, *Cochrane Database Syst Rev* (3):CD000213, 2003.

Wipke-Tevis DD, Stotts NA, Williams DA et al: Tissue oxygenation, perfusion, and position in patients with venous leg ulcers, *Nurs Res* 50(1):24, 2001.

Wojner AW, El-Mitwalli A, Alexandrov AV: Effect of head positioning on intracranial blood flow velocities in acute ischemic stroke: a pilot study, *Crit Care Nurs Q* 24(4):57, 2002.

Zafar MU, Farkouh ME, Chesebro JH: A practical approach to lower-extremity arterial disease, *Patient Care* 30:96, 2000.


T

# Impaired Transfer ability

*Brenda Emick-Herring*

## NANDA

### Definition

Limitation of independent movement between two nearby surfaces

### Defining Characteristics

Impaired ability to transfer: from bed to chair and chair to bed/on or off toilet or commode/between uneven levels/from chair to car or car to chair/from chair to floor or floor to chair/from standing to floor or floor to standing

### Related Factors (r/t)

Intolerance to activity, decreased strength and endurance, pain or discomfort, perceptual or cognitive impairment, neuromuscular impairment, musculoskeletal impairment, depression, severe anxiety

Suggested functional level classifications include the following:
0—Completely independent
1—Requires use of equipment or device
2—Requires help from another person for assistance, supervision, or teaching
3—Requires help from another person and equipment or device
4—Dependent—does not participate in activity

## NOC

### Outcomes (Nursing Outcomes Classification)

#### Suggested NOC Outcomes

Balance; Body Positioning: Self-Initiated; Transfer Performance

**Example NOC Outcome with Indicators**

**Transfer Performance** as evidenced by the following indicators: Transfers from bed to chair and back/Transfers from chair to commode and back/Transfers from wheelchair to car and back (Rate each indicator of **Transfer Performance:** 1 = severely compromised, 2 = substantially compromised, 3 = moderately compromised, 4 = mildly compromised, 5 = not compromised [see Section I].)

### Client Outcomes

**Client Will (Specify Time Frame):**

- Transfer from bed to chair and back successfully
- Transfer from chair to chair successfully



T

- Transfer from wheelchair to toilet and back successfully
- Transfer from wheelchair to car and back successfully

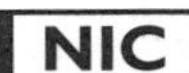

## Interventions (Nursing Interventions Classification)

### Suggested NIC Interventions

Exercise Promotion: Strength Training; Exercise Therapy: Muscle Control

**Example NIC Activities—Exercise Promotion: Strength Training**

Obtain medical clearance for initiating a strength-training program, as appropriate; assist client in setting realistic short- and long-term goals and taking ownership of the exercise plan

## Nursing Interventions and Rationales

▲ Request a consult for a physical therapist (PT) and/or occupational therapist (OT) to develop an exercise and strengthening program early in the client's recovery. *Lower extremity and trunk strength will be key for doing partial or full weight-bearing transfers; upper extremity and trunk strength will be important for slide-board transfers.*

▲ Obtain a consult for a PT, OT, or orthotist to evaluate, measure, and fit the client with the proper orthoses, braces, splints, collars and walking aids before sitting and standing clients. *Equipment and walking aids must be individualized to help clients move and function safely, comfortably, and as independently as possible (Hoeman, 2002).*

▲ Ergonomically assess the client's dependence level, weight, strength, movement ability, balance, tolerance to position change, sensation, behavior, and cognition, as well as available equipment and staff ratio/experience, to decide whether to perform a manual transfer or device-assisted lift. (If PT has identified a specific transfer method and it is compatible with the nursing assessment, then use it.) **EBN:** *Use of a wheelchair ramp or hoist scale to weigh clients reduced perceived stress on employees' shoulders and backs and objectively reduced compressive and shear forces at the L5 to S1 discs (Owen & Garg, 1994). Staff reported that work fatigue, demands, and back and shoulder pain decreased, and safety increased after they received education on a "safe lifting" and "no strenuous lifting" approach to lift and transfer hospitalized clients; musculoskeletal injuries did not change (Yassi et al, 2001). A pilot study using a trained nursing lift team to transfer clients needing maximal assistance successfully transferred numerous clients, prevented nursing injury, and was positively evaluated by staff (Caska, Patnode, & Clickner, 1998).*

T

- Do not use the under-axilla method to transfer, move, or weigh a physically dependent client. Rather, use mechanical devices such as hydraulic or battery-operated mechanical lifts, stand-assist lifts, and bed or wheelchair ramp scales. **EBN:** *Researchers concluded that under-axilla lifts can cause overexertion back injuries to nursing staff and that clients may be more physically and psychologically comfortable when lifted with mechanical devices, yet nurse educators still teach and staff nurses still use the under-axilla method (Owen, Welden, & Kane, 1999).*
- Apply a gait or walking belt to client's low back, or under the axilla if an abdominal wound or tube is present, before transferring them. Keep the belt and client close to

you during the transfer. *A gait belt counteracts weakness and unsteadiness. If the belt is used incorrectly (e.g., at arm's length), it moves the client's base of support away from staff, prevents support of the client, and places staff at risk for back and arm injury (Minor & Minor, 1999).* **EBN:** *Research showed use of a gait belt decreased staff exertion, back stress, and compressive force at L5 to S1 (Owen & Garg, 1993). Garg et al (1991) concluded that two staff using a walking belt, a rocking motion to gain momentum, and a pulling motion to transfer clients into and out of a wheelchair and shower chair, was preferred by staff and clients over four other methods.*

- Remind clients to comply with weight-bearing restrictions ordered by their physician.
- Assist client to don/doff orthoses, braces, collars, prostheses, immobilizers, and abdominal binders while in bed. *Devices stabilize and align body parts during motion. Abdominal binders help prevent postural hypotension.*
- Adjust transfer surfaces so they are similar in height. For example, lower a hospital bed to equal the height of a commode. **EB:** *Equal heights between seat surfaces require much less upper extremity muscular effort during transfers (Wang et al, 1994).*
- Help clients don shoes or socks with nonskid soles before transfers. *A client may fall if wearing footwear with smooth or slick soles. Educate diabetic clients to consistently wear shoes or slippers because their feet heal poorly if injured (Yetzer, 2002).*
- Remove or swivel the wheelchair arm rests, leg rests, and footplates off to the side especially if clients do a squat or slide board transfer. *This gives the clients and nurses feet space in which to maneuver and provides fewer obstacles to trip over (Minor & Minor 1999; Ossman & Campbell, 1990).*
- Place the wheelchair, commode, or shower chair at a slight angle toward the surface to which the client will transfer onto. *An angle positions the two surfaces close to one another yet allows room for client and caregiver to adjust the client's movements during the transfer (Hoeman, 2002; Kumagai, 1998; Ossman & Campbell, 1990).*
- Teach the client to consistently lock the brakes on the wheelchair, commode, shower chair, or bed before transferring. *Portable devices often have wheels that will roll if not locked, thus creating high risk for falls. Pneumatic wheelchair tires must be adequately inflated for the brakes to lock effectively (Minor & Minor, 1999).*
- Position walking aids logistically so that the client can grasp and use them once he or she is standing. *Walking aids provide support, balance, and stability to help the client stand and step safely (Bohannon, 1997).* **EB:** *Elders with peripheral neuropathy had less risk of losing their balance while standing on an unstable (tilting) surface in normal and low light when using a cane in the nondominant hand (Ashton-Miller et al, 1996).*
- Reinforce that clients are to place one hand on the walker and to push with the other hand on the arm of the chair or on the surface on which they are sitting, to arise. *Placing both hands on the walker may cause it to tip and the client to lose balance.*
- Give clear, simple instructions, allow time to process the information, and let the client do as much of the transfer as possible.

▲ Implement and document on the team plan of care, the type of transfer (slide board, squat, and so on), weight-bearing status (non–, partial, full), equipment (lift, walker, and so on), level of assistance (standby, moderate, and so on), and type of assistance to provide (manual guidance, balance control, verbal cueing, and so on). *Team communication and consistency plus repeated instructions are critical for clients learning,*

T

*motor recovery, and safety. Collaboration allows team members to monitor the client's progress and update the transfer as needed. (Rehabilitation Nursing Standards Task Force, 2000; Kumagai, 1998).* **EBN:** *Researchers concluded there is a positive relationship between nurses' skill in performing patient transfers, and quality of care as measured by patient safety and comfort while being lifted up in bed, and transferred from bed to wheelchair (Kjellberg et al, 2004).*

- Incorporate set position before transferring clients (e.g., sitting on the edge of the bed/seat with bilateral weight bearing on the buttocks, hips and knees flexed, front [balls] of the feet aligned under the knees, and the head in midline). *These are the normal postures that prepare humans for weight bearing. They permit shifting of weight from the pelvis to the feet as the center of gravity changes as one arises (Kumagai, 1998; Gee & Passarella, 1985).*
- Recognize the normal sequence of movements for standing (e.g., hips and knees flex; back extends; trunk, head, and knees then lean well forward over the feet; the weight shifts to the feet, thus lifting up the hips and buttocks—standing occurs as the knees, hips, and trunk extend). *Familiarity with the normal movements involved in standing may help nurses identify key points to verbally and physically emphasize as they assist clients (Kumagai, 1998; Gee & Passarella, 1985).*
- Support and stabilize the client's knee(s) by placing one or both of your knees next to or encircling the client's knee(s), rather than "blocking" the client's knee(s). *This allows the client to flex the knee(s) and to lean forward during transfers.* Refer to Gee and Passarella (1985), Ossman and Campbell (1990), Kumagai (1998), and Minor and Minor (1999) for information and sketches/photographs of various transfer techniques. Three methods are briefly summarized below.
  1. Squat transfer—the client leans well forward and slightly raises flexed hips off the surface, then pivots and sits down on the new surface. Use for clients with poor muscle control and slight weight bearing ability.
  2. Standing pivot transfer—the client leans forward with hips flexed and pushes up with hands from the seat surface or arms of the chair, then stands erect and pivots toward the new surface and sits down. Use with clients who have at least partial weight bearing ability.
  3. Slide board transfer—client should have on pants, or a pillowcase should be placed over the board. Remove arm and leg rest from the chair and slightly angle it toward the new surface. Have client lean sideways, thus shifting his/her weight so the transfer board can be placed under the upper thigh of the leg next to the new surface. Make sure the board is safely angled across both surfaces. Instruct client to return to neutral alignment and place one hand on the board and the other hand on the seat surface. Remind the client to perform a series of pushups with the arms while leaning forward and lifting (not sliding) the hips in small increments, with each pushup. One or more nurses may need to help the client by using the gait belt and lifting up the hips during each pushup. *It benefits clients who have little to no weight-bearing ability (Hoeman 2002; Minor & Minor 1999).* **EBN:** *The ability to perform bed transfers was shown to be the most important factor in enabling frail elderly clients to live independently (Seidenfeld, Eberle, & Potter, 2000).*

- ▲ Extra staff may be needed to transfer debilitated bariatric (extremely obese) clients. Place their beds against a corner wall and lock the brakes. Assist them to establish balance as they sit up onto the edge of the bed and help them get into the set position by placing both knees level with their thighs (feet may need to be placed up on a stool). Help or remind client to lean well forward during the transfer. *Walls and brakes prevent the bed from moving. Center-of-gravity and balance skills must be learned so the client is willing to lean forward; staff use this momentum to help transfer the client. Fear of falling is a grave concern because past falls may have evoked embarrassment. Level knees prevent the feet (and weight) from drifting downward (Daus, 2001).*
- ▲ Investigate and use devices and equipment to safely transfer the bariatric population. Transfer aids may include: air mattress overlay, Gore-Tex or silicone transfer sheet, 60-inch-long gait belt or two regular gait belts strapped together, supine sliding or roller board, bedside sling-lift or standing-lift device, overhead ceiling-mounted lift, or overhead A-frame lift (Dionne, 2000, 2002). Special equipment may include high-low chair, 1000-pound load limit manual or powered wheelchair, wide and durable commode, and shower chair (Daus, 2001, 2003).
- ▲ Administer bilevel or continuous airway pressure therapy at night to bariatric clients, as ordered. *Obesity is a causative factor in obstructive sleep apnea, which can contribute to poor endurance and activity intolerance (Daus, 2001).*

## Home Care

- ▲ Obtain referral for OT and PT to develop a home exercise program and safe transfer routine and to evaluate for needed modifications such as ramps; wide doorways; safe floor surfaces; grab bars; tub seats; commode; clutter elimination; adequate lighting; and proper chairs. *Therapists and nurses can help families understand, choose, access, and evaluate needed assistive technology to promote independence (Aiello et al, 2001; Berry & Ignash, 2003).* **EB:** *Finlayson & Havixbeck, (1992) concluded that nonuse of prescribed equipment could be prevented by ensuring that home visits were made by therapists prior to discharge; they also found tub transfers were frightening and difficult at home even if clients had received instructions prior to hospital discharge. A different study indicated that canes and crutches reduced the number of hours of care a person needed with ADLs, but walkers and wheelchairs only supplemented; they did not replace human assistance (Allen, 2001).*
- ▲ Assess for optimum furniture placement for functional activities and maneuverability while using an assistive device, and for stability in getting up in case of a fall. Fitted bedspreads are necessary so clients do not trip over them. *Home evaluations meet the unique mobility needs of clients (Aiello et al, 2001).*
- ▲ Involve a therapist, social worker, and/or nurse case manager to educate the client and family about assistive technology availability and costs, financial benefits, and regulations associated with Medicare, Medicaid, and third-party payers, as well as local community options for securing aids and home care services. *Such information helps families understand options for assistive technology and support services, and their financial implications (Berry & Ignash, 2003).*
- • Implement ergonomic approaches for home care staff and family to safely handle and transfer clients in their homes. *Risk of back, shoulder, and neck injury is high because*

*home health care staff work alone, often without mechanical aids, in crowded spaces, without adjustable beds and chairs, and in awkward postures as they move and care for clients (Galinsky, Waters, & Malit, 2001).*

- For further information, refer to care plans for **Impaired physical Mobility** and **Impaired Walking.**

## Client/Family Teaching

- ▲ Begin discharge planning as soon as possible along with a case manager or social worker to assess the need for home care services.
- • Assess client and family readiness to learn and use teaching modalities conducive to their personal learning styles. *Learning varies, but may be enhanced with visual, auditory, tactile, and cognitive stimulus (Allen 2002).*
- ▲ Coordinate with therapists to reinforce client and family education on safe and effective transfer methods; application and skin checks associated with braces, splints, immobilizers, and so on; and proper fit, use, and care of transfer devices. *Repetition and consistency reinforce learning and follow-through. Basic principles for transfers are constant from surface to surface; however, individuals often need special instruction from a therapist to individualize the approaches for home (Gee & Passarella, 1985; Ossman & Campbell, 1990).*
- • Schedule supervised practice sessions accordingly, where client and family use gait belts, do the specified transfer or return, and demonstrate proper use of lifts or other devices. *Correct transfer techniques and devices help prevent back injuries in family and enhance safety. Overassistance by the family may decrease learning, self-esteem, and independence of the client.*
- • Teach, model, and then monitor client's and family's consistent performance of safety precautions for transfers, including wearing proper shoes, placing equipment and chairs correctly, locking brakes, swiveling leg rests out of the way, and so on. *Such actions will help prevent falls and injury to clients and caregivers.*
- ▲ Teach the client and family how to check brakes on chairs to make sure they engage and how to check so that tires have adequate air pressure. Recommend routine inspection and annual tune-up of the wheelchair. *Long-term use may loosen brakes or cause them to slip. The brakes work only if they make sound contact with the tire or wheel; therefore it is important that pneumatic tires be adequately inflated (Minor & Minor, 1999).*
- ▲ Offer information on safe use of shower and commode chairs to prevent serious complications such as discomfort, pressure ulcers, falls during transfer or transport, and inaccessibility for bowel care and hygiene (bowel care may take 30 minutes to 3 hours in persons with neurogenic bowel). **EBN:** *Three shower/bowel care chairs were evaluated by clients and caregivers for comfort, safety transportability, accessibility for bowel care and showering, and repeated use in the shower. Many inadequacies and unsafe features were identified, especially regarding pressure ulcers and falls (Malassigne´ et al, 1993). Based on this data the research team designed, tested, and marketed a new shower/bowel chair to minimize such risks and client error in using the chair (Nelson et al, 2000).*
- • For further information, refer to the care plans for **Impaired physical Mobility** and **Impaired Walking.**

T

## evolve WEBSITES FOR EDUCATION

See the EVOLVE website for World Wide Web resources for client education.

## REFERENCES


Aiello DD et al: Safety in the home, *Rehab Manag* 14(5):54, 2001.

Allen JC: Outcome-directed client and family education. In Hoeman SP, editor: *Rehabilitation nursing: process, application, and outcomes,* ed 3, St Louis, 2002, Mosby.

Allen SM: Canes, crutches and home care services: the interplay of human and technological assistance, *Cent Home Care Policy Res Policy Briefs* (4):1, 2001.

Ashton-Miller JA et al: A cane reduces loss of balance in patients with peripheral neuropathy: results from a challenging unipedal balance test, *Arch Phys Med Rehabil* 77:446, 1996.

Berry BE, Ignash S: Assistive technology: Providing independence for individuals with disabilities, *Rehab Nurs* 28(1):6, 2003.

Bohannon RW: Gait performance with wheeled and standard walkers, *Percept Mot Skills* 85:1185, 1997.

Caska BA, Patnode RE, Clickner D: Feasibility of a nurse staffed lift team, *AAOHN J* 46(6):283, 1998.

Daus C: Rehab and the bariatric patient, *Rehab Manag* 14(9):42, 2001.

Daus C: The right fit, *Rehab Manag* 16(7):32, 2003.

Dionne M: Maximizing efficiency with minimum effort: transferring the bariatric patient, *Rehab Manag* 13(6):64, 2000.

Dionne M: Ten tips for safe mobility in the bariatric population, *Rehab Manag* 15(8):28, 2002.

Finlayson M, Havixbeck K: A post-discharge study on the use of assistive devices, *Can J Occup Ther* 59(4):201, 1992.

Galinsky T, Waters T, Malit B: Overexertion injuries in home health care workers and the need for ergonomics, *Home Health Care Serv Q* 20(3):57, 2001.

Garg A et al: A biomechanical and ergonomic evaluation of patient transferring tasks: wheelchair to shower chair and shower chair to wheelchair, *Ergon* 34(4):407, 1991.

Gee AL, Passarella PM: *Nursing care of the stroke patient: a therapeutic approach,* Pittsburgh, 1985, Harmarville Rehabilitation Center.

Hoeman SP: Movement, functional mobility, and activities of daily living. In Hoeman SP, editor: *Rehabilitation nursing: process, application, and outcomes,* ed 3, St Louis, 2002, Mosby.

Kjellberg K, Lagerstrom M, Hagberg M: Patient safety and comfort during transfers in relation to nurses' work technique, *J Adv Nurs* 47(3):251, 2004.

Kumagai KAS: Physical management of the neurologically involved client: techniques for bed mobility and transfers. In Chin PA, Finocchiaro D, Rosebrough A, editors: *Rehabilitation nursing practice,* New York, 1998, McGraw-Hill

Malassigne´ P et al: Toward the design of a new bowel care chair for the spinal cord injured: a pilot study, *SCI Nurs* 10(3):84, 1993.

Minor MAD, Minor SD: *Patient care skills,* ed 4, Stamford, Conn, 1999, Appleton and Lange.

Nelson A et al: Promoting safe use of equipment for neurogenic bowel management, *SCI Nurs* 17(3):119, 2000.

Ossman NJH, Campbell M: *Adult positions, transitions, and transfers: reproducible instruction cards for caregivers,* Therapist Guide No. 4166, Tucson, Ariz, 1990, Therapy Skill Builders.

Owen BD, Garg A: Back stress isn't part of the job, *Am J Nurs* 93(2):48, 1993.

Owen BD, Garg A: Reducing back stress through an ergonomic approach: weighing a patient, *Int J Nurs Stud* 31(6):511, 1994.

Owen BD, Welden N, Kane J: What are we teaching about lifting and transferring patients? *Res Nurs Health* 22(1):3, 1999.

Rehabilitation Nursing Standards Task Force: *Standards and scope of rehabilitation nursing practice,* ed 2, Glenview, Ill, 2000, Association of Rehabilitation Nurses.

Seidenfeld SE, Eberle CM, Potter JF: Functional abilities of frail elderly that enable return to the community, *Home Health Care Consult* 7(8):29, 2000.

Wang YT et al: Reaction force and EMG analyses of wheelchair transfers, *Percep Mot Skills* 79:763, 1994.

Yassi A et al: A randomized controlled trial to prevent patient lift and transfer injuries of health care workers, *Spine* 26(16):1739, 2001.

Yetzer EA: Causes and prevention of diabetic foot skin breakdown, *Rehabil Nurs* 27(2):52, 2002.




T

# Risk for Trauma

*Michele Walters*

**NANDA**

## Definition

Accentuated risk of accidental tissue injury (e.g., wound, burn, fracture)

## Risk Factors

### External

High-crime neighborhood and client vulnerability; pot handles facing toward front of stove; knives stored uncovered; inappropriate call-for-aid mechanisms for bed-resting client; inadequately stored combustibles or corrosives (e.g., matches, oily rags, lye); highly flammable children's toys or clothing; obstructed passageways; high beds; large icicles hanging from roof; nonuse or misuse of seat restraints; overexposure to sun, sunlamps, or radiotherapy; overloaded electrical outlets; overloaded fuse boxes; play or work near vehicle pathways (e.g., driveways, lane ways, railroad tracks); playing with fireworks or gunpowder; unlocked storage of guns or ammunition; contact with rapidly moving machinery, industrial belts, or pulleys; litter or liquid spills on floors or stairways; defective appliances; bathing in very hot water (e.g., unsupervised bathing of young children); bathtub without hand grip or antislip equipment; children's playing with matches, candles, cigarettes, or sharp-edged toys; children's playing at top of stairs without gates; children's riding in front seat of car; delayed lighting of gas burner or oven; contact with intense cold; collection of grease waste on stove; operation of mechanically unsafe vehicle; driving after use of alcoholic beverages or drugs; driving at excessive speeds; entry into unlighted rooms; experimentation with chemicals or gasoline; exposure to dangerous machinery; faulty electrical plugs; frayed wires; contact with acids or alkalis; unsturdy or absent stair rails; use of unsteady ladders or chairs; use of cracked dishware or glasses; wearing of plastic apron or flowing clothes around open flame; lack of screening on fires or heaters; unsafe window protection in homes with young children; sliding on coarse bed linen or struggling within bed restraints; use of thin or worn potholders; unanchored electric wires; misuse of necessary headgear for motor cyclists or young children carried on adult bicycles; gas leaks; unsafe road or road-crossing conditions; slippery floors (e.g., wet or highly waxed); smoking in bed or near oxygen-delivery system; snow or ice on stairs or walkways; unanchored rugs; driving without necessary visual aids



### Internal

Lack of safety education, insufficient finances to purchase safety equipment or effect repairs, history of trauma, lack of safety precautions, poor vision, reduced temperature and/or tactile sensation, balancing difficulties, cognitive or emotional difficulties, reduced large or small muscle coordination, weakness, reduced hand-eye coordination

## Related Factors (r/t)

See Risk Factors.

**NOC**

## Outcomes (Nursing Outcomes Classification)

### Suggested NOC Outcomes

Risk Control, Fall Prevention Behavior

**Example NOC Outcome with Indicators**

Accomplishes **Risk Control** as evidenced by the following indicators: Monitors environmental risk factors/Develops effective risk control strategies/Modifies lifestyle to reduce risk (Rate each indicator of **Risk Control:** 1 = never demonstrated, 2 = rarely demonstrated, 3 = sometimes demonstrated, 4 = often demonstrated, 5 = consistently demonstrated [see Section I].)

## Client Outcomes

### Client Will (Specify Time Frame):

- Remain free from trauma
- Explain actions that can be taken to prevent trauma

**NIC**

## Interventions (Nursing Interventions Classification)

### Suggested NIC Interventions

Environmental Management: Safety; Skin Surveillance

**Example NIC Activities—Environmental Management**

Provide family/significant other with information about making home environment safe for client; remove harmful objects from environment

## Nursing Interventions and Rationales

- Screen clients using a fall risk factor assessment tool to identify those at risk for falls. **EBN:** *This may reduce the incidence of client falls and provides an opportunity to offer health education to high-risk clients (Hsu et al, 2004).*
- Provide vision aids for visually impaired clients. *A client with a sensory loss must be protected from injury; therefore the visually impaired client must use vision aids (Potter & Perry, 2003).*
- Assist the client with ambulation. *Allow the client to use assistive devices in ADLs as needed. Assistive devices can augment the client's ability to perform ADLs (Potter & Perry, 2003).*
- Have a family member evaluate water temperature for the client. *A client with a tactile*

T

*sensory impairment resulting from age or psychological or physiological factors must be protected from burns (Potter & Perry, 2003).*

- Assess the client for causes of impaired cognition. **EB:** *Clients with dementia have a higher rate of injurious falls than those without dementia (Doorn et al, 2003).* **EB:** *Fall prevention programs will be more beneficial to clients with a higher level cognition by decreasing the number of falls (Jensen et al, 2003).*
- Keep walkways clear of snow, debris, and household items. *Cluttered walkways impair mobility and are a hazard for falls (Beers & Berkow, 2000).*
- Provide assistive devices in bathrooms (e.g., hand rails, nonslip decals on the floor of the shower and bathtub). **EB:** *Home hazard assessment and modification are personal safety measures to prevent falls (Gillespie et al, 2003).*
- Ensure that call-light systems are functioning and that the client is able to use them. *Hospital injuries often result from a client's attempt to get out of bed and use the bathroom when a caregiver cannot be contacted (Hammond & Levine, 1999).*
- Use a nightlight after dark. *A nightlight provides some light in the room to assist in orientation and improves visual acuity (Beers & Berkow, 2000).*
- Teach the client to observe safety precautions in high-crime neighborhoods (e.g., lock doors, do not leave home at night without a companion, keep entryways well lighted). *Adequate lighting helps protect the home and its inhabitants from crime (Potter & Perry, 2003).*

▲ Instruct the client not to drive under the influence of alcohol or drugs. Assess for a substance abuse problem and refer to appropriate resources for drug and alcohol education. **EB:** *The use of alcohol or drugs (benzodiazepines, cocaine, or opiates) places increased risk for motor vehicle accidents. Alcohol and drug combinations were at the highest risk of experiencing injurious road accidents (Movig et al, 2004).*

▲ Review drug profile for potential side effects that may inhibit performance of ADLs. *Over-the-counter medication (antihistamines) and prescriptive medications (benzodiazepines and opioid analgesic) may affect performance (Beers & Berkow, 2000).* **EB:** *Benzodiazepines have a fivefold increase injury risk for drivers (Movig et al, 2004).*

▲ See Nursing Interventions and Rationales in the care plans for **Risk for Aspiration, Impaired Home maintenance, Risk for Injury, Risk for Poisoning,** and **Risk for Suffocation.**

## Pediatric

T

- Assess the client's social economic status. **EB:** *Pediatric clients living in poverty are at higher risk for injury (Shenassa et al, 2004).*
- Never leave young children unsupervised around water or cooking areas. *Young children are at risk for drowning even in small amounts of water. Heat and fire from cooking are a hazard to young children (Potter & Perry, 2003).*
- Keep flammable and potentially flammable articles out of the reach of young children.
- Lock up harmful objects such as guns. *Increased access to guns and limited parental supervision significantly increase the risk of youths' exposure to gun violence (Slovak, 2002).*

## Geriatric

- Assess the geriatric client's level of functioning both at admission and periodically.

- Perform a home safety assessment and recommend the following preventive measures: keep electrical cords out of the flow of traffic; remove small rugs or make sure they are slip resistant; increase lighting in hallways and other dark areas; place a light in the bathroom; keep towels, curtains, and other items that might catch fire away from the stove; store harmful products away from food products; provide at least one grab bar in tubs and showers; check prescribed medications for appropriate labels; store medications in original containers or in a dispenser of some type (e.g., egg carton, seven day plastic dispenser); if the client cannot administer medications according to directions, secure someone to administer medications. **EB:** *Home hazard assessment and modification are personal safety measures to prevent falls (Gillespie et al, 2003). Identifying risks and implementing changes decreases risk of injury (National Center for Injury Prevention and Control, 2003).*
- Mark stove knobs with bright colors (yellow or red), and outline the borders of steps. *Easily visible markings are helpful for clients with decreased depth perception (Potter & Perry, 2003).*
- Discourage driving at night. *A decline in depth perception, slower recovery from glare, and night blindness are common in the elderly and make night driving a difficult and unsafe task (Beers & Berkow, 2000).*
- Encourage the client to participate in resistance and impact exercise programs as tolerated. **EB:** *Muscle strengthening and balance retraining are beneficial in preventing falls (Gillespie et al, 2003). These types of exercise have been found to delay bone loss in the hip (Snow et al, 2000).*
- Implement fall and injury prevention strategies in residential care facilities. **EB:** *An interdisciplinary and multifactorial prevention program targeting residents, staff, and the environment may reduce falls and femoral fractures (Jensen et al, 2002).*

## Client/Family Teaching

- Educate the family regarding age-appropriate child safety precautions, environmental safety precautions, and intervention in an emergency. **EB:** *Infants and toddlers are more likely to be injured than older children regardless of setting (Waibel & Ranjita, 2003).*
- Teach the family to assess the childcare provider's knowledge regarding child safety, environmental safety precautions, and assistance of a child in an emergency. **EB:** *Infants and toddlers are more likely to be injured than older children regardless of setting (Waibel & Ranjita, 2003).*
- Educate the client and family regarding helmet use during recreation and sports activities. *Each year 1.5 million people sustain traumatic brain injuries, which account for one third of all injury deaths (National Center for Injury Prevention and Control, 2002).*
- Encourage the use of proper car seats and safety belts. *The risk of fatal injury in motor vehicle accidents is decreased by 45% when a shoulder and lap safety belt is worn (Segui-Gomez, 2000). Every state requires that children ride buckled up and using a car safety seat or belt correctly can prevent injuries to children (American Academy of Pediatrics, 2002).*
- Teach how to plan safe prom and graduation parties. *Guests can have fun and live to tell about it (Mothers Against Drunk Driving, 2002).*

- Teach parents the importance of monitoring youths after school. *Firearm injuries increase after school and violent crimes by youths peak between 3 pm and 4 pm (Slovak, 2002).*
- Teach firearm safety. Encourage the family to keep firearms and ammunition in locked storage. **EB:** *Behavioral skills training programs are effective for teaching children to perform gun-safety skill during supervised role play, but the skills were not used when the children were assessed through real-life assessments. More research is needed to determine the most effective way to promote the use of the skills outside the training sessions (Himle et al, 2004).*
- ▲ Educate that the use of psychotropic medications may increase the risk of falls and that withdrawal of psychotropic medications should be considered. **EB:** *Withdrawal of psychotropic medication decreased risk of falls in the elderly (Gillespie et al, 2003).*
- For further information, refer to care plans for **Risk for Aspiration, Impaired Home maintenance, Risk for Injury, Risk for Poisoning,** and **Risk for Suffocation.**

## evolve WEBSITES FOR EDUCATION

See the EVOLVE website for World Wide Web resources for client education.

## REFERENCES

American Academy of Pediatrics: *Car safety seats: a guide for families,* 2002. Available at www.aap.org/advocacy/releases/car.html, accessed on June 23, 2003.

Beers M, Berkow R: *The Merck manual of geriatrics*, ed 3, Whitehouse Station, NJ, 2000, Merck.

Doorn C, Gruber-Baldini A, Zimmerman S et al: Dementia as a risk factor for falls and fall injuries among nursing home residents, *J Am Geriatr Soc* 51:1213-1218, 2003.

Gillespie LD, Gillespie WJ, Robertson MC et al: Interventions for preventing falls in elderly people *Cochrane Database Syst Rev* (4):CD000340, 2003.

Hammond M, Levine JM: Bedrails: choosing the best alternative, *Geriatr Nurs* 20(6):297, 1999.

Himle M, Miltenberger R, Gatheridge B et al: An evaluation of two procedures for training skills to prevent gun play in children, *Pediatrics* 113(1):70-77, 2004.

Jensen J, Nyberg L, Gustafson Y et al: Fall and injury prevention in residential care: effects in residents with higher and lower levels of cognition, *J Am Geriatr Soc* 51:627-635, 2003.

Jensen J, Lundin-Olsson L, Nyberg L et al: Fall and injury prevention in older people living in residential care facilities, *Ann Intern Med* 136(10):733, 2002.

Hsu S, Lee C, Wang S et al: Fall risk factors assessment tool: enhancing effectiveness in falls screening, *J Nurs Res* 12(3):169-178, 2004.

Movig K, Mathijssen M, Nagel P et al: Psychoactive substance use and the risk of motor vehicle accidents, *Accid Anal Prev* 36:631-636, 2004.

Mothers Against Drunk Driving: *Prom/graduation party guide,* 2002. Available at www.madd.org/madd_programs/0,1056,1494,00.html, accessed on January 11, 2003.

National Center for Injury Prevention and Control: *Traumatic brain injury,* 2002. Available at www.cdc.gov/ncipc/factsheets/tbi.htm, accessed on January 11, 2003.

National Center for Injury Prevention and Control: *Falls and hip fractures among older adults,* Available at www.cdc.gov/ncipc/factsheets/falls.htm, accessed on June 23, 2003.

Potter P, Perry A: *Basic nursing: essentials for practice,* St Louis, 2003, Mosby.

Segui-Gomez M: Evaluating worksite-based interventions that promote safety belt use, *Am J Prev Med* 18(4S):11, 2000.

Shenassa E, Stubbendick A, Brown M: Social disparities in housing and related pediatric injury: A multilevel study, *Am J Pub Health* 94(4):633-640, 2004.

Slovak K: Gun violence and children: factors related to exposure and trauma, *Health Soc Work* 27(2):104, 2002.

T

Snow CM, Shaw JM, Winters KM et al: Long-term exercise using weighted vests prevents hipbone loss in postmenopausal women, *J Gerontol* 55(9):M489, 2000.

Waibel R, Ranjita M: Injuries to preschool children and infection control practices in childcare programs, *J School Health* 73(4): 167-172, 2003.

# Readiness for enhanced Urinary elimination

*Mikel Gray*

## NANDA

### Definition

A pattern of urinary functions that is sufficient for meeting eliminatory needs and can be strengthened

### Defining Characteristics

Expresses willingness to enhance urinary elimination, urine is straw colored with no odor, specific gravity is within normal limits, amount of output is within normal limits for age and other factors, positions self for emptying of bladder, fluid intake is adequate for daily needs

## NOC

### Outcomes (Nursing Outcomes Classification)

#### Suggested NOC Outcomes

Urinary Continence, Urinary Elimination

**Example NOC Outcome with Indicators**

**Urinary Continence** as evidenced by the following indicators: Voids >150 mL each time/Empties bladder completely/Absence of postvoid residual or residual volume is <100–200 mL (Rate each indicator of **Urinary Continence:** 1 = never demonstrated, 2 = rarely demonstrated, 3 = sometimes demonstrated, 4 = often demonstrated, 5 = consistently demonstrated [see Section I].)

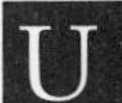

### Client Outcomes

#### Client Will (Specify Time Frame):

- Eliminate or reduce incontinent episodes
- Recognize sensory stimulus indicating readiness for urine elimination
- Respond to prompts for toileting

NIC

## Interventions (Nursing Interventions Classification)

### Suggested NIC Intervention

Urinary Elimination Management

**Example NIC Activities—Urinary Elimination Management**

Monitor urinary elimination—including frequency, consistency, odor, volume, and color—as appropriate; teach client signs and symptoms of urinary tract infection (UTI)

## Nursing Interventions and Rationales

- Assess the client for readiness for improving urine elimination patterns, focusing on need for physical assistance to access toilet, cognitive awareness of sensations indicating readiness for urine elimination and current continence status (bladder management strategy, frequency of incontinent episodes). *Definitions of urinary continence and incontinence applied to ambulatory adults must be modified for the frail, elder client who is homebound or who resides in a long-term care setting (Palmer et al, 1997).*
- Complete a bladder diary of diurnal and nocturnal urine elimination patterns and patterns of urinary leakage. *A bladder diary provides a more objective verification of urine elimination patterns than a history (Resnick et al, 1994).* **EBN:** *A bladder diary is an integral portion of the evaluation of urinary incontinence in the client who is homebound or residing in a long-term setting, and it provides a baseline against which outcomes of treatment can be evaluated (Pfister, 1999).*
- Begin a scheduled toileting program (usually every 2–3 hours) for the client who is normally continent (recognizes cues to toilet and expresses readiness to toilet) but requires physical assistance to access the toilet.
- Remove environmental barriers to toilet access.
- Provide a urinal or bedside toilet as indicated.
- Assist client to remove clothing, transfer to the toilet, cleanse the perineal skin, and redress as indicated.
- Ensure that toileting opportunities are offered both during daytime hours and during hours of sleep. *Certain clients who are homebound or reside in a long-term care facility have the potential for continence but experience urine loss because they lack adequate physical assistance needed to access the toilet, remove clothing, and redress after toileting is finished. The level of assistance varies significantly and depends on the client's mobility and dexterity, as well as the availability of bedside toileting aids (Palmer et al, 1997).*

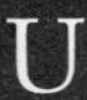

- For the client experiencing urinary incontinence who has mild cognitive deficits, begin a prompted voiding program or patterned urge response toileting program. Begin a prompted toileting program based on the results of bladder log over a period of 2–3 days, using a check and change system as indicated.
  - Approach the client and briefly explain that it is time to toilet.
  - Assist the client to the toilet, provide assistance removing clothing and urine-containment devices (pads, adult urine-containment briefs), and check for urinary leakage since the last scheduled toileting.

- ■ Praise the client when toileting occurs with prompting.
- ■ If the client does not toilet or has evidence of an incontinence episode, refrain from praise, gently inform the client of the urine loss, remove and replace the soiled containment device, and assist the client to redress and rejoin activities or return to bed.

**EBN:** *A meta-analysis of available research provides weak evidence that prompted voiding increases successful, self-initiated voiding episodes and diminishes incontinent episodes (Eustice et al, 2000).*

- • Institute regular use of incontinence-containment devices combined with routine perineal skin care for the client with severe cognitive impairment, significant functional impairment, or no reduction in urinary incontinence frequency or severity with a scheduled or prompted toileting program. (Refer to **Total urinary Incontinence.**) *Urine-containment products include a variety of absorptive pads, incontinent briefs, underpads for bedding, absorptive inserts that fit into specially designed undergarments, and condom catheters. Careful selection of an absorptive device and education concerning its use maximizes its effectiveness in controlling urine loss in a particular individual (Dunn et al, 2002).*

## evolve WEBSITES FOR EDUCATION

See the EVOLVE website for World Wide Web resources for client education.

## REFERENCES

Dunn S, Kowanko I, Paterson J et al: Systematic review of the effectiveness of urinary continence products, *J Wound Ostomy Continence Nurs* 29(3):129, 2002.

Eustice S, Roe B, Paterson J: Prompted voiding for the management of urinary incontinence in adults, *Cochrane Database Syst Rev* (2):CD002113, 2000.

Palmer MH et al: Urinary outcomes in older adults: research and clinical perspective, *Urol Nurs* 17(1):2, 1997.

Pfister SM: Bladder diaries and voiding patterns in older adults, *J Gerontol Nurs* 25(3):36, 1999.

Resnick NM, Beckett LA, Branch LG et al: Short term variability of self-report of incontinence in older persons, *J Am Geriatr Soc* 42:202, 1994.

# Impaired Urinary elimination

evolve

*Mikel Gray*

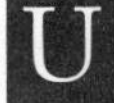

**NANDA**

### Definition

Disturbance in urine elimination

NOTE: This broad diagnosis may be used to describe many dysfunctional voiding conditions. Refer to **Functional urinary Incontinence**, **Reflex urinary Incontinence**, **Stress urinary Incontinence**, **Total urinary Incontinence**, **Urge urinary Incontinence**, and **Urinary retention** for information on these more specific diagnoses.

## Defining Characteristics

The term *lower urinary tract symptoms* (LUTS) is now used to describe the variety of complaints associated with disorders of bladder filling/storage or altered patterns of urine elimination (Jackson, 1999). Bothersome bladder filling/storage symptoms include diurnal frequency (voiding more than every 2 hours), infrequent urination (voiding less then every 6 hours), and nocturia (arising from sleep more than twice to urinate). Our understanding of the physiologic desire is incomplete, but the term *urgency* has been defined as "a sudden and strong desire to urinate that is not easily deferred" (Abrams et al, 2002). Lower urinary tract pain may present as dysuria (pain associated with micturition), burning, pressure, or cramping discomfort during bladder filling and storage. Voiding symptoms may include reduced force of the urinary stream, intermittency, hesitancy, and the need to strain to evacuate the bladder. Other voiding symptoms are postvoid dribbling, feelings of incomplete bladder emptying, or the total inability to urinate (acute urinary retention).

Urinary incontinence is the uncontrolled loss of urine of sufficient magnitude to constitute a problem for the client, family, or caregivers (Abrams et al, 2002). Stress urinary incontinence is the loss of urine with physical exertion. Urge urinary incontinence is the loss of urine associated with overactive detrusor contractions and a precipitous desire to urinate. It is part of a larger symptom syndrome called *overactive bladder*. The overactive bladder is characterized by bothersome urgency and typically associated with frequent daytime voiding and nocturia. Approximately 37% of patients with overactive bladder dysfunction experience urge urinary incontinence (Stewart et al, 2003).

Reflex urinary incontinence is urine loss associated with neurogenic detrusor overactivity, diminished or absent sensations of bladder filling, and dyssynergia between the detrusor and striated urethral sphincter muscles. Functional urinary incontinence is urine loss associated with deficits of mobility, dexterity, cognition, or environmental barriers to timely toileting. Urine loss from an extraurethral source can be defined as total incontinence, and urinary retention is the condition where the client is unable to completely evacuate urine from the bladder despite micturition. Chronic urinary retention is defined as the inability to completely evacuate urine from the bladder after voiding, and acute urinary retention is the inability to urinate (Gray, 2000).

## Related Factors (r/t)

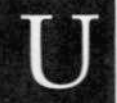


Bothersome LUTS (urological disorders, neurological lesions, gynecological conditions, dysfunction of bowel elimination); incontinence (refer to specific diagnosis); urinary retention (refer to specific diagnosis); acute urinary retention (refer to **Urinary retention**)

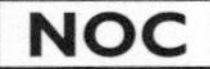


## Outcomes (Nursing Outcomes Classification)

### Suggested NOC Outcomes

Urinary Continence; Urinary Elimination; Knowledge: Medication

**Example NOC Outcome with Indicators**

**Urinary Continence** as evidenced by the following indicators: Has no urine loss with physical activity or exertion, coughing, sneezing, or other maneuvers that precipitously raise abdominal pressure/Voids in appropriate receptacle/Is able to move to toilet after strong desire to urinate perceived/Keeps underclothing dry during day/Keeps underclothing or bedding dry during night (Rate each indicator of **Urinary Continence:** 1 = never demonstrated, 2 = rarely demonstrated, 3 = sometimes demonstrated, 4 = often demonstrated, 5 = consistently demonstrated [see Section I].)

## Client Outcomes

### Client Will (Specify Time Frame):

- Demonstrate diurnal frequency no more than every 2 hours
- Demonstrate nocturia two times or less per night
- Be able to postpone voiding until toileting facility is accessed and clothing is removed
- Be able to perceive and recognize cues for toileting, move to toilet or use urinal or portable toileting apparatus, and remove clothing as necessary for toileting
- Demonstrate postvoiding residual volumes less than 150 mL–200 mL or 25% of total bladder capacity
- State absence of pain or excessive urgency during bladder storage or during urination

NIC

## Interventions (Nursing Interventions Classification)

### Suggested NIC Intervention

Urinary Elimination Management

**Example NIC Activities—Urinary Elimination Management**

Monitor urinary elimination—including frequency, consistency, odor, volume, and color—as appropriate; teach client signs and symptoms of UTI

## Nursing Interventions and Rationales

- Routinely screen all adult women and aging men for urinary incontinence or LUTS including bothersome urgency. *Urinary incontinence and overactive bladder dysfunction are prevalent problems, particularly among women and aging males in the sixth decade of life or older (Gray, 2003). Routine screening is justified because urinary incontinence is prevalent, negatively affects physical health and psychosocial function, and is amenable to treatment (Gray, 2003).*
- Assess bladder function using the following techniques:
  - Take a focused history including duration of bothersome LUTS, characteristics of symptoms, patterns of diurnal and nocturnal urination, frequency and volume of

U

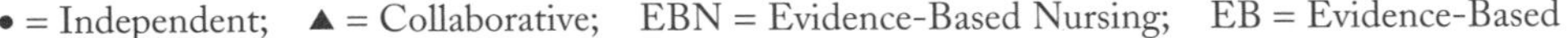

urine loss, alleviating and aggravating factors, and exploration of possible causative factors.
- ■ Perform a focused physical assessment of perineal skin integrity, evaluation of the vaginal vault, evaluation of urethral hypermobility, and neurological evaluation including bulbocavernosus reflex and perineal sensations.
- ■ Review results of urinalysis for the presence of urinary infection, polyuria, hematuria, proteinuria, and other abnormalities, or obtain urine for analysis.

*A history, focused physical assessment, and urinalysis are the essential components of evaluation for any client with dysfunctional voiding complaints (Shull et al, 2002; Urinary Incontinence Guideline Panel, 1996).*

- • Complete a more detailed assessment on selected clients including a bladder log and functional/cognitive assessment. (Refer to **Functional urinary Incontinence, Reflex urinary Incontinence**, **Stress urinary Incontinence**, **Total urinary Incontinence**, and **Urge urinary Incontinence**.)
- • Assess the client for urinary retention. (Refer to **Urinary retention**.)
- • Teach the client general guidelines for bladder health:
  - ■ Clients should avoid dehydration and its irritative effects on the bladder; fluid consumption for the ambulatory, normally active adult should be approximately 30 mL/kg of body weight (0.5 oz per pound per day).
  - ■ Clients with storage LUTS, overactive bladder dysfunction, or urinary incontinence should reduce or cease caffeine intake (Gray, 2001).
  - ■ Clients with lower urinary tract pain or interstitial cystitis should be encouraged to eliminate multiple potential bladder irritants including caffeine, alcohol, aspartame, carbonated beverages, alcohol, citrus juices, chocolate, vinegar, and highly spiced foods such as those flavored with curries or peppers (Bade, Peeters, & Mensink, 1997; Interstitial Cystitis Association, 1999). These foods should be reintroduced singly to the diet to determine their effect (if any) on bothersome LUTS.
  - ■ All clients should be counseled about measures to alleviate or prevent constipation including adequate consumption of dietary fluids, dietary fiber, exercise, and regular bowel elimination patterns.
  - ■ All clients should be strongly advised to stop smoking.

*Dehydration increases irritating voiding symptoms and may enhance the risk of urinary infection. Constipation predisposes the individual to urinary retention, and it increases the risk of urinary infection. Smoking may increase the severity and risk of stress incontinence, and it is clearly linked with an increased risk for bladder cancer (Tampakoudis et al, 1995).*
**EBN:** *Multiple randomized clinical trials and noncontrolled clinical trials demonstrate that client education, alteration of fluid volume intake, reduction of caffeine consumption, and bladder training and pelvic floor muscle training administered by generic and advanced practice nurses reduce the frequency of urinary incontinence, pad use, and perceived severity of bothersome LUTS (Borrie et al, 2002; Dougherty et al, 2002; Dowd, Kolcaba, & Steiner, 2000; Sampselle et al, 2000).*

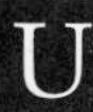


▲ Consult the physician for culture and sensitivity testing and antibiotic treatment in the individual with evidence of a urinary infection. *UTI is a transient, reversible condition that is associated with urge urinary incontinence and overactive bladder syndrome (Brown*

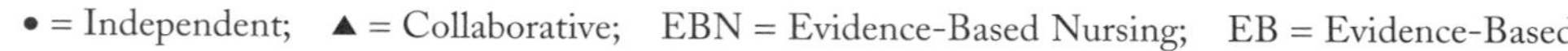

*et al, 2001). Although the precise nature of this relationship remains unclear, it is known that eradication of UTI will alleviate or reverse LUTS including suprapubic pressure and discomfort, bothersome urgency, daytime voiding frequency, and dysuria (Malterud & Baerheim, 1999).*

▲ Refer the individual with chronic lower urinary tract pain to a urologist or specialist in the management of pelvic pain. *Bladder pain and storage symptoms, in the absence of an acute urinary infection, may indicate the presence of interstitial cystitis, a chronic condition requiring ongoing treatment (Gray, Hufstuttler, & Albo, 2002).*

▲ Teach the client to recognize symptoms of UTI (dysuria that crescendos as the bladder nears complete evacuation; urgency to urinate followed by micturition of only a few drops; suprapubic aching discomfort; malaise; voiding frequency; sudden exacerbation of urinary incontinence with or without fever, chills, and flank pain). *Qualitative research focusing on women with a history of recurring UTIs reveals a variety of typical and unexpected symptoms (Malterud & Baerheim, 1999).*

▲ Teach the client to recognize hematuria and to seek help promptly if hematuria occurs. *Hematuria in the presence of irritative voiding symptoms typically indicates urinary infection; however, gross or microscopic, in the absence of an existing UTI it raises the risk for urinary system tumor and requires further investigation (Mazhari & Kimmel, 2002).*

▲ Assist the individual with urinary leakage to select a product that adequately contains urine, avoids soiling clothing, is not apparent when worn under clothing, and protects the underlying skin. (Refer to **Total urinary Incontinence.**)

▲ Teach perineal care including judicious use of soaps and use of vaginal douches only under special circumstances. (Refer to **Total urinary Incontinence.**)

## Geriatric

- Provide an environment that encourages toileting for the elderly client cared for in the home or in acute care, long-term care, or critical care units. *Insufficient toileting opportunities, medications, acute or chronic illnesses, and environmental factors may contribute to functional incontinence or exacerbate other forms of urinary leakage in the elderly client (Gray & Burns, 1996; Jirovec & Wells, 1990; Morris, Browne, & Saltmarche, 1992).*
- Perform urinalysis in all elderly persons who experience a sudden change in urine elimination patterns, lower abdominal discomfort, acute confusion, or a fever of unclear origin. *Elderly persons, particularly adults aged 80 years and older, often experience atypical symptoms with a UTI or pyelonephritis (Bostwick, 2000; Suchinski et al, 1999).*
- Encourage elderly women to drink at least 10 oz of cranberry juice daily, regularly consume one to two servings of fresh blueberries, or supplement the diet with cranberry concentrate capsules (usually taken in 500 mg doses with each meal). **EBN:** *Systematic literature review reveals that consumption of 400 mg of cranberry tablets, 8–10 oz of cranberry juice or an equivocal portion of foods containing whole cranberries or blueberries exerts a bacteriostatic effect on Escherichia coli, the most common pathogen associated with urinary infection among community-dwelling adult women. Mixed evidence tends to support a reduction in UTI risk among community-dwelling women, although no beneficial*

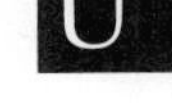

*effect has been found in patients with neurogenic bladder dysfunction who are managed by intermittent or indwelling catheters (Gray, 2002).*

## Client/Family Teaching

- Provide all clients with the basic principles for optimal bladder function.
- Teach the community and health care providers that urinary incontinence is not a normal part of aging and that incontinence can be corrected or managed with proper evaluation and care.
- Provide information to health care providers and the community about the signs, symptoms, and management of UTIs and interstitial cystitis.
- Teach all persons the signs and symptoms of UTI and its management.
- Teach all persons to recognize hematuria and to promptly seek care if this symptom occurs.

## evolve WEBSITES FOR EDUCATION

See the EVOLVE website for World Wide Web resources for client education.

## REFERENCES


Abrams P, Cardozo L, Fall M et al: The standardization of terminology of lower urinary tract function: report from the Standardization Subcommittee of the International Continence Society, *Am J Obste Gynecol* 187(1):116-126, 2002.

Bade JJ, Peeters JM, Mensink HJ: Is the diet of patients with interstitial cystitis related to their disease? *Eur Urol* 32:179, 1997.

Borrie MJ, Bawden M, Speechley M et al: Interventions led by nurse continence advisers in the management of urinary incontinence: a randomized controlled trial, *Can Med Assoc J* 166(10):1267, 2002.

Bostwick JM: The many faces of confusion. Timing and collateral history often hold the key to diagnosis, *Postgrad Med* 108(6):60, 2000.

Brown JS et al: Heart and Estrogen/Progestin Replacement Study Research Group. Urinary tract infections in postmenopausal women: effect of hormone therapy and risk factors, *Obstet Gynecol* 98(6):1045, 2001.

Dougherty MC, Dwyer JW, Pendergast JF et al: A randomized trial of behavioral management for continence with older rural women, *Res Nurs Health* 25:3, 2002.

Dowd T, Kolcaba K, Steiner R: Using cognitive strategies to enhance bladder control and comfort, *Holist Nurs Pract* 14(2):91, 2000.

Gray M: Urinary retention: management in the acute care setting. I. *Am J Nurs* 100:40, 2000.

Gray M: Caffeine and urinary incontinence, *J Wound Ostomy Continence Nurs* 28:66, 2001.

Gray M: Are cranberry juice or cranberry products effective in the prevention or management of urinary tract infection? *J Wound Ostomy Continence Nurs* 29:122, 2002.

Gray M: The importance of screening, assessing and managing urinary incontinence in primary care, *J Am Acad Nurse Practit* 15(3):102, 2003.

Gray ML, Burns SB: Continence management, *Crit Care Clin North Am* 8:29, 1996.

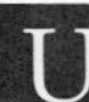

Gray M, Hufstuttler S, Albo M: Interstitial cystitis: a guide to recognition, evaluation and management for the nurse practitioner, *J Wound Ostomy Continence Nurs* 29:93, 2002.

Hunskaar S et al: Epidemiology and natural history of urinary incontinence. In Abrams P, Khoury S, Wein A, editors: *Incontinence,* Plymouth, UK, 1999, Plymbridge, Health Publications.

Interstitial Cystitis Association: *Interstitial cystitis and diet,* Rockville, Md, 1999, The Association.

Jackson S: Lower urinary tract symptoms and nocturia in men and women: prevalence, etiology and diagnosis, *Br J Urol Int* 84(suppl 1):5, 1999.

Jirovec MM, Wells TJ: Urinary incontinence in nursing home residents with dementia: the mobility-cognition paradigm, *Appl Nurs Res* 3:11, 1990.

Malterud K, Baerheim A: Peeing barbed wire. Symptom experiences in women with lower urinary tract infection, *Scand J Prim Health Care* 17(1):49, 1999.

Mazhari R, Kimmel PL: Hematuria: an algorithmic approach to finding the cause, *Cleve Clin J Med* 69(11): 870, 2002.
Morris A, Browne G, Saltmarche A: Urinary incontinence among cognitively impaired elderly veterans, *J Gerontol Nurs* 18:33, 1992.
Parazzini F, Colli E, Origgi G et al: Risk factors for urinary incontinence in women, *Eur Urol* 37(6):637, 2000.
Sampselle CM, Wyman JF, Thomas KK et al: Continence for women: evaluation of AWHONN's third research utilization project. Association of Women's Health Obstetric and Neonatal Nurses, *J Obstet Gynecol Neonatal Nurs* 29(1):9, 2000.
Shull BL et al: Physical examination. In Abrams P, Khoury S, Wein AJ, editors: *Incontinence: 2nd International Consultation on Incontinence,* ed 2, Plymouth, UK, 2002, Plymbridge, Health Publications.
Suchinski GA, Piano MR, Rosenberg N et al: Treating urinary tract infections in the elderly, *Dimens Crit Care Nurs* 18(1):21, 1999.
Stewart WF, Van Rooyen JB, Cundiff GW et al: Prevalence and burden of overactive bladder in the United States, *World J Urol* 20(6):327-336, 2003.
Tampakoudis P, Tantanassis T, Grimbizis G et al: Cigarette smoking and urinary incontinence in women—a new calculative method of estimating the exposure to smoke, *Eur J Obstet Gynecol Reprod Biol* 63(1):27, 1995.
Urinary Incontinence Guideline Panel: Urinary incontinence in adults: clinical practice guideline, ed 2, Rockville, Md, 1996, Agency for Health Care Policy and Research.

# Urinary retention

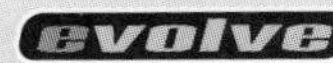

*Mikel Gray*

**NANDA**

## Definition

Incomplete emptying of the bladder

## Defining Characteristics

Measured urinary residual greater than 150–200 mL or 25% of total bladder capacity; obstructive LUTS (poor force of stream, intermittency of stream, hesitancy of urination, postvoiding dribbling, feelings of incomplete bladder emptying); often accompanied by storage LUTS (urgency, day and nighttime voiding frequency); occasionally accompanied by overflow incontinence (dribbling urine loss caused when intravesical pressure overwhelms the sphincter mechanism)

## Related Factors (r/t)

Bladder outlet obstruction (benign prostatic hyperplasia [BPH], prostate cancer, prostatitis, acute prostatic congestion and inflammation after implantation of irradiated seeds, urethral stricture, bladder neck dyssynergia, bladder neck contracture, detrusor striated sphincter dyssynergia, pseudodyssynergia or high tome pelvic floor muscle dysfunction, obstructing cystocele or urethral distortion, urethral tumor, urethral polyp, posterior urethral valves, postoperative complication)

Deficient detrusor contraction strength (sacral level spinal lesions, cauda equina syndrome, peripheral polyneuropathies, herpes zoster or simplex affecting sacral nerve roots, injury or extensive surgery causing denervation of pelvic plexus, medication side effect, complication of illicit drug use, impaction of stool)

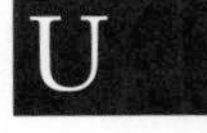

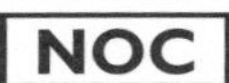

## Outcomes (Nursing Outcomes Classification)

### Suggested NOC Outcomes

Urinary Continence, Urinary Elimination

**Example NOC Outcome with Indicators**

**Urinary Continence** as evidenced by the following indicators: Absence of urinary leakage between catheterizations or containment of micturition by condom catheter and drainage bag/Absence of UTI (negative leukocytes and bacterial growth negative or >100,000 CFU/mL)/Underclothing dry during day/Underclothing or bedding dry during night (Rate each indicator of **Urinary Continence:** 1 = never demonstrated, 2 = rarely demonstrated, 3 = sometimes demonstrated, 4 = often demonstrated, 5 = consistently demonstrated [see Section I].)

CFU, Colony-forming units; UTI, urinary tract infection.

## Client Outcomes

### Client Will (Specify Time Frame):

- Consistent ability to urinate when desire to void is perceived or via timed schedule; measured urinary residual volume is <150–200 mL or 25% of total bladder capacity (voided volume plus urinary residual volume)
- Experience correction or relief from obstructive symptoms
- Experience correction or alleviation of irritative symptoms
- Be free of upper urinary tract distress (renal function remains sufficient; febrile urinary infections are absent)

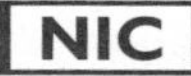

## Interventions (Nursing Interventions Classification)

### Suggested NIC Interventions

Urinary Catheterization, Urinary Retention Care

**Example NIC Activities—Urinary Retention Care**

Perform a comprehensive urinary assessment focusing on incontinence (e.g., urinary output, urinary voiding pattern, cognitive function, preexistent urinary problems); use the power of suggestion by running water or flushing the toilet

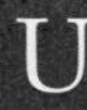

## Nursing Interventions and Rationales

- Obtain a focused urinary history emphasizing the character and duration of lower urinary symptoms. Query the client about episodes of acute urinary retention (complete inability to void) or chronic retention (documented elevated postvoid residual volumes). *Although the presence of obstructive or irritative voiding symptoms is not diag-*

*nostic of urinary retention (Roehrborn et al, 2002), a focused nursing history can provide clues to the likely cause of retention and its management (Gray, 2000a).*

- Question the client concerning specific risk factors for urinary retention including:
  - Disorders affecting the sacral spinal cord such as spinal cord injuries of vertebral levels T12–L2, disk problems, cauda equina syndrome, tabes dorsalis
  - Acute neurological injury causing sudden loss of mobility such as spinal shock or ischemic stroke
  - Metabolic disorders such as diabetes mellitus, chronic alcoholism, and related conditions associated with polyuria and peripheral polyneuropathies
  - Herpetic infection involving the sacral skin and underlying spinal dermatomes
  - Heavy-metal poisoning (lead, mercury) causing peripheral polyneuropathies
  - Advanced stage human immunodeficiency virus (HIV)
  - Medications including antispasmodics/parasympatholytics, alpha-adrenergic agonists, antidepressants, sedatives, narcotics, psychotropic medications, illicit drugs
  - Recent surgery requiring general or spinal anesthesia
  - Bowel elimination patterns, history of fecal impaction, encopresis
  - Current or recent surgical procedures

  *Urinary retention is related to multiple factors affecting either detrusor contraction strength or urethral obstruction (Acheson & Mudd, 2004; Anders & Goebel, 1998; Darabi et al, 2004; Ginsberg et al, 1998; Gray, 2000a; Kong et al, 2000; Kruse, Bray, & deGroat, 1995; Pertek & Haberer, 1995).* **EBN:** *Multiple factors in the surgical patient are associated with an increased risk of postoperative urinary retention including preoperative voiding difficulty, advanced age, total amount of fluid replacement during a 24-hour postoperative period, type of anesthesia, pain management medications, and route and length of medication administration (Wynd et al, 1996).*

▲ Perform a focused physical assessment or review results of a recent physical including perineal skin integrity; inspection, percussion, and palpation of the lower abdomen for obvious bladder distention; a neurological examination including perineal skin sensation and the bulbocavernosus reflex; and vaginal vault examination in women and digital rectal examination in men. *The physical assessment provides clues to the likely cause of urinary retention and its management.*

▲ Determine the urinary residual volume by catheterizing the client immediately after urination or by obtaining a bladder ultrasound after micturition. *Although catheterization provides the most accurate method to determine urinary residual volume, it is invasive, produces discomfort, and carries a risk of infection (Gray, 2000b).* **EBN:** *Two studies of 30 and 176 patients, respectively, treated in acute care and geriatric rehabilitation units found that postvoid bladder ultrasound, performed by registered nurses provided reasonable estimates of postvoid residual bladder volumes (Borrie et al, 2001; O'Farrell et al, 2001). In addition, one study (O'Farrell et al, 2001) found that the results of the ultrasonic measurement changed nursing practice in 51% of instances, reducing unneeded catheterizations by 32%.*

- Complete a bladder log including patterns of urine elimination, urine loss (if present), nocturia, and volume and type of fluids consumed for a period of 3–7 days. *The bladder log provides an objective verification of urine elimination patterns and allows comparison*

U

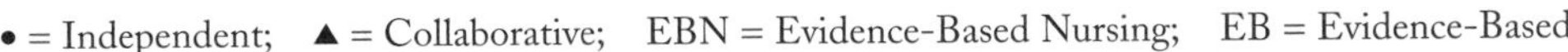

*of fluids consumed vs. urinary output during a 24-hour period (Nygaard & Holcomb, 2000).*

- ▲ Consult with the physician concerning eliminating or altering medications suspected of producing or exacerbating urinary retention. *Medication side effects may cause or greatly exacerbate urinary retention in susceptible individuals (Gray, 2000a,b).*
- • Teach the client with mild to moderate obstructive symptoms to double void by urinating, resting in the bathroom for 3–5 minutes, and then trying again to urinate. *Double voiding promotes more efficient bladder evacuation by allowing the detrusor to contract initially and then rest and contract again (Gray, 2000b).*
- • Teach the client with urinary retention and infrequent voiding to urinate by the clock. *Timed or scheduled voiding may reduce urinary retention by preventing bladder overdistention (Gray, 2000b).*
- • Advise the male client with urinary retention related to BPH to avoid risk factors associated with acute urinary retention as follows:
  - ■ Avoid over-the-counter cold remedies containing a decongestant (alpha-adrenergic agonist).
  - ■ Avoid taking over-the-counter dietary medications (frequently contain alpha-adrenergic agonists).
  - ■ Discuss voiding problems with a health care provider before beginning new prescription medications.
  - ■ After prolonged exposure to cool weather, warm the body before attempting to urinate.
  - ■ Avoid overfilling the bladder by regular urination patterns and refrain from excessive intake of alcohol.

  *These modifiable factors predispose the client to acute urinary retention by overdistending the bladder and compromising detrusor contraction strength or by increasing outlet resistance (Gray, 2000b). One study of 8418 elder men with prostatic enlargement found that medications with antimuscarinic or alpha-adrenergic agonistic effects increased the risk for acute urinary retention (Meigs et al, 1999).*
- ▲ Teach the elderly male client with BPH to self-administer a 5 alpha-reductase inhibitor, such as finasteride or *dutasteride,* or an alpha-adrenergic–blocking agent, such as *tamsulosin, alfuzosin,* doxazosin, or terazosin, as directed. Provide careful instruction concerning the dose, administration schedule, and side effects of these drugs, including possible adverse side effects (postural hypotension) when multiple doses are inadvertently missed. *Finasteride is a 5-alpha-reductase inhibitor that reduces the risk of acute urinary retention when taken by men with BPH over a prolonged period (McConnell et al, 1998). The magnitude of obstruction associated with BPH is also reduced by routine administration of alpha-adrenergic–blocking agents including tamsulosin, terazosin, or doxazosin. However, these agents must be taken regularly to reduce the risk of side effects including postural hypotension (Narayan & Tewari, 1998; Lepor et al, 1997, 1998). Some agents must be titrated, and a risk for postural hypotension increases if doses are missed; other agents do not require titration and are associated with a reduced risk of postural hypotension (Schulman, 2003).*

- ▲ Teach the client who is unable to void specific strategies to manage this potential medical emergency as follows:
  - ■ Attempt urination in complete privacy.
  - ■ Place the feet solidly on the floor.
  - ■ If unable to void using these strategies, take a warm sitz bath or shower and void (if possible) while still in the tub or shower.
  - ■ Drink a warm cup of coffee or tea to stimulate the bladder, which may promote voiding.
  - ■ If unable to void within 6 hours or if bladder distention is producing significant pain, seek urgent or emergency care.

  *Attempting urination in complete privacy and placing the feet solidly on the floor help relax the pelvic muscles and may encourage voiding. Warm water also stimulates the bladder and may produce voiding; the cooling experienced by leaving the tub or shower may again inhibit the bladder (Gray, 2000b).*
- ▲ Remove the indwelling urethral catheter at midnight in the hospitalized client to reduce the risk of acute urinary retention. **EBN:** *A systematic literature review demonstrated that removal of indwelling catheters at midnight offers several advantages to "morning removal," including a larger initial voided volume and earlier hospital discharge with no increased risk for readmission compared with those undergoing morning removal (Griffiths et al, 2004).*
- ▲ Consult the physician about bladder stimulation in the client with urinary retention caused by deficient detrusor contraction strength. **EBN:** *High-frequency transvaginal electrical stimulation of the bladder neck has been shown to be beneficial in a small case series involving women with chronic urinary retention owing to deficient detrusor contraction strength (Bernier & Davila, 2000).*
- ▲ Teach the client with significant urinary retention to perform self-intermittent catheterization as directed. **EBN:** *Intermittent catheterization allows regular, complete bladder evacuation without serious complications (Horsley, Crane, & Reynolds, 1982).*
- • Advise clients who undergo intermittent catheterization that bacteria are likely to colonize the urine but that this condition does not indicate a clinically significant urinary tract infection. *Bacteriuria frequently occurs in the client undergoing intermittent catheterization; only symptoms producing infections warrant treatment (Wyndaele, 2002).*
- • Insert an indwelling catheter for the individual with urinary retention who is not a suitable candidate for intermittent catheterization. *An indwelling catheter provides continuous drainage of urine; however, the risks of serious urinary complications with prolonged use are significant (Anson & Gray, 1993; Weld et al, 2000).*
- • Advise clients with indwelling catheters that bacteria in the urine is an almost universal finding after the catheter has remained in place for a period of 30 days or longer and that only symptomatic infections warrant treatment. *The long-term indwelling catheter is inevitably associated with bacterial colonization. Most bacteriuria does not produce significant infection, and attempts to eradicate bacteriuria often produce subsequent morbidity because resistant bacteria are encouraged to reproduce while more easily managed strains are eradicated (Gray, 2004).*

- Use the following strategies to reduce the risk for catheter associated UTI whenever feasible:
  - Insert a silver impregnated catheter for short-term indwelling catheterization (<30 days).
  - Maintain a closed drainage system whenever feasible.
  - Change the catheter every 4-6 weeks whenever possible, more frequent catheter changes should be reserved for patients who experience catheter encrustation and blockage.
  - Place patients managed in an acute or long-term care facility with a catheter associated UTI in a separate room from others managed by an indwelling catheter to reduce the risk of spreading the offending pathogen.
  - Educate staff about the risks of catheter associated UTI and specific strategies to reduce this risk.

  **EBN:** *A systematic review of the literature found that these strategies are supported by sufficient evidence to recommend routine use. Strategies that lack sufficient evidence to support routine use include (1) aseptic technique when replacing a long-term indwelling catheter, (2) routine meatal care, (3) application of antimicrobial ointments or creams to the urethral meatus, (4) adding hydrogen peroxide or silver sulfadiazine or slow releasing silver ions to the catheter drainage bag, (5) frequent drainage bag changes, or (6) one way catheter valves (Gray, 2004).*

## Geriatric

- Aggressively assess elderly clients, particularly those with dribbling urinary incontinence, UTIs, and related condition for urinary retention. *Elderly women (and men) may experience urinary retention of 1500 mL or more with few or no apparent symptoms; a urinary residual volume and related assessments are necessary to determine the presence of retention in this population (Williams, Wallhagen, & Dowling, 1993).*
- Assess elderly clients for impaction when urinary retention is documented or suspected. *Fecal impaction and urinary retention frequently coexist in elderly clients and, unless reversed, may lead to acute delirium, UTI, or renal insufficiency (Waale, Bruijns, & Dautzenberg, 2001).*
- Assess elderly male clients for retention related to BPH or prostate cancer. *Prostate enlargement in elderly men increases the risk of acute and chronic urinary retention (Loh & Chin, 2002; McNeill & Hargreave, 2000).*

## Home Care

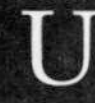


- The interventions listed previously may be adapted for home care use.
- Encourage the client to report any inability to void. *Pathophysiological factors of urinary retention require follow-up.*

▲ Maintain an up-to-date medication list; evaluate side effect profiles for risk of urinary retention. *New medications or changes in dose may cause urinary retention.*

▲ Refer the client for physician evaluation if urinary retention. *Identification of cause is important. Left untreated, urinary retention may lead to UTI or kidney failure.*

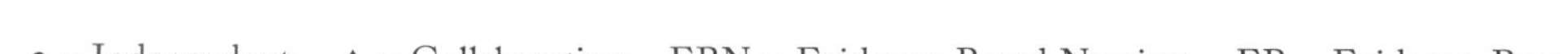

## Client/Family Teaching

- Teach techniques for intermittent catheterization including use of clean rather than sterile technique, washing using soap and water or a microwave technique, and reuse of the catheter.
- Teach the client with an indwelling catheter to assess the tube for patency, maintain the drainage system below the level of the symphysis pubis, and routinely cleanse the bedside bag.
- Teach the client with an indwelling catheter or undergoing intermittent catheterization the symptoms of a significant urinary infection including hematuria, acute-onset incontinence, dysuria, flank pain, or fever.

## evolve WEBSITES FOR EDUCATION

See the EVOLVE website for World Wide Web resources for client education.

## REFERENCES


Acheson J, Mudd D: Acute urinary retention attributable to sacral herpes zoster, *Emerg Med J* 21(6):752-753, 2004.

Anders HJ, Goebel FD: Cytomegalovirus polyradiculopathy in patients with AIDS, *Clin Infect Dis* 27:345, 1998.

Anson C, Gray ML: Secondary complications after spinal cord injury, *Urol Nurs* 13:107, 1993.

Bernier F, Davila GW: The treatment of nonobstructive urinary retention with high-frequency transvaginal electrical stimulation, *Urol Nurs* 20(4):261-264, 2000.

Borrie MJ, Campbell K, Arcese ZA et al: Urinary retention in patients in a geriatric rehabilitation unit: prevalence, risk factors, and validity of bladder scan evaluation, *Rehab Nurs* 26(5):187-191, 2001.

Darabi K, Segal AM, Torres G: Herpes zoster infection: a rare cause of urinary retention, *Can J Urol* 11(4):2314, 2004.

Ginsberg PC, Harkaway RC, Elisco AJ III et al: Rare presentation of acute urinary retention secondary to herpes zoster, *J Am Osteopath Assoc* 98(9):508, 1998.

Gray M: What nursing interventions reduce the risk of symptomatic urinary tract infection in the patient with an indwelling catheter? *J Wound Ostomy Continence Nurs* 31(1):3-13, 2004.

Gray M: Urinary retention: management in the acute care setting. I. *Am J Nurs* 100(7):40, 2000a.

Gray M: Urinary retention: management in the acute care setting. II. *Am J Nurs* 100(8):36, 2000b.

Griffiths RD, Fernandez RS, Murie P: Removal of short-term indwelling urethral catheters: the evidence, *J Wound, Ostomy Continence Nurs* 31(5):299-308, 2004.

Horsley JA, Crane J, Reynolds MA: *Clean intermittent catheterization: conduct and utilization of research in nursing project,* New York, 1982, Grune & Stratton.

Kong K, Young S: Incidence and outcome of poststroke urinary retention: a prospective study, *Arch Phys Med Rehabil* 81(11): 1464-1467, 2000.

Kruse MN, Bray LA, deGroat WC: Influence of spinal cord injury in the morphology of bladder afferent and efferent neurons, *J Autonom Nerv Sys* 54:215, 1995.

Lepor H, Kaplan SA, Klimberg I et al: Doxazosin for benign prostatic hyperplasia: long-term efficacy and safety in hypertensive and normotensive patients, *J Urol* 157:525, 1997.

Lepor H, Williford WO, Barry MJ et al: The impact of medical therapy due to symptoms, quality of life and global outcome, and factors predicting response, *J Urol* 160:1358, 1998.

Loh SY, Chin CM: A demographic profile of patients undergoing transurethral resection of the prostate for benign prostate hyperplasia and presenting in acute urinary retention, *Br J Urol Int* 89(6):531, 2002.

McConnell JD, Bruskewitz R, Walsh P et al: The effect of finasteride on the risk of acute urinary retention and the need for surgical treatment among men with benign prostatic hyperplasia. Finasteride Long-Term Efficacy and Safety Study Group, *N Engl J Med* 338(9):557, 1998.


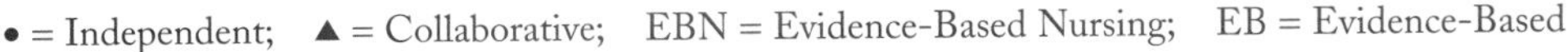

McDonald C, Thompson J: A comparison of midnight versus early morning removal of urinary catheters following transurethral resection of the prostate, *J Wound Ostomy Continence Nurs* 26:94, 1999.
McNeill SA, Hargreave TB: Efficacy of PSA in the detection of carcinoma of the prostate in patients presenting with acute urinary retention, *J R Coll Surg Edinb* 45(4):227, 2000.
Meigs JB, Barry MJ, Giovannucci E et al: Incidence rates and risk factors for acute urinary retention: the health professionals follow-up study, *J Urol* 162(2):376-382, 1999.
Moore KN, Rayome RG: Problem solving and troubleshooting: the indwelling catheter, *J Wound Ostomy Continence Nurs* 22:242, 1995.
Narayan P, Tewari A: A second phase III multicenter placebo study of 2 dosages of modified release tamsulosin in patients with symptoms of benign prostatic hyperplasia. United States 93-01 study group, *J Urol* 160:1701, 1998.
Nygaard I, Holcomb R: Reproducibility of the seven day voiding diary in women with stress urinary incontinence, *Int Urogynecol J Pelvic Floor Dysfunct* 11:15, 2000.
O'Farrell B, Vandervoort MK, Bisnaire D et al: Evaluation of portable bladder ultrasound: accuracy and effect on nursing practice in an acute neuroscience unit, *J Neurosci Nurs* 33(6):301, 2001.
Pertek JP, Haberer JP: Effects of anesthesia on postoperative micturition and urinary retention, *Ann Fr Anesth Reanim* 14(4):340, 1995.
Roehrborn CG et al: Storage (irritative) and voiding (obstructive) symptoms as predictors of benign prostatic hyperplasia progression and related outcomes, *Eur Urol* 42(1):1, 2002.
Schulman CC: Lower urinary tract symptoms/benign prostatic hyperplasia: minimizing morbidity caused by treatment, *Urology* 62(3 Suppl 1):24-33, 2003.
Waale WH, Bruijns E, Dautzenberg PJ: Delirium due to urinary retention: confusing for both the patient and the doctor, *Tijdschr Gerontol Geriatr* 32(3):100, 2001.
Weld KJ, Wall BM, Mangold TA et al: Influences on renal function in chronic spinal cord injured patients, *J Urol* 164(5):1490, 2000.
Williams MP, Wallhagen M, Dowling G: Urinary retention in elderly hospitalized women, *J Gerontol Nurs* 19:7, 1993.
Wynd CA, Wallace M, Smith KM et al: Factors influencing postoperative urinary retention following orthopaedic surgical procedures, *Orthop Nurs* 15(1):43, 1996.
Wyndaele JJ: Complications of intermittent catheterization: their prevention and treatment, *Spinal Cord* 40(10):536, 2002.

# Impaired spontaneous Ventilation

*Elizabeth A. Henneman*

**NANDA**

## Definition

Decreased energy reserves result in an individual's inability to maintain breathing adequate for supporting life

## Defining Characteristics

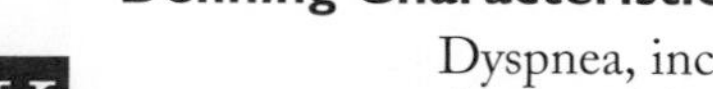

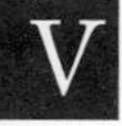

Dyspnea, increased metabolic rate, increased heart rate, decreased $Po_2$, increased $Pco_2$, decreased $Sao_2$, increased restlessness, apprehension, increased use of accessory muscles, decreased tidal volume, decreased cooperation

## Related Factors (r/t)

Metabolic factors, respiratory muscle fatigue

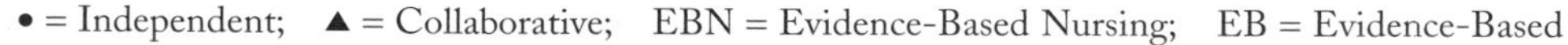

**NOC**

## Outcomes (Nursing Outcomes Classification)

### Suggested NOC Outcomes

Neurological Status: Central Motor Control; Respiratory Status: Gas Exchange, Ventilation

**Example NOC Outcome with Indicators**

Achieves appropriate **Respiratory Status: Ventilation** as evidenced by the following indicators: Respiratory rate/Respiratory rhythm/Depth of inspiration/Chest expansion symmetrical/Ease of breathing/Moves sputum out of airways/Accessory muscle use not present/Adventitious breath sounds not present/Chest retraction not present/Auscultated breath sounds/Tidal volume/Vital capacity (Rate each indicator of **Respiratory Status: Ventilation:** 1 = severely compromised, 2 = substantially compromised, 3 = moderately compromised, 4 = mildly compromised, 5 = not compromised [see Section I].)

## Client Outcomes

### Client Will (Specify Time Frame):

- Maintain arterial blood gases within safe parameters
- Remain free of dyspnea or restlessness
- Effectively maintain airway
- Effectively mobilize secretions

**NIC**

## Interventions (Nursing Interventions Classification)

### Suggested NIC Interventions

Artificial Airway Management; Mechanical Ventilation; Respiratory Monitoring; Resuscitation: Neonate; Ventilation Assistance

**Example NIC Activities—Mechanical Ventilation**

Monitor for respiratory muscle fatigue; consult with other health care personnel in selection of a ventilator mode

## Nursing Interventions and Rationales

▲ Collaborate with the client, family, and physician regarding possible intubation and ventilation. Ask whether the client has advanced directives and, if so, integrate them into the plan of care in conjunction with clinical data regarding overall health and reversibility of the medical condition. **EB:** *Patient preferences must be acknowledged when planning care. Advanced directives protect patient autonomy and help to ensure that the patient's wishes are respected (Garas & Pantilat, 2001).*

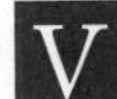

- Assess and respond to changes in the client's respiratory status. Monitor the client for dyspnea, increasing respiratory rate, use of accessory muscles, intercostal retractions, flaring of nostrils, and subjective complaints. **EBN:** *It is essential to monitor for these signs of impending respiratory failure or inability to tolerate mechanical ventilation/weaning (Earven et al, 2004).*
- Have the client use a numerical scale (0–10) to rate dyspnea before and after interventions. **EBN:** *The numerical rating scale is a valid measure of dyspnea. This allows measurement of the intensity, progression, and resolution of dyspnea (Gift & Narsavage, 1998).*
- Assess for history of chronic respiratory disorders when administering oxygen. *With chronic obstructive pulmonary disease (COPD) the respiratory drive is primarily in response to hypoxia, not hypercarbia; oxygenating too aggressively can result in respiratory depression. When managing acute respiratory failure in clients with COPD, use caution in administering oxygen because hyperoxygenation can lead to respiratory depression.*

▲ Collaborate with the physician and respiratory therapists in determining the appropriateness of noninvasive positive pressure ventilation (NPPV) for the decompensated client with COPD.

- Assist with implementation, client support, and monitoring if NPPV is used. EB: *In a client with exacerbation of COPD, NPPV can be as effective as intubation with use of a ventilator or if the client has other complications such as hypotension or severely impaired mental status (Perkins & Shortall, 2000; Pierson, 2002). The use of continuous positive airway pressure (CPAP) and bilevel positive airway pressure (bi-PAP) has been shown to improve oxygenation and decrease the rate of endotracheal intubation in patients with acute pulmonary edema (Park, Sangean, & Volpe, 2004).*
- If the client has apnea, pH <7.25, Pa$CO_2$ >50 mm Hg, Pa$O_2$ <50 mm Hg, respiratory muscle fatigue, or somnolence, prepare the client for intubation and placement on a ventilator. **EBN:** *These indicators are predictive of the need for invasive mechanical ventilation (Burns, 2001; Pierson, 2002).*

## Ventilator Support

▲ Explain the intubation intervention to the client and family as appropriate and, during the procedure, administer sedation for client comfort according to the physician's orders. **EBN:** *Explanation of the procedure decreases anxiety and increases understanding; premedication allows for a more controlled intubation with decreased incidence of insertion problems (Burns, 2001).*

- Secure the endotracheal tube in place using either tape or a device, auscultate bilateral breath sounds, use a $CO_2$ detector, and obtain a chest radiograph to confirm endotracheal tube placement. **EBN:** *Secure taping is needed to prevent inadvertent extubation. Nursing studies have shown conflicting results regarding the preferable way to secure the endotracheal tube (Barnason et al, 1998; Clarke et al, 1998; Kaplow & Bookbinder, 1994).* **EB:** *Auscultation alone is an unreliable method for checking endotracheal tube placement. A $CO_2$ detector can be used to confirm tube placement in the trachea; however, correct position of the endotracheal tube in the trachea (3–5 cm above the carina) must be confirmed by CXR (Burns, 2001; Henneman, Ellstrom, & St. John, 1998).*

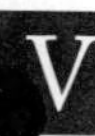


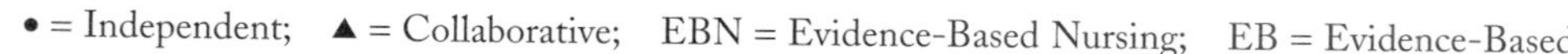

- Suction as needed, and hyperoxygenate and hyperventilate according to policy. Refer to **Ineffective Airway clearance** for further information on suctioning.
- Ensure activation of all monitor alarms each shift. *This action helps ensure client safety (Burns, 2001).*
- Respond to ventilator alarms promptly. If unable to rapidly locate the source of alarm, use a manual self-inflating resuscitation bag to ventilate the client while waiting for assistance. *Common causes of a high-pressure alarm include secretions, condensation, biting of the endotracheal tube, decreased compliance of the lungs, and tubing compression. Common causes of a low-pressure alarm are ventilator disconnection, leaks in the circuit, and changing compliance and resistance. Using a manual self-inflating resuscitation bag with supplemental oxygen, the nurse can provide immediate ventilation and oxygenation as needed (Burns, 2001).*
- Prevent unplanned extubation by maintaining stability of endotracheal tube and using soft wrist restraints on the client if needed and ordered. *Use only when other methods are ineffective, such as orienting patient, allowing family at bedside.*
- Drain collected fluid from condensation out of ventilator tubing as needed. *This action reduces the risk of infection by decreasing potential inhalation of contaminated fluid (Burns, 2001).*
- Note ventilator settings of flow of inspired oxygen, peak inspiratory pressure, tidal volume, and alarm activation at intervals and when removing the client from the ventilator for any reason. *Checking the settings ensures that safety measures are taken and that the client is not left on 100% oxygen after suctioning (Burns, 2001).*

▲ Administer analgesics and sedatives as needed with a defined protocol to facilitate client comfort and rest. Use pain and sedation scales to provide a consistent way of monitoring sedation levels and ensuring that therapeutic outcomes are being met (Consensus Conference on Sedation Assessment, 2004). **EBN:** *A study demonstrated that a nurse-implemented sedation protocol decreased the number of days of intubation, the need for a tracheotomy, and the length of hospital stay (Brook et al, 1999).* **EB:** *Avoid over sedation; use of continuous IV sedative infusions is associated with longer duration of mechanical ventilation compared with bolus sedation (Kress et al, 2000; Brook et al, 1999). Oral intubation and inadequate sedation have been noted to be indicators for unplanned extubation (Chevron et al, 1998).*

- To decrease anxiety, use music therapy with selections of client's choice played on headphones at intervals. **EBN:** *A study demonstrated that playing music that was chosen by the client decreased anxiety and increased relaxation as shown by reduced heart and respiratory rate in intubated adults (Chlan, 1998).*
- Analyze and respond to arterial blood gas results, end-tidal $CO_2$ levels, and pulse oximetry values. *Ventilatory support must be closely monitored to ensure adequate oxygenation and acid-base balance.* **EBN:** *End-tidal $CO_2$ monitoring is best used as an adjunct to direct patient observation (St. John, 2003).*

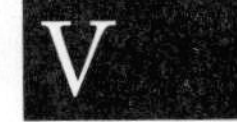

- Use an effective means of communication with the client. Use nonverbal communication, an electronic voice output communication aid, an alphabet board, a picture board, a computer, or a writing slate. Ask the client for input into care as able. Ensure client's human rights are met. **EBN:** *Inability to communicate can lead to client frustra-*

*tion, insecurity, and sometimes panic (Happ, 2001). Patients have reported a high level frustration in communicating their needs while being mechanically ventilated (Patak et al, 2004).* **EB:** *Use of a voice-output communication device was shown to be effective in a group of intubated surgery clients (Costello, 2000).* **EBN:** *Use of a picture board increased nurse-client communication in intubated cardiothoracic surgical clients (Stovsky, Rudy, & Dragonette, 1988). Practitioner behaviors reported to facilitate communication include being kind, informative, and physically present at the bedside (Patak et al, 2004).*

- Move the endotracheal tube from side to side every 24 hours, and tape it or secure it with a device. Assess and document client's skin condition, and ensure correct tube placement at lip line. *These steps help prevent skin breakdown at the lip line resulting from endotracheal tube pressure (Chang, 1995).*
- Provide oral care every 4 hours and PRN. **EB**: *Most episodes of ventilator-associated pneumonia (VAP) are thought to result from aspiration of oropharyngeal secretions containing potentially pathogenic organisms (Collard et al, 2003).*
- Use endotracheal tubes that allow for the continuous aspiration of subglottic secretions (CASS) (if available). **EB:** *The accumulation of contaminated oropharyngeal secretions above the endotracheal tube may contribute to the risk of aspiration. Two studies have suggested a decrease in the rate of VAP in patients requiring mechanical ventilation for > 3 days when CASS was used (Mahul et al, 1992; Valles et al, 1995).*
- Position the client in a semirecumbent position with the head of the bed at a 45-degree angle to decrease the aspiration of gastric secretions. **EB:** *Studies have shown that mechanically ventilated clients have a decreased incidence of pneumonia if the client is positioned at a 45-degree semirecumbent position as opposed to a supine position (Collard, Saint, & Matthay, 2003; Drakulovic et al, 1999; Torres et al, 1992).*
- Turn the client from side to side every 2 hours or more often if possible. Use rotational bed therapy in patients for whom side-to-side turning is contraindicated or difficult. **EBN:** *Changing position frequently decreases the incidence of atelectasis, pooling of secretions, and resultant pneumonia (Burns, 2001).* **EB:** *Continuous, lateral rotational therapy has been to improve oxygenation, decrease the incidence of VAP (Wang, Chuang, & Lin, 2003).*
- Assess bilateral anterior and posterior breath sounds every 2–4 hours and prn; respond to any relevant changes.
- Assess responsiveness to ventilator support; monitor for subjective complaints and sensation of dyspnea (Ferrin & Tino, 1997).

▲ Collaborate with the interdisciplinary team in treating patients with acute respiratory failure. **EB:** *A collaborative approach to caring for mechanically ventilated patients has been demonstrated to reduce length of time on the ventilator and length of stay in the ICU (Henneman et al, 2002; Henneman et al, 2001). The mechanical ventilator is usually a temporary support until the underlying pathology can be effectively resolved.*

## Geriatric

- Recognize that elderly have a high rate of morbidity when mechanically ventilated. *Implement interventions to prevent decline such as positioning, nutrition maintenance early to prevent decline (Phelan, Cooper, & Sangkachand, 2002).*

## Home Care

- ▲ Some of the interventions listed previously may be adapted for home care use. Begin discharge planning as soon as possible with the case manager or social worker to assess the need for home support systems, assistive devices, and community or home health services.
- ▲ With help from a medical social worker, assist the client and family to determine the fiscal affect of home care vs. an extended care facility.
- • Assess the home setting during the discharge process to ensure the home can safely accommodate ventilator support (e.g., adequate space and electricity).
- • Have the family contact the electric company and place the client residence on a high-risk list in case of a power outage. *Some home-based care requires special conditions for safe home administration.*
- • Assess the caregivers for commitment to support a ventilator-dependent client in the home. *Commitment to care and valuing home as a healing place provides meaning for participating in caregiving and decrease caregiver role strain (Boland & Sims, 1996).*
- • Be sure that the client and family or caregivers are familiar with operation of all ventilation devices, know how to suction if needed, are competent in doing tracheostomy care, and know schedules for cleaning equipment. Have the designated caregiver or caregivers demonstrate care before discharge. *Some home-based care involves specialized technology and requires specific skills for safe and appropriate care.*
- • Assess client and caregiver knowledge of the disease, client needs, and medications to be administered via ventilation-assistive devices. Avoid analgesics. Assess knowledge of how to use equipment. Teach as necessary. *A client receiving ventilation support may not be able to articulate needs. Respiratory medications can have side effects that change the client's respiration or level of consciousness.*
- • Establish an emergency plan and criteria for use. Identify emergency procedures to be used until medical assistance arrives. Teach and role play emergency care. *A prepared emergency plan reassures the client and family and ensures client safety.*
- ▲ Institute case management of frail elderly clients to support continued independent living. *Respiratory difficulties represent and can lead to increasing need for assistance in using the health care system effectively. Case management combines nursing activities of the client and family assessment, planning and coordination of care among all health care providers, delivery of direct nursing care, and monitoring of care and outcomes. These activities are able to address continuity of care, mutual goal setting, behavior management, and prevention of worsening health problems (Guttman, 1999).*

## Client/Family Teaching

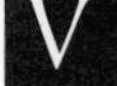


- • Explain to the client the potential sensations that will be experienced including relief of dyspnea, the feeling of lung inflations, the noise of the ventilator, and the reality of alarms. **EBN:** *Knowledge of potential sensations and experiences before they are encountered can help to decrease anxiety (Johnson, 1972).*
- • Explain to the client and family about being unable to speak, and work out an alternative system of communication. See previous intervention.

- Demonstrate to the family how to perform simple procedures such as suctioning the mouth with a tonsil-tip catheter, providing range-of-motion exercises, and reconnecting the ventilator immediately if it becomes disconnected. *Families often need to be part of the client's care (Burns, 2001) and may be present at the bedside for prolonged periods of time.*
- Offer both the client and family explanations of how the ventilator works and answer any questions asked. *Having questions answered is often cited as an important need of clients and families when a client is on a ventilator (Burns, 2001).*

## evolve WEBSITES FOR EDUCATION

See the EVOLVE website for World Wide Web resources for client education.

## REFERENCES


Barnason S, Graham J, Wild MC et al: Comparison of two endotracheal tube securement techniques on unplanned extubation, oral mucosa, and facial skin integrity, *Heart Lung* 27(6):409, 1998.

Boland D, Sims S: Family caregiving at home as a solitary journey, *Image* 28:1, 1996.

Brook AD, Ahrens TS, Schaiff R et al: Effect of a nursing-implemented sedation protocol on the duration of mechanical ventilation, *Crit Care Med* 27(12):2609, 1999.

Burns SM: Ventilatory management—volume and pressure modes. In Lynn-McHale DJ, Carolson KK, editors: *AACN procedure manual for critical care,* ed 4, Philadelphia, 2001, WB Saunders.

Chang V: Protocol for prevention of complications of endotracheal intubation, *Crit Care Nurs* 15:19, 1995.

Chevron V, Menard JF, Richard JC et al: Unplanned extubation risk factors of development and predictive criteria for reintubation, *Crit Care Med* 26(6):1049, 1998.

Chlan L: Effectiveness of a music therapy intervention on relaxation and anxiety for patients receiving ventilatory assistance, *Heart Lung* 27(3):169, 1998.

Clarke T, Evans S, Way P et al: A comparison of two methods of securing an endotracheal tube, *Aust Crit Care* 11(2):45, 1998.

Collard HR, Saint S, Matthay MA: Prevention of ventilator-associated pneumonia: an evidence-based systemic review, *Ann Intern Med* 138(6):494, 2003.

Consensus Conference on Sedation Assessment. Abbott Laboratories, American Association of Critical Care Nurses, St. Thomas Health System, *Critical Care Nurse* 24:33, 2004.

Costello JM: AAC intervention in the intensive care unit: the Children's Hospital Boston model, *Augment Alternative Comm* 16, 2000.

Drakulovic MB, Torres A, Bauer TT et al: Supine body position as a risk factor for nosocomial pneumonia in mechanically ventilated patients: a randomized trial, *Lancet* 354(9193):1851, 1999.

Earven S, Fisher C, Lewis R et al: The experience of four outcomes managers: an institutional approach to weaning patients from long-term mechanical ventilation, *Crit Care Nurs Clin N Am* 16:395, 2004.

Ferrin MS, Tino G: Acute dyspnea, *AACN Clin Issues* 8(3):398, 1997.

Garas N, Pantilat SZ: Advance planning for end-of-life care. In Shojania KG, Duncan BW, McDonald KM et al, editors: *Making healthcare safer: a critical analysis of patient safety practices. Evidence report/technology assessment No. 43* (Prepared by the University of California at San Francisco-Stanford Evidence-based Practice Center under Contract No. 290-97-0013), AHRQ Publication No. 01-E058, Rockville, Md, July 2001, Agency for Healthcare Research and Quality, p 561.

Gift A, Narsavage G: Validity of the numeric rating scale as a measure of dyspnea, *Am J Crit Care* 7(3):200, 1998.

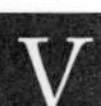

Guttman R: Case management of the frail elderly in the community, *Clin Nurs Spec* 13(4):174, 1999.

Happ MB: Communicating with mechanically ventilated patients: state of the science, *AACN Clin Issues* 12(2):247, 2001.

Henneman EA, Ellstrom KE, St. John RE: *Airway management. AACN practice protocol.* Aliso Viejo, Calif, 1998, American Association of Critical Care Nursing.

Henneman EA, Dracup K, Ganz T et al: Effect of a collaborative weaning plan on patient outcome in the critical care setting, *Crit Care Med* 29:297, 2001.

Henneman EA, Dracup K, Ganz T et al: Using a collaborative weaning plan to decrease duration of mechanical ventilation and length of stay in the intensive care unit for patients receiving long-term ventilation, *AJCC* 11:132, 2002.

Johnson J: Effects of structuring patient's expectations on their reactions to threatening events, *Nurs Res* 21(6):499, 1972.

Kaplow R, Bookbinder M: A comparison of four endotracheal tube holders, *Heart Lung* 23:59, 1994.
Kress JP, Pohlman AS, O'Connor MF et al: Daily interruption of sedative infusions in critically ill patients undergoing mechanical ventilation, *N Eng J Med* 342:1471, 2000.
Mahul P, Auboyer C, Jospe R et al: Prevention of nosocomial pneumonia in intubated patients: respective role of mechanical subglottic secretions drainage and stress ulcer prophylaxis, *Intensive Care Medicine* 18:20, 1992.
Park M, Sangean MC, Volpe MS et al: Randomized, prospective trial of oxygen, continuous positive airway pressure and bilevel positive airway pressure by face mask in acute cardiogenic pulmonary edema, *Crit Care Med* 32:2407, 2004.
Patak L, Gawlinski A, Fung NI et al: Patient's reports of healthcare practitioner interventions that are related to communication during mechanical ventilation, *Heart Lung* 33:308, 2004.
Perkins LA, Shortall SP: Ventilation without intubation, *RN* 63(1):34, 2000.
Phelan BA, Cooper DA, Sangkachand P: Prolonged mechanical ventilation and tracheostomy in the elderly, *AACN Clin Issues* 13:1, 2002.
Pierson DJ: Indications for mechanical ventilation in adults with acute respiratory failure, *Respir Care* 47:3, 2002.
St. John RE: End-tidal carbon dioxide monitoring, *Crit Care Nurse* 23:83, 2003.
Stovsky B, Rudy E, Dragonette P: Comparison of two types of communication methods used after cardiac surgery with patients with endotracheal tubes, *Heart Lung* 17(3):281, 1988.
Torres A, Serra-Batlles J, Ros E et al: Pulmonary aspiration of gastric contents in patients receiving mechanical ventilation: the effect of body position, *Ann Intern Med* 116:540, 1992.
Valles J, Artigas A, Rello J et al: Continuous aspiration of subglottic secretions in preventing ventilator-associated pneumonia, *Ann Intern Med.* 122:179, 1995.
Wang JY, Chuang PY, Lin CJ et al: Continuous lateral rotational therapy in the medical intensive care unit, *J Formos Med Association* 102:788, 2003.

# Dysfunctional Ventilatory weaning response

*Elizabeth A. Henneman*

**NANDA**

## Definition

Inability to adjust to lowered levels of mechanical ventilator support that interrupts and prolongs the weaning process

## Defining Characteristics

### Severe

Deterioration in arterial blood gases from current baseline; respiratory rate increases significantly from baseline; increase from baseline blood pressure (20 mm Hg); agitation; increase from baseline heart rate (20 beats/min); paradoxical abdominal breathing; adventitious breath sounds, audible airway secretions; cyanosis; decreased level of consciousness; full respiratory accessory muscle use; shallow, gasping breaths; profuse diaphoresis; breathing uncoordinated with the ventilator

### Moderate

Slight increase from baseline blood pressure (<20 mm Hg); baseline increase in respiratory rate (<5 breaths/min); slight increase from baseline heart rate (<20 beats/

min); pale, slight cyanosis; slight respiratory accessory muscle use; inability to respond to coaching; inability to cooperate; apprehension; color changes; decreased air entry on auscultation; diaphoresis; eye widening, wide-eyed look; hypervigilance to activities

### Mild

Warmth, restlessness, slight increase of respiratory rate from baseline, queries about possible machine malfunction, expressed feelings of increased need for oxygen, fatigue, increased concentration on breathing

## Related Factors (r/t)

### Physiological

Ineffective airway clearance, sleep pattern disturbance, inadequate nutrition, uncontrolled pain or discomfort

### Psychological

Knowledge deficit of the weaning process and client role, perceived inefficacy about the ability to wean, decreased motivation, decreased self-esteem, moderate or severe anxiety or fear, hopelessness, powerlessness, insufficient trust in nurse

### Situational

Uncontrolled episodic energy demands or problems, inappropriate pacing of diminished ventilator support, inadequate social support, adverse environment (e.g., noise, activity, negative events in the room), low nurse-client ratio, extended nurse absence from bedside, unfamiliar nursing staff, history of ventilator dependence for >4 days–1 week, history of multiple unsuccessful weaning attempts

**NOC**

## Outcomes (Nursing Outcomes Classification)

### Suggested NOC Outcomes

Respiratory Status: Gas Exchange, Ventilation

**Example NOC Outcome with Indicators**

**Respiratory Status: Ventilation** as evidenced by the following indicators: Respiratory rate/Respiratory rhythm/Depth of inspiration/Chest expansion symmetrical/Ease of breathing/Moves sputum out of airways/Accessory muscle use not present/Adventitious breath sounds not present/Chest retraction not present/Auscultated breath sounds/Tidal volume/Vital capacity (Rate each indicator of **Respiratory Status: Ventilation:** 1 = extremely compromised, 2 = substantially compromised, 3 = moderately compromised, 4 = mildly compromised, 5 = not compromised [see Section I].)

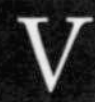

## Client Outcomes

**Client Will (Specify Time Frame):**
- Wean from ventilator with adequate arterial blood gases
- Remain free of unresolved dyspnea or restlessness
- Effectively clear secretions

**NIC**

## Interventions (Nursing Interventions Classification)

### Suggested NIC Interventions

Mechanical Ventilation, Mechanical Ventilatory Weaning

**Example NIC Activities—Mechanical Ventilatory Weaning**

Monitor for optimal fluid and electrolyte status; monitor to ensure client is free of significant infection before weaning

## Nursing Interventions and Rationales

- Assess client's readiness for weaning as evidenced by the following:
  - Physiological readiness: (Brochard et al, 1994; Dries, 1997; Esteban et al, 1995; Lessard & Brochard, 1996; Mancebo, 1996)
    - ❑ Resolution of initial medical problem that led to ventilator dependence
    - ❑ Hemodynamic stability
    - ❑ Normal hemoglobin levels
    - ❑ Absence of fever
    - ❑ Normal state of consciousness
    - ❑ Metabolic, fluid, and electrolyte balance
    - ❑ Adequate nutritional status with serum albumin levels >2.5 g/dL
    - ❑ Adequate sleep

  **EB:** *Adequate respiratory parameters include the following: adequate gas exchange ($PaO_2$/ $FiO_2$ ratio >200); respiratory rate </= 35 breaths/min; a negative inspiratory pressure <-20 cm, positive expiratory pressure >+30 cm $H_2O$, spontaneous tidal volume >5 mL/kg, vital capacity >10–15 mL/kg.* **EBN:** *These respiratory predictors of weaning success have proven to be of limited value in the management of patients receiving long-term mechanical ventilation (Burns, 2004).*
  - Psychological readiness: There has been little research devoted to the study of psychological readiness to wean. **EBN:** *An in-depth qualitative nursing research study has provided new insight into the weaning process and suggests that three key criteria give an indication of a patients' psychological readiness: (1) being orientated, (2) mental ease, and (3) a positive attitude (Logan & Jenny, 1997).*

  *For best results ensure that the client is in an optimal physiological and psychological state before introducing the stress of weaning (Burns, 2004; Earven et al, 2004; MacIntyre, 2004; Martensson & Fridlund, 2002; Blackwood, 2000). For more information on*

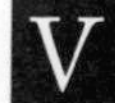

*weaning assessment, please refer to the Burns Weaning Assessment Program (Burns, 2001).*

- Use evidence-based weaning protocol if available. **EB:** *Protocol directed weaning has been demonstrated to be safe and effective (Crocker, 2002; Kress et al, 2000; Brook et al, 1999; Kollef et al, 1997; Ely et al, 1996). They appear to work by decreasing practice variation (Burns, 2004). Two, large randomized studies have demonstrated that no one method or mode of mechanical ventilation has been demonstrated to be superior in weaning patients (Esteban et al, 1995; Brochard et al, 1994).*
- Identify reasons for previous unsuccessful weaning attempts, and include that information in development of the weaning plan. **EBN:** *Analyzing client responses after each weaning attempt prevents repeated unsuccessful weaning trials (Burns, 2004; Henneman et al, 2002; Henneman et al, 2001; Henneman, 2001).*

▲ Collaborate with an interdisciplinary team (physician, nurse, respiratory therapist, physical therapist, and dietician) to develop a weaning plan with a timeline and goals; revise this plan throughout the weaning period. Use a communication device such as a weaning board or flow sheet. **EBN:** *Effective interdisciplinary collaboration can positively affect client outcomes (Baggs et al, 1992). Collaborative weaning plans using dry-erase boards and flow sheets have been demonstrated to decrease ventilator days and length of stay in the intensive care unit (Henneman et al, 2002; Henneman et al, 2001).*

- Assist client to identify personal strategies that result in relaxation and comfort (e.g., music, visualization, relaxation techniques, reading, television, family visits). Support implementation of these strategies. **EBN:** *Personal strategies for relaxation are effective (Gift, Moore, & Soeken, 1992). A study demonstrated that playing music that was relaxing decreased anxiety and increased relaxation as shown by reduced heart and respiratory rate in intubated adults (Chlan, 1998).*
- Provide a safe and comfortable environment. Stay with the client during weaning if at all possible. If unable to stay, make the call light button readily available and assure the client that needs will be met responsively. **EBN:** *A client who feels safe and trusts the health care providers can focus on the immediate work of weaning; support from the nurse helps decrease anxiety (Blackwood, 2000; Burns, 2004; Logan & Jenny, 1997).*

▲ Coordinate pain and sedation medications to minimize sedative effects. **EB:** *Appropriate use of sedation is key to successful weaning. Use of continuous IV sedation is associated with longer duration of mechanical ventilation compared with bolus sedation (Brook, Ahrens, & Schaiff, 1999; Kress et al, 2000).*

- Schedule weaning periods for the time of day when the client is most rested. Cluster care activities to promote successful weaning. Avoid other procedures during weaning: keep the environment quiet and promote restful activities between weaning periods. *It is important that the client receive adequate rest between weaning periods. Control of external noises and stimuli can promote restful periods (Cropp et al, 1994).*
- Promote a normal sleep-wake cycle, allowing uninterrupted periods of nighttime sleep (Higgins, 1998). *Limit visitors during weaning to close and supportive persons; ask visitors to leave if they are negatively affecting the weaning process.*
- During weaning, monitor the client's physiological and psychological responses; acknowledge and respond to fears and subjective complaints. Validate that the client

V

is doing the work of weaning. **EBN:** *Weaning is a stressful experience that requires active participation by the client. The client's work needs to be understood and supported by clinicians to facilitate recovery from mechanical ventilation and weaning (Blackwood, 2000; Logan & Jenny, 1997).*

- • Monitor subjective and objective data (breath sounds, respiratory pattern, respiratory effort, heart rate, blood pressure, oxygen saturation per oximetry, amount and type of secretions, anxiety, and energy level) throughout weaning to determine client tolerance and responses. **EBN:** *Continued assessment and maintenance of airway clearance throughout weaning supports client comfort, safety, and trust (Carroll & Milikowski, 1996).*
- • Coach the client through episodes of increased anxiety. Remain with client or place a supportive and calm significant other in this role. Give positive reinforcement, and with permission use touch to communicate support and concern. *It is not unusual for a client with lung disease to experience self-limiting episodes of increased shortness of breath. Supporting and coaching a client through such episodes allows weaning to continue.*
- • Terminate weaning when the client demonstrates predetermined criteria or when the following signs of weaning intolerance occur:
  - ■ Tachypnea, dyspnea, or chest and abdominal asynchrony
  - ■ Agitation or mental status changes
  - ■ Decreased oxygen saturation: $SaO_2$ <90%
  - ■ Increased or decreased pulse rate or blood pressure or presence of new onset of dysrhythmias

  **EBN:** *Continuing the weaning trial when the client has intolerance leads to fatigue and possible cardiovascular failure (Burns, 2001).*
- ▲ If the dysfunctional weaning response is severe, consider slowing weaning to brief increments of time (e.g., 5 minutes). Continue to collaborate with the team to determine whether an untreated physiological cause for the dysfunctional weaning pattern remains. Consider an alternative care setting (subacute, rehabilitation facility, home) for clients with prolonged ventilator dependence as a strategy that can positively affect outcomes. **EB:** *One study indicated that half of the clients admitted to a rehabilitation facility were weaned from the ventilator (Modawal et al, 2002).*

## Geriatric

- • Recognize that older clients may require longer periods of time to wean. **EBN:** *A study demonstrated that older clients required a longer period of time to wean, especially if they were older than 80 years (Epstein, Modadem, & Peerless, 2002).*

## Home Care

NOTE: Weaning from a ventilator at home should be based on client stability and comfort of the client and caregivers under an intermittent care plan. The client and/or family may be more comfortable having the client rehospitalized for the process.

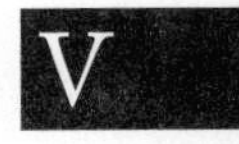


- • Assess comfort and coping ability of the client and/or family to wean at home, as well as fiscal implications and home care coverage. *Compromises in respiratory function are frightening for clients and family who perceive the availability of a high-technology, structured environment as a more appropriate environment for weaning (Sevick et al, 1997).*

- Establish an emergency plan and methods of implementation. Include emergency aeration and reestablishment of the ventilation assistive device. *Having a prepared emergency plan reassures the client and family and provides for client safety.*
- ▲ Obtain orders for alternative routes of medication administration when medications have been administered via a ventilation device. Instruct the client and family in changes.

## evolve WEBSITES FOR EDUCATION

See the EVOLVE website for World Wide Web resources for client education.

## REFERENCES


Baggs JG, Ryan SA, Phelps CE et al: The association between interdisciplinary collaboration and patient outcomes in a medical intensive care unit, *Heart Lung* 21(1):18, 1992.

Blackwood B: The art and science of predicting patient readiness for weaning from mechanical ventilation, *Int J Nurs Stud* 37:145, 2000.

Brochard L, Rauss A, Benito S et al: Comparison of three methods of gradual withdrawal from ventilatory support during weaning from mechanical ventilation, *Am J Resp Crit Care Med* 150:896, 1994.

Brook AD, Ahrens TS, Schaiff R et al: Effect of a nursing-implemented sedation protocol on the duration of mechanical ventilation, *Crit Care Med* 27:2609, 1999.

Burns SM: Standard weaning criteria. In Lynn-McHale DJ, Carolson KK, editors: *AACN procedure manual for critical care,* ed 4, Philadelphia, 2001, WB Saunders.

Burns SM: The science of weaning: when and how? *Crit Care Nurs Clin North Am* 16:379, 2004.

Carroll P, Milikowski K: Getting your patient off a ventilator, *RN* 96(6):42, 1996.

Chlan L: Effectiveness of a music therapy intervention on relaxation and anxiety for patients receiving ventilatory assistance, *Heart Lung* 27(3):169, 1998.

Crocker C: Nurse-led weaning from ventilatory and respiratory support, *Intens Crit Care Nurs* 18:272, 2002.

Cropp AJ, Woods LA, Raney D et al: Name that tone: the proliferation of noise in the intensive care unit, *Chest* 105:1217, 1994.

Dries DJ: Weaning from mechanical ventilation, *J Trauma* 43:372, 1997.

Earven S, Fisher C, Lewis R et al: The experience of four outcomes managers: an institutional approach to weaning patients from long-term mechanical ventilation, *Crit Care Nurs Clin North Am* 16:395, 2004.

Ely EW, Baker AM, Dunagan DP et al: Effect on the duration of mechanical ventilation of identifying patients capable of breathing spontaneously, *N Engl J Med* 335:1864, 1996.

Epstein CD, El-Modadem N, Peerless JR: Weaning older patients from long-term mechanical ventilation: a pilot study, *Am J Crit Care* 11:4, 2002.

Esteban A, Frutos F, Tobin MJ et al: A comparison of four methods of weaning patients from mechanical ventilation, *N Eng J Med* 332:345, 1995.

Gift A, Moore T, Soeken K: Relaxation to reduce dyspnea and anxiety in COPD patients, *Nurs Res* 41:242, 1992.

Henneman EA: Liberating patients from mechanical ventilation, a team approach, *Crit Care Nurs* 21(3):25, 2001.

Henneman EA, Dracup K, Ganz T et al: Effect of a collaborative weaning plan on patient outcome in the critical care setting, *Crit Care Med* 29:297, 2001.

Henneman EA, Dracup K, Ganz T et al: Using a collaborative weaning plan to decrease duration of mechanical ventilation and length of stay in the intensive care unit for patients receiving long-term ventilation, *Am J Crit Care* 11:132, 2002.

Higgins P: Patient perception of fatigue while undergoing long term mechanical ventilation: incidence and associated factors, *Heart Lung* 27:177, 1998.

Kollef MH, Levy NT, Ahrens TS et al: The use of continuous IV sedation is associated with prolongation of mechanical ventilation, *Chest* 114(2):541, 1998.

Kollef MH, Shapiro SD, Silver P et al: A randomized controlled trial of protocol-directed versus physician-directed weaning from mechanical ventilation, *Crit Care Med* 25(4):567, 1997.

Kress JP, Pohlman AS, O'Connor MF et al: Daily interruption of sedative infusions in critically ill patients undergoing mechanical ventilation, *N Engl J Med* 342:1471, 2000.

Lessard MR, Brochard LJ: Weaning from mechanical support, *Clin Chest Med* 17:475, 1996.
Logan J: Qualitative analysis of patient's work during mechanical ventilation and weaning, *Heart Lung* 26:140, 1997.
Logan J, Jenny J: Qualitative analysis of patients' weaning work during mechanical ventilation and weaning, *Heart Lung* 26:140, 1997.
MacIntyre NR: Evidence-based guidelines for weaning and discontinuing ventilatory support, *Respir Care* 47(1):69, 2004.
Mancebo J: Weaning from mechanical ventilation, *Eur Resp J* 9:1923, 1996.
Martensson IE, Fridlund B: Factors influencing the patient during weaning from mechanical ventilation: a national survey, *Intensive Crit Care Nurs* 18:223, 2002.
Modawal A, Candadai NP, Mandell KM et al: Weaning success among ventilator-dependent patients in a rehabilitation facility, *Arch Phys Med Rehabil* 83(2):154, 2002.
Sevick MA, Bradham DD: Economic value of caregiver effort in maintaining long term ventilatory assisted individuals, *Heart Lung* 26(2):148, 1997.

# Risk for other-directed Violence

*Kathleen L. Patusky*

**NANDA**

## Definition

At risk for behaviors in which an individual demonstrates that he or she can be physically, emotionally, and/or sexually harmful to others

## Risk Factors

Body language: rigid posture, clenching of fists and jaw, hyperactivity, pacing, breathlessness, threatening stances; history of violence against others (e.g., hitting someone, kicking someone, spitting at someone, scratching someone, throwing objects at someone, biting someone, attempted rape, rape, sexual molestation, urinating/defecating on someone); history of threats of violence (e.g., verbal threats against property, verbal threats against person, social threats, cursing, threatening notes/letters, threatening gestures, sexual threats); history of violent antisocial behavior (e.g., stealing, insistent borrowing, insistent demanding of privileges, insistent interrupting of meetings, refusing to eat, refusing to take medication, ignoring instructions); history of violence, indirect (e.g., tearing off clothes, ripping objects off walls, writing on walls, urinating on floor, defecating on floor, stamping feet, displaying temper tantrum, running in corridors, yelling, throwing objects, breaking a window, slamming doors, making sexual advances); neurological impairment (e.g., positive EEG, CAT, or MRI; head trauma; positive neurological findings; seizure disorders); cognitive impairment (e.g., learning disabilities, attention deficit disorder, decreased intellectual functioning); history of childhood abuse; history of witnessing family violence; cruelty to animals; fire setting; prenatal/perinatal complications or abnormalities; history of drug or alcohol abuse; pathological intoxication; psychotic symptomatology (e.g., auditory, visual, command hallucinations; paranoid delusions; loose, rambling, or illogical thought processes); motor vehicle offenses (e.g., frequent traffic violations, use of a motor vehicle to release anger); suicidal behavior; impulsivity; availability/possession of weapon(s)

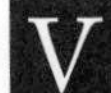

# NOC

## Outcomes (Nursing Outcomes Classification)

### Suggested NOC Outcomes

Abuse Cessation; Abusive Behavior Self-Restraint; Aggression Self-Control; Distorted Thought Self-Control; Impulse Self-Control; Parenting: Psychosocial Safety; Risk Detection

**Example NOC Outcome with Indicators**

**Aggression Self-Control** as evidenced by the following indicators: Refrains from harming others/Communicates needs and feelings appropriately/Identifies when angry (Rate each indicator of **Aggression Self-Control:** 1 = never demonstrated, 2 = rarely demonstrated, 3 = sometimes demonstrated, 4 = often demonstrated, 5 = consistently demonstrated [see Section I].)

## Client Outcomes

### Client Will (Specify Time Frame):

- Stop all forms of abuse (physical, emotional, sexual; neglect; financial exploitation)
- Have cessation of abuse reported by victim
- Display no aggressive activity
- Refrain from verbal outbursts
- Refrain from violating others' personal space
- Refrain from antisocial behaviors
- Maintain relaxed body language and decreased motor activity
- Identify factors contributing to abusive/aggressive behavior
- Demonstrate impulse control or state feelings of control
- Identify impulsive behaviors
- Identify feelings/behaviors that lead to impulsive actions
- Identify consequences of impulsive actions to self or others
- Avoid high-risk environments and situations
- Identify and talk about feelings; express anger appropriately
- Express decreased anxiety and control of hallucinations as applicable
- Displace anger to meaningful activities
- Communicate needs appropriately
- Identify responsibility to maintain control
- Express empathy for victim
- Obtain no access or yield access to harmful objects
- Use alternative coping mechanisms for stress
- Obtain and follow through with counseling
- Demonstrate knowledge of correct role behaviors

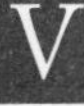

### Victim (and Children If Applicable) Will (Specify Time Frame):

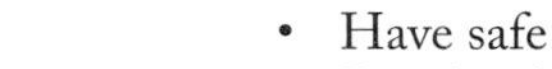

- Have safe plan for leaving situation or avoiding abuse
- Resolve depression or traumatic response

**Parent Will (Specify Time Frame):**

- Monitor social/play contacts
- Provide supervision and nurturing environment
- Intervene to prevent high-risk social behaviors

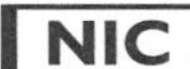

## Interventions (Nursing Interventions Classification)

### Suggested NIC Interventions

Abuse Protection Support; Anger Control Assistance; Behavior Management; Calming Technique; Coping Enhancement; Crisis Intervention; Delusion Management; Dementia Management; Distraction; Environmental Management: Violence Prevention; Mood Management; Physical Restraint; Seclusion; Substance Use Prevention

**Example NIC Intervention—Environmental Management: Violence Prevention**

Remove other individuals from the vicinity of a violent or potentially violent client; provide ongoing surveillance of all client access areas to maintain client safety; therapeutically intervene as needed

## Nursing Interventions and Rationales

### Client Violence

▲ Monitor the environment, evaluate situations that could become violent, and intervene early to deescalate the situation. Enlist support from other staff rather than attempting to handle the situation alone. *Violent situations can arise any time that anger or frustration occurs and need not limit participation to clients. Family members or other staff can initiate violence, especially around disagreements over a client's treatment plan or if kept waiting for prolonged periods (Duncan, Estabrookes, & Reimer, 2000). Most psychiatric facilities identify specific policies and offer training in crisis intervention or conflict resolution. Participation in such training for all staff is highly recommended.* **EBN:** *One study suggested that systematic risk assessment, aggression management training, and decreasing nurses' coercive responses to clients could reduce coercion and client violence (Needham et al, 2004).*

▲ Know and follow institution's policies and procedures concerning violence. *Being familiar with and following policies and procedures of the department prevents violence. Policies should be developed, and training programs should be provided in proper use and application of restraints. All nursing units should develop a proactive plan for dealing with violent situations.*

• Initiate client assessment by distinguishing the broadest categories of causes of aggression: social versus biological. *A nursing concept analysis of aggression examined the causes of aggression, identifying social causes (learned behavior, frustration) and biological causes (brain dysfunction, high levels of testosterone, low levels of serotonin, birth complications, nutrition deficiency). Knowledge of the source of aggression is important in applying and developing the most appropriate interventions (Liu, 2004).*

- ▲ Assess the client for risk factors of violence including those in the following categories: psychiatric disorders (particularly paranoid or bipolar disorders, substance abuse), neurological disorders (e.g., head injury, temporal lobe epilepsy), psychological precursors (e.g., low tolerance for stress, impulsivity), coping difficulties (e.g., inability to plan solutions or see long-term consequences of behavior), and personal history (e.g., past violent behavior). *All of these risk factors have been implicated in aggressive, agitated, or violent behavior. Additional potential triggers include confusion, anxiety/frustration, boredom, heat, excessive or constant noise, lack of information, having no right or appeal, lack of choice, lack of space, or group/peer pressure (Graham, 2001). Medical history and physical findings should be considered carefully for elements that may decrease the client's anger threshold or influence the client's thought processes (e.g., chronic medical condition, neoplasm) (Citrome & Volavka, 1999).*
- ▲ Assess for potential indicators of impending violence against others: frequent medication change, high use of sedative drugs, past violent behavior, a *Diagnostic and Statistical Manual of Mental Health IV* diagnosis of antisocial personality or borderline personality disorder, and long hospitalization. Other indicators include hypervigilance, hostility, substance use, and lack of adherence to medication regimen. *A study indicated that behaviors and situations in the first list are the most powerful predictors of violence (Soliman & Reza, 2001). Knowing, recognizing, and promptly intervening in early precipitating factors prevents violence.*
- • Assess the client with history of previous assaults. Listen to and acknowledge feelings of anger, observe for increased motor activity, and prepare to intervene if the client becomes aggressive. **EBN:** *In one study, physically assaultive clients had significantly more previous assaults and more difficulty appropriately verbalizing angry feelings on their units than did control group members. Before the assault, assaultive clients were more verbally hostile and showed more increased motor activity than control subjects (Lanza et al, 1996).*
- • Assess for the client's experience of physiological signs and for external signs of anger. *Internal signs of anger include increased pulse, respirations, and blood pressure; chills; prickly sensations; numbness; choking sensation; nausea; and vertigo. External signs include increased muscle tone, changes in body posture (clenched fists, set jaw), eye changes (eyebrows lower and drawn together, eyelids tense, eyes assuming a "hard" appearance), lips pressed together, flushing or pallor, goose bumps, twitching, and sweating (Harper-Jacques & Reimer, 2002).*
- • A brief self-report measures may aid in the assessment of violence risk. **EB**: *The Broset violence checklist (BVC) has been developed for short-term prediction of violence in psychiatric inpatients. Some false-positive cases were met with preventive measures, which may have avoided violence (Abderhalden et al, 2004).*

- • Assess for the presence of hallucinations. *Command hallucinations may direct the client to behave violently, and assessment of their presence is important when evaluating the risk for violence in clients with major mental disorders (McNeil, Eisner, & Binder, 2000).*
- • Determine the presence and degree of homicidal risk. A number of questions will elicit the necessary information:
  - ■ Have you been thinking about harming someone? If yes, who?
  - ■ How often do you have these thoughts, and how long do they last?

- ■ Do you have a plan? What is it?
- ■ Do you have access to the means to carry out that plan?
- ■ What has kept you from hurting the person until now?

*Psychotherapists are required to report harm or threats of harm to another person; this is referred to as the duty to warn. State laws and mental health codes should be checked to determine local mandates for threat reporting by specific types of health care professionals.*

- • Take action to minimize personal risk:
  - ■ Use nonthreatening body language.
  - ■ Respect personal space and boundaries.
  - ■ Do not allow the client to block access to an exit.
  - ■ If speaking with the client alone, keep the door to the room open.
  - ■ Be aware of where other staff is at all times.
  - ■ Notify other staff of where you are at all times.
  - ■ Take verbal threats seriously, and notify other staff.
  - ■ Wear clothing and accessories that are not restricting and that will not be dangerous (e.g., sandals or shoes with heels can lead to twisted ankles; necklaces or dangling earrings could be grabbed).

  *Actions must be taken by nurses to minimize personal risk if they are to be available to respond to violence (Harper-Jacques & Reimer, 2002). Other staff must be notified so they can also take proper precautions and be alert to the potential for violence.*
- • Maintain at least an arm's length distance from the client; do not touch the client without permission (unless physical restraint is the goal). *Encroaching on the client's personal space is likely to increase fear, anger, or paranoia and thus increase the magnitude of the reaction. Touching may be perceived as initiation of an attack; the client may strike out in self-defense.*
- • Remove potential weapons from the environment. Be prepared to remove obstructions to staff response from the environment. *Clients prone to violence may use available weapons opportunistically. If client restraint becomes necessary, environmental hazards (e.g., chairs, wastebaskets) should be moved out of the way to prevent injuries.*
- • Search the client and his or her belongings for weapons or potential weapons on admission to the hospital as appropriate. *Clients prone to violence may carry a weapon routinely (e.g., knife). Weapons should be removed for safety of clients and staff.*
- • Inform the client of unit expectations for appropriate behavior and the consequences of not meeting these expectations. Emphasize that the client must comply with the rules of the unit. Give positive reinforcement for compliance. *Clients benefit from clear guidance regarding behavioral expectations and consequences, providing much-needed structure and emphasizing client responsibility for his or her own behavior. It is important to reinforce appropriate behavior to encourage repetition. The unit serves as a microcosm of the client's outside world, so adherence to social norms while on the unit models adherence upon discharge, while providing the client with staff support to learn appropriate coping skills and alternative behaviors.*
- • Increase surveillance of the hospitalized client at smoking, meal, and medication times. **EBN:** *A study of temporal patterns of physical control use (mechanical restraint and locked seclusion) at a state psychiatric hospital revealed that the use of control increased at cli-*

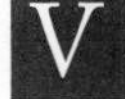

*ents' smoking, meal, and medication times. Increased demands on clients, difficulty adjusting to shifts in activity, close proximity to other clients, or denial of privileges (e.g., smoking) may have accounted for the increases (Vittengl, 2002).*

- Assign a single room to the client with a potential for violence toward others. *The client will be able to take time away from unit stimulation to calm self as needed. Another client will not be placed at risk as a roommate.*
- Maintain a secluded area for the client to be placed when violent. Ensure that staff are continuously present and available to client during seclusion. *The violent client is removed from a potentially overstimulating environment. Violence on a unit can frighten other persons present.* **EBN:** *Clients perceived seclusion to be punishment; however, the main negative effect reported by clients was that seclusion intensified preexisting feelings of exclusion, rejection, abandonment, and isolation. Staff presence is necessary to prevent the harmful effects of social isolation and to honor clients' motivation to connect with staff (Holmes, Kennedy, & Perron, 2004).*
- Maintain a calm attitude in response to the client. *Anxiety is contagious.*
- Provide a low level of stimulation in the client's environment; place the client in a safe, quiet place, and speak slowly and quietly. *A safe, quiet environment that provides structure decreases the outside stimuli that may be precipitating violent behavior (Citrome & Volavka, 1999).*
- Redirect possible violent behaviors into physical activities (e.g., walking, jogging) if the client is physically able. *Using a punching bag or hitting a pillow may not be indicated because they are not calming activities and they continue patterning violent behavior. However, activities that distract while draining excess energy help to build a repertoire of alternative behaviors for stress reduction.*
- Provide sufficient staff if a show of force is necessary to demonstrate control to the client. *When staff responds to an escalating or violent situation, it can reassure clients that they will not be allowed to lose control. On the other hand, leave immediately if the client becomes violent and you are not trained to handle it.*
- Protect other clients in the environment from harm. Remove other individuals from the vicinity of a violent or potentially violent client. Follow safety protocols of the department. *Proper preparation, training, and implementation of strict protocols can save nurses' and others' lives when violence occurs. Others can be injured during a violent outburst; therefore their safety must be considered. The risk of a violent client to others in the area (other clients, visitors) should be anticipated, even as efforts proceed to deescalate the situation with the client.*

▲ Use chemical restraints as ordered. Obtain an order for medication, and administer it immediately. *Medications should be offered before physical restraints or seclusion is considered; the medications used most often are haloperidol (Haldol) and lorazepam (Ativan).*

▲ Use mechanical restraints if ordered and as necessary. *Physical restraint can be therapeutic to keep the client and others safe.*

- Follow institution's protocol for releasing restraints. Observe client closely, remain calm, and provide positive feedback as client's behavior becomes controlled. *The period during which restraints are removed can be dangerous for staff if they do not recognize that the client may choose to reinitiate violence. Protocols will specify safe procedures for removing restraints.*

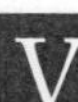

- If restraints are necessary, provide the client with musical tapes and a headset. *Music can provide a distraction from negative thoughts or auditory hallucinations.* **EBN:** *Use of taped music via a headset can decrease negative behaviors. Listening to music of their own choosing may help produce positive behaviors in previously restrained clients (Janelli & Kanski, 1997).*
- Encourage clients to eat a balanced diet instead of junk food. *In clients with a poor dietary history, particularly indigent clients or clients with alcoholism, deficiencies of thiamine and niacin may lead to irritability, disorientation, and paranoia (Harper-Jacques & Reimer, 2002).*
- Form a therapeutic alliance with the client, identifying the source of anger as external to both nurse and client. *The development of a therapeutic relationship before aggressive behavior occurs provides an alternative for working through anger and frustration. Assisting the client to identify a source of anger or frustration that is external to both the nurse and client prevents the need for defensiveness by both and directs energy at solving an external problem.*
- Allow and encourage the client to verbalize feelings either one on one or in a group setting. *When clients' feelings are not addressed, intense emotions can obstruct the ability to consider alternatives to violence (Wright & Leahey, 2000). Violence is a physical manifestation of feelings (e.g., anger, frustration, fear). When clients verbalize their feelings, they are exercising a more appropriate means of expressing feelings and entering into an opportunity to examine the source of those feelings. Clients can then problem solve to determine a more effective way to address the situation.*
- Recognize that anger is generally purposeful and situation dependent. Actively listen to the client; explore the source of the client's anger, and negotiate resolution when possible. *Anger can be a normal response when an individual feels threatened or experiences delay or denial of gratification. Concern arises when anger escalates to the extent that it becomes intimidating or behavioral control may be lost. Conflict resolution before anger is expressed behaviorally is the goal of listening to the individual. A paranoid client who is becoming agitated because he or she believes another client is watching him or her generally calms when encouraged to discuss his or her fears and is reassured that staff will keep him or her safe.*
- Teach healthy ways to express feelings/anger, appropriate gender roles, and how to communicate needs appropriately. *Instruction that expands young men's conceptions of manhood and appropriate gender roles can reduce the likelihood of their engaging in sexually or physically violent behavior (Hong, 2000). Clients may become violent if their perceived needs are thwarted. Instruction that prepares them to express their needs appropriately, while recognizing that others are under no obligation to meet their needs, prepares them to defuse this anger trigger.*
- Help the client identify when anger develops. Have the client keep an anger diary and discuss alternative responses together. Teach cognitive-behavioral techniques. *Clients with anger management difficulties may not be alert to physiological changes or cues that they are becoming angry. They may not be aware of any time delay between the stimulus and their angry response. Instruction in cognitive-behavioral techniques and review of the diary with staff assists clients in identifying thought processes leading to anger and the space between stimulus and response.*

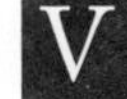

- Identify stimuli that initiate violence and means of dealing with the stimuli. *Assisting the client to identify situations and people that upset him or her provides information needed for problem solving. The client may then identify alternative responses (e.g., leaving the stimulus; using relaxation techniques, such as deep breathing; initiating thought stopping; initiating a distracting activity; responding assertively rather than aggressively).*
- Emphasize that the client is responsible for his or her choices and behavior. Introduce descriptions of possible effects of client's aggressive/violent behavior on others. *In most cases clients are capable of learning to control angry impulses. In many cases clients operate from a worldview that perceives others as instruments of the clients' gratification. A difficult but important insight that clients must gain is that they are dealing with other human beings who experience pain. Clients' behaviors influence how others respond to them.*
- ▲ Always follow up a violent episode with a debriefing of clients and staff. *Allowing discussion of a violent episode, either individually or in a group, among other clients present reveals clients' responses to the event and provides the opportunity for staff to offer reassurance and support. Clients may have concerns that staff will attempt to restrain them without reason or may feel uncertain whether staff can keep them safe. Staff debriefing offers a calming influence while providing the opportunity to evaluate the effectiveness of the reaction to violence and to brainstorm any necessary changes in procedure. Recent evidence has suggested that more extensive psychological debriefing, of the type used for individuals who experience extreme trauma, may not be warranted for all individuals. Providing comfort, support, and information and meeting immediate practical needs is useful; assumptions that global psychological debriefing would prevent subsequent psychopathology (e.g., posttraumatic stress disorder [PTSD]) have not been supported. Intervention beyond the initial screening and psychological first aid should be individualized (Litz et al, 2002).*

## Domestic Violence

NOTE: Before implementation of interventions in the face of domestic violence, nurses should examine their own emotional responses to abuse, their knowledge base about abuse, and systemic elements within the emergency department (ED) to ensure that interventions will be compassionate and appropriate. Particular attention to the influence of domestic violence on children and adolescents is warranted. **EBN:** *A study of two hospital emergency units revealed that stereotypical thinking, a focus on physical problems, and rapid patient turnover obscured treatment of women who were victims of abuse. Nurses frequently did not recognize abuse or reported a range of witnessed scenarios of providers from actively offering choices to doing nothing to attempting to impose solutions on abuse victims. If victims returned to the ER without having implemented the solution, they were seen as undeserving of additional assistance (Varcoe, 2001). The ability of nurses to provide effective care was found to be compromised by a lack of knowledge about the influence of domestic abuse on the mental health of children and adolescents (De Wit & Davis, 2004).*

- Screen for possible abuse in women or children with a pattern of multiple injuries, particularly if any suspicion exists that the physical findings are inconsistent with the explanation of how the injuries were incurred. **EBN:** *A study of women (N = 1313) at five clinics found that 98% believed it was a "good idea" to screen for domestic violence. Of 30 women who found the process uncomfortable, 77% still agreed that it was a good idea to*

*screen (Webster, Stratigos, & Grimes, 2001). A group of women approaching the justice system for domestic violence actions (filing charges, restraining orders) were asked about their last health care visit. Although 86% of the women had health care visits in the previous year, only 24% had been assessed for interpersonal violence. Universal screening for interpersonal violence was urged (Willson et al, 2001).*

▲ Report suspected child abuse to Child Protective Services. Refer women suspected of being in a spouse abuse situation to an area crisis center and provide phone number of area crisis hotline. Rapid screening tools are helpful to identify intimate partner violence. *All nurses are required by law to report suspected child abuse.* **EB:** *A study found that hotline, advocacy, counseling, and shelter services for domestic violence were effective in achieving positive outcomes (Bennett et al, 2004). Screening for battering was demonstrated as an effective tool in this study (Coker et al, 2001).*

• With women who repeatedly experience injuries from domestic violence, maintain a nonjudgmental approach and continue to offer resources/referrals. If the woman voices a willingness to leave her situation, assist with developing an emergency plan that will consider all contingencies possible (e.g., safe location, financial resources, care of children, when to leave safely). *Women in domestic violence situations may change their minds several times before actually leaving. Proactive organization of an emergency plan helps to increase the possibility that women will be able to leave safely. The most dangerous time of a domestic violence situation is when the spouse tries to leave.* **EB:** *Forgiveness of the partner for abusive behavior and willingness to let go of anger has been found to be a more reliable predictor of intention to return to the relationship than severity of violence, attributions regarding violence, or psychological constraints or investments (Gordon, Burton, & Porter, 2004).*

▲ In cases where spouse or child abuse accompanies substance abuse, refer the abusive client to a substance abuse treatment program and refer the spouse receiving abuse to Al-Anon, children to Al-Ateen. *Use of drugs or alcohol decreases impulse control and aggravates abusive behavior.* **EB:** *A study found that marital violence decreased significantly after the husband received substance abuse treatment (Stuart et al, 2003).*

▲ In cases where an adult reveals a history of unresolved/untreated sexual abuse as a child, referral to a local Adults Molested as Children (AMAC) group may be helpful. **EB:** *Childhood sexual abuse has been associated with adult depression, attempted suicide, self-harm, and higher risk for later interpersonal violence (Gladstone et al, 2004). Interventions tailored to the AMAC experience may be helpful. Refer to care plans for* **Risk for Suicide, Self-mutilation**, and **Risk for Self-mutilation**.

▲ In dealing with abused wives, maintain a nonjudgmental response when clients return to husbands or refuse to leave them. *An estimated 90%–95% of abused partners are women battered by men (Sisley et al, 1999). Reasons for remaining in or returning to the relationship include economic concerns (especially with children), socialization about the women's role, political or legal obstacles, traumatic bonding that leaves the woman feeling powerless, and realistic fear of retaliation or death (Boyd & Mackey, 2000; Wallace, 1999).* **EB:** *A study found that interventions with victims of domestic violence that focus on dysphoria, hopelessness, or self-esteem are unlikely to be effective unless issues of perceived control and coping are also addressed (Clements, Sabourin, & Spiby, 2004). Refer to care plan for* **Powerlessness.**

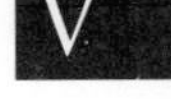

- • Women with physical or mental disabilities require extended assessment if abuse is suspected or present to determine unique ways in which they may experience abuse. In addition to an assessment of the usual power and control concerns, a comprehensive functional assessment should be conducted along with attention to cultural issues and the nature of the disability. *Women with disabilities are abused at rates equal to or greater than nondisabled women. Functional limitations rather than diagnosis provide important information regarding the risk of abuse and its triggers (e.g., the woman's inability to perform certain household functions) (Gilson, DePoy, & Cramer, 2001).*
- ▲ Women with disabilities who experience abuse may require referral to disability service providers, along with domestic violence services. **EB:** *A study of services used by disabled women in abusive situations noted the need for collaboration to ensure that the women's unique needs are met (Chang et al, 2003).*
- ▲ Women with disabilities may experience abuse from multiple sources, and may have fewer resources and options to draw on. Particular attention should be paid to needs for resource referrals and the additional emotional stresses for these women. **EBN:** *The limitations of disabilities can mean that women cannot leave the home situation without much difficulty; shelters may not be prepared to accommodate the disabilities; and nursing home placement may be an undesirable option (Curry, Hassouneh-Phillips, & Johnston-Silverberg, 2001). Women with disabilities may be vulnerable to abuse from any caregiver delivering care, including personal-assistance providers. Themes expressed by women with disabilities included (1) confusion of social and personal boundaries (e.g., intrusiveness into client's personal business); (2) challenging power dynamics (e.g., client as employer but dependent upon assistance); (3) additional forms of abuse (e.g., financial, neglectful); (4) inability of client to confront abusive behavior (fear of retaliation, potential loss of care provider) (Saxton et al, 2001).*
- ▲ In cases of potential child abuse, refer the parent to parenting classes or a parental counseling support group. *Early intervention may prevent abuse from occurring. Young parents in particular may have difficulty dealing with the stresses of parenthood combined with other life stresses; sharing their concerns with others can help normalize the stress. Support from others can help prevent the need to displace anger and frustration onto the child.*

## Social Violence

- ▲ Assess the support network of women who become victims of violent crime and refer for appropriate levels of assistance. **EB:** *In a national study of female crime victims, three help-seeking strategies were identified: (1) minimal or no help seeking, (2) family and friend help seeking, and (3) substantial help seeking (from family, friends, psychiatrists, social service providers, and police) (Kaukinen, 2004). Of particular concern would be women who do not have family or friends to provide support or who have difficulty accessing other types of assistance.*
- • Be aware that hate crime is increasing, particularly toward transgendered individuals, and it requires support and advocacy for victims. *The growth of hate crimes toward transgendered individuals has been noted, and more research is needed to understand the influence of hate crimes on gay males (Thomas, 2004; Willis, 2004).*

- ▲ Victims of violence seen in the ED should receive an assessment for needed services and assignment to case management. Establishment of linkages with social service agencies can provide important services for referral. **EB:** *An ED study provided linkages with internal services providing such services as primary care, gang-related tattoo removal, psychiatric services, substance abuse treatment, and dental care; and with a social service agency providing such services as programs in personal development and education, comprehensive employment preparation, computer skills, and others. Outside agencies were also used for legal assistance, spiritual counseling, GED classes, and financial assistance. A random assignment of victims of interpersonal violence aged 10–24 years seen for treatment were enrolled in the study. With case management initiated in the ED as the key element, the number of resources used by young victims of interpersonal violence as compared with controls was significantly increased (Zun, Downey, & Rosen, 2003).*

## Pediatric

- • Assess for dating violence among adolescent girls. Additional assessments may be required for sexually transmitted diseases and pregnancy. **EB:** *Dating violence has been found to be prevalent among U.S. adolescent girls. Adolescent girls who have been intentionally hurt by a date in the previous year were found to be more likely to experience sexual health risks and pregnancy (Silverman, Raj, & Clements, 2004). A high rate of dating violence by both male and female university students has been found worldwide (Straus, 2004).*
- • Pregnant teens should be assessed for abuse, particularly if they are with an older partner. **EBN:** *In a study of predominantly African-American pregnant teens, 13% reported domestic violence during pregnancy. Teens with adult partners (4 or more years older) were twice as likely to report abuse as teens with similar age partners (Harner, 2004).*
- ▲ When physical abuse by parents is present, parent-child interaction therapy (PCIT) may be helpful. **EB:** *PCIT is an empirically supported treatment that has been shown to reduce abuse (Chaffin et al, 2004; Chambless & Ollendick, 2000).*
- ▲ In the case of child abuse or neglect, refer for early childhood home visitation. **EB:** *Home visits during a child's first 2 years of life have been found to be effective in preventing child abuse and neglect (Hahn et al, 2003).*

## Geriatric

- • Be alert to the potential for elder abuse in clients. *Although awareness of elder abuse has increased, sufficient attention is still not paid to this concern. Only the most severe cases are reported (Gordon & Brill, 2001). Abuse may occur along a continuum, from neglect to physical or sexual abuse. Family and strangers may commit financial exploitation. Look for signs of bruising, malnutrition, and fearful responses to or around caregivers.*
- • Assess for changes in physiological functions (e.g., constipation, dehydration) or impairment of the ability to meet basic needs (e.g., inadequate toileting, decreased mobility). *In older adults subtle physiological changes can lead to observable changes in behavior, including agitation. Interruptions of or changes in routine can unsettle the older adult and be expressed as frustration or anger. Fears about medical disorders or potential loss of independence can be transformed into anger, irritability, or agitation.* **EB:** *Agitation in nursing home patients was found to be predicted independently by cognitive impairment, vi-*

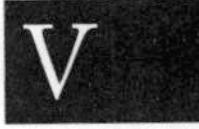

• = Independent; ▲ = Collaborative; EBN = Evidence-Based Nursing; EB = Evidence-Based

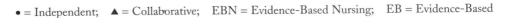

*sion and hearing impairment, and gender. Individuals with significant hearing impairment were more likely to become agitated than less impaired individuals (Vance et al, 2003).*

- • Observe for dementia and delirium. *Clients with dementia or delirium may strike out if they are frustrated or if they have the sense that their personal space is being violated. However, this may not occur within a cognitive capacity that permits discussion of the behavior.*
- • Assess sensory impairments and the influence they may have on the client's behavior. *Agitation and striking out may be precipitated in older adults who are experiencing either sensory impairment or difficulty communicating (Allen, 1999).*
- • Observe for signs of fear, anxiety, anger, and agitation, and intervene immediately. *Gerontology nurses can prevent the incidence of assault by recognizing the potential risks, preventing clients' fear and anxiety, reducing the outburst of anger, and decreasing clients' agitation (Chou, Kaas, & Richie, 1996).*
- ▲ Monitor for paradoxical drug reactions, and report any to the physician. *Violent behavior can be stimulated by a medication intended to calm the client.*
- ▲ Assess for brain insults such as recent falls or injuries, strokes, or transient ischemic attacks. *Clients with brain injuries need specific interventions such as stimulus control, problem solving, social skills training, relaxation training, and anger management to reduce aggressive behaviors (Teichner, Golden, & Giannaris, 1999). Maintenance of a structured environment limits confusing external stimuli. Brain injuries, which are related to ambivalence, lowered impulse control, and reduced coping, can cause violent reactions to self or others. Brain injury symptoms may be mistaken for mental illness.*
- • Decrease environmental stimuli if violence is directed at others. *Removal of the client to a quiet area can reduce violent impulses. Use a calm voice to "talk down" the client.*
- • Provide hand or back rubs and calming music when elderly client experiences agitation. **EBN:** *In a study of older adults in nursing homes, calming music, and hand massage were found to soothe agitation for up to 1 hour. No additional benefit was found from combining the two interventions (Remington, 2002).*
- ▲ If abuse or neglect of an elderly client is suspected, report the suspicion to a local Adult Protective Services agency. *The telephone number for the Adult Protective Services office can be found by checking the blue governmental section of the phone book or by calling directory assistance and asking for the department of social services or aging services. It is essential to call the office with jurisdiction over the geographical area where the client lives.*

## Home Care

- • Be alert to the potential for violent behavior in the home setting. Respond to verbal aggression with interventions to deescalate negative emotional states. *Violence is a process that can be recognized early. Deescalation involves reducing client stressors, responding to the client with respect, acknowledging the client's feeling state, and assisting the client to regain control. If deescalation does not work, the nurse should leave the home (Distasio, 2000).* **EB:** *Verbal aggression was shown to be a predictor of negative psychological outcomes (Bussing & Hoge, 2004).*
- • Assess family members or caregivers for their ability to protect the client and themselves. *The safety of the client between home visits is a nursing priority. Caregivers often need assistance with recognizing or admitting fear of or danger from a loved one.*

- Include an initial and ongoing assessment and evaluation of potential abuse and neglect. Photograph evidence of abuse or neglect when possible. *Victims of abuse perceive themselves to be powerless to change the situation. Indeed, the abuser fosters this perception and may threaten violence or death if the victim attempts to leave. Chronic abuse and neglect by a spouse or other family among the elderly is often hidden until home care is actively involved. Refer to the care plan for* **Powerlessness.**
- ▲ If neglect or abuse is suspected, identify an emergency plan that addresses the problem immediately, ensures client safety, and includes a report to the appropriate authorities. Discuss when to use hotlines and 911. Role play access to emergency resources with the client and caregivers. *Client safety is a nursing priority. An emergency plan should address either immediate removal to a safe environment or identification of appropriate steps to take in the event of abuse and the securing of resources for the anticipated action (e.g., available phone, packed bag, alternative living arrangements). Reporting is a legal requirement of health care workers.*
- Encourage appropriate safety behaviors in abused women; call the client at intervals during a 6-month period to determine whether safety behaviors are being carried out. **EBN:** *A study of telephone contacts to women who sought help through the district attorney's office demonstrated that safety behaviors increased dramatically. Safety behaviors included hiding money; hiding an extra set of house and car keys; establishing a code for abuse occurrence with family or friends; asking neighbors to call police if violence occurred; removing weapons; keeping available family social security numbers, rent and utility receipts, family birth certificates, identification or drivers licenses, bank account numbers, insurance policies and numbers, marriage license, valuable jewelry, important phone numbers, and a hidden bag with extra clothing (McFarlane et al, 2002).*
- Assess the home environment for harmful objects. Have the family remove or lock objects as able. *The safety of the client and caregivers is a nursing priority.*
- ▲ Refer for homemaker or psychiatric home health care services for respite, client reassurance, and implementation of a therapeutic regimen. *Responsibility for a person who may become violent provides high caregiver stress. Respite decreases caregiver stress. The presence of caring individuals is reassuring to both the client and caregivers, especially during periods of client anxiety. Violent behaviors can respond to the interventions described previously, modified for the home setting.*
- ▲ If the client is taking psychotropic medications, assess client and family knowledge of medication and its administration and side effects. Teach as necessary. *Knowledge of the medical regimen supports compliance.*
- ▲ Evaluate effectiveness and side effects of medications. *Accurate clinical feedback improves physician ability to prescribe an effective medical regimen specific to client needs.*
- If client displays mildly intensifying aggressive behavior, attempt to diffuse anger or violence (e.g., ask for a glass of water to distract client). Later in the visit explain that aggressive behavior is not acceptable and present consequences of continued aggressive behavior (i.e., right of agency to discontinue services). *Mild aggression can be diffused safely. Confronting the client before severe aggression is evident places responsibility on the client and family for respectful partnership in care.*
- Document all acts or verbalizations of aggression. *Safety of the staff is a primary responsibility of home health agencies. Law enforcement intervention may be necessary.*

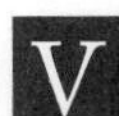

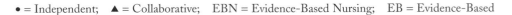

- ▲ If client verbalizes or displays threatening behavior, notify supervisor and plan to make joint visits with another staff person or a security escort. *Having a second person at the visit is a show of power and control used to subdue aggressive behavior.*
- ▲ If the client behaves in such a manner as to make the nurse uncomfortable without overt threat, a meeting may be held outside the home in sight of others (e.g., front porch). *The nurse should trust a "gut" reaction that prompts concern regarding the client's potential for aggressive or violent behavior. Such intuitive reactions are often the result of subliminal cues that are not readily voiced.*
- ▲ Never enter a home or remain in a home if aggression threatens your well-being.
- ▲ Never challenge a show of force such as a gun threat. Leave and notify your supervisor and the appropriate authorities. Document the incident. *Safety of the staff is a primary responsibility of home health agencies. Law enforcement intervention may be necessary.*
- ▲ If client behaviors intensify, refer for immediate mental health intervention. *The degree of disturbance and ability to manage care safely at home determines the level of services needed to protect the client.*

## Client/Family Teaching

- • Teach relaxation and exercise as ways to release anger.
- • Teach cognitive-behavioral activities such as active problem solving, reframing (reappraising the situation from a different perspective), or thought stopping (in response to a negative thought, picture a large stop sign and replace the image with a prearranged positive alternative). Teach the client to confront his or her own negative thought patterns (or cognitive distortions) such as catastrophizing (expecting the very worst), dichotomous thinking (perceiving events in only one of two opposite categories), magnification (placing distorted emphasis on a single event), or unrealistic expectations (e.g., "I should get what I want when I want it."). *Aggressive clients often have negative, even paranoid, perceptions of others and unrealistic expectations of how they should be treated, leading to their anger. The client may or may not be capable of empathy for others. Cognitive-behavioral activities address clients' assumptions, beliefs, and attitudes about their situations, fostering modification of these elements to be as realistic as possible. Through cognitive-behavioral interventions, clients become more aware of their cognitive choices in adopting and maintaining their belief systems, thereby exercising greater control over their own reactions (Hagerty & Patusky, 2003; Sinclair et al, 1998).*
- • For religious couples, encourage the use of prayer. *Prayer may invoke a couple-God system, which significantly influences couple interaction during conflict. Prayer appears to be a significant "softening" event for religious couples, facilitating reconciliation and problem solving. It deescalates hostile emotions and reduces emotional reactivity (Butler, Gardner, & Bird, 1998).*

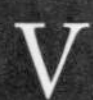

- ▲ Refer to individual or group therapy.
- • Teach the adolescent client violence prevention and encourage him or her to become involved in community service activities. *School programs that couple community service with classroom health instruction can have a measurable effect on violent behaviors of young adolescents at high risk for being both the perpetrators and victims of peer violence. Community service programs may be an effective supplement to curricular interven-*

*tions and a valuable component of multicomponent violence-prevention programs (O'Donnell et al, 1999).*

- • Teach caregivers and family members of clients with dementia to use expressive physical touch and verbalization (EPT/V) when caring for these clients. **EBN:** *One study found that (1) anxiety is lower immediately after EPT/V, and (2) EPT/V causes decreasing episodes of dysfunctional behavior. It is cost-effective and simple to learn and practice, and it is most effective in improving and maintaining a client's high quality of life (Kim & Buschmann, 1999).*
- ▲ Teach the use of appropriate community resources in emergency situations (e.g., hotline, community mental health agency, ED, 911 in most places in the United States, the toll-free National Domestic Violence Hotline [1-800-799-SAFE]). *Internet resources are increasing and should be made available to clients (Hopkins et al, 2003). It is necessary to get immediate help when violence occurs.*
- ▲ Encourage the use of self-help groups in nonemergency situations.
- ▲ Inform the client and family about medication actions, side effects, target symptoms, and toxic reactions.

## evolve WEBSITES FOR EDUCATION

See the EVOLVE website for World Wide Web resources for client education.

## REFERENCES


Abderhalden C, Needham I, Miserez B et al: Predicting inpatient violence in acute psychiatric wards using the Broset violence checklist: a multicenter prospective cohort study, *J Psychiatr Men Health Nurs* 11(4):422, 2004.

Allen LA: Treating agitation without drugs, *Am J Nurs* 99(4):36, 1999.

Bennett L, Riger S, Schewe P et al: Effectiveness of hotline, advocacy, counseling, and shelter services for victims of domestic violence, *J Interpers Violence* 19(7):815, 2004.

Boyd MR, Mackey M: Alienation from self and others: the psychosocial problem of rural alcoholic women, *Arch Psychiatr Nurs* 14:134, 2000.

Bussing A, Hoge T: Aggression and violence against home care workers, *J Occup Health Psychol* 9(3):206, 2004.

Butler MH, Gardner BC, Bird MH: Not just a time-out: change dynamics of prayer for religious couples in conflict situations, *Fam Process* 37(4):451, 1998.

Chaffin M, Silovsky JF, Funderburk B et al: Parent-child interaction therapy with physically abusive parents: efficacy for reducing future abuse reports, *J Consult Clin Psychol* 72(3):500, 2004.

Chambless DL, Ollendick TH: Empirically supported psychological interventions: controversies and evidence, *Ann Rev Psychol* 52:685, 2000.

Chang JC, Martin SL, Moracco KE et al: Helping women with disabilities and domestic violence: strategies, limitations, and challenges of domestic violence programs and services, *J Womens Health* 12(7):699, 2003.

Chou K, Kaas M, Richie M: Assaultive behavior in geriatric patients, *J Gerontol Nurs* 22(11):30, 1996.

Citrome L, Volavka J: Violent patients in the emergency setting, *Psychiatr Clin North Am* 22(4):789, 1999.

Clements CM, Sabourin CM, Spiby L: Dysphoria and hopelessness following battering: the role of perceived control, coping, and self-esteem, *J Fam Violence* 19(1):25, 2004.

Coker AL, Pope BO, Smith PH et al: Assessment of clinical partner violence screening tools, *J Am Med Womens Assoc* 56(1):19, 2001.

Curry MA, Hassouneh-Phillips D, Johnston-Silverberg A: Abuse of women with disabilities: an ecological model and review, *Violence Against Women* 7(1):60, 2001.

De Wit K, Davis K: Nurses' knowledge and learning experiences in relation to the effects of domestic abuse on the mental health of children and adolescents, *Contemp Nurs* 16(3):214, 2004.


V

Distasio CA: Violence against home care providers. Stop it before it starts, *Caring* 19(10):14, 2000.
Duncan S, Estabrookes CA, Reimer M: Violence against nurses, *Alberta RN* 56(2):13, 2000.
Gilson SF, DePoy E, Cramer EP: Linking the assessment of self-reported functional capacity with abuse experiences of women with disabilities, *Violence Against Women* 7(4):418, 2001.
Gladstone GL, Parker GB, Mitchell PB et al: Implications of childhood trauma for depressed women: an analysis of pathways from childhood sexual abuse to deliberate self-harm and revictimization, *Am J Psychiatry* 161(8):1417, 2004.
Gordon KC, Burton S, Porter L: Predicting the intentions of women in domestic violence shelters to return to partners: does forgiveness play a role? *J Fam Psychol* 18(2):331, 2004.
Gordon RM, Brill D: The abuse and neglect of the elderly, *Intl J Law Psychiatry* 24:183, 2001.
Graham P: Understanding and dealing with anger, aggression and violence, *Nurs Stand* 16:37, 2001.
Hagerty B, Patusky K: Mood disorders: depression and mania. In Fortinash KM, Holoday-Worret PA, editors: *Psychiatric mental health nursing,* ed 3, St Louis, 2003, Mosby.
Hahn RA, Bilukha OO, Crosby A et al: First reports evaluating the effectiveness of strategies for preventing violence: early childhood home visitation, *MMWR Recomm Rep* 52(RR-14):1, 2003.
Harner HM: Domestic violence and trauma care in teenage pregnancy: does paternal age make a difference? *J Obstet Gynecol Neonatal Nurs* 33(3):312, 2004.
Harper-Jacques S, Reimer M: Management of aggression. In Boyd MA, editor: *Psychiatric nursing. Contemporary practice,* ed 2, Philadelphia, 2002, Lippincott.
Holmes D, Kennedy SL, Perron A: The mentally ill and social exclusion: a critical examination of the use of seclusion from the patient's perspective, *Issues Ment Health Nurs* 25:559, 2004.
Hong L: Toward a transformed approach to prevention: breaking the link between masculinity and violence, *J Am Coll Health* 48(6):269, 2000.
Hopkins K, Sleet DA, Mickalide A et al: Internet resources for injury and violence prevention, *Am J Health Educ Supplement* 34(5): S-62, 2003.
Janelli LM, Kanski GW: Music intervention with physically restrained patients, *Rehabil Nurs* 22(1):14, 1997.
Kaukinen C: The help-seeking strategies of female violent crime victims, *J Interpers Violence* 19(9):967, 2004.
Kim EJ, Buschmann MT: The effect of expressive physical touch on patients with dementia, *Int J Nurs Stud* 36(3):235, 1999.
Lanza ML, Kayne HL, Pattison I et al: The relationship of behavioral cues to assaultive behavior, *Clin Nurs Res* 5(1):6, 1996.
Litz BT, Gray MJ, Bryant RA et al: Early intervention for trauma: current status and future directions, *Clin Psychol Sci Pract* 9(2): 112, 2002.
Liu J: Concept analysis: aggression, *Issues Ment Health Nurs* 25:693, 2004.
McFarlane J, Malecha A, Gist J et al: An intervention to increase safety behaviors of abused women: results of a randomized clinical trial, *Nurs Res* 51:347, 2002.
McNeil DE, Eisner JP, Binder RL: The relationship between command hallucinations and violence, *Psychiatr Serv* 51(10):1288, 2000.
Needham I, Abderhalden C, Meer R et al: The effectiveness of two interventions in the management of patient violence in acute mental inpatient settings: report on a pilot study, *J Psychiatr Ment Health Nurs* 11(5):595, 2004.
O'Donnell L, Stueve A, San Doval A et al: Violence prevention and young adolescents' participation in community youth service, *J Adolesc Health* 24(1):28, 1999.
Remington R: Calming music and hand massage with agitated elderly, *Nurs Res* 51:317, 2002.
Saxton M, Curry MA, Powers L et al: "Bring my scooter so I can leave you": a study of disabled women handling abuse by personal assistance providers, *Violence Against Women* 7(4):393, 2001.
Silverman JG, Raj A, Clements K: Dating violence and associated sexual risk and pregnancy among adolescent girls in the United States, *Pediatrics* 114(2):220, 2004.
Sinclair VG, Wallston KA, Dwyer KA et al: Effects of a cognitive-behavioral intervention for women with rheumatoid arthritis, *Res Nurs Health* 21:315, 1998.
Sisley A, Jacobs LM, Poole G et al: Violence in America: a public health crisis—domestic violence, *J Trauma* 46:1105, 1999.
Soliman AE, Reza H: Risk factors and correlates of violence among acutely ill adult psychiatric inpatients, *Psychiatr Serv* 52(1):75, 2001.
Straus MA: Prevalence of violence against dating partners by male and female university students worldwide, *Violence Against Women* 10(7):790, 2004.
Stuart GL, Ramsey SE, Moore TM et al: Reductions in marital violence following treatment for alcohol dependence, *J Interpers Violence* 18(10):1113, 2003.

Teichner G, Golden CJ, Giannaris WJ: A multimodal approach to treatment of aggression in a severely brain-injured adolescent, *Rehabil Nurs* 24(5):207, 1999.
Thomas SP: Rising violence against transgendered individuals (editorial), *Issues Ment Health Nurs* 25:557, 2004.
Vance DE, Burgio LD, Roth DL et al: Predictors of agitation in nursing home residents, *J Gerontol* 58B(2):P129, 2003.
Varcoe C: Abuse obscured: an ethnographic account of emergency nursing in relation to violence against women, *Can J Nurs Res* 32(4):95, 2001.
Vittengl JR: Temporal regularities in physical control at a state psychiatric hospital, *Arch Psychiatr Nurs* 16:80, 2002.
Wallace H: *Family violence: legal, medical, and social perspectives,* ed 2, Boston, 1999, Allyn & Bacon.
Webster J, Stratigos SM, Grimes KM: Women's responses to screening for domestic violence in a health-care setting, *Midwifery* 17:289, 2001.
Willis D: Hate crimes against gay males: an overview, *Issues Ment Health Nurs* 25:115, 2004.
Willson P, Cesario S, Fredland N et al: Primary healthcare provider's lost opportunity to help abused women, *J Am Acad Nurs Pract* 13(12):565, 2001.
Wright LM, Leahey M: *Nurses and families: a guide to family assessment and intervention,* ed 3, Philadelphia, 2000, FA Davis.
Zun LS, Downey LV, Rosen J: Violence prevention in the ED: linkage of the ED to a social service agency, *Am J Emerg Med* 21(6):454, 2003.

# Risk for self-directed Violence

*Kathleen L. Patusky*

**NANDA**

## Definition

At risk for behaviors in which an individual demonstrates that he or she can be physically, emotionally, and/or sexually harmful to self

## Risk Factors

Body language: rigid posture, clenching of fists and jaw, hyperactivity, pacing, breathlessness, threatening stances; history of violence against others (e.g., hitting someone, kicking someone, spitting at someone, scratching someone, throwing objects at someone, biting someone, attempted rape, rape, sexual molestation, urinating/defecating on someone); history of threats of violence (e.g., verbal threats against property, verbal threats against person, social threats, cursing, threatening notes/letters, threatening gestures, sexual threats); history of violent antisocial behavior (e.g., stealing, insistent borrowing, insistent demanding of privileges, insistent interrupting of meetings, refusing to eat, refusing to take medication, ignoring instructions); history of violence, indirect (e.g., tear-

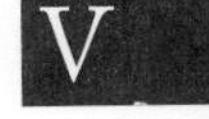

ing off clothes, ripping objects off walls, writing on walls, urinating on floor, defecating on floor, stamping feet, displaying temper tantrum, running in corridors, yelling, throwing objects, breaking a window, slamming doors, making sexual advances); neurological impairment (e.g., positive EEG, CAT, or MRI; head trauma; positive neurological findings; seizure disorders); cognitive impairment (e.g., learning disabilities, attention deficit disorder, decreased intellectual functioning); history of childhood abuse; history of witnessing family violence; cruelty to animals; fire setting; prenatal/perinatal complications or abnormalities; history of drug or alcohol abuse; pathological intoxication; psychotic symptomatology (e.g., auditory, visual, command hallucinations; paranoid delusions; loose, rambling, or illogical thought processes); motor vehicle offenses (e.g., frequent traffic violations, use of a motor vehicle to release anger); suicidal behavior; impulsivity; availability/possession of weapon(s)

**NOC**

## Outcomes (Nursing Outcomes Classification)

### Suggested NOC Outcomes

Depression Self-Control, Distorted Thought Self-Control, Impulse Self-Control, Loneliness Severity, Mood Equilibrium, Risk Detection, Self-Mutilation Restraint, Suicide Self-Restraint

**Example NOC Outcome with Indicators**

**Suicide Self-Restraint** as evidenced by the following indicators: Expresses feelings and seeks help when feeling self-destructive/Verbalizes and controls suicidal ideas and impulses (Rate each indicator of **Suicide Self-Restraint:** 1 = never demonstrated, 2 = rarely demonstrated, 3 = sometimes demonstrated, 4 = often demonstrated, 5 = consistently demonstrated [see Section I].)

## Client Outcomes

### Client Will (Specify Time Frame):

- Refrain from self-injury
- State appropriate ways to cope with increased psychological or physiological tension
- Talk about feelings; express anger appropriately
- Seek help when feeling self-destructive or having urges to self-mutilate
- Maintain self-control without supervision
- Use appropriate community agencies when caregivers are unable to attend to emotional needs
- Maintain connectedness in relationships
- Express decreased anxiety and control of impulses
- Refrain from using mood-altering substances
- Obtain no access to harmful objects
- Yield access to harmful objects
- Maintain self-control without supervision

## NIC

### Interventions (Nursing Interventions Classification)

#### Suggested NIC Interventions

Anger Control Assistance; Anxiety Reduction; Behavior Management: Self-Harm; Calming Technique; Coping Enhancement; Crisis Intervention; Mood Management; Substance Use Prevention; Suicide Prevention; Surveillance

**Example NIC Activities—Suicide Prevention**

Determine presence and degree of suicide risk; encourage client to seek out care providers to talk as urge to harm self occurs

### Nursing Interventions and Rationales

- Refer to care plan for **Risk for Suicide.**
- Refer to care plans for **Self-mutilation** and **Risk for Self-mutilation.**

# Impaired Walking

*Brenda Emick-Herring*

## NANDA

### Definition

Limitation of independent movement within the environment on foot (or artificial limb)

### Defining Characteristics

Impaired ability to climb stairs, walk on uneven surface, walk required distances, walk on even surfaces, walk on an incline or decline, navigate curbs

### Related Factors (r/t)

Intolerance to activity, decreased strength and endurance, pain or discomfort, perceptual or cognitive impairment, neuromuscular impairment, musculoskeletal impairment, depression, severe anxiety

NOTE: These are the same as the etiologies for **Impaired physical Mobility** with the addition of lower extremity amputation.

Suggested functional level classifications follow:
0—Completely independent
1—Requires use of equipment or device
2—Requires help from another person for assistance, supervision, or teaching
3—Requires help from another person and equipment device
4—Dependent (does not participate in activity)

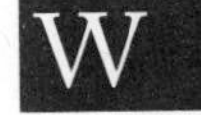

**NOC**

## Outcomes (Nursing Outcomes Classification)

### Suggested NOC Outcomes

Ambulation; Mobility

**Example NOC Outcome with Indicators**

**Ambulation** as evidenced by the following indicators: Walks with effective gait/Walks at moderate pace/Walks up and down steps/Walks moderate distance (Rate each indicator of **Ambulation:** 1 = severely compromised, 2 = substantially compromised, 3 = moderately compromised, 4 = mildly compromised, 5 = not compromised [see Section I].)

## Client Outcomes/Goals

**Client Will (Specify Time Frame):**

- Demonstrate optimal independence and safety in walking
- Demonstrate the ability to direct others on how to assist with walking
- Demonstrate the ability to properly and safely use and care for assistive walking devices

**NIC**

## Interventions (Nursing Interventions Classification)

### Suggested NIC Intervention

Exercise Therapy: Ambulation

**Example NIC Activities—Exercise Therapy: Ambulation**

Assist client to use footwear that facilitates walking and prevents injury; encourage client to sit in bed, on side of bed ("dangle"), or in chair, as tolerated

## Nursing Interventions and Rationales

▲ Reinforce or request physical therapy (PT) consult to teach "bridging" (lifting the hips up); have client use the technique to move side to side in bed and to raise buttocks off bed. *This activity prepares a person for walking because it involves hip extension with simultaneous weight bearing through the lower extremity. It is particularly helpful for hemiplegics (Bobath, 1978; Gee & Passarella, 1985).*

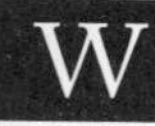


▲ Explain progressive mobilization (gradual elevation of head of bed, tilt table, reclined chair, sitting, standing, and so on) to immobilized clients. *Helps clients adapt to upright position changes. The tilt table incrementally allows passive standing in physical therapy (PT); cardiopulmonary assessment is critical while on it (Hoeman, 2002).*

• Apply antiembolic stockings, elastic wraps, and abdominal binders; raise head of bed in small increments, teach client to sit up and change positions slowly and sit on the

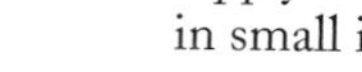

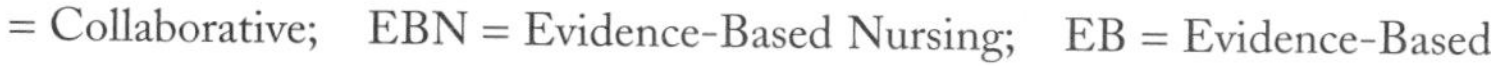

edge of the bed a few minutes before standing to prevent orthostatic hypotension. *Promotes circulatory redistribution to prevent blood frompooling in the legs (Halm, 2001; Irvin & White, 2004).*

- ▲ If suspected, monitor for orthostatic hypotension by comparing lying, sitting, and standing blood pressures and pulse. If systolic blood pressure falls 20 mm Hg or diastolic pressure decreases 10 mm Hg from lying to standing position within three minutes, and/or if light headedness, weakness, syncope, or unexplained falls occur, consult physician (Bradley & Davis, 2003; Irvin & White, 2004). *Detection is key to fall prevention. If blood pressure falls and pulse increases upon arising, adjustment of medications, especially antihypertensives, and psychotropics, may be needed (Irvin & White, 2004).* **EB:** *Medical research found persons with orthostatic hypotension are commonly symptomatic and experience postprandial (after meal) hypotension and heart rate variability (Ejaz et al, 2004).*
- ▲ Administer oral water and medications as prescribed by physician to treat orthostatic hypotension. *Water tends to have a pressor effect in those with autonomic orthostatic hypotension (Shannon et al, 2002).* **EB:** *Results from a small study of seated persons with severe orthostatic and postprandial hypotension indicated that rapid oral ingestion of 500 mL of water raised blood pressure (Shannon et al, 2002).*
- • Place clients supine and elevate legs to oppose postprandial syncope. *Allows for cerebral reperfusion (Sherman, 2003).*
- ▲ Employ prophylaxis for deep vein thrombosis (DVT) and pulmonary emboli (PE) in clients with prolonged immobility, recent lower extremity or major surgery, stroke, and in the aged (Aronow, 2004). Refer to care plan for **Ineffective Tissue perfusion.**
- • Vigilantly apply antiembolic or elastic stockings and intermittent pneumatic compression devices on persons at risk for DVT and PE (Aronow, 2004; Proctor & Greenfield, 2001).
- ▲ Follow physician orders for activity and ambulation in persons diagnosed with DVT and PE since early ambulation versus bed rest may be recommended. *Authors summarized a literature search of five clinical trials on when to ambulate clients with DVT: They suggested early ambulation (24 to 48 hours after anticoagulants are started) is safe in those who have ". . . adequate cardiopulmonary reserve and no evidence of PE" (Aldrich & Hunt, 2004, p 272 ).*
- ▲ Remind clients of physician's orders for weight-bearing limitations during walking (e.g., non–weight bearing on left foot). *Weight bearing may retard bone healing in fractured extremities.*
- ▲ As weight-bearing resumes after prolonged bed-rest, teach clients to ingest protein, avoid nonsteroidal anti-inflammatory drugs (NSAIDs) for 7 days, prevent exposure to infections, and realize that depression is possible. *Protein is needed for muscle repair. NSAIDs may delay muscle recovery. Soreness is from release of prostaglandins and kinins that occurs with muscle damage. Depression relates to short-term soreness and fatigue (St. Pierre & Flaskerud, 1995).* **EBN:** *Animal studies showed that muscle fiber damage occurred with non–weight bearing (e.g., macrophages increased, and myofiber changes occurred through the seventh day of recovery) (St. Pierre & Tidball, 1994).*
- • Encourage patients to stand and walk frequently. *Weight bearing and skeletal muscle*

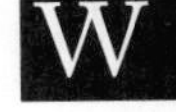

*contraction stimulate bone growth and calcium resorption, thus helping maintain bone density; it prevents disuse osteoporosis and increases oxygen-carrying capacity (International Food Information Council Foundation, 2002; Sims & Olson, 2002).* **EB:** *The risk of hip fracture was reduced 20% to 40% in elders who were physically active (Gregg, Pereira, & Casperson, 2000). Micro-computed tomography imaging of bone suggests antiresorptive medications affect the arrangement and quality (not just strength) of bone to prevent osteoporosis (Boone et al, 2004).*

- • Assist clients to properly apply orthoses, immobilizers, splints, and braces before walking. *Devices maintain joint stability, immobilization, and alignment during out-of-bed movement (Hoeman, 2002).*
- • Teach clients with leg amputations to correctly don sheath, stump socks, liner, and prosthesis before walking. *Prostheses increase functional ability to walk and cosmetically look similar to limbs. A thin nylon sheath prevents the limb from turning in the socket of the prosthesis. Stump socks establish a proper fit between limb and socket. A liner is donned last, before applying the prosthesis. The stump should not touch the bottom of the socket because a pressure ulcer may form (Kipnis, 1993; Yeltzer, 1998).*
- ▲ Use individualized assistive devices (as recommended by PT) when walking a client, including gait belts, walkers, crutches, and canes. *Snug gait belts provide a safe surface for staff to grasp to steady a client as long as the client is close to staff. Devices give support and help compensate for poor balance, coordination, and weakness (Minor & Minor, 1999).* **EBN:** *Use of a gait belt decreased staff exertion, back stress, and compressive force from L5 to S1 of the spine (Owen & Garg, 1993).* **EB:** *Study results suggested that elderly living in a residential facility with high activity and use of a walking aid had less falls (Graafmans et al, 2003). Two-wheeled walkers allowed persons with lower limb amputations who wore prosthetics, to walk more quickly and halt less often than did four-footed walkers (Tsai et al, 2003). Walkers slowed walking speed of persons with Parkinson's and did not decrease freezing time; authors concluded a wheeled vs. standard walker was preferred (Cubo et al, 2003).*
- • Obtain the appropriate number of assistants to walk clients. One team member should give short, simple instructions (e.g., ask client to raise the head, and so on). *Adequate helpers prevent falls and lessen client fear and anxiety, which can cause hypertonicity (Gee & Passarella, 1985). One spokesperson giving directions prevents confusion and mixed messages. Walking requires concentration, visualization, and thinking, especially if the client is learning new information.* **EB:** *Researchers found that stroke survivors who engaged in a verbal cognitive task as they walked had poorer balance and gait velocity (Bowen et al, 2001). Study results indicated elderly subjects lost balance and swayed as they stood when an auditory task was introduced, especially when sensory cues were removed (Shumway-Cook & Woollacott, 2000).*
- ▲ Ask the PT where to stand in relation to the client. Assistants commonly stand slightly behind and to the side of the client, holding onto the gait belt with one supinated hand. The other hand rests on the client's closest shoulder. *The assistant needs to be nearby but should not stand so close as to interferes with the client's movements. The forearms have more strength when supinated (Minor & Minor, 1999).*
- • Strategically place obstacles in the walking path as the client's balance, gait, endurance, and concentration improve. *This prepares clients for walking in real-life situations.*

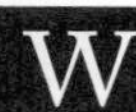

- Document on the care plan how many assistants are needed to walk the client, level of assistance needed (e.g., maximum, standby, and so on), type of assistance needed (e.g., physical support, verbal cues, balance control, and so on), and assistive devices used. *Communication promotes a consistent approach to care; practice allows repetition and rehearsal, both strategies promote motor relearning.*
- Collect a baseline pulse rate and rhythm before walking the client, and reassess it 5 minutes after walking. If abnormal, let the client sit and rest 5 minutes before taking the pulse again. If still abnormal, walking may need to be done more slowly, with more help, or for a shorter period. *Pulse indicates cardiac tolerance to walking. If the pulse rises too high after a few walking trials, it is probably too difficult a task, and the physician should be notified (Radwanski & Hoeman, 1996).*
- ▲ Monitor the client's tolerance for walking. Initiate a 5-minute rest period if any of the following are noted: shortness of breath, use of accessory muscles to breathe, chest pain, nausea, cold sweat, pale or flushed skin, dizziness, syncope, or mental confusion. If signs persist, notify the physician. For more information, refer to the care plan for **Activity intolerance.**
- ▲ Perform initial and subsequent screening to detect clients at high risk for falls. *Fall assessments tools help identify persons at risk for falling (Browne et al, 2004; Hendrich et al, 2003).* **EBN:** *Many falls occurred in client rooms trying to get to the bathroom; use of bed side-rails and restraints did not prevent falls (Hendrich et al, 1995). Assessment and root cause analysis indicated inpatients who fell, were confused, had gait problems, and were attempting self-toileting; individualizing fall preventions decreased fall rates (Gowdy & Godfrey, 2003). Researchers tested and validated the Hendrich Fall Risk Model tool to use on inpatients (Hendrich et al, 2003).*
- Individualize interventions to prevent falls and overuse of restraints and bedrails, including scheduled toileting, lower extremity balance and strength training, sleep hygiene, education on risk of medication and alcohol's relationship to falls, removal of hazards, and detection and treatment of underlying medical problems (Browne et al, 2004; Resnick & Junlapeeya, 2004). **EBN:** *Balance and fear of falling improved in elderly nursing home residents after ankle strengthening and walking programs were implemented (Schoenfelder & Rubensteim, 2004). Retrospective analysis of hospitalized patients indicated falls with bed rails up were equal or higher than when rails were not up; one death occurred from falling over bedrails (van Leeuwen et al, 2001).*

## Geriatric

- Monitor pulse, respirations, and blood pressure before and 5 minutes after a new activity. Stop activity if any of the following occur: resting heart rate >100 beats/min, exercise heart rate 35% greater than resting rate, exercise systolic blood pressure >25 to 35 mm Hg above resting pressure, or a decrease in systolic blood pressure of >20 mm Hg (Radwanski & Hoeman, 1996). *Teach the benefits of walking, and recognize aged adults will have a slow gait. Muscle strength in the hip extensors, abductors, and plantar flexors decrease and knee flexion contractures are not uncommon. Declining visual acuity and balance, foot pain, and fear of falling also slow their walking speed (Jones, 2001; Sims & Olson, 2002).*

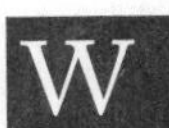


- Recognize that use of a walking aid increases energy and therefore may raise pulse and blood pressure. *Devices give stability and support to clients with lower extremity weakness and poor balance, or weight-bearing restrictions (Jones, 2001).* **EB:** *Elderly subjects with peripheral neuropathy had less risk of losing balance standing on a tilting surface in normal and low-light conditions when using a cane in the nondominant hand (Ashton-Miller et al, 1996).*

▲ Implement safety and fall precautions, e.g., visual identification (arm bands, and so on) of clients at high risk for falling; call system placed within reach and repeated reminders given to call for help before standing; bed/chair alarm or one-to-one observation, obstacle clearance; assistive devices that are specifically chosen and measured for clients; and avoidance of all side rails up. *Safety measures are imperative because many elders experience impaired balance and unsteadiness when moving, postural control and visual disturbances, and adverse effects from multiple medications (Alexander, 1994; Ulfarsson & Robinson, 1997).* **EB:** *After falling, elderly persons were placed in an intervention group in which education about fall prevention, safety at home, and environmental modification and equipment were compared with a control group. The intervention group had significantly fewer recurrent falls the next year (Close et al, 1999). Lower limb weakness and poor tandem walk ability were predictive for elderly hospitalized clients who fell; these two tests could potentially be used to screen those at risk for falls (Chu et al, 1999).*

• Assess for swaying, poor balance and short first step length during standing and the walking of elders. *These gait parameters may reflect postural instability.* **EB:** *Researchers found that elders prone to falling had a shorter first step as they began to walk; this may be a factor to help identify postural problems (Mbourou, 2003).*

• If the client experiences dizziness from orthostatic hypotension when arising, teach compensatory methods mentioned above. Have someone present or a stable support surface to hold onto while arising. *The elderly develop arterial stiffness and reduced autonomic nervous system functioning thus their baroreceptors respond more slowly and have less ability to maintain blood pressure when standing (Fluckiger et al, 1999).*

• Emphasize the importance of wearing firm, low-heeled shoes with nonskid and nonfriction soles and seeking medical care for foot pain, problems, and diabetes. **EB:** *Elderly women had more foot problems than men. Persons with foot pain did worse with leaning, stair climbing/descent, alternate step up, and timed 6-meter walk testing (Menz & Lord, 2001).*

▲ Introduce and reinforce positive perceptions of old age. **EB:** *A study of older adults exposed to positive and negative stereotypes of aging reported significant improvements in gait were associated with positive images; no change was seen with negative stereotypes (Hausdorff, Levy, & Wei, 1999). There was a positive association of two variables—living alone and high mastery (belief in self)—with walking, even if clients had physical difficulty (Simonsick, Guralnik, & Fried, 1999).*

## Home Care

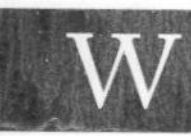


• Assess the client and obtain a complete history with reference to reasons for walking impairments. *Promotes accurate determination of client needs and individualized care.*

• Explain the importance of adequate lighting day and night; tacking carpet edges down, removing throw rugs from high-traffic areas and having nonskid backings on those that are used; applying nonskid wax on floors; and removing clutter from the floor. *Prophylaxis and removal of potential hazards is a means of preventing falls (Ulfarsson & Robinson, 1997).*

- • Assess the home environment for all barriers to walking.
- • Assess client's support system for emergency and contingency care (e.g., Lifeline). *Impaired walking mobility may pose a life threat during a crisis (e.g., falls, fire, orthostatic episode).*
- ▲ Refer clients at risk for falls to physical therapy (PT) and occupational therapy (OT) for skill and strength building; resistive training; and stretching and exercising programs, especially those with osteoporosis and postural problems. *A multidisciplinary approach supports total needs assessment and intervention planning (Hertel & Trahiotis, 2001; Sloan, Haslam, & Foret, 2001).*
- ▲ Refer to home health aide services as appropriate for assistance with activities of daily living (ADLs). *Mobility impairments may serve as a barrier to self-care.*
- ▲ Provide support to the client and caregivers. Refer to case manager, or medical social services or mental health/support group services as necessary. *Long-term impairment may necessitate role changes and create anger and frustration. Counseling and support groups provide validation of feelings and alternative methods of problem solving.*
- ▲ Ensure that the client has information on advocacy, environmental accessibility, assistive technology and related issues under the Americans with Disabilities Act. *The more informed a person is, the more potential he or she has for being independent (Berry & Ignash, 2003; Minor & Minor, 1999).*
- • Teach client and family to check assistive devices to keep them in safe working order (e.g., replace rubber tips if worn and remove dirt in grooves of walkers, crutches, and canes), otherwise they will not grip the floor. Check push button locks on walkers with telescoping legs (Minor & Minor, 1999). Inspect and repair prostheses for cracks, rough spots inside the socket, and odd noises or movement at the joints or foot (Yeltzer, 1998).
- ▲ Recommend daily weight-bearing activities, walking, calcium and vitamin D supplementation, and avoidance of smoking to prevent or manage, to men and women with osteoporosis and hip fractures. Strongly encourage clients to drink milk at mealtime. Estrogen-replacement and antiresorptive therapy is also therapeutic, so clients should consult their physicians (Franzen-Korzendorfer, 2002). **EB:** *Fifty of 52 studies concluded that high calcium intake increased accumulation of bone, prevented bone loss in elderly persons, and lessened risk of fractures (Heaney, 2000); Results from surveys of elders surviving hip fractures showed men rarely received antiresorptive therapy nor did they take calcium or vitamin D supplements (Kiebzak et al, 2002).*

## evolve WEBSITES FOR EDUCATION

See the EVOLVE website for World Wide Web resources for client education.

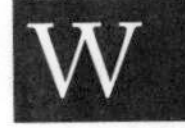

## REFERENCES

Aldrich D, Hunt DP: When can the patient with deep venous thrombosis begin to ambulate? *Physical Therapy* 84(3):268, 2004.

Alexander NB: Postural control in older adults, *J Am Geriatr Soc* 42(1):93, 1994.

Aronow WS: The prevention of venous thromboembolism in older adults: guidelines, *J Gerontol* 59A(1):42, 2004.

Ashton-Miller JA, Yeh MW, Richardson JK et al: A cane reduces loss of balance in patients with peripheral neuropathy: results from a challenging unipedal balance test, *Arch Phys Med Rehabil* 77:446, 1996.
Berry BE, Ignash SL: Assistive technology: providing independence for individuals with disabilities, *Rehabil Nurs* 28(1):6, 2003.
Bobath B: *Adult hemiplegia: evaluation and treatment,* London, 1978, William Heinemann.
Boone S, et al: Preventing osteoporotic fractures with antiresorptive therapy: implications of microarchitectural changes, *J Intern Med* 255:1, 2004.
Bowen A, Wenman R, Mickelborough J et al: Dual-task effects of talking while walking on velocity and balance following stroke, *Age Ageing* 30(4):319, 2001.
Bradley JG, Davis KA: Orthostatic hypotension, *Am Fam Physician* 68(12):2393, 2003.
Browne JA, Covington BG, Davila Y et al: Using information technology to assist in redesign of a fall prevention program, *J Nurs Care Qual* 19(3):218, 2004.
Chu LW, Pei CK, Chiu A et al: Risk factors for falls in hospitalized older medical patients, *J Gerontol* 54(1):M38, 1999.
Close J, Ellis M, Hooper R et al: Prevention of falls in the elderly trial (PROFET): a randomised controlled trial, *Lancet* 353(9147):93, 1999.
Cubo E, Moore CG, Leurgans S et al: Wheeled and standard walkers in Parkinson's disease patients with gait freezing, *Parkinsonism Relat Disord* 10(1):9, 2003.
Ejaz AA, Haley WE, Wasiluk A et al: Characteristics of 100 consecutive patients presenting with orthostatic hypotension, *Mayo Clin Proc* 79(7):890, 2004.
Fluckiger L, Boivin JM, Quilliot D et al: Differential effects of aging on heart rate variability and blood pressure variability, *J Gerontol* 54(5):B219, 1999.
Franzen-Korzendorfer H: The silent disease, *Rehabil Manage* 15(8):30, 2002.
Gee ZL, Passarella PM: *Nursing care of the stroke patient: a therapeutic approach,* Pittsburgh, 1985, AREN.
Gowdy M, Godfrey S: Using tools to assess and prevent inpatient falls, *Jt Comm J Qual Saf* 29(7):363, 2003.
Graafmans WC, Lips P, Wijlhuizen GJ et al: Daily physical activity and the use of a walking aid in relation to falls in elderly people in a residential care setting, Z *Gerontol Geriatr* 36(1):23:2003.
Gregg EW, Pereira MA, Casperson CJ: Physical activity, falls, and fractures among older adults: a review of the epidemiologic evidence, *J Am Geriatr Soc* 48:883, 2000.
Halm M: Altered tissue perfusion. In Maas ML et al, editors: *Nursing care of older adults: diagnosis, outcomes, and interventions,* St Louis, 2001, Mosby.
Hamers JP, Gulpers MJ, Strik W et al: Use of physical restraints with cognitively impaired nursing home residents, *J Adv Nurs* 45(3):246, 2004.
Hausdorff JM, Levy BR, Wei JY: The power of ageism on physical function of older persons: reversibility of age-related gait changes, *J Am Geriatr Soc* 47:1346, 1999.
Heaney RP: Calcium, dairy products and osteoporosis, *J Am Coll Nutr* 19:835, 2000.
Hendrich A, Nyhuis A, Kippenbrock T et al: Hospital falls: development of a predictive model for clinical practice, *Appl Nurs Res* 8(3):129, 1995.
Hendrich AL, Bender PS, Nyhuis A: Validation of the Hendrich II Fall Risk Model: a large concurrent case/control study of hospitalized patients, *Appl Nurs Res* 16(3):203, 2003.
Hertel KL, Trahiotis MG: Exercise in the prevention and treatment of osteoporosis, *Nurs Clin North Am* 36(3):441, 2001.
Hoeman SP: Movement, functional mobility, and activities of daily living. In Hoeman SP, editor: *Rehabilitation nursing: process, application, and outcomes,* ed 3, St Louis, 2002, Mosby.
International Food Information Council Foundation (IFIC): *IFIC review: physical activity, nutrition and bone health,* available online at *http://ific.org/healthybones,* April 2002.
Irvin DJ, White M: The importance of accurately assessing orthostatic hypotension, *Geriatri Nurs* 25(2):99, 2004.
Jones DA: Successful aging: maintaining mobility in a geriatric patient population, *Rehabil Manage* 14(9):46, 2001.
Kiebzak GM, Beinart GA, Perser K et al: Undertreatment of osteoporosis in men with hip fracture, *Arch Intern Med* 162(19):2217, 2002.
Kipnis ND: Musculoskeletal/orthopedic disorders. In McCourt A, editor: *The specialty practice of rehabilitation nursing: a core curriculum,* ed 3, Skokie, Ill, 1993, Rehabilitation Foundation.
Menz HB, Lord SR: Foot pain impairs balance and functional ability in community-dwelling older people, *J Am Podiatr Med Assoc* 91(5):222, 2001.
Minor MAD, Minor SD: *Patient care skills,* ed 4, Stamford, Conn, 1999, Appleton & Lange.
Mbourou GA, Lajoie Y, Teasdale N: Step length variability at gait initiation in elderly fallers and anon-fallers, and young adults, *Gerontology* 49(1):21, 2003.

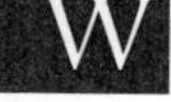

Proctor MC, Greenfield LJ: Thromboprophylaxis in an academic medical center, *Cardiovasc Surg* 9(5):426, 2001.
Owen BD, Garg A: Back stress isn't part of the job, *Am J Nurs* 93(2):48, 1993.
Radwanski MB, Hoeman SP: Geriatric rehabilitation nursing. In Hoeman SP, editor: *Rehabilitation nursing: process and application,* ed 2, St Louis, 1996, Mosby.
Resnick B, Junlapeeya P: Falls in a community of older adults: findings and implications for practice, *App Nurs Res* 17(2):81, 2004.
Schoenfelder DP, Rubenstein LM: An exercise program to improve fall-related outcomes in elderly nursing home residents, *Appl Nurs Res* 17(1):21, 2004.
Shannon JR, Diedrich A, Biaggioni I et al: Water drinking as a treatment for orthostatic syndromes, *Am J Med* 112(5):355, 2002.
Sherman FR: The art and science of syncope in the aged, *Geriatrics* 58(5):12, 2003.
Shumway-Cook A, Woollacott M: Attention demands and postural control: the effect of sensory context, *J Gerontol A Biol Sci Med Sci* 55(1):M10, 2000.
Simonsick EM, Guralnik JM, Fried LP: Who walks? Factors associated with walking behavior in disabled older women with and without self-reported walking difficulty, *J Am Geriatr Soc* 47(6):672, 1999.
Sims GL, Olson RS: Muscle and skeletal function. In Hoeman SP, editor, *Rehabilitation nursing: process, application, and outcomes,* ed 3, St Louis, 2002, Mosby.
Sloan HL, Haslam K, Foret CM: Teaching the use of walkers and canes, *Home Health Nurs* 19:241, 2001.
St. Pierre BA, Flaskerud JH: Clinical nursing implications for the recovery of atrophied skeletal muscle following bed rest, *Rehabil Nurs* 20(6):314, 1995.
St. Pierre BA, Tidball JG: Differential response of macrophage subpopulations to soleus muscle reloading after rat hindlimb suspension, *J Appl Physiol* 77:290, 1994.
Tsai HA, Kirby RL, MacLeod DA et al: Aided gait of people with lower-limb amputations: Comparisons of 4-footed and 2-wheeled walkers, *Arch Phys Med Rehabil* 84(4):584, 2003.
Ulfarsson J, Robinson BE: Falls and falling. In Ham RJ, Sloane PD, editors: *Primary care geriatrics: a case-based approach,* ed 3, St Louis, 1997, Mosby.
van Leeuwen M, Bennett L, West S et al.: Patient falls from bed and the role of bedrails in the acute care setting, *Aust J Adv Nurs* 19(2):8, 2001.
Yeltzer EA: Care of the client with an amputation. In Chin PA, Finocchiaro D, Rosebrough A, editors: *Rehabilitation nursing practice,* New York, 1998, McGraw-Hill.

# Wandering

evolve

*Donna Algase*

NANDA

## Definition

Meandering; aimless or repetitive locomotion that exposes the individual to harm; frequently incongruent with boundaries, limits, or obstacles

## Defining Characteristics

Frequent or continuous movement from place to place, often revisiting the same destinations; persistent locomotion in search of "missing" or unattainable people or places; haphazard locomotion; locomotion in unauthorized or private spaces; locomotion resulting in unintended leaving of a premise; long periods of locomotion without an apparent destination; fretful locomotion or pacing; inability to locate significant landmarks in a familiar setting; locomotion that cannot be easily dissuaded or redirected; following behind or shadowing a caregiver's locomotion; trespassing; hyperactivity; scanning, seeking,

W

or searching behaviors; periods of locomotion interspersed with periods of nonlocomotion (e.g., sitting, standing, sleeping); getting lost

## Related Factors (r/t)

Cognitive impairment, specifically memory and recall deficits, disorientation, poor visuoconstructive (or visuospatial) ability, and language (primarily expressive) defects; cortical atrophy; premorbid behavior (e.g., outgoing, sociable personality); premorbid dementia; separation from familiar people and places; sedation; emotional state, especially frustration, anxiety, boredom, or depression (agitation); overstimulating/understimulating social or physical environment; physiological state or need (e.g., hunger/thirst, pain, urination, constipation); time of day

**NOC**

## Outcomes (Nursing Outcomes Classification)

### Suggested NOC Outcomes

Caregiver Home Care Readiness; Fall Prevention Behavior; Falls Occurrence

**Example NOC Outcome with Indicators**

**Caregiver Home Care Readiness** as evidenced by the following indicators: Knowledge of recommended treatment regimen/Knowledge of prescribed activity/Knowledge of emergency care/Confidence in ability to manage care at home (Rate each indicator of **Caregiver Home Care Readiness:** 1 = not adequate, 2 = slightly adequate, 3 = moderately adequate, 4 = substantially adequate, 5 = totally adequate [see Section I].)

## Client Outcomes

### Client Will (Specify Time Frame):

- Decrease incidence of falls (preferably free of falls)
- Decrease incidence of elopements
- Maintain appropriate body weight

### Caregiver Will (Specify Time Frame):

- Be able to explain interventions he or she can use to provide a safe environment for a care receiver who displays wandering behavior

**NIC**

## Interventions (Nursing Interventions Classification)

### Suggested NIC Intervention

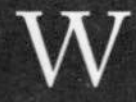

Dementia Management

**Example NIC Activities—Dementia Management**

Place identification bracelet on the client; provide space for safe pacing and wandering

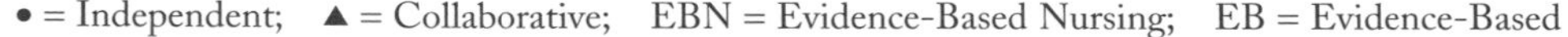

• = Independent; ▲ = Collaborative; EBN = Evidence-Based Nursing; EB = Evidence-Based

## Nursing Interventions and Rationales

- Assess and document the amount (frequency and duration), pattern (random, lapping, or pacing), and 24-hour distribution of wandering behavior over a 3-day interval. **EBN:** *Assessment over time provides a baseline against which behavior change can be evaluated (Algase et al, 1997). Such assessment can also reveal the time of day when wandering is greatest and when surveillance or other precautionary measures are most necessary.*
- Document particular aspects of wandering that are troubling. **EBN:** *Instruments such as the Algase Wandering Scale (Version 2) (Algase et al, 2001, 2004) can indicate whether the behavior is persistent, spatially disordered, or prone to elopement. Such information can direct caregivers toward more appropriate intervention strategies.*
- Obtain a history of personality characteristics and behavioral responses to stress. **EBN and EB:** *Information about long-standing behavioral tendencies may reveal circumstances under which wandering will occur and can aid in interpreting both positive and negative meanings of wandering behavior of the client (Kolanowski, Strand, & Whall, 1997; Monsour & Robb, 1982; Thomas, 1997).*
- Evaluate for neurocognitive strengths and limitations, particularly language, attention, visuospatial skills, and perseveration. **EBN:** *Wanderers may have expressive language deficits that hamper their ability to communicate needs (Algase, 1992; Dawson & Reid, 1987).* **EBN and EB:** *Knowledge of attentional and visuospatial deficits, which may account for certain patterns of wandering or way-finding deficits and can lead to identification of appropriate environmental modifications that could enhance functional ambulation such as elimination of distractions and enhancement of cues marking desired destinations (Chiu, 2002; Fischer, Marterer, & Danielczyk, 1990; Henderson, Mack, & Williams, 1989; Passini et al, 1995, 2000).* **EB:** *The presence of perseveration may indicate that the wanderer is unable to voluntarily stop his or her behavior (Passini et al, 1995; Ryan et al, 1995), thus calling for nursing judgment as to when wandering should be interrupted to enhance the wanderer's safety, comfort, or well-being.*
- Assess for physical distress or needs such as hunger, thirst, pain, discomfort, or elimination. **EBN:** *Although physical needs have not been documented in relation to wandering, the Need-Driven Dementia-Compromised Model hypothesizes this relationship (Algase et al, 1996).*
- Assess for emotional or psychological distress such as anxiety, fear, or feeling lost. **EB:** *Anxiety and depression frequently accompany wandering (Teri et al, 1999).*
- Observe wandering episodes for antecedents and consequences. **EBN and EB:** *People, events, or circumstances surrounding the onset or conclusion of wandering may provide cues about triggers or rewards that are stimulating or reinforcing wandering behavior (Heard & Watson, 1999; Hirst & Metcalf, 1989; Hussian, 1981, 1982).*
- Apply observed consequences of wandering such as personal attention, food, and so forth at times when the person is *not* wandering, and withhold them while the person is wandering. **EB:** *Differential reinforcement of other behavior (non-wandering) can reduce wandering episodes by 50% to 80% (Heard & Watson, 1999).*

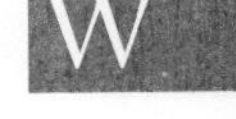


- Assess regularly for the presence of or potential for negative outcomes of wandering such as declining social skills, falls, and elopement. **EB:** *Wanderers are at greater risk for falls than other cognitively impaired persons (Kippenbrock & Soja, 1993; Morse, Tylko, &*

*Dixon, 1987). Wanderers have also shown greater loss in social skills over time than nonwandering counterparts (Cornbleth, 1977).*

- Weigh client at defined intervals to detect onset of weight loss and watch for symptoms associated with inadequate food intake including constipation, dehydration, muscle wasting, and starvation. *Wandering behavior can affect the client's ability to eat, where the client is unable to sit at a table for the time needed to eat a meal (Beattie & Algase, 2002).*
- For the client who displays wandering behavior during meal times, use behavioral interventions to shape behavior, including verbal statements, nonverbal social behavior, and systematic extinguishing of undesirable client behavior. **EBN:** *Results of a study using behavior interventions demonstrated that it was effective in increasing sitting at the table behavior, and in the client eating more food (Beattie, Algase, & Song, 2004).*
- Provide for safe ambulation with comfortable and well-fitting clothes, shoes with nonskid soles and foot support, and any necessary walking aids (e.g., a cane, walker, or Merry-Walker). **EB:** *Falls in persons with advanced dementia are often related to a decline in vigor in persons who had been previously active (Brody et al, 1984).*
- Provide safe and secure surroundings that deter accidental elopements using perimeter control devices, camouflage, or electronic tracking systems. **EBN:** *Eloping can have hazardous outcomes, including death (Rowe & Glover, 2001).* **EB:** *Perimeter control devices can effectively reduce or prevent exiting behavior (Negley, Molla, & Obenchain, 1990).* **EBN and EB:** *However, under some circumstances, these devices are viewed as unnecessarily restrictive, and more passive means such as camouflage have been substituted. Camouflage techniques such as masking the doorknob or creating striped floor patterns in front of exits have been used with success (Namazi, Rosner, & Calkins, 1989; Hussian & Brown, 1987), particularly in subjects with Alzheimer's disease (Hewewasam, 1996), but the effectiveness may be mitigated by other architectural features of the setting (Hamilton, 1993; Chafetz, 1990). A Cochrane review found that no randomized controlled trials have been done to validate the effectiveness of subjective barriers to prevent wandering in cognitively impaired clients (Price, Hermans, & Grimley, 2005). Newer electronic monitoring and tracking systems are highly effective and reduce caregiver burden (Altus et al, 2000; Nelson et al, 2004).*
- During periods of inactivity, position the wanderer so that desirable destinations (e.g., bathroom) are within the client's line of vision and undesirable destinations (e.g., exits or stairwells) are out of sight. **EBN and EB:** *Functional, nonwandering ambulation is possible even into late-stage dementia and may be facilitated by keeping appropriate visual cues accessible (Passini et al, 2000; Algase, 1999; Martino-Saltzman et al, 1991).*
- If wandering takes a random or haphazard route, reduce environmental distractions and increase relevant environmental cues. Note and eliminate stimuli that distract the wanderer while in route. Provide afternoon rest periods if assessment reveals that random-pattern wandering worsens as the day progresses. **EBN:** *Random-pattern wandering may be affected by environmental stimuli (Algase, 1999). The proportion of wandering that is random increases as the day progresses (Algase et al, 1997; Algase, 1999) and may indicate fatigue.*
- Enhance institutional settings with areas that provide interesting views and opportunities to sit. **EB:** *Enhanced environments can improve mood, and they encourage wanderers*

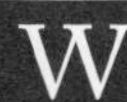

*to linger or sit more than purely institutional surroundings do (Cohen-Mansfield & Werner, 1998).*

- Engage wanderers in social interaction and structured activity, especially when wanderers appear distressed or otherwise uncomfortable or their wandering presents a challenge to others in the setting. **EBN and EB:** *Wandering and social interaction are inversely related. Wanderers often have an outgoing or sociable personality and also have deficits in expressive language skills. Thus while they may prefer social interaction, their ability to initiate it may be compromised (Algase, 1992; Thomas, 1997).*
- If wandering has a pacing quality, attempt to identify and address any underlying problems or concerns. Offer stress-reducing approaches such as music, massage, or rocking. Attempts to distract or redirect the pacing wanderer may worsen wandering. **EBN:** *Pacing, as a wandering pattern, is not associated with level of cognitive impairment and may reflect anxiety, agitation, pain, or another internal process (Algase, Beattie, & Therrien, 2001; Gerdner, 2000; Snyder & Olson, 1996).*
- If wandering is a new or recently acquired behavior or if it increases in intensity over previous levels, evaluate for constipation, pneumonia, or acute physical problems. **EBN and EB:** *Persons who first exhibit wandering within 3 months after admission to a nursing home are more likely than others to have developed physical problems that stimulate wandering (Keily, Morris, & Algase, 2000).*
- If wandering has a lapping or circuitous pattern, signs or labels may be effective. Substitute another repetitive activity such as folding or rocking if lapping becomes problematic or excessive. **EBN:** *Not all wanderers display lapping-pattern wandering, and when it does occur, it tends to occur early in the day or to follow rest periods. Thus it may be a more functional pattern than random wandering and may indicate a slightly better level of cognitive function for the individual, even if transient. Thus wanderers who lap may be better able to make use of information in the environment (Algase, Beattie, & Therrien, 2001).* **EB:** *However, this pattern of wandering may also be a form of perseveration, and therefore the person may be unable to disengage voluntarily (Passini et al, 1995; Ryan et al, 1995).*
- Provide a regularly scheduled and supervised exercise or walking program, particularly if wandering occurs excessively during the night or at times that are inconvenient in the setting. **EBN and EB:** *Although exercise or walking programs do not reduce daytime wandering, they have been shown to reduce or eliminate nighttime wandering (Carillon Nursing and Rehabilitation Center, 2000; Robb, 1987) and to decrease general agitation levels (Holmberg, 1997).*
- Use slow-stroke, hand, or foot massage before the times of day or events that induce wandering. **EBN and EB:** *Various massage techniques have been shown to reduce wandering and diffuse agitation in persons with dementia (Kilstoff & Chenoweth, 1998; Malaquin-Pavan, 1997; Rowe & Alfred, 1999; Snyder, Egan, & Burns, 1995; Sutherland Reakes, & Bridges, 1999).*

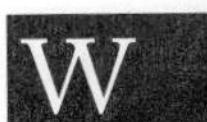


## Multicultural

- Assess for the influence of cultural beliefs, norms, and values on the family's understanding of wandering behavior. **EBN:** *Latina dementia caregivers delay institutionalization significantly longer than female Caucasian caregivers. In addition, Latino cultural* *values and positive views of the caregiving role are important factors that may significantly influence their decision to institutionalize loved ones with dementia (Mausbach et al, 2004). Another study found that black and Latino community-dwelling patients with moderate to severe dementia have a higher prevalence of wandering and other dementia related behaviors (Sink et al, 2004).*

▲ Refer the family to social services or other supportive services to assist with the impact of caregiving for the wandering client. **EBN:** *African-American caregivers of dementia clients may evidence less desire than other caregivers to institutionalize their family members and are more likely to report unmet service needs (Hinrichsen & Ramirez, 1992). African-American and white families of dementia clients may report restricted social activity (Haley et al, 1995).*

• Encourage the family to use support groups or other service programs. **EBN:** *Studies indicate that minority families of clients with dementia use few support programs even though these programs could have a positive impact on caregiver well-being (Cox, 1999).*

• Validate the family's feelings regarding the impact of client wandering on family lifestyle. **EBN:** *Validation is a therapeutic communication technique that lets the client know that the nurse has heard and understands what was said (Heineken, 1998).*

## Home Care

• Help the caregiver set up a plan to deal with wandering behavior using the interventions mentioned in Nursing Interventions and Rationales.

• Assess the home environment for modifications that will protect the client and prevent elopement. *Security devices are available to notify the caregiver of the client's movements (e.g., alarms at doors, bed alarms).*

• Assist the family to set up a plan of exercise for the client, including safe walking. *Walking is a valuable source of exercise, even for clients with dementia (Oddy, 2004).*

▲ Enroll wanderers in the Safe Return Program of the Alzheimer's Association, and help the caregiver develop a plan of action to use if the client elopes. **EBN:** *The Safe Return Program has assisted in locating numerous persons who have eloped from their homes or other residential care settings. Mortality rates are high if there is failure to locate elopers within the first 24 hours (Rowe & Glover, 2001).*

• Help the caregiver develop a plan of action to use if the client elopes.

▲ Institute case management of frail elderly clients to support continued independent living. *Wandering behavior represents and can lead to increasing needs for assistance in using the health care system effectively. Case management combines nursing activities of client and family assessment, planning and coordination of care among all health care providers, delivery of direct nursing care, and monitoring of care and outcomes. These activities are able to address continuity of care, mutual goal setting, behavior management, and prevention of worsening health problems (Guttman, 1999).*

▲ Refer for homemaker or psychiatric home health care services for respite, client reassurance, and implementation of a therapeutic regimen. Refer to the care plan for **Caregiver role strain.** *Responsibility for a person at high risk for wandering provides high caregiver stress. Respite care decreases caregiver stress. The presence of caring individuals is reassuring to both the client and caregivers, especially during periods of client anxiety. Wan-*

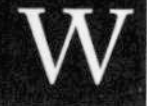

*dering behavior can make use of the interventions described above, modified for the home setting.*

## Client/Family Teaching

- Inform the client and family of the meaning of and reasons for wandering behavior. An understanding of wandering behavior will enable the client and family to provide the client with a safe environment.
- Teach the caregiver/family methods to deal with wandering behavior using the interventions mentioned in Nursing Interventions and Rationales.

## evolve WEBSITES FOR EDUCATION

See the EVOLVE website for World Wide Web resources for client education.

## REFERENCES


Algase DL: Cognitive discriminants of wandering among nursing home residents, *Nurs Res* 41(2):78, 1992.

Algase DL: Wandering: a dementia-compromised behavior, *J Gerontol Nurs* 25(9):10, 1999.

Algase DL et al: Validation of the Algase Wandering Scale: version 2 in a cross cultural sample, *Aging Ment Health* 8(2):133, 2004.

Algase DL, Beattie ERA, Therrien B: Impact of cognitive impairment on wandering behavior, *West J Nurs Res* 23:283, 2001.

Algase DL et al: Need-driven dementia-compromised behavior: an alternative view of disruptive behavior, *Am J Alzheimers Dis* 11(6):10, 1996.

Algase DL et al: Estimates of stability of daily wandering behavior among cognitively impaired long-term care residents, *Nurs Res* 46(3):172, 1997.

Algase DL et al: The Algase Wandering Scale: initial psychometrics of a new caregiver reporting tool, *Am J Alzheimers Dis Other Demen* 16(3):141, 2001.

Altus DE et al: Evaluating an electronic monitoring system for people who wander, *Am J Alzheimers Dis* 15(2):121, 2000.

Beattie ERA, Algase DL: Improving table-sitting behavior of wanderers via theoretic substruction, *J Geront Nurs* 28(10):6, 2002.

Beattie ERA, Algase DL, Song J: Keeping wandering nursing home residents at the table: improving food intake using a behavior communication intervention, *Aging Ment Health* 8(2):109, 2004.

Brody E et al: Predictors of falls among institutionalized females with Alzheimer's disease, *J Am Geriatr Soc* 32: 877, 1984.

Carillon Nursing and Rehabilitation Center: Nature walk: from aimless wandering to purposeful walking, *Nurs Homes Long Term Care Manage* 49(11):50, 2000.

Chafetz PK: Two dimensional grid is ineffective against demented patients' exiting through glass doors, *Psychol Aging* 5:146, 1990.

Chiu Y: *Getting lost behavior and directed attention impairments in Taiwanese patients with early Alzheimer's disease* (unpublished doctoral dissertation), Ann Arbor, 2002, University of Michigan.

Cochran M: Tears have no color, *Am J Nurs* 98(6):53, 1998.

Cohen-Mansfield J, Werner P: The effects of an enhanced environment on nursing home residents who pace, *Geronotologist* 38(2): 199, 1998.

Cornbleth T: Effects of a protected hospital ward area on wandering and non-wandering geriatric patients, *J Gerontol* 32:573, 1977.

Cox C: Race and caregiving: patterns of service use by African American and white caregivers of persons with Alzheimer's, *J Gerontol Soc Work* 32(2):5, 1999.

Dawson P, Reid DW: Behavioral dimensions of patients at risk for wandering, *Gerontologist* 27:104, 1987.

Doswell W, Erlen J: Multicultural issues and ethical concerns in the delivery of revising care interventions, *Nurs Clin North Am* 33(2):353, 1998.

Fischer P, Marterer A, Danielczyk W: Right-left disorientation in dementia of the Alzheimer's type, *Neurology* 40:1619, 1990.

Gerdner LA: Effects of individualized versus classical "relaxation" music on the frequency of agitation in elderly persons with Alzheimer's disease and related disorders, *Int Psychogeriatr* 12(1):49, 2000.


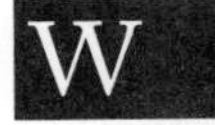

Guarnaccia P: Multicultural experiences of family caregiving: a study of African American, European American, and Hispanic American families, *New Direct Ment Health Serv* 77:45, 1998.

Guttman R: Case management of the frail elderly in the community, *Clin Nurs Spec* 13(4):174, 1999.

Haley WE et al: Psychological, social, and health impact of caregiving: a comparison of black and white dementia family caregivers and noncaregivers, *Psychol Aging* 10(4):540, 1995.

Hamilton C: *The use of tape patterns as an alternative method for controlling wanderers' exiting behavior in a dementia care unit* (unpublished master's thesis), Blacksburg, Va, 1993, Virginia Polytechnic Institute and State University.

Heard K, Watson TS: Reducing wandering by persons with dementia using differential reinforcement, *J Appl Behav Anal* 32(9): 381, 1999.

Heineken J: Patient silence is not necessarily client satisfaction: communication in home care nursing, *Home Healthc Nurse* 16(2): 115, 1998.

Henderson V, Mack W, Williams BW: Spatial disorientation in Alzheimer's disease, *Arch Neurol* 46:391, 1989.

Hewewasam L: Floor patterns limit wandering of people with Alzheimer's, *Nurs Times* 92:41, 1996.

Hinrichsen GA, Ramirez M: Black and white dementia caregivers: a comparison of their adaptation, *Gerontologist* 32(3):375, 1992.

Hirst ST, Metcalf BJ: Whys and whats of wandering, *Geriatr Nurs Am J Care Aging* 10(5):237, 1989.

Holmberg SK: Evaluation of a clinical intervention for wanderers on a geriatric nursing unit, *Arch Psychiatr Nurs* 11:21, 1997.

Hussian RA: Psychotherapeutic intervention: organic mental disorders. In Hussian RA: *Geriatric psychology: a behavioural perspective,* New York, 1981, Van Nostrand Reinhold.

Hussian RA: Stimulus control in the modification of problematic behavior in elderly institutionalized patients, *Int J Behav Geriatr* 1:33, 1982.

Hussian RA, Brown DC: Use of two dimensional grid patterns to limit hazardous ambulation in demented patients, *J Gerontol* 42: 558, 1987.

Keily DK, Morris JN, Algase DL: Resident characteristics associated with wandering in nursing homes, *Int J Geriatr Psychiatry* 15: 1013, 2000.

Kilstoff K, Chenoweth L: New approaches to health and well-being for dementia day-care clients, family carers and day care staff, *Int J Nurs Pract* 4(2):72, 1998.

Kippenbrock T, Soja M: Preventing falls in the elderly: interviewing patients who have fallen, *Geriatr Nurs* 14:205, 1993.

Kolanowski AM, Strand G, Whall A: A pilot study of the relation in premorbid characteristics to behavior in dementia, *J Gerontol Nurs* 23:21, 1997.

Leininger MM, McFarland MR: *Transcultural nursing: concepts, theories, research and practices,* ed 3, New York, 2002, McGraw-Hill.

Malaquin-Pavan E: Therapeutic benefit of touch-massage in the overall management of demented elderly, *Recherche en Soins Infirmiers* 49:11, 1997.

Martino-Saltzman D et al: Travel behavior of nursing home residents perceived as wanderers and nonwanderers, *Gerontologist* 31: 666, 1991.

Mausbach BT, Coon DW, Depp C et al: Ethnicity and time to institutionalization of dementia patients: a comparison of Latina and Caucasian female family caregivers, *J Am Geriatr Soc* 52(7):1077-1084, 2004.

Monsour N, Robb S: Wandering behavior in old age: a psychosocial study, *Soc Work* 27:411, 1982.

Morse J, Tylko S, Dixon H: Characteristics of the fall-prone patient, *Gerontologist* 27:516, 1987.

Namazi KH, Rosner TT, Calkins MP: Visual barriers to prevent ambulatory Alzheimer's patients from exiting through an emergency door, *Gerontologist* 29:699, 1989.

Negley E, Molla PM, Obenchain J: No exit: the effects of an electronic security system on confused patients, *J Gerontol Nurs* 16: 21, 1990.

Nelson A et al: Technology to promote safe mobility in the elderly, *Nurs Clin North Am* 39(3):649, 2004.

Oddy R: Walk this way: Assisted exercise for all people with dementia, *J Dement Care* 12(1):21, 2004.

Passini R et al: Wayfinding in dementia of the Alzheimer's type: planning abilities, *J Clin Exp Neuropsychol* 17:820, 1995.

Passini R et al: Wayfinding in a nursing home for advanced dementia of the Alzheimer's type, *Environ Behav* 32(5):684, 2000.


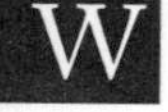


Price JC, Hermans DG, Grimley EV: Subjective barriers to prevent wandering of cognitively impaired people, *The Cochrane Library*, CD001932, 2005.

Robb SS: Exercise treatment for wandering. In Altman HJ, editor: *Alzheimer's disease: problems, prospects, and perspectives,* New York, 1987, Plenum.

Rowe M, Alfred D: The effectiveness of slow stroke massage in diffusing agitated behaviors in individuals with Alzheimer's disease, *J Gerontol Nurs* 25(6):22, 1999.
Rowe MA, Glover JC: Antecedents, descriptions and consequences of wandering in cognitively-impaired adults and the Safe Return (SR) program, *Am J Alzheimers Dis* 16(6):344, 2001.
Ryan JP et al: Graphomotor perseveration and wandering in Alzheimer's disease, *J Geriatr Psychiatry Neurol* 8:209, 1995.
Sink KM, Covinsky KE, Newcomer R et al: Ethnic differences in the prevalence and pattern of dementia-related behaviors, *J Am Geriatr Soc* 52(8):1277-1283, 2004.
Snyder M, Egan E, Burns K: Interventions for decreasing agitation behaviors in persons with dementia, *J Gerontol Nurs* 21(7):34, 1995.
Snyder M, Olson J: Music and hand massage interventions to produce relaxation and reduce aggressive behaviors in cognitively impaired elders: a pilot study, *Clin Gerontol* 17(1):64, 1996.
Sutherland JA, Reakes J, Bridges C: Foot acupressure and massage for patients with Alzheimer's disease and related dementias, *J Nurs Sch* 31(4):34, 1999.
Teri L et al: Anxiety of Alzheimer's disease: prevalence and comorbidity, *J Gerontol A Biol Sci Med Sci* 54(7): M348, 1999.
Thomas DW: Understanding the wandering patient: a continuity of personality perspective, *J Gerontol Nurs* 23(1):16, 1997.

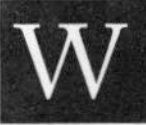

# APPENDIX A

## Nursing Diagnoses Arranged by Maslow's Hierarchy of Needs

Because human beings adapt in many ways to establish and maintain the self, health problems are much more than simple physical matters. Maslow's Hierarchy of Needs (see diagram below) is a system of classifying human needs. Maslow's hierarchy is based on the idea that lower-level physiological needs must be met before higher-level, abstract needs can be met.

For nurses, Maslow's hierarchy has special significance in decision making and planning for care. By considering need categories as you identify client problems, you will be able to provide more holistic care. For example, a client who demands frequent attention for a seemingly trivial matter may require help with self-esteem needs. Need levels vary from client to client. If a client is short of breath, the client is probably not interested in or capable of discussing spirituality. In addition, a client's need level may change throughout planning and intervention, so you will need to be vigilant in your assessment.

Read the descriptions of each category in the diagram, and see how you would relate them to nursing diagnoses. Compare your evaluation with how the authors categorized the nursing diagnoses according to this hierarchy. Be sure to assess clients for potential problems at all levels of the pyramid, regardless of their initial complaint.

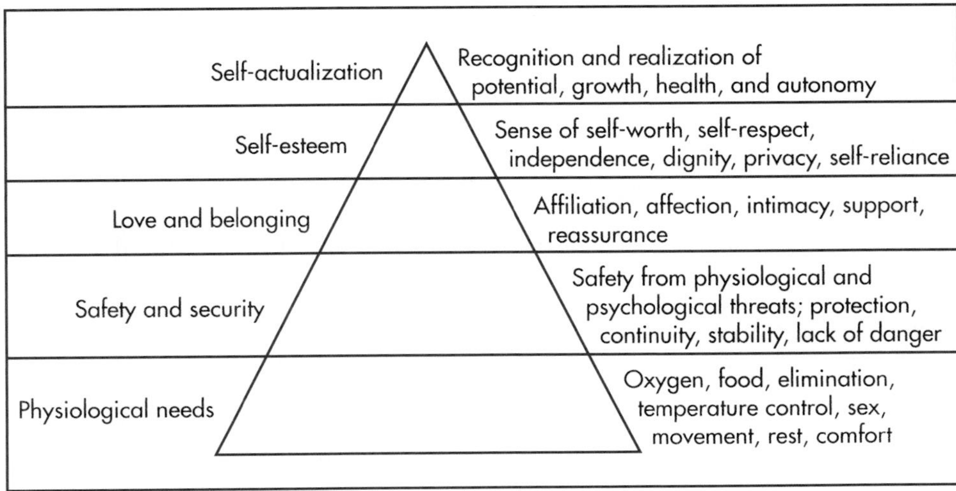

### Physiological Needs

Activity intolerance
Activity intolerance, risk for
Airway clearance, ineffective
Allergy response, latex
Aspiration, risk for
Body temperature, risk for imbalanced
Bowel incontinence
Breastfeeding, effective
Breastfeeding, ineffective
Breastfeeding, interrupted
Breathing pattern, ineffective
Cardiac output, decreased
Comfort, impaired
Constipation
Constipation, perceived
Constipation, risk for
Dentition, impaired
Diarrhea
Fatigue
Fluid balance, readiness for enhanced
Fluid volume, deficient
Fluid volume, excess
Fluid volume, risk for deficient
Fluid volume, risk for imbalanced
Gas exchange, impaired
Hyperthermia
Hypothermia
Incontinence, functional urinary
Incontinence, reflex urinary
Incontinence, risk for urge urinary
Incontinence, stress urinary
Incontinence, total urinary
Incontinence, urge urinary
Infant behavior, disorganized
Infant behavior, readiness for enhanced organized
Infant behavior, risk for disorganized
Infant feeding pattern, ineffective
Intracranial adaptive capacity, decreased
Mobility, impaired bed
Mobility, impaired physical
Mobility, impaired wheelchair
Nausea
Nutrition, imbalanced: less than body requirements
Nutrition, imbalanced: more than body requirements
Nutrition, imbalanced: risk for more than body requirements
Oral mucous membrane, impaired
Pain, acute
Pain, chronic
Protection, ineffective
Self-care deficit, bathing/hygiene
Self-care deficit, dressing/grooming
Self-care deficit, feeding
Self-care deficit, toileting
Sensory perception, disturbed (specify): visual, auditory, kinesthetic, gustatory, tactile, olfactory
Sexual dysfunction
Sexuality patterns, ineffective
Skin integrity, impaired
Skin integrity, risk for impaired
Sleep deprivation
Sleep pattern, disturbed
Sleep, readiness for enhanced
Surgical recovery, delayed
Swallowing, impaired
Thermoregulation, ineffective
Thought processes, disturbed
Tissue integrity, impaired
Tissue perfusion, ineffective (specify type): cerebral, renal, cardiopulmonary, gastrointestinal, peripheral
Transfer ability, impaired
Urinary elimination, readiness for enhanced
Urinary elimination, impaired
Urinary retention
Ventilation, impaired spontaneous
Ventilatory weaning response, dysfunctional
Walking, impaired

### Safety and Security Needs

Allergy response, risk for latex
Anxiety
Anxiety, death
Autonomic dysreflexia
Autonomic dysreflexia, risk for
Communication, readiness for enhanced
Communication, impaired verbal

Confusion, acute
Confusion, chronic
Death syndrome, risk for sudden infant
Disuse syndrome, risk for
Environmental interpretation syndrome, impaired
Falls, risk for
Family role performance, supportive
Family processes, dysfunctional: alcoholism
Fear
Grieving, anticipatory
Grieving, dysfunctional
Grieving, risk for dysfunctional
Growth, risk for disproportionate
Health maintenance, ineffective
Home maintenance, impaired
Infection, risk for
Injury, risk for
Perioperative-positioning injury, risk for
Knowledge, deficient
Knowledge of (specify), readiness for enhanced
Memory, impaired
Neglect, unilateral
Peripheral neurovascular dysfunction, risk for
Poisoning, risk for
Religiosity impaired
Religiosity, risk for impaired
Sorrow, chronic
Suffocation, risk for
Therapeutic regimen management, ineffective
Therapeutic regimen management, ineffective community
Therapeutic regimen management, ineffective family
Therapeutic regimen management, readiness for enhanced
Trauma, risk for
Wandering

## Love and Belonging Needs

Anxiety
Attachment, risk for impaired parent/infant/child
Caregiver role strain
Caregiver role strain, risk for
Conflict, parental role
Coping, compromised family
Coping, disabled family
Coping, readiness for enhanced
Coping, readiness for enhanced family
Failure to thrive, adult
Family processes, interrupted
Family processes, readiness for enhanced
Grieving
Loneliness, risk for
Parenting, impaired
Parenting, readiness for enhanced
Parenting, risk for impaired
Relocation stress syndrome
Relocation stress syndrome, risk for
Social interaction, impaired
Social isolation

## Self-Esteem Needs

Adjustment, impaired
Body image, disturbed
Conflict, decisional
Coping, defensive
Coping, ineffective
Coping, ineffective community
Coping, readiness for enhanced community
Denial, ineffective
Diversional activity, deficient
Hopelessness
Identity, disturbed personal
Noncompliance
Post-trauma syndrome
Post-trauma syndrome, risk for
Powerlessness
Powerlessness, risk for
Rape-trauma syndrome
Rape-trauma syndrome: compound reaction
Rape-trauma syndrome: silent reaction
Role performance, ineffective
Self-esteem, chronic low
Self-esteem, situational low
Self-esteem, risk for situational low
Self-mutilation
Self-mutilation, risk for
Suicide, risk for
Violence, risk for other-directed
Violence, risk for self-directed

## Self-Actualization Needs

Development, risk for delayed
Energy field, disturbed

Growth and development, delayed
Health-seeking behaviors
Nutrition, readiness for enhanced
Religiosity readiness for enhanced
Sedentary lifestyle
Self-concept, readiness for enhanced
Spiritual distress
Spiritual distress, risk for
Spiritual well-being, readiness for enhanced
Therapeutic regimen management, effective

# APPENDIX B

## Nursing Diagnoses Arranged by Gordon's Functional Health Patterns[1]

### Health-Perception-Health-Management

Latex Allergy response
Risk for latex Allergy response
Risk for Sudden Infant Death syndrome
Disturbed Energy field
Risk for Falls
Supportive Family role performance
Health-seeking behaviors (specify)
Ineffective Health maintenance
Risk for Infection
Risk for Injury
Risk for perioperative-positioning Injury
Deficient Knowledge (specify)
Readiness for enhanced Knowledge of (specify)
Noncompliance
Risk for Poisoning
Ineffective Protection
Risk for Suffocation
Effective Therapeutic regimen management
Ineffective Therapeutic regimen management
Ineffective community Therapeutic regimen management
Ineffective family Therapeutic regimen management
Readiness for enhanced Therapeutic regimen management
Risk for Trauma
Wandering

### Nutritional-Metabolic

Risk for Aspiration
Risk for imbalanced Body temperature
Effective Breastfeeding
Ineffective Breastfeeding
Interrupted Breastfeeding
Impaired Dentition
Readiness for enhanced Fluid balance
Deficient Fluid volume
Excess Fluid volume
Risk for deficient Fluid volume
Risk for imbalanced Fluid volume
Hyperthermia
Hypothermia
Nausea
Readiness for enhanced Nutrition
Imbalanced Nutrition: less than body requirements
Imbalanced Nutrition: more than body requirements
Risk for imbalanced Nutrition: more than body requirements
Ineffective Infant feeding pattern
Impaired Oral mucous membrane
Impaired Skin integrity
Risk for impaired Skin integrity
Impaired Tissue integrity
Ineffective Thermoregulation
Impaired Swallowing

### Elimination

Bowel Incontinence
Perceived Constipation
Constipation
Risk for Constipation
Diarrhea
Functional urinary Incontinence
Reflex urinary Incontinence
Stress urinary Incontinence
Total urinary Incontinence
Urge urinary Incontinence
Risk for urge urinary Incontinence
Altered Urinary elimination
Readiness for enhanced Urinary elimination
Impaired Urinary elimination
Urinary Retention

### Activity-Exercise

Activity intolerance

[1]As updated by Gail Ladwig to incorporate the 2005-2006 NANDA-I Nursing Diagnoses.

Risk for Activity intolerance
Ineffective Airway clearance
Autonomic dysreflexia
Risk for Autonomic dysreflexia
Ineffective Breathing pattern
Decreased Cardiac output
Risk for delayed Development
Risk for Disuse syndrome
Deficient Diversional activity
Adult Failure to thrive
Fatigue
Impaired Gas exchange
Delayed Growth and development
Risk for disproportionate Growth
Impaired Home maintenance
Disorganized Infant behavior
Risk for disorganized Infant behavior
Readiness for enhanced organized Infant behavior
Impaired bed Mobility
Impaired physical Mobility
Impaired wheelchair Mobility
Sedentary lifestyle
Risk for peripheral Neurovascular dysfunction
Bathing/hygiene Self-care deficit
Dressing/grooming Self-care deficit
Feeding Self-care deficit
Toileting Self-care deficit
Delayed Surgical recovery
Ineffective Tissue perfusion (specify type)
Impaired Transfer ability
Impaired spontaneous Ventilation
Dysfunctional Ventilatory weaning response
Impaired Walking

## Sleep-Rest

Sleep deprivation
Disturbed Sleep patterns
Readiness for enhanced Sleep

## Cognitive-Perceptual

Impaired Comfort
Decisional Conflict (specify)
Acute Confusion
Chronic Confusion
Impaired Environmental interpretation syndrome
Decreased Intracranial adaptive capacity
Impaired Memory
Unilateral Neglect
Acute Pain
Disturbed Sensory perception
Disturbed Thought processes

## Chronic Pain Self-Perception-Self-Concept

Anxiety
Death Anxiety
Disturbed Body image
Fear
Hopelessness
Disturbed personal Identity
Risk for Loneliness
Powerlessness
Risk for Powerlessness
Readiness for enhanced Self-concept
Self-esteem Disturbance
Chronic low Self-esteem
Situational low Self-esteem
Risk for situational low Self-esteem
Self-mutilation
Risk for Self-mutilation

## Role-Relationship

Risk for impaired parent/infant/child Attachment
Caregiver role strain
Risk for Caregiver role strain
Impaired verbal Communication
Readiness for enhanced Communication
Parental role Conflict
Dysfunctional Family processes: alcoholism
Interrupted Family processes
Readiness for enhanced Family processes
Anticipatory Grieving
Dysfunctional Grieving
Impaired Parenting
Risk for impaired Parenting
Readiness for enhanced Parenting
Relocation stress syndrome
Risk for Relocation stress syndrome
Social Isolation
Impaired Social Interaction
Chronic Sorrow
Risk for other-directed Violence
Risk for self-directed Violence

## Sexuality-Reproductive

Rape trauma syndrome
Rape trauma syndrome: compound reaction
Rape trauma syndrome: silent reaction
Sexual dysfunction
Ineffective Sexuality patterns

## Coping-Stress-Tolerance

Impaired Adjustment
Compromised family Coping
Defensive Coping
Disabled family Coping
Ineffective Coping
Ineffective community Coping
Readiness for enhanced Coping
Readiness for enhanced community Coping
Readiness for enhanced family Coping
Ineffective Denial
Post-trauma syndrome
Risk for Post-trauma syndrome
Risk for Suicide

## Value-Belief

Impaired religiosity
Readiness for enhanced Religiosity
Risk for impaired Religiosity
Spiritual distress
Risk for Spiritual distress
Readiness for enhanced Spiritual well-being

# Recommended Childhood and Adolescent Immunization Schedule UNITED STATES • 2005

| Vaccine ▼ / Age ▶ | Birth | 1 month | 2 months | 4 months | 6 months | 12 months | 15 months | 18 months | 24 months | 4–6 years | 11–12 years | 13–18 years |
|---|---|---|---|---|---|---|---|---|---|---|---|---|
| Hepatitis B[1] | HepB # 1 | | HepB #2 | | | HepB #3 | | | | | HepB Series | |
| Diphtheria, Tetanus, Pertussis[2] | | | DTaP | DTaP | DTaP | | DTaP | | | DTaP | Td | Td |
| *Haemophilus influenzae* type b[3] | | | Hib | Hib | Hib | Hib | | | | | | |
| Inactivated Poliovirus | | | IPV | IPV | | IPV | | | | IPV | | |
| Measles, Mumps, Rubella[4] | | | | | | MMR #1 | | | | MMR # 2 | MMR #2 | |
| Varicella[5] | | | | | | | Varicella | | | | Varicella | |
| Pneumococcal[6] | | | PCV | PCV | PCV | PCV | | | PCV | | PPV | |
| Influenza[7] | | | | | | Influenza (Yearly) | | | | | Influenza (Yearly) | |
| — · — · — · — Vaccines below red line are for selected populations — · — · — · — | | | | | | | | | | | | |
| Hepatitis A[8] | | | | | | | | | | | Hepatitis A Series | |

This schedule indicates the recommended ages for routine administration of currently licensed childhood vaccines, as of December 1, 2004, for children through age 18 years. Any dose not given at the recommended age should be given at any subsequent visit when indicated and feasible.

■ Indicates age groups that warrant special effort to administer those vaccines not previously given. Additional vaccines may be licensed and recommended during. Licensed combination vaccines may be used whenever any components of the combination are indicated and the vaccine's other components are not contraindicated. Providers should consult the manufacturers' package inserts for detailed recommendations. Clinically significant adverse events that follow immunization should be reported to the Vaccine Adverse Event Reporting System (VAERS). Guidance about how to obtain and complete a VAERS form can be found on the Internet: **www.vaers.org** or by calling **800-822-7967**.

**Range of recommended ages**

**Preadolescent assessment**

**Only if mother HBsAg(–)**

**Catch-up immunization**

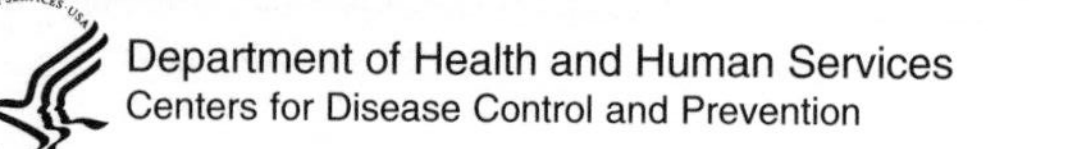

Department of Health and Human Services
Centers for Disease Control and Prevention

CDC SAFER · HEALTHIER · PEOPLE™

**The Childhood and Adolescent Immunization Schedule** is approved by:
Advisory Committee on Immunization Practices www.cdc.gov/nip/acip
American Academy of Pediatrics www.aap.org
American Academy of Family Physicians www.aafp.org

# Footnotes
## Recommended Childhood and Adolescent Immunization Schedule
UNITED STATES 2005

1. **Hepatitis B (HepB) vaccine.** All infants should receive the first dose of hepatitis B vaccine soon after birth and before hospital discharge; the first dose may also be given by age 2 months if the infant's mother is hepatitis B surface antigen (HBsAg) negative. Only monovalent HepB can be used for the birth dose. Monovalent or combination vaccine containing HepB may be used to complete the series. Four doses of vaccine may be administered when a birth dose is given. The second dose should be given at least 4 weeks after the first dose, except for combination vaccines which cannot be administered before age 6 weeks. The third dose should be given at least 16 weeks after the first dose and at least 8 weeks after the second dose. The last dose in the vaccination series (third or fourth dose) should not be administered before age 24 weeks.

   **Infants born to HBsAg-positive mothers** should receive HepB and 0.5 mL of Hepatitis B Immune Globulin (HBIG) within 12 hours of birth at separate sites. The second dose is recommended at age 1–2 months. The last dose in the immunization series should not be administered before age 24 weeks. These infants should be tested for HBsAg and antibody to HBsAg (anti-HBs) at age 9–15 months.

   **Infants born to mothers whose HBsAg status is unknown** should receive the first dose of the HepB series within 12 hours of birth. Maternal blood should be drawn as soon as possible to determine the mother's HBsAg status; if the HBsAg test is positive, the infant should receive HBIG as soon as possible (no later than age 1 week). The second dose is recommended at age 1–2 months. The last dose in the immunization series should not be administered before age 24 weeks.

2. **Diphtheria and tetanus toxoids and acellular pertussis (DTaP) vaccine.** The fourth dose of DTaP may be administered as early as age 12 months, provided 6 months have elapsed since the third dose and the child is unlikely to return at age 15–18 months. The final dose in the series should be given at age ≥4 years. **Tetanus and diphtheria toxoids (Td)** is recommended at age 11–12 years if at least 5 years have elapsed since the last dose of tetanus and diphtheria toxoid-containing vaccine. Subsequent routine Td boosters are recommended every 10 years.

3. ***Haemophilus influenzae* type b (Hib) conjugate vaccine.** Three Hib conjugate vaccines are licensed for infant use. If PRP-OMP (PedvaxHIB or ComVax [Merck]) is administered at ages 2 and 4 months, a dose at age 6 months is not required. DTaP/Hib combination products should not be used for primary immunization in infants at ages 2, 4 or 6 months but can be used as boosters following any Hib vaccine. The final dose in the series should be given at age ≥12 months.

4. **Measles, mumps, and rubella vaccine (MMR).** The second dose of MMR is recommended routinely at age 4–6 years but may be administered during any visit, provided at least 4 weeks have elapsed since the first dose and both doses are administered beginning at or after age 12 months. Those who have not previously received the second dose should complete the schedule by the visit at age 11–12 years.

5. **Varicella vaccine.** Varicella vaccine is recommended at any visit at or after age 12 months for susceptible children (i.e., those who lack a reliable history of chickenpox). Susceptible persons aged ≥13 years should receive 2 doses, given at least 4 weeks apart.

6. **Pneumococcal vaccine.** The heptavalent **pneumococcal conjugate vaccine (PCV)** is recommended for all children aged 2–23 months. It is also recommended for certain children aged 24–59 months. The final dose in the series should be given at age ≥12 months. **Pneumococcal polysaccharide vaccine (PPV)** is recommended in addition to PCV for certain high-risk groups. See *MMWR* 2000;49(RR-9):1-35.

7. **Influenza vaccine.** Influenza vaccine is recommended annually for children aged ≥6 months with certain risk factors (including but not limited to asthma, cardiac disease, sickle cell disease, HIV, and diabetes), healthcare workers, and other persons (including household members) in close contact with persons in groups at high risk (see *MMWR* 2004;53[RR-6]:1-40) and can be administered to all others wishing to obtain immunity. In addition, healthy children aged 6–23 months and close contacts of healthy children aged 0–23 months are recommended to receive influenza vaccine, because children in this age group are at substantially increased risk for influenza-related hospitalizations. For healthy persons aged 5–49 years, the intranasally administered live, attenuated influenza vaccine (LAIV) is an acceptable alternative to the intramuscular trivalent inactivated influenza vaccine (TIV). See *MMWR* 2004;53(RR-6):1-40. Children receiving TIV should be administered a dosage appropriate for their age (0.25 mL if 6–35 months or 0.5 mL if ≥3 years). Children aged ≥8 years who are receiving influenza vaccine for the first time should receive 2 doses (separated by at least 4 weeks for TIV and at least 6 weeks for LAIV).

8. **Hepatitis A vaccine.** Hepatitis A vaccine is recommended for children and adolescents in selected states and regions and for certain high-risk groups; consult your local public health authority. Children and adolescents in these states, regions, and high-risk groups who have not been immunized against hepatitis A can begin the hepatitis A immunization series during any visit. The 2 doses in the series should be administered at least 6 months apart. See *MMWR* 1999;48(RR-12):1-37.

# Recommended Immunization Schedule for Children and Adolescents Who Start Late or Who Are More Than 1 Month Behind

UNITED STATES 2005

The tables below give catch-up schedules and minimum intervals between doses for children who have delayed immunizations. There is no need to restart a vaccine series regardless of the time that has elapsed between doses. Use the chart appropriate for the child's age.

## CATCH-UP SCHEDULE FOR CHILDREN AGED 4 MONTHS THROUGH 6 YEARS

| Vaccine | Minimum Age for Dose 1 | Minimum Interval Between Doses | | | |
|---|---|---|---|---|---|
| | | Dose 1 to Dose 2 | Dose 2 to Dose 3 | Dose 3 to Dose 4 | Dose 4 to Dose 5 |
| Diphtheria, Tetanus,Pertussis | 6 wks | 4 weeks | 4 weeks | 6 months | 6 months |
| Inactivated Poliovirus | 6 wks | 4 weeks | 4 weeks | 4 weeks[2] | |
| Hepatitis B[3] | Birth | 4 weeks | 8 weeks (and 16 weeks after first dose) | | |
| Measles, Mumps, Rubella | 12 mo | 4 weeks[4] | | | |
| Varicella | 12 mo | | | | |
| *Haemophilus influenzae* type b[5] | 6 wks | **4 weeks** if first dose given at age <12 months<br>**8 weeks (as final dose)** if first dose given at age 12–14 months<br>**No further doses needed** if first dose given at age ≥15 months | **4 weeks**[6] if current age <12 months<br>**8 weeks (as final dose)**[6] if current age ≥12 months and second dose given at age <15 months<br>**No further doses needed** if previous dose given at age ≥15 mo | **8 weeks (as final dose)** This dose only necessary for children aged 12 months–5 years who received 3 doses before age 12 months | |
| Pneumococcal[7] | 6 wks | **4 weeks** if first dose given at age <12 months and current age <24 months<br>**8 weeks (as final dose)** if first dose given at age ≥12 month sor current age 24–59 months<br>**No further doses needed** for healthy children if first dose given at age ≥24 months | **4 weeks** if current age <12 months<br>**8 weeks (as final dose)** if current age ≥12 months<br>**No further doses needed** for healthy children if previous dose given at age ≥24 months | **8 weeks (as final dose)** This dose only necessary for children aged12 months–5 years who received 3 doses before age 12 months | |

## CATCH-UP SCHEDULE FOR CHILDREN AGED 7 YEARS THROUGH 18 YEARS

| Vaccine | Minimum Interval Between Doses | | |
|---|---|---|---|
| | Dose 1 to Dose 2 | Dose 2 to Dose 3 | Dose 3 to Booster Dose |
| **Tetanus, Diphtheria** | **4 weeks** | **6 months** | **6 months**[8] if first dose given at age <12 months and current age <11 years<br>**5 years**[8] if first dose given at age ≥12 months and third dose given at age <7 years and current age ≥11 years<br>**10 years**[8] if third dose given at age ≥7 years |
| **Inactivated Poliovirus**[9] | **4 weeks** | **4 weeks** | **IPV**[2,9] |
| **Hepatitis B** | **4 weeks** | **8 weeks** (and 16 weeks after first dose) | |
| **Measles, Mumps, Rubella** | **4 weeks** | | |
| **Varicella**[10] | **4 weeks** | | |

## Footnotes

### Children and Adolescents Catch-up Schedules

**UNITED STATES • 2005**

1. **DTaP.** The fifth dose is not necessary if the fourth dose was given after the fourth birthday.
2. **IPV.** For children who received an all-IPV or all-oral poliovirus (OPV) series, a fourth dose is not necessary if third dose was given at age ≥4 years. If both OPV and IPV were given as part of a series, a total of 4 doses should be given, regardless of the child's current age.
3. **HepB.** All children and adolescents who have not been immunized against hepatitis B should begin the HepB immunization series during any visit. Providers should make special efforts to immunize children who were born in, or whose parents were born in, areas of the world where hepatitis B virus infection is moderately or highly endemic.
4. **MMR.** The second dose of MMR is recommended routinely at age 4–6 years but may be given earlier if desired.
5. **Hib.** Vaccine is not generally recommended for children aged ≥5 years.
6. **Hib.** If current age <12 months and the first 2 doses were PRP-OMP (PedvaxHIB or ComVax [Merck]), the third (and final) dose should be given at age 12–15 months and at least 8 weeks after the second dose.
7. **PCV.** Vaccine is not generally recommended for children aged ≥5 years.
8. **Td.** For children aged 7–10 years, the interval between the third and booster dose is determined by the age when the first dose was given. For adolescents aged 11–18 years, the interval is determined by the age when the third dose was given.
9. **IPV.** Vaccine is not generally recommended for persons aged ≥18 years.
10. **Varicella.** Give 2-dose series to all susceptible adolescents aged ≥13 years.

**Report adverse reactions to vaccines through the federal Vaccine Adverse Event Reporting System. For information on reporting reactions following immunization, please visit www.vaers.org or call the 24-hour national toll-free information line 800-822-7967. Report suspected cases of vaccine-preventable diseases to your state or local health department.**

**For additional information about vaccines, including precautions and contraindications for immunization and vaccine shortages, please visit the National Immunization Program Web site at www.cdc.gov/nipor call the National Immunization Information Hotline at 800-232-2522 (English) or 800-232-0233 (Spanish).**

# INDEX

Boldface entries indicate care plan titles; page numbers in italics indicate care plan locations.

## C

## Q



## R